Retreatments

Solutions for Periapical Diseases of Endodontic Origin

PIO **BERTANI**
MASSIMO **GAGLIANI**
FABIO **GORNI**

Calogero **Bugea**
Filippo **Cardinali**
Enrico **Cassai**
Arnaldo **Castellucci**
Francesca **Cerutti**
Roberto **Fornara**
Paolo **Generali**
Massimo **Giovarruscio**
Davide **Guglielmi**
Marco **Martignoni**
Tiziano **Testori**
Riccardo **Tonini**

Retreatments

Solutions for Periapical Diseases of Endodontic Origin

edra

STYLE ITALIANO ENDODONTICS

Books Publishing Manager: Arianna Ribichesu
Book Editor: Paola Sammaritano
Books Production Manager: Michele Ribatti
Graphic design and cover: JDT, Milan

ISBN 978-88-214-5093-8
eISBN 978-88-214-5094-5

Medicine is an ever-evolving science. Research and clinical experience are constantly expanding our knowledge, especially in relation to therapeutic modalities and pharmacology. Where the text refers to the dosage or contraindications of a medicinal product, the reader can be assured that the authors, editors, and publisher have made every effort to ensure that such references are consistent with the state of knowledge at the time of publication of the book. However, the reader is advised to read the medicinal product's package leaflet carefully to personally check whether the recommended dosages or contraindications specified differ from what is indicated in the text. This is particularly important in the case of medicinal products that are rarely used or were only recently placed on the market.

Edra S.p.A.
Via G. Spadolini 7, 20141 Milano
Tel. 02 881841
www.edizioniedra.it

Printed in Italy
Printed in March 2020 by "Printer Trento" S.r.l., Trento, Italy

(*) Edra S.p.A. is part of LSWR GROUP

Editors

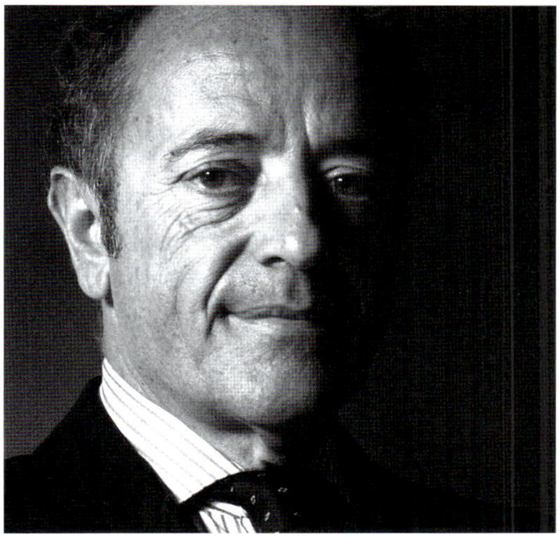

piobertani@piobertani.com

Pio Bertani

Surgeon, Specialist in Dentistry.
Adjunct Professor of Conservative Dentistry at the University of Modena and Reggio Emilia from 2003 to 2008.
Teacher of the Postgraduate Course in Conservative Dentistry in 2004 to 2005 at the University of Modena and Reggio Emilia.
Teacher of Advanced Training Course in Prosthetics from 2009 to 2013 at the University of Bologna.
Adjunct Professor of Endodontics at the University of Parma. Active Member of the Italian Academy of Aesthetic Dentistry. Active Member of the Italian Society of Endodontics (SIE), of which he is the Past President.
Active Member of the European Society of Endodontics. Co-author of the book "Illustrated Manual of Endodontics" (Masson, 2003) and of the "Manual of Endodontics" (Edra, 2013).

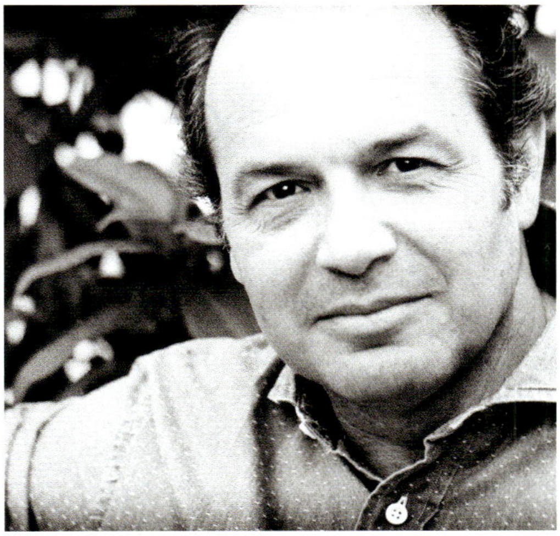

massimo.gagliani@unimi.it

Massimo Gagliani

He graduated in Medicine and dedicated himself to Dentistry, in particular Conservative Dentistry and Endodontics, as part of the degree course in Dentistry and Dental Prosthetics at the University of Milan. Associate Professor of Dentistry Diseases since 2000 at the University of Milan. He practices at the "Giorgio Vogel" Dental Practice in Milan.
He is the author of numerous scientific publications in national and international journals, including *International Endodontic Journal*, *Journal of Endodontics*, and *Giornale Italiano di Endodonzia*.
He is the Editorial Coordinator of the EDRA Group for Dentistry, former Editor-in-Chief of *Giornale Italiano di Endodonzia*, and Founding Partner of the Digital Dental Academy (www.digitaldentalacademy.it).

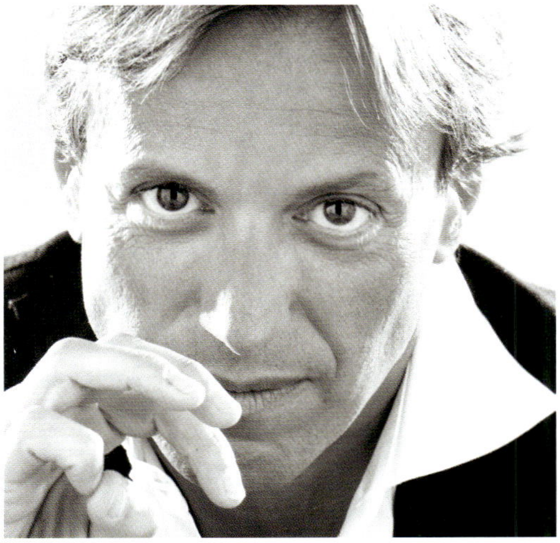

fabiogorni@dentalservicesanzio.it

Fabio Gorni

He graduated in Dentistry and Dental Prosthetics from the University of Milan in 1984. Former Adjunct Professor in Endodontics at the University of Milan, Ospedale San Paolo. Adjunct Professor holder of teaching in Perioral Aesthetics of the Degree Course in Dentistry and Dental Prosthetics, Università Vita-Salute San Raffaele, Milan.
Active Member of the Italian Society of Endodontics (SIE) and the Italian Academy of Microscopic Dentistry, Specialist Member of the European Society of Endodontology, and Member of the American Association of Endodontists. Speaker in Italy and abroad in numerous courses and congresses, author of several publications in national and international journals. In collaboration with C.J. Ruddle, he published a video-series entitled "The Endodontic Game," distributed in Europe, USA, Canada, Australia, and Asia. Co-founder of StyleItaliano Endodontics.

Authors

Calogero Bugea

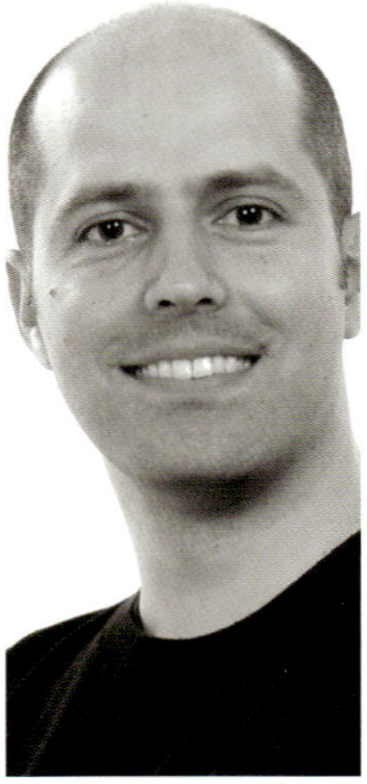

Degree in Dentistry and Specialization in Oral Surgery at "G. d'Annunzio" University of Chieti-Pescara. Active Member of the International Piezoelectric Surgery Academy (IPA). Member of StyleItaliano Endodontics. Active Member of the Italian Society of Endodontics (SIE). Author of national and international publications on Implantology and Endodontics.

Filippo Cardinali

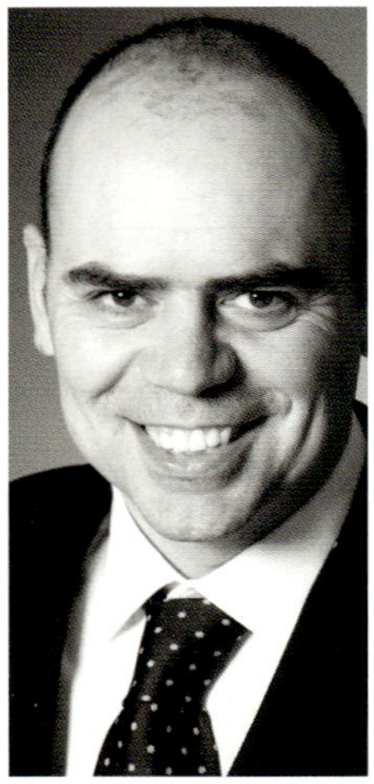

He graduated in Dentistry and Dental Prosthetics from the University of Ancona in 1992. Active Member of the Italian Society of Endodontics. Certified Member of the European Society of Endodontology. Specialist Member of the American Association of Endodontists. Gold Member of StyleItaliano Endodontics. Speaker at courses and congresses in Italy and abroad. He practices his profession dedicating himself above all to Endodontics and Conservative Dentistry and is the author of publications on the subject in specialist national and international journals.

Enrico Cassai

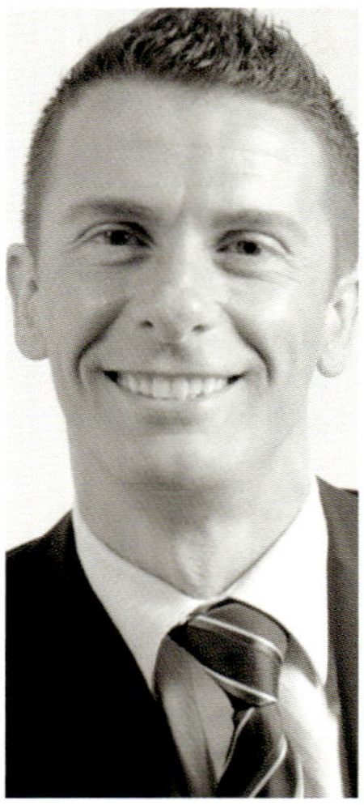

He graduated with honors in Dentistry and Dental Prosthetics from the University of Ferrara in 1999. Active Member of the Italian Society of Endodontics and of the Italian Academy of Microscopic Dentistry. Associate Member of the American Association of Endodontists and of the European Society of Endodontology. Member of the SIE Cultural Commission from 2017 to 2019. Speaker at courses and congresses in Italy and abroad. Author of numerous publications in national and international journals.

Arnaldo Castellucci

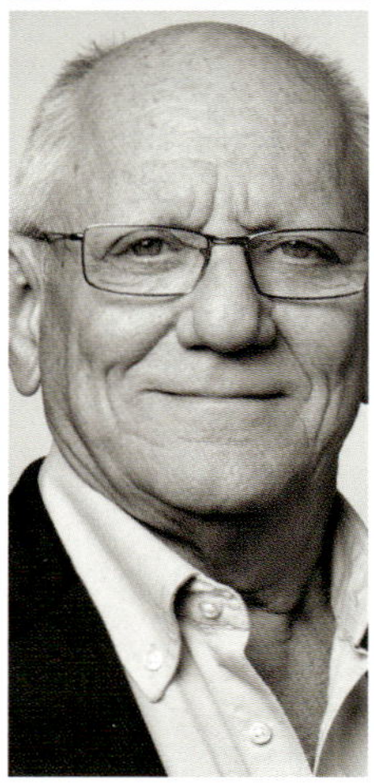

Past President of the Italian Society of Endodontics and the International Federation of Endodontic Associations. Active Member of the American Association of Endodontists. Active Member of the European Society of Endodontology. Editor-in-Chief of *Giornale Italiano di Endodonzia* and *L'Informatore Endodontico*. Author of "Endodonzia" (Ed. Martina, Bologna) and "Microendodonzia Chirurgica" (Edra, Milan, in print). Founder and President of Centro per l'Insegnamento della Microendodonzia. International speaker.

Francesca Cerutti

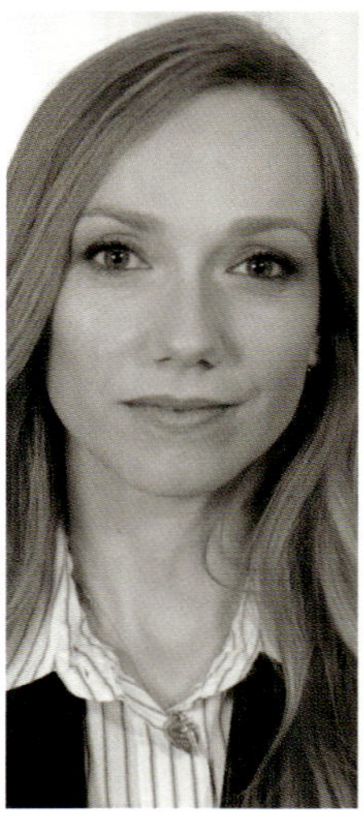

She graduated from the University of Brescia (2007), where she also obtained her PhD (2013). Adjunct Professor at the University of Milan. Member of the Italian Society of Endodontics (SIE) and Silver Member of StyleItaliano Endodontics. Editorial Coordinator of *Giornale Italiano di Endodonzia* (2008-2011). Reviewer for international journals and author of articles and texts on restorative dentistry and Endodontics. Speaker on topics regarding Conservative Dentistry and Endodontics.

Roberto Fornara

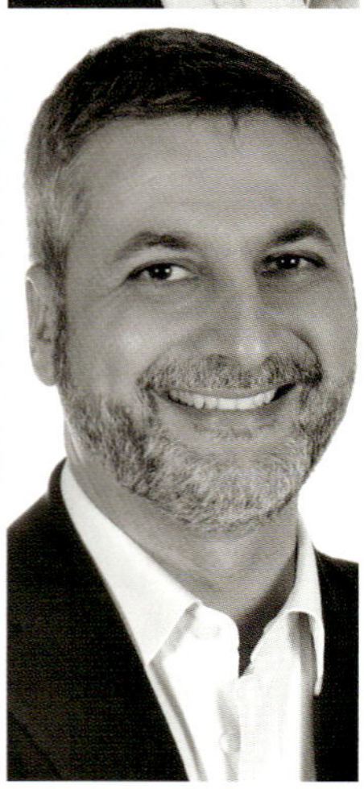

He graduated with honors in Dentistry and Dental Prosthetics in 1995 from the University of Pavia. Since 2003, Active Partner of the Italian Society of Endodontics (SIE) and current Chairman-Elect of the SIE. Since 2010, Certified Member of the European Society of Endodontics (ESE). Active Member of the Digital Dental Society (DDS). Member of the Editorial Committee of *Giornale Italiano di Endodonzia*. Author of scientific articles in national and international journals. Speaker at national and international congresses and lecturer in theoretical and practical courses.

Paolo Generali

He graduated with honors in Medicine and Surgery and specialized in Dentistry. Full Member of Amici di Brugg, Active Member of the Italian Society of Endodontics (SIE). Member of the ANDI. Author of texts, articles, and reports at Congresses in Italy and abroad. Lecturer in Conservative Dentistry at CLSOPD, former lecturer in postgraduate and master courses. Lecturer at the 2nd Level Master's Degree in Endodontics and Restorative Dentistry at the University of Siena.

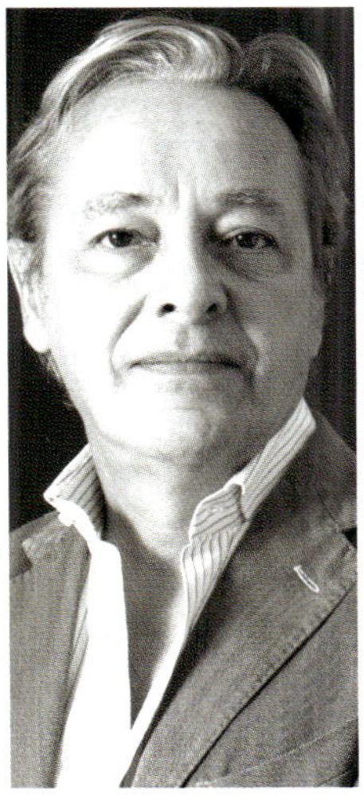

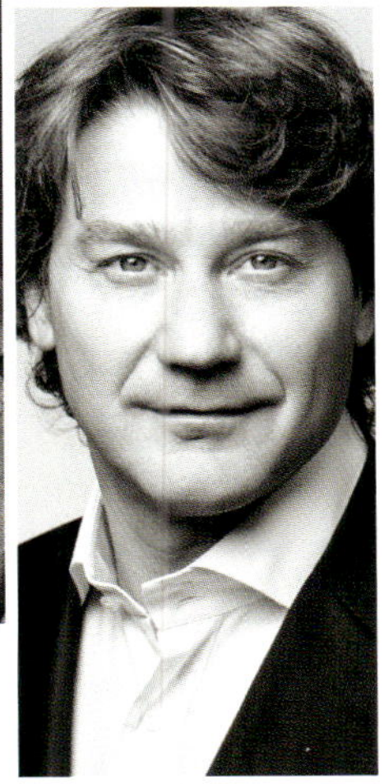

Massimo Giovarruscio

He graduated with honors from the "Tor Vergata" University of Rome in 1995. Active Member of the Italian Society of Endodontics and the Italian Academy of Microscopic Dentistry.
Member of the European Society of Endodontology and the British Endodontic Society. Visiting Professor in 2005 at New York University (Dir. Prof. Paul Rosenberg). Since 2010, Specialist Clinical Teacher at the King's College London Institute and Guy's Hospital in London.
Author of clinical works in *Giornale Italiano di Endodonzia*. Speaker at national and international congresses.

Davide Guglielmi

He graduated with honors from the University of Insubria in Varese in 2010. Master's degree in Periodontology and Postgraduate degree in Oral Surgery. Member of the Italian Society of Periodontology and Implantology (SIdP) and Italian Society of Endodontics (SIE) and Silver Member of Styleitaliano Endodontics. Collaborator at the Department of Periodontology (Dir. Prof. M. de Sanctis) of Ospedale Vita-Salute San Raffaele and of Prof. F. Gorni. Winner of the Giorgio Lavagnoli SIE Award in 2018.

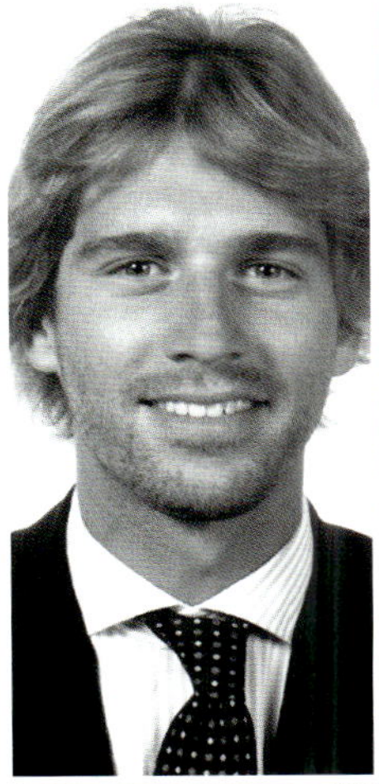

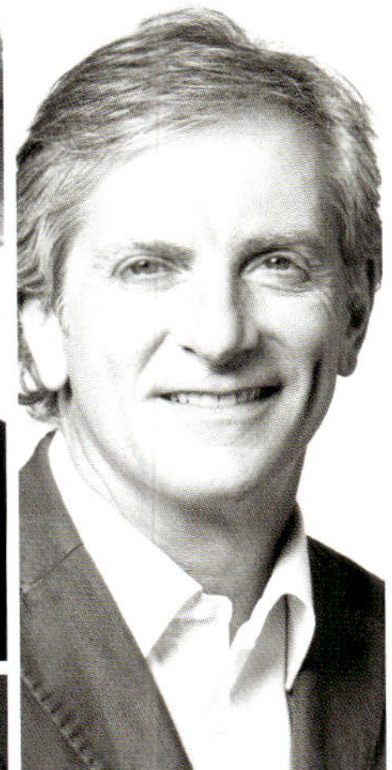

Marco Martignoni

He graduated with honors from the University of Chieti in 1988. Chairman of the European Society of Endodontology Congress for ESE-Rome 2011.
Past President of the Italian Society of Endodontics. Professor at Steinbeis Transfer Institute Hochschule Berlin. Visiting Professor at the International Master in Endodontics and Restorative Dentistry, University of Siena. Founder of the Italian Academy of Microscopic Dentistry and Honorary Member of the French Endodontics Society. Speaker at national and international level.

Tiziano Testori

He graduated in Medicine and Surgery in 1981, specializing in Dentistry in 1984 and Orthodontics in 1986 at the University of Milan. Head of the Department of Implantology and Oral Rehabilitation Dental Clinic (Dir. Prof. Francetti), IRCCS Istituto Ortopedico Galeazzi, University of Milan. Adjunct Clinical Associate Professor, Dept. of Periodontics and Oral Medicine, University of Michigan, School of Dentistry. Author of 123 scientific articles indexed on PubMed.

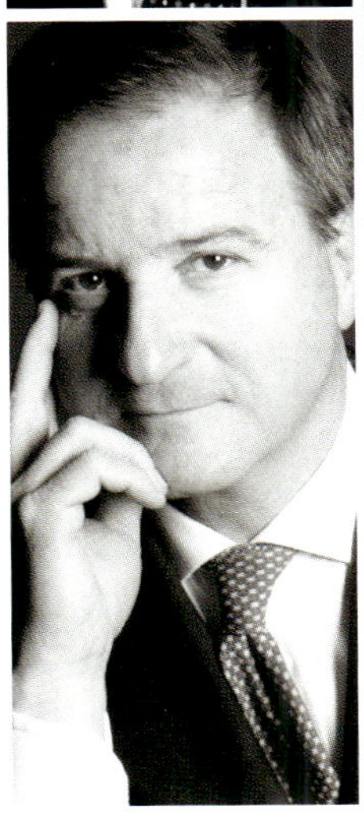

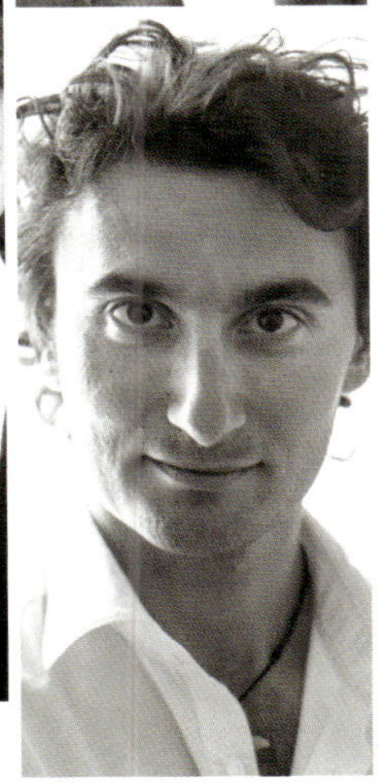

Riccardo Tonini

D.D.S., M.Sc, he graduated from the University of Brescia in 2004. In 2007, he obtained a Master's Degree in Endodontics from the University of Verona. Since 2010, he has been an Active Member of the Italian Society of Endodontics (SIE) and the Italian Society of Microscopic Dentistry.
Member of StyleItaliano Endodontics.
He runs private practice, committed to Endodontics, in Brescia.

Co-authors

Zaher Al-Taqi

He graduated in Dentistry from the Syrian Private University (SPU), College of Dentistry in Syria. Post-graduate degree in Endodontics from Damascus University, College of Dentistry, Syria and member of the the Syrian Board of Endodontics within the Syrian commission for health specialists. He is a member of the editorial board of *International Dental and Medical Journal of Advanced Research*. He lectures internationally in the clinical approach to microscopic endodontics. He conducts international private courses and modules on Modern Endodontics. Gold member of StyleItaliano Endodontics. His private practice in Riyadh, Saudi Arabia is committed to microscopic endodontic treatment.

Ahmed Alwaidh

He graduated with a BDS from the University of Baghdad in 2008. Specialized in microscopic endodontics. In 2017, he enrolled in the MSc in Endodontics at King's College London. He has conducted many courses in microscopic endodontics. He's also a KOL at Fanta Dental, Scientific Advisor at Teimdent, Finland and Silver member of StyleItaliano Endodontics. CEO and owner of BurJuman Dental Polyclinic, in Najaf, Iraq (private sector). His practice is committed to microscopic endodontics and aesthetic dentistry.

Mostafa Anwar

BDS, DHHM, MDSc, PhD Researcher. He is Fellow Assistant Lecturer of Endodontics at The British University in Egypt (BUE) and Certified Healthcare & Hospital Management Specialist at the American University in Cairo (AUC). Member of the Editorial Board of *EC Dental Science Journal* and Silver Member of StyleItaliano Endodontics. Endodontics Specialist at the Whity Dental Center. His private practice is committed to microscopic endodontic treatment.

Khalid Jamal Attar

He graduated from the Faculty of Dentistry of University of Basrah in 2010. He worked in the first specialist center in the province of Basrah. He has about 9 years'experience in the field of root fillings. Member of the Iraqi Endodontic Society and certified Silver member of StyleItaliano Endodontics since 2018. His private practice is committed to microscopic endodontic and restorative treatment.

Errico Bucci

He graduated in Medicine from the University of L'Aquila, Italy in 1984. He specialized in dentistry in 1987 and orthodontics in 1991 at the University of Milan, Italy. He has always dedicated himself to the practice of orthodontics and to the recovery and preservation of severely compromised teeth. Member of the following scientific societies: the Italian Society of Endodontics (SIE), the Italian Society of Orthodontics (SIDO).

Federico Ceroni

He graduated from the University of Milan, Italy in 2013.
He has always dedicated himself to the practice of minimally-invasive aesthetic dentistry and to the recovery and preservation of severely compromised teeth. He has spoken at national and international conferences on conservative dentistry and endodontics. He is the co-author of several publications. Member of the following scientific societies: the Italian Society of Endodontics (SIE), the Italian Academy of Conservative dentistry (AIC), Silver member of StyleItaliano Endodontics and Shade Guide.

Gilberto Debelian

He received his DMD degree from the University of Sao Paulo, Brazil in 1987. He specialized in Endodontics at the University of Pennsylvania, USA in 1991. Clinical instructor and Associate professor at the endodontic program at the University of Oslo (UIO), Norway 1991-2010. Adjunct visiting professor at the post-graduate program in endodontics,

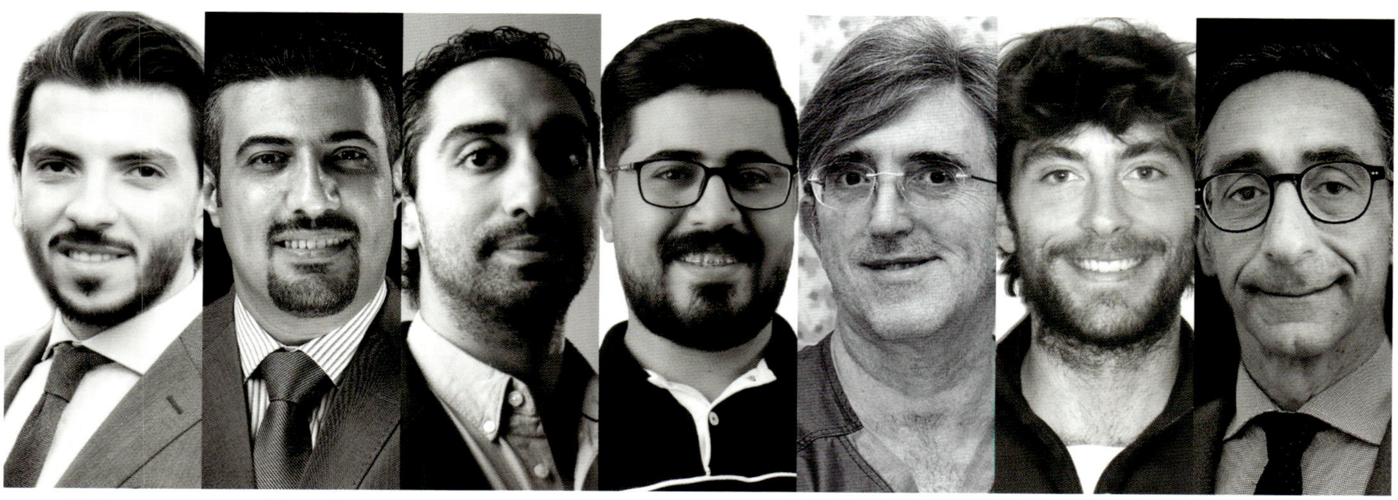

Zaher Al-Taqi | Ahmed Alwaidh | Mostafa Anwar | Khalid Jamal Attar | Errico Bucci | Federico Ceroni | Gilberto Debelian

University of North Carolina in Chapel Hill 2006-2015. Adjunct visiting professor at the post-graduate program in endodontics at the University of Pennsylvania.
He runs a private practice committed to endodontics and he is the director of the advanced endodontic microscopy center – ENDO INN in Oslo, Norway.
He has authored 7 chapters in books on Endodontics, one book on Endodontics and written more than 80 scientific and clinical papers.

Matteo Deflorian

He graduated with honours in Dentistry and Dental Prosthetics from University of Milan in 2007. Tutor at the Department of Implantology and Oral Rehabilitation (Head Prof. T. Testori), University of Milan, Department of Biomedical, Surgical and Dental Sciences, IRCCS Istituto Ortopedico Galeazzi, Servizio di Odontostomatologia (Dir. Prof. L. Francetti). I&J's Scientific Co-Director. Active Member of the Italian Academy of Osseointegration (IAO).

Massimo Del Fabbro

Degree in Biological Sciences, PhD in Human Physiology, Associate professor at University of Milan, Department of Biomedical, Surgical, Dental Sciences. Coordinator of research activities of the Dental Clinic, IRCCS Istituto Ortopedico Galeazzi, Milan. Director of the Oral Health Research Centre from 2011 to 2016. Coordinator of the PhD in Dentistry from 2015 to 2018. Over 300 indexed articles.

Alexandru Gliga

He graduated from "Carol Davila" University of Medicine Bucharest in 2013 with a Bachelor's Degree in Dentistry and MSc Endodontics Programme at King's College London with distinction. Member of the European Society of Endodontology since 2017 and Silver member of StyleItaliano Endodontics since 2018. Member of the British Endodontic Society since 2020. In 2015 he was elected councillor and advisor of Bucharest College of Dentists. Lecturer in national and international conferences and private theoretical and practical courses on Endodontology.
His private practice has been committed to endodontics and restorations since 2010.

Mark Habib

He graduated in Dentistry with honors from the Saint Joseph University of Beirut, where he also obtained a Master's in Endodontics and a Master's in Biomaterials for the oral cavity. Clinical Assistant at the endodontics department in the School of dentistry and Senior Lecturer at the Endodontic University Diploma program at the Saint Joseph University. Member of the European Society of Endodontology and of the Italian Society of Endodontics (SIE). Silver member of StyleItaliano Endodontics. Speaker at conferences and workshops in Lebanon and abroad. His private practice at Beirut Endodontic Clinic is committed to Endodontics.

Konstantinos Kalogeropoulos

He graduated from Athens Dental School in 2005. He did his three-year post graduate studies at the same University and received a Master of Science in Endodontics.
He has run a private practice committed to Endodontics in Athens, Greece, since 2008. He lectures both nationally and internationally. His clinical cases have been published in endodontic journals and text books around the world. He is a Silver member of StyleItaliano Endodontics.

Marc K. Kaloustian

He graduated in Dental Surgery at the Saint Joseph University, Lebanon, where he also obtained a Master's in Endodontics and Master's in Biomaterials. He is senior lecturer in the Endodontic department of the Saint Joseph University Dental School, Lebanon. Active member iof the board of the Lebanese Society of Endodontology,

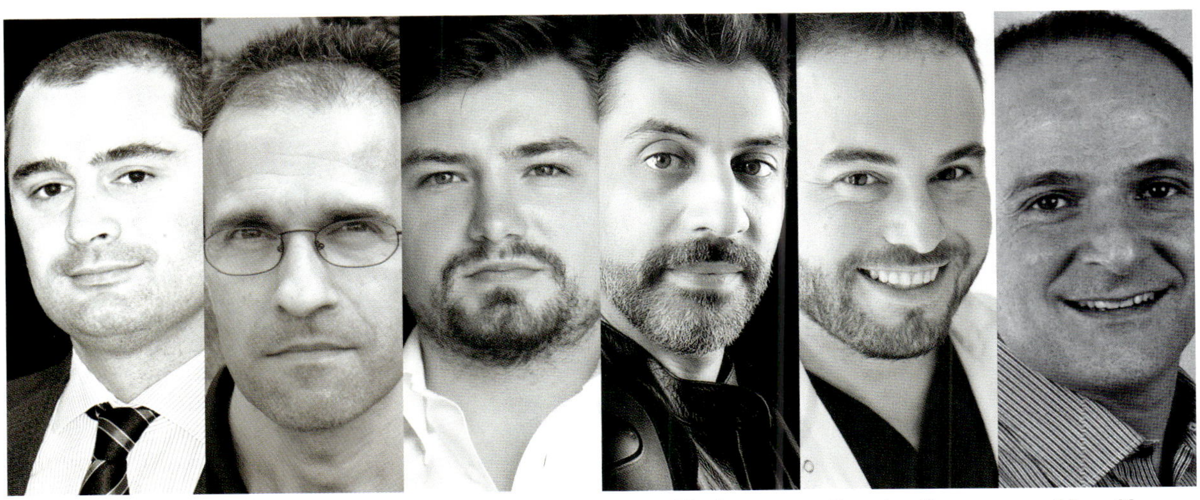

Matteo Deflorian | Massimo Del Fabbro | Alexandru Gliga | Mark Habib | Konstantinos Kalogeropoulos | Marc K. Kaloustian

Silver member of StyleItaliano Endodontics. He commits his private practice to Endodontics. He is an international lecturer in various aspects of endodontic and has published several scientific publications in indexed journals.

Waleed Kurdi

He graduated with honours in Oral and Dental Medicine B.D.S (2009) and obtained a Master's in Endodontics M.D.S (2013) from Cairo University. Endodontist and owner of the BW Dental Clinics since 2013. Clinician, researcher and lecturer in the development of strategies and guidance on root canal treatment and dental hygiene. Lecturer and course director of the Endo-Dam team. Silver member of StyleItaliano Endodontics.

Marco Maraldi

DDS, he graduated with honors in Dentistry and Dental Prosthesis from the University of Milan in 1997. Teacher of the practical-theoretical course "Esthetic rehabilitation of anterior teeth with porcelain veneers", and has his own private practice besides being an endodontics and prosthodontics consultant. Ordinary member of the Italian Society of Endodontics (SIE) and of the Italian Academy of Conservative Dentistry (AIC).

João Meirinhos

DDS, MsC (Endodontics). Integrated Master's in Dental Medicine from Instituto Superior de Ciências da Saúde do Norte (2014); Endodontics and Rehabilitation at RPCEndo 2014; Endodontics Specialty Program at the University of Lisbon.
Teacher of Basic and Advanced Endodontics at RPCEndo. Author and co-author of scientific articles published in national and international journals. Speaker at national and international conferences and author of several presentations and posters on Endodontics. Member of the Portuguese Society of Endodontology (PSE), of the European Society of Endodontology (ESE) and of StyleItaliano Endodontics.
His practice is committed to Endodontics.

Ivan Mirovic

He graduated from from University of Belgrade, School of Dentistry, Serbia, in 2008 (DDS, Master of Science). In 2009, he completed his one-year general practice residency. From 2009 he completed advanced training in endodontics attending the continuing education in endodontics courses by leading international experts in the field, as well as national and international congresses. Since 2012 he has committed his professional career to endodontics. In 2018 he was promoted to Silver member of StyleItaliano Endodontics. Dr. Mirovic runs a private practice committed to endodontics in Belgrade, Serbia.

Dennis Quintero Santos

He graduated from the Latin University of Costa Rica. National and international speaker. Constant participation in continuing education events.
Active member of the international group StyleItaliano Endodontics.

Renzo Raffaelli

He graduated in Medicine from the University of Pavia in 1981 and specialized in Dentistry and Prosthodontics in 1985. He specialized in Endodontics and in Implantology at the University of Verona. He taught the course in Ergonomics - Degree in Dental Hygene - at the University of Verona. Active Member of the Italian Society of Endodontics (SIE) and of the Italian Academy of Microdentistry (AIOM).
He runs a private practice in Rovereto (Italy). He has been a speaker at various courses and conferences in Italy.
He authored a chapter on urgencies in endodontics in "Manual of Endodontics" by SIE.

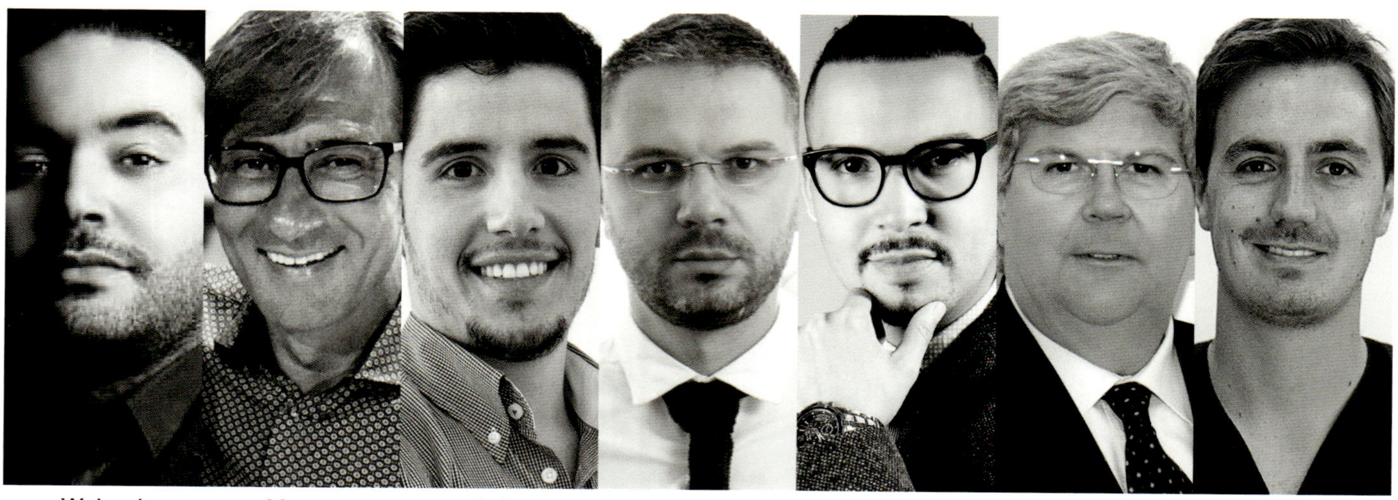

Waleed Kurdi | Marco Maraldi | João Meirinhos | Ivan Mirovic | Dennis Quintero Santos | Renzo Raffaelli | Gabriele Ragucci

Gabriele Ragucci

He graduated in Dentistry at the Universidad Europea de Valencia and obtained the Diploma in Conservative Aesthetic Dentistry at the Universidad Pubblica de Valencia. He is an ordinary under 32 member of the Italian Society of Endodontics (SIE), as well as junior member of the Italian Academy of Conservative and Restorative Dentistry. He runs private practice at Studio Burdick-Ragucci in Milan, and Studio Allegri Verona, Italy.

Riccardo Scaini

He graduated in Dentistry and Dental Prosthetics from University of Milan, where he also specialized in Dental Surgery. Tutor at the Department of Implantology and Oral Rehabilitation (Head Prof. T. Testori), University of Milan, Department of Biomedical, Surgical and Dental Sciences, IRCCS Istituto Ortopedico Galeazzi, Servizio di Odontostomatologia (Head Prof. L. Francetti). I&J's Scientific Co-Director. Active Member of the Italian Academy of Osseointegration (IAO).

Fitim Shabani

He graduated as a dental technician in Tetovo, North Macedonia.
He graduated in Medicine and Dentistry from the University of Prishtina, Kosovo in 2011. Lecturer in Switzerland and abroad. Private practice in Switzerland since 2012. His main areas of interest are endodontology, restoration, prosthetics and surgery.

Marino Sutedjo

He graduated with a DDS from Trisakti University (Jakarta-Indonesia) course in 2003. Postgraduate in Conservative Dentistry and Endodontics.
He is currently a KOL and a speaker and instructor in Endodontics both nationally and internationally. In 2016, he became the first Asian dentist to join StyleItaliano Endodontic and is now a certified Gold member. He runs a private practice in Surabaya-Indonesia.

Silvio Taschieri

Assistant Professor at University of Milan, Department of Biomedical, Surgical and Dental Sciences, Dental Clinic of IRCCS Istituto Ortopedico Galeazzi, Milan. Associate Professor at the Sechenov State University in Moscow. Reviewer of the Restorative Expert Panel, Cochrane Oral Health Group, University of Manchester. Associate Editor Section of Implantology of *Journal of Investigative and Clinical Dentistry*. Author of more than 200 international publications.

Yoshitsugu Terauchi

He earned his DDS in 1993 and completed his residency at Tokyo Medical & Dental University in 1995, where he also received his PhD from the Department of Endodontics. He has published several articles in national and international peer-reviewed journals.
He also has authored several chapters in textbooks including the 11th ed. of "Pathways of the Pulp" and "Endodontics: the 6th edition of Principles and Practice" He has lectured nationally and internationally and has appeared twice on National TV for modern endodontics. He is a part-time lecturer at Tokyo Medical & Dental University and has run a private practice committed to endodontics in Tokyo since 1998.

Mohamad Zaafrany

Certified speaker for DentSply Sirona Endodontics. He is KOL for Zumax Medical CO. He is also Official DSD team member and director of the Endodontic Program MEDLINK DTC. His practice is committed to microendodontics.
He is a Gold member of Styleitaliano Endodontics.

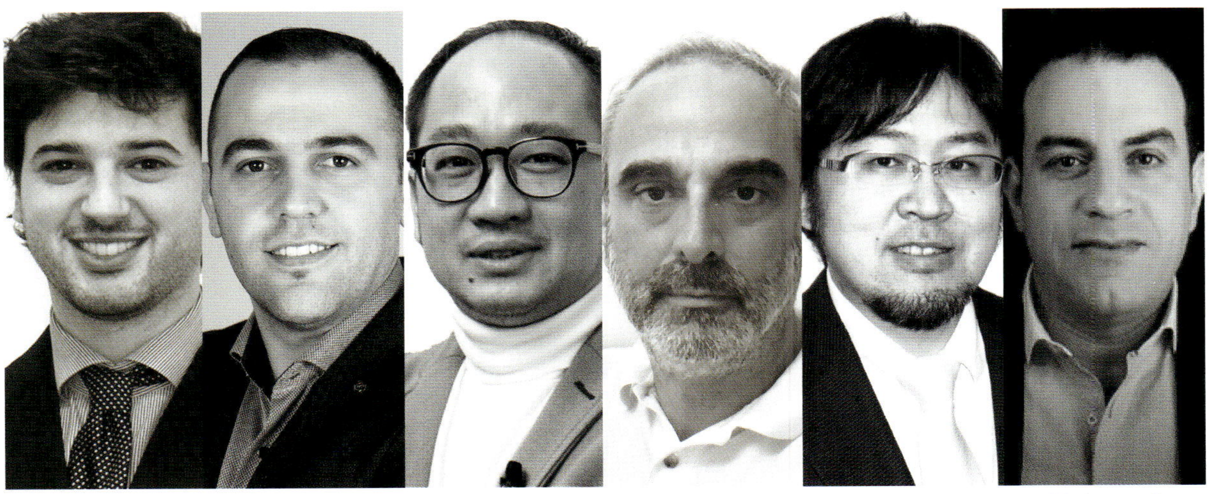

Riccardo Scaini · Fitim Shabani · Marino Sutedjo · Silvio Taschieri · Yoshitsugu Terauchi · Mohamad Zaafrany

Table of Contents

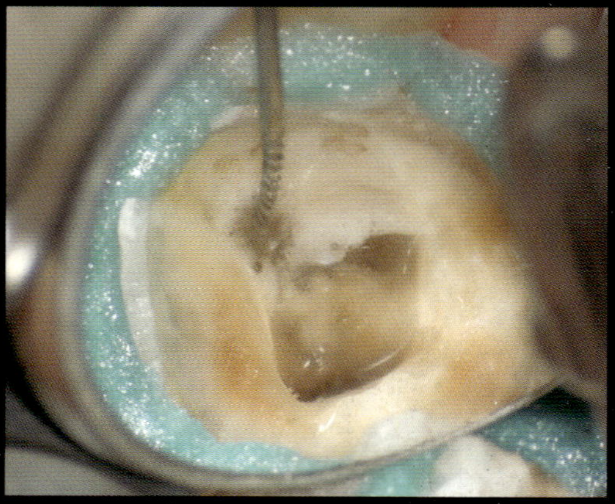

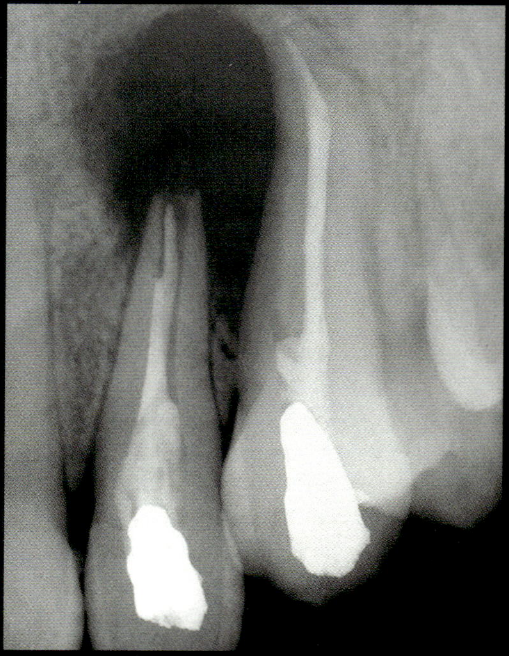

Acknowledgements

The authors would like to thank the following: Dr. Anna Maria Pirovano for the images on pages XVII and 189; Dr. Luciano Giardino for the histological images on page 44; Dr. Nicola Perrini for the histological image on page 45; Prof. Eugenio Brambilla for the numerous electron microscopy images on pages 6, 46, and 47 and for the endodontic microbiology section; Dr. Mario Badino for the advice on Chapter 2; Prof. Marco Scarpelli for the boxes on pages 214 and 215; Dr. Marco Femia and Dr. Sara Berri for the case report on page 78; Dr. Francesca Carrara for the figures on

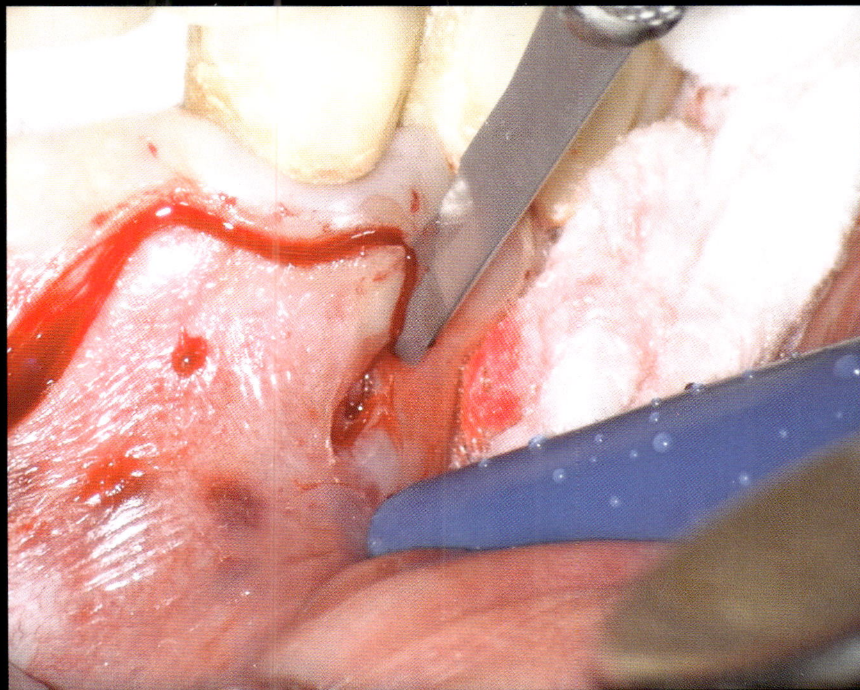

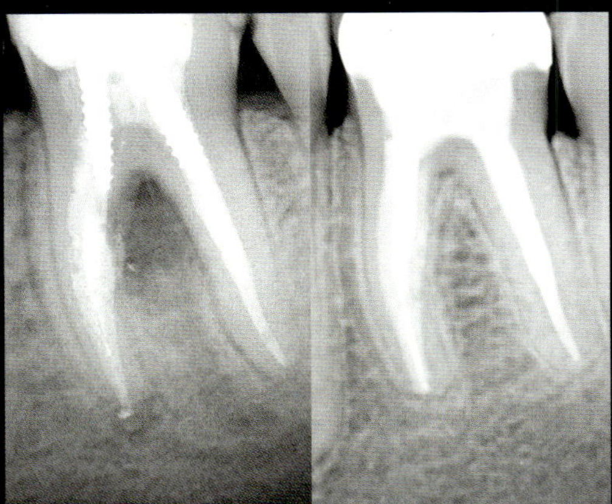

page 257 (4.4a,b); Dr. Federico Berton for the SEM images on pages 284, 289, and 306; Dr. Alessandra Abbà and Giulia Palandrani for the images on pages 324 and 325.

Calogero Bugea would also like to thank Dr. Maurizio Porcino, Dr. Roberto Placella, Dr. Vittoria Eleonora Mazza, Dr. Roberto Luongo, Dr. Vanessa Villani, Dr. Ketty Bugea, Dr. Nicola Basile, Ms. Caterina De Giorgi, and Dr. Jordi P. Manauta.

Preface

The need to write a text concerning the treatment of inflammatory periapical diseases of endodontic origin—that is, disease affecting the supporting tissues of the tooth that was not resolved resolved by or following endodontic treatment—seems to us to be relevant, since the occurrence of these clinical situations in the population is very common.

Although epidemiological data are not uniform worldwide, the percentage of endodontically treated teeth with visible radiographic inflammatory reactions is not negligible, despite not being high; however, given the number of patients who are affected by this kind of disease, the extent of this phenomenon is immediately obvious, since millions of people have, or have had, periradicular disease of endodontic origin. Hence, it is important to perform a therapy on a tooth that has this type of disease, with the ambition of restoring effective and lasting masticatory function.

To achieve this result, the clinician must perform a comprehensive examination—from the general health of the patient's oral cavity, to all the aspects of the dental branch—following a path that is shared with the patient; this will lead us to the diagnosis and choice of the treatment plan with the patient's acceptance.

Insisting on the analysis of clinical parameters is a key factor in reaching the final decision as to whether or not to perform a retreatment procedure. The complexity of the phenomenon requires a very thorough examination, which includes not only assessments of the tooth itself but also of the surrounding tissues.
The therapeutic choice to undertake

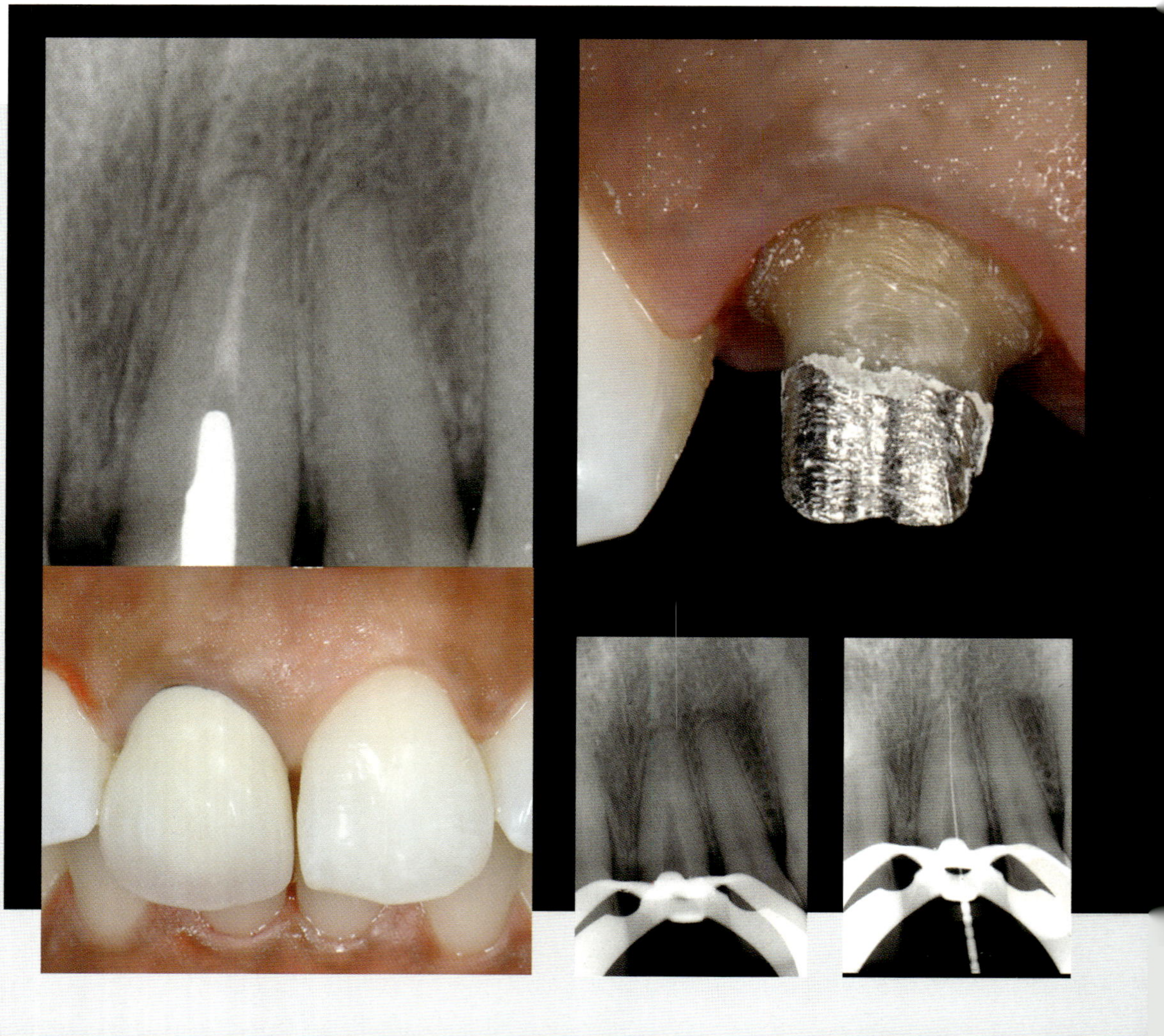

a new root canal therapy is, today, favored by the techniques for removing the materials that were previously inserted into the canal lumen and by the materials that can be used to seal the endodontium; in addition, the need and willingness—on the patients' part—to preserve their teeth appear to be a further determining factor for motivating this choice.

These are very often patients who, as life expectancy increases, present with these types of problems when they are elderly—and have a number of concomitant systemic conditions, treated with a large number of drugs, not without their own side effects. This last aspect, far from being negligible, is of great interest to the ethical sphere of the dental profession, aimed primarily at preserving the dental and periodontal structures of people affected by these diseases while respecting the general health of the patient. The path to carrying out retreatment is therefore full of pitfalls that may often not be obvious to the less experienced operator; neglecting them would mean running into uncertainties that could be unpleasant and predicting them is a moral obligation.

It is the specific objective of this text to provide the clinician with a reasoned guide to the diagnostic approach to and the performance of endodontic retreatment, with the clear intention of providing all the discriminating elements for dealing with this operation with peace of mind and skill and essential elements in order to obtain the best possible result for the overall oral health of the patient.

The editors

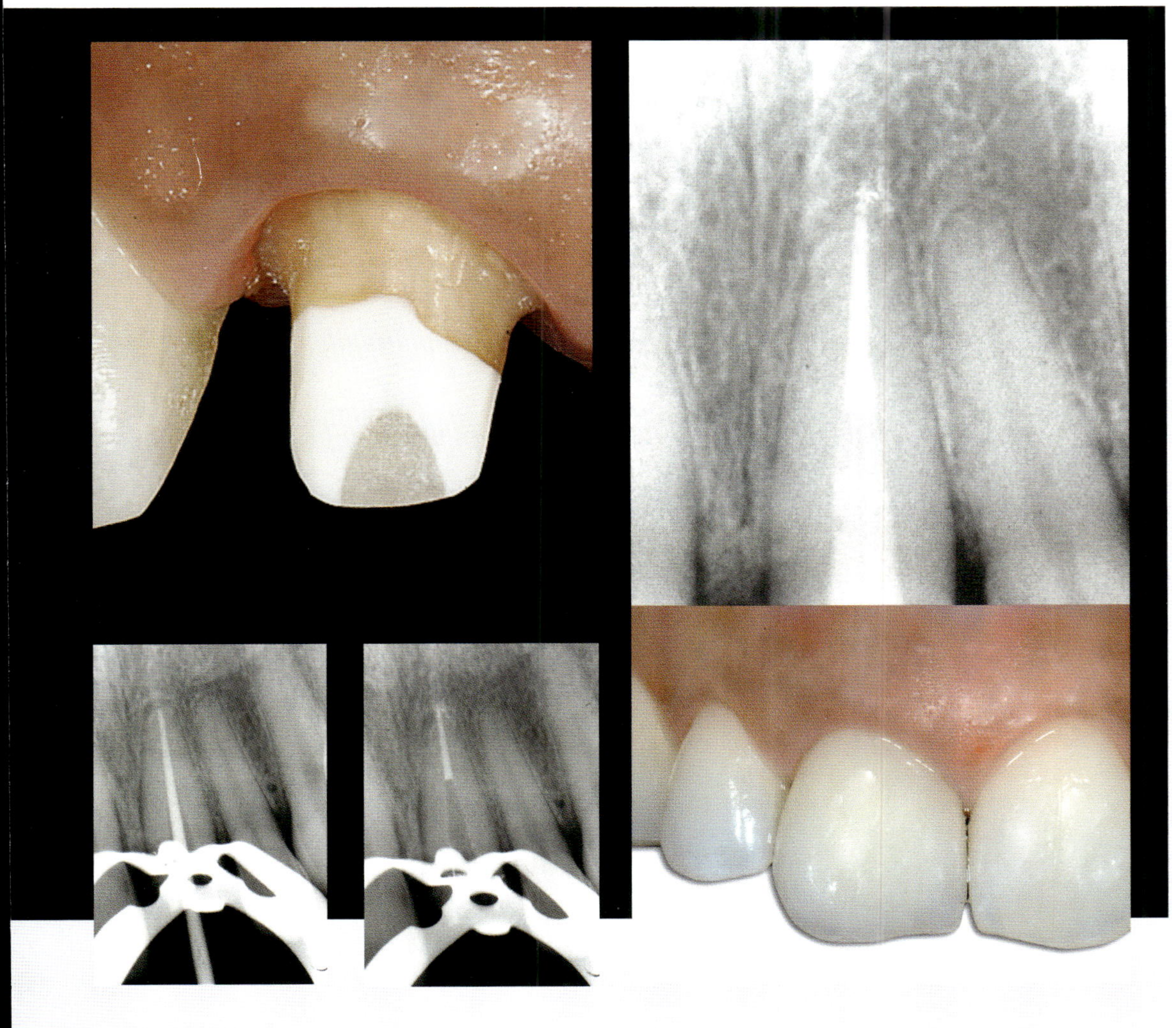

10 questions when endodontic treatment fails

These ten simple questions are just some of the questions we intend to answer; there are no absolute truths in this regard, but solid indications from the literature are available for each of the questions posed.

It will be up to the clinician to understand the contents and translate them with careful and scrupulous application, an essential element for any dental and stomatological therapy to obtain an effective result.

1

WHEN IS AN ENDODONTIC IN ORDER TREATMENT CONSIDERED INEFFECTIVE?

2

HOW CAN ENDODONTIC FAILURES BE IDENTIFIED RADIOLOGICALLY?

3

IS RETREATMENT ALWAYS INDICATED? (CONSIDERATIONS REGARDING IMPLANTOLOGY AND ENDODONTIC SURGERY)

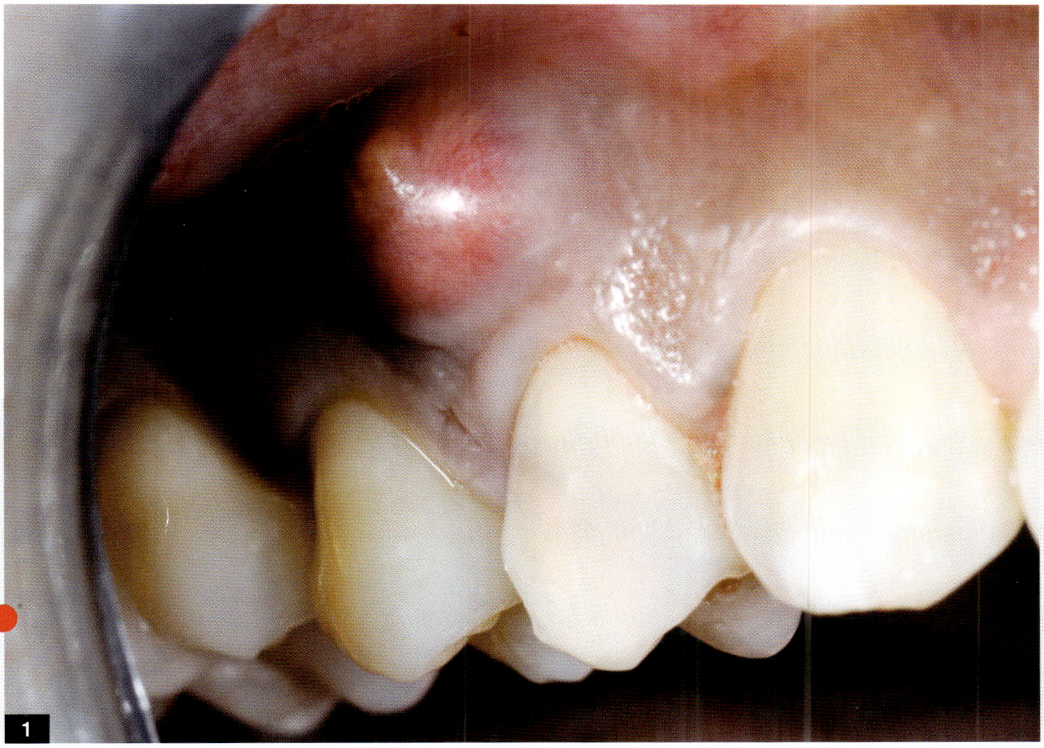

Fig. 1: The presence of a painful swelling is often one of the clinical signs characteristic of periapical lesions of endodontic origin.

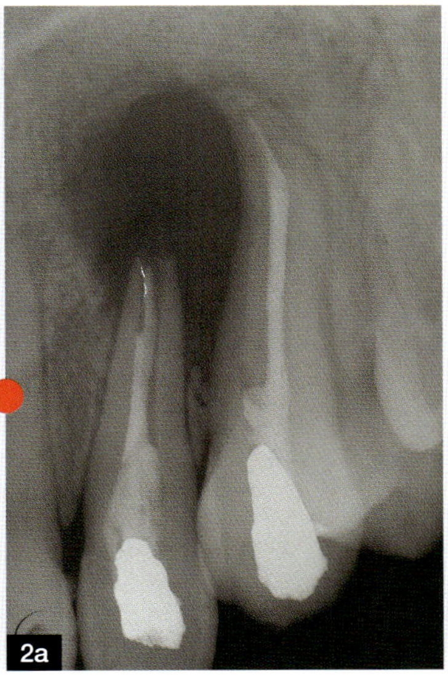

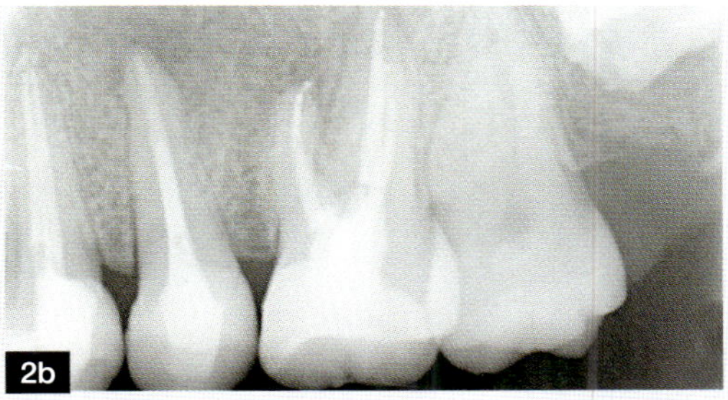

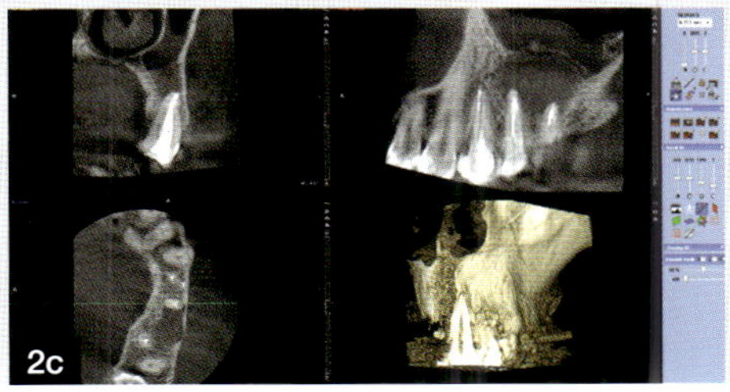

Fig. 2a: Radiotransparent bone fractures: a typical scenario of endodontic infections. In these cases, diagnosis is straightforward.

Fig. 2b: Pathological images often appear more blurred, and the two-dimensional radiography cannot accurately identify the extent of the lesions.

Fig. 2c: The use of three-dimensional radiological examinations (CBCT) makes it possible to clarify the magnitude of bone rarefaction.

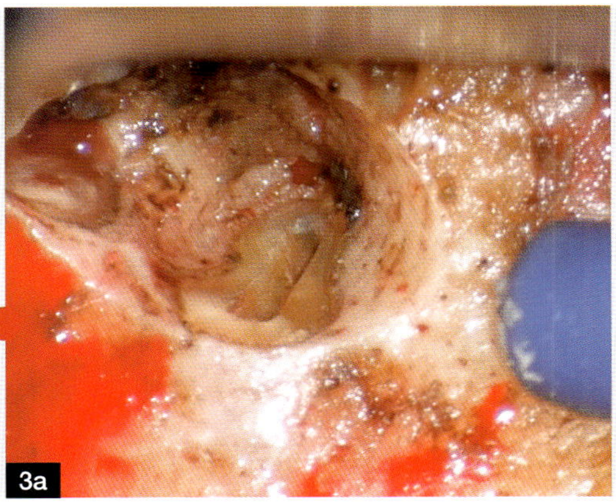

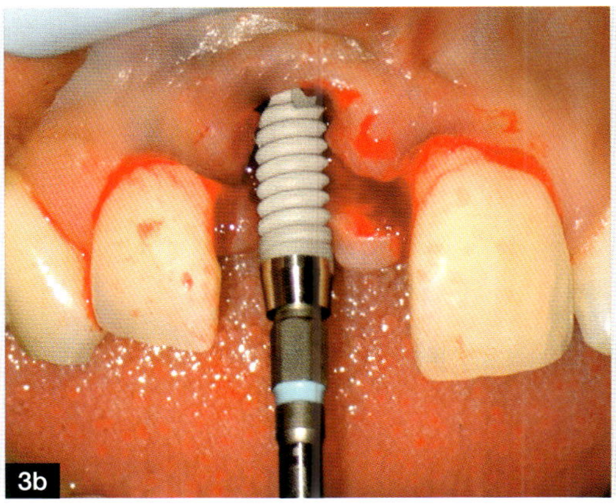

Fig. 3a: Surgical endodontics, performed with suitable methods and materials, is a very effective alternative to orthograde retreatment.

Fig. 3b: The implantology option must always be considered with the right timing, so as not to lose useful bone structure implant placement.

4

WHAT ARE THE BEST SOLUTIONS FOR PERFORMING CORRECT IRRIGATION IN RETREATMENTS?

5

WHAT ARE THE BEST FILLING TECHNIQUES IN RETREATMENT?

6

WHEN DO WE KNOW THAT A PERIAPICAL LESION OF ENDODONTIC ORIGIN IS HEALING?

7

IS IT ALWAYS NECESSARY TO REMOVE THE CORONAL RESTORATION?

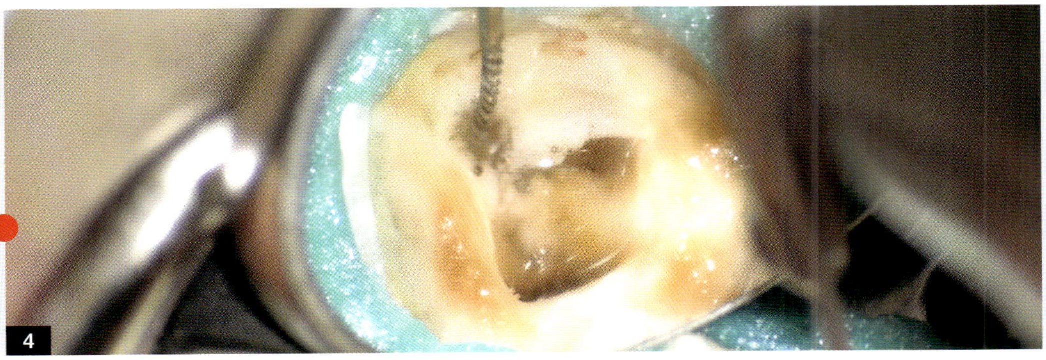

4

Fig. 4: The use of suitable irrigators, combined with appropriate techniques, is the essential requirement for achieving effective endodontium disinfection.

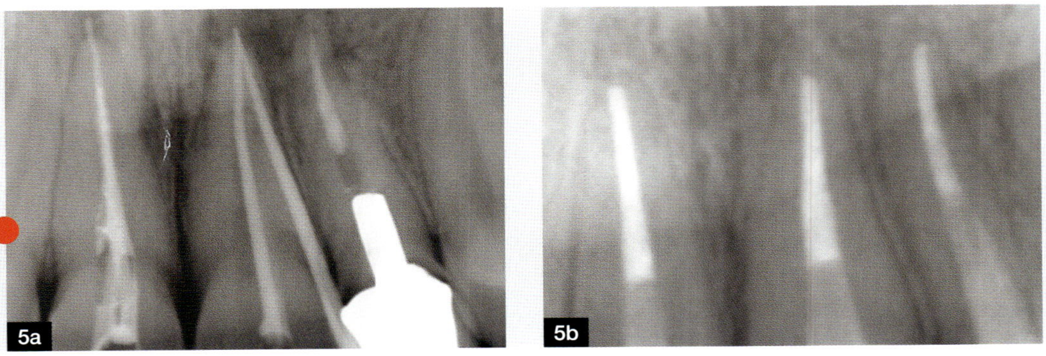

5a 5b

Fig. 5a-b: The clinician must be familiar with a number of different filling techniques in order to achieve good results in both the short and the long term.

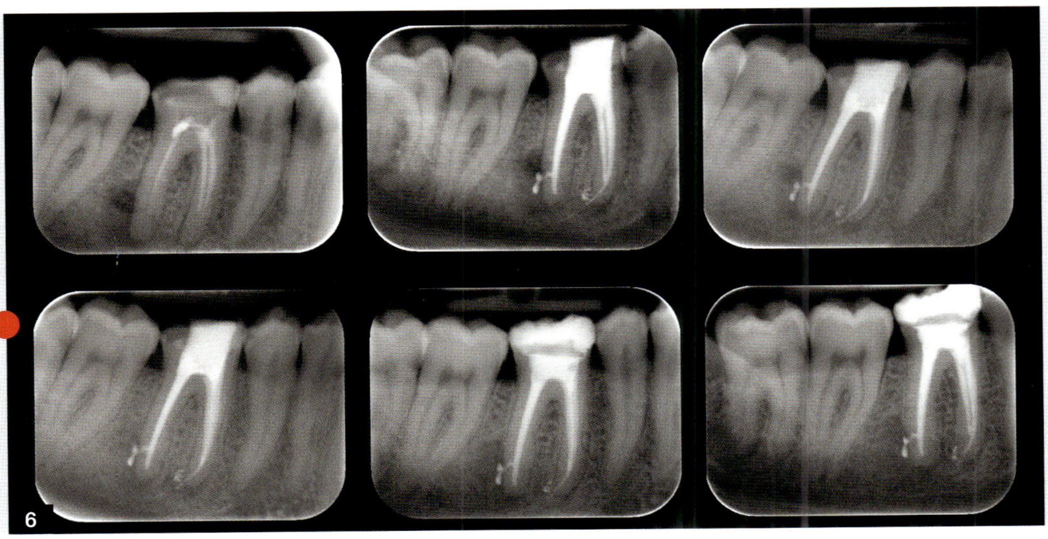

6

Fig. 6: The time required for the body to repair a periapical lesion of endodontic origin varies greatly; medium- and long-term follow-up is therefore mandatory.

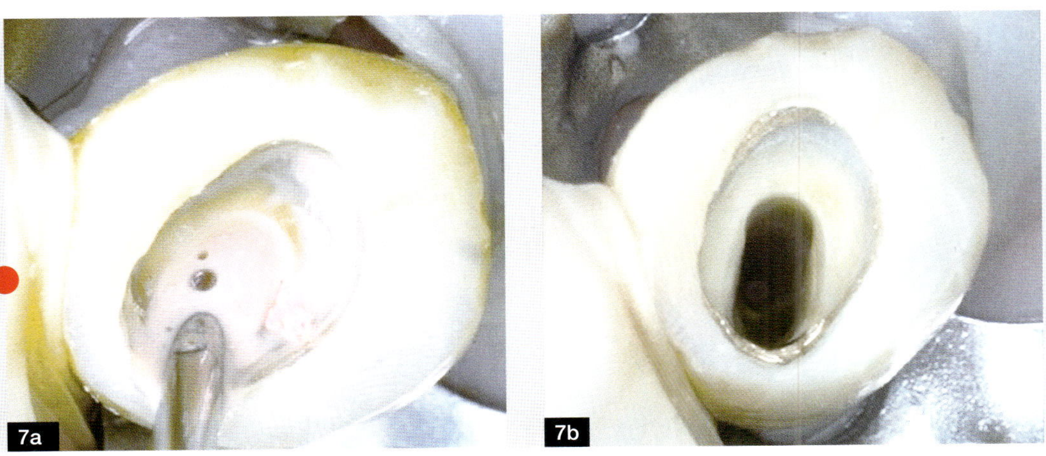

7a 7b

Fig. 7a-b: Saving the patient's restorations can be useful in the early stages in order to assess the evolution of therapy.

8 WHAT TECHNIQUES ARE USED TO REMOVE FILLING MATERIALS FROM THE ROOT CANALS?

9 SINGLE OR MULTIPLE TREATMENT SESSIONS FOR A RETREATMENT?

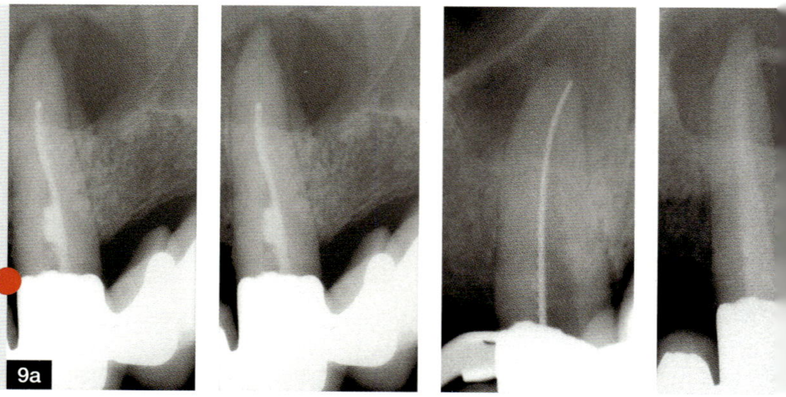

9a

10 WHAT SOLUTIONS TO ADOPT FOR THE RESTORATION OF ENDODONTICALLY-TREATED TEETH?

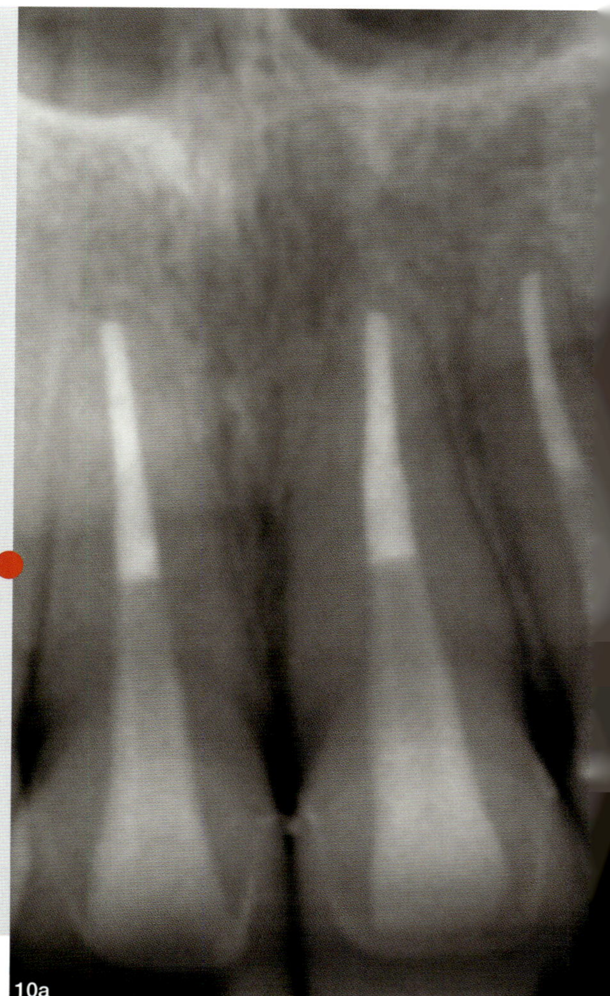

10a

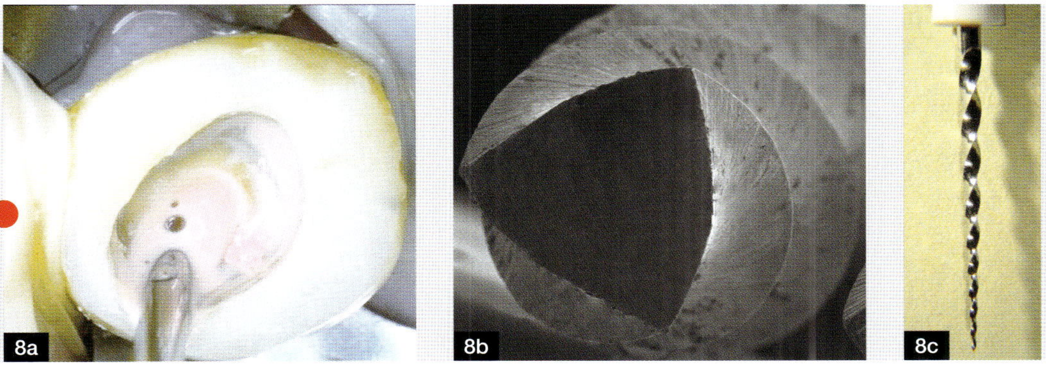

Fig. 8a-c: The emptying of endodontic space is one of the essential steps for achieving decontamination; new generation instruments and technical solutions are now available for completing this vital phase.

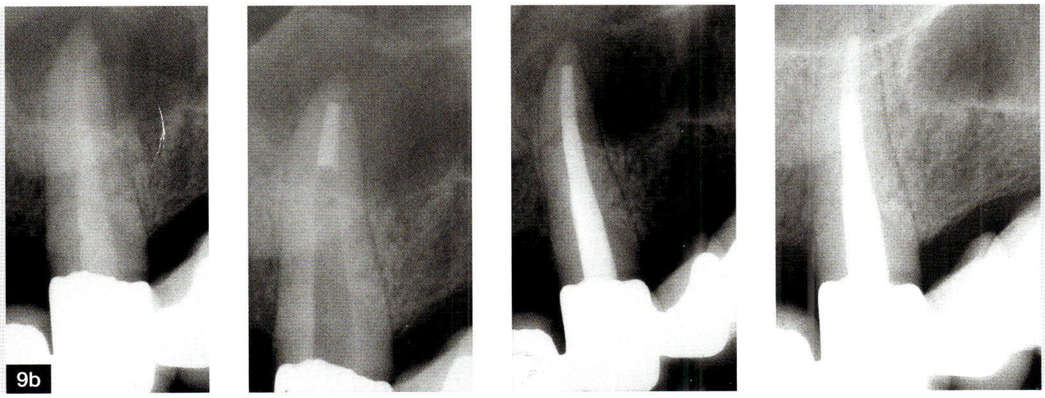

Fig. 9a-b: The retreatment of teeth associated with large and complex lesions calls for the application of intermediate dressings.

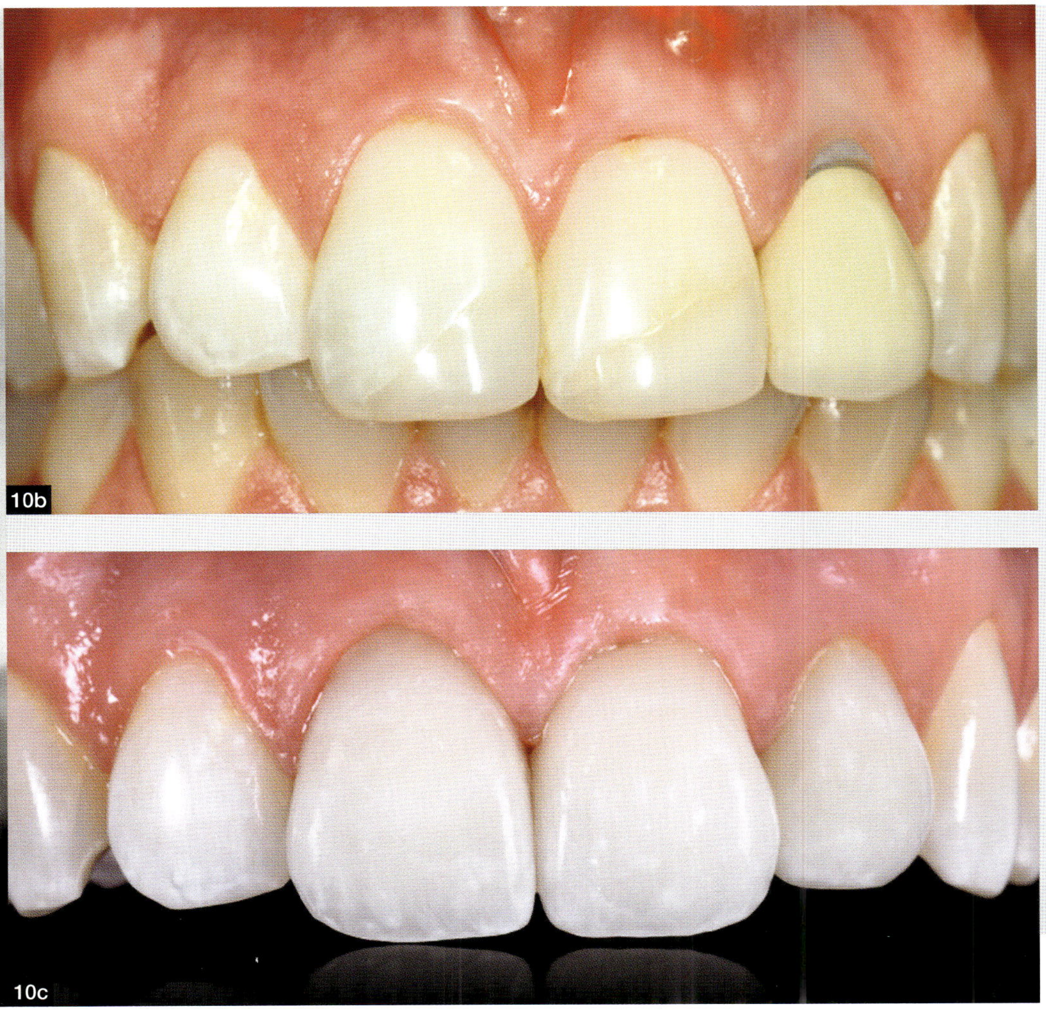

Fig. 10a-c: The reconstruction solution on endodontically – treated teeth ensures the quality of retreatment and provides the opportunity to transform the function and the aesthetics of the patient.

Retreatments: clinical pathways

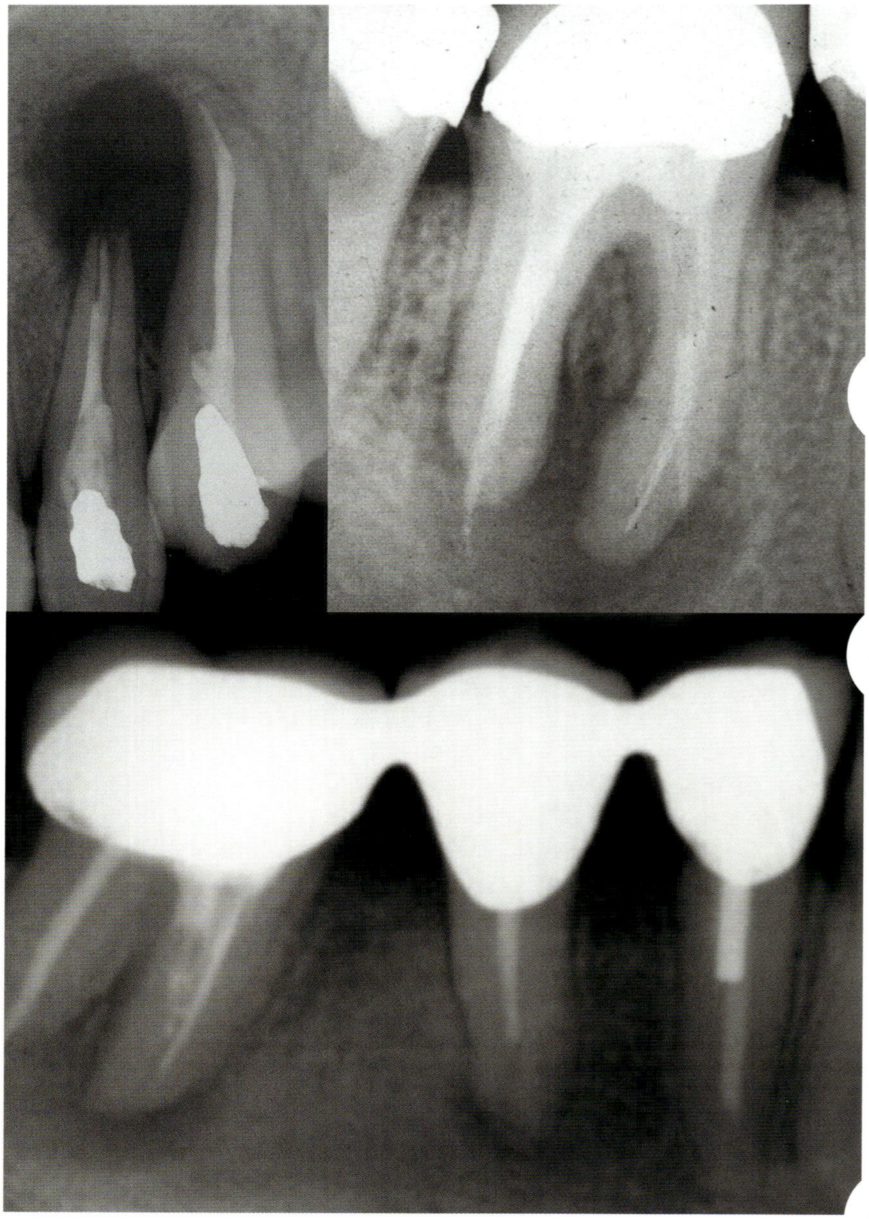

Periapical lesion of secondary endodontic origin or not resolved by previous endodontic treatment

RETREATMENT

SURGICAL ENDODONTICS

RETREATMENT AND SURGICAL ENDODONTICS

EXTRACTION

Immediate post-extraction implant placement

Healing

Prosthesic option

When the clinician encounters a condition such as that described above, and decides to intervene, the clinical implications are so numerous as to involve several areas of dentistry, as sufficiently-refined expertise is required to deal with the periodontal, restorative, and prosthetic, as well as endodontic aspects.

The overall view of the case to be treated, combined with skills in the use of uncommon instruments, such as the surgical microscope, becomes essential in oder to obtain a clear picture of the paths that can lead to the desired result: the oral health of the patient.

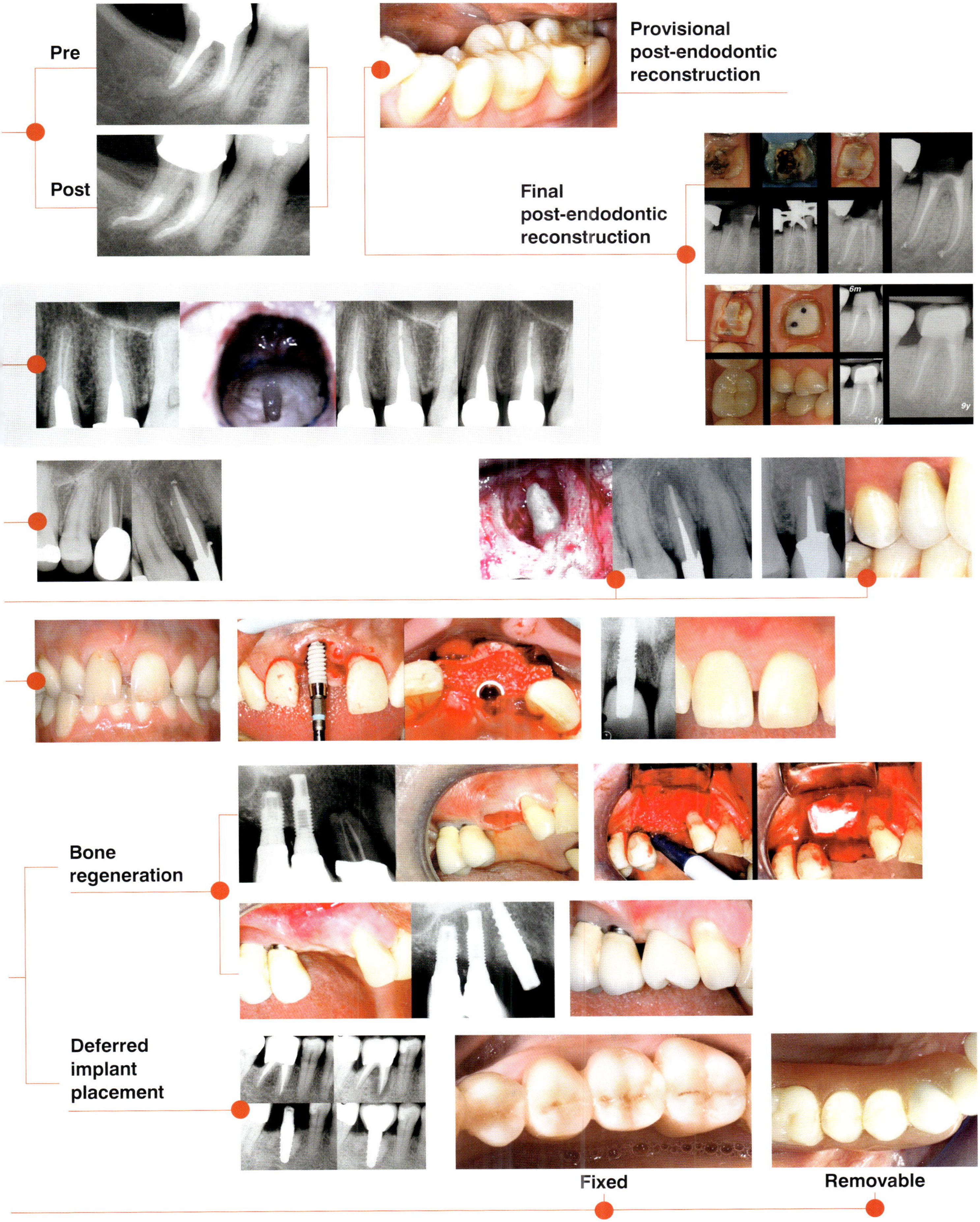
Pre
Post
Provisional post-endodontic reconstruction
Final post-endodontic reconstruction
6m
1y
9y
Bone regeneration
Deferred implant placement
Fixed
Removable

- Perform a thorough review of the epidemiological scope of **periapical diseases of endodontic origin**, and, in particular, their social implications.
- Describe the pathogenetic agents and the pathophysiological evolution of the disease, secondary to **failure of root canal therapy**.
- Identify the favorable and unfavorable prognostic factors resulting from longitudinal studies, as they form the basis for a confident management of the **diagnostic and therapeutic process**.

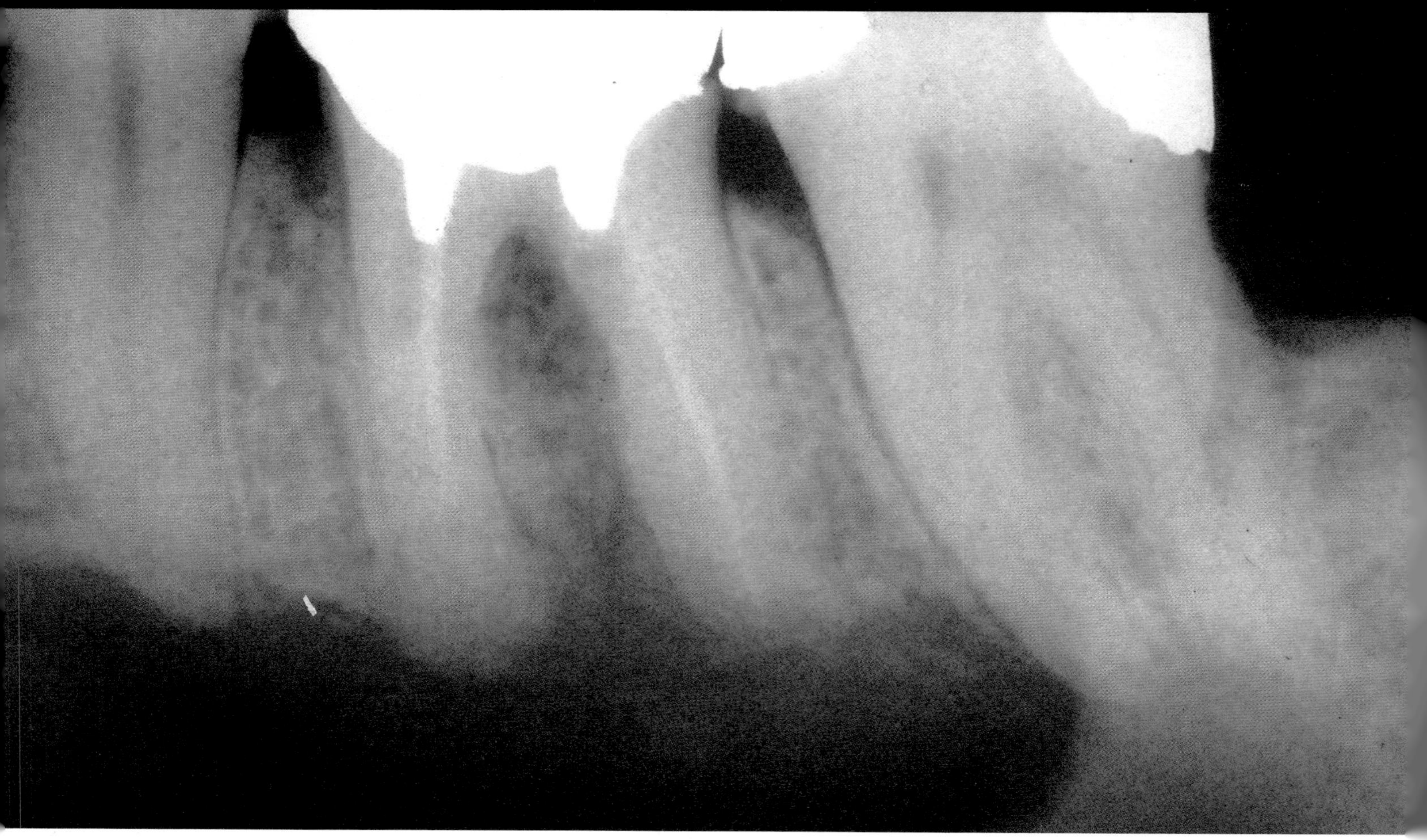

Massimo Gagliani, Fabio Gorni,
Marco Martignoni

01

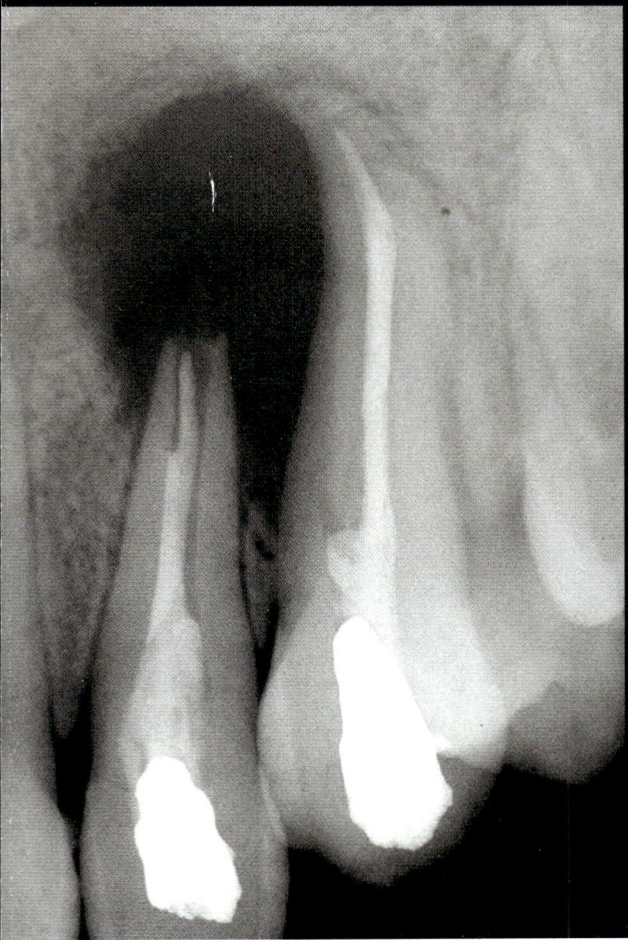

Failures in endodontics

An epidemiological and clinical analysis

General considerations on failure in endodontics

Being able to talk, in an absolute sense, about success or failure in a dental surgical discipline, such as endodontics, would be a great advantage; however, as our research methods become increasingly sophisticated, the cut-off between success and failure becomes increasingly difficult to establish, due to constant changes in the parameters used. The simplest, but not for that matter simplistic, solution would be to observe and comply with the guidelines drawn up by major international scientific societies in the endodontic field.[1a] In this sense, many scientific societies have endeavored to exemplify clinical situations pertaining the sector and closer attention will be dedicated to this aspect later in this chapter.
Periapical disease of endodontic origin is identified by X-ray.
Figures 1.1-1.8 provide an emblematic overview. As the clinical findings are often separated from radiographic evidence available, the possibility of these scenarios providing discordant results makes it even

Figs. 1.1-1.8: These images represent radiographic scenarios typical of periapical lesions of endodontic origin, secondary to treatment failure. The common denominator is that of a radio - transparent area of variable entity, around the apical limit of each tooth, associated with insufficient canal filling in terms of both length and width. In some cases, the endodontium has not been explored, whereas in others (Fig. 1.5), the fracture of an instrument leads to the suspension of the treatment.

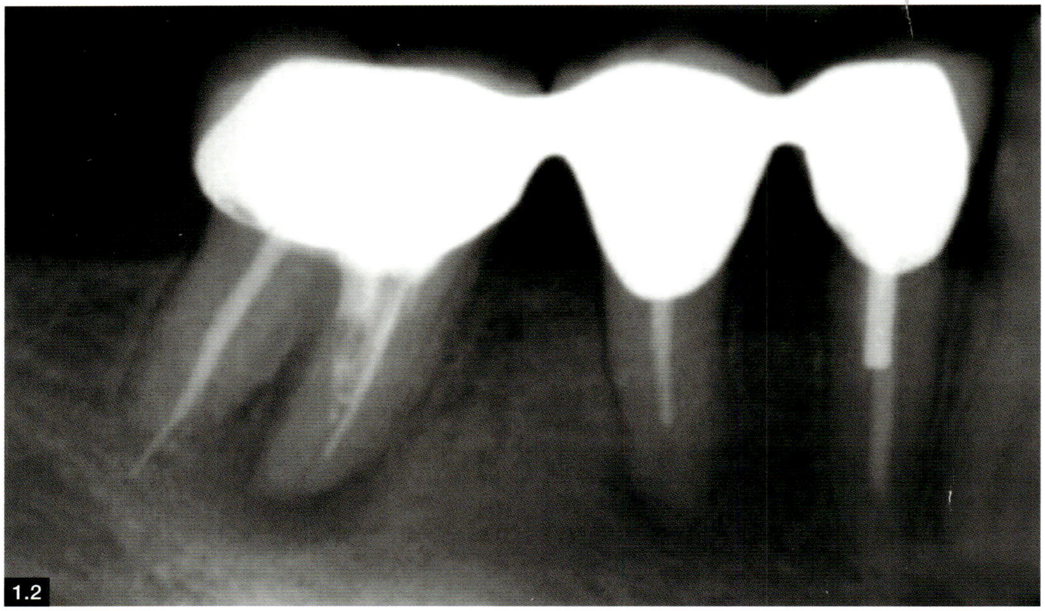
1.2

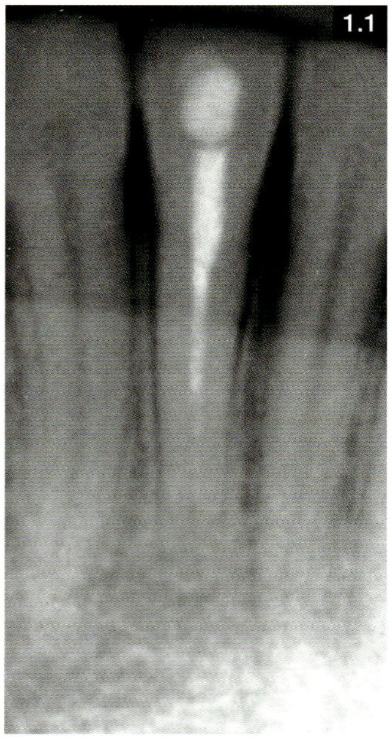
1.1

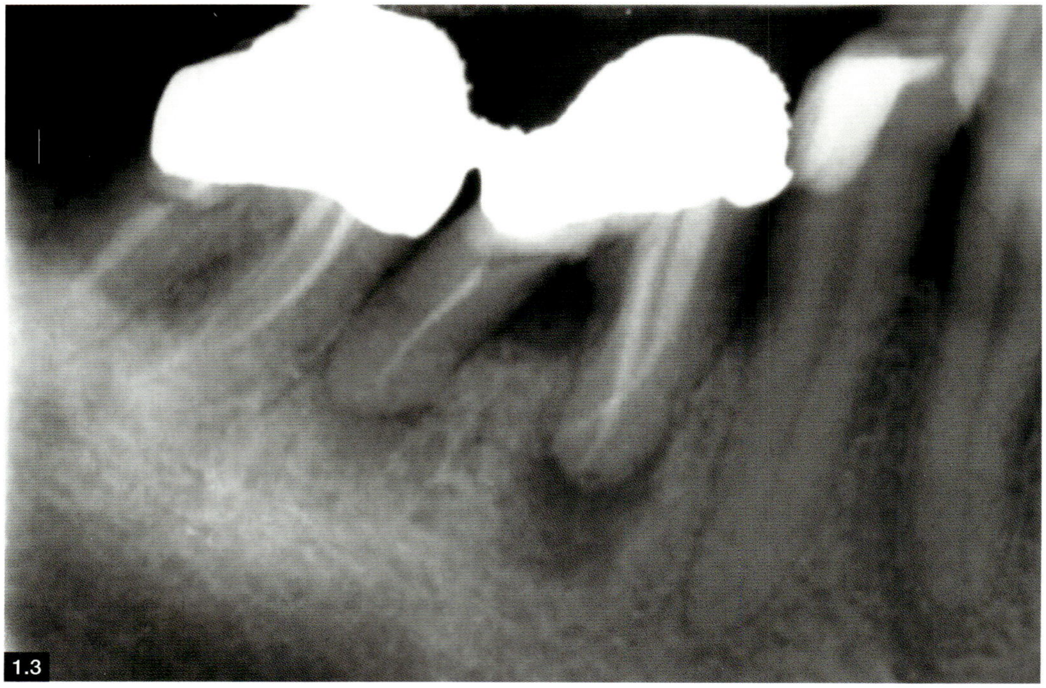
1.3

more difficult for the practitioner to formulate a diagnosis and, to an even greater degree, to establish a treatment plan compatible with a favorable prognosis.
In this volume, we will review the inflammatory periapical diseases of endodontic origin[1] that are caused rather than solved by previous treatments – be they apparently correct or incorrect – based on dental elements using an exclusively clinical approach (Figs. 1.9-1.12).
This choice precludes an exhaustive consideration of the issues associated with the pathophysiology of the supporting tissues and with the microbiology underlying development of "posttreatment disease"[2, 3] or disease after endodontic treatment or, in a broader sense, disease not solved by endodontic treatment[4]. This condition involves a bacterial component inside or even outside the root canal[5-7], which represents one of the determining etiological elements (Figs. 1.13-1.14); and concomitant causes associated with the microorganisms present inside the root may play a secondary role in the maintenance of the disease. The term "post-treatment disease" could be considered rather simplistic, since root canal therapy is frequently carried

▶ continue to page 6

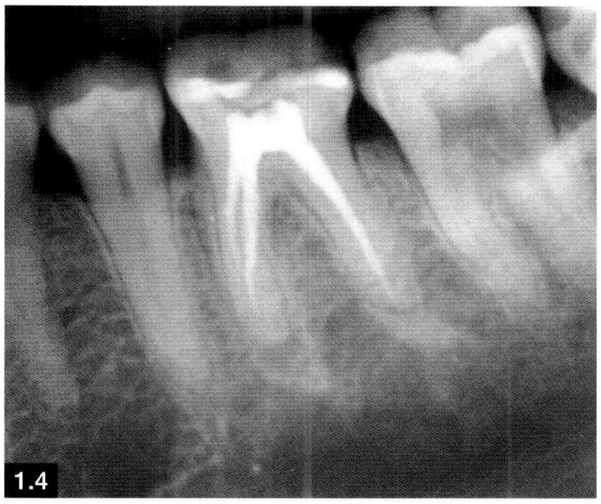
1.4

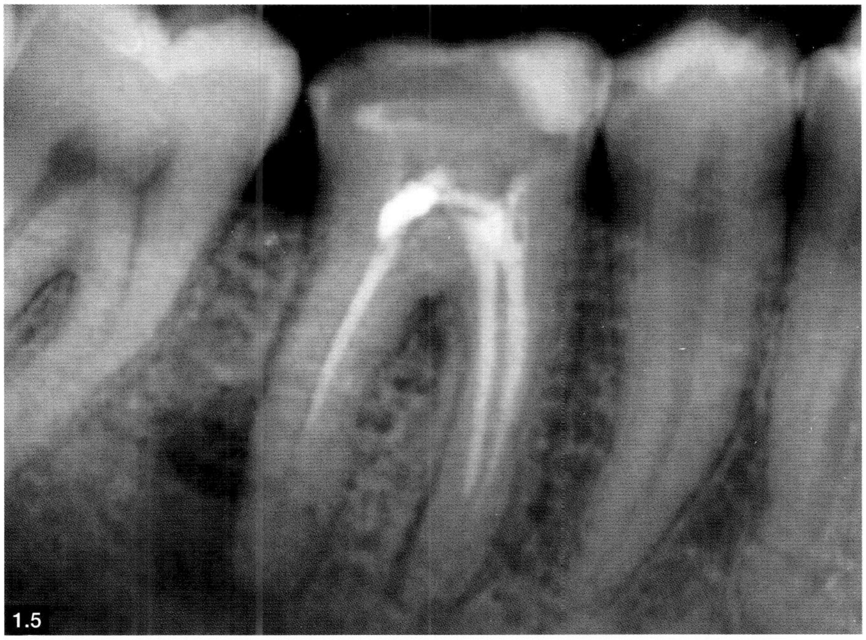
1.5

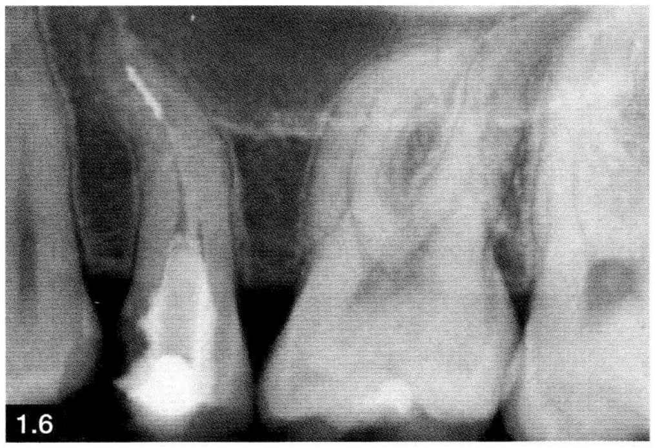
1.6

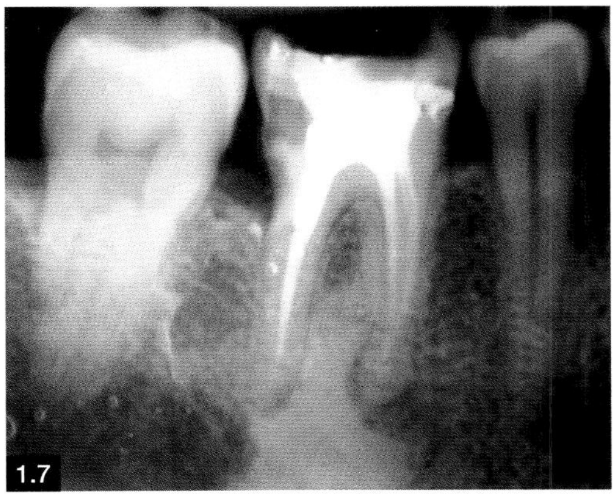
1.7

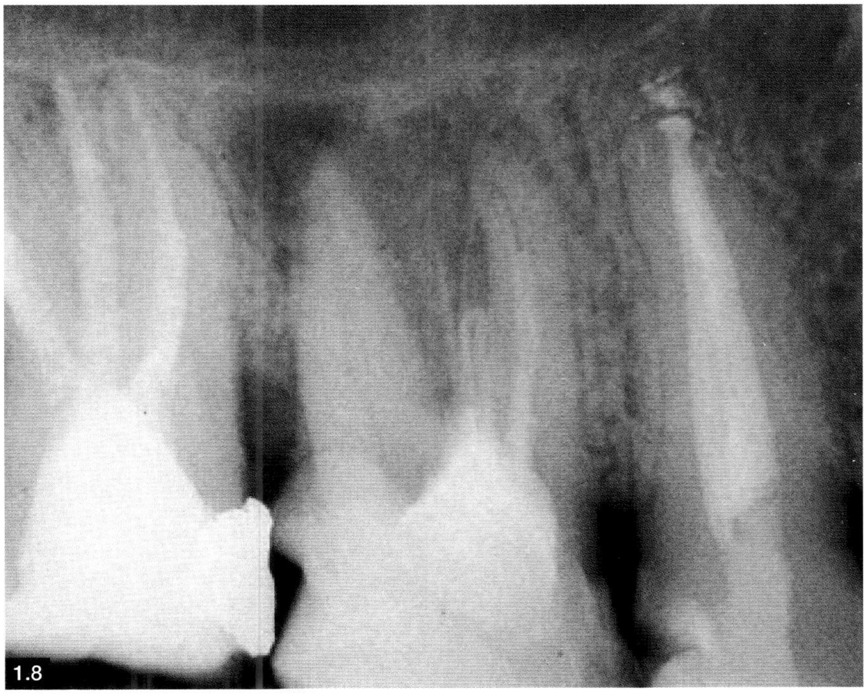
1.8

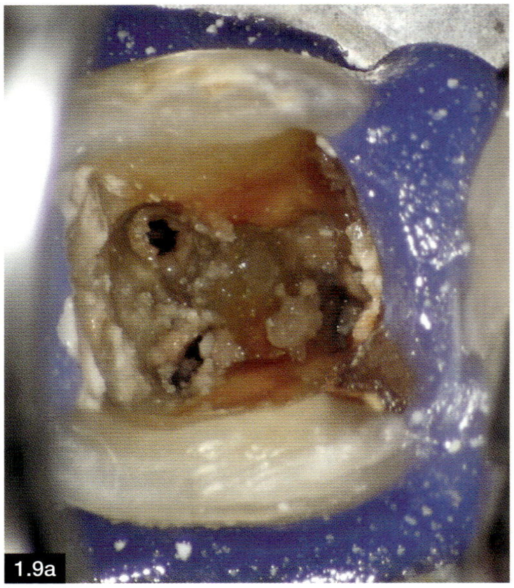
1.9a

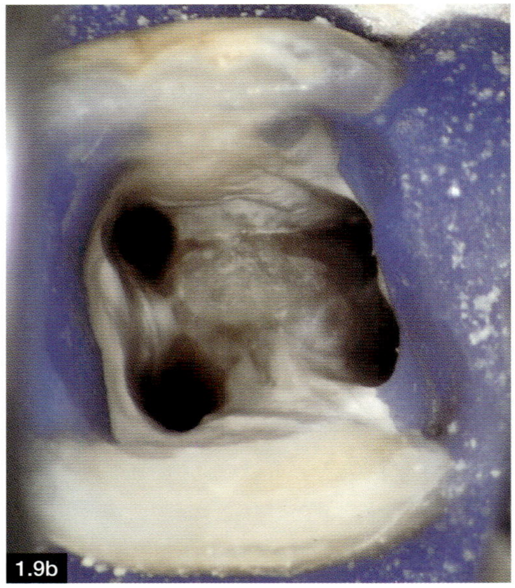
1.9b

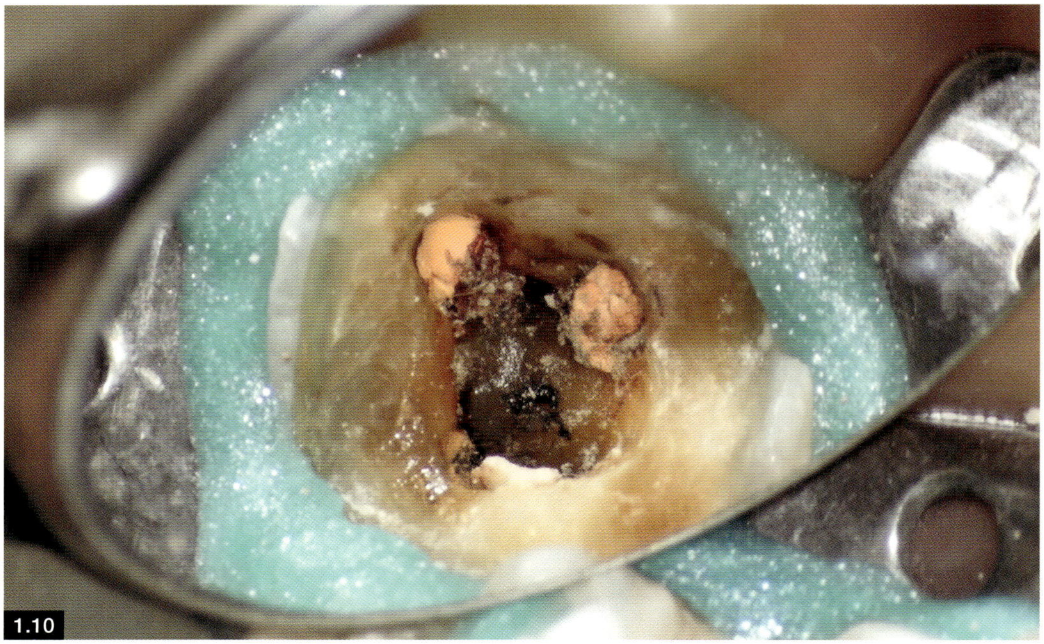
1.10

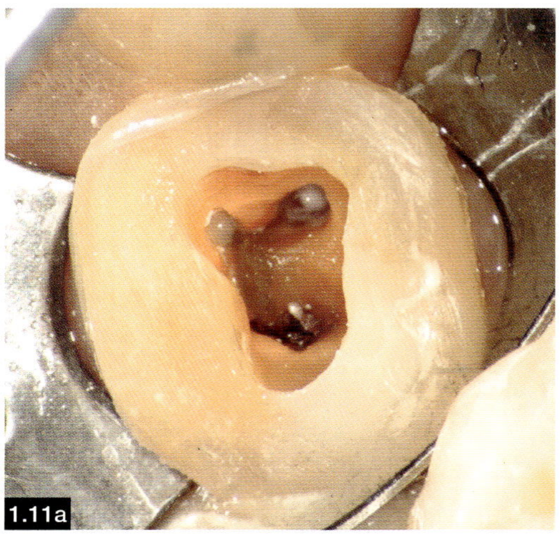
1.11a

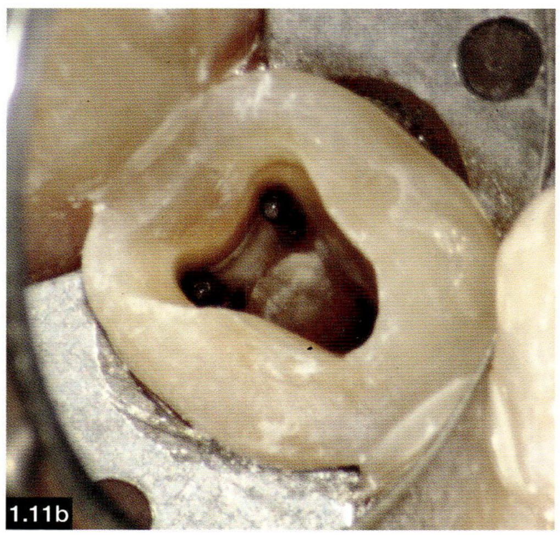
1.11b

Figs. 1.9-1.12: The clinical scenario of the teeth, which develop periapical disease as a result of sub-optimum endodontic treatment, is often characterized by unsatisfactory pulp chamber openings, the presence of carious tissues in the coronal compartment and a receptacle of bacterial plaque, and lack of correct vision.

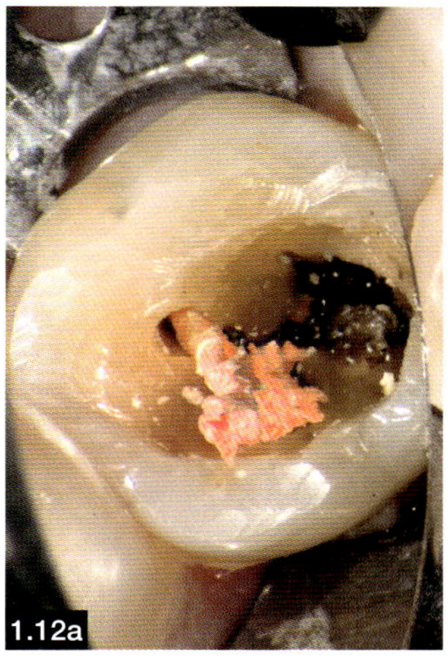

1.12a

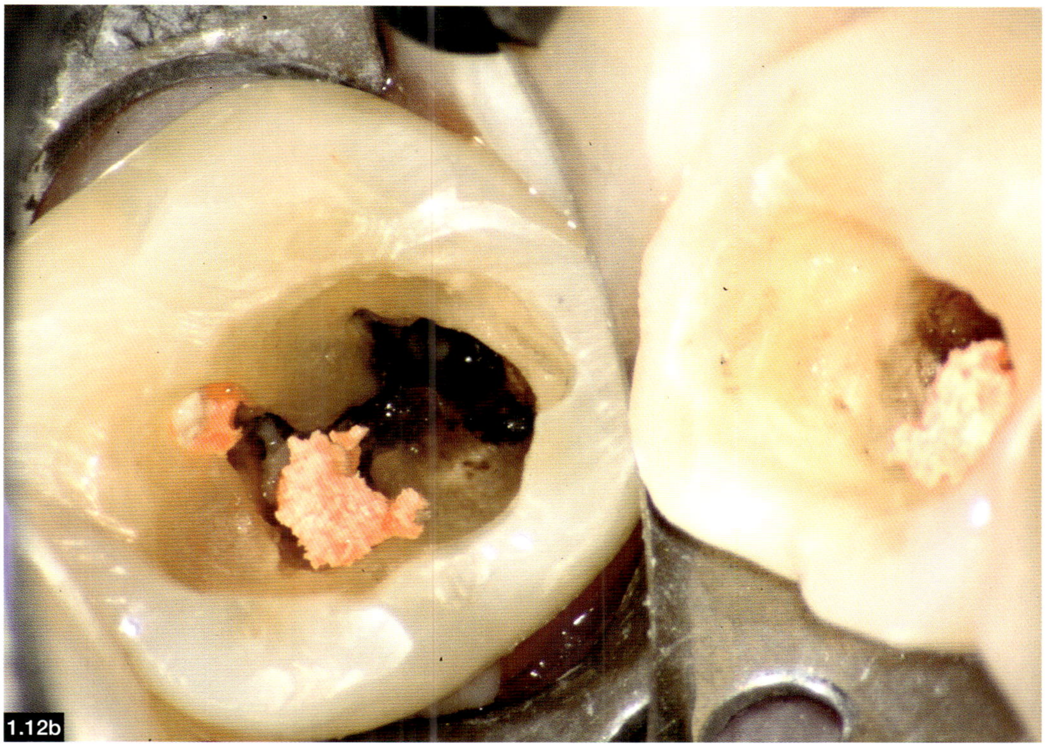

1.12b

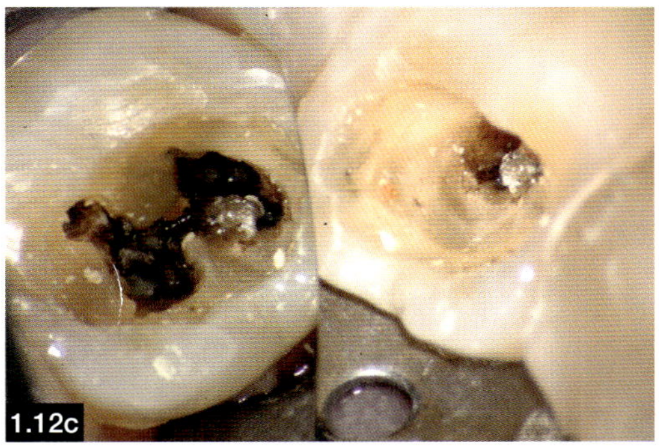

1.12c

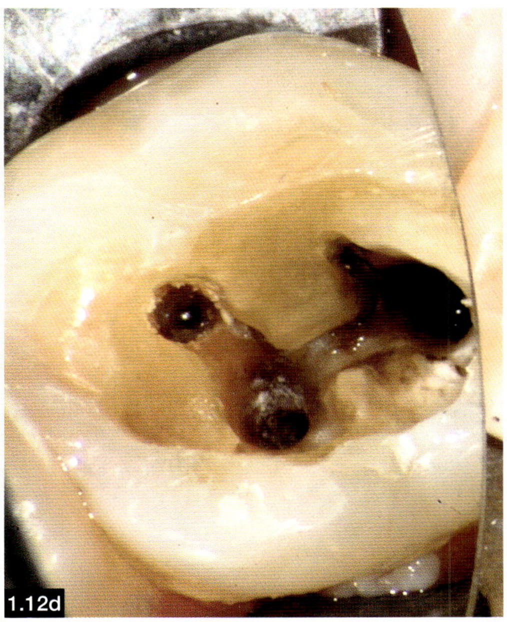

1.12d

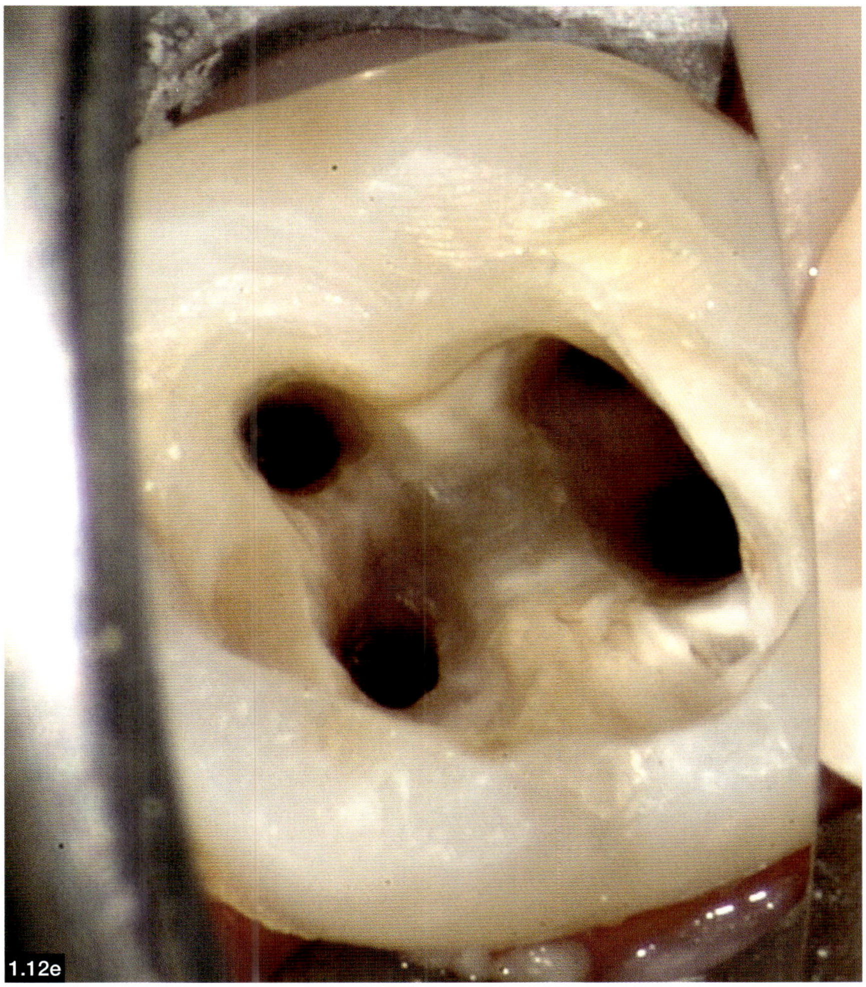

1.12e

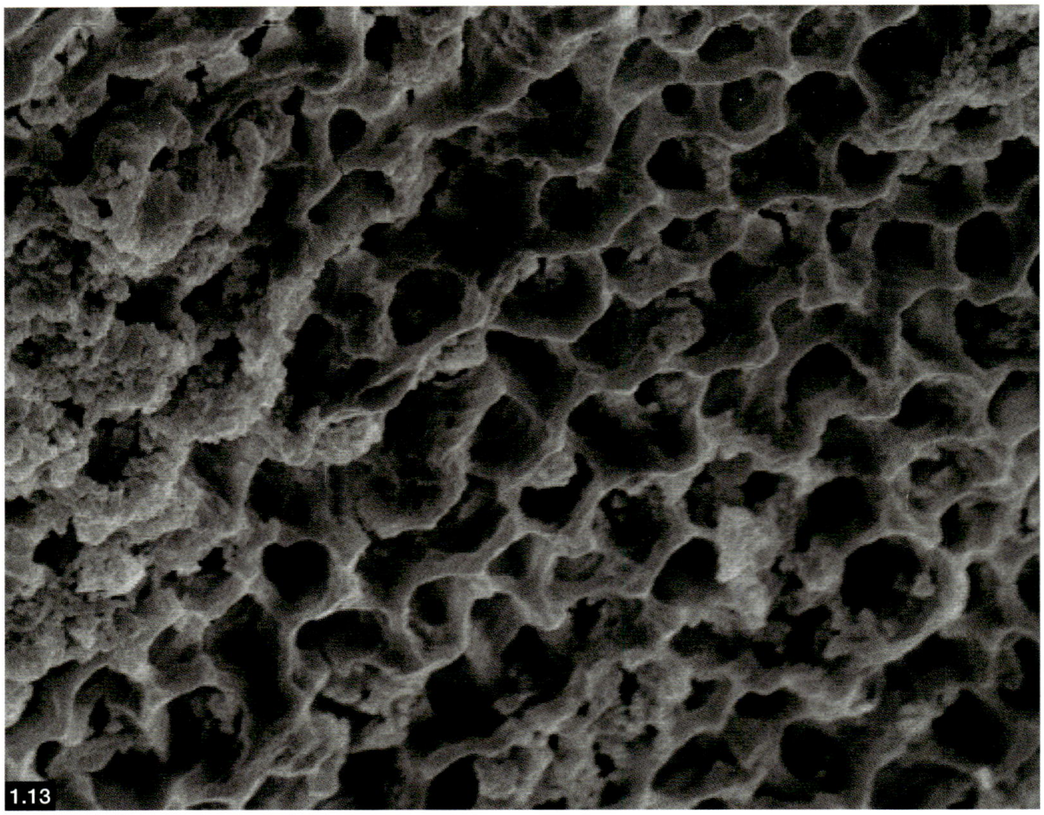

Fig. 1.13: Canal lumen with proliferating bacterial population that is not yet aggregated into biofilm.

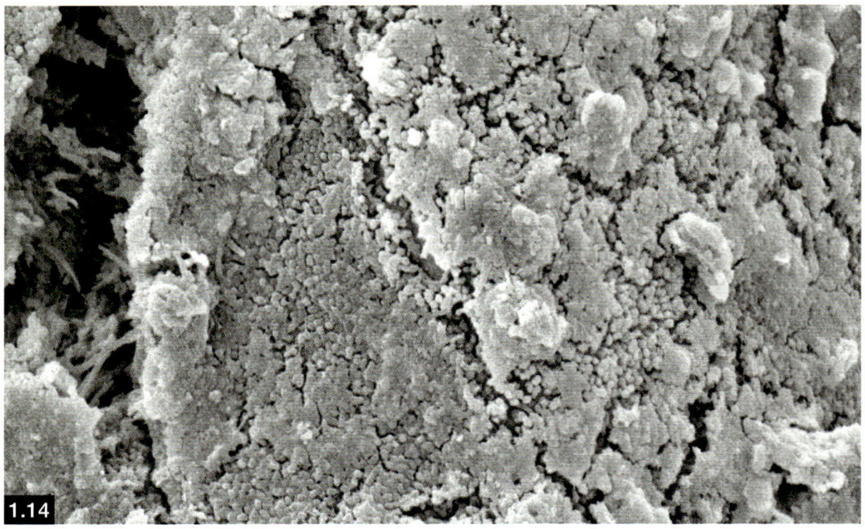

Fig. 1.14: Canal wall with consistent bacterial biofilm and dentin mud.

out in previously untreated teeth.
The content of the root canal is generated by a chronic periapical inflammatory reaction. Therefore, the operational causes that make it impossible to achieve the desired effect cannot always be determined (Figs. 1.15-1.18). Failure remains intrinsic to the clinician's inability to completely remove the *pathogenic noxa* responsible for the radiographically detectable periapical reaction, regardless of whether it is clinically evident. With regard to the microbiological issues, the causes of failure are simultaneously simple and complex. The studies conducted by Kakehashi et al.[8, 9] clarified the etiology of apical periodontitis beyond all reasonable doubt by demonstrating that the vast majority of cases are mainly caused by bacteria.
In the absence of bacteria, the periapical reaction in dental elements that have been deprived of their pulp does not develop.
This finding was extensively corroborated by subsequent studies by Sjogren[10], Sundqvist[11-13], Moller et al.[14], and Nair[15, 16]. More recently, important contributions were made by Siqueira[17-19] and Ricucci[20, 21].
In some cases, the presence of bacteria inside the root canal may not be the only trigger of periapical diseases, because their proliferation in the ecological niches of the periapical contour[20] may be just one contributing factor for the development of a chronic inflammatory reaction in the periapical tissues that is difficult to treat using conventional orthograde therapies.
Having pointed out that the microbiological aspect is the prevailing factor, whether it is already present in the phases of the primary

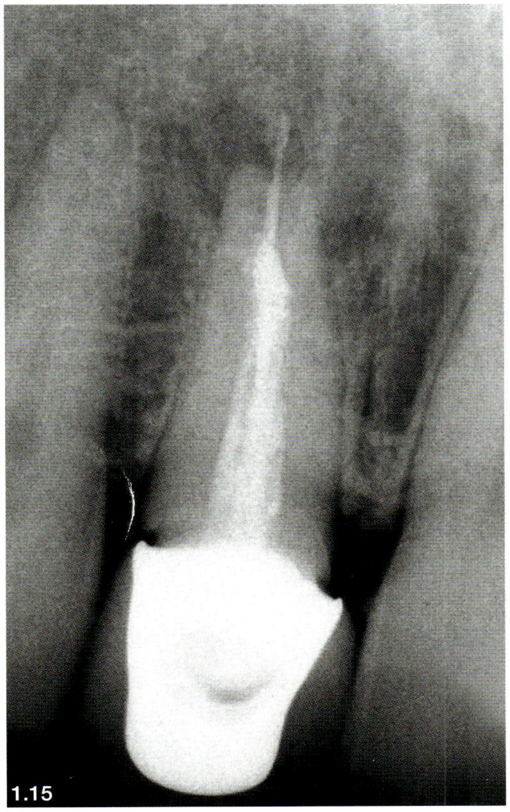

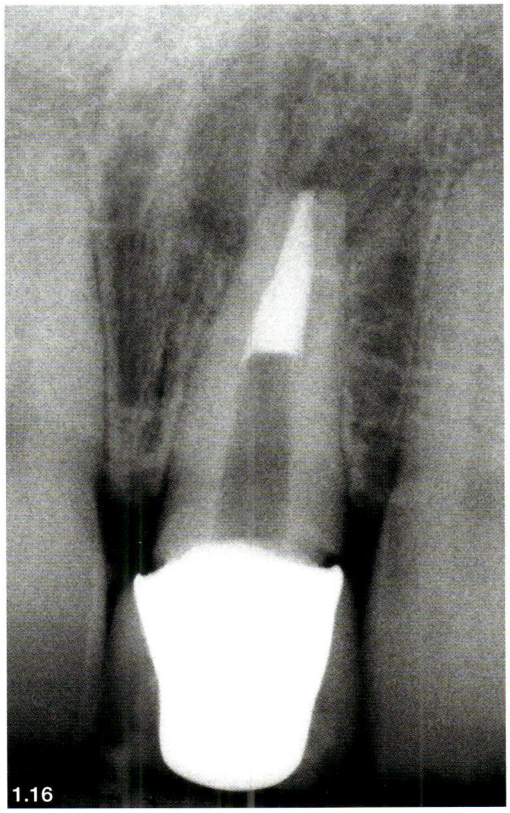

Fig. 1.15: Typical situation of a periapical disease secondary to an incorrect endodontic treatment; a poor relationship exists between the canal lumen and filler material at apical level.

Fig. 1.16: Retreatment performed with a different quality of shaping and filling of the apical limit.

Fig. 1.17: Radiotransparent periapical lesion in the upper premolar.

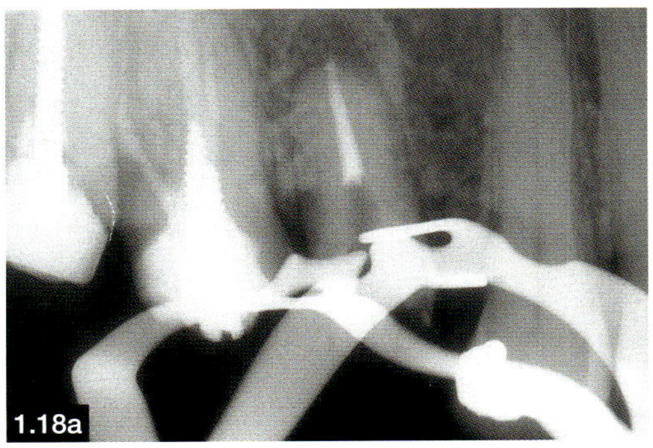

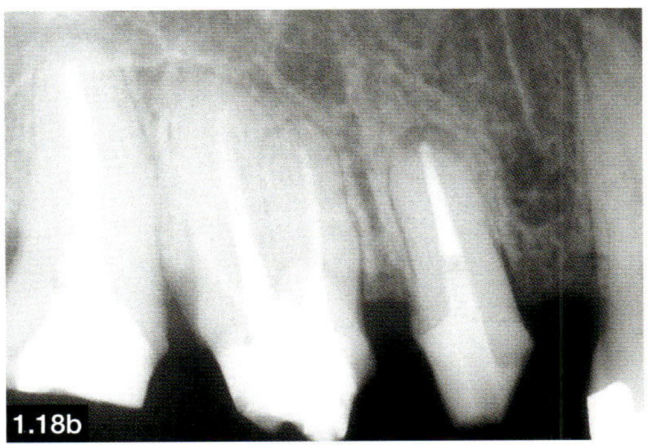

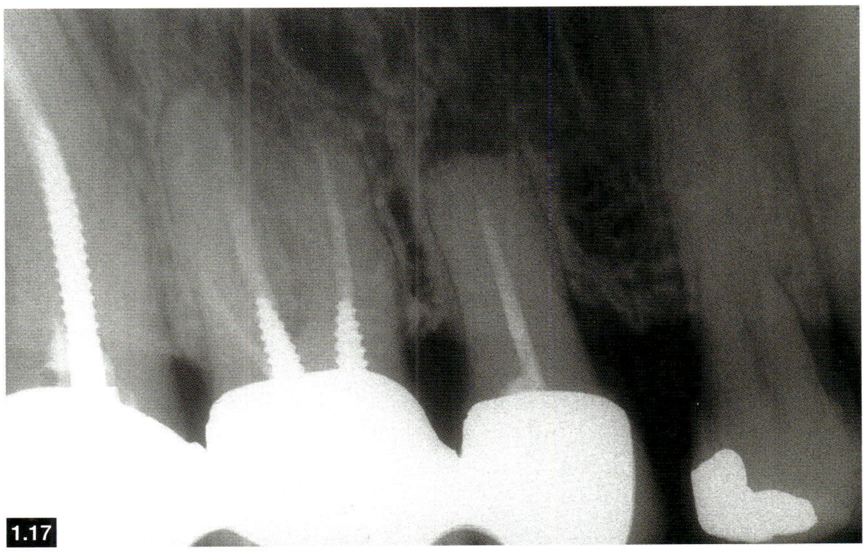

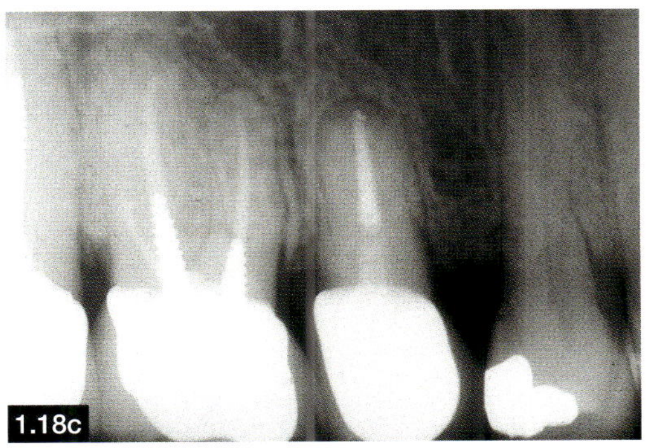

Fig. 1.18a-c: Retreatment and evaluation at two different time points; the final outcome is clinically satisfactory but the radiographic study, although better than at the beginning, has not given the expected result approximately one year later.

treatment or it is the result of inadequate treatment carried out in the first instance, other factors, such as the concomitant presence of viruses[22, 23] and yeasts (Candida albicans)[24-26] cannot be ignored.
It is also important to remember that foreign body reactions, caused by the filling materials used previously, may occur[27].
A recent systematic review (A) described the role of the apical extrusion of the sealer, reporting a 32% higher risk of contributing to a nonhealing outcome in teeth with extrusion than in those without. In an analogous study, Mello et al. (B) obtained similar final considerations, although the quality of the studies included was not of the highest possible level.
It goes without say that the presence of a rich bacterial flora in the early stages of treatment makes a satisfactory result in the first endodontic treatment less likely[27-29]. This notwithstanding, the practitioner's inability of clinicians to remove the entire bacterial component from the endodontic compartment remains the primary cause of failure, and one that cannot be eradicated with sufficient certainty, regardless of the endodontic procedure adopted. In some cases, once the associated risks and benefits have been weighed up, clinicians find themselves in the position of having to consider retreatment, primarily for clinical reasons. An emblematic situation is shown in Figures 1.19-1.24.
The patient was referred given the need to perform prosthetic work due to the loss of masticatory function in quadrant four. After a thorough clinical examination, mild pain was observed when chewing in the right lower quadrant at the last molar; the x-ray showed slight ectasia of the periodontal space of element 47.
The proposed therapeutic solution is to retreat this tooth and to rehabilitate the arch to guarantee restored function to the whole area. The clinical and radiographic scenario shows the steps of the retreatment, the steps of the treatment carried out on element 45, and the evolution over time from 3 to 18 years later. In the pages that follow, similar successful cases are reported up to almost 20 years.

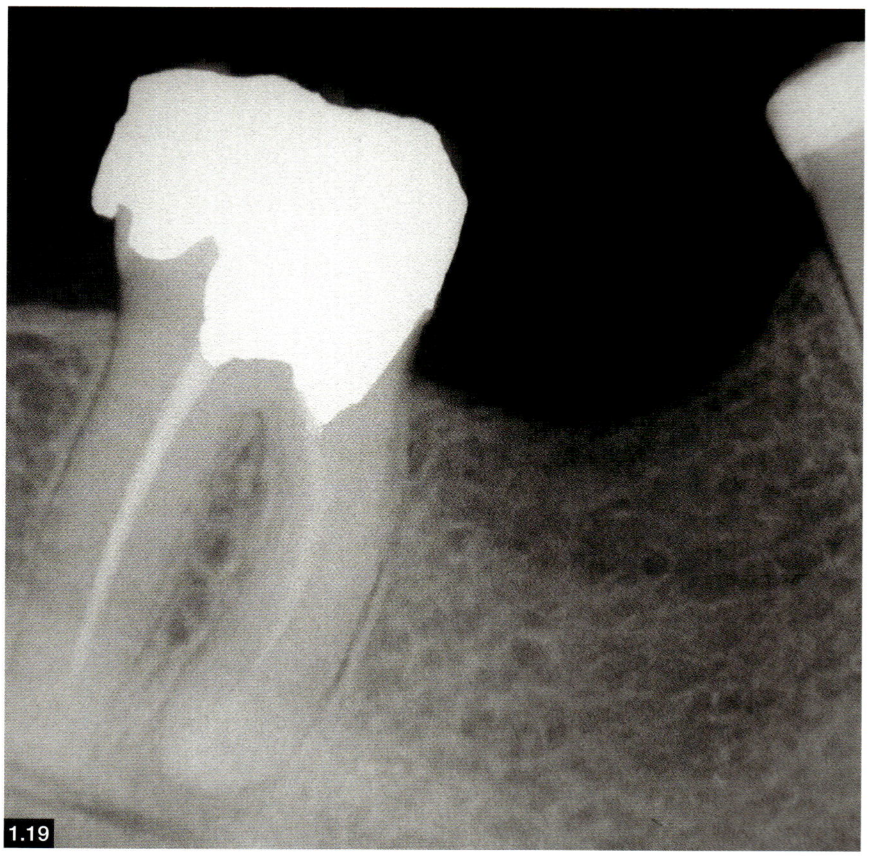

1.19

Fig. 1.19: The two-dimensional radiographic study shows a slight ectasia of the mesial periapical space of element 47; radiotransparency in this area is only intuitable but not quantifiable.

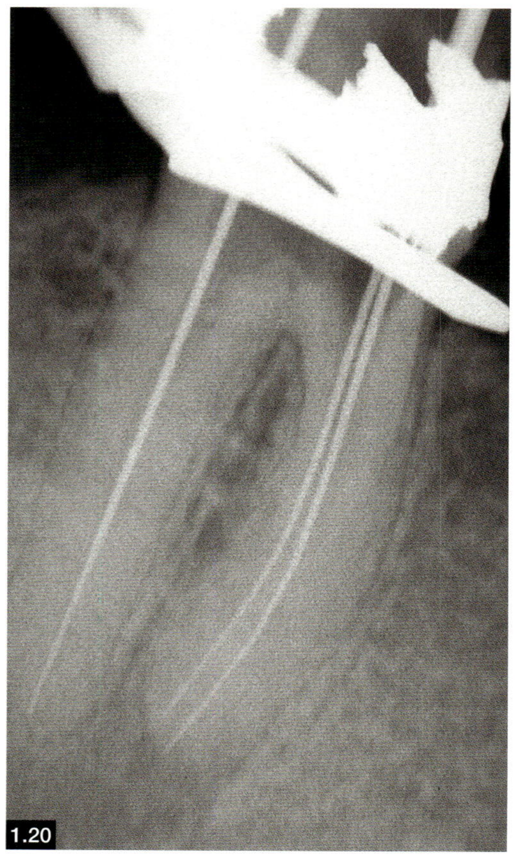

1.20

Fig. 1.20: Work length achieved better than that of the previous endodontic treatment.

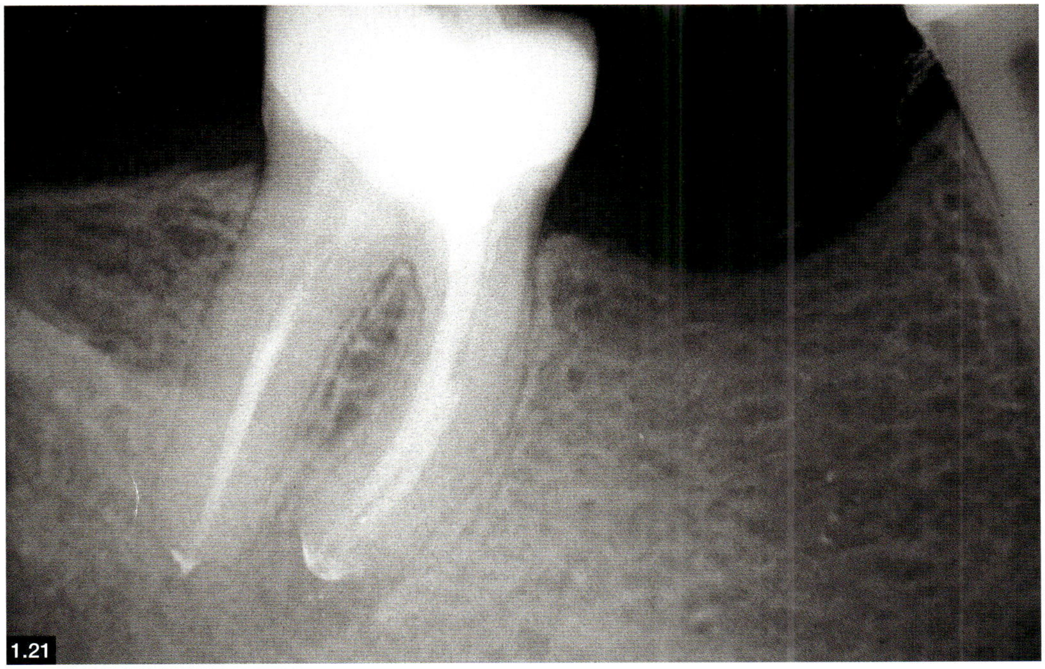

Fig. 1.21: Filling of the endodontic space with its composite reconstruction; long-term temporary restoration to reevaluate symptomatology and functionality over time.

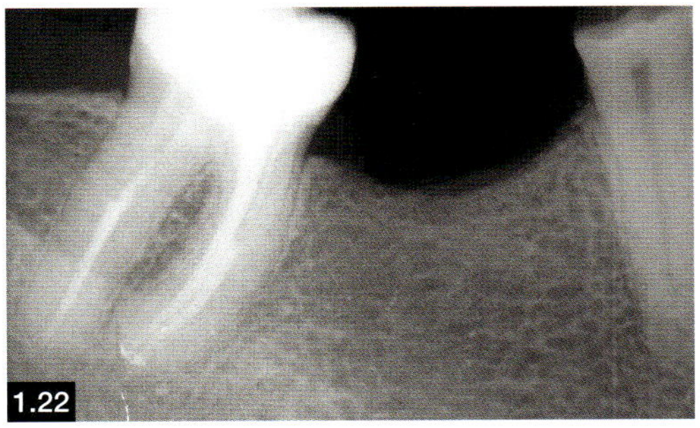

Fig. 1.22: Follow-up x-ray after 1 year warranting the preparation of a bridge.

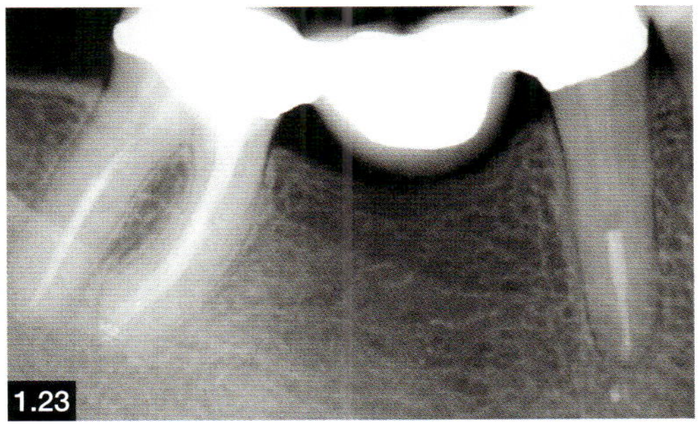

Fig. 1.23: Follow-up x-ray of the bridge after 3 years.

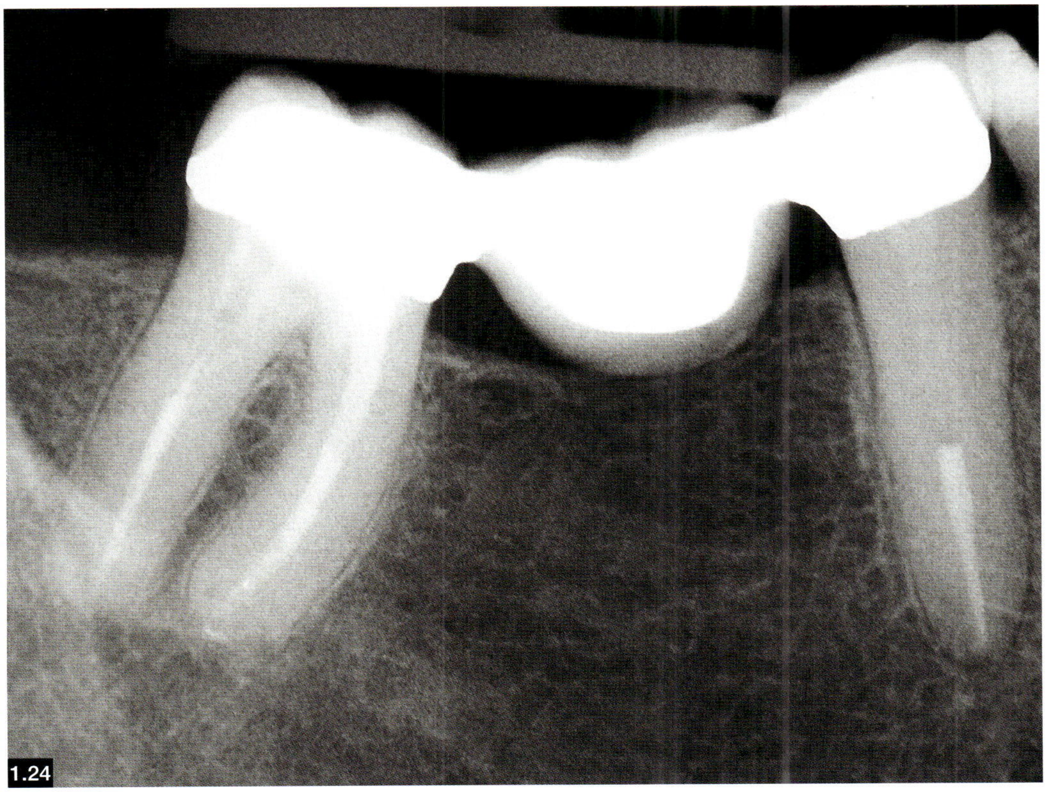

Fig. 1.24: Same prosthetic artifact x-rayed after 18 years.

CASE REPORT 1

Severe root resorption: result after 18 years

The analysis of the case, from the very first consult, seemed to be very complex; the tooth in question had been reconstructed several times with little success. The continuous contamination of the endodontic space with salivary fluids resulted in a consistent periapical reaction that was extrinsic with extensive root resorption at the expense of the distal root canal.

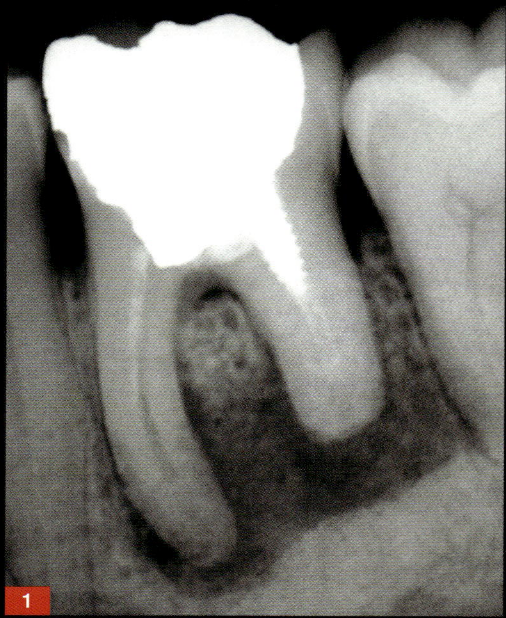

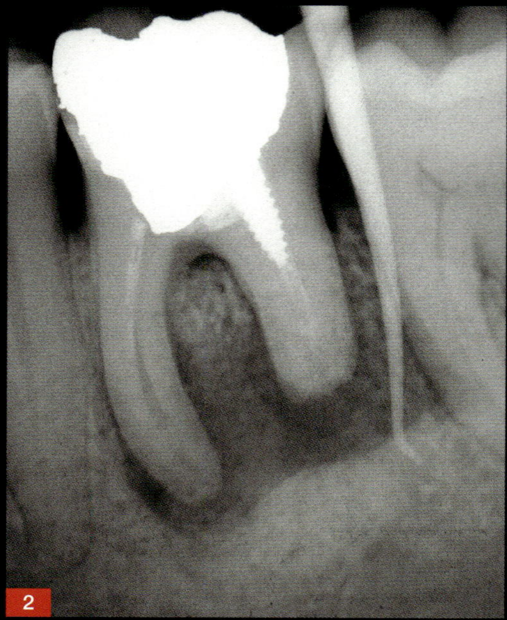

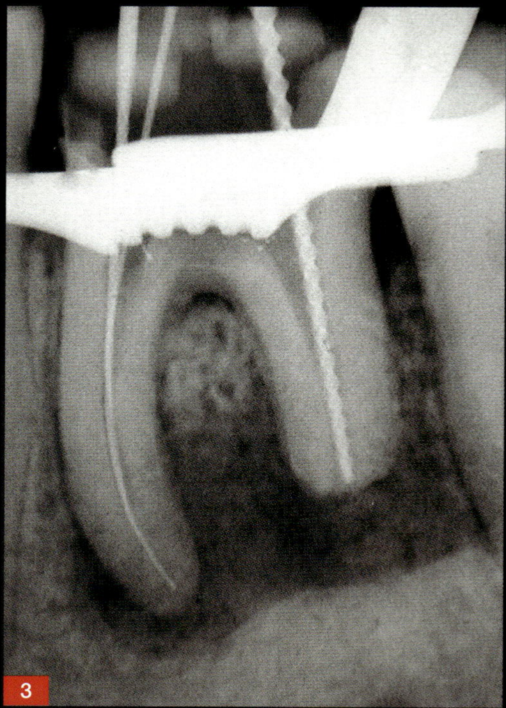

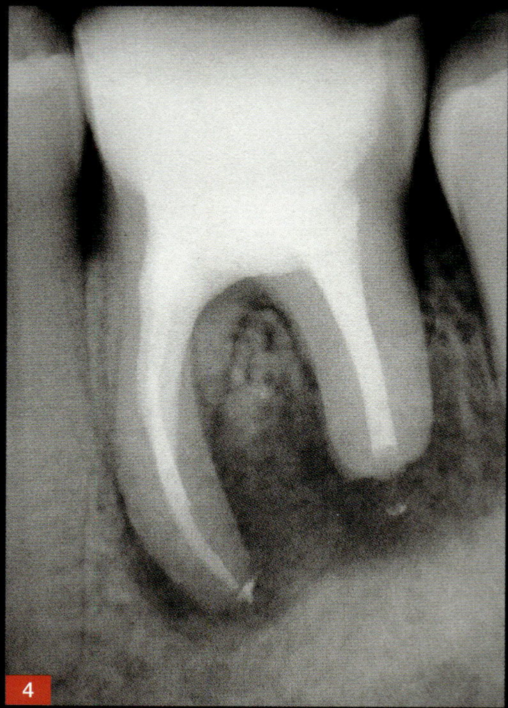

Figure 1: The diagnostic x-ray that shows a clear and extensive pariapical lesion with massive resorption of the distal root of the lower molar; the mesial canals do not appear to have been shaped, and it is possible to observe that part of the distal root canal has not been instrumented.

Figure 2: The clinically-evident fistula is traversed by a cone of gutta-percha to establish the congruence between the periapical lesion and the fistuolous path: the radiograph confirms this contiguity.

Figure 3: Once the root canal content has been emptied, the length of the root canals is measured.

Figure 4: The new endodontic treatment was completed with direct coronal reconstruction; due to the poor reliability of the tooth element, no further reconstruction was planned.

At the time, there was no pathological periodontal probing or dental mobility such as to suggest an impairment of the supporting tissues. This encouraged the clinician to pursue the path of orthograde retreatment. Although during the examinations carried out, the clinician has always suspected a chronic situation below the lesion, but the absence of clinical symptoms always comforted both the doctor and the patient, until the desired end result was achieved.

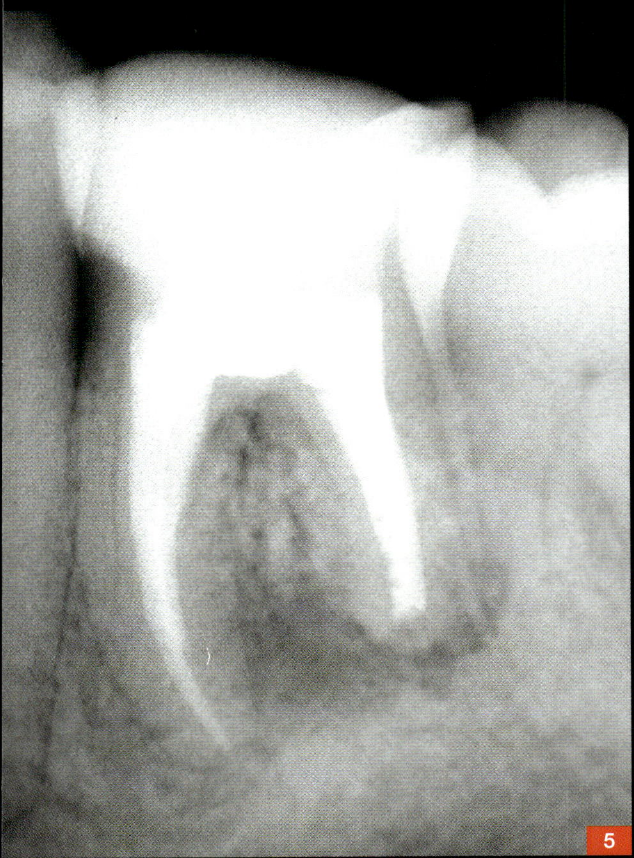

5

Figure 5: Although the 1-year x-ray shows a drastic reduction in radio-transparency, it has not completely resolved.

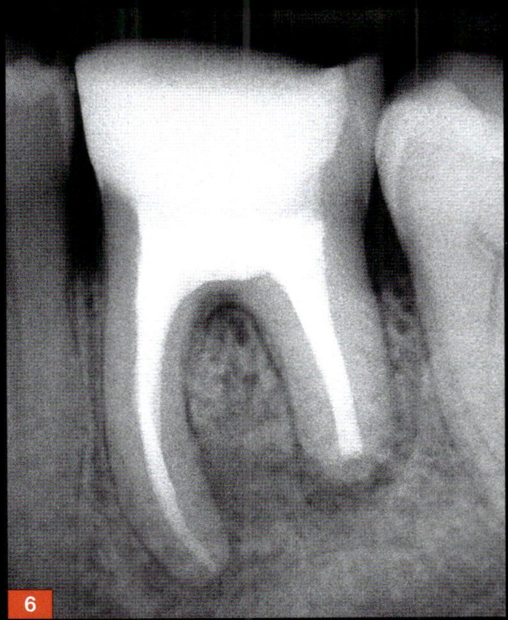

6

Figure 6: The same tooth three years later.

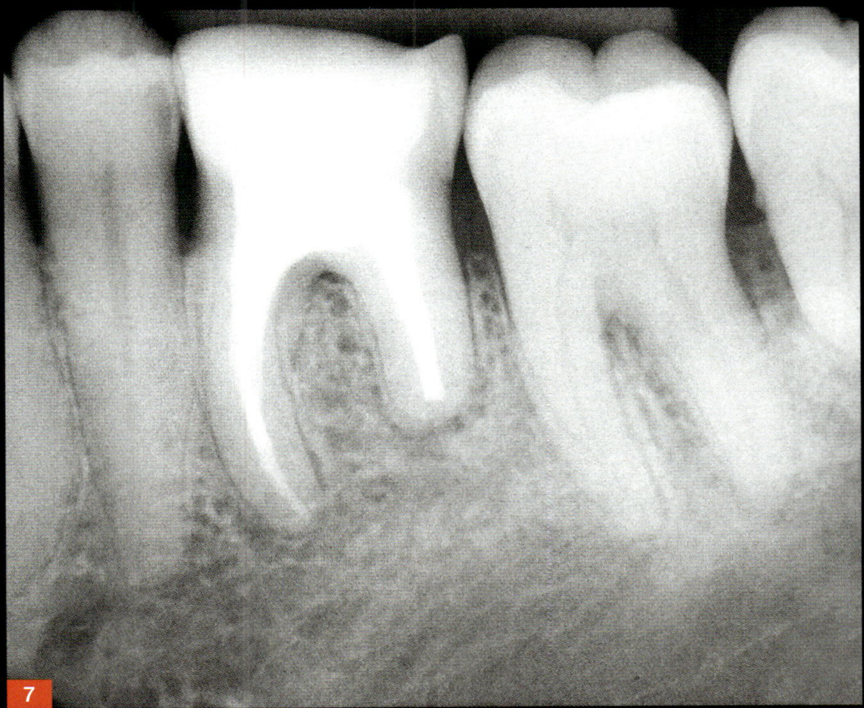

7

Figure 7: The x-ray at 18 years shows the satisfactory resolution of a condition that, at first glance, could have led to the clinician to extract the tooth.

CASE REPORT 2

Lower molars with different anatomies

Although these two cases are similar in terms of clinical condition, they differ greatly in terms of the anatomical features taken into consideration, since they are all lower molars. Anatomical variations often play a decisive role in the evolution of periapical disease and misinterpretations can lead to relevant parts of the endodontium being overlooked.

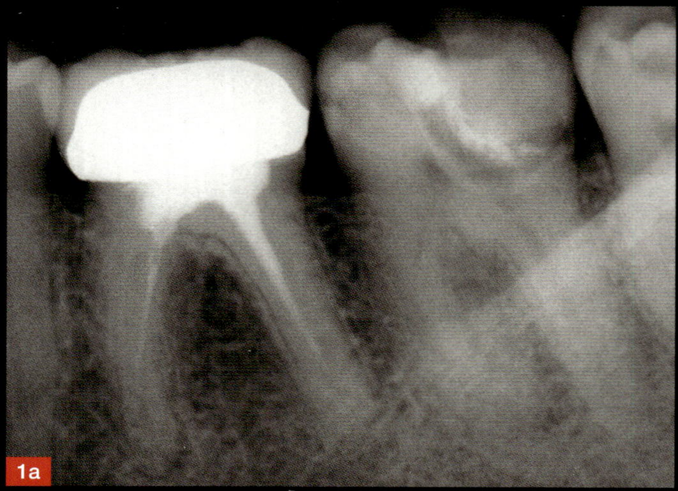

Figure 1a: A diabetic, patient with well-controlled general health comes in for an appointment complaining of pain in quadrant 4. Two endodontic lesions are observed, a primary lesion in tooth no. 47 and a secondary lesion in tooth no. 46.

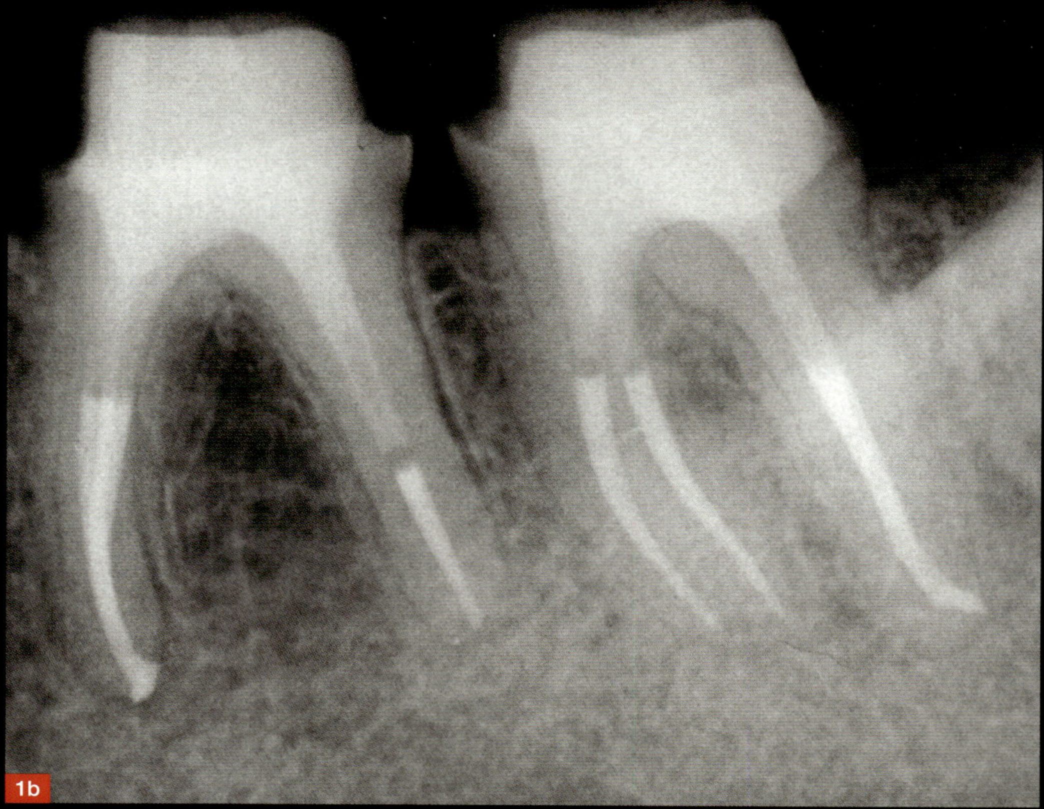

Figure 1b: Resolution after 1 year, the patient still has temporary restorations.

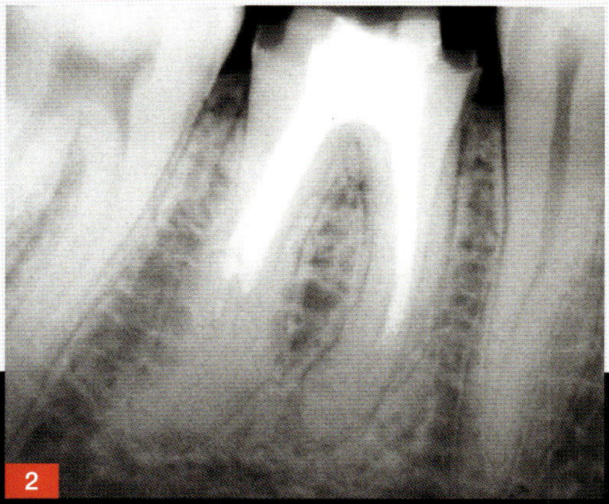

Figure 2: Radiographic view of the lower molar with periapical disease; note the inadequate length of the treatment.

Figure 3: Coronal access and an adequate apical shape have made it possible to retrace the entire endodontic space, to seal it properly and to design a correct reconstruction with adhesive techniques.

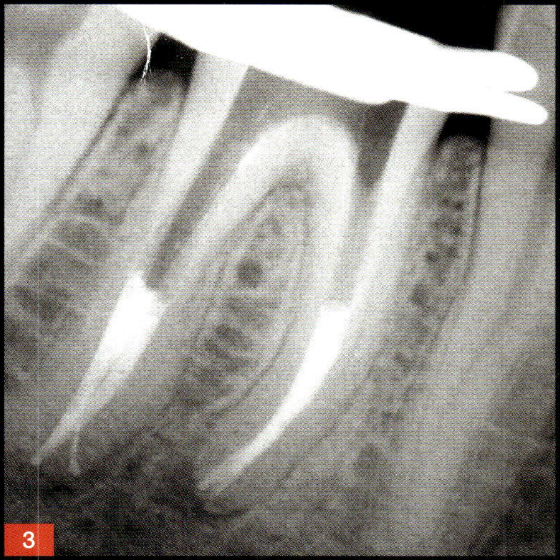

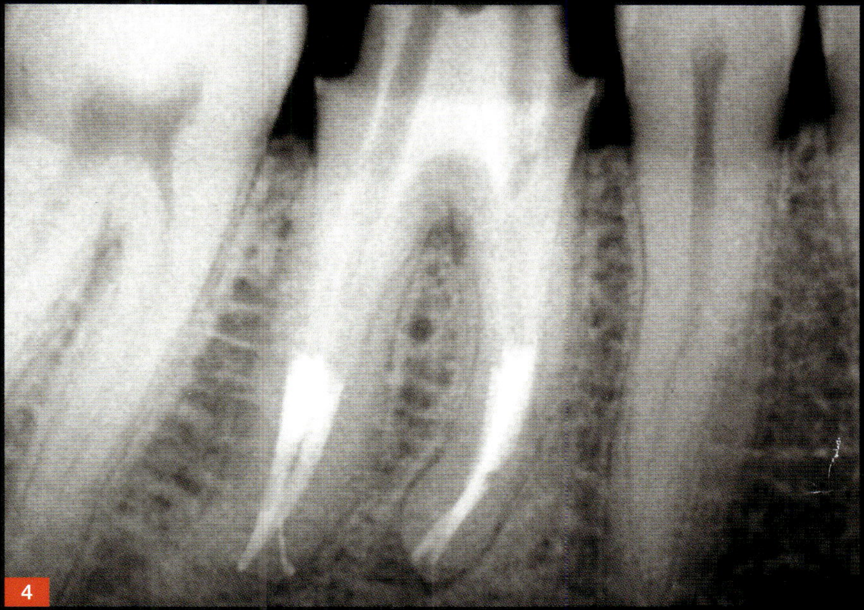

Figure 4: The scenario at the end of the reconstruction with fiber root canal posts.

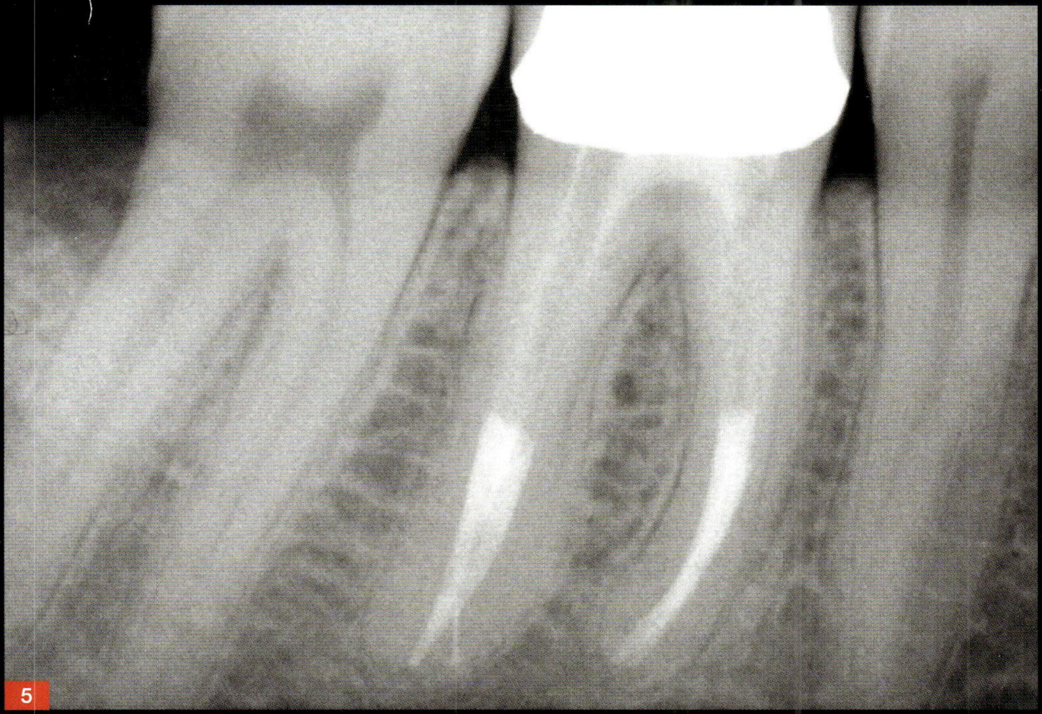

Figure 5: A 10-year X-ray reveals complete reconstruction of the periapical bone and excellent integration of the restoration.

The epidemiology of periapical disease

Chronic inflammatory diseases of endodontic origin in the maxillary bones are a far from negligible event; recent findings indicate that approximately 10% of the population has at least one tooth with endodontic problems[30]. The epidemiological data on periapical disease vary significantly depending on the approach to dental care, resulting in a low prevalence in some countries, and a higher prevalence in others (Table 1.1). In Italy, few related findings have been published; however, on the basis of the studies conducted in the last decade, the observations reported in Box 1.1 have been highlighted. Many of these studies are based on observations performed on panoramic x-rays (Figs. 1.25-1.26) whereas, others use different imaging techniques, including Cone-Beam Computed Tomography (CBCT)[31], a description of which is provided in the next chapter (Figs. 1.27-1.30).

Recent studies have been carried out using this technique, which is more sensitive in detecting periapical disease of endodontic origin. The results are provided below.

Paes da Silva et al.[32] selected a sample of about 300 images and reported a 35% prevalence of periapical rarefactions related to inadequate endodontic treatments.

Table 1.1 **EPIDEMIOLOGICAL DATA ON THE PREVALENCE OF PERIAPICAL DISEASES IN VARIOUS POPULATIONS WORLDWIDE**

	Year	Imaging technique employed	Patients	Teeth analyzed	Treated teeth present and examined	% apical periodontitis out of all teeth	% of treated teeth out of all examined teeth	% of correctly treated teeth with periapical lesions	% of incorrectly treated teeth with periapical lesions	Country
Jimenez-Pinzon et al.	2004	OPT*	180	4453		4.2	2.1		64.5	Spain
Kabak et al.	2005	OPT	1423	8632		12			45	Belarus
Siqueira et al.	2005	OPT		2051	2051		100	18	71	Brazil
Tercas et al.	2006	OPT	200	5008	553	5.9	11		42.5	Brazil
Estrela et al.	2008	OPT		1372	1372		100	12.1	71.7	Brazil
Frisk et al.	2008	OPT	490				23	36	24.5	Sweden
Georgopoulou et al.	2008	OPT						39.2	67.6	Greece
Tavares et al.	2009	OPT		1035	1035		100	19	93.5	France
Peters L.B. et al.	2010	OPT	178	4594		7	4.8	24.1	55.8	Netherlands
Kim S.	2010	OPT			896	22.8			29.3	Korea
Santos et al.	2010	OPT			291		100	11	19	Brazil
Al-Omari et al.	2011	OPT	294	7390	4655	11.6	5.7		87	Jordan
Chala et al.	2011	OPT				63.79			39.5	Morocco
Kamberi et al.	2011	OPT	193	4131	95	12.3	2.3		46.3	Kosovo
Lopez-Lopez et al.	2012	OPT	397			34	59	23	42	Spain
Kalender et al.	2013	Periapical OPT and Rx	1006	24730	7986	7.01	9.4		62	Cyprus
Jersa et al.	2013	OPT	312	7065		7	18		78	Lithuania
Berlinck et al.	2015	Rx periapicali	1126	25292		7			16.7	Brazil
Huumonen et al.	2017	OPT	5335	120635	32571	4.42	5.3		15.3	Finland
Kielbassa et al.	2017	OPT	1000	22586	2504	6.4	11.1		42.6	Austria

*OPT: orthopantomographic radiogram.

Box 1.1 PREVALENCE OF CHRONIC INFLAMMATORY DISEASES OF ENDODONTIC ORIGIN IN ITALY

Few epidemiological studies have been carried out in Italy (Table 1.2). Generali et al. reported that the prevalence of apical periodontitis was equal to 6.6% of the teeth involved; 10.8% of all the elements presented evidence of endodontic treatment. In 45.8% of the latter, a periapical lesion was observed. Hence, the percentage of apical periodontitis was higher in endodontically treated teeth than in untreated teeth, and no close correlation was observed between the quality of canal fillings and the prevalence of apical periodontitis. In the same year, Cotti et al. analyzed 318 patients and found that periapical pathologies were attributable to endodontium infections in 7.9% of the teeth examined; of which, more than 50% were found in endodontically treated teeth. Similar findings were confirmed by Covello et al. In a study on 214 subjects using digital panoramic x-rays, the authors observed that almost half of endodontically treated teeth had a radiologically visible periapical inflammatory reaction. More recently, in a preliminary study conducted in 2014 in the Milan area, Fini et al. reported similar results. Dolci et al. described a more optimistic scenario using similar methods but with a more significant sample.

Table 1.2 ITALIAN EPIDEMIOLOGICAL DATA

	Year	Imaging technique employed	Patients	Teeth examined	Treated teeth present and examined	% of apical periodontitis out of all teeth	% of treated teeth out of all the teeth analyzed	% of teeth correctly treated with periapical lesions	% of incorrectly treated teeth with periapical lesions	Country
Generali et al.	2007	OPT*	214	4707	226	6.6	10.8	29.3	71.7	Italy
Cotti et al.	2007	OPT	318	7287	293	7.8	4.1	50.8	62.3	Italy
Covello et al.	2010	OPT	384	9423	1081	8.3	11.4	-	41.6	Italy
Fini et al.	2014	OPT	108	1284	318	9.4	24.8	19	47	Italy
Dolci et al.	2016	Periapical Rx	312	8101	534	1.3	6.6	-	17	

*OPT: orthopantomographic radiogram.

Cotti E, Lusso D, Baroni C, Dettori C. *Valutazione sullo stato di salute periapicale di un campione di popolazione sarda*. G It Endo. 2007;21(1):1-8.

Covello F et al. *Prevalence of apical periodontitis and quality of endodontic treatment in an Italian adult population*. Oral Implantol. 2010 Oct-Dec; 3(4):9-14.

Dolci M et al. *Prevalence and distribution of endodontic treatments and apical periodontitis in an Italian population sample*. European Journal of Inflammation. 2016;(14)1:48-53.

Fini M and Grassi M .*Prevalence of* periapical pathologies in a sample of adults in the Milan area. In Cardinali F, Fornara R, Gorni F, Gagliani M. La risoluzione delle complessità nei ritrattamenti. Dental Cadmos. 2014;(10)2-24.

Generali P et al. *Prevalenza di parodontiti apicali croniche e qualità dei trattamenti endodontici in una popolazione adulta italiana*. G It Endo. 2007;21(1):35-40.

Van der Veken et al.[33] conducted the most extensive study with CBCT tests in a large sample of patients (631). In this study, the prevalence of periapical diseases is approximately 6%, which is in line with the results of other studi conducted in neighboring countries. More than half of all endodontically treated teeth had inadequate canal filling, a result that is consistent with recent studies (Table 1.3). One of the most important findings is the prevalence of periapical lesions in endodontically treated teeth; almost half of the treatments had problems, suggesting that this treatment is not performed using the correct criteria by most dentists worldwide. In short, post-treatment endodontic disease – or that with a persistent aetiology involving a periapical lesion of endodontic origin – does not look set to decrease over time and, despite the fact that, in percentage terms, it involves a limited number of dental elements, it affects a large part of the population. Indeed, although, on the one hand, the number of affected teeth per individual are

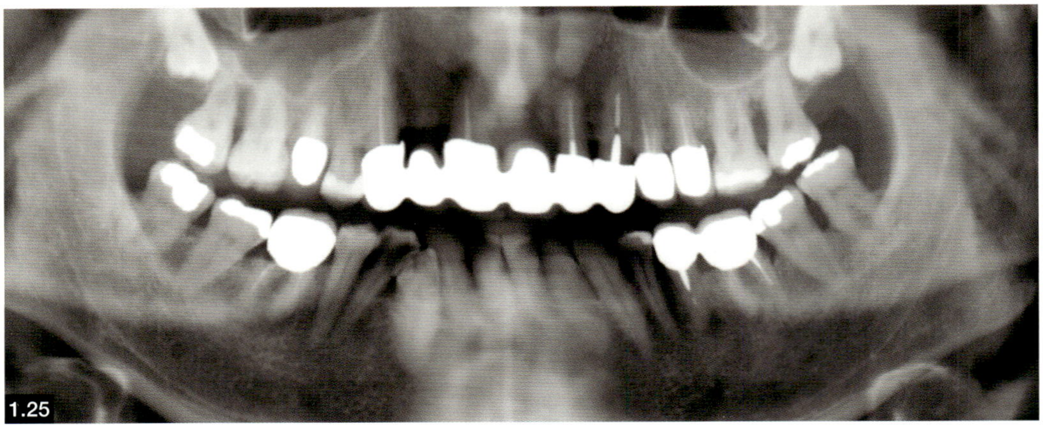

Fig. 1.25: Orthopantomographic scenario in patients suffering from various periapical pathologies; the degree of definition of individual lesions is barely noticeable.

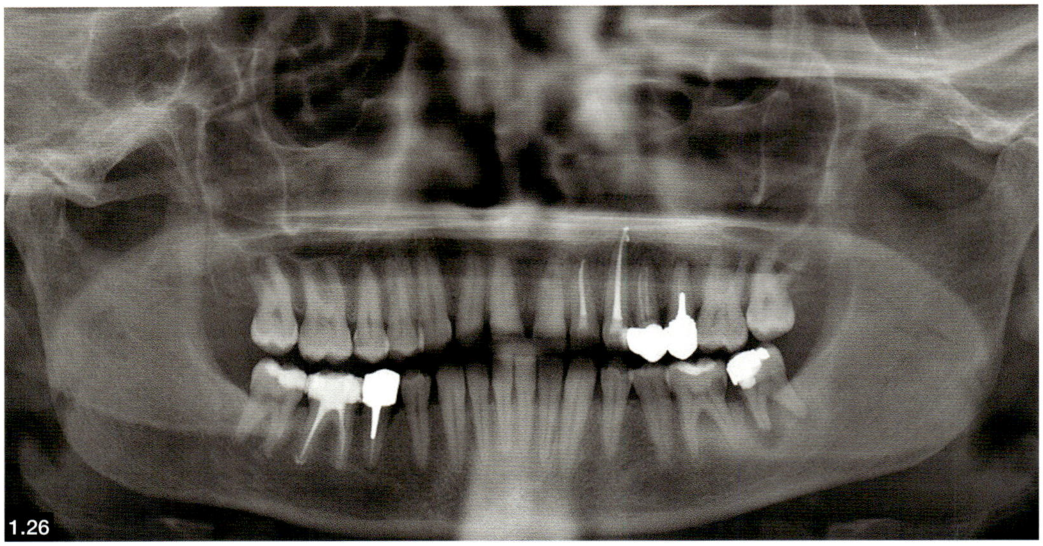

Fig. 1.26: Similar scenario to the previous but with manifestations of more evident periapical lesions; notice on the upper canine left the apical overfilling.

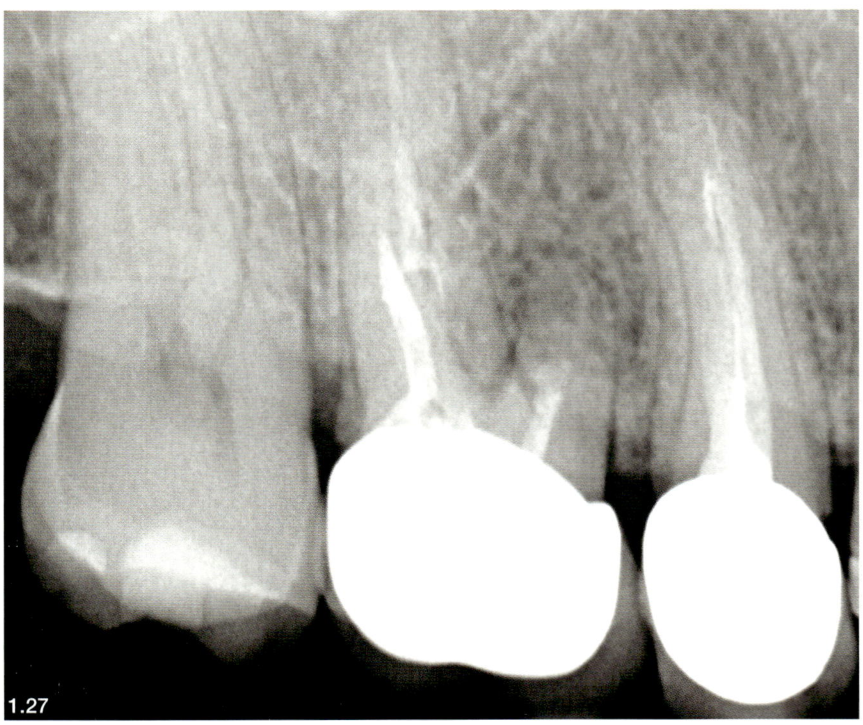

Fig. 1.27: Intraoral x-ray presenting an area of radiotransparency at the mesial root of tooth 16 and a suspected lesion on tooth 15.

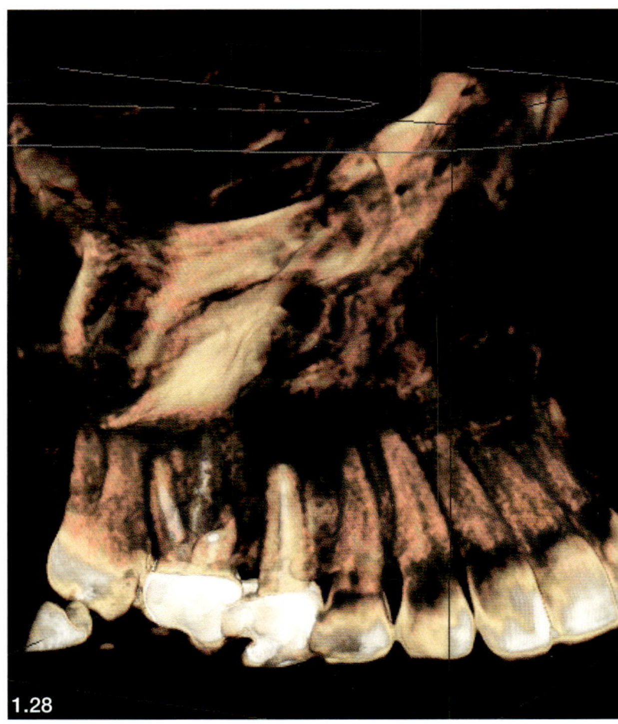

Fig. 1.28: A three-dimensional image (Cone-Beam Computed Tomography, CBCT) makes it possible to obtain an optimum view of the periapical tissues.

Table 1.3 **EPIDEMIOLOGICAL DATA COLLECTED BY CONE-BEAM COMPUTERIZED TOMOGRAPHY (CBCT)**

	Year	Imaging technique used for analysis	Patients	Teeth examined	Treated teeth present and examined	% of apical periodontitis out of all teeth	% of treated teeth out of all analyzed teeth	% of teeth correctly treated teeth with periapical lesions	% of incorrectly treated teeth with periapical lesions	Country
Paes da Silva et al.	2013	CBCT	300	5585	-	7	8.9	-	35.4	Brazil
Dutta et al.	2014	CBCT	245	3595	-	5.8	4.8	-	47.4	UK
Lemagner et al.	2015	CBCT	100	2368	431	8.6	8.6	-	40.8	France
Karabucak et al.*	2016	CBCT	1397	1137	1137	59.5	-	-	82.8	-
Van der Veken et al.	2017	CBCT	804	11117	1357	5.9	12.2	22.8	46.6	Belgium

* The Authors examine only the teeth affected by periapical disease and check for the presence of unidentified canals (consequently, untreated): among the teeth with lesion, those with unidentified canals-not treated were found to be 23.04%.

Paes da Silva Ramos Fernandes LM et al. *Prevalence of apical periodontitis detected in cone beam CT images of a Brazilian subpopulation*. Dentomaxillofac Radiol. 2013;42(1): 80179163.

Dutta A et al. *Prevalence of periradicular periodontitis in a Scottish subpopulation found on CBCT images*.Int Endod J. 2014 Sep;47(9):854-63.

Lemagner F et al. *Prevalence of Apical Bone Defects and Evaluation of Associated Factors Detected with Cone-beam Computed Tomographic Images*. J Endod. 2015 Jul;41(7):1043-7.

Karabucak B et al. *Prevalence of Apical Periodontitis in Endodontically Treated Premolars and Molars with Untreated Canal: A Cone-beam Computed Tomography Study*. J Endod. 2016 Apr;42(4):538-41.

Van der Veken D et al. *Prevalence of apical periodontitis and root filled teeth in a Belgian subpopulation found on CBCT images*. Int Endod J. 2017;50(4):317-29.

Burklein S, Schafer E, Johren HP, Donnermeyer D. Quality of root canal fillings and prevalence of apical radiolucencies in a German population: a CBCT analysis. Clin Oral Investig 2019 (on-line pre-press).

few; on the other, the epidemiological evidence available suggests that this problem may affect millions of people.
Pak et al.[34] conducted a very thorough study that moved in this direction; they clarified through the joint analysis of several community studies, they clarified that about 5% of the teeth presented endodontic periapical disease.
About 10% of the teeth had received nonsurgical endodontic treatments; of the 30,000 treated teeth incorporated in the systematic review, about 36% of them had a periapical lesion of endodontic relevance. Almost all of the patients involved in the study had a periapical lesion associated with unsuccessful root canal therapy. The most worrying fact is that, instead of being eradicated, the disease persists, even in settings where the quality level of dental care is presumed to be high, as reported by a number of authors[35-37];

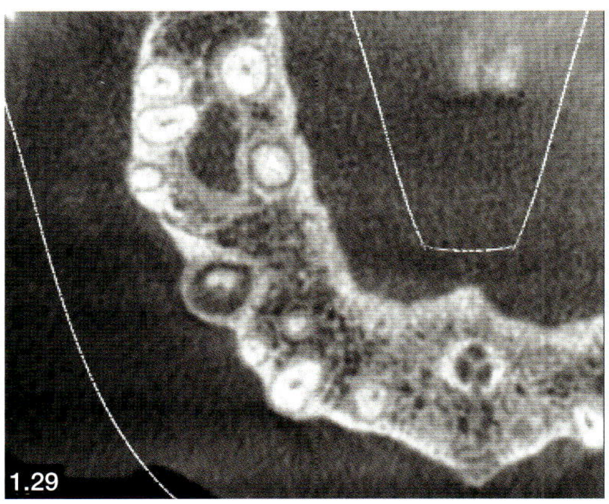

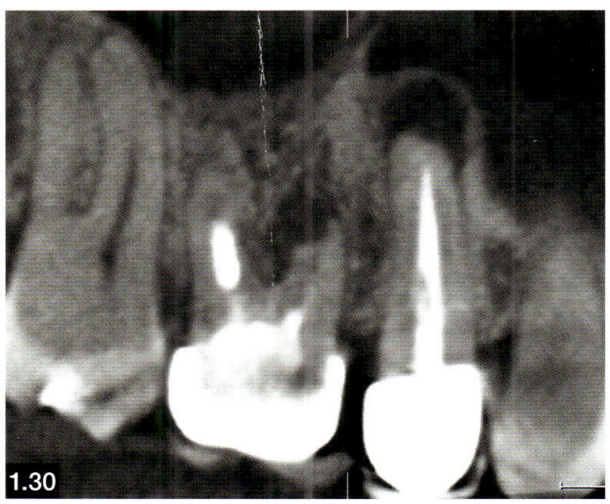

Fig. 1.29: Axial image providing the best possible view of the two lesions.

Fig. 1.30: Sectional lateral vision showing the extent of the disease (the case is presented in an aesthetic way in Chapter 2 on page 101).

Box 1.2 PREVALENCE OF PERIAPICAL DISEASE OF ENDODONTIC ORIGIN

The periapical disease of endodontic origin appears to be of little relevance in percentage terms considering the teeth involved (on average less than 10%), but is of far greater importance if we consider the number of patients involved (more than 60% of the population attending dental appointments).

certain paradoxical situations have been highlighted. In studies comparing groups of patients who underwent endodontic treatment 20 years ago and those treated in more recent times, there was little difference in the percentage of subjects with periapical diseases of endodontic origin and the quality of the treatments administered, suggesting that although the techniques available to practitioners have changed, the variable associated with the practitioner and his/her expertise in this setting is still a key factor for the achievement of an optimal result. New and old techniques do not appear to differ greatly in terms of the achievement of satisfactory clinical and radiological results. Kirkevang et al.[38] compared two groups of Danish patients undergoing endodontic treatments at different times and observed that patients trends were similar with regard to both the periapical lesions and the therapies used to treat them. The authors deduced that the advent of *new surgical technologies* had not helped them to reach significantly better results. Similar conclusions were reported by another study conducted in a Dutch population reported the same conclusions by comparing groups of patients about 20 years apart[37]. Based on a recent study in a German population, a limited improvement was observed over a timespan of 20 years, but data were insufficient to affirming that new technologies might radically improve the outcomes of the root canal treatment (D). Therefore, the prevalence of periapical inflammatory diseases of endodontic origin is not decreasing, and new technologies are unable to address clinicians-related issues and the objective difficulties in the eradication of bacteria proliferating in biofilm within the endodontium.

EVOLUTION

New techniques have no clear advantages in terms of success of endodontic therapies.

Periapical diseases and systemic diseases

As discussed in the previous paragraphs, the percentage of endodontically treated teeth affected by periapical problems is not very high; however, if we consider the prevalence of the condition in population terms, it affects millions of people.
This fact has always attracted the interest of researchers not only because of the local effects but also the potential systemic effects. A number of studies[39, 40] have attempted to establish potential relationships between systemic disease and chronic periapical infection problems[41, 42]. As the population continues to age[43-45], the likelihood that these jaw bone conditions may affect other body tissues does not seem remote[46].
In a systematic review[43] of studies on a population over 65 years of age, the percentages of periapical lesions (Fig. 1.31) and endodontically treated teeth were high; given that the latter was less affected by inflammatory periradicular conditions, age did not affect the likelihood of a successful endodontic retreatment. In other words, a periapical disease is equally likely to heal once the endodontic bacterial component has been eliminated in both young and old individuals; indeed, several studies have confirmed that the prognosis is not influenced by the age variable[47, 48].
Treatment of endodontic periapical diseases is therefore possible at all ages, provided thorough patient assessments are performed. Diagnostic work-up and treatment plan assessments will be discussed later in this chapter. With regard to the correlations between systemic and periapical disease, a number of situations of a general nature can be associated with periapical diseases of endodontic origin; for example,

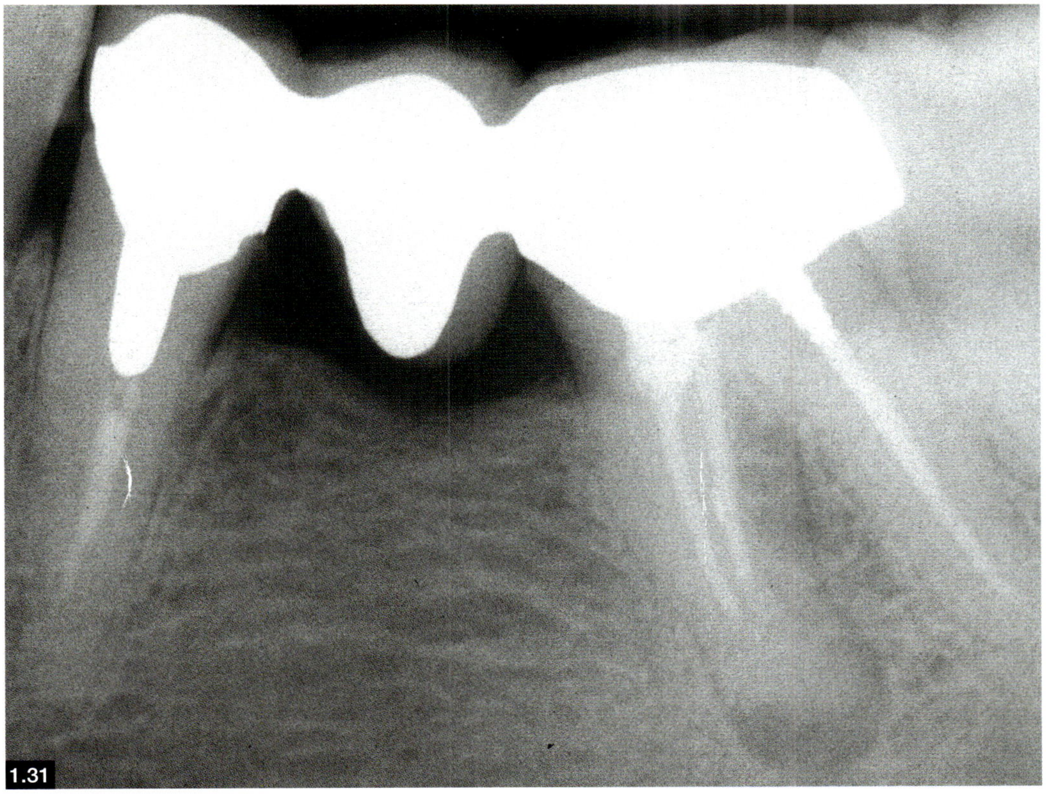

Fig. 1.31: Radiographic scenario in a patients of more than 80 years of age. The lesion is not symptomatic; given the general situation, the patient should have an annual x-ray to monitor the progress of the lesion.

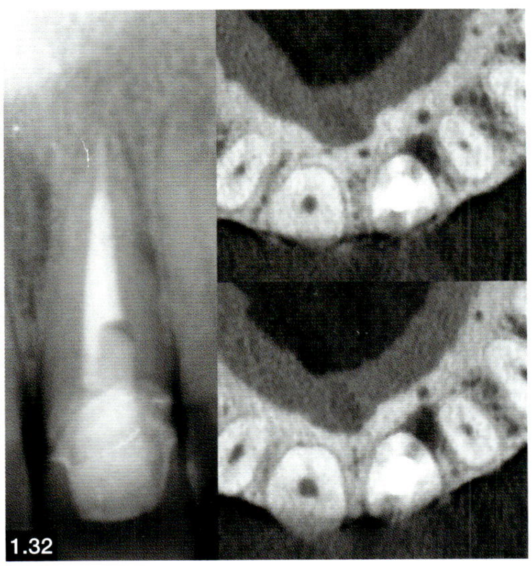

Fig. 1.32: In a patient with juvenile diabetes, nuanced symptoms are present at tooth 21; the radiographic scenario suggests a recrudescence of the periapical lesion, but the CBCT study shows a fracture. The therapeutic treatment option is not practical because of the patient's general health.

patients with insulin-dependent diabetes mellitus have an increased risk of developing endodontic disease[49, 50] (E-F-G) (Fig. 1.32). Hypertension, on the other hand, does not play a fundamental role in the development of periapical diseases[51]. Other chronic diseases, such as rheumatoid arthritis[39, 52], have not shown any significant correlation with periapical endodontic lesions. Undoubtedly, certain health conditions or overt diseases are unfavorable factors in the success of an endodontic treatment (Table 1.4); however, this fact alone does not allow a definitive decision in favor of the most radical solution, i.e. extraction, and numerous viable alternatives are available.

Table 1.4 **MEDICAL AND SYSTEMIC FACTORS CONDITIONING THE SUCCESS OF ENDODONTIC TREATMENT**

• NUTRITIONAL DEFICIENCIES	• HORMONAL IMBALANCES
• DIABETES	• AUTOIMMUNE DISEASES
• KIDNEY DISEASE	• OPPORTUNISTIC INFECTIONS
• BLOOD DISORDERS	• STEROID THERAPY

Correlation between periapical disease and cardiovascular diseases

Cardiovascular conditions and periapical inflammations of endodontic origin deserve serious evaluation. In a recent study, Virtanen et al.[53] reported the correlation between *cardiovascular diseases* and the presence of periapical lesions linked or not to unsuccessfull endodontic treatments. The findings appeared to be noteworthy and thus should be considered particularly in adult patients.

CARDIOVASCULAR DISEASES

The relationship between cardiovascular diseases and periapical lesions of endodontic origin has been supported by preliminary clinical evidence.

A systematic review of literature[54] on this subject revealed that cardiovascular diseases can coincide with periapical lesions of endodontic origin; by examining a number of studies, the authors found positive correlations, but of mild evidence, in more than 70% of the works analyzed. This opinion is shared by Cotti and coll.[55] who examined the issue several times, not merely from a cardiological point of view. Pasqualini et al.[56] highlighted the positive correlation between cardiovascular disease and the number of missing teeth or teeth with periradicular inflammatory diseases. Hence, inflammatory situations in dental elements must be considered (Fig. 1.33a-d) not only with regard to the local issues but also to the systemic implications.
These implications are indicative of a complex setting to which due attention must be dedicated; once again we are aware of the need to integrate our observations as dental surgeons with those of the general practitioners responsible for the patient's general health.

Pharmacological therapies and retreatments

In addition to nondental disease, pharmacological therapies can also play a decisive role in the development or nonresolution of periapical lesions of endodontic origin because they interfere with bone metabolism to some extent.

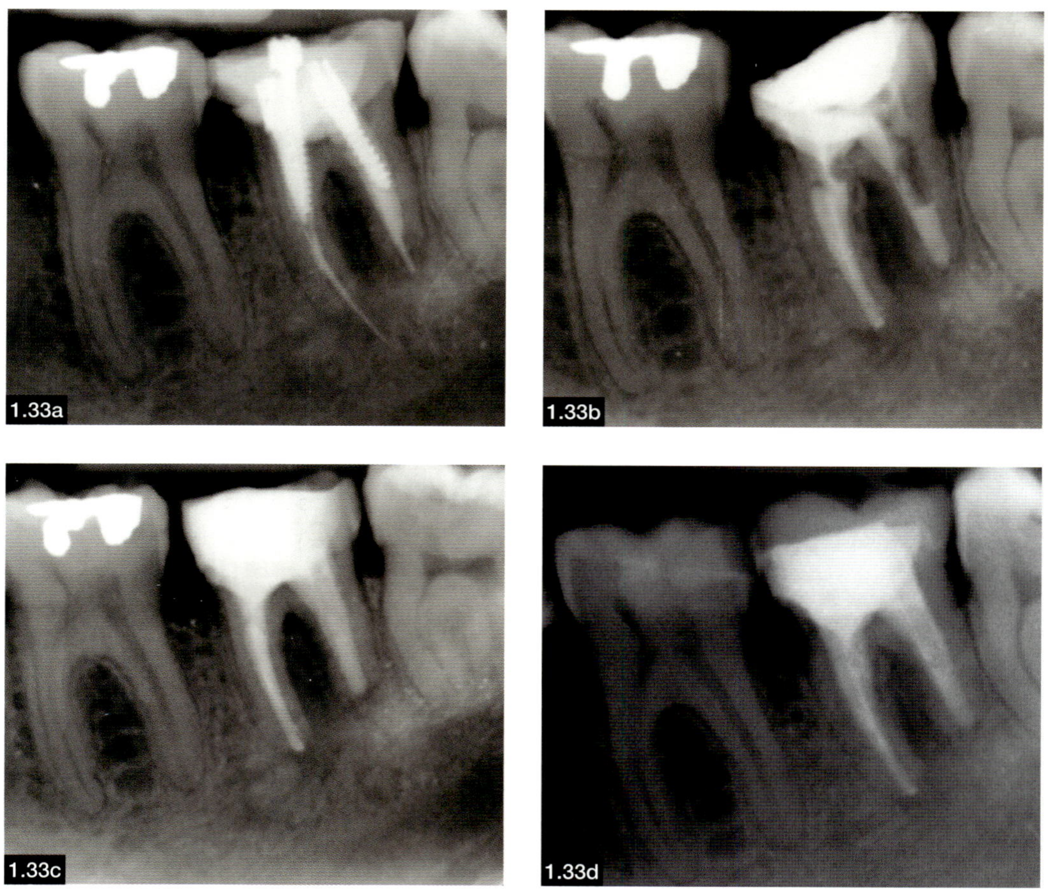

Fig. 1.33a-d: A cardiopathic patient who came in for observation with pain in tooth 47. The x-ray (a) shows a periapical lesion and poor-quality endodontic treatment. Once the previous filling had been removed, the tooth was resealed (b-c). The 5-year follow-up (d) showed a perfect reintegration of the periapical tissues of the tooth.

Table 1.5 **EXAMPLES OF COMMERCIALLY AVAILABLE BISPHOSPHONATES**

Active substance	Trade name	Nitrogen content	Route of administration	Relative potency	Common use
Alendronate	Fosamax®	Yes	Oral	700	Osteoporosis
Clodronate	Bonefos® Clasteon®	No	Oral	10	Hypercalcemia secondary to neoplastic diseases
Ethylated	Didronel®	No	Oral and IV	1	Paget's disease
Ibandronate	Boniva®	Yes	Oral and IV	4000	Osteoporosis
Pamidronate	Aredia®	Yes	Oral and IV	325	Cancer
Risedronato	Actonel®	Yes	Ora	2000	Osteoporosis
Tiludronate	Skelid®	No	Oral	10	Hypercalcemia secondary to neoplastic diseases
Zoledronate	Zometa®	Yes	IV	700	Cancer
Zoledronate	Reclast®	Yes	IV (once/year)	700	Osteoporosis

Source: AAE POSITION STATEMENT – Endodontic Implications of Bisphosphonate-Associated Osteonecrosis of the Jaws. https://www.aae.org/specialty/wpcontent/uploads/sites/2/2017/07/bisphosonatesstatement.pdf

In addition, the need to carry out treatment in elderly subjects with concomitant health problems must always be a cause for concern for the clinician, who is faced with the prospect of a clinical session that frequently neither easy nor short). We will take a closer look at certain pharmacological aspects of general interest:

1. endodontic treatments in patients on bisphosphonate therapy;
2. which patients require prophylactic antibiotic treatment;
3. analgesic strategies prior to root canal therapy and the use of anesthetics in retreatments.

Basic rules, supported by scientific evidence, will be provided on these issues, which are increasingly frequently observed in patients, especially the elderly.
The use of antibiotics can also contribute to the exacerbation of periapical diseases immediately after the retreatment. Segura-Egea et al.[57] stress that antibiotics should only be used when necessary and at the lowest effective dose during the postoperative period.

This aspect should therefore be carefully pondered in terms of the patient's general condition, concomitant medication, and potential interactions.

Bisphosphonates and endodontic retreatments

Patients who are receiving treatment or have been treated with bisphosphonates are increasingly frequent.
In recent times, bisphosphonates have been used in myriad ways for the short- or long-term treatment of many conditions affecting the bone and bone marrow and for breast and prostate cancer[58].
Bisphosphonates can be classified according to whether they are administered orally or intravenously, and their dosage and the duration of therapy depend on the method of administration.
Tables 1.5 and 1.6 show the conditions for which *bisphosphonates* are used on a continuous basis and clarify the boundaries within which the highest level of attention is required.

BISPHOSPHONATES

The clinical situations that should be focused on are those that develop in patients who received high-dose IV therapies.

Table 1.6 **PATIENTS RECEIVING TREATMENT WITH BISPHOSPHONATES: DEGREE OF RISK FOR RELEVANT ENDODONTIC PROCEDURES**

Patients at risk		
High	**Medium**	**Low**
Prolonged intravenous therapies for neoplasms (multiple myeloma, prostate or breast cancer, lymphomas, leukemia) or Paget's disease	Intensive care for the treatment of osteoporosis lasting more than three years, both intravenously and intraorally	Oral therapies for the treatment of osteoporosis

Source: AAE POSITION STATEMENT – Endodontic Implications of Bisphosphonate-Associated Osteonecrosis of the Jaws. https://www.aae.org/specialty/wpcontent/uploads/sites/2/2017/07/bisphosonatesstatement.pdf

Bisphosphonate therapy is considered to be responsible for osteonecrosis of the jaws, as first reported by Ruggiero and Marx[58-61].

In other studies[62, 63], maxillary osteonecrosis is more common in the mandible than in the maxilla and is associated with prolonged, high-dose use of these medicinal products.

This posology is associated with a number of diseases such as multiple myeloma, metastatic forms of prostate and breast cancer, and certain forms of leukemia and/or lymphomas, Paget's disease, and severe osteoporosis.

As intravenous administration is common, the anamnestic finding is already in itself decisive with regard to the potential development of osteonecrosis of the jaws, despite its extremely low prevalence, which varies according to the source consulted and is less than one in ten thousand in the most favorable situations, and never more than 2% of treated cases in situations of greater severity.

Osteonecrosis of the maxilla is frequently associated with traumatic events, first and foremost dental extractions, particularly for those in whom the anamnestic risk, i.e., use of high-dose intravenous bisphosphonates, was not considered or was overlooked.

In the endodontic field, Moinzadeh et al.[64] reported that the potential development of osteonecrosis, following contingent canal treatment maneuvers, can be related to two main factors: lesions of the marginal periodontium during the positioning of the clasp for the fixation of the rubber dam and the extrusion of the infected material beyond the root apex during the maneuvers involving the shaping and cleansing of the endodontic space.

The use of anesthetics without vasoconstrictors is also recommended.

For example, in a patient who has received or is currently receiving bisphosphonates therapy for cancer (Table 1.6), the osteonecrosis issue should be addressed with the utmost caution. In other cases, the normal precautions will be more than sufficient for preventing undesirable side effects.

No clear consensus has been reached with regard to the possible effectiveness of antibiotic prophylaxis.

Considering inconsequential problems related to bacterial resistance that could develop in conjunction with the prophylactic regimen, conventional antibiotic prophylaxis (Table 1.7) is recommended for all subjects undergoing root canal treatment, especially in those cases in which the disease has already progressed at periapical level.

The above authors[64] recommend, in particularly severe cases, performing root canal therapy and permanently sealing the canal lumen, even in teeth that should logically be extracted.

This approach would result in a lower risk than that of an extraction.

Endodontic surgery deserves separate consideration.

Despite not being without its risks, the procedure can be performed with relative peace of mind in patients with a limited risk, provided adequate antibiotic prophylaxis is prescribed and the therapy is continued according to conventional regimens, where necessary. It should only be performed when strictly required in subjects with a high or medium risk, in whom, as mentioned previously, duly-controlled orthograde therapies can be considered[65] instead of surgery,

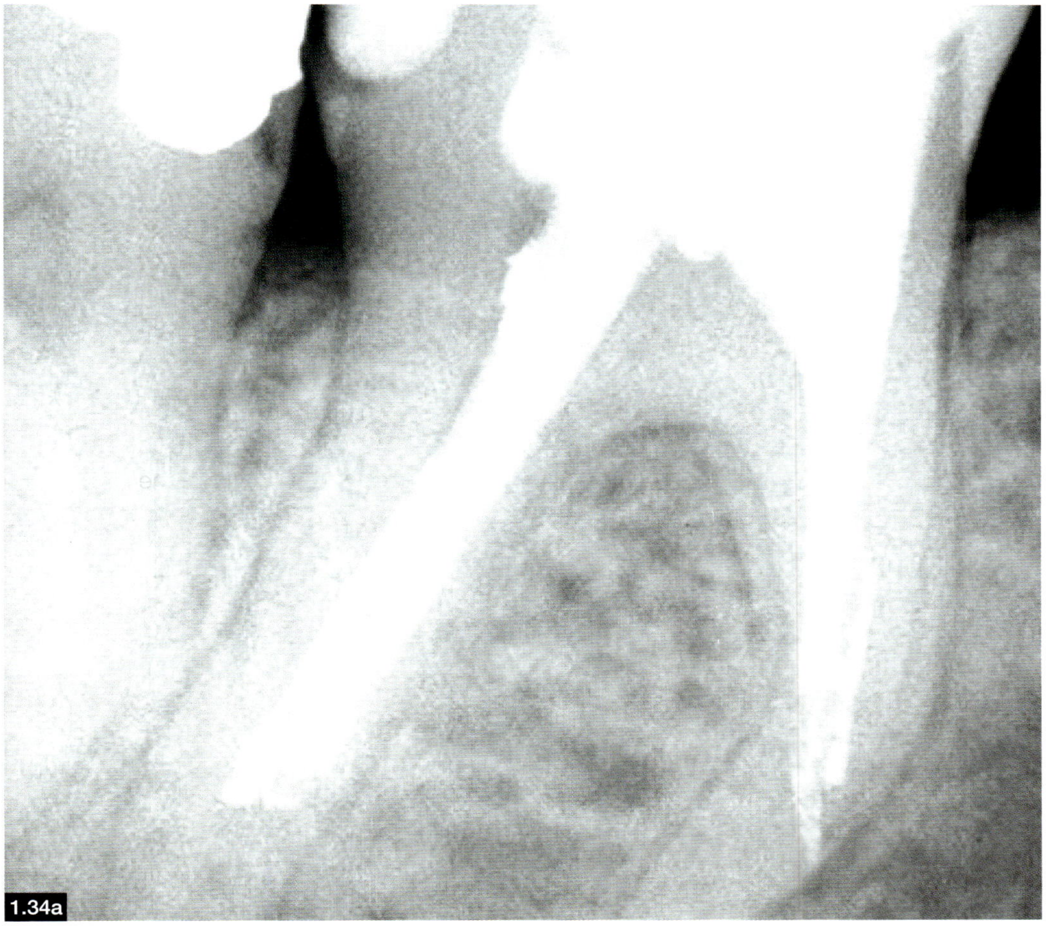

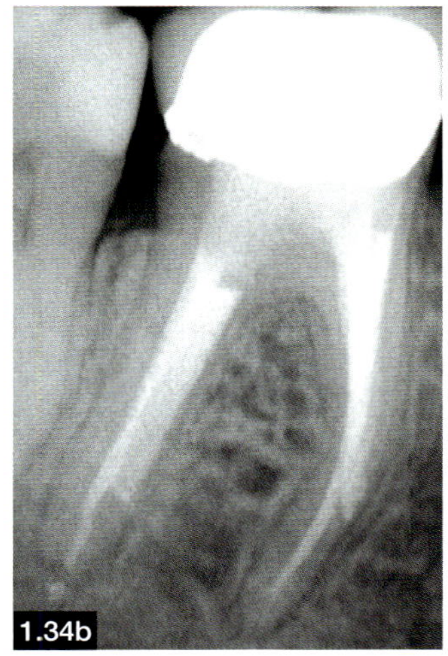

Fig. 1.34a-b: A lower molar with a number of problems associated with inappropriate treatment of the apical third is reviewed and resealed. The response of the periradicular tissues confirms success of the therapy.

precisely to avoid tooth extraction, which is reported by several authors[66, 67] as being one of the main sources of osteonecrosis of the jaws.

In any case, endodontic surgery – provided the early stages are performed correctly by sculpting a flap to obtain effective final suture without mucous dehiscence – would be preferable to extraction, which, as mentioned previously, is one of the main sources of jaw osteonecrosis.

Antibiotic prophylaxis

As retreatment is a surgical procedure that, to a greater or lesser extent, can transfer bacteria into the periapical tissues and, consequently, into the bloodstream, antibiotic prophylaxis must always be considered.

The need to administer it is specifically expressed for certain well-defined groups of patients (Box 1.3).

Attempts to use antibiotic prophylaxis to improve the success rate, however, have not proved ineffective because success is the result of a series of factors of which the spread of bacteria beyond the root apex is thought to be one of the least important[68].

Antibiotic therapy should, in any case, be considered an option in the postoperative phase in the case of infective exacerbations (which do not exceed 6%-7% of the cases treated) in the lifetime of individuals undergoing treatment, despite the presence, in almost half of all cases, of mild or moderate pain not warranting the use of a medicinal product (Chapter 6).

We also refer the reader to Chapter 6 on the use of antibiotics in pre-or postendodontic retreatment period, stressing the percentage of events that deserve this kind of therapy should not exceed 6% of the total number of cases[69].

Box 1.3 **ANTIBIOTIC PROPHYLAXIS**

The European Society of Endodontology (ESE) "Position statement": "the use of antibiotics in endodontics with regard to the use of antibiotic prophylaxis"

Antibiotic prophylaxis should be seriously considered in all patients who may develop bacterial endocarditis as a result of particularly bloody oral interventions.

These include, subjects who have:

- **congenital heart defects**
- **natural and mechanical heart valves**
- **previous history of bacterial endocarditis.**

The general definition of invasive dental procedure is yet to be established. This category may include all clinical procedures that lead to the violation of the gingival margin and surgeries performed to solve periapical diseases of endodontic origin.
All of the following may be added to these conditions leading to perforation of the alveolar mucosa. For example, this category should include all patients who have undergone orthopedic surgery with prosthetic replacement, i.e., hip or knee prostheses. Antibiotic prophylaxis should be considered in patients who have had radiation therapy on the maxillary bones and undergone treatment with bisphosphonates at the recommended doses for cancer (see paragraph *Bisphosphonates and endodontic retreatment*).

TYPES OF PATIENTS	INDICATIONS
Decompensated immune function (leukemia, HIV/AIDS, irreversible renal dysfunction, dialysis, uncontrollable diabetes, chemotherapy, treatment with corticosteroids or immunosuppressive drugs post-transplantation, genetic defects)	Absolute both in endodontic surgery and in orthodontic endodontic treatments taking into account: a) general health of the patient b) related risk of further infection c) risk of cross-reactions with other drugs or side effects
Subjects at risk for the development of bacterial endocarditis (patients with congenital heart defects, heart valves, heart defects and a history of past endocarditis)	Orthograde endodontics and surgery
Patients with hip or knee prostheses	Orthograde and surgical endodontic treatment if within three months of treatment
Exposed to high-dose radiation therapies, especially to the maxillary bones	Orthograde endodontics and surgical treatment
Exposed to high IV doses of bisphosphonates	Endodontic surgery

Montefusco V, Gay F, Spina F, et al. (2008) *Antibiotic prophylaxis before dental procedures may reduce the incidence of osteonecrosis of the jaw in patients with multiple myeloma treated with bisphosphonates*. Leukemia and Lymphoma 49, 2156-2162.

European Society of Endodontology developed by: Segura-Egea JJ, Gould K, , Hakan-Sen B, Jonasson P, Cotti E, Mazzoni A, Sunay H, Tjäderhane L, Dummer PMH.

European Society of Endodontology position statement: the use of antibiotics in endodontics. International Endodontic Journal, 51, 20-25, 2018.

* Segura-Egea JJ, Gould K, Hakan-Sen B et al. (2017) *Antibiotics in Endodontics:* a review. International Endodontic Journal 50, 1169-1184.

Sollecito TP, Abt E, Lockhart PB, et al. (2015) *The use of prophylactic antibiotics prior to dental procedures in patients with prosthetic joints: evidence-based clinical practice guideline for dental practitioners–a report of the American Dental Association Council on Scientific Affairs*. Journal of the American Dental Association 146, 11-16.e8.

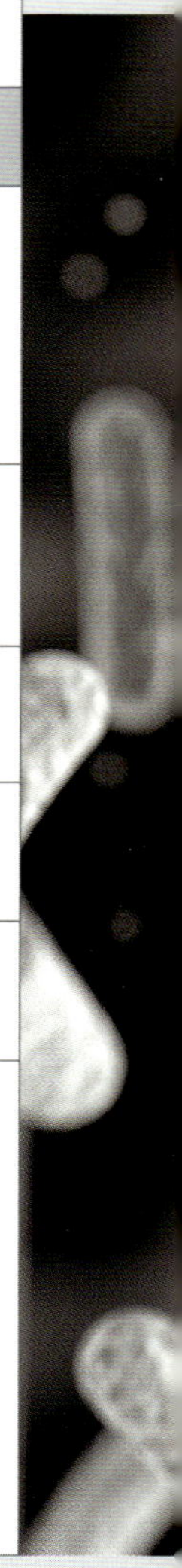

Table 1.7 **RECOMMENDED ANTIBIOTIC PROPHYLAXIS REGIME IN ENDODONTICS***

Patient group	Antibiotic	Route of administration	Dosage		Time before the procedure
			Adults	Children	
Standard general prophylaxis	Amoxicillin	Oral	2 g	50 mg kg^{-1}	1 h
Unable to take oral medications	Ampicillin	IV or IM	2 g	50 mg kg^{-1}	Within 30 min
Allergic to penicillins	Clindamycin Cefalexin or cefadroxil Azithromycin or clarithromycin	Oral Oral Oral	600 mg 2 g 500 mg	20 mg kg^{-1} 50 mg kg^{-1} 15 mg kg^{-1}	1 h 1 h 1 h
Allergic to penicillins/amoxicillins/ampicillin and unable to take oral medications	Clindamycin Cefazolin	IV IV	600 mg 1 g	20 mg kg^{-1} 25 mg kg^{-1}	Within 30 min Within 30 min

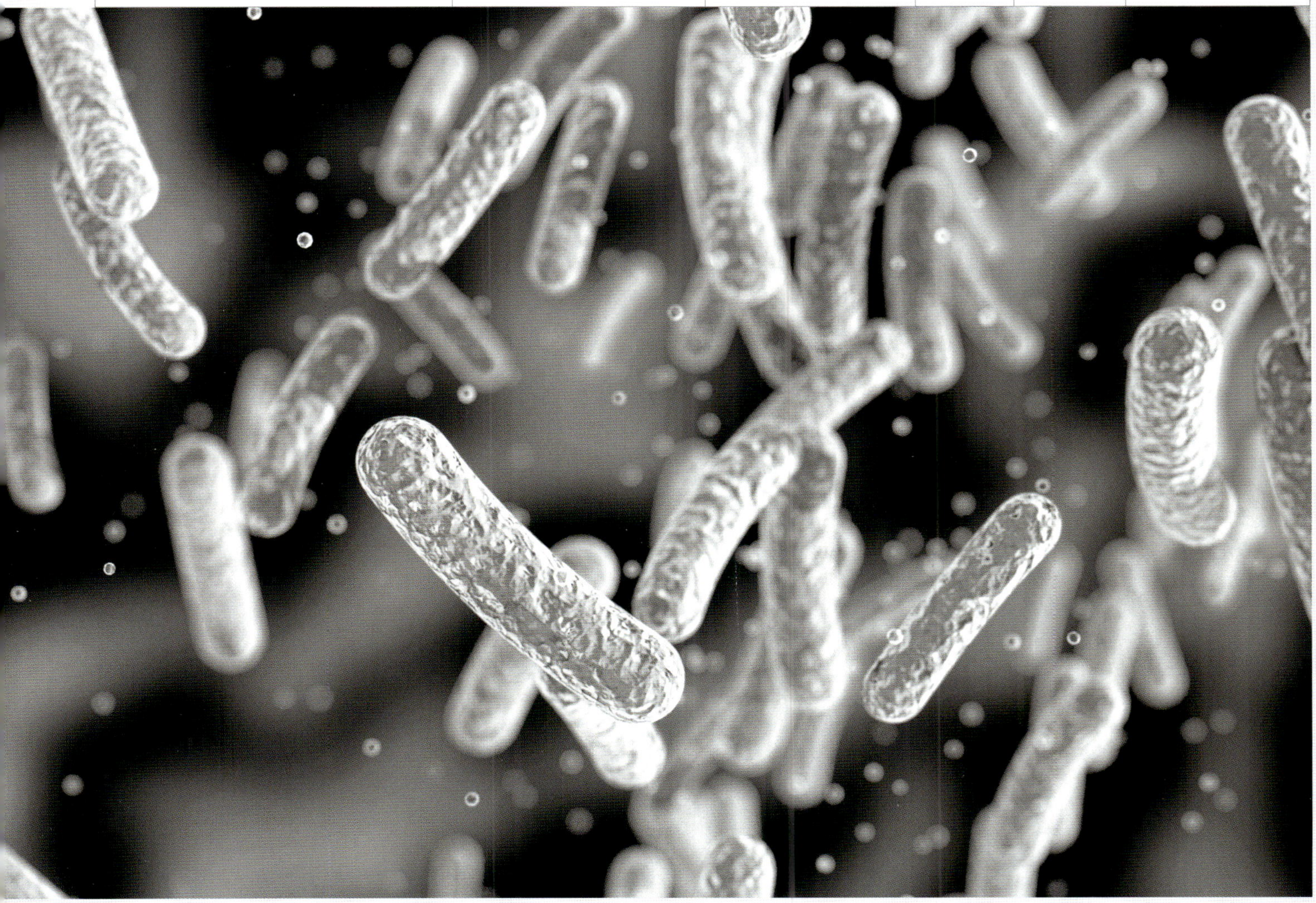

Box 1.4 ASSESSMENT OF CANAL TREATMENT OUTCOMES ACCORDING TO THE EUROPEAN SOCIETY OF ENDODONTOLOGY (ESE)

Root canal treatment should be evaluated at least after 1 year and subsequently if necessary. The following results indicate favorable outcomes: absence of pain, swelling, and other symptoms; absence of fistula; no loss of function; and radiological evidence of normal periodontal ligament space around the root.
The root canal treatment has an uncertain outcome if the radiographs reveal that a radiotransparent lesion remains, that is, has the same size or has decreased but it has not disappeared completely. In this case, the lesion should be further evaluated for a minimum of 4 years until it resolves. If a lesion persists after 4 years, then the root canal treatment is considered responsible for the endodontic post-treatment disease; whether it precedes the treatment itself and therefore is not resolved, or it is the result of it, in any case, it has not achieved the desired results.

The canal treatment has unfavorable outcomes when the following occurs:

1. The tooth shows signs and symptoms of infection.
2. A radiologically visible radiolucent lesion appears after treatment or a pre-existing lesion has increased in size.
3. A lesion has remained the same size or only decreases in size during the 4-year follow-up.
4. Signs of root resorption are present.

In this case, additional treatments should be carried out.

Source: European Society of Endodontology. Quality guidelines for endodontic treatment: consensus report of the European Society of Endodontology. International Endodontic Journal, 2006;39,921-930.

Endodontic pretreatment analgesic strategies and anesthesia

Although true anesthesia is not necessary during retreatment, as the dental pulp is no longer present in the root canal, the patient should be placed in a state of absolute relaxation during the procedure, which can be long and complex. This type of treatment causes anxiety especially in females[70]. Cho et al.[71] reported that in particularly anxious patients, the mere application of an anesthetic ointment can be effective in establishing a good state of analgesia due to the infiltration of articaine as anesthetic[72].
In cases where surgery is required, submucosal administration of tramadol (50 mg) may be sufficient, since the analgesic effect generated by the anesthetic, especially in the lower arch, is likely to be potent[73].
This drug also increases the effect of anesthetics, which are particularly effective when used synergistically in many instances.
In conclusion, the use of anesthetics seems advisable in these cases, despite the absence of dental pulp in most cases.
The use of specific analgesics or anesthetics is recommended for patients who are in pain.

Success and failure: what clinical and radiographic parameters?

We come now to the core of this chapter, that is, how to judge, with sufficient precision, the success or failure of endodontic therapy and how to assess whether a tooth should be retreated.
In previous paragraphs of this chapter, we have dealt with general issues.
In subsequent chapters, we will perform a thorough examination of the clinically relevant factors that result in the development of chronic periapical inflammatory diseases or failure to resolve them.
A sufficiently approximative approach should therefore be adopted when establishing a cut-off between success and failure.
This is no mean feat, given the existence of a vast range of intermediate situations that should be better defined and outlined.
Defining success and failure is the key to approaching this problem.

Box 1.5 ASSESSMENT OF TREATMENT OUTCOME ACCORDING TO THE AMERICAN ASSOCIATION OF ENDODONTISTS (AAE)

To further confirm the data in Box 1.4, numerous detailed and exhaustive documents are available from the website of the American Association of Endodontists, the results of which can be summarized with a series of clinical and radiological considerations that do not differ greatly from those expressed by the European Society of Endodontology. These considerations include correct procedures for the isolation and disinfection of the endodontic space, correct filling within 2 mm of the radiological apical limit, and appropriate posttreatment reconstruction. For detailed reading, please refer to the sitemap below.

https://www.aae.org/specialty/wpcontent/uploads/sites/2/2018/04/TreatmentStandards_Whitepaper.pdf
https://www.aae.org/specialty/wpcontent/uploads/sites/2/2017/06/2014treatmentoptionsguidefinalweb.pdf

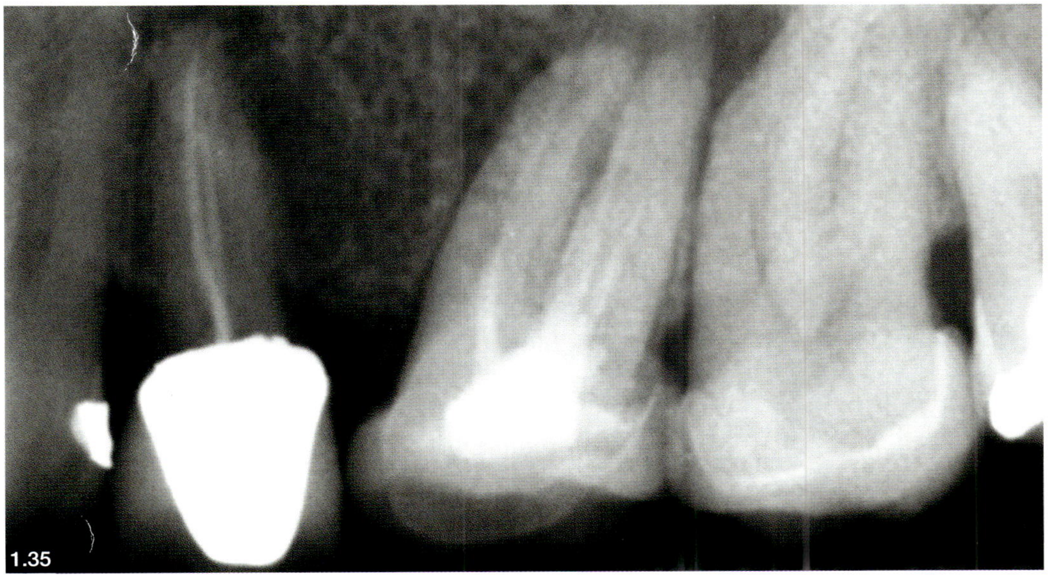

1.35

Fig. 1.35: An upper premolar and an upper molar with prosthetic reconstructions both present poor endodontic treatments that have caused significant periapical damage.

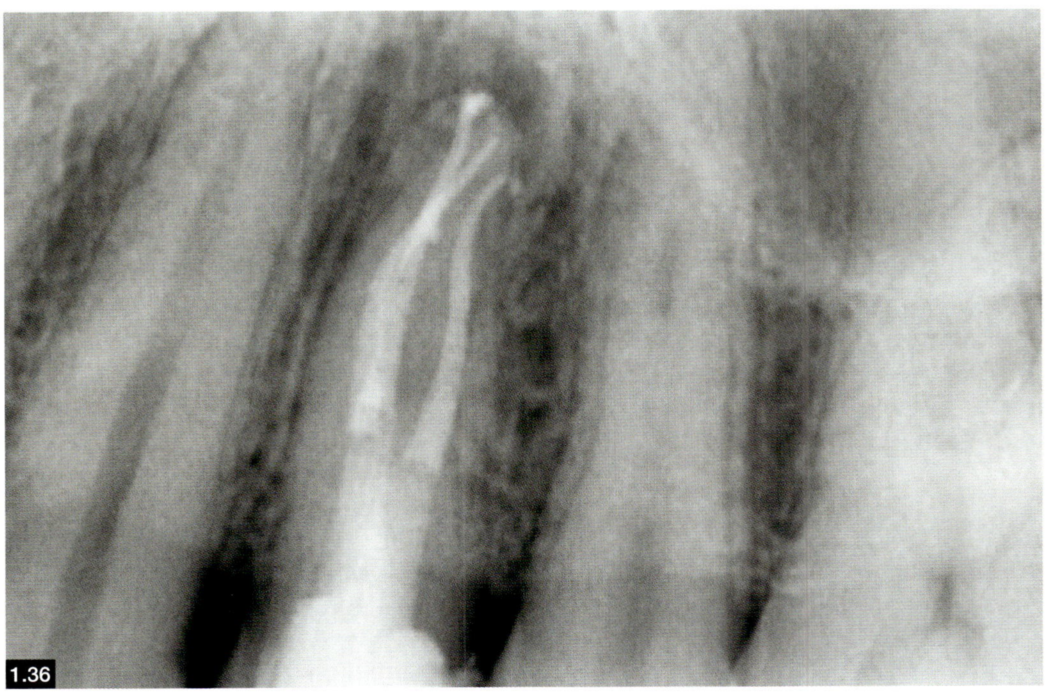

1.36

Fig. 1.36: An upper premolar with a complex anatomy (three canals) has been correctly shaped and blocked; the continuous black line surrounding the apical portion of the tooth confirms the success of treatment.

Some authors[74] have minimized the radiological aspect, while others have emphasized the clinical aspect[75]. The need for the two scenarios to be concordant would lead to further subdivision into four categories: from clinical and radiological success to failure for both categories, passing through the two intermediate scenarios in which the clinical and radiological aspect present two different scenarios. The function of the tooth has been proposed as a central element for evaluation; however, not all scholars agree that a clinically asymptomatic tooth should be considered in any case free of post-treatment diseases[2, 4]. To solve this question, the only viable solution is to adopt the guidelines of the European Society of Endodontology (ESE, reported in Box 1.4) and the American Association of Endodontists (AAE, reported in Box 1.5). By summarizing the guidelines of the major international scientific societies and drawing on other studies, can we realistically define the cut-offs between health and disease? When faced with a patient who has received poorly-managed endodontic therapy, would we have all the information needed to make the right decisions? The answer, it would seem, is no; indeed, there is a large body of evidence confirming the substantial discordance of therapeutic choices depending on the level of the respondents' professional expertise[76-80]. Clinical factors that are relevant to the absolute indication for retreatment include impossibility of chewing or onset of acute events, such as abscess.

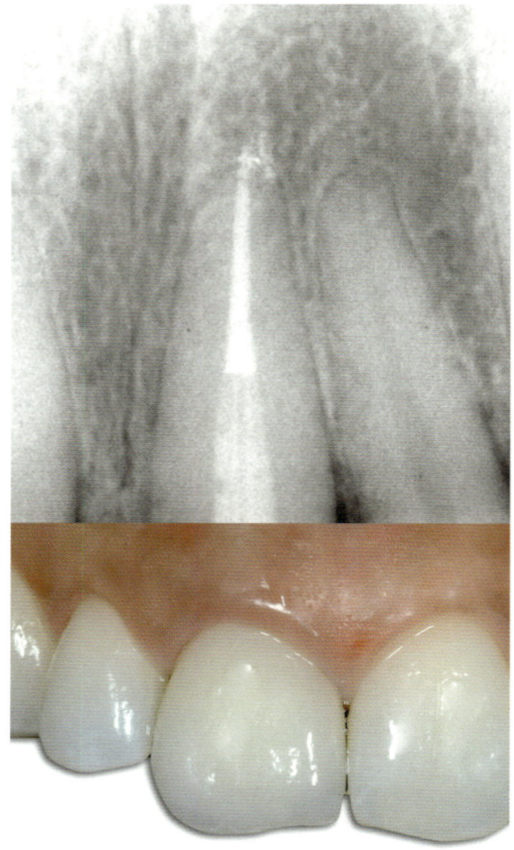

Box 1.6 **CLINICAL AND RADIOLOGICAL NORMALITY**

NORMAL FRAMEWORK TO CLINICS

Absence of:

- spontaneous pain;
- pain caused by chewing or percussion;
- mobility;
- redness or swelling in the adherent mucosa;
- localized periradicular periodontalfistulas orprobes.

Dental structure without dyschromia or of the normal tooth-restoration whole, in a mucous context also free from suspicious chromaticisms.

NORMAL FRAMEWORK TO RADIOLOGICAL

- Uniform periradicular margin.
- Periodontal ligament space not exceeding one millimeter.
- Hard foil circumscribing and clearly delimits the periodontal space.
- Absence of:
  - root resorption;
  - radiotransparent areas periradicular in contiguity with the roots themselves.

As regards the reconstruction of deficient treatments, in the presence of secondary caries or fractures on previously treated teeth, the signs of periapical suffering, from a radiological point of view, urge the clinician to consider endodontic retreatment as the first step toward tooth restoration. The following phase involves a thorough discussion with the patient regarding the different therapeutic options in reconstructive settings and the possible consequences associated with the procedures listed. If it is well-designed, this therapeutic agreement will protect each of its parties from any possible misunderstanding. Numerous elements of judgment come into play, moving away from the tooth in the stricter sense towards the broader context of patient care and guidelines for the therapeutic decision-making, primarily in relation to those local factors that, in the final analysis, we will consider to in order to decide whether to address the retreatment procedure or whether to start the operational choice in other surgical fields, not least the tooth extraction.

Box 1.7 **WHAT TO LOOK FOR ON AN X-RAY**

Coronal

1 Coronal seal

2 Reconstruction material

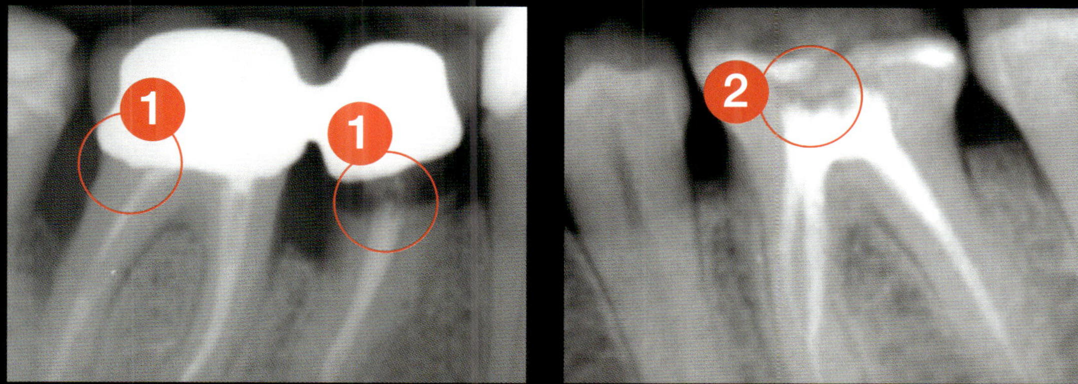

Radicular

Presence of obstacles inside the canal:

3 Tools

4 Blocks

5 Pins

6 Voids

7 Trunk-taper

8 Length of the filling

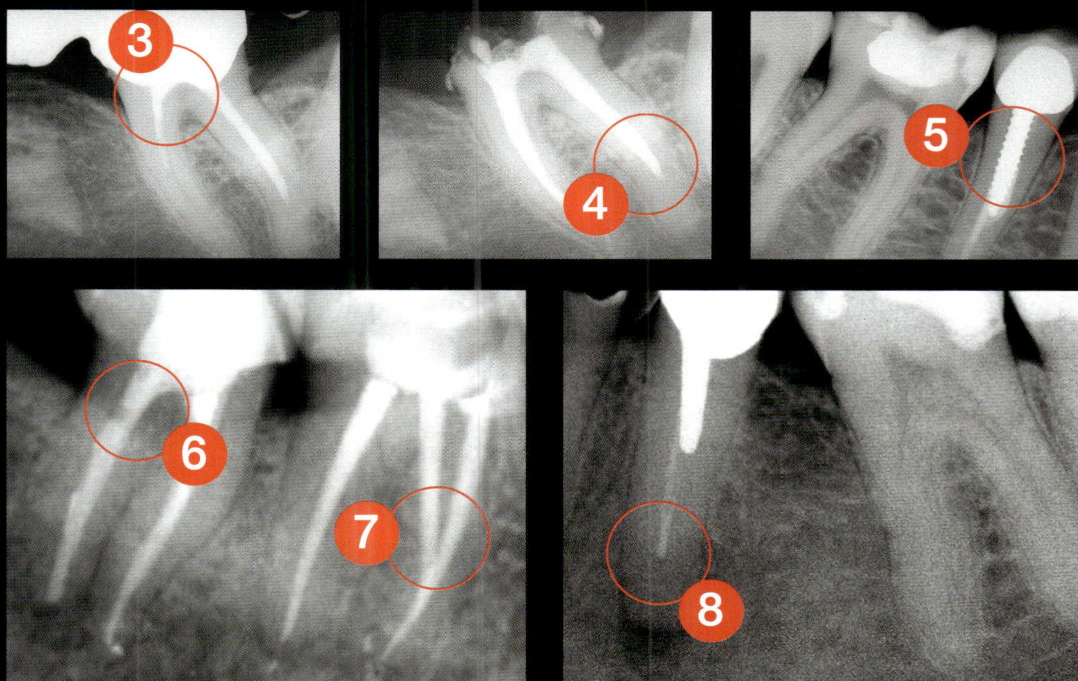

Periradicular

9 Extension along the root of the radiolucent area

9 Amplitude of the radiotransparent area

10 Overfill

11 Appearance of the periradicular ligament

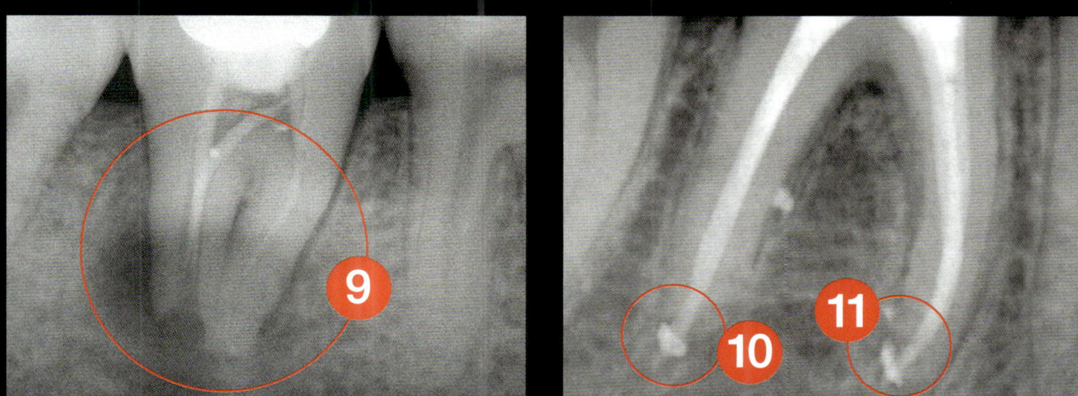

CASE REPORT 3

Suspected periapical lesion in the case of endodontic retreatment

The information provided by two-dimensional X-ray images is often very limited and the pathological state of the tooth must be investigated with three-dimensional X-ray studies. Three-dimensional radiographic x-ray techniques are essential for formulating a diagnosis of chronic apical periodontitis with maxillary sinus involvement.

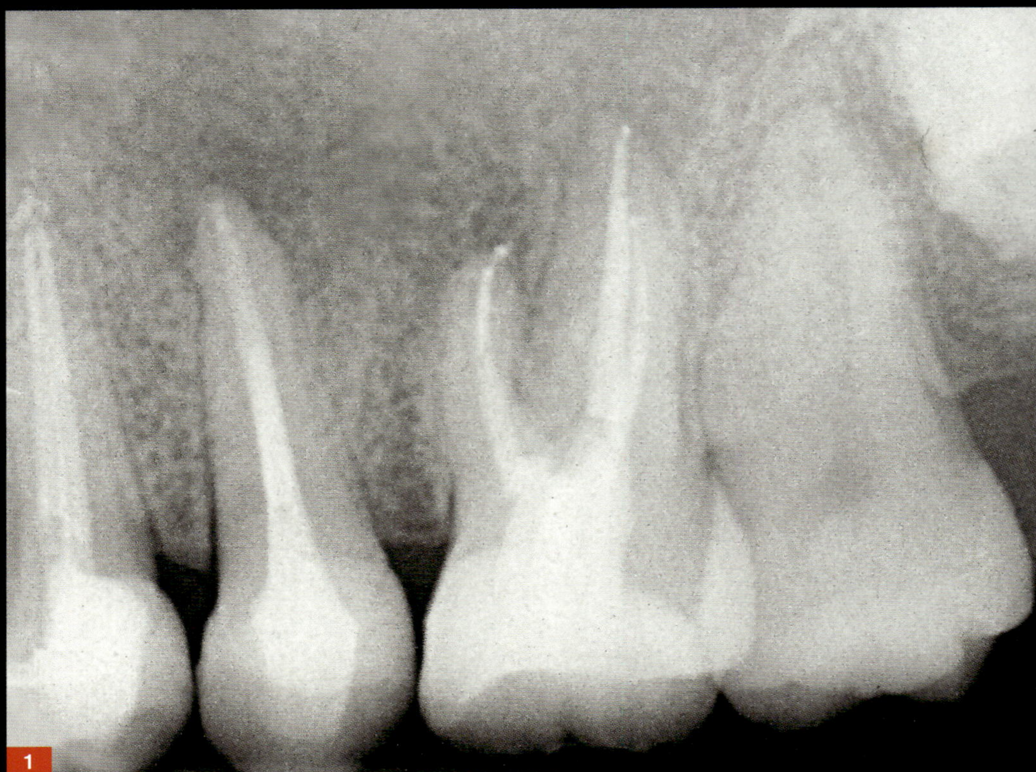

Figure 1: The two-dimensional x-ray view does not show a very large lesion in the same tooth, the endodontic treatment appears correct, although it shows a modest overfilling.

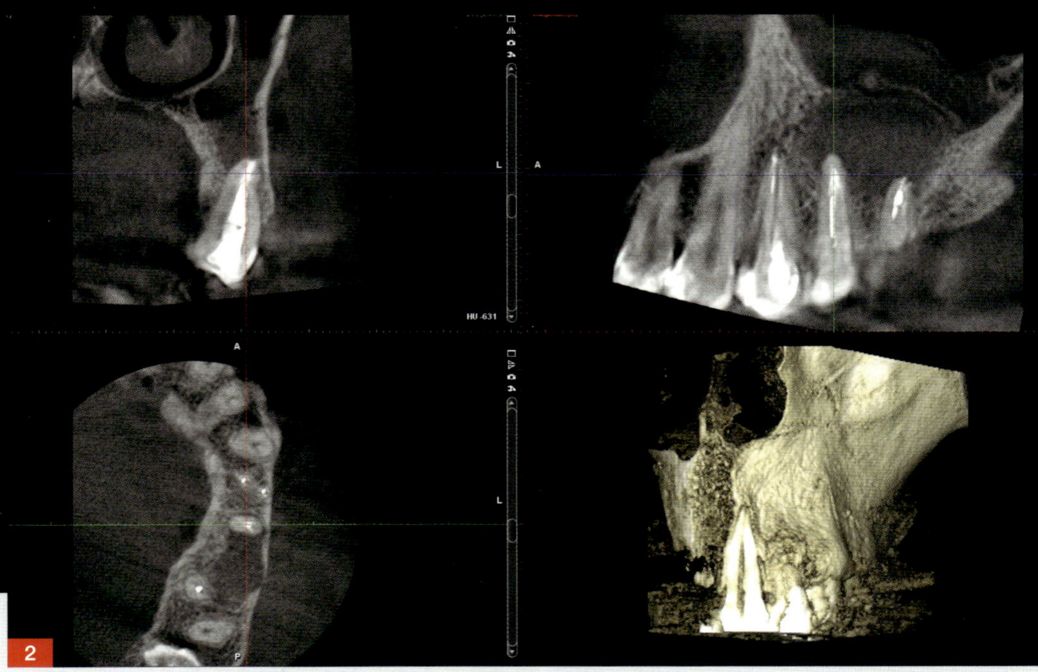

Figure 2: The CBCT image highlights a very large lesion affecting both the premolar and the molar and extends to the floor of the upper sinus.

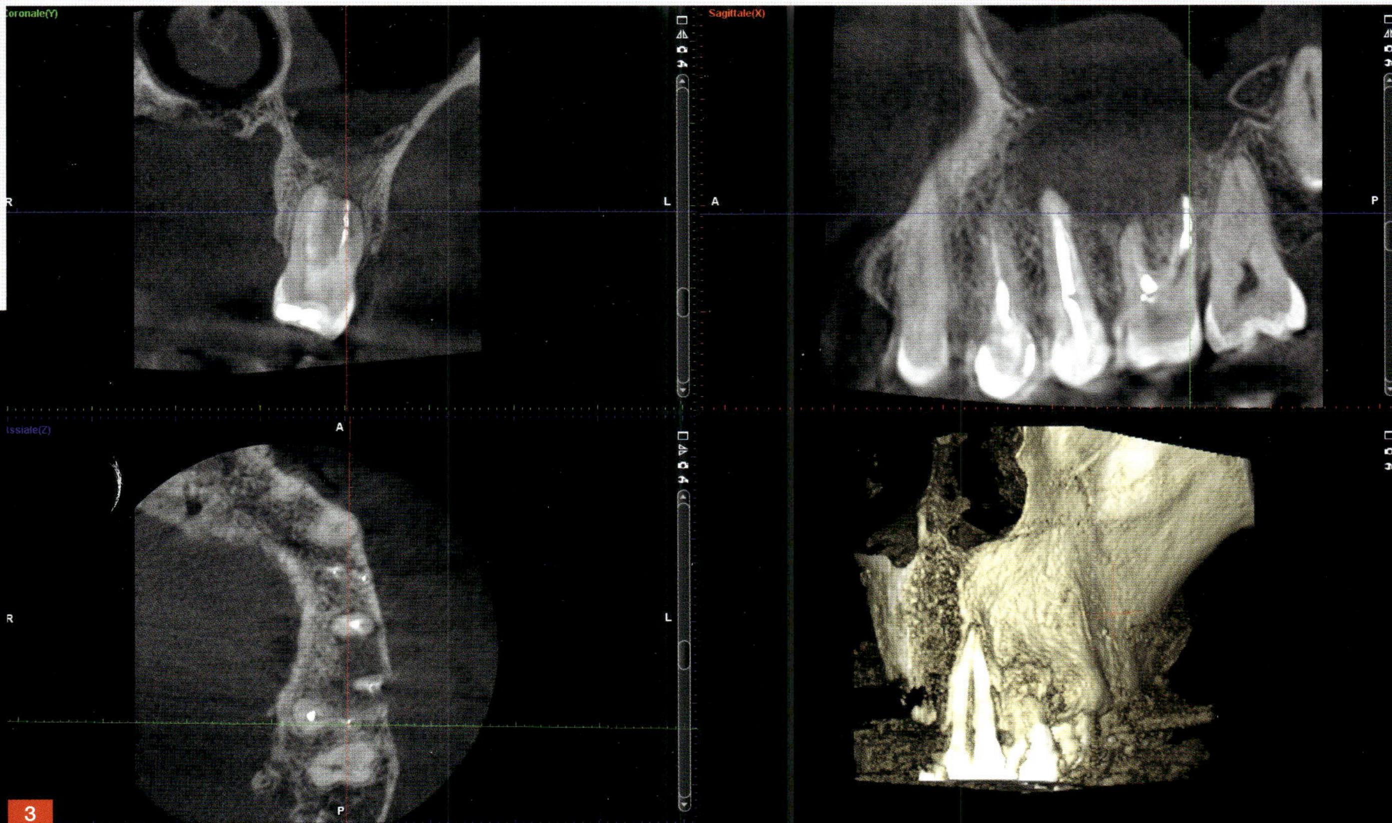

3

Figure 3: The same scenario seen from a different angle.

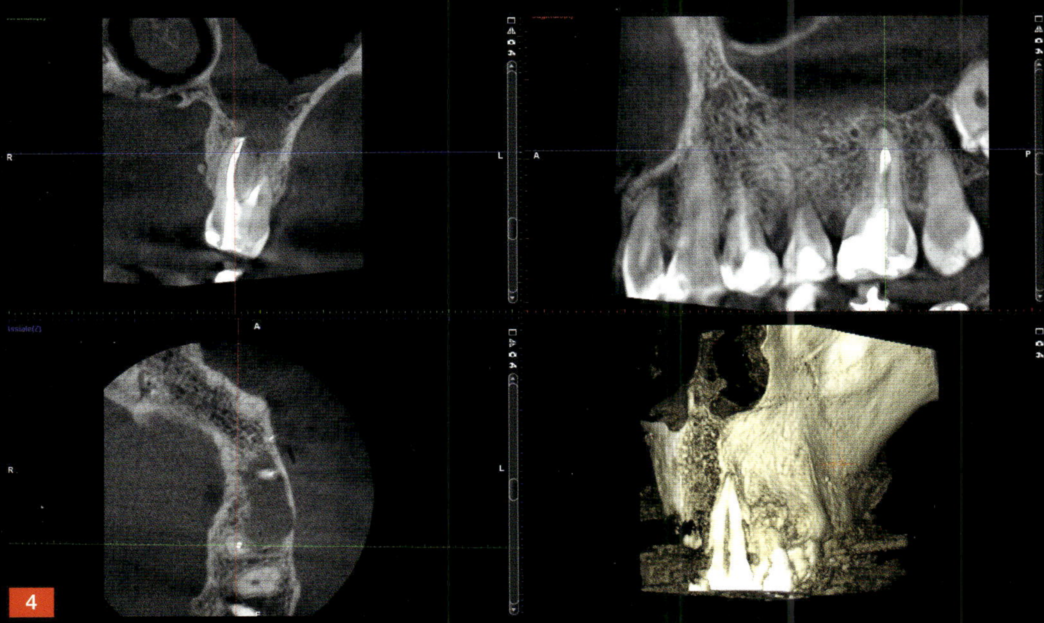

4

Figure 4: These images clearly show the massive involvement of the maxillary sinus, which could underlie the very severe symptoms reported by the patient. An extra-radicular infection (see next section) could be hypothesized, given the excellent congruence between the canal lumen and the filling material.

CASE REPORT 4

Upper premolar with prosthetic reconstruction: integrated endodontic-orthodontic-prosthetic treatment

The second upper premolar presents clinically and radiologically evident infiltration (Fig. 1); the prosthetic restoration will lead to a reduction in root size and the need to place a root canal post.

Figure 1: Second upper premolar with clinically and radiologically evident infiltration.

Figure 2: The case before retreatment.

Figure 3: After retreatment.

Figure 4 and 5: The newly inserted orthodontic appliance and the final result one year later.

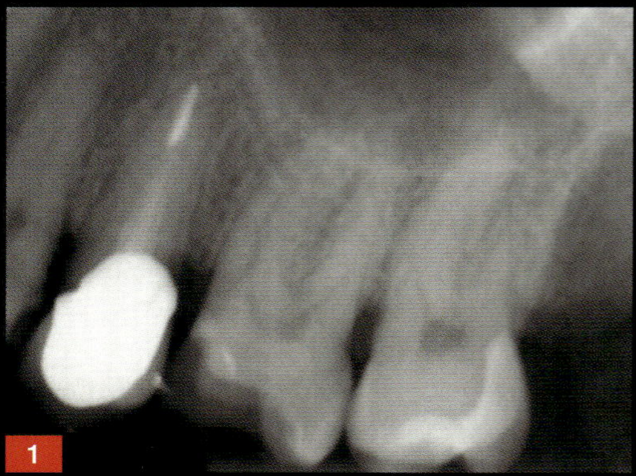

1

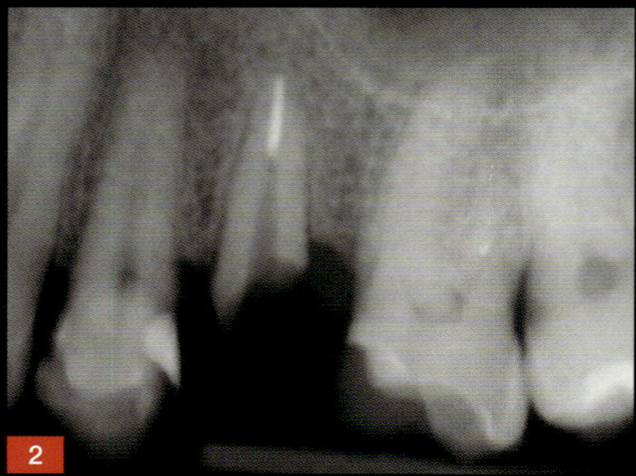

2

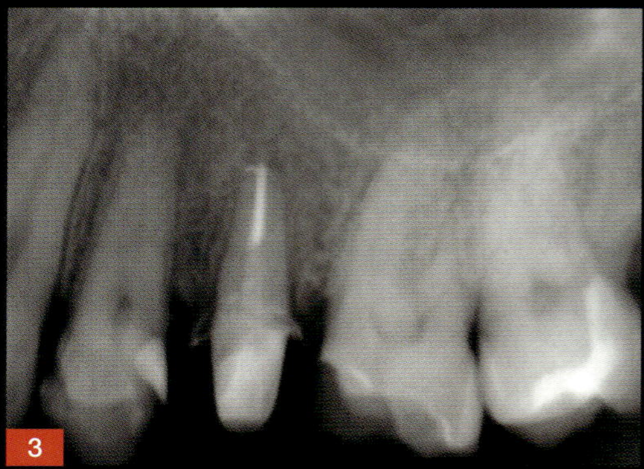

3

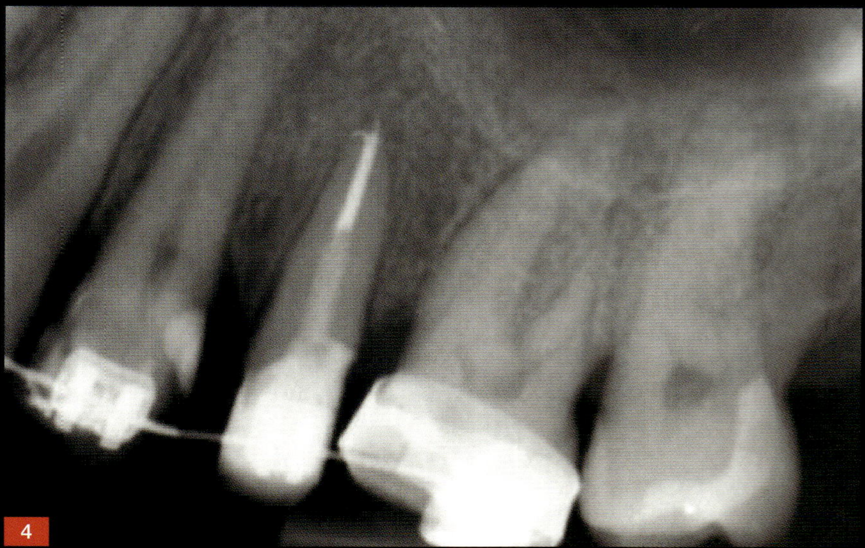

4

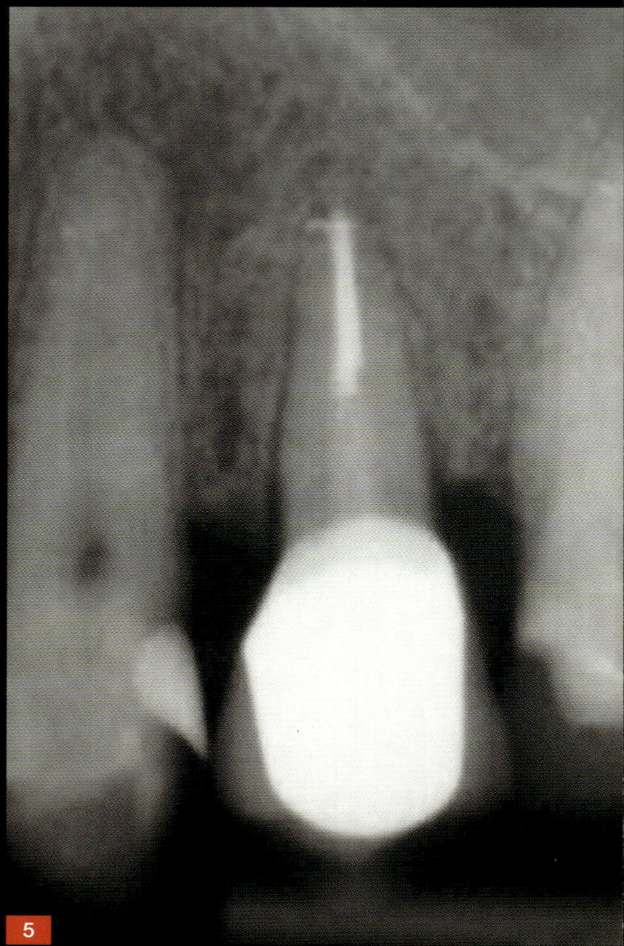

5

In addition, the reduced amount of supporting tissues and the root size encouraged the practitioner, when formulating the treatment plan, to perform retreatment and a root extrusion procedure (Figs. 2-5).
The violation of the coronal seal and of the previous filling bode in favor of the retreatment procedure even in the presence of a periradicular aspect that, despite not being overtly pathological, considering the underestimation of the 2D x-ray, seems increasingly advisable in clinical settings such as those represented in this case (Figs. 6-7).

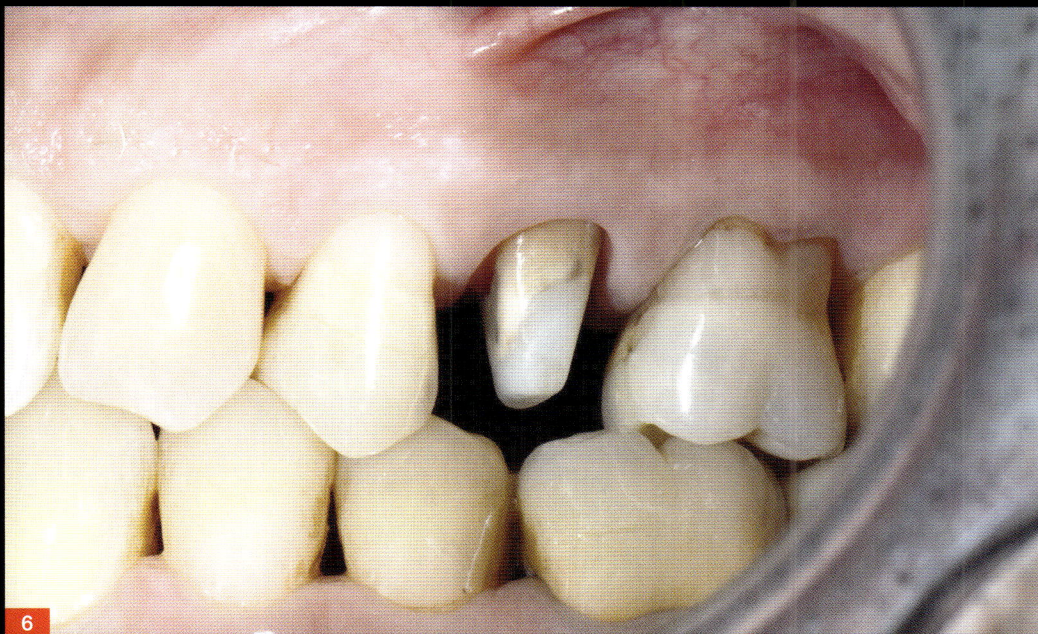

6

Figure 6: The abutment on the day of cementation: note the good condition of periodontal tissues.

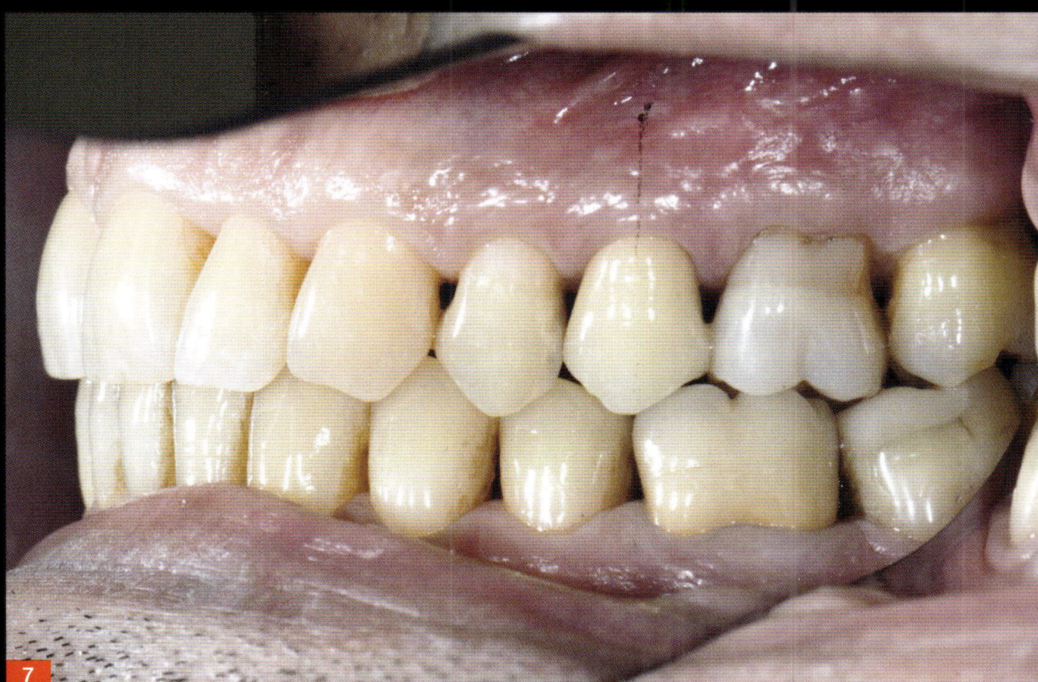

7

Figure 7: The 1-year follow-up shows perfect integration with the supporting tissues and neighboring teeth.

Periapical disease classification systems based on x-ray and CBCT images

Based on their analysis of x-rays, a number of scholars have attempted to classify the pathological aspects and the damages caused by previous endodontic treatments to the tooth and/or the supporting tissues, using numerical indices. These include the periapical index, commonly known as the PAI[81] (Box 1.8), which primarily classifies the periapical state of teeth affected by diseases of that district, and the classification proposed by Elyas et al.[82] (Box 1.9). The former index has a significant historical value, whereas the latter reconciles the dental problems and those regarding the supporting tissues to quantify the complexity of any retreatment procedure. The content of this classification system proposed for the analysis of pathological scenarios using CBCT (Box 1.10) is different. The possibility of obtaining a better radiographic detail leads to a redefinition of classification systems; three of those discussed in current literature are reviewed here.

Box 1.8 **PERIAPICAL INDEX SCORE (PAI)**

Developed by Ørstavik et al. the periapical index (often abbreviated to PAI) is a system for radiologically classifying the apical and periapical situation of a tooth affected by inflammatory reactions of endodontic origin using 2D x-rays. The figure below provides a brief description of the classification system that has been used in endodontics to classify the initial conditions as well as the results after endodontic treatment in teeth that are affected or not affected by periapical problems.

Ørstavik D, Kerekes K, Eriksen HM. The periapical index: a scoring system for radiographic assessment of apical periodontitis. *Endodontics & Dental Traumatology 1986;2:20-34.*

1

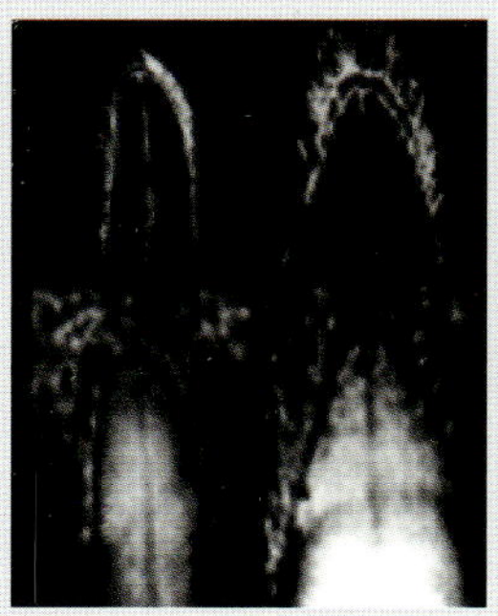

Apical and periapical structures in normal conditions, periodontal ligaments surrounded by the lamina dura

2

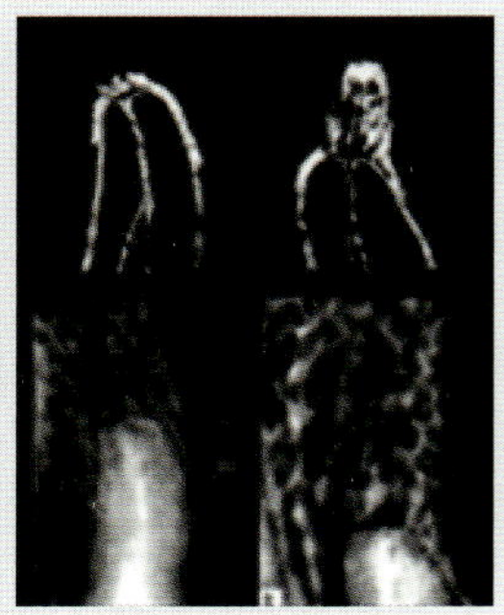

Very slight alterations in the bone structure with limited radiotransparency at the periodontal ligament

3

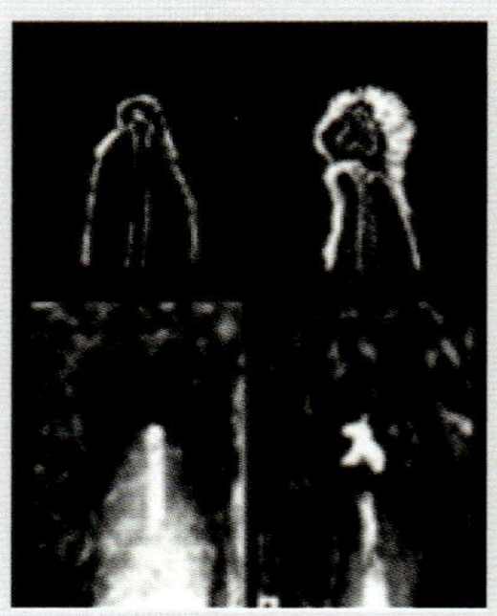

Alterations in the bone structure with slight radiotransparency

4

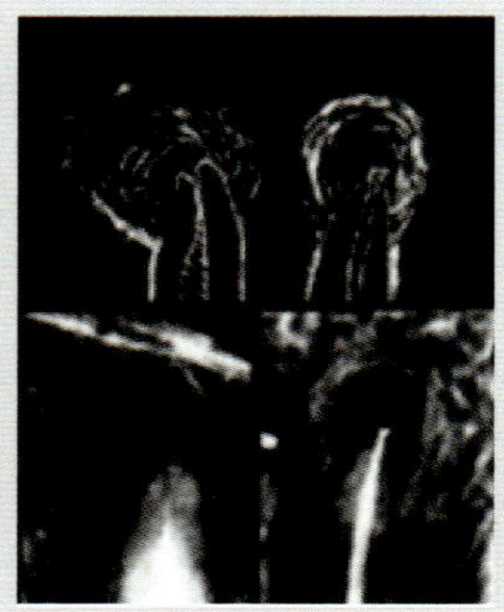

Well-defined area of radiotransparency, indicating overt periodontitis

5

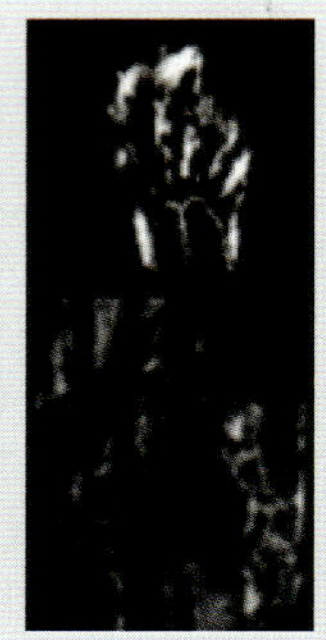

Very severe periodontitis with very well-defined radiotransparency

In clinical studies, conditions 1 and 2 are often associated with normal scenarios; cases with such a radiographic appearance are classified as healthy.

In clinical studies, conditions with an index greater than or equal to 3 are considered to be abnormal and are incorporated into the groups of cases that are either overtly pathological (usually at the beginning of longitudinal studies) or that do not achieve the desired effect if treated during a longitudinal study.

Box 1.9 X-RAY STUDY: IDENTIFICATION OF THE TEETH AND RATING OF TREATMENT ADEQUACY

X-ray studies play a key role whenever the success of root canal therapy is to be judged. The practitioner must be perfectly aware of the aspects to be examined and considered and forming connections between these findings is not an easy exercise. This makes it essential to establish a sequence of aspects on which to base the analysis, which, in this particular case, consists in assigning a score to each of the elements examined.
This was the aim of the study conducted by Elyas et al., who attributed a dichotomous value to each single item in the list below (1 point if the item is present, 0 if the item is not present) to obtain numerical score. The scores obtained indicate the quality of the treatment, i.e., the higher the score, the poorer the quality of treatment.

The items considered are:

1. Shaping errors

- wrong access;
- steps or hourglass morphologies;
- perforations or erosion of the root wall;
- root canal blocking;
- fractured instruments;
- undetected root canals.

2. Filling errors

- morphological discontinuity and poor-conicity;
- presence of voids;
- presence of bubbles;
- filling limit, short (if more than 2 mm from the radiological apex) or long (if clearly oversized).

Despite the limitations of abstract classifications, this method provides a rough guide for judging the quality of treatment; if the quality is poor, then the tooth should be retreated. Otherwise, in the presence of an endodontic periapical lesion in a well-treated tooth, alternative therapeutic procedures, such as endodontic surgery, should be initiated.

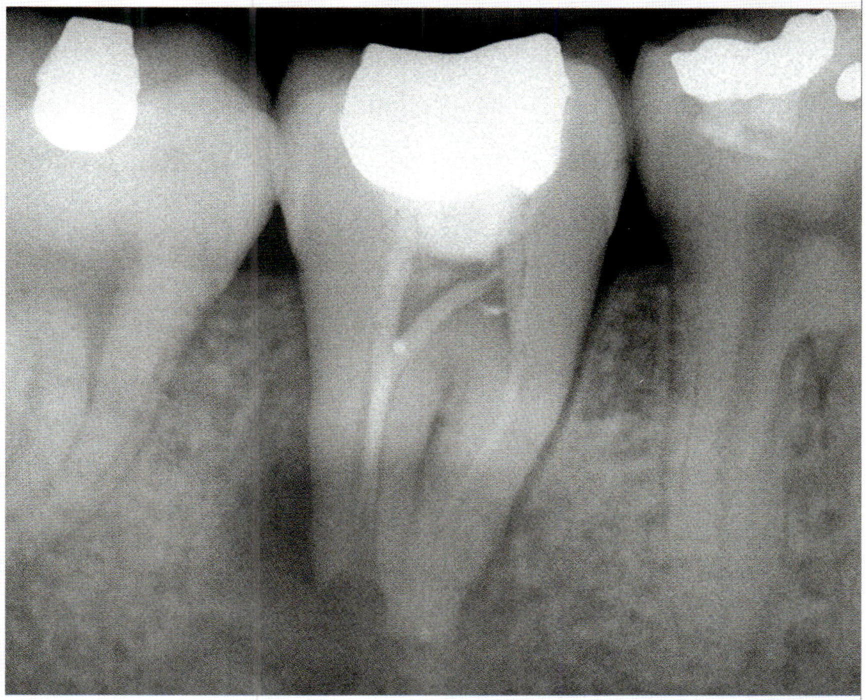

Using on the indices considered, the case has four points for procedural errors in shaping and as many points for errors in the filling phase (a total of 8 out of 10 points).

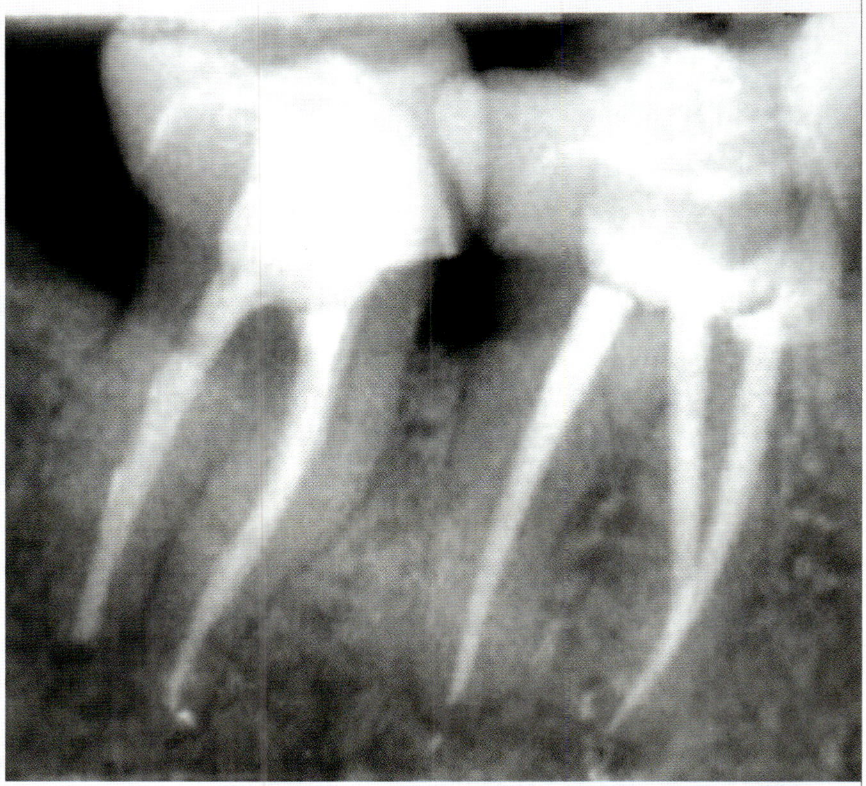

Using the same scoring system, the x-ray does not score any points for the first part; in the filling errors part, one point can be attributed for the presence of clinically irrelevant voids in the distal root. The total score is 1 out of 10, which confirms the correctness of the treatment.

Eliyas et al. Technical skills in Endodontics. International Endodontic Journal 2017;50;652-66.

Box 1.10 **CBCT-BASED ANALYSIS**

The progress achieved in two-dimensional digital radiological techniques (digital subtraction) (L) and, in particular, the introduction of the CBCT technique in the endodontic field, have called for new indices for evaluating the initial pathological situation (Table 1.8) and parameters for analyzing the success or failure of treatment.
Through analysis with CBCT before and after retreatment therapy, Davies et al.[99] highlighted the sensitivity of this technique in identifying pathological radiotransparency at periapical level; the classification of successful or unsuccessful measures proposed by the authors provides an optimum classification of periapical disease that is otherwise impossible with two-dimensional x-rays. Two cases are given as examples.

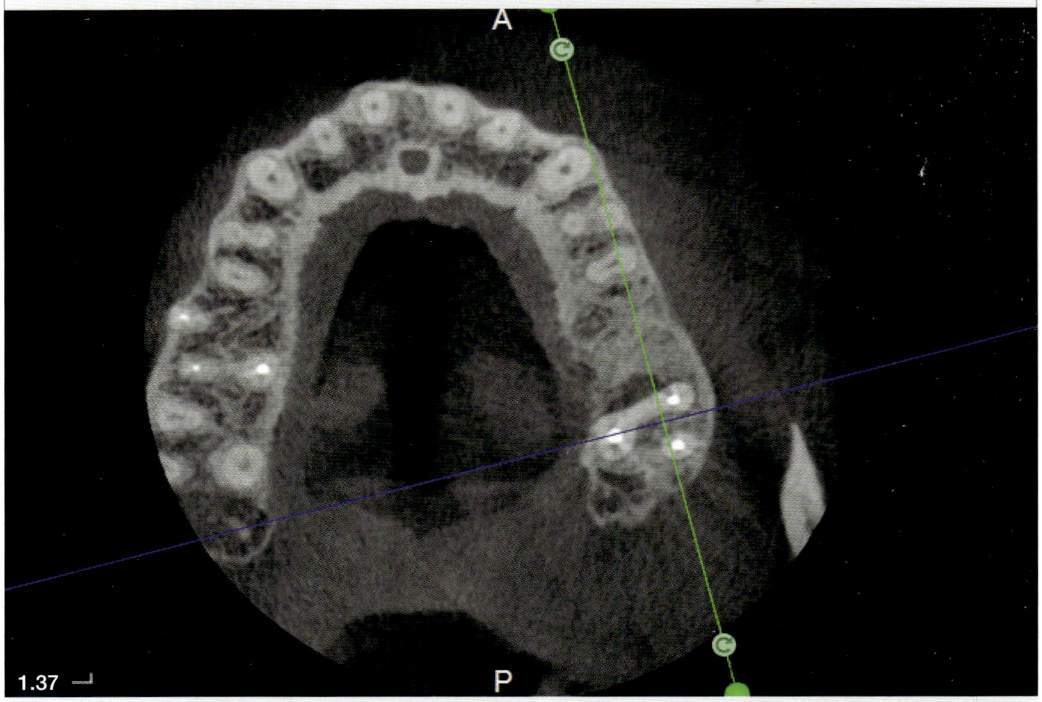

Fig.1.37: Typical CBCT image for dental use, an indispensable tool for making a detailed diagnosis of the problems afflicting the apical periodontium of endodontically treated teeth.

Table 1.8 **CBCT-BASED IMAGING SYSTEMS**

Score	Estrela et al.[(1)]	Torabinejad et al. (Eri Score)[(2)]
	Periapical radiotransparency	**Periapical radiotransparency**
0	Absent	Absent
1	0.5-1 mm	< 0.5 mm
2	1-2 mm	0.5-1.0 mm
3	2-4 mm	1.0-1.5 mm
4	4-8 mm	1.5-2.0 mm
5	> 8 mm	2.0-2.5 mm
6		> 2.5 mm
E	Expansion of the periapical cortical bone	
D	Destruction of the periapical cortical bone	

(1) Index to classify periapical diseases identified by CBCT. C. Estrela et al., A New Periapical Index Based on Cone-Beam Computed Tomography. J Endod 2008;34:1325-1331.

(2) ERI (Endodontic Radiolucency Index) for CBCT analysis. M.Torabinejad et al., Incidence and Size of Periapical Radiolucencies Using Cone-beam Computed Tomography in Teeth without Apparent Intraoral Radiographic Lesions: A New Periapical Index with a Clinical Recommendation. J Endod 2018;44:389-394.

Radiological doubt solved with 3D x-ray

CASE REPORT 5

Despite effective retreatment, an upper molar presents a nuanced but persistent symptoms; combined use of multiple investigation techniques alone will lead to the desired diagnostic result.

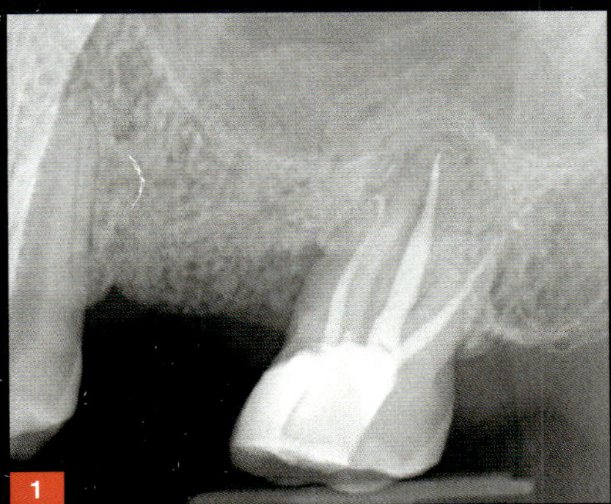

1

Figure 1: The intraoral x-ray shows good closure of the root canals; however, the clinical symptoms remain abnormal.

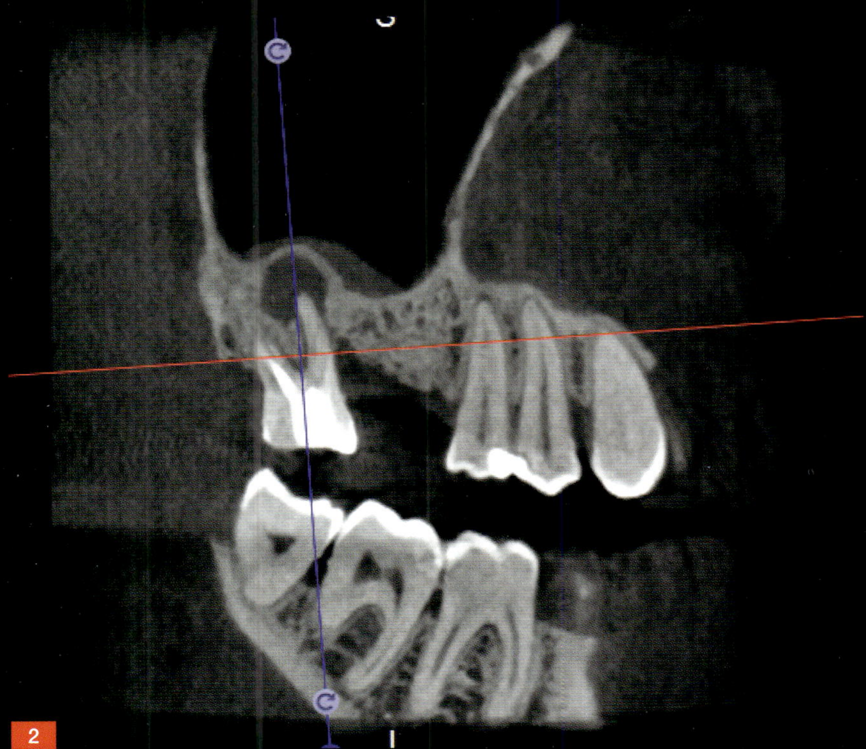

2

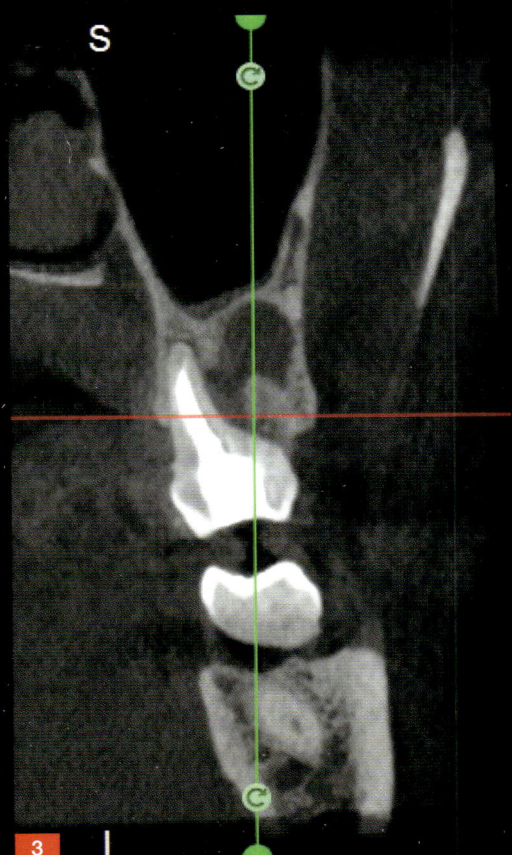

3

Figure 2: The two images show overt periapical disease that can most likely be attributed, to an extra-radicular infection (see next section).

Figure 3: The same situation with a posteroanterior view.

CASE REPORT 6

Severe periapical lesion with perforation on lateral incisor

The patient, a 26-year-old female, had undergone root canal treatment on tooth 12 as a result of a traumatic event; after about 2 years after treatment, a narrow vestibular fistula was observed on the same tooth.

Figure 1: The fistula in the vestibular area tooth 12.

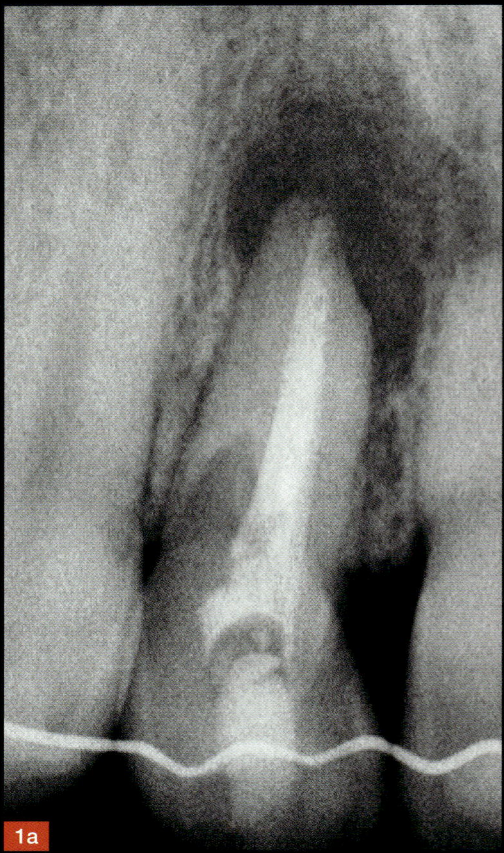

1a

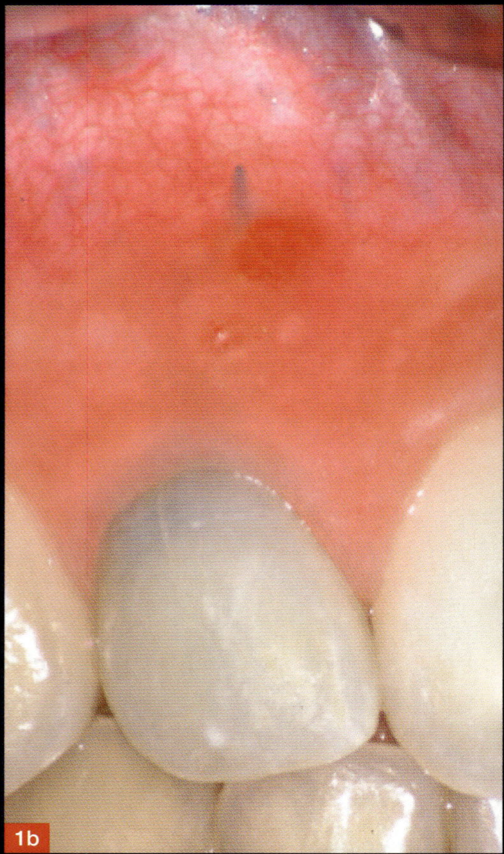

1b

Figure 2: The radiographic study shows a very extensive lesion secondary to a non-exceptional but acceptable endodontic treatment.

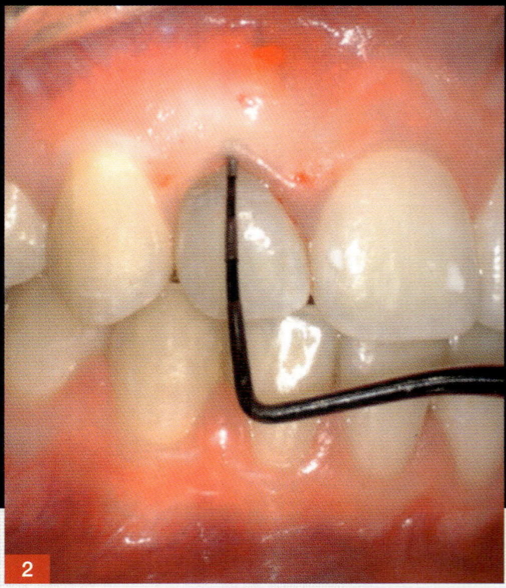

2

This kind of evolution must always lead to a suspicion of periodontal impairment and, in this specific case, must attract the attention of the clinician who, in such cases, with young patients, has double responsibilities, be they diagnostic or therapeutic.

Figure 3a: The CBCT image brings to light a radically different scenario, because it is the result of a perforation of the middle third with extrusion of the filling material.

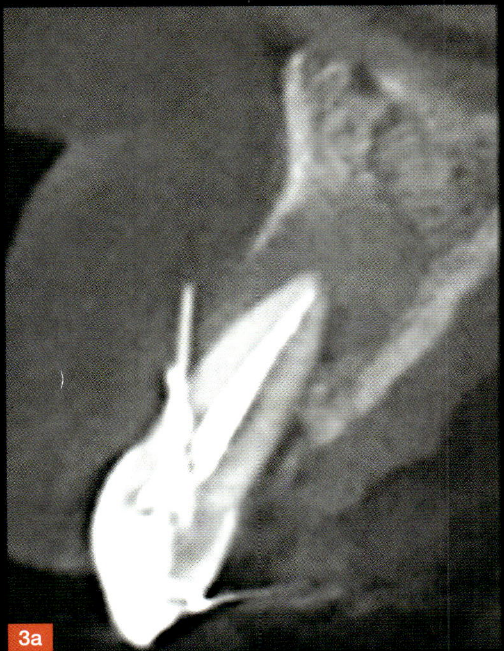

3a

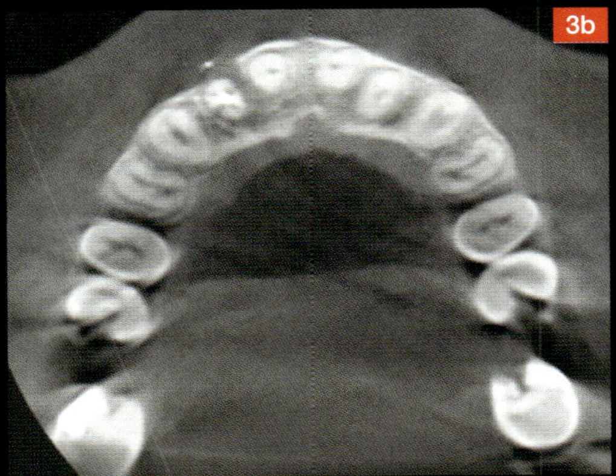

3b

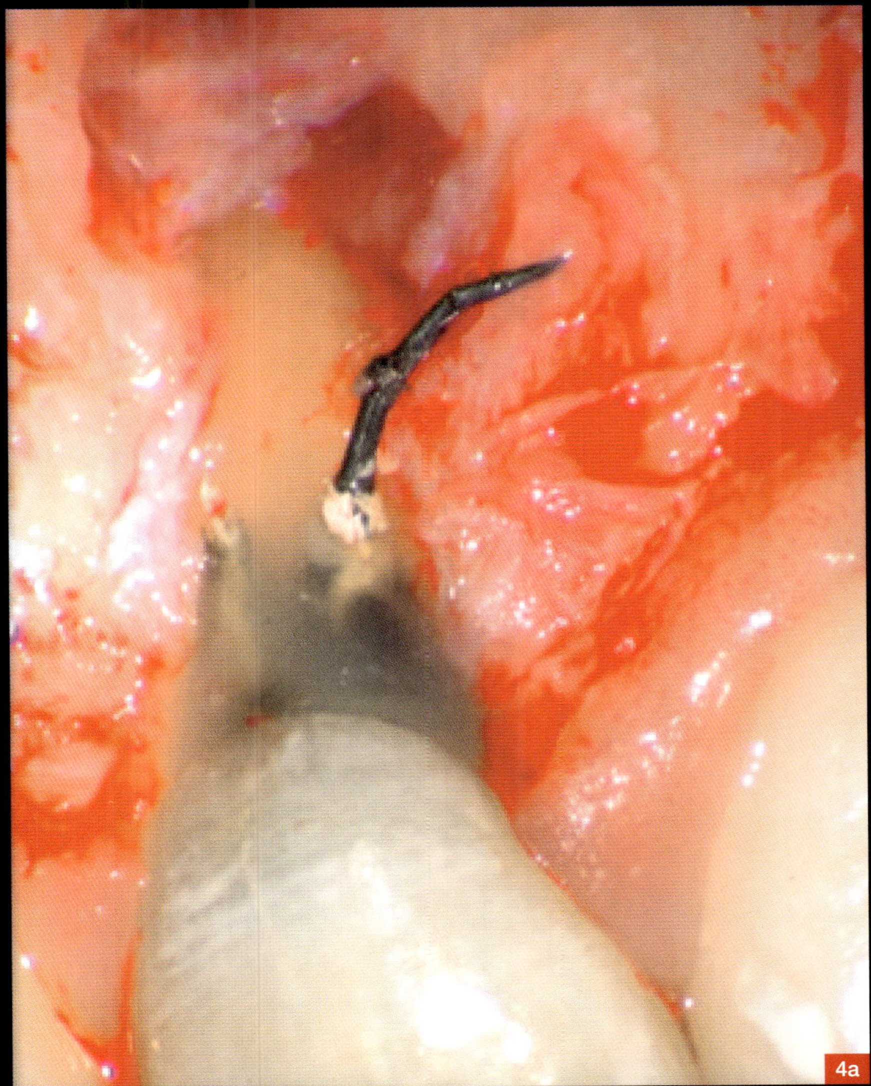

4a

Figure 3b: CBCT image, the occlusal view does not appear to reveal further impairment; a consistent lack of vestibular cortical bone tissue at tooth no. 12 is also evident.

Figure 4a: The three-dimensional images confirmed the clinically observed pathological condition.

Figure 4b-c: Two initial phases of the intervention, the gutta-percha in the perforation was cut and revealed further perforations.

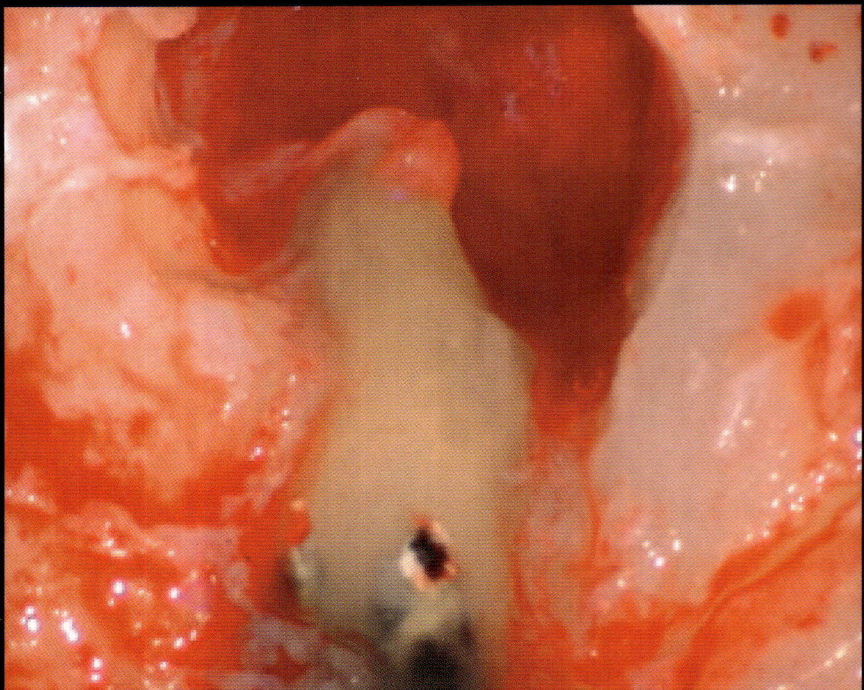

4b

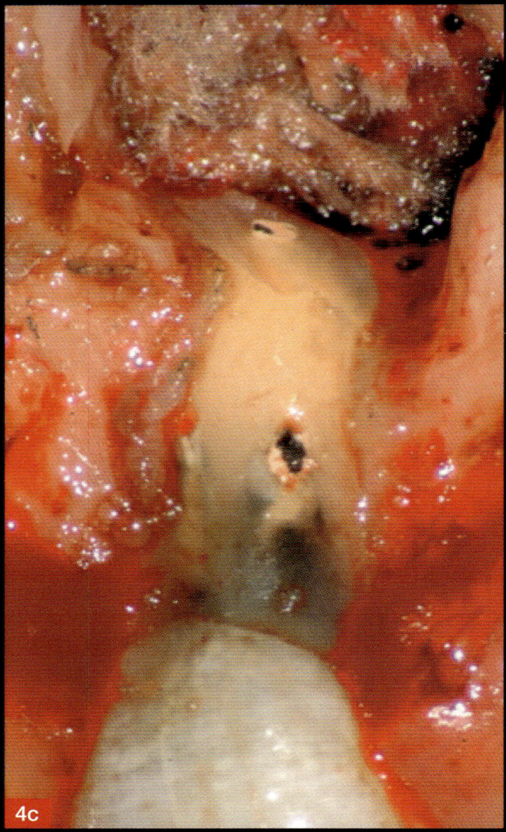

4c

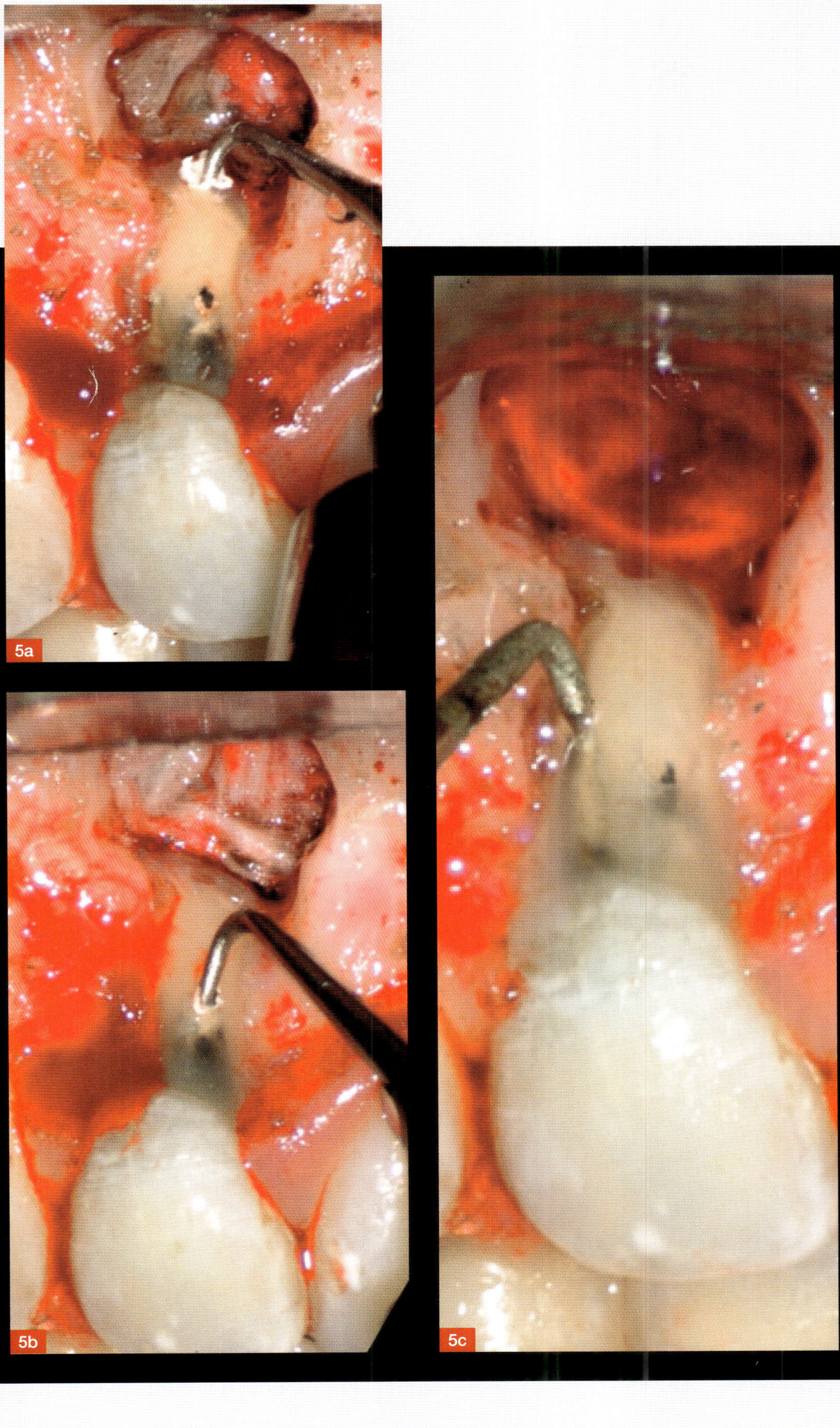

Figure 5a-c: Some phases of endodontic and periodontal surgery aimed at sealing the perforations.

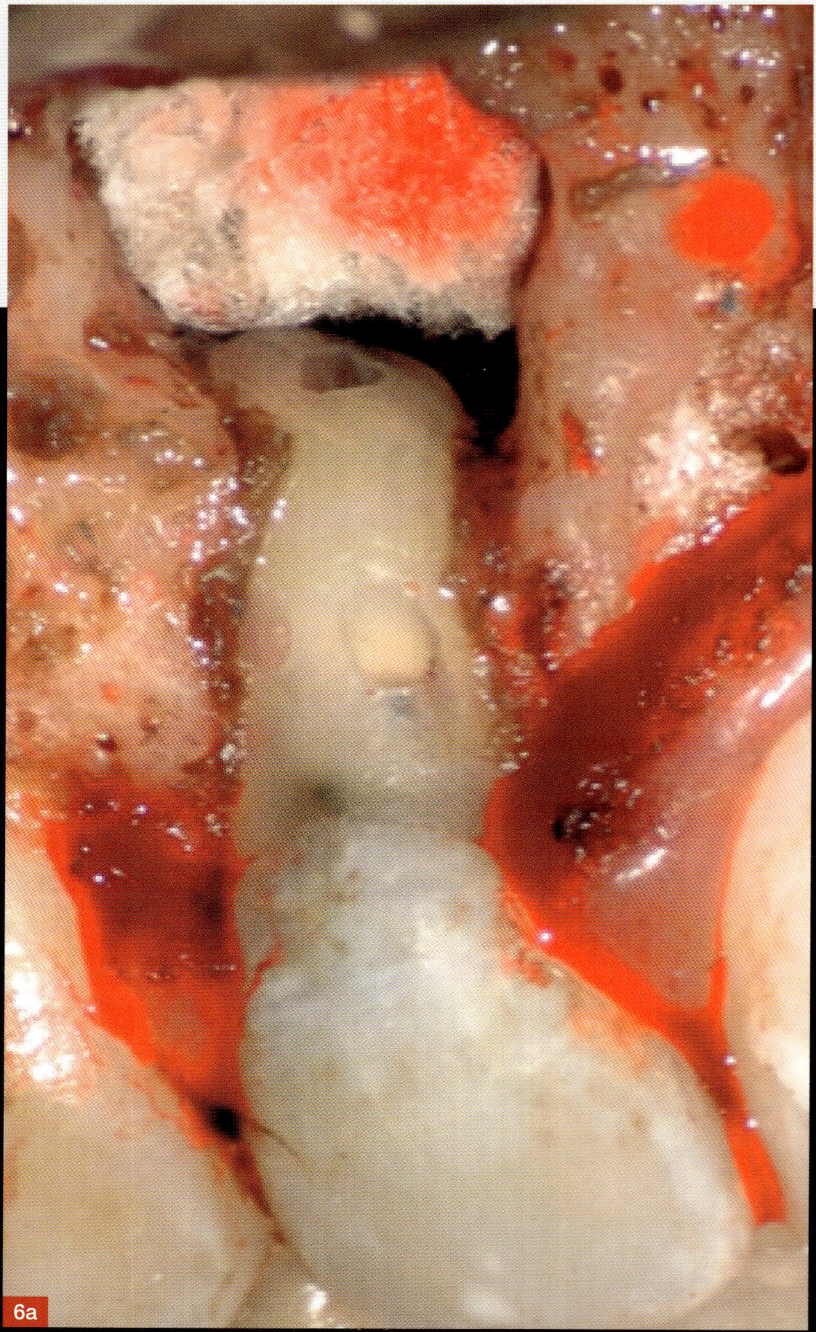

6a

Figure 6a-b: The perforations are perfectly sealed with biocompatible material and the retrograde cavity is finished to the limit of the apical lesion.

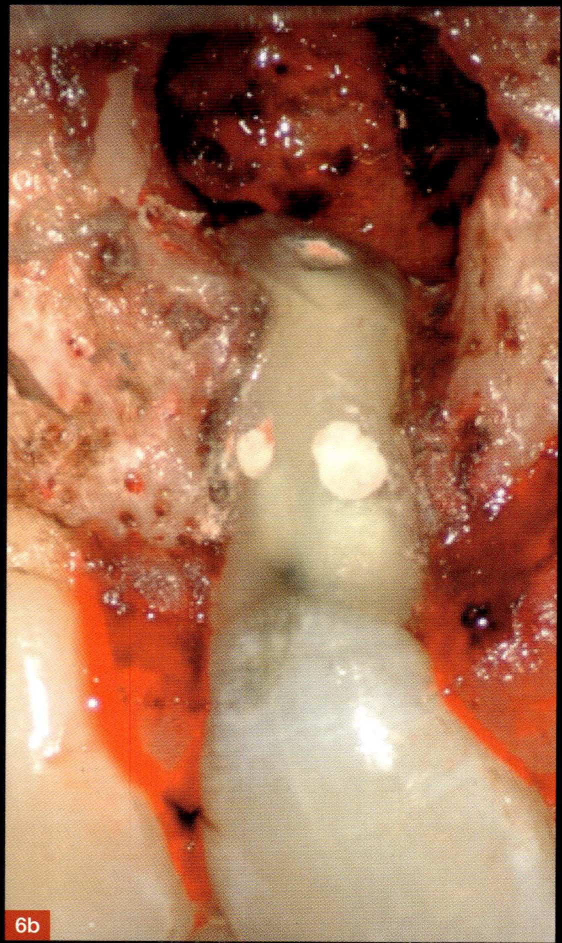

6b

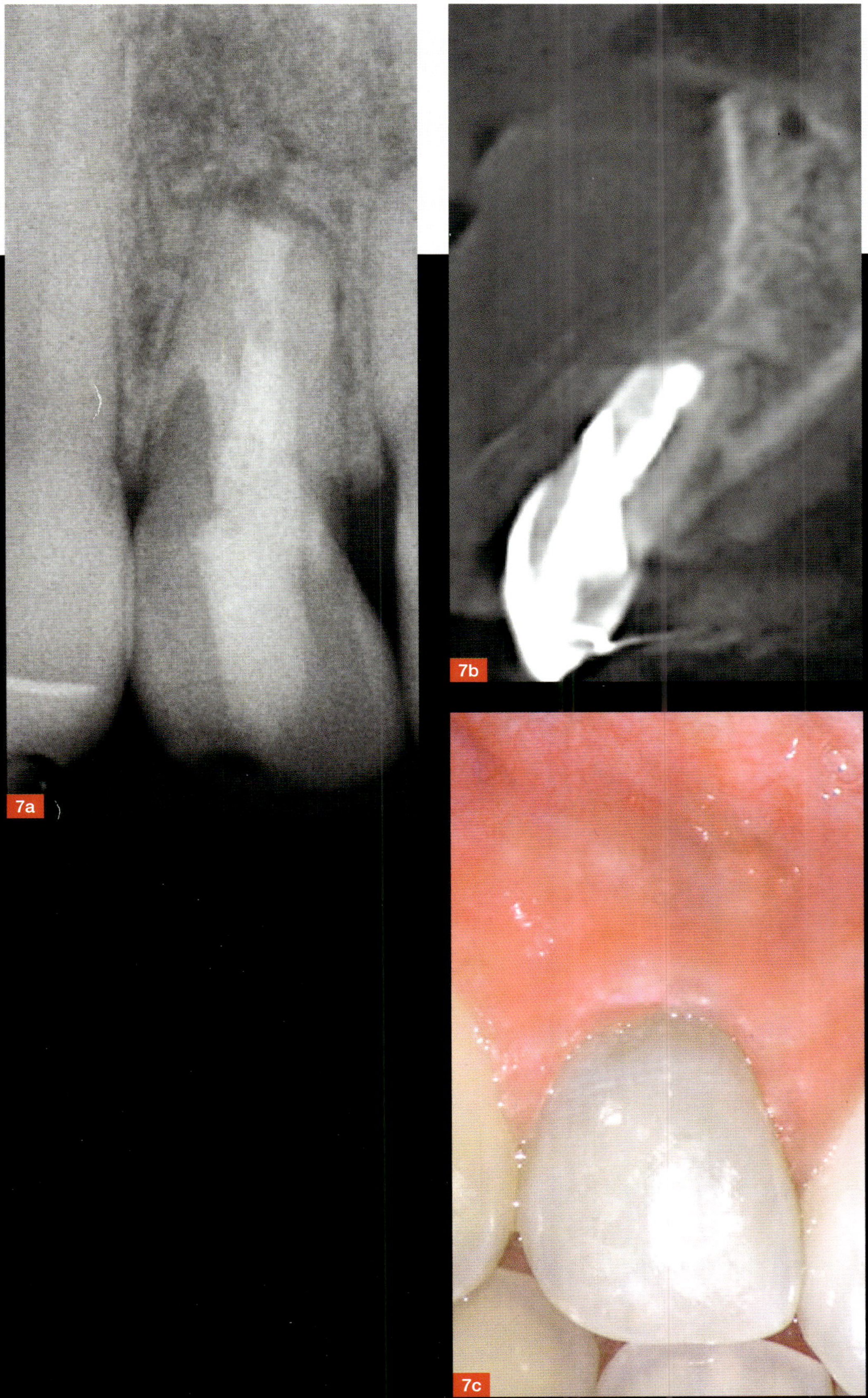

Figure 7a-c: Two- and three-dimensional images confirming the full success of the intervention. The dyschromia remains, but the cosmetic problem can be brilliantly solved at a later time.

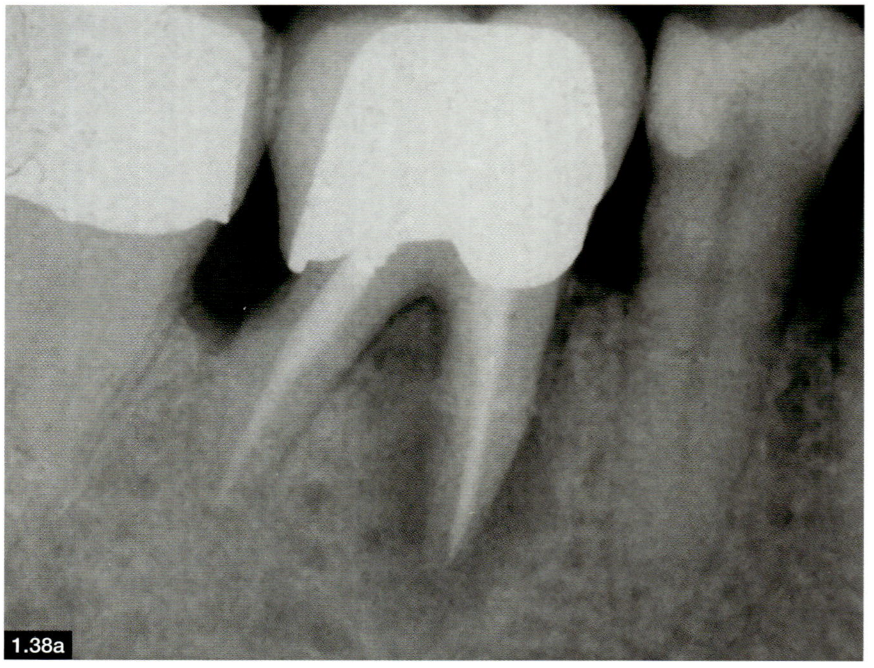

1.38a

Fig. 1.38a: Injury to the mesial root of the lower molar, in which the periapical disease developed suddenly, suggesting a concomitant root lesion.

Failures: which determinants?

Four factors are responsible for endodontic periapical diseases:

1. intraradicular infections (Fig. 1.38a-d);
2. extraradicular infections (Fig. 1.39);
3. foreign bodyreactions (Fig. 1.40);
4. cyst with cholesterol crystals (Fig. 1.41).

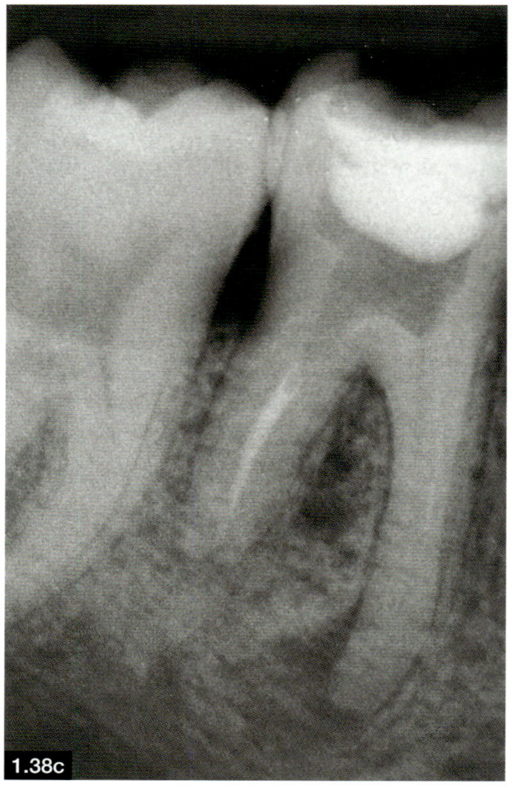

1.38c

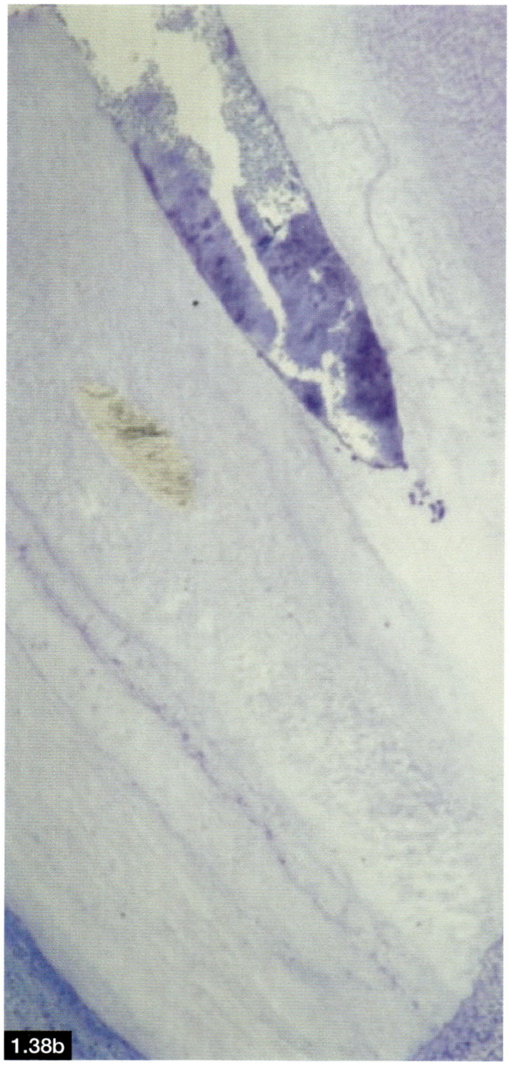

1.38b

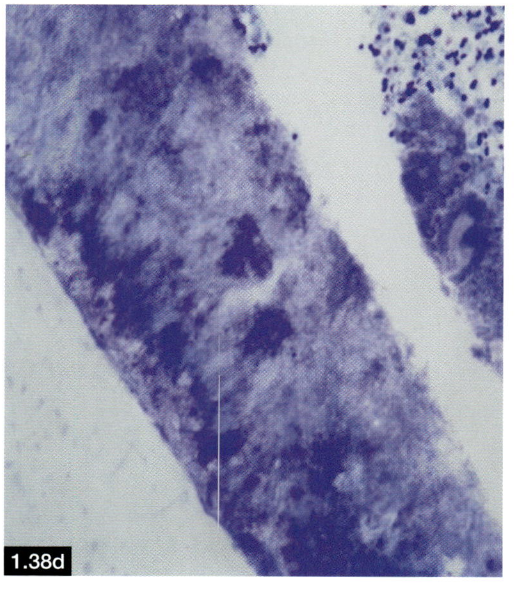

1.38d

Fig. 1.38b-d: Intracanal bacterial aggregation in the form of biofilm.

Fig. 1.38c: Lower molar with partial root canal therapy and poor coronal reconstruction: the essential prerequisite for failure of the treatment.

Considering cases 3 and 4 as marginal in percentage terms and easy to identify, practitioners must focus on the microbiological aspect, as the first two causes are, by definition, infectious. From a microbiological point of view, the bacterial colonization of the endodontic space is carried out by microorganisms organized in biofilms (Box 1.11). These entities are represented by bacterial cells immersed in an extracellular matrix that protects them from external agents and makes them extremely resistant to interventions aimed at eradicating the infection. This result is very difficult to achieve in tissues with a complex structure, such as dentin, which is rich in collagen fibers deeply embricated into the characteristic tubular structure.

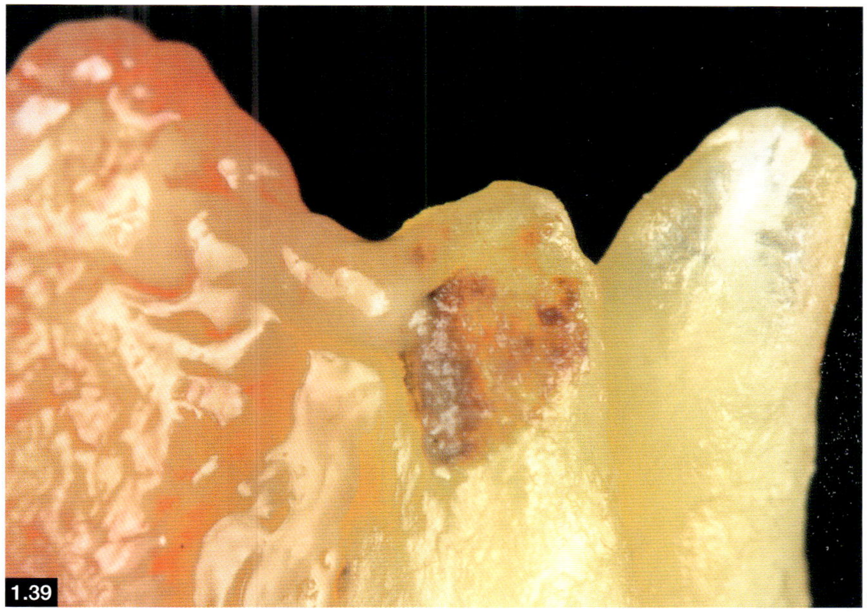

1.39

Fig. 1.39: Extraradicular calcifications exemplifying lesions generated by extraradicular infections.

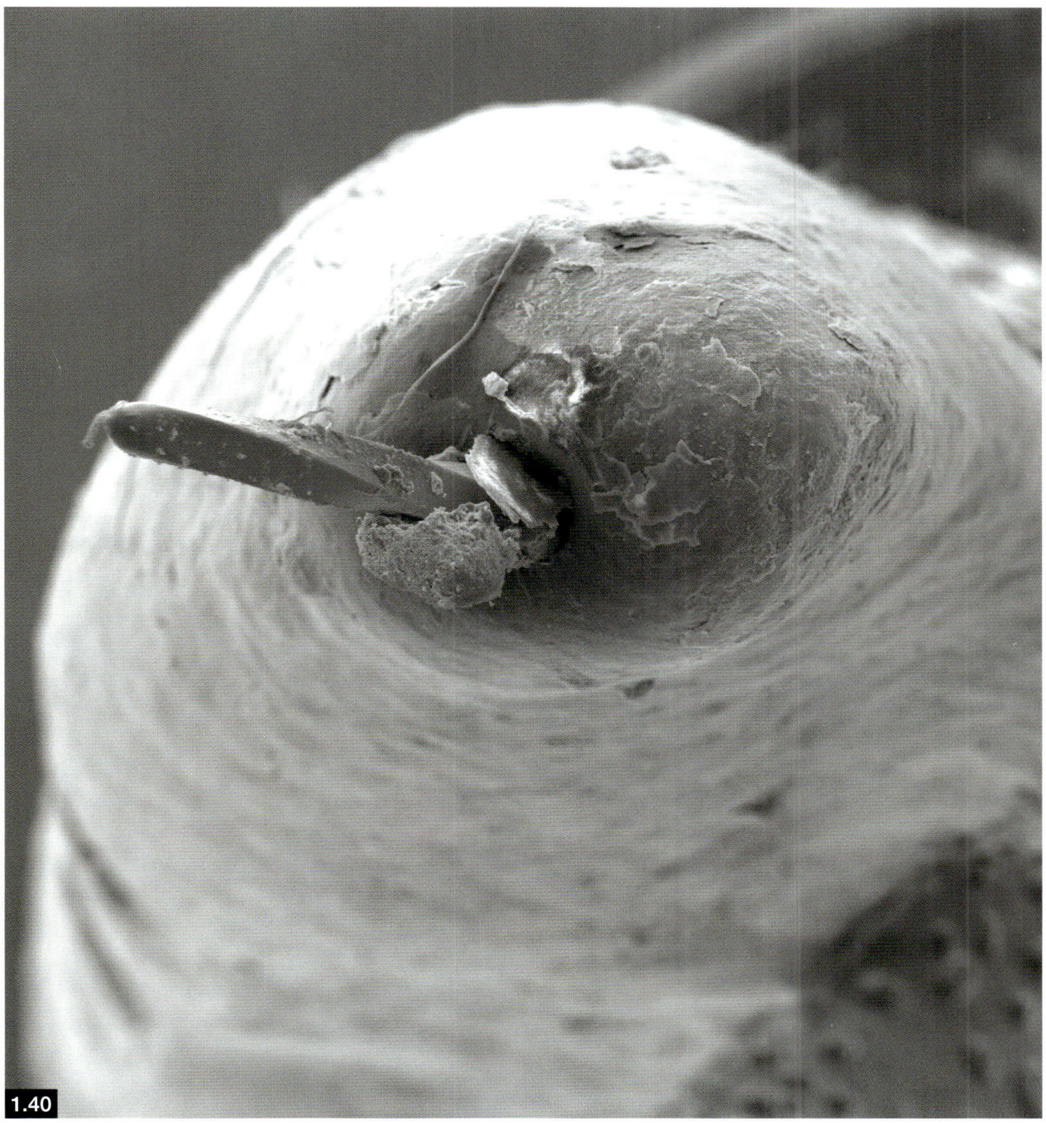

1.40

Fig. 1.40: An instrument extruded beyond the apical limit generated a foreign body granuloma and led to the avulsion of the tooth.

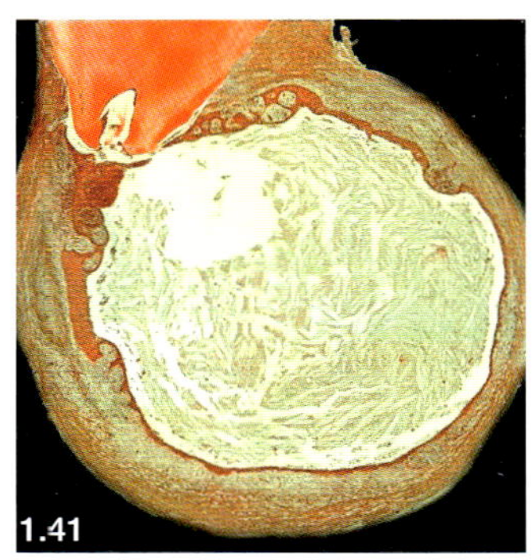

1.41

Fig. 1.41: Typical appearance of root cysts filled with cholesterol crystals.

Box 1.11 **ENDODONTIC MICROBIOLOGY**

DETERMINANTS OF PERIAPICAL DISEASE: BACTERIA

In a purely clinical context, including too much material regarding endodontic microbiology seems inappropriate given the many bacterial species are involved in this process[83].
Some studies[84] have established the need to thoroughly investigate the specific composition of the flora and its structural aspects in order to identify strategies for eliminating, limiting, and controlling the bacterial colonization of the endodontium[85].
As has been extensively demonstrated, certain bacterial species have a representative role due to their ability to withstand long periods of low nutrient availability and colonize unfavorable environments, such as previously treated root canals[86].
This aggregation leads to the formation of a biofilm, which is very difficult to violate using root canal cleansing procedures (Figs. 1.42a-e).
The endodontic space cannot be sterilized and sealed without involving the presence of bacterial cells, albeit with a far lower load.
Likewise, in many clinical situations, it is impossible to obtain a perfectly durable coronal seal.
The bacterial species involved (most of which are Gram positive) are able to grow in environments that are almost completely devoid of oxygen[87].
Yeast findings are frequent, and, according to very specific literature, viruses[88, 89] are not given adequate consideration.
The bacteria present in infections of previously treated dental elements are mainly Gram positive, and only a minority are Gram negative[90].
Peptostreptococcus and *Streptococcus* would appear to be prevalent. *Porphyromonas* is found in unsuccessfully treated canals. *Enterococcus faecali*, *S. sanguis*, *S. salivarius*, *P. endodontalis* together with *A. odontolyticus*, and *Peptostreptococcus* are present in treated and untreated teeth.
Despite the lack of universal agreement, *Enterococcus faecalis* is the most commonly observed bacterial species[91] in the endodontium of endodontically treated teeth and generates periapical distress. This process is due to the intrinsic ability of this bacterium to resist depleted nutrient supplies and to the ability to deeply colonize the dentinal tubules, thereby ensuring protection from the irrigation agents used to disinfect the root canal.

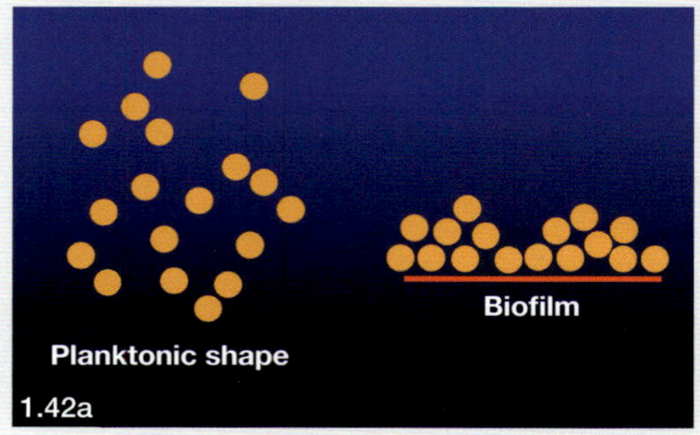

1.42a

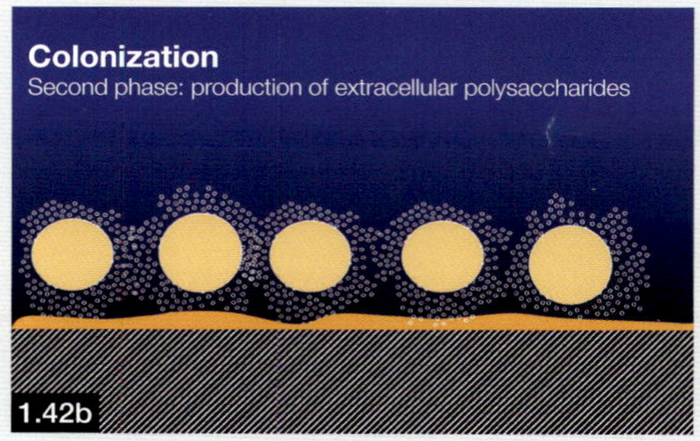

1.42b

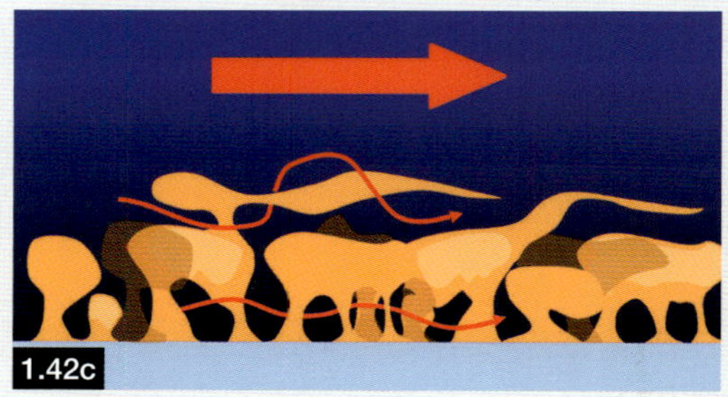
1.42c

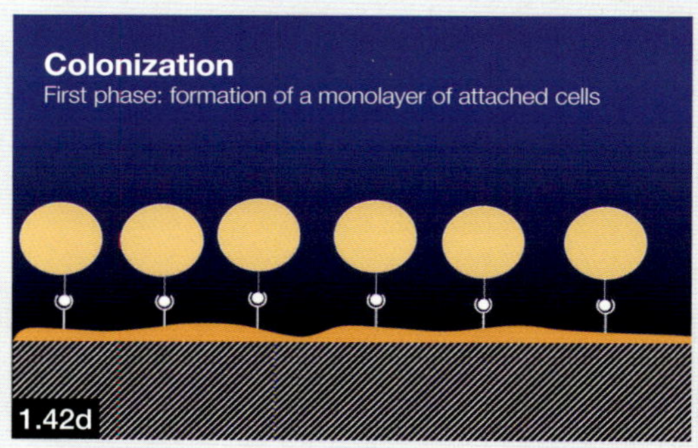

1.42d

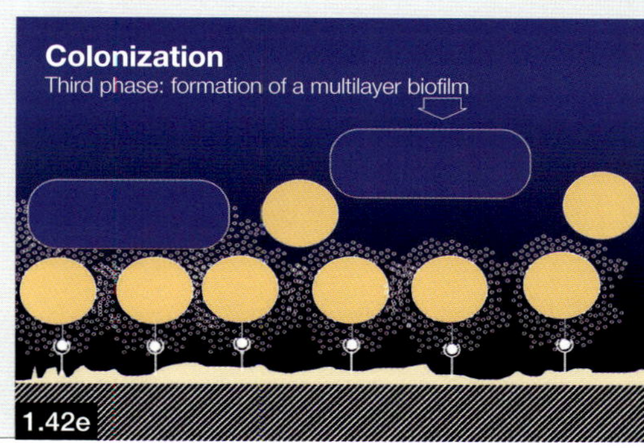

1.42e

Viruses and yeasts in periapical diseases

Although it is yet to be clarified, the presence of *Candida albicans* in teeth with previously treated periapical lesions could represent a cofactor in the development of the disease, as suggested by a number of studies reporting an association with *E. faecalis*. However, this finding is yet to be clarified. In other cases, herpes and cytomegalo viruses have been assumed to be involved in the development of acute periapical diseases secondary to failed endodontic treatments. However, their role within the pathogenetic mechanism is unclear, confirming the fact that although the evolution of periapical problems secondary to infections of endodontic origin is clear in terms of its general contours, the finer details remain somewhat hazy.

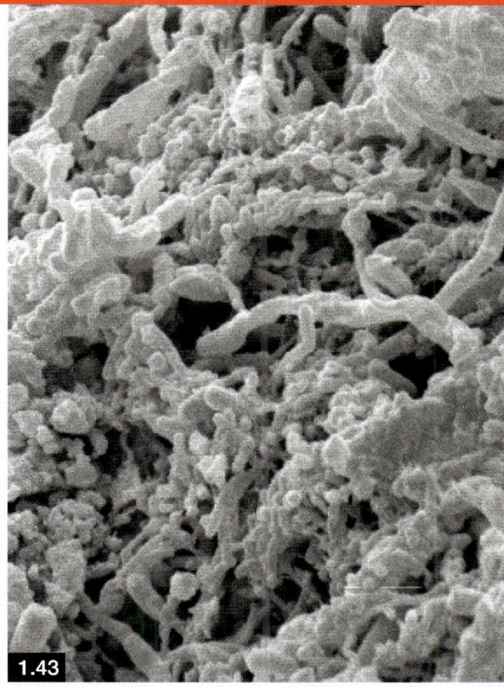

1.43

Fig. 1.43: Bacterial biofilm inside the root canal (1800x).

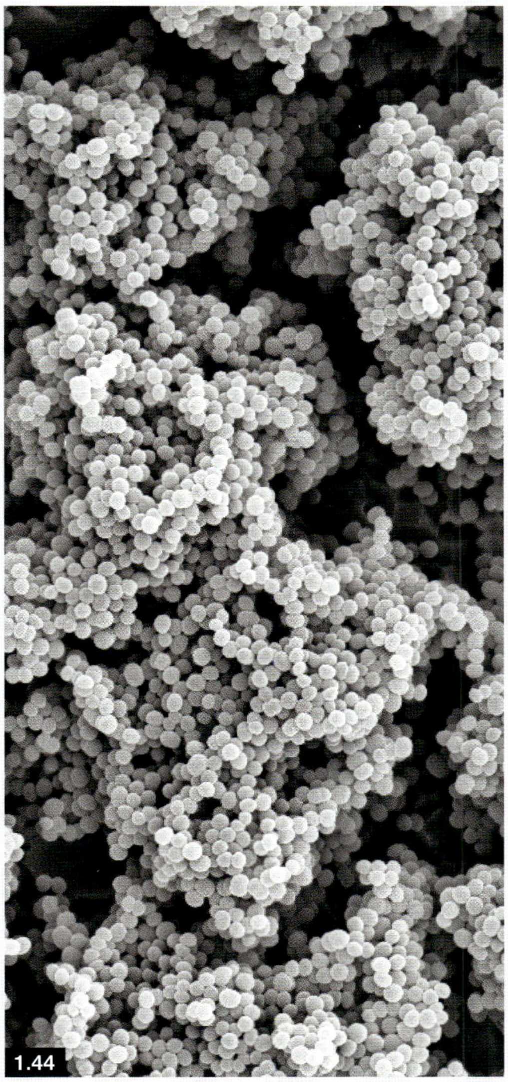

1.44

Fig. 1.44: Biofilm of *E. faecalis* in necrotic root canal (2000x).

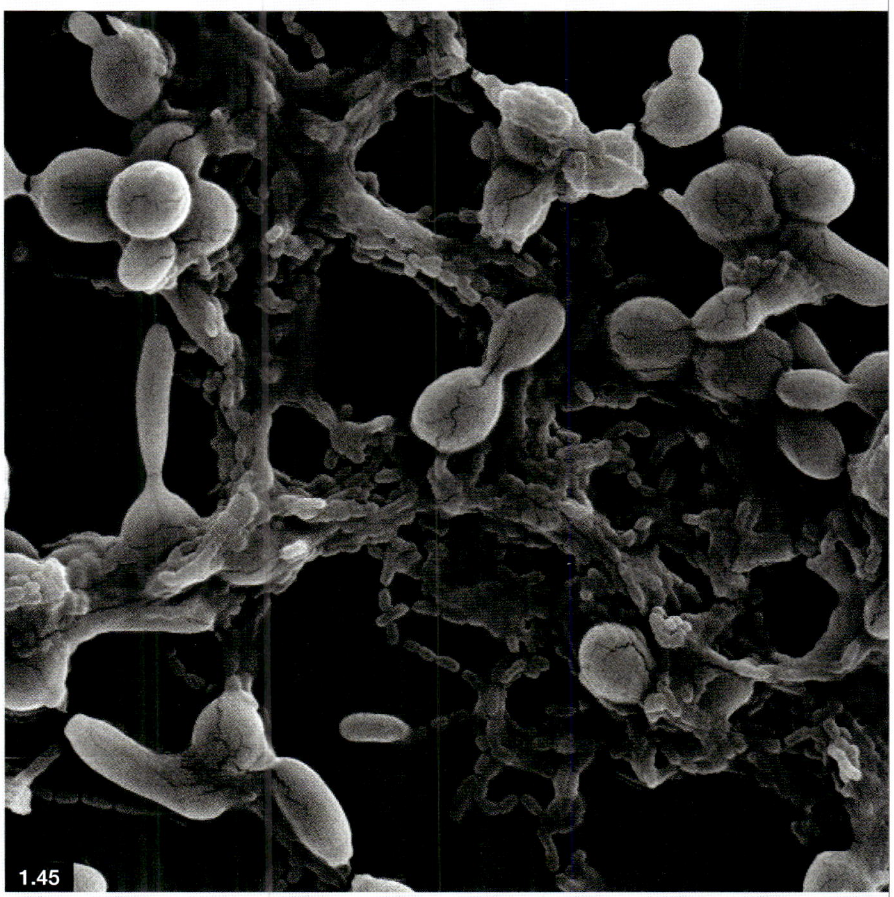

1.45

Fig. 1.45: Coaggregation of *C. albicans* and *Enterococcus faecalis* (2000x).

Extraradicular infections

Extraradicular infection, as was well described by Ricucci et al.[7, 20], deserves separate consideration.

Although the identification of an extraradicular infection can only be assumed[92], there are a number of clinical and radiological signs that suggest such involvement. One such parameter is the presence of a suppurating fistula, which is very often associated with the bacterial colonization of the apical root surface[21].

The microorganisms that are most commonly isolated in this type of infection are *Actinomyces israelii* and *P. propionicum*. These microorganisms invade the root surface and aggregate to form well-organized biofilms, making their elimination by the immune system very unlikely.

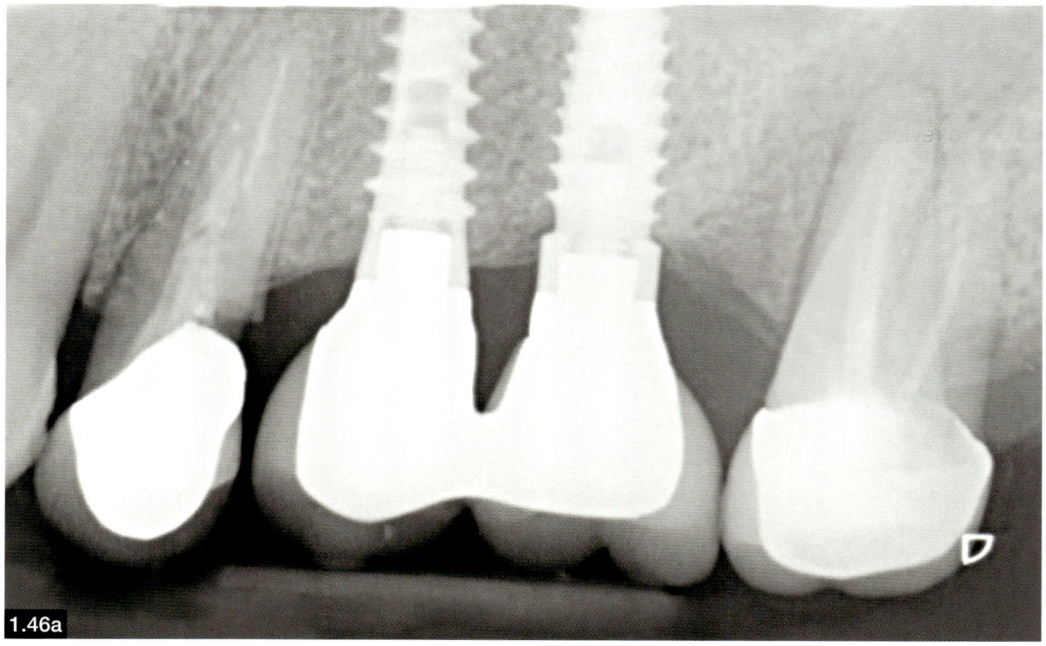

Fig. 1.46a: The second upper molar still causes pain when chewing, although the radiographic scenario is reassuring, except for a clear ectasia of the mesial canal. Subsequent periodontal evaluations lead to tooth extraction.

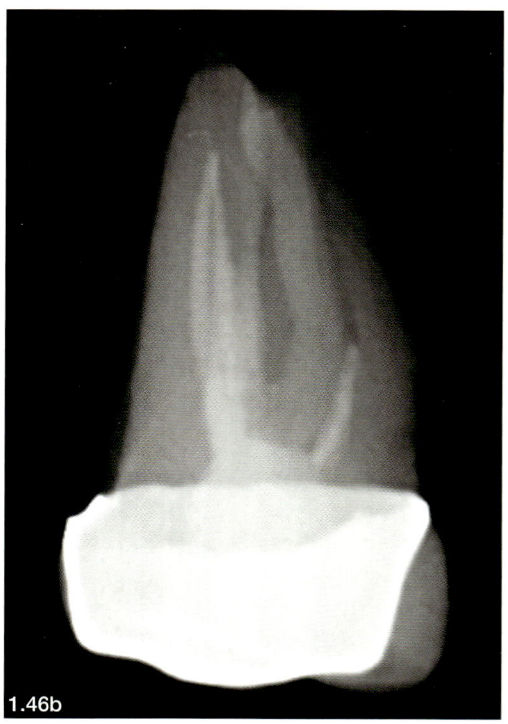

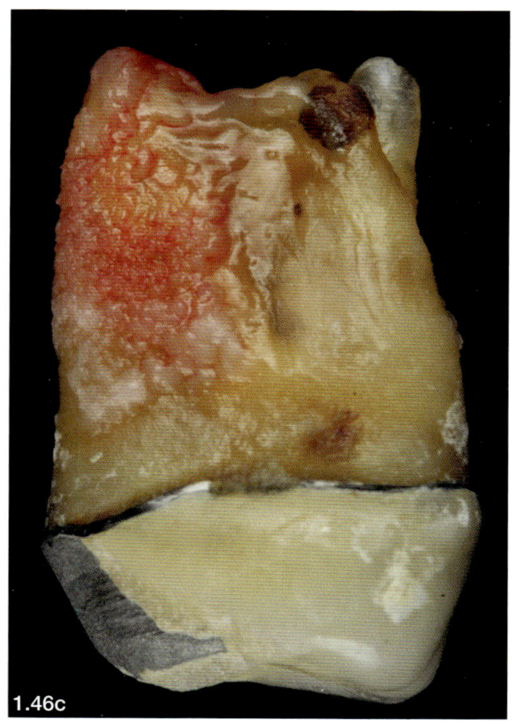

Fig. 1.46b: X-ray investigation shows an ineffective endodontium filling.

Fig. 1.46c: Anatomical finding reveals an obvious calcific aggregation on the surface of the entire root of the molar, thereby justifying the clinical scenario.

Prognosis of retreatments

The likelihood of successful retreatment depends to a large extent on the initial condition of the tooth concerned and a myriad of factors that can often not be precisely quantified.
As pointed out by Farzaneh et al.[93] and De Chevigny et al.[94], periapical health, the degree of canal filling, and the presence of transformations in canal anatomy, such as perforations, play a crucial role in the success of retreatment.
Referring to the well-consolidated systematic literature reviews conducted by Ng et al.[95-97] (Table 1.9), it can be said that the success rate of retreatment, be it judged by selective or less specific criteria, is greater than 80% of the dental elements considered.
The variables that affect the success rate are as follows:

- the presence or absence of an area of radiographic periapical radiotransparency visible on 2D x-rays;
- the size of this area, which coincides with the size of the inflamed periapical lesion;
- the extent of the canal filling, regardless of whether it respects the apical limit.

Among the cofactors, the lack of a correct coronal seal was seen to be one of the most relevant elements in this section.
Conversely, the following were seen to be elements that favored tooth survival:

- the reconstruction with a crown after treatment;
- the presence of elements that were mesial and distal to the treated tooth;
- the absence of fixed or removable prosthetic devices;
- the type of tooth, molars having the highest risk of failure.

These results are consistent with the findings of Torabinejad et al.[98], who reported a success rate of 77.8% in all the works examined.
More recently, Davies et al.[99] used CBCT as an investigation technique, i.e., an imaging method that can accurately identify inflammatory periapical lesions of endodontic origin; the results showed that the one-year success rate was approximately 93% when analyzed with normal endodontic x-rays, but dropped to 77% in cases in which CBCT was used.
He et al.[75] showed that the success rate can increase considerably when retreatment is tackled using more modern technologies, a finding that partly contradicts many epidemiological studies.
However, this last fact must make us think, as this evidence brings to light a number of non-negligible facts, not least that concerning the study in question, exist. The authors used rather lax criteria to judge the final result and the so-called complete healings at two years did not exceed 75%. This finding once again shows the difficulty in obtaining a realistic estimation of the likelihood of success that can be achieved in cases in which retreatment is performed.
In the early 2000s, Gorni and Gagliani[100] examined a sample of more than 400 retreated teeth and concluded that the success rate was around 68% (Box 1.12).
Recent studies have emphasized the prognostic value of the preoperative status of the tooth, which can be divided into two separate categories: clinical and radiographic.
With regard to the radiographic status, Kirkevang et al.[74] used a previously defined radiographic scoring system, namely the PAI (Box 1.8), and correlated its initial score with the 5-year result.

Table 1.9 **PROGNOSIS FOR ENDODONTICALLY TREATED TEETH**

Survival (years)	Percentage	95% confidence interval
2-3	86%	75-98
4-5	93%	92-94
8-10	87%	82-92

Box 1.12 **ANALYSIS OF SUCCESS IN THE RETREATMENT OF TEETH WITH DIFFERENT MORPHOLOGICAL ALTERATIONS OF TH**

In a sample of 425 patients, more than 250 molars,100 premolars and 91 front teeth were retreated. Depending on the type of retreatment, they were classified into two broad categories:

A. dental elements, in which the anatomy of the root canal was respected by the previous treatment;

B. teeth in which the previous treatment modified the structure of the endodontium.

Group A. Canal morphology respected by the previous treatment

This group, an example of which is given in case 1, includes the following categories:

A.1 APICAL CALCIFICATIONS OR STOPS

A.2 FRACTURE OF ENDODONTIC INSTRUMENTS

A.3 ROOT CANALS NOT FILLED IN TERMS OF VOLUME AND LENGTH

A.1

Apical calcifications and obliterations (stops) are most likely two sides of the same coin; indeed, they represent two canal configurations, in which the root canal is not visible as far as the radiological apex. This may be due to the closure of the canal by the root pulp of the canal lumen and the proliferation of the root cement; both are signs of a reaction to bacterial infection, which is probably mild in its virulent component, and causes a sufficient or self-limiting defensive response for itself. In such cases, disinfection and closure of the residual endodontic space, in which the microorganisms responsible for the periapical inflammatory reaction are located, may be sufficient to ensure a favorable end result.

A.2

One chapter of great interest is that regarding fractured endodontic instruments, an area that is almost always represented by dental elements, in which root canal treatment was started but had to be discontinued when the instrument broke. Consequently, the endodontic anatomy of these teeth is rarely modified because instrument fractures often occur in the early stages of the treatment.
With sophisticated systems, such as ultrasonic tips and special excavators (Chapter 3), fractured instruments can be extracted from root canals, which can be shaped in the most appropriate way.

A.3

Root canals that are inadequately filled in terms of volume and length are extremely common and constitute the majority of referred cases because they are prone to periapical disease of endodontic origin.
In these cases, shaping did not change the size and shape of the canal, because the reaming work was not adequately extensive; sub-instrumentation, as shaping that does not include the entire root canal is known, is also a finding with recently-proposed instrumentation techniques, as reported in the studies published by Peters[37]. Not infrequently in these teeth, the second canal of the mesial root of the upper molars and the middle canal of the mesial root of the lower molars are not considered in the treatment.
Lingual canals should not be overlooked in the lower incisors.

Group B.
Canal morphology not respected by the previous treatment

This second group (an example of which is given in case 2) includes the following

B.1 EXTERNAL OR INTERNAL APEX TRANSPORT

B.2 DRILLING AND/OR STRIPPING

B.3 INTERNAL ROOT RESORPTION

B.1

Canal anatomy transport is one of the major causes of endodontic treatment failure. Transport means an outwards or inwards deviation of the curvature; it is often due to an incorrect opening of the pulp chamber and insufficient reaming of the coronal third of the root canal and results in an action of the instruments at apical level that does not respect this nerve area of the root canal.
Even when flexible, endodontic instruments are unable to properly interpret the curvatures of this area and, inevitably, tend to "rest" against the outer side of the curvature, thereby shaping, at apical limit level, that side of the canal without intervening on the inner part.
This leads to the creation of an so-called "hourglass morphology", which makes mechanical cleansing ineffective, leaves debris in the inner part of the canal's curvature and creates a final shape that cannot be effectively sealed using any technique. Moreover, this type of shaping has a traumatic effect on the periapical tissues.

B.2

Drilling and stripping are two events of iatrogenic origin caused by incorrect canal maneuvers inside the root canal that lead to undesirable endoparodontal communications.
There is an evident alteration in the anatomy of the root canal, whose perforation, as clearly illustrated in Chapter 7, may occur at various levels within the canal.

B.3

Apical root resorption is a common finding in teeth with severe periapical disease (clinical case 8, page 54); in other cases, chronic pulp disease has resulted in an uneven enlargement of the root canal to create a space in the middle of the canal itself (Chapter 2, clinical case 8).

Conclusion

Once these subdivisions had been established, all cases were subjected to orthograde treatment. The results are summarized in Table 1.10. The best results were found in dental elements with unaltered canal morphology and without radiologically visible periapical lesions. In general terms, the best results were obtained in teeth with preserved root canal morphology, with a successful rate close to 90% in group A and with a consistent difference from that obtained in teeth attributed to group B.

Gorni F & Gagliani The Outcome of Endodontic Retreatment: A 2-yr Follow-up; Journal of Endodontics 2004;30(1):1-4.

Table 1.10 **CASE STUDY PROPOSED BY GORNI AND GAGLIANI**

	Controlled patients	Mean age	Males	Females	Teeth included in the study	Duration of follow-up	
	425	40.5 (11.6)	211	214	452	24 months	
		No. of teeth	**Healed**	**Recovering**	**Failures**	**Success rate**	**Failure rate**
Teeth with preserved root canal morphology	Undamaged	83	76	0	7	91.6	8.4
	Damaged	167	136	4	27	83.8	16.2
Teeth with unrestored root canal morphology	Undamaged	32	27	0	5	84.4	15.6
	Damaged	170	56	12	102	40	60

Source: Gorni e Gagliani, 2004.

CASE REPORT 7

Retreatment on a tooth with preserved canal anatomy

The lower molar being retreated has an almost normal anatomy; following the fracture of an instrument in both the mesial and distal roots, the clinician referred the case to a specialist.

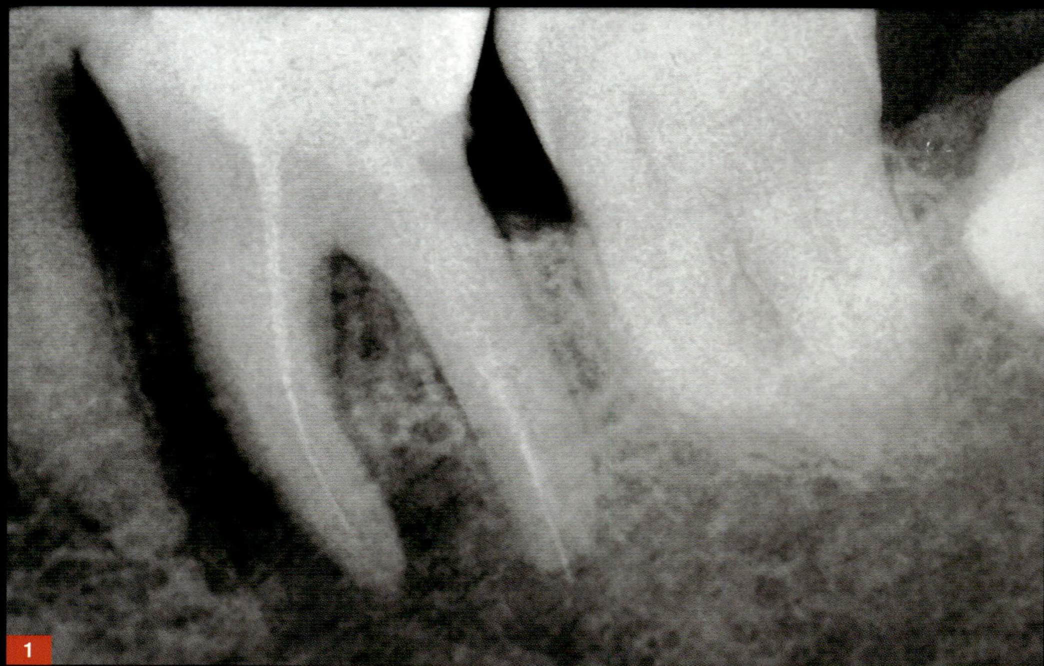

Figure 1: Initial situation.

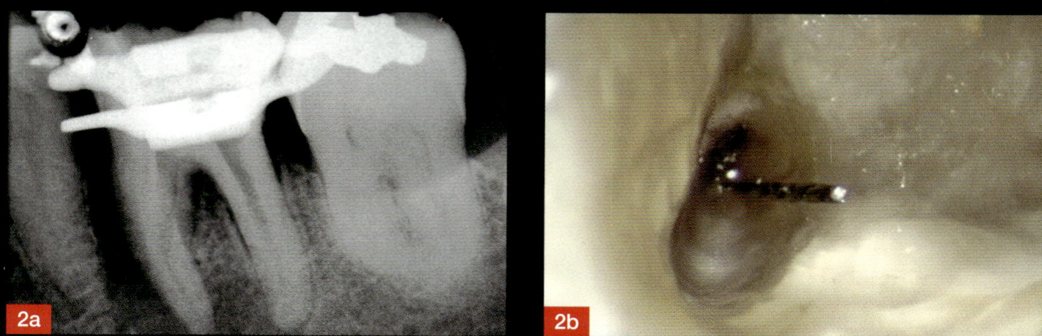

Figure 2a-b: Opening and extraction of instruments using ultrasonic tips and a surgical microscope.

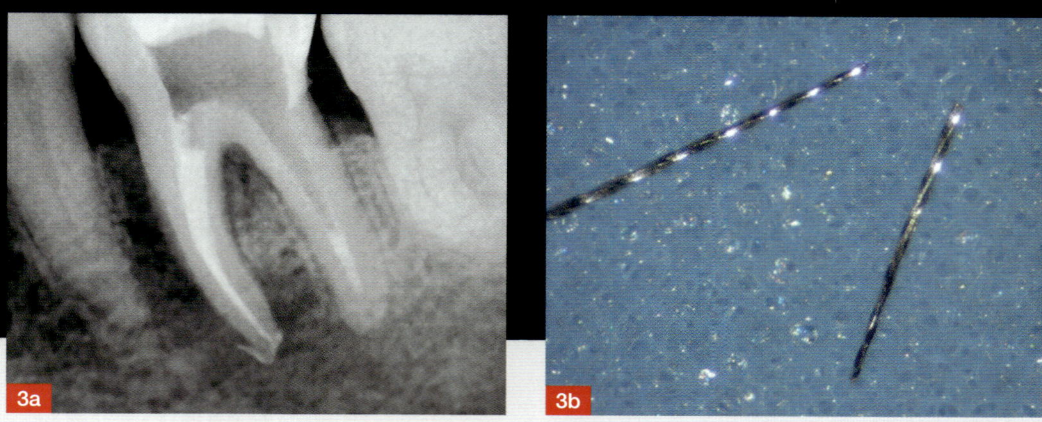

Figure 3a-b: The two broken instruments were extracted and the canal was closed with an apical cap in MTA on the distal root.

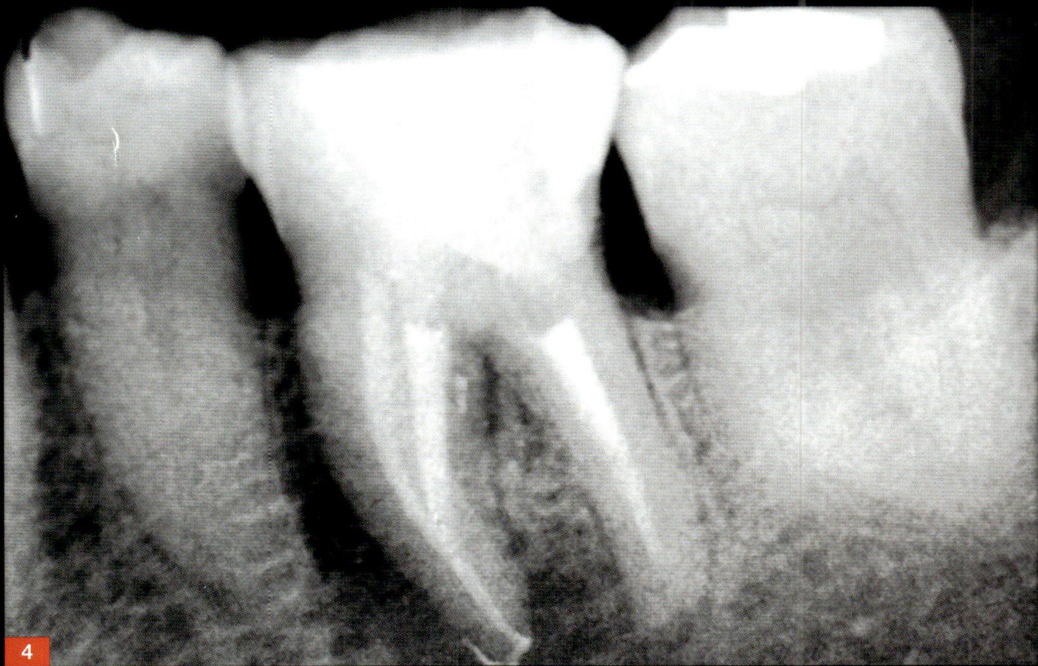

Figure 4: Case completed.

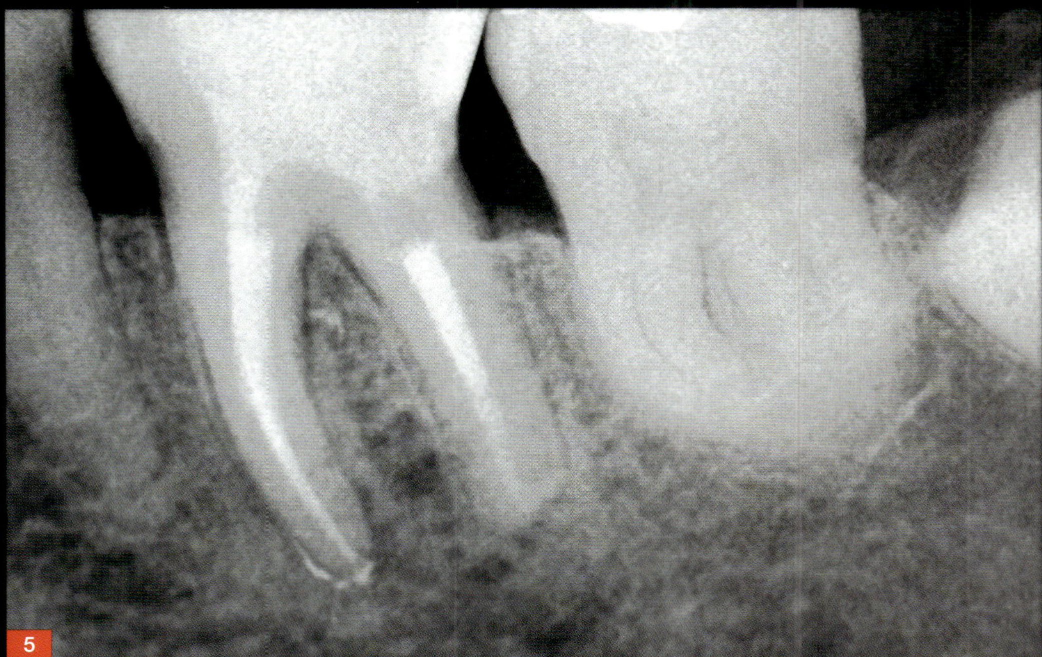

Figure 5: Follow-up at 1 year.

CASE REPORT 8

Retreatment of a tooth with unpreserved root canal anatomy

The anatomy of the lower molar being retreated is greatly altered; the apical lesion is very large and the clinically detectable fistulous path provides another reason to proceed with retreatment. Although the retreatment was performed despite the poorly preserved anatomy of the root canal, unfortunately, it did not show good results at subsequent follow-up.

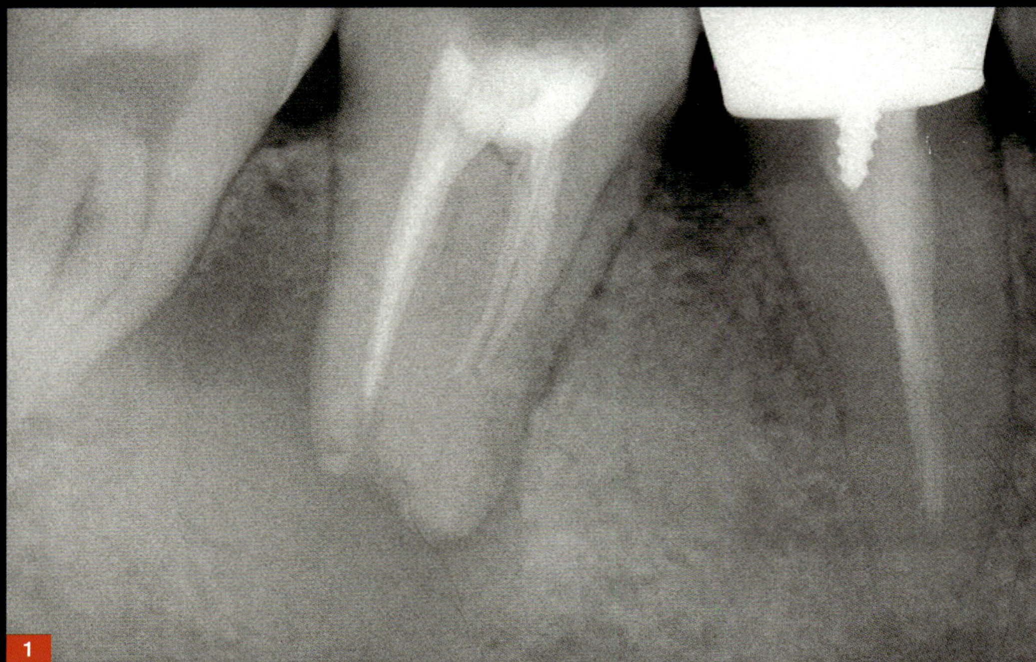

Figure 1: The initial situation. Note the extent of periapical radiotransparency and the inconsistency of the canal filling.

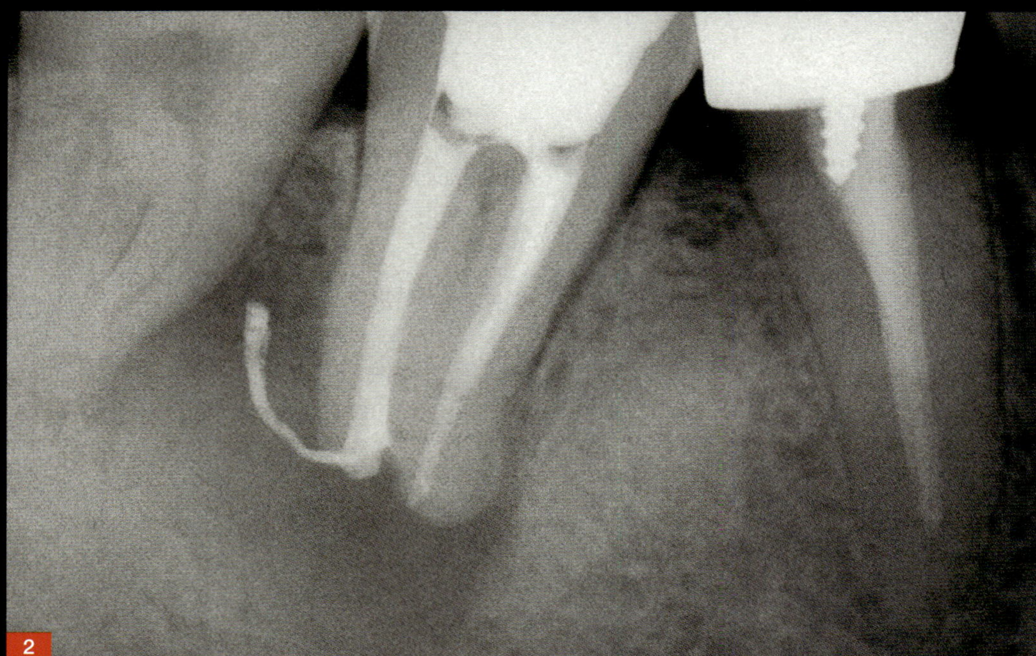

Figure 2: The filling, due to a large erosion of the distal root apex, is not perfectly contained within the endodontium.

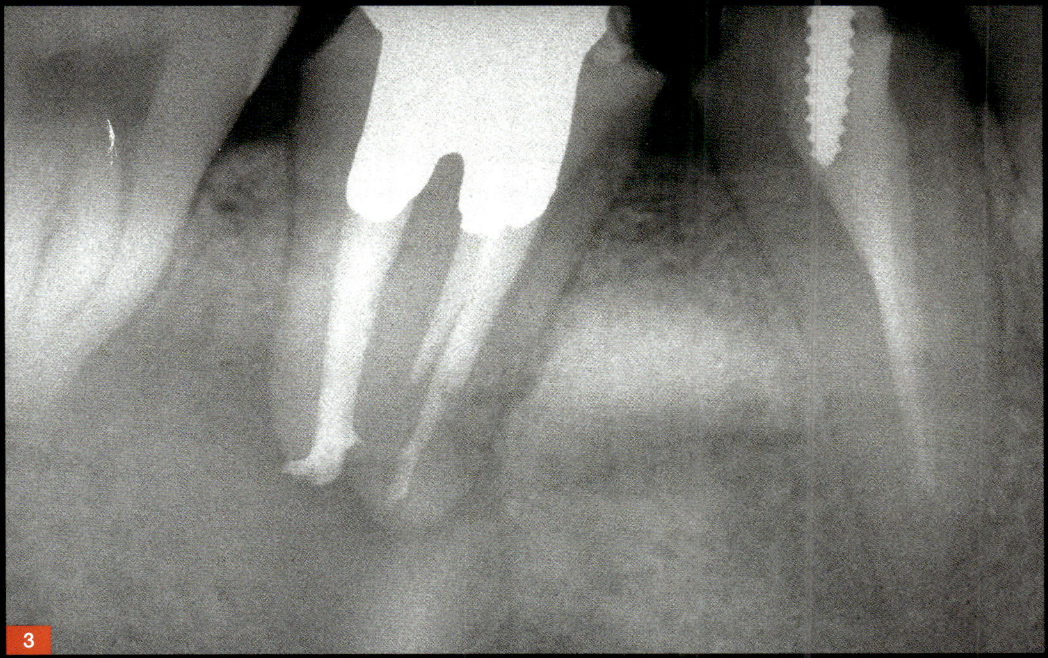

3

Figure 3: At 6 months, although the excess cement has been reabsorbed, the lesion remains.

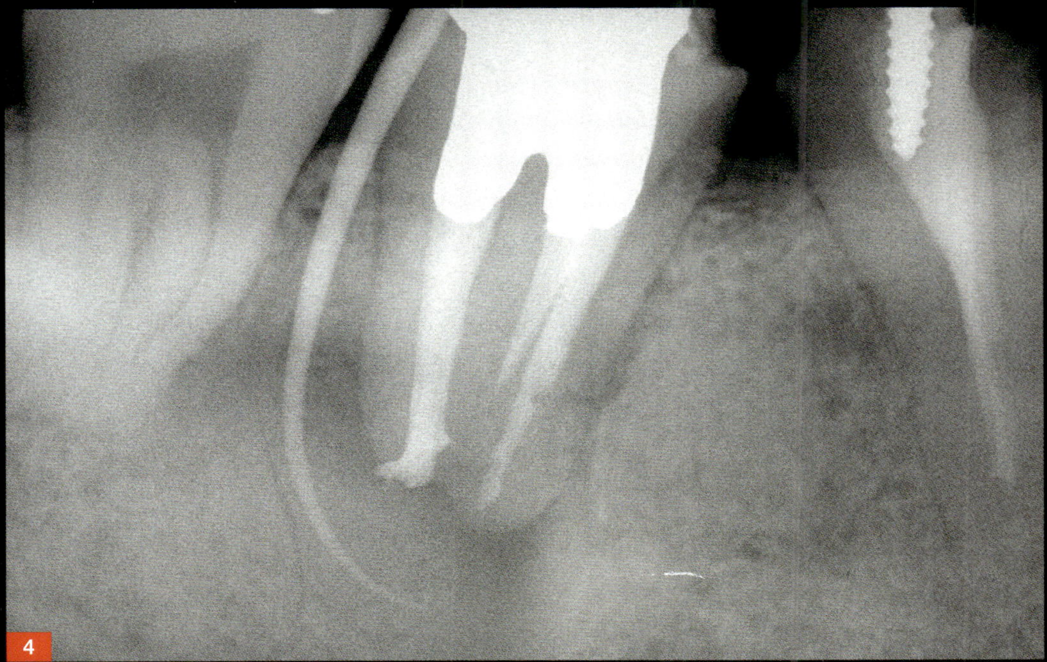

4

Figure 4: One year later, the appearance of a supportive fistula leads us to consider this case as a failure; the case is referred for endodontic surgery.

On the basis of the findings on 143 patients, the authors concluded that each initial PAI score could result in a largely corresponding PAI score at the end of the 5-years observation period; i.e., a given initial score was prognostically more or less favorable.
From a clinical point of view, Al-Nuaimi et al.[101, 102] analyzed 137 posterior teeth using CBCT to accurately assess the extent of the periapical problem, as well as intraoral scanners to quantify the volume of the residual dental crown; they concluded that a residual dental structure of less than 30% was a highly unfavorable prognostic factor for retreatment success.
The success rates 1 year after the treatment were 82% with CBCT imaging and 88% with two-dimensional x-rays, confirming that the latter tends to overestimate healing.
As highlighted by the excellent study conducted by Ricucci et al.[7, 103], the presence of suppurative fistulae suggests the presence of extraradicular bacterial arborescence, which is difficult to control with normal orthograde retreatment procedures.
Fonzar et al.[104] performed a study on almost 500 patients (a total of 1175 teeth) treated by a group of highly qualified specialists; a 10-year success rate of 94% was observed for retreatment, equivalent to approximately 40% of the sample examined.
Preoperative symptoms and the presence of a considerable radiologically-evident lesion emerged as the two main factors for failure. In a 5-year cohort study conducted in Korea, a success rate of 88.4% was observed for retreatment, whereas the treatment outcome in previously untreated teeth was 90.8%. (H) Pirani et al. (I) used a different filling technique and achieved a slightly lower rate.
To conclude, the success rate is – according to the data discussed above – approximately 80% and the influencing factors are the degree of involvement of the periapical tissue, followed by canal morphology and the entity of the residual crown. Seen with a broader treatment perspective, this percentage can be increased by adopting the endodontic surgery solution.
A combination of the two therapeutic techniques, which are closely related to the skill of the operator (see below), will lead to excellent results.

Fig. 1.47: Upper molar with endodontic treatment that seems to be correct in the two vestibular roots but has a different conicity in the palatine root. In such cases, frank symptoms can lead to retreatment; otherwise, the watchful waiting is the best choice.

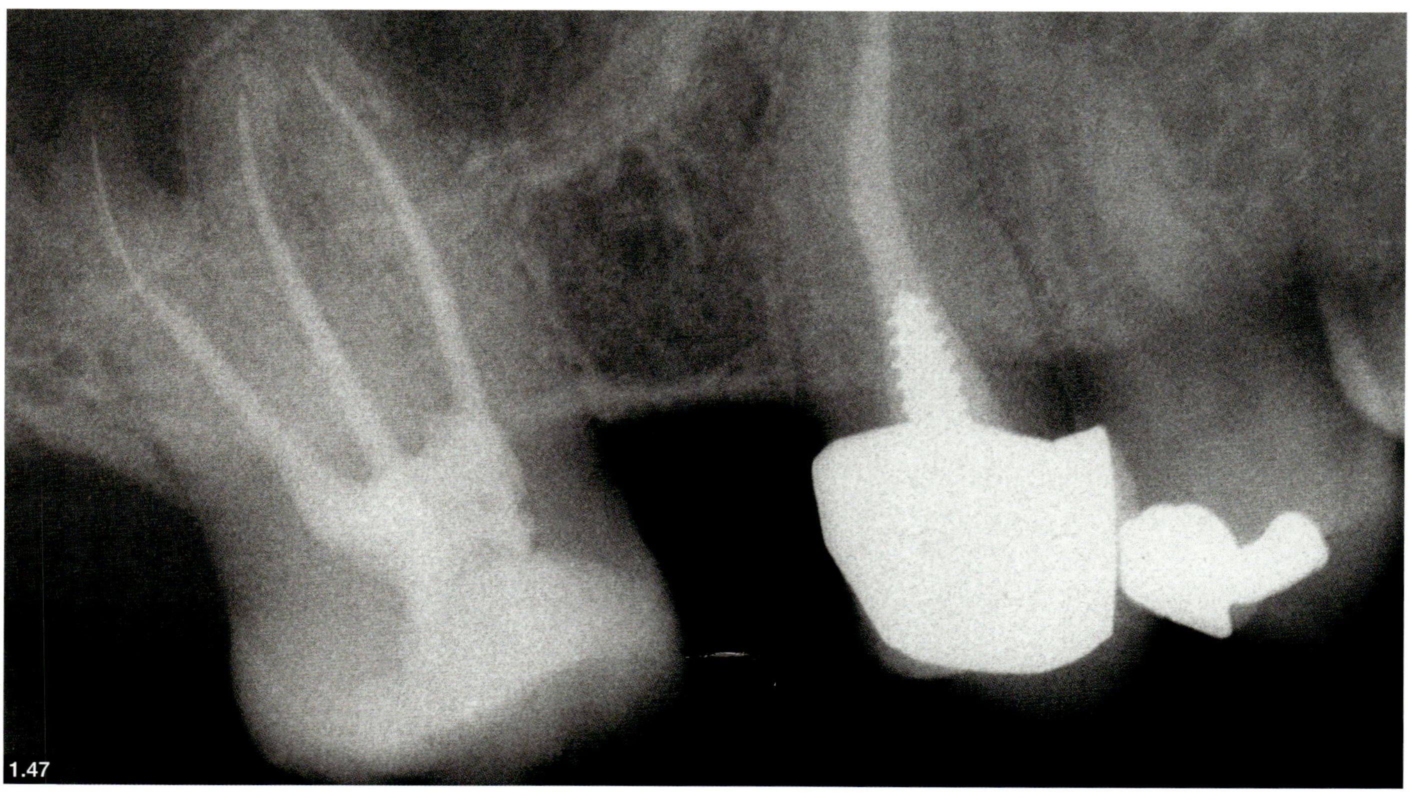

1.47

Why to perform or not perform a retreatment: Preliminary considerations

The discovery of endocontic periapical disease is often an incidental finding. This issue is far from irrelevant, particularly when we consider that the finding of asymptomatic disease that may or may not generate local or systemic disease presents the clinician with the dilemma of whether or not to perform retreatment.

As pointed out by Wesselink[105], it is not uncommon for an endodontical x-ray or an orthopantomographic x-ray – for reasons others than those for which the patient was referred – to present a radiolucent area near a root apex of a previously treated tooth. As indicated in the behavior patterns (page 64), the main factor on which retreatment decision-making is based is a negative transformation of the lesion. In the study conducted by Yu et al.[69], less than 6% of the lesions

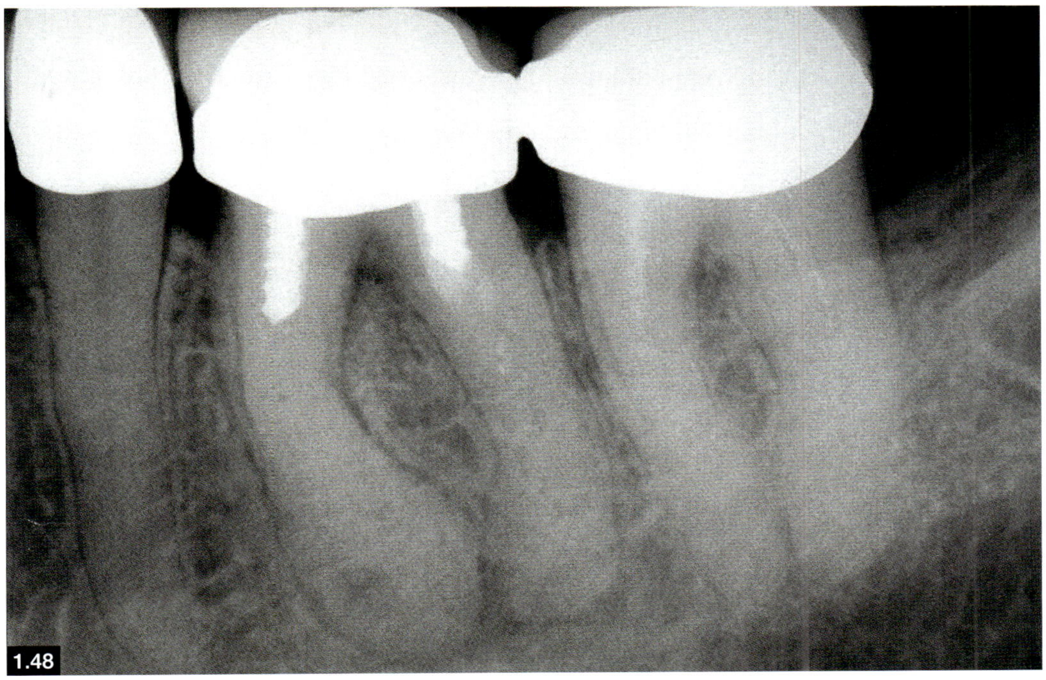

1.48

Fig. 1.48: Typical case of a self-limiting periapical reaction, caused by an enormous proliferation of root cement; the canal lumens are obliterated. Retreatment is strongly discouraged.

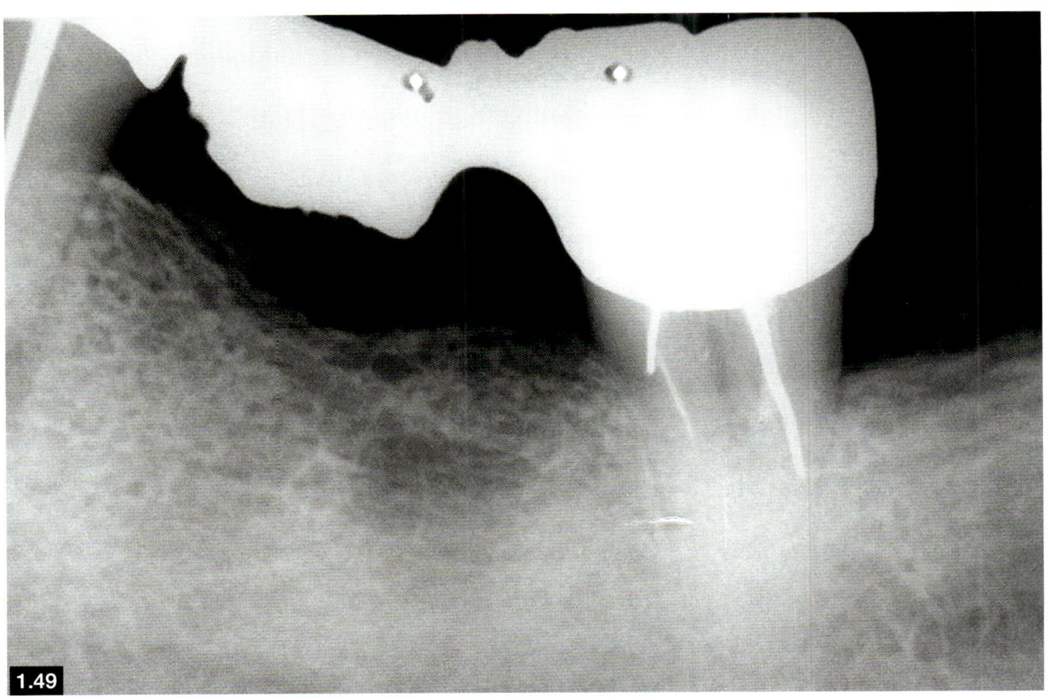

1.49

Fig. 1.49: Similar case with a treatment that did not cause a periapical lesion but that totally occluded the canal lumen: retreatment would be impossible.

Fig. 1.50a: Inappropriate endodontic treatment at the expense of tooth 16 and a frank periapical lesion on tooth 15 determine the need for endodontic surgery.

Fig. 1.50b: Reconstructions that ineffective in terms of sealing and are worn.

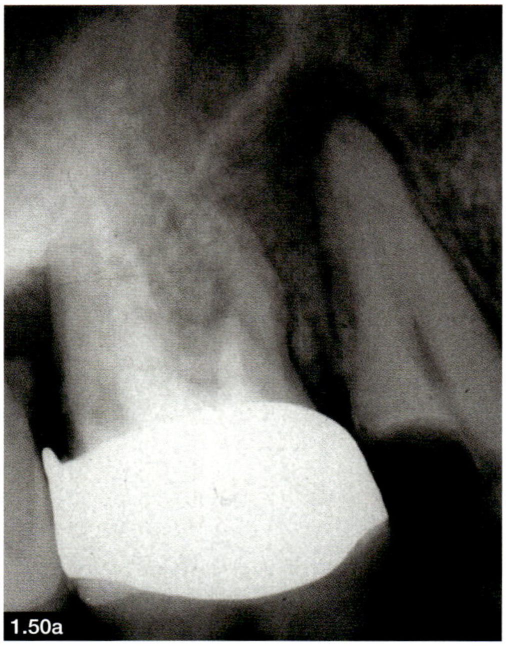

1.50a

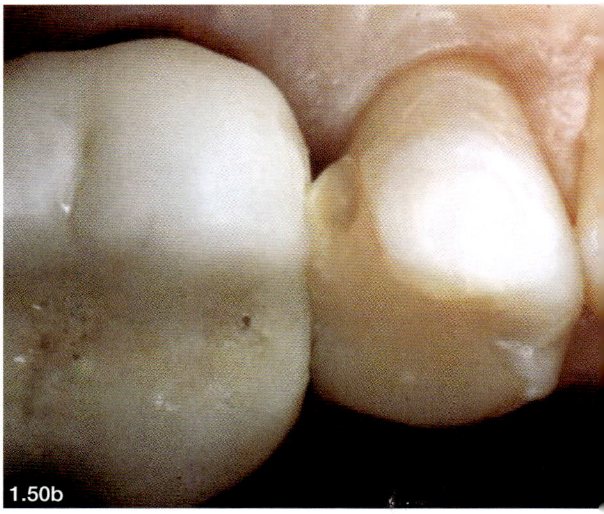

1.50b

Fig. 1.51a: Two reconstructions made of ceramic-metallic material.

Fig. 1.51b: After 6 months, the treatment of tooth 15 had already achieved the expected result, whereas tooth 16 was examined but was not considered to be retreatable.

Fig. 1.52a: Follow-up x-ray after 22 years, confirming the appropriateness of the therapeutic choice, that is, watchful waiting on the tooth 16 and intervention on tooth 15.

Fig. 1.52b: Same images from different angles.

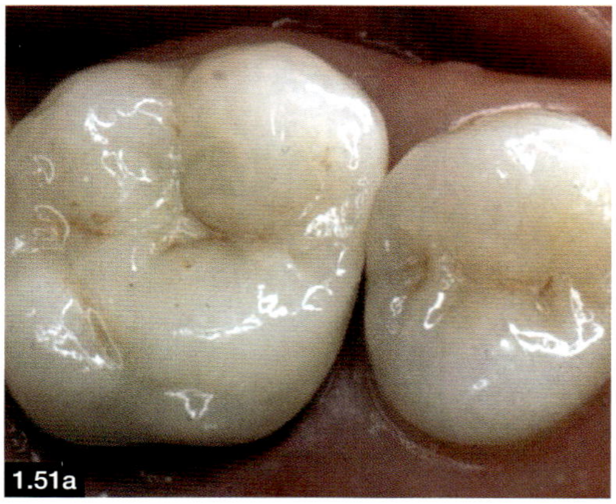

1.51a

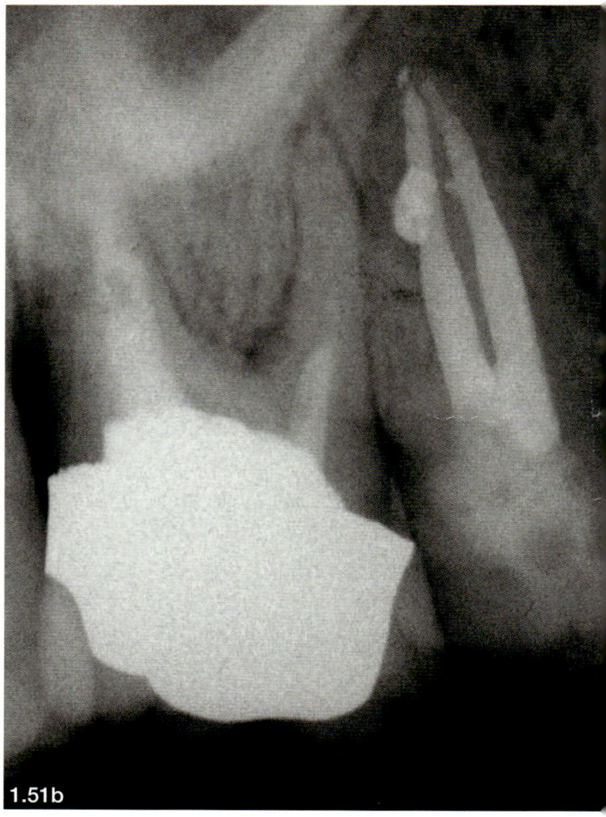

1.51b

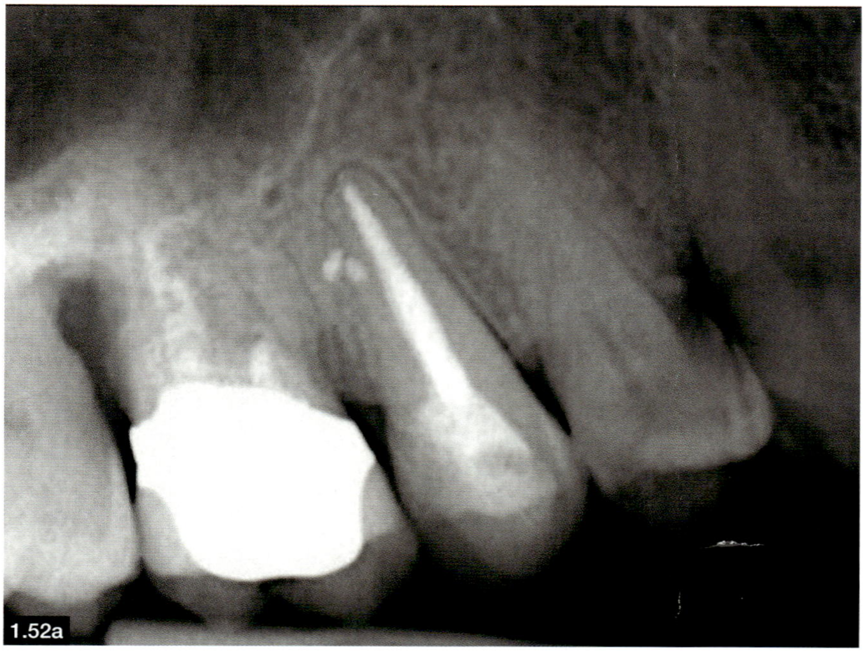

1.52a

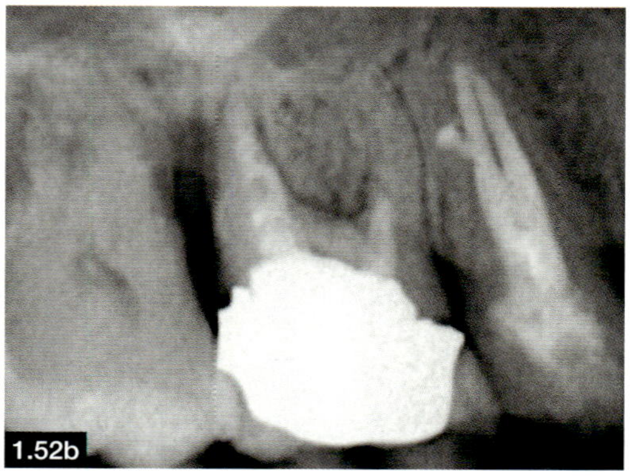

1.52b

over a 20-year period, become more acute, i.e., they cause significant infection that requires an emergency dental and stomatological procedure. However, almost one in two teeth present pain over the same period, without impacting the patient's quality of life. It was therefore decided to deal with this topic in a separate chapter because, although it refers to other procedures already described or to others described later, this allows us to make a number of specific considerations. Some of these have been taken from contributions from literature that we consider worthy of note; one

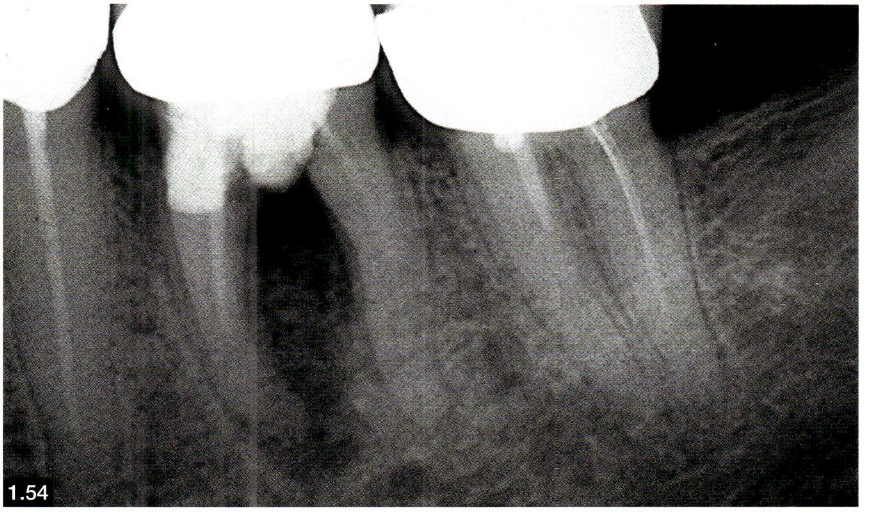

1.54

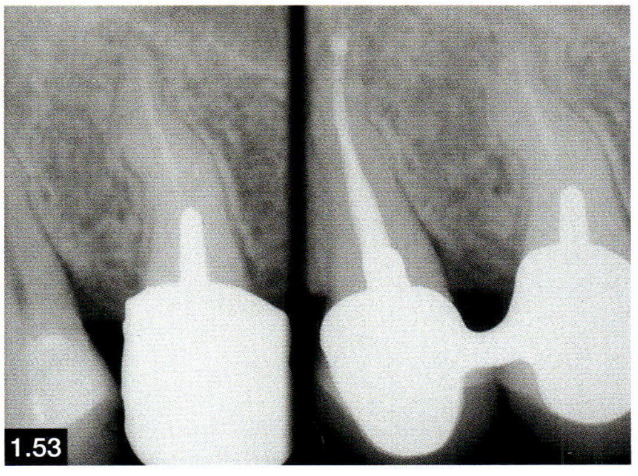

1.53

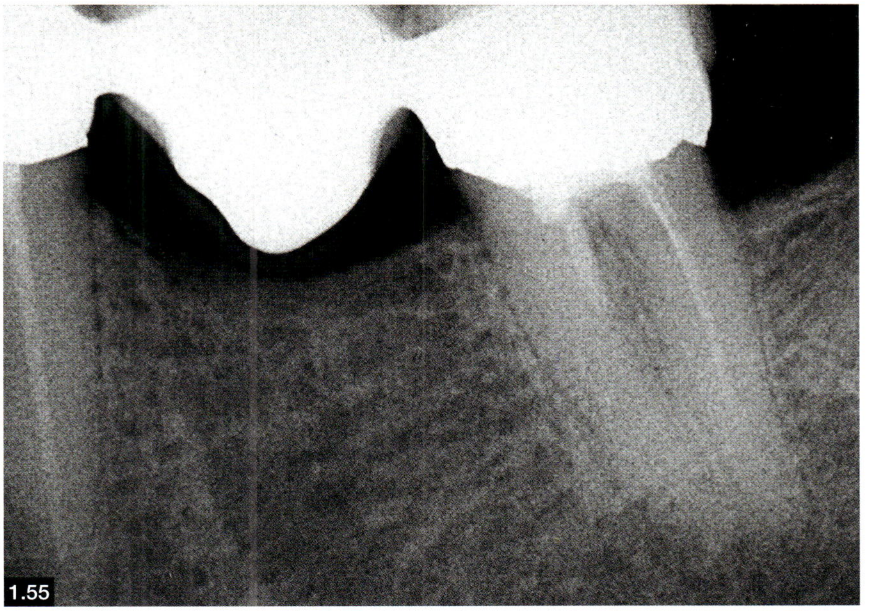

1.55

non-negligible aspect is that relating to costs. A study conducted by Schwendicke & Stolpe[106], focuses on the economic aspect that this kind of consideration involves. The authors used an economic model employed in healthcare cost-effectiveness analyses to evaluate the various types of retreatment; they compared all these settings (reconstruction with filling, with a prosthetic crown or with a root canal post and a prosthetic crown) by simulating the results that could be obtained without retreatment and after performing the retreatment. The complications and problems were classified according to data available in the literature, and the results at a distance were recorded. The results of the study would appear to be discouraging, as performing a reconstruction on a failed root canal treatment even in the presence of a periapical lesion, in the absence of clinical symptoms, causes - from an economic point of view - far fewer problems than would have to be faced if it were decided to perform a retreatment before performing a restoration or a direct filling. Although it is not entirely satisfactory, as it is based on a virtual simulation that does not consider natural circumstances, such as poor root canal treatment associated with a periapical radiographic lesion; the study deserves great consideration because it deals with an aspect of clinical practice that is particularly relevant today. This aspect, which textbooks and literature in general often mystify, can represent a significant decision-making factor, not only for the patient but also for the dentist: the cost of managing the inconveniences generated by complications typical of retreatment.

Fig. 1.53: Premolar with a complicated canal anatomy kept under observation (second follow-up at 5 years); retreatment would be poorly indicated given the operational complexity.

Fig. 1.54: Lost tooth leads to the decision of extraction; the neighboring teeth, although not well treated were not retreated.

Fig. 1.55: Follow-up at 5 years, confirming the validity of the choice.

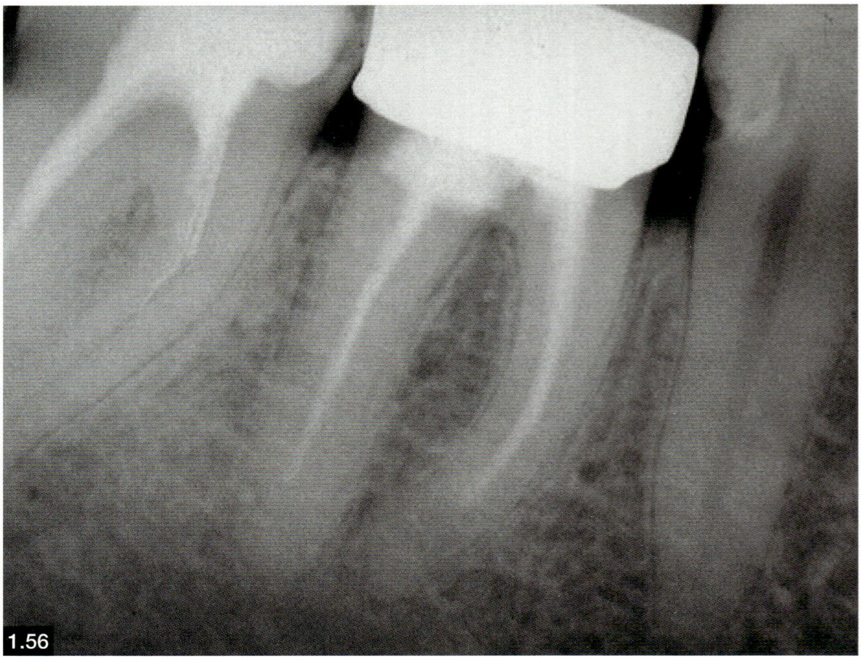

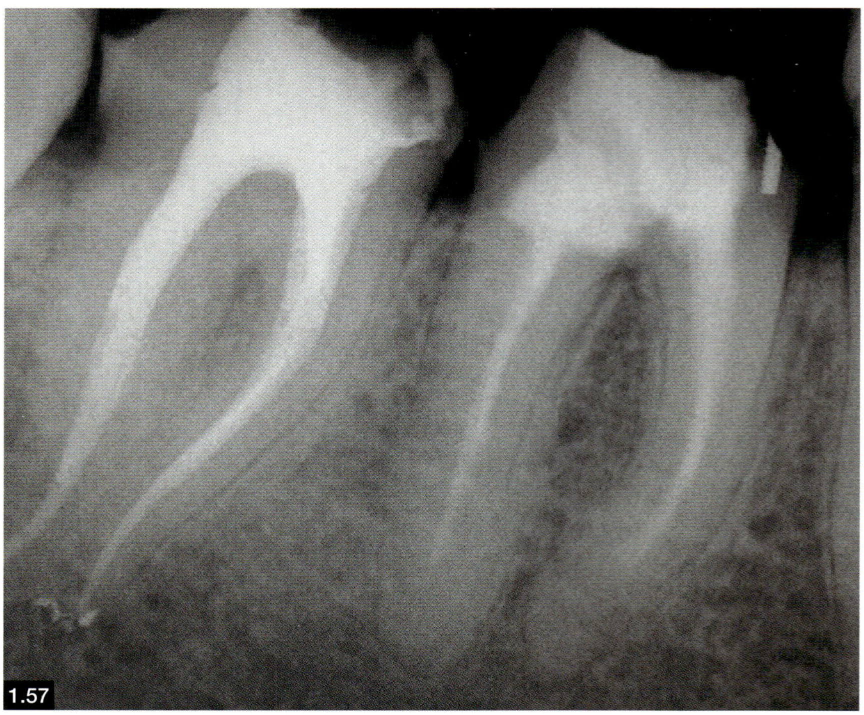

Figs. 1.56-1.57: Pair of lower molars with an inappropriate treatment. In 47, the vision of the root canal beyond the previous filling suggests an easier retreatment; on the other hand, 46 is characterized by the obliteration of the remaining part of the canal, which advises against retreatment.

Endodontic periapical diseases could affect the general health of patients and, therefore, any further reasoning in this regard would largely take second place.
However, the economic aspect also emphasizes on the treatment alternatives, i.e., endodontic surgery extraction, and implants, even if it is granted that the "wait and see" approach is the best solution provided there is no clear evidence that periapical disease can play a very different role to that currently attributed to them.
Therefore, at the preliminary examination, purely as a learning exercise, we considered it useful to explore all the alternatives that treatment decision-making may present not only for the dentist, but also for the patient.
Tifooni et al. (x) proposed a more sophisticated prognostic index, which supported the idea that a score-based decision-making process might be useful in predicting favorable or negative outcomes.
To conclude, we believe that providing the patient with full knowledge of the facts is a further aspect required to foster a solid bond of trust, the essential basis for establishing a relationship that refers to the "therapeutic alliance," of which there is much talk but which, in situations like this, is often relegated to a few words that only regard the practitioners' duties toward their patients.
The patient should be informed that an infection, albeit asymptomatic, has been found. Intervention is required for the reasons described above, but it is equally true that non-intervention can be the solution in certain cases. The costs of the therapy will not be negligible, because of the need for further reconstructions.
Complications may arise, and, whilst they are almost always manageable, they are still unpleasant. Undesirable alternatives, such as extraction, should not be overlooked, although this should be seen as an extreme solution. One possible alternative is watchful waiting, or identifying the most appropriate time for intervention, when it is required, such as when it is necessary to replace an obsolete restoration or provide more extensive rehabilitation. The main risk associated with waiting is that of a violent exacerbation, which often makes it impossible to carry out a retreatment and calls for solutions that are more radical and destructive and involves the need for more expensive rehabilitation. It is important to remember that intervening with reconstructive or prosthetic solutions on a previously-treated tooth involves the assumption of full responsibility by the last operator.

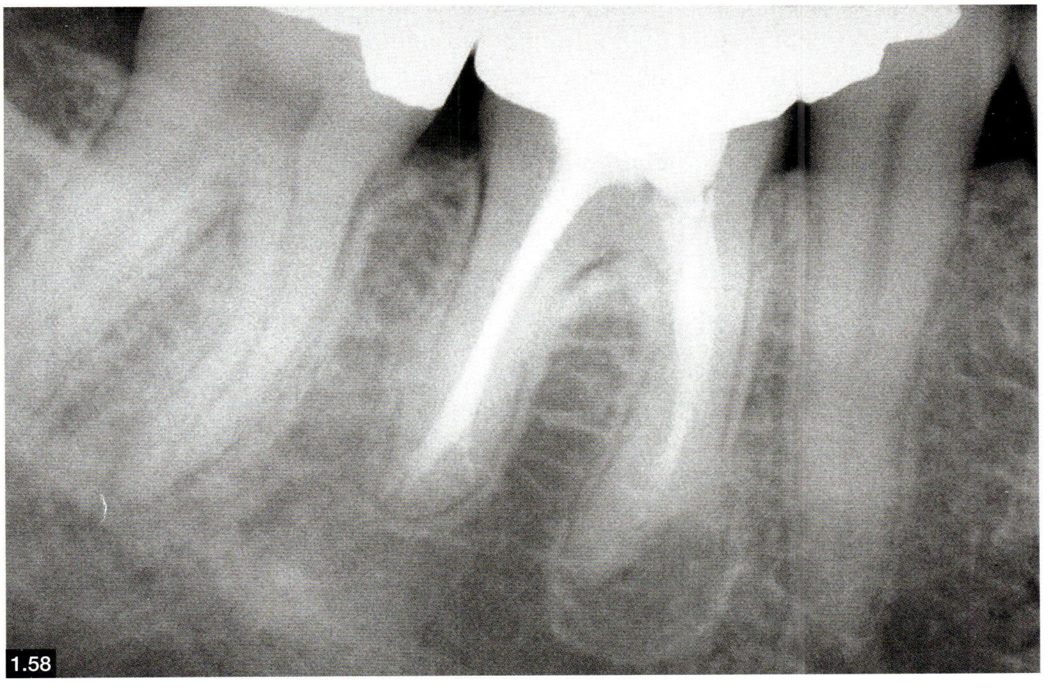

1.58

Fig. 1.58: The large lesion on the lower molar cannot be eliminated unless with endodontic surgery; the patient asked to postpone the treatment.

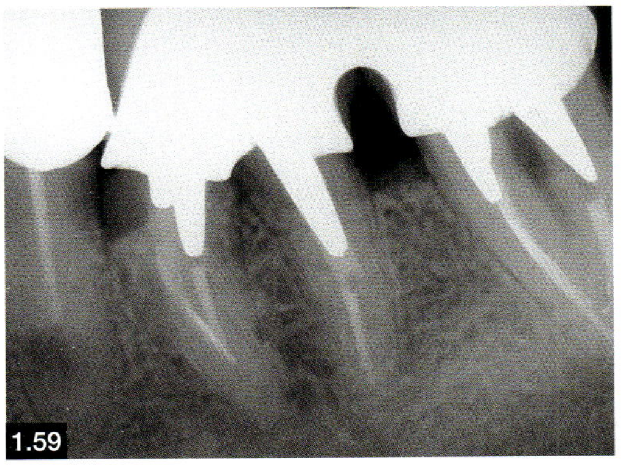

1.59

Fig. 1.59: The presence of root canal posts discourages a retreatment.

Figs. 1.60-1.61: Replacement of a crown on a previously treated tooth without periapical lesions.

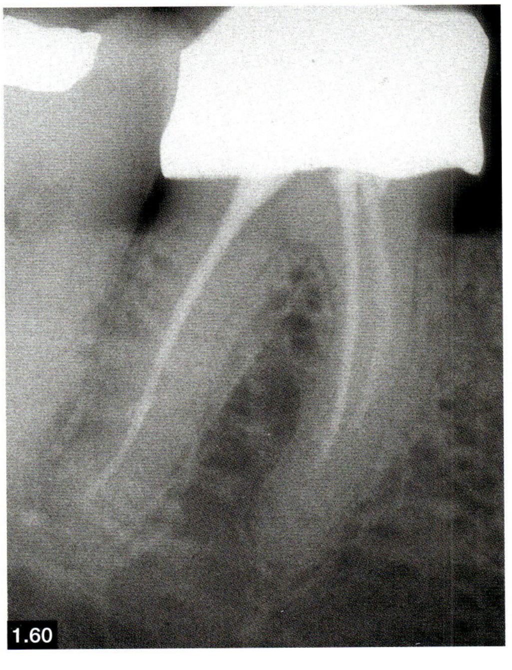

1.60

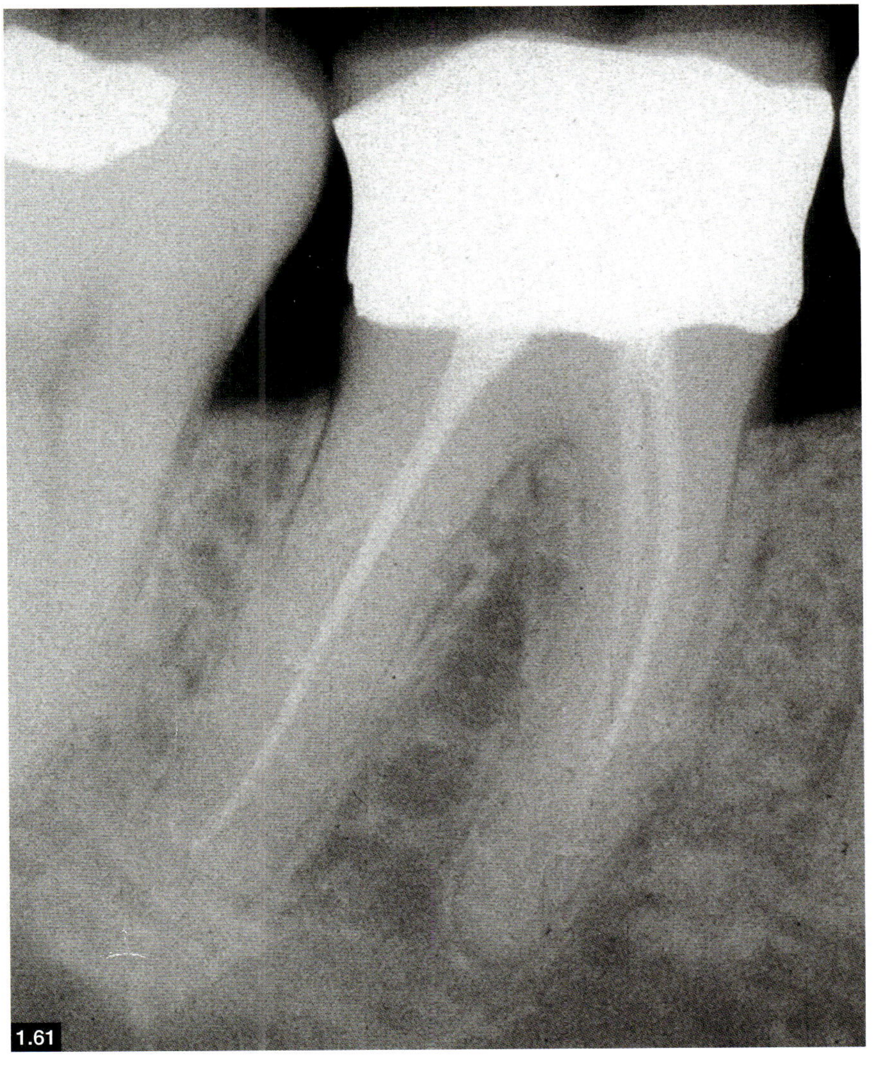

1.61

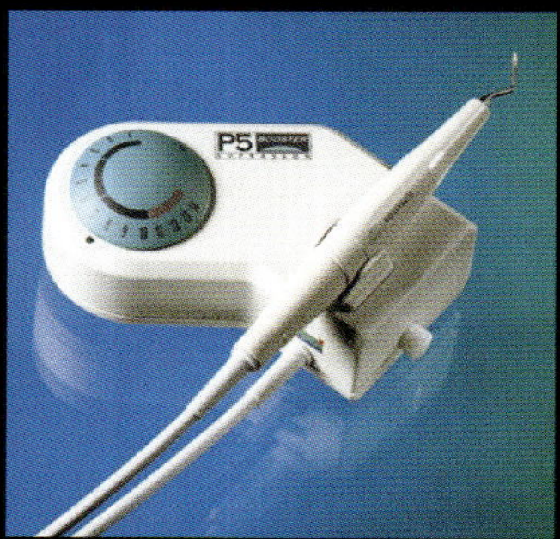

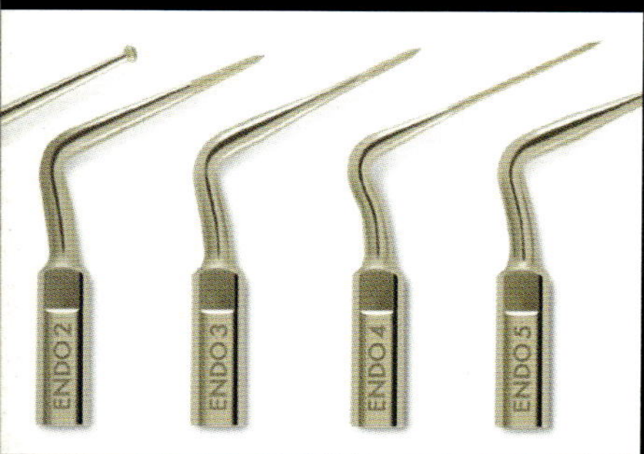

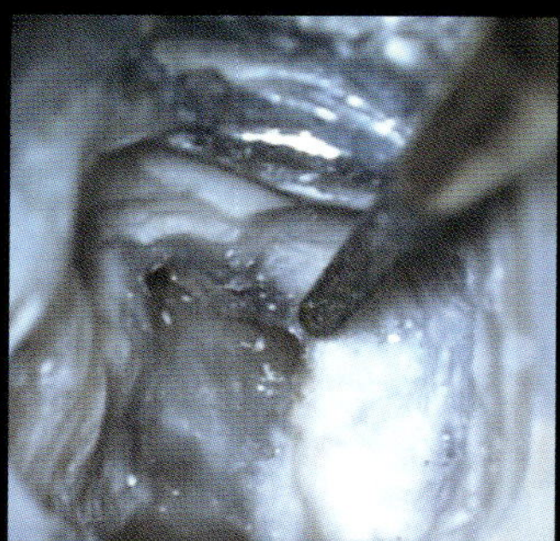

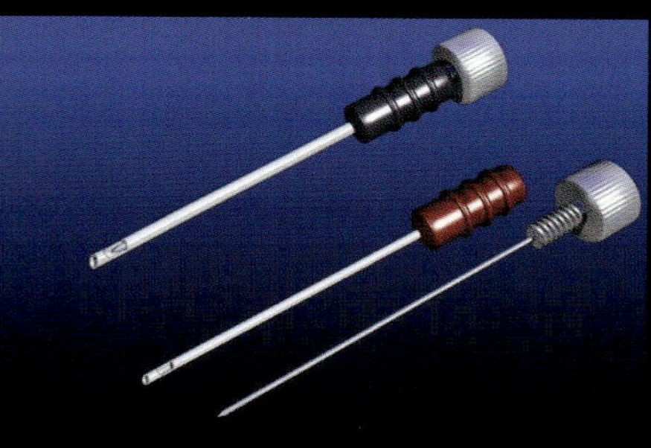

Retreatment: the role of the specialist

As discusssed in these opening paragraphs, retreatment is an extremely demanding clinical procedure that must be performed by a experienced clinician[107].
This makes it essential for the practitioner to have a full awareness, from the outset, of his/her technical limits as well as the availability of the tools needed to solve all the problems imposed by retreatment that may occur once the procedure is under way.
As reported by the American Association of Endodontists (AAE) (Box 1.5), a long list of clinical situations, previously considered unapproachable by less experienced clinicians, can now be contemplated.
Consequently, once a correct diagnosis has been established, deciding to conduct complex endodontic treatment becomes much easier; at this stage, careful consideration by the dentist will lead to the decision as to whether to carry out the procedure personally or to refer the matter to a colleague with greater experience in the field and who is likely to have more refined instrumentation that is suitable for solving the case in the best possible way.

In a study of treatments performed by endodontic specialists and general dentists, the former achieved better results than the latter on molar teeth[108]. Many scholars[109-113] have reiterated that the use of a surgical microscope could be an important aid for achieving the desired clinical results[114-117]. Lee et al.[118] compared practitioners belonging to institutional associations and general practitioners and found a higher success rate amongst the former; this finding indicates the contribution that the number of cases treated in environments with a high workflow can have in maintaining a high quality
Ramey et al.[119] performed a retrospective study on more than 2000 treatments and reported a close correlation between endodontic success and the quality of the operator's training; the treatments carried out by colleagues with postgraduate training from courses or in specialization programs had better results. Savani et al.[120] emphasized that the younger generations are more sensitive to the use of new technologies, but that the degree of attention to endodontics cannot be measured on the basis of the training courses attended.
Ultimately, the clinician's level of expertise would appear to be a significant factor in the success of root canal treatment and retreatment and this factor could also affect the final result of complex procedures.

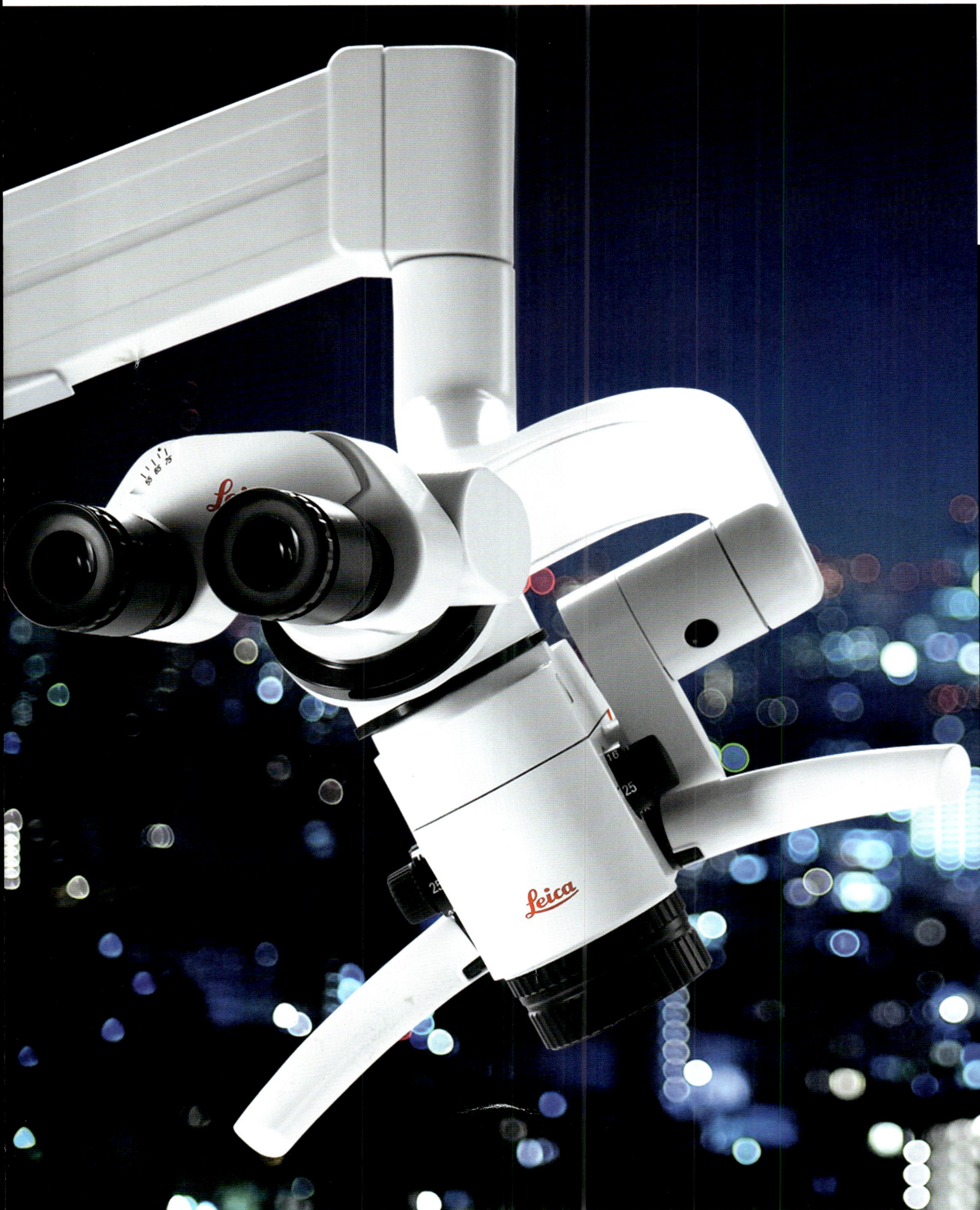
Leica

BEHAVIOR PATTERNS

The following is a sequence of the four phases that precede the performance of retreatment and represent key moments of analysis that the clinician must perform before formulating a prognosis and starting treatment.

1.

ASPECTS TO BE CONSIDERED IN A RETREATMENT

Factors influencing the prognosis

- Preoperative status of periapical tissues
- Size of periradicular lesion
- Canal anatomy
- Coronal or root fractures
- Iatrogenic factors (see below)
- Quality of the post-endodontic restoration
- Time elapsed since first treatment
- Microbiology
- Observation period

Iatrogenic errors leading to retreatment

- Fractured instruments
- Blocked canals - steps or plugs
- Perforations
- Incomplete root canal fillings in terms of extent and quality
- Overlooked canals
- Extent of filling beyond the apical limit

General factors to be considered in retreatment

- General patient health
- Operator experience
- Available instruments
- Diagnosis and treatment plan
- Radiographic interpretation
- Canal anatomy
- Quality and extension of the canal seal
- Quality of endodontic post-retreatment restoration

Contraindications for retreatment

Endodontic retreatment inevitably leads to a weakening of the tooth root, a fact that must be considered in the diagnostic phase; practitioners must also consider that root warming caused by the use of drills or ultrasound can cause damage to and weaken the surrounding periodontium, particularly the structure that supports the tooth.

2

CASE SELECTION

The following issues may contraindicate retreatment and make endodontic surgery a preferable option:

- Patient reluctancy
- Clinical history of of recurrent infections
- Presence of extensive periodontal lesion
- Presence of adjacent erupting teeth
- Occlusal trauma
- Unfavorable root-to-crown ratio
- Complex canal anatomies
- External root resorption
- Root fractures
- Quality of filling
- Relationship between the size of the lesion and the quality of the filling
- Overfilling or overextension of root canal fillings

3

SEQUENCE OF ANALYSIS BEFORE PERFORMING RETREATMENT

1. Patient **2.** Oral cavity **3.** Quadrant **4.** Tooth

PRETREATMENT CONSIDERATIONS

Elements to consider when evaluating the need for a new endodontic treatment procedure

- Asymptomatic patient
- Strategic importance of the element in question
- Real effectiveness of retreatment

SEAT TIME AND RELATED COSTS

- Removal and new fabrication of prosthetic restorations
- Technical difficulties
- Hypothetical quality of the future result

SUCCESS OR FAILURE OF A RETREATMENT: THE DETERMINANTS

Elements that do not determine the failure of retreatment

- Type and position of the tooth
- Age and sex of the patient
- Number of appointments for therapy
- Type of filling material
- Pre- or postoperative-operative pain

Elements leading to the failure of retreatment

- Persistence of infection
- Incorrect shaping - canal transport (hemorrhage)
- Irritation of periapical tissues with chemical agents
- Minor and major iatrogenic errors (blocks and/or perforations)

References

1. Cardinali F, et al., *La risoluzione delle complessitè nei ritrattamenti.* Dental Cadmos, 2014. 82(10): p. 690-712.
2. Friedman S, *Considerations and concepts of case selection in the management of post-treatment endodontic disease (treatment failure).* Endodontic Topics, 2002. 5(1): p. 54-78.
3. Haapasalo MSY, Ricucci D, *Reasons for persistent and emerging post-treatment endodontic disease.* Endodontic Topics, 2011. 18(1): p. 31-50.
4. Abbott P, *Diagnosis and management planning for root-filled teeth with persisting or new apical pathosis.* Endodontic Topics, 2008. 19(1): p. 1-21.
5. Dofour DL, V Leung, Levesque, CM, *Bacterial biofilm: structure, function, and antimicrobial resistance.* Endodontic Topics, 2010. 22(1): p. 2-16.
6. Ricucci D and G Bergenholtz, *Bacterial status in root-filled teeth exposed to the oral environment by loss of restoration and fracture or caries-a histobacteriological study of treated cases.* Int Endod J, 2003. 36(11): p. 787-802.
7. Ricucci D, et al., *Extraradicular infection as the cause of persistent symptoms: a case series.* J Endod, 2015. 41(2): p. 265-273.
8. Kakehashi S, HR Stanley, and R Fitzgerald, *The exposed germ-free pulp: effects of topical corticosteroid medication and restoration.* Oral Surg Oral Med Oral Pathol, 1969. 27(1): p. 60-67.
9. Kakehashi S, HR Stanley, and RJ Fitzgerald, *The Effects of Surgical Exposures of Dental Pulps in Germ-Free and Conventional Laboratory Rats.* Oral Surg Oral Med Oral Pathol, 1965. 20: p. 340-349.
10. Sjogren U, et al., *Factors affecting the long-term results of endodontic treatment.* J Endod, 1990. 16(10): p. 498-504.
11. Sundqvist G, *Ecology of the root canal flora.* J Endod, 1992. 18(9): p. 427-430.
12. Sundqvist G, *Taxonomy, ecology, and pathogenicity of the root canal flora.* Oral Surg Oral Med Oral Pathol, 1994. 78(4): p. 522-530.
13. Sundqvist G and D Figdor, *Life as an endodontic pathogen. Ecological differences between untreated and root-filled root canals.* Endodontic Topics, 2003. 6: p. 3-28.
14. Moller AJ, et al., *Influence on periapical tissues of indigenous oral bacteria and necrotic pulp tissue in monkeys.* Scand J Dent Res, 1981. 89(6): p. 475-484.
15. Nair PN, *Pathogenesis of apical periodontitis and the causes of endodontic failures.* Crit Rev Oral Biol Med, 2004. 15(6): p. 348-381.
16. Nair PN, *Pathobiology of Apical Periodontitis*, in *Essential Endodontology*, D. Orstavik and T.R. Pitt Ford, Editors. 2008, Blackwell Munksgaard Ltd: Oxford, UK. p. 81-123.
17. Siqueira JF, Jr., *Endodontic infections: concepts, paradigms, and perspectives.* Oral Surg Oral Med Oral Pathol Oral Radiol Endod, 2002. 94(3): p. 281-293.
18. Siqueira Jr, JFR, IN Rôças, Ricucci D, *Biofilms in endodontic infection.* Endodontic Topics, 2010. 22(1): p. 33-49.
19. Siqueira Jr, JFR, IN Rôças, *Present status and future directions in endodontic microbiology.* Endodontic Topics, 2014. 30(1): p. 3-22.
20. Ricucci D and JF Siqueira, Jr., *Apical actinomycosis as a continuum of intraradicular and extraradicular infection: case report and critical review on its involvement with treatment failure.* J Endod, 2008. 34(9): p. 1124-1129.
21. Ricucci D and JF Siqueira, Jr., *Biofilms and apical periodontitis: study of prevalence and association with clinical and histopathologic findings.* J Endod, 2010. 36(8): p. 1277-1288.
22. Sabeti M, et al., *Cytomegalovirus and Epstein-Barr virus active infection in periapical lesions of teeth with intact crowns.* J Endod, 2003. 29(5): p. 321-323.
23. Sabeti M and J Slots, *Herpesviral-bacterial coinfection in periapical pathosis.* J Endod, 2004. 30(2): p. 69-72.
24. Egan MW, et al., *Prevalence of yeasts in saliva and root canals of teeth associated with apical periodontitis.* Int Endod J, 2002. 35(4): p. 321-329.
25. Siqueira JF, Jr. and BH Sen, *Fungi in endodontic infections.* Oral Surg Oral Med Oral Pathol Oral Radiol Endod, 2004. 97(5): p. 632-641.
26. Waltimo TM, et al., *Yeasts in apical periodontitis.* Crit Rev Oral Biol Med, 2003. 14(2): p. 128-37.
27. Nair PN, *On the causes of persistent apical periodontitis: a review.* Int Endod J, 2006. 39(4): p. 249-281.
28. Aminoshariae A, Kulild JC. *The impact of sealer extrusion on endodontic outcome: A systematic review with meta-analysis*. Aust Endod J, 2019 (in-press).
29. Mello, F. W., et al., *The influence of apical extent of root canal obturation on endodontic therapy outcome: a systematic review*. Clin Oral Investig, 2019. 23(5).
30. Sakamoto M, et al., *Molecular analysis of bacteria in asymptomatic and symptomatic endodontic infections.* Oral Microbiol Immunol, 2006. 21(2): p. 112-122.
31. Lang MLZ, Zhu L, Kreth J, *Keeping the bad bacteria in check: interactions of the host immune system with oral cavity biofilms* Endodontic Topics, 2010. 22(1): p. 17-32.
32. Hülsmann M, *Epidemiology of post-treatment disease.* Endodontic Topics, 2016. 34(1): p. 42-63.
33. Tsai P, et al., *Accuracy of cone-beam computed tomography and periapical radiography in detecting small periapical lesions.* J Endod, 2012. 38(7): p. 965-970.
34. Paes da Silva Ramos Fernandes LM, et al., *Prevalence of apical periodontitis detected in cone beam CT images of a Brazilian subpopulation.* Dentomaxillofac Radiol, 2013. 42(1): 80179163.
35. Van der Veken D, et al., *Prevalence of apical periodontitis and root filled teeth in a Belgian subpopulation found on CBCT images.* Int Endod J, 2017. 50(4): p. 317-329.

36. Burklein S, Schafer E, Johren HP, Donnermeyer D. *Quality of root canal fillings and prevalence of apical radiolucencies in a German population: a CBCT analysis*. Clin Oral Investig, 2019 (on-line pre-press).
37. Pak JG, S Fayazi, and SN White, *Prevalence of periapical radiolucency and root canal treatment: a systematic review of cross-sectional studies.* J Endod, 2012. 38(9): p. 1170-1176.
38. Kirkevang L, *Root canal treatment and apical periodontitis: What can be learned from observational studies?* Endodontic Topics, 2011. 18(1): p. 51-61.
39. Kirkevang LL, M Vaeth, and A Wenzel, *Ten-year follow-up of root filled teeth: a radiographic study of a Danish population.* Int Endod J, 2014. 47(10): p. 980-988.
40. Peters LB, et al., *Prevalence of apical periodontitis relative to endodontic treatment in an adult Dutch population: a repeated cross-sectional study.* Oral Surg Oral Med Oral Pathol Oral Radiol Endod, 2011. 111(4): p. 523-528.
41. Kirkevang LL, M Vaeth, and A Wenzel, *Ten-year follow-up observations of periapical and endodontic status in a Danish population.* Int Endod J, 2012. 45(9): p. 829-839.
42. Connert, T., et al, *Changes in periapical status, quality of root fillings and estimated endodontic treatment need in a similar urban German population 20 years later*. Clin Oral Investig, 2019. 23(3): p. 1373-1382.
43. Murray CA and WP Saunders, *Root canal treatment and general health: a review of the literature.* Int Endod J, 2000. 33(1): p. 1-18.
44. Cotti E, et al., *An overview on biologic medications and their possible role in apical periodontitis.* J Endod, 2014. 40(12): p. 1902-1911.
45. Aminoshariae A, et al., *Association between Systemic Diseases and Endodontic Outcome: A Systematic Review.* J Endod, 2017. 43(4): p. 514-519.
46. Aminoshariae A, JC Kulild, and AF Fouad, *The Impact of Endodontic Infections on the Pathogenesis of Cardiovascular Disease(s): A Systematic Review with Meta-analysis Using GRADE.* J Endod, 2018. 44(9): p. 1361-1366 e3.
47. Hamedy R, et al., *Prevalence of root canal treatment and periapical radiolucency in elders: a systematic review.* Gerodontology, 2016. 33(1): p. 116-127.
48. Hamedy R, B Shakiba, and SN White, *Essential elder endodontics.* Gerodontology, 2016. 33(4): p. 433.
49. Shakiba B, et al., *Influence of increased patient age on longitudinal outcomes of root canal treatment: a systematic review.* Gerodontology, 2017. 34(1): p. 101-109.
50. Segura-Egea, JJ, J. Martin-Gonzalez, and L Castellanos-Cosano, *Endodontic medicine: connections between apical periodontitis and systemic diseases.* Int Endod J, 2015. 48(10): p. 933-951.
51. Allen PF, JM Whitworth, *Endodontic considerations in the elderly.* Gerodontology, 2004. 21: p. 185-194.
52. Rutz da Silva F, et al., *Relationship between quality of root canal obturation and periapical lesion in elderly patients: a systematic review.* Gerodontology, 2016. 33(3): p. 290-298.
53. Lopez-Lopez J, et al., *Periapical and endodontic status of type 2 diabetic patients in Catalonia, Spain: a cross-sectional study.* J Endod, 2011. 37(5): p. 598-601.
54. Segura-Egea JJ, et al., *High prevalence of apical periodontitis amongst type 2 diabetic patients.* Int Endod J, 2005. 38(8): p. 564-569.
55. Cabanillas-Balsera, D., et al., *Association between diabetes and non-retention of root filled teeth: a systematic review and meta-analysis*. Int Endod J, 2019. 52(3): p. 297-306.
56. Laukkanen, E., et al,. *Impact of systemic diseases and tooth-based factors on outcome of root canal treatment*. Int Endod J, 2019. 52(10): p. 1417-1426.
57. Nagendrababu, V., et al., *Association between diabetes and the outcome of root canal treatment in adults: An umbrella review*. Int Endod J, 2019. (in press)
58. Segura-Egea JJ, et al., *Hypertension and dental periapical condition.* J Endod, 2010. 36(11): p. 1800-1804.
59. Jalali P, et al., *Prevalence of Periapical Rarefying Osteitis in Patients with Rheumatoid Arthritis.* J Endod, 2017. 43(7): p. 1093-1096.
60. Virtanen E, et al., *Apical periodontitis associates with cardiovascular diseases: a cross-sectional study from Sweden.* BMC Oral Health, 2017. 17(1): p. 107.
61. Berlin-Broner Y, M Febbraio and L Levin, *Association between apical periodontitis and cardiovascular diseases: a systematic review of the literature.* Int Endod J, 2017. 50(9): p. 847-859.
62. Cotti E, et al., *Association of endodontic infection with detection of an initial lesion to the cardiovascular system.* J Endod, 2011. 37(12): p. 1624-1629.
63. Pasqualini D, et al., *Association among oral health, apical periodontitis, CD14 polymorphisms, and coronary heart disease in middle-aged adults.* J Endod, 2012. 38(12): p. 1570-1577.
64. Segura-Egea JJ, et al., *Antibiotics in Endodontics: a review.* Int Endod J, 2017. 50(12): p. 1169-1184.
65. Marx RE, JE Cillo Jr, and JJ Ulloa, *Oral bisphosphonate-induced osteonecrosis: risk factors, prediction of risk using serum CTX testing, prevention, and treatment.* J Oral Maxillofac Surg, 2007. 65(12): p. 2397-2410.
66. Price N, et al., *Prevention and management of osteonecrosis of the jaw associated with bisphosphonate therapy.* Support Cancer Ther, 2004. 2(1): p. 14-17.
67. Ruggiero SL, et al., *Osteonecrosis of the jaws associated with the use of bisphosphonates: a review of 63 cases.* J Oral Maxillofac Surg, 2004. 62(5): p. 527-534.
68. Sawatari Y and RE Marx, *Bisphosphonates and bisphosphonate induced osteonecrosis.* Oral Maxillofac Surg Clin North Am, 2007. 19(4): p. 487-498, v-vi.
69. Assael LA, *Oral Bisphosphonates as a Cause of Bisphosphonate-Related Osteonecrosis of the Jaws: Clinical Findings, Assessment of Risks, and Preventive Strategies.* Journal of Oral Maxillofacial Surgery, 2009. 67: p. 35-43.

70. Fantasia JE, *Bisphosphonates - What the Dentist Needs to Know: Practical Considerations.* Journal of Oral Maxillofacial Surgery, 2009. 67: p. 53-60.
71. Moinzadeh AT, et al., *Bisphosphonates and their clinical implications in endodontic therapy.* Int Endod J, 2013. 46(5): p. 391-398.
72. Hsiao A, G Glickman and J He, *A retrospective clinical and radiographic study on healing of periradicular lesions in patients taking oral bisphosphonates.* J Endod, 2009. 35(11): p. 1525-1528.
73. Alsalleeh F, et al., *Bisphosphonate-associated osteonecrosis of jaw reoccurrence after methotrexate therapy: a case report.* J Endod, 2014. 40(9): p. 1505-1507.
74. Ruggiero SLC, ER Carlson, LA Assael, *Comprehensive Review of Bisphosphonate Therapy: Implications for the Oral and Maxillofacial Surgery Patient.* Journal of Oral Maxillofacial Surgery, 2009. 67: p. 1.
75. Segura-Egea JJ, et al., *European Society of Endodontology position statement: the use of antibiotics in endodontics.* Int Endod J, 2018. 51(1): p. 20-25.
76. Yu VS, et al., *Incidence and impact of painful exacerbations in a cohort with post-treatment persistent endodontic lesions.* J Endod, 2012. 38(1): p. 41-46.
77. Carter AE, G Carter, and R George, *Pathways of fear and anxiety in endodontic patients.* Int Endod J, 2015. 48(6): p. 528-532.
78. Cho SY, et al., *Effect of Topical Anesthesia on Pain from Needle Insertion and Injection and Its Relationship with Anxiety in Patients Awaiting Apical Surgery: A Randomized Double-blind Clinical Trial.* J Endod, 2017. 43(3): p. 364-369.
79. Monteiro MR, et al., *4% articaine buccal infiltration versus 2% lidocaine inferior alveolar nerve block for emergency root canal treatment in mandibular molars with irreversible pulpits: a randomized clinical study.* Int Endod J, 2015. 48(2): p. 145-152.
80. De Pedro-Munoz A and J Mena-Alvarez, *The effect of preoperative submucosal administration of tramadol on the success rate of inferior alveolar nerve block on mandibular molars with symptomatic irreversible pulpitis: a randomized, double-blind placebo-controlled clinical trial.* Int Endod J, 2017. 50(12): p. 1134-1142.
81. Kirkevang LL, et al., *Prediction of periapical status and tooth extraction.* Int Endod J, 2017. 50(1): p. 5-14.
82. He J, et al., *Clinical and Patient-centered Outcomes of Nonsurgical Root Canal Retreatment in First Molars Using Contemporary Techniques.* J Endod, 2017. 43(2): p. 231-237.
83. Burns LE, et al., *Long-term Evaluation of Treatment Planning Decisions for Nonhealing Endodontic Cases by Different Groups of Practitioners.* J Endod, 2018. 44(2): p. 226-232.
84. Foltyn P, *Ethical decision making in aged care.* Gerodontology, 2017. 34: p. 289-290.
85. Alani A, K Bishop, and S Djemal, *The influence of specialty training, experience, discussion and reflection on decision making in modern restorative treatment planning.* Br Dent J, 2011. 210(4): p. E4.
86. Re D, et al., *Natural tooth preservation versus extraction and implant placement: patient preferences and analysis of the willingness to pay.* Br Dent J, 2017. 222(6): p. 467-471.
87. Mounce R and JD Moody, *The decision fork in the road; When to treat, when to refer, and when it's time for titanium.* Dent Today, 2013. 32(11): p. 98-103.
88. Orstavik D, K Kerekes and HM Eriksen, *The periapical index: a scoring system for radiographic assessment of apical periodontitis.* Endod Dent Traumatol, 1986. 2(1): p. 20-34.
89. Eliyas S, et al., *Development of quality measurement instruments for root canal treatment.* Int Endod J, 2017. 50(7): p. 652-666.
90. Del Fabbro M, et al., *Analysis of the secondary endodontic lesions focusing on the extraradicular microorganisms: an overview.* J Investig Clin Dent, 2014. 5(4): p. 245-254.
91. Rocas IN and JF Siqueira Jr, *Characterization of microbiota of root canal-treated teeth with posttreatment disease.* J Clin Microbiol, 2012. 50(5): p. 1721-1724.
92. Zhu X, et al., *Prevalence, phenotype, and genotype of Enterococcus faecalis isolated from saliva and root canals in patients with persistent apical periodontitis.* J Endod, 2010. 36(12): p. 1950-1955.
93. Rocas IN, M. Hulsmann, and J.F. Siqueira, Jr., *Microorganisms in root canal-treated teeth from a German population.* J Endod, 2008. 34(8): p. 926-931.
94. Siqueira JF, Jr. and IN Rocas, *Bacterial pathogenesis and mediators in apical periodontitis.* Braz Dent J, 2007. 18(4): p. 267-280.
95. Li H, et al., *Herpesviruses in endodontic pathoses: association of Epstein-Barr virus with irreversible pulpitis and apical periodontitis.* J Endod, 2009. 35(1): p. 23-29.
96. Chen V, et al., *Herpesviruses in abscesses and cellulitis of endodontic origin.* J Endod, 2009. 35(2): p. 182-188.
97. Schirrmeister JF, et al., *New bacterial compositions in root-filled teeth with periradicular lesions.* J Endod, 2009. 35(2): p. 169-174.
98. Wang QQ, et al., *Prevalence of Enterococcus faecalis in saliva and filled root canals of teeth associated with apical periodontitis.* Int J Oral Sci, 2012. 4(1): p. 19-23.
99. Signoretti FG, et al., *Persistent extraradicular infection in root-filled asymptomatic human tooth: scanning electron microscopic analysis and microbial investigation after apical microsurgery.* J Endod, 2011. 37(12): p. 1696-1700.
100. Farzaneh M, S Abitbol, and S Friedman, *Treatment outcome in endodontics: the Toronto study. Phases I and II: Orthograde retreatment.* J Endod, 2004. 30(9): p. 627-633.
101. De Chevigny C, et al., *Treatment outcome in endodontics: the Toronto study--phases 3 and 4: orthograde retreatment.* J Endod, 2008. 34(2): p. 131-137.

102. Ng YG K, et al.;, *Outcome of non-surgical re-treatment.* Endodontic Topics, 2008. 18(1): p. 3-30.
103. Ng YL, V Mann and K. Gulabivala, *Outcome of secondary root canal treatment: a systematic review of the literature.* Int Endod J, 2008. 41(12): p. 1026-1046.
104. Ng YL, V Mann and K. Gulabivala, *Tooth survival following non-surgical root canal treatment: a systematic review of the literature.* Int Endod J, 2010. 43(3): p. 171-189.
105. Torabinejad M, et al., *Outcomes of nonsurgical retreatment and endodontic surgery: a systematic review.* J Endod, 2009. 35(7): p. 930-937.
106. Davies A, et al., *The detection of periapical pathoses using digital periapical radiography and cone beam computed tomography in endodontically retreated teeth - part 2: a 1 year post-treatment follow-up.* Int Endod J, 2016. 49(7): p. 623-635.
107. Gorni FG and MM Gagliani, *The outcome of endodontic retreatment: a 2-yr follow-up.* J Endod, 2004. 30(1): p. 1-4.
108. Al-Nuaimi N, et al., *A prospective study assessing the effect of coronal tooth structure loss on the outcome of root canal retreatment.* Int Endod J, 2017. 50(12): p. 1143-1157.
109. Al-Nuaimi N, et al., *Pooled analysis of 1-year recall data from three root canal treatment outcome studies undertaken using cone beam computed tomography.* Int Endod J, 2018. 51 Suppl 3: p. e216-e226.
110. Ricucci DG, D et al.;, *The compromised tooth: conservative treatment or extraction?* Endodontic Topics, 2006. 13(1): p. 108-122.
111. Fonzar F, et al., *The prognosis of root canal therapy: a 10-year retrospective cohort study on 411 patients with 1175 endodontically treated teeth.* Eur J Oral Implantol., 2009. 2(3): p. 201-208.
112. Kwak, Y., et al., *The 5-Year Survival Rate of Nonsurgical Endodontic Treatment: A Population-based Cohort Study in Korea*. J Endod, 2019. 45(10): pp. 1192-1199.
113. Pirani, C., et al., *Outcome of secondary root canal treatment filled with Thermafil: a 5-year follow-up of retrospective cohort study*. Clin Oral Investig, 2018. 22(3): pp. 1363-1373.
114. Wesselink PR, *The incidental discovery of apical periodontitis.* Endodontic Topics, 2014. 30(1): p. 23-28.
115. Schwendicke F and M Stolpe, *Secondary Treatment for Asymptomatic Root Canal Treated Teeth: A Cost-effectiveness Analysis.* J Endod, 2015. 41(6): p. 812-816.
116. Tifooni, A., et al.,*Validation of the effectiveness of the Dental Practicality Index in predicting the outcome of root canal retreatments*. Int Endod J, 2019.52(10): pp. 1403-1409.
117. Torabinejad M, et al., *Levels of evidence for the outcome of nonsurgical endodontic treatment.* J Endod, 2005. 31(9): p. 637-646.
118. Burry, J.C., et al., *Outcomes of Primary Endodontic Therapy Provided by Endodontic Specialists Compared with Other Providers.* J Endod, 2016. 42(5): p. 702-705.
119. Iandolo A, et al., *Modern technologies in Endodontics.* Giornale Italiano di Endodonzia, 2016. 30(1): p. 2-9.
120. Lababidi EA, *Discuss the impact technological advances in equipment and materials have made on the delivery and outcome of endodontic treatment.* Aust Endod J, 2013. 39(3): p. 92-97.
121. Rampado ME, et al., *The benefit of the operating microscope for access cavity preparation by undergraduate students.* J Endod, 2004. 30(12): p. 863-867.
122. Rapani M, et al., *Influenza del microscopio operatorio nella diagnosi intraoperatoria e nel ritrattamento chirurgico endodontico: studio clinico e radiografico con follow-up a un anno.* Dental Cadmos, 2011. 79(8): p. 533-543.
123. Riccitiello F, et al., *Microscopio operatorio: diffusione e limiti.* Giornale Italiano di Endodonzia, 2012. 26(2): p. 67-72.
124. Del Fabbro M and S Taschieri, *Endodontic therapy using magnification devices: a systematic review.* J Dent, 2010. 38(4): p. 269-275.
125. Del Fabbro M, et al., *Magnification devices for endodontic therapy.* Cochrane Database Syst Rev, 2009(3): p. CD005969.
126. Taschieri S, et al., *Magnification in modern endodontic practice.* Refuat Hapeh Vehashinayim (1993), 2010. 27(3): p. 18-22, 61.
127. Taschieri S, et al., *Magnifying loupes versus surgical microscope in endodontic surgery: a four-year retrospective study.* Aust Endod J, 2013. 39(2): p. 78-80.
128. Lee CB, et al., *Association of Failed Root Canal Treatment with Dentist and Institutional Volumes: A Population-based Cohort Study in Taiwan.* J Endod, 2017. 43(10): p. 1628-1634.
129. Ramey K, J Yaccino, and J Wealleans, *A Retrospective, Radiographic Outcomes Assessment of 1960 Initial Posterior Root Canal Treatments Performed by Endodontists and Dentists.* J Endod, 2017. 43(8): p. 1250-1254.
130. Savani GM, et al., *Current trends in endodontic treatment by general dental practitioners: report of a United States national survey.* J Endod, 2014. 40(5): p. 618-624.

Sitography

[1a] https://www.aae.org/specialty/wp-con-tent/uploads/sites/2/2017/06/2006casedifficultyassessmentformb_edited2010.pdf

[1b] American Association of Endodontists (2005) Endodontic Case Difficulty Assessment and Referral. https:// www.aae.org/uploadedfiles/dental_professionals/endodontic_case_assessment/2006casedifficultyassessmentformb_edited 2010.pdf. [accessed on 24 April 2016].

[1c] https://www.endodonzia.it/articoli-scientifici/cose-un-granuloma/

[1d] https://www.e-s-e.eu/publications/index.html

> State the **diagnostic procedures** used in the endodontic field with particular reference to patients suspected of having a periapical lesion.

> Identify the most effective and accurate **diagnostic tools** for examining cases of inflammatory disease of the periapical tissues.

> Describe the **diagnostic tests**, such as cone beam computed tomography, which may be decisive in formulating a correct diagnosis and treatment plan.

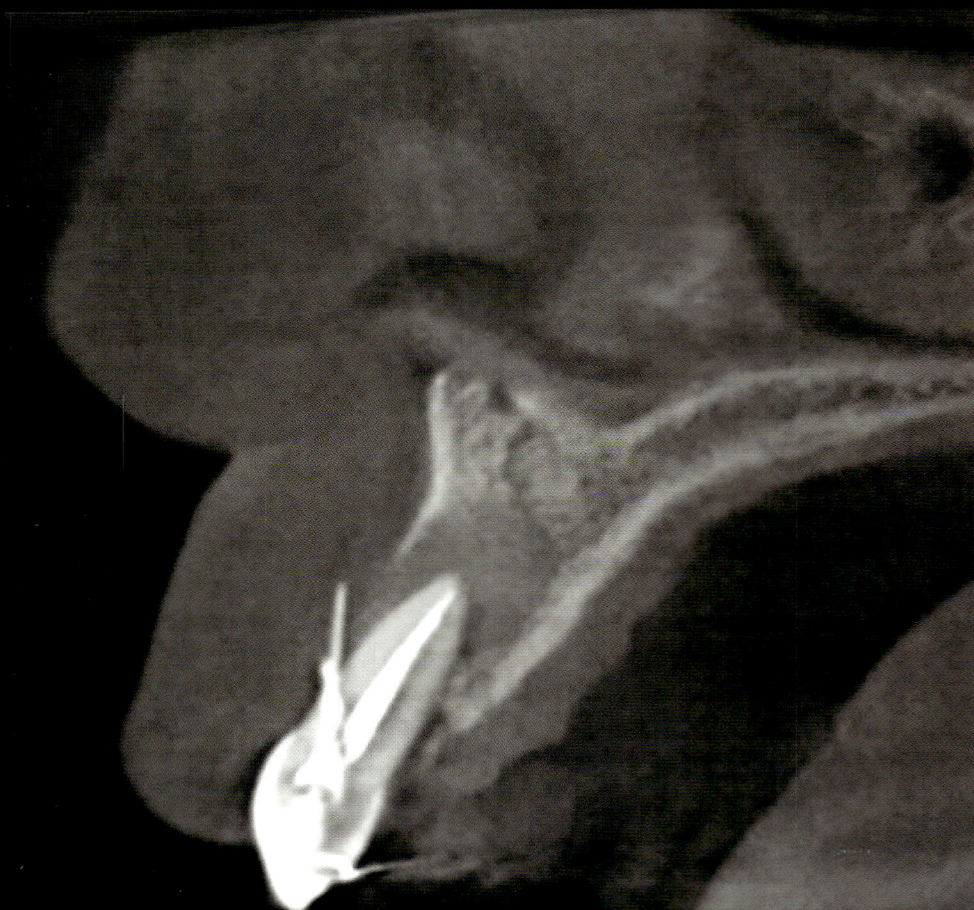

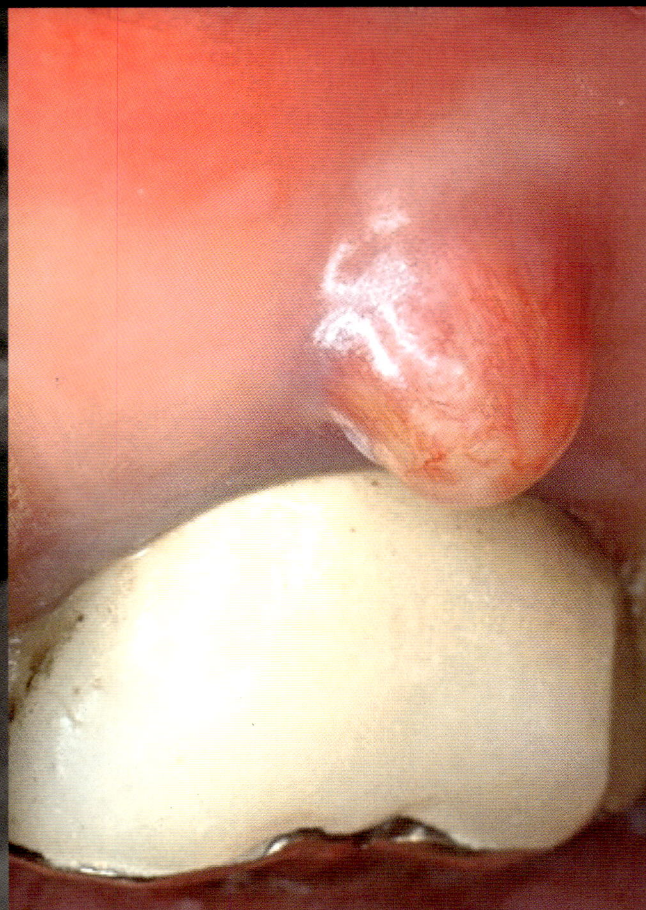

Roberto Fornara, Filippo Cardinali

02

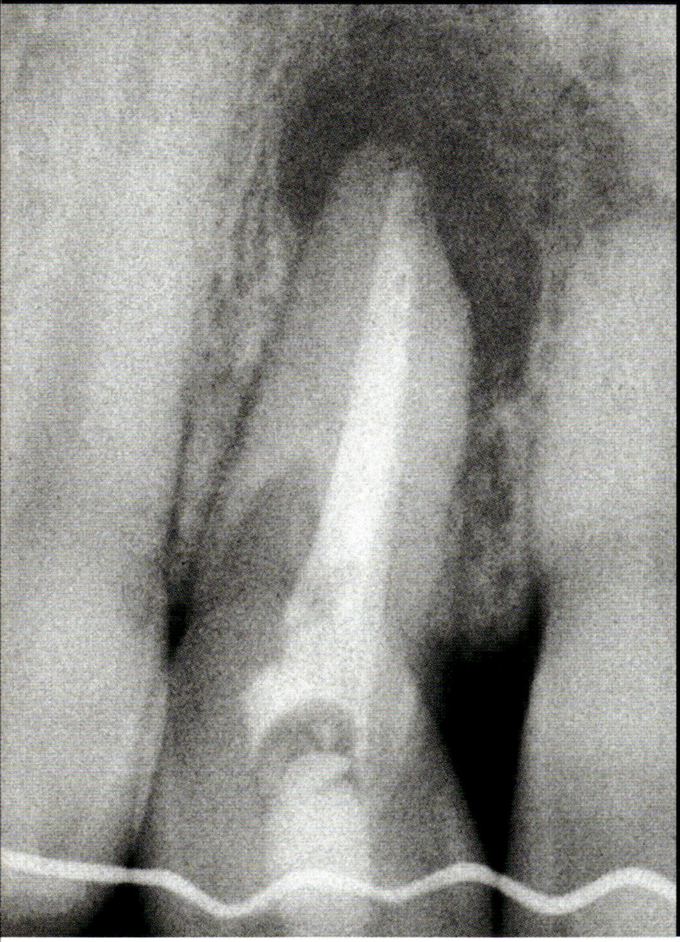

Diagnostic procedures for endodontic failure

Clinical and radiological examinations useful for identifying periapical lesions

Preliminary remarks

This chapter presents the numerous situations in which a previous endodontic treatment and reconstruction of the tooth has created the conditions for an inflammatory reaction of the tissues at the apex, be they acute or chronic[1]. It focuses on cases for which endodontic treatment did not have the desired effect regardless of the starting conditions. Root canal treatment prevents the onset of periapical problems, but improper administration of this treatment leads to the development of endodontic periapical disease. This type of problem includes cases in which a root canal treatment performed in the presence of a periapical lesion of endodontic origin has not achieved, or is yet to achieve the desired outcome.[2, 3]
In other words, they are two very distinct initial situations that present to the dentist examining them for the first time as the same clinical situation.[4]
Any diagnostic tool used must therefore consider the variables involved and facilitate the formulation of a correct, technically flawless treatment plan, supported by the most favorable prognostic framework possible. Abbott divided periapical problems into two separate categories.[5, 6]

Fig. 2.1a: Radiographic analysis must be considered in every detail, including the coronal aspect, the root canal content, and the texture of the alveolar bone. Slight imperfections can be observed clinically; the x-ray shows a treatment with slight imperfections but not worthy of retreatment because the tooth is completely asymptomatic.

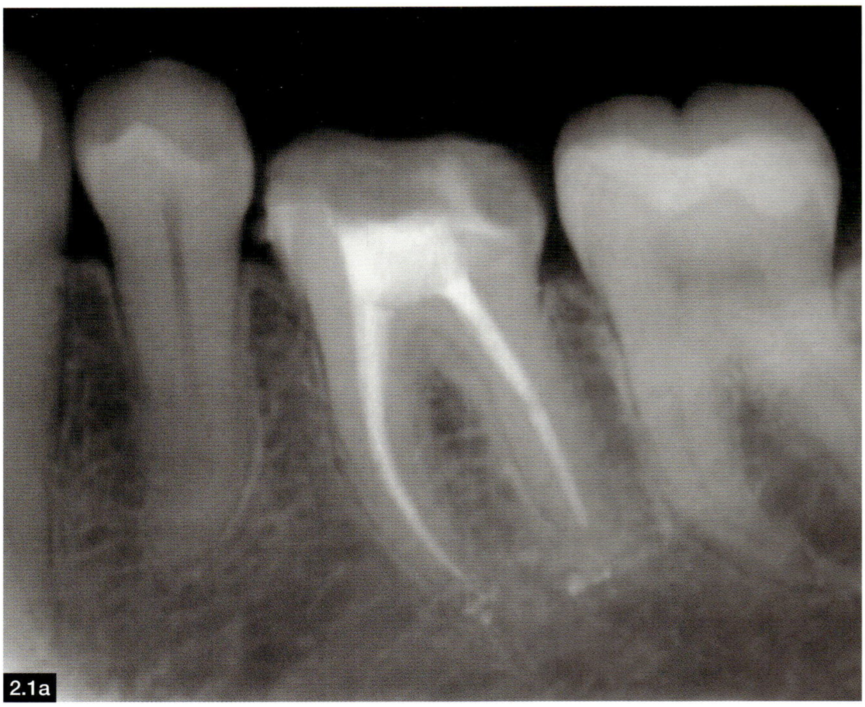
2.1a

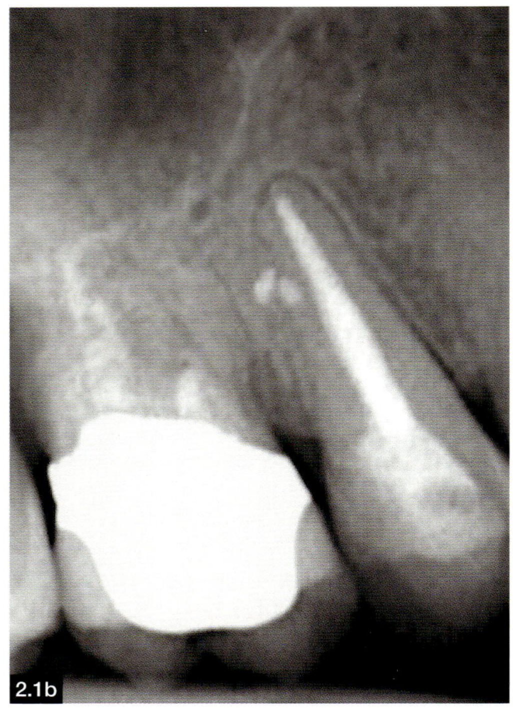
2.1b

Fig. 2.1b: The same criteria must be considered when observing the X-ray results at subsequent follow-up.

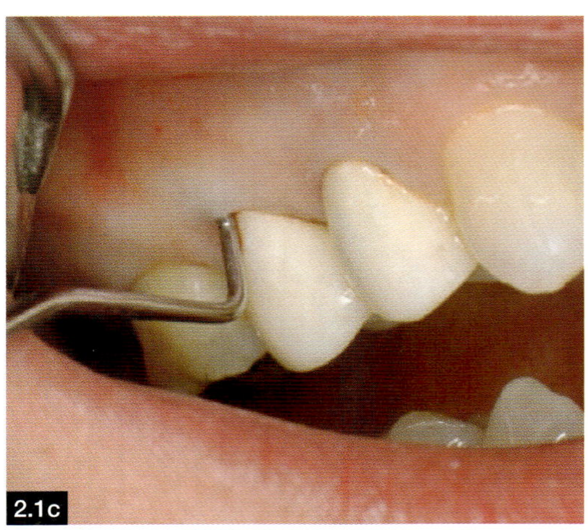
2.1c

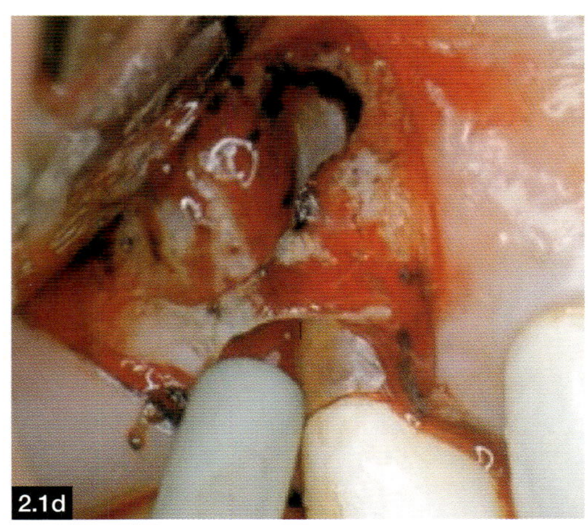
2.1d

Fig. 2.1c-d: When disease is suspected at the first clinical examination, an exploratory flap examination is often performed with (example of root fracture that is not radiographically visible).

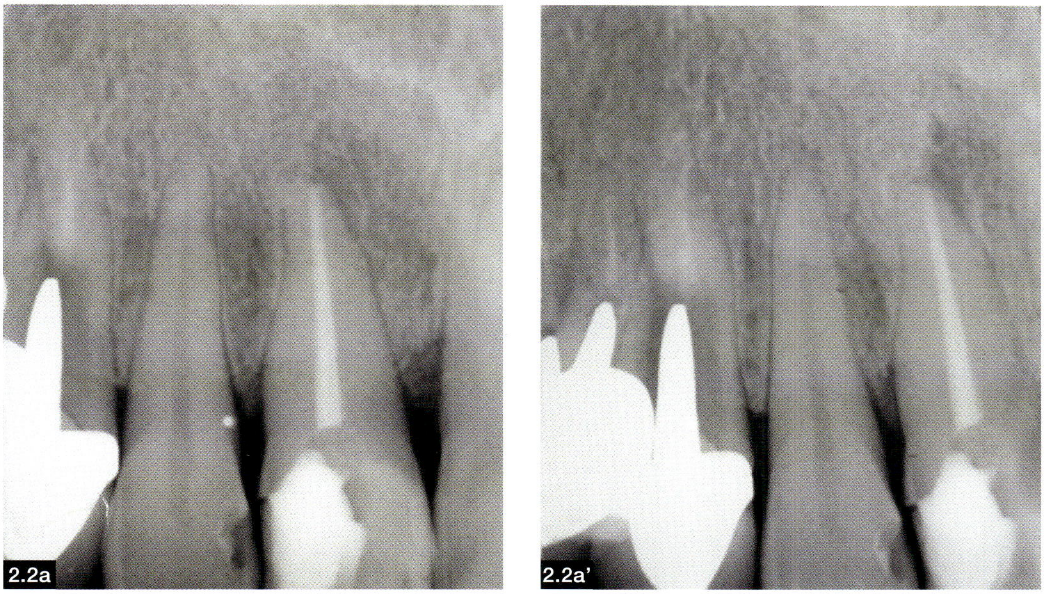

Fig. 2.2a-a': A simple change of projection can reveal the presence of a radio-transparent area which, when superimposed on the root, is not evident.

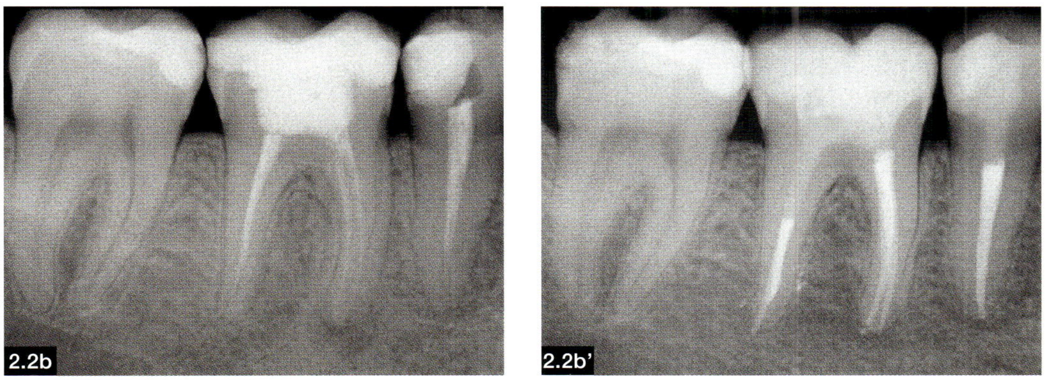

Fig. 2.2b: Associating radiolucent bone lesions with endodontic treatments is inappropriate.

Fig. 2.2b': Radiographic healing on both teeth: the performance of two x-rays with the same projection allows a correct evaluation.

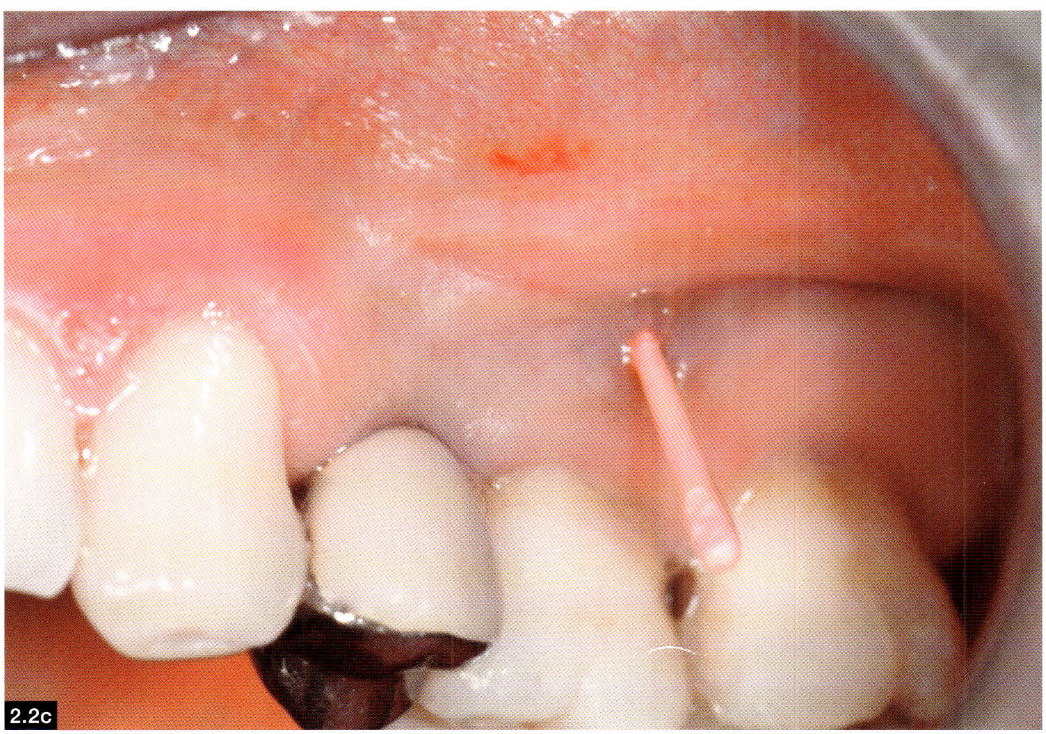

Fig. 2c-c': The presence of a fistula often leads to the insertion of a gutta-percha cone in order to identify the tooth responsible for the chronic inflammatory process; integration between clinic and radiology findings.

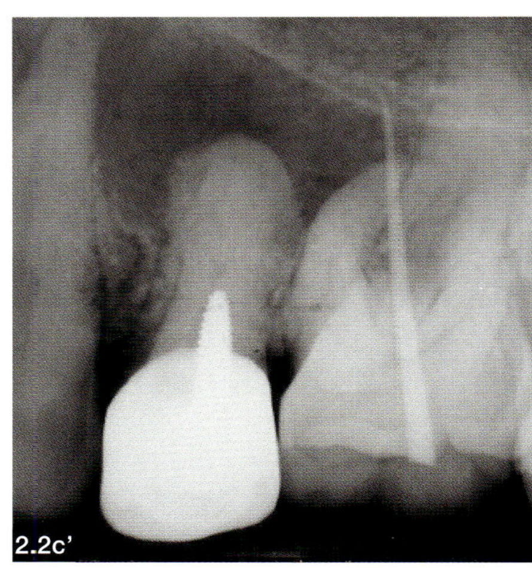

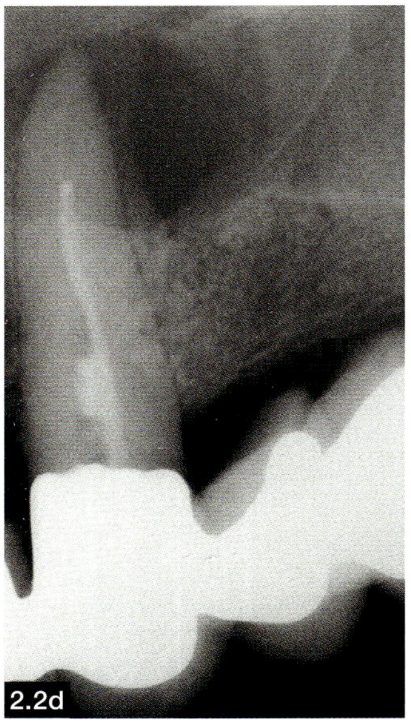

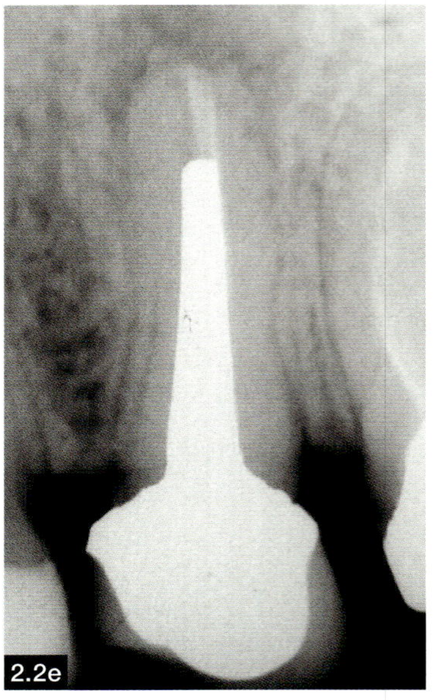

Fig. 2.2d-e: Two similar cases with different therapeutic results; the tooth without a post will be treated directly, while the other cannot be retreated.

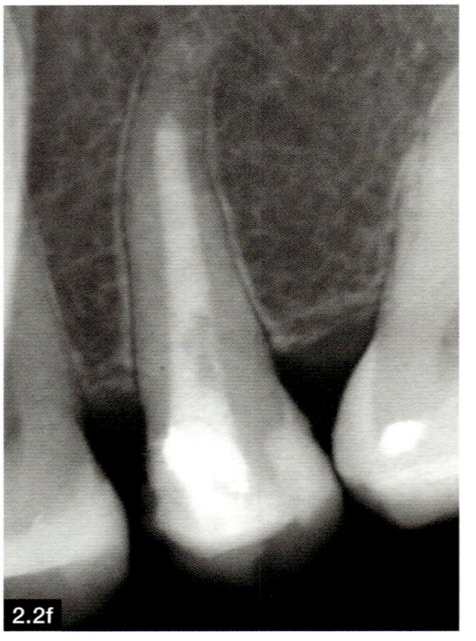

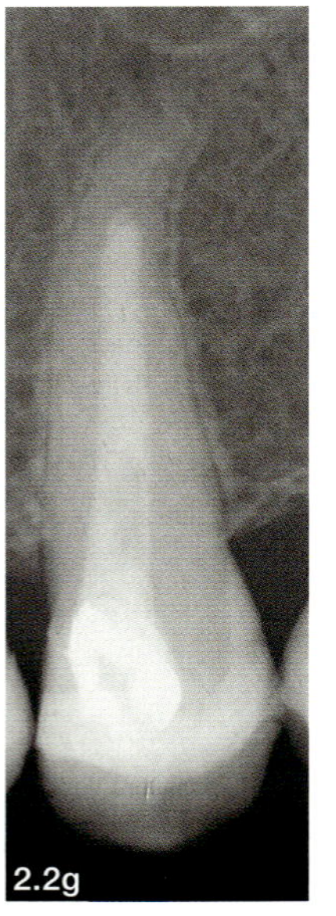

Fig. 2.2f-g: The initial X-ray image provides conflicting information, in that it shows a treatment that, despite not having been performed correctly, did not produce any radiologically appreciable results. Analysis of the path to be followed to perform the retreatment suggests not performing the procedure. The 5-year x-ray image does not show any anomalies.

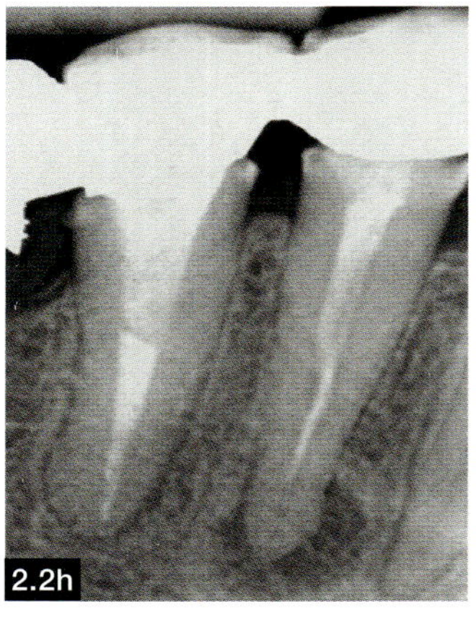

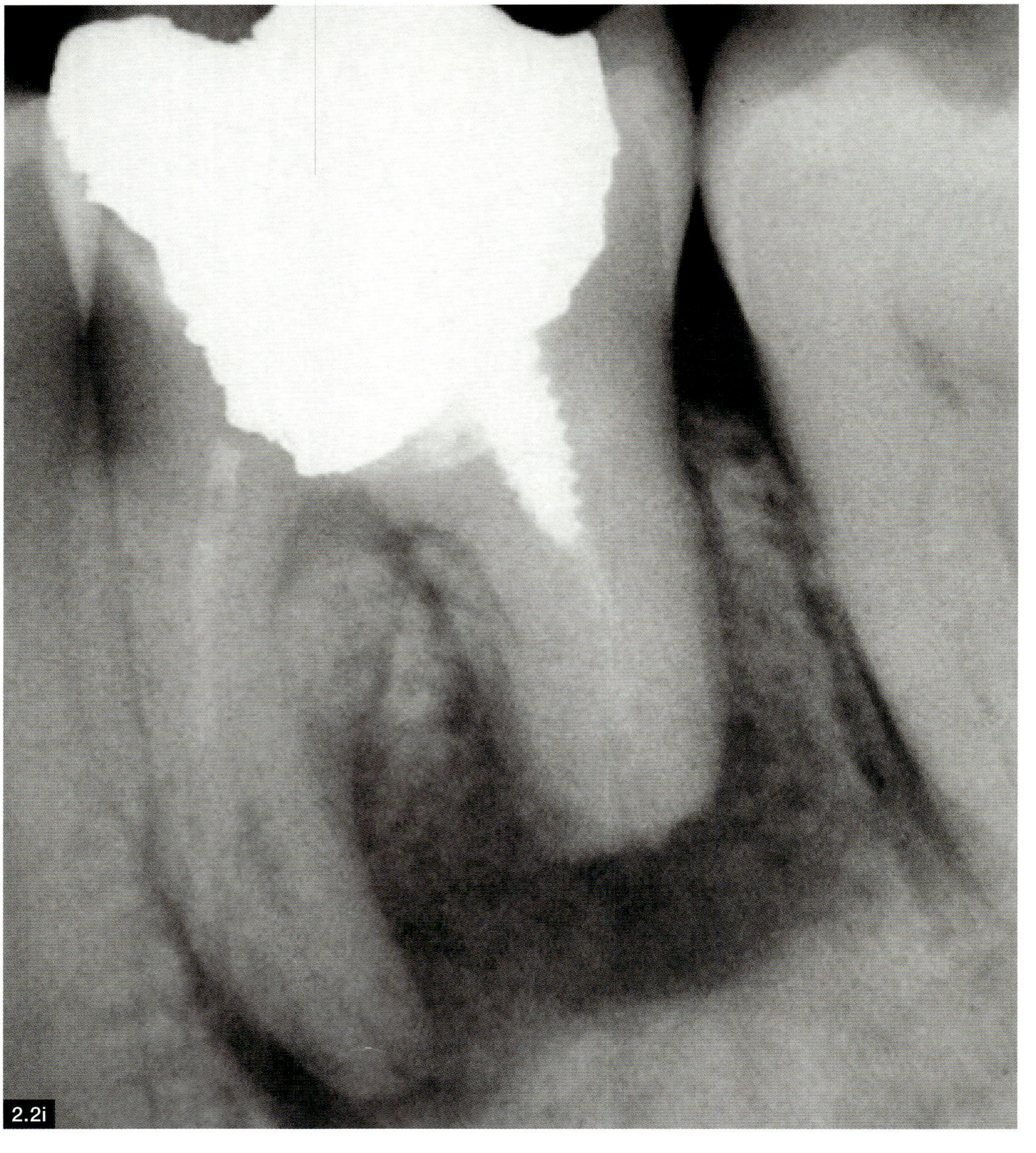

Fig. 2.2h-i: Clear radiographic images of periapical lesions of endodontic origin; the size and damage caused at the root level suggest a different prognosis in the two cases.

Failure analysis

When we talk about the failure of an endodontic therapy, we venture into a field full of pitfalls: what are the parameters that indicate, with reasonable certainty, failure? The clinical parameters may be the patient's symptoms or the radiographic examination. Clinical findings, in accordance with the guidelines of the major international scientific societies, are the fundamental elements for reaching a verdict.
Two-dimensional and three-dimensional radiographic examinations provide detailed information on the actual state of disease and provide a rough guide as to whether to perform endodontic treatment to decontaminate a bacterially infected space. Legitimate considerations can be made in these clinical cases, but the response of the body may vary.
Certain conditions lead to favorable or unfavorable results; consequently, a therapeutic choice or alternative often has the same weight in the balance, preventing a final correct decision.
In the preliminary phase, the authors believe that the clinical element of spontaneous or provoked, is a prevailing condition for starting the operations that lead to the retreatment of the endodontic space. This pain must persist over time, as evidenced by a lack of chewing, and must be related to a reasonably long interval of time from the performance of the treatment.
Finally, the pain symptoms should have a negative evolution, even mild, and worsen over time.
The rest of the decision-making will be left to radiographic examination, which will better define the state of the tooth and, depending on the clinical findings to be considered for that tooth, will make the dentist choose an endodontic evaluation or wait.
In summary, the elements taken from classical literature[2, 4, 6] make us consider three parameters, namely:

1. clinical data
2. radiographic feedback
3. histological certification

The latter could undoubtedly testify the disease process in progress but, unfortunately, it is not practical except in cases where the endodontic surgery option is chosen. This aspect will be examined in Chapter 9. Therefore, two clinical aspects should be considered: the clinical scenario and/or the three-dimensional radiographic image.

History and informed consent

The diagnostic phase, before any medical or surgical intervention, is based on the collection of the patient's medical history. In surgical procedures, as endodontic procedures should be considered, the patient's history may be fundamental for establishing a diagnosis and the collection of information by the clinician should be as thorough as possible.
This series of information, which is crucial for obtaining a precise characterization of the disease, will have to be combined with other, equally fundamental, elements, in order to establish a correct treatment plan.
At this stage, the patient's expectations, the desire to preserve the affected teeth and the willingness to undergo treatments that require some time become fundamental.
It is not essential, but may be advisable, to explain to the patient the possible complications that can be encountered if the intervention fails; however, it will be necessary to obtain consent to act not only with regard to the strictly necessary endodontic maneuvers but also to be able to proceed with any alternative solutions.
One emblematic example is when it is impossible to obtain a good result with an endodontic treatment: if the patient has already been anesthetized, the clinician can proceed with the removal of the tooth without having to seek further consent from the patient. All these eventualities must be included and illustrated in an informed consent form, which must be signed by the patient and be prepared in compliance with local regulations.

Clinical examination

Each clinical examination must be preceded by a thorough medical history.
As in any medical procedure, anamnesis plays a fundamental role in understanding the clinical discomforts experienced by the patient, the attitude of the patient toward his teeth, and whether the timing of any retreatment is compatible with its availability.
Contact with the patient and contextualizing of the disease is fundamental[7].
Indeed, the most relevant elements must be established at an early stage, in order to alleviate the patient's pain or preventing it from occurring, if the finding of the periapical disease is incidental (further details will be provided later), is the first fundamental step towards establishing the therapeutic alliance required by complex procedures, such as those of retreatment.
In this regard, the scheme proposed by Friedman[8] is a good guide with which to proceed (Table 2.1).
Given the general conditions of the patient and the absolute contraindications to exploratory dental procedures in the presence of intercurrent systemic disease (see Chapter 1), treatment must start with a specific anamnesis linked to the tooth or the teeth presumably affected by the symptoms.
In these cases, not infrequently, the pain is non-specific, intermittent, and not always possible to locate with precision.
However, pain when chewing or at the mere contac in maximum intercuspation, that is clearly definable by the patient, or pain due to the position in the dental arch immediately leads to a suspicion of periapical disease of endodontic origin.
The patient's testimony is important for reconstructing the timing with which the symptoms developed; postoperative pain cannot be considered in the same way as pain that occurs some time after treatment or that has always accompanied an endodontic treatment performed more than 6 months previously.
The literature[9-12] defined a case in which the treatment was performed on a tooth that had a periapical disorder. In this case, an evolving periapical lesion can be reasonably suspected[5].
The elements obtained in the anamnestic phase must then be validated in the subsequent inspection phase, which is essential for completing the clinical examination that will precede the radiological phase.

Extraoral examination

An extraoral examination should always be carried out to identify swelling or lymph node reactions, which are often the first warning sign of inflammatory diseases of the teeth.

Table 2.1 **MEDICAL HISTORY-RELATED CONSIDERATIONS FOR CASE SELECTION**

	No	**Yes**
Patient's motivation to preserve the tooth	Extraction	Endodontic retreatment/ surgery
Patient's motivation to achieve the best long-term result	Endodontic surgery	Retreatment
Time issues	Retreatment	Endodontic surgery
Economic issues	Retreatment	Endodontic surgery

Source: Friedman S. *Considerations and concepts of case selection in the management of post-treatment endodontic disease (treatment failure)*. Endodontic Topics, 2002;1:54-78.

Extraoral palpation

Swelling

Swelling is typical of acute cases and permit a diagnosis at the mere sight of the patient; acute scenarios place emphasis on the seriousness of the pathological process underway and advise a careful assessment of the infected tooth. This complication does not always have to be considered as an unfavorable prognostic element, but it certainly arouses reservations regarding the type of treatment to be undertaken on this tooth. For the treatment of emergencies, the authors recommend consulting, in addition to Box 2.1, Chapter 6 and Box 1.3 on page 24.

Box 2.1 EMERGENCIES INVOLVING ACUTE EVENTS

Emergencies related to acute abscesses can take different forms, from simple swelling, to phlegmon, through to the most unfavorable situation affecting the whole body, with fever involving the entire organism with feverish rise and generalized sense of malaise.

Although rare, certain cases of negative developments putting the patient's health at risk are described in the literature. Pharmacological therapy involves the use of broad-spectrum antibiotics at appropriate doses (see Chapter 6).

Non-steroidal anti-inflammatory drugs, such as ibuprofen at doses of over 400 mg, with or without paracetamol 1000 mg, may be helpful. Abscess drainage may also be useful in order to prevent complications and speed up the resolution of the acute condition. Once the septic situation is under control, the diagnostic–prognostic procedure concerning the tooth involved can be resumed, bearing in mind that the acute episode must guide the choice of therapy.

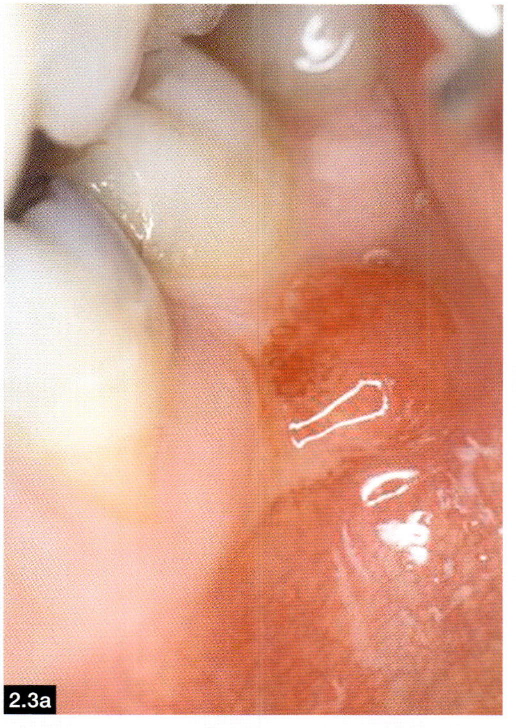

2.3a

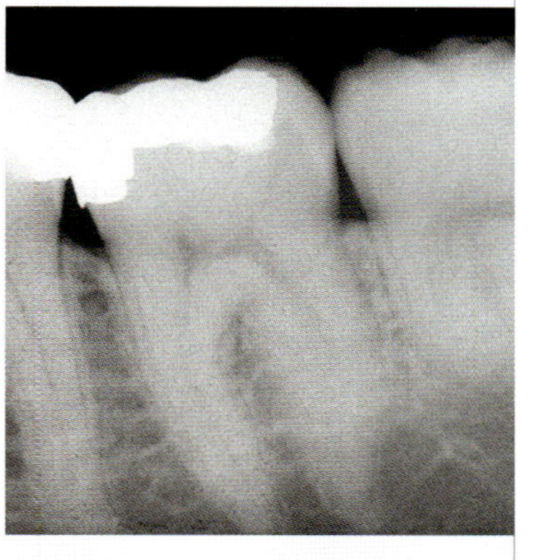

Fig. 2.3a: A sample taken in the area of 37 suggests septic involvement of the endodontium. A thorough medical history and a proper clinical examination suggest the involvement of 38 secondary to overt dysodontiasis.

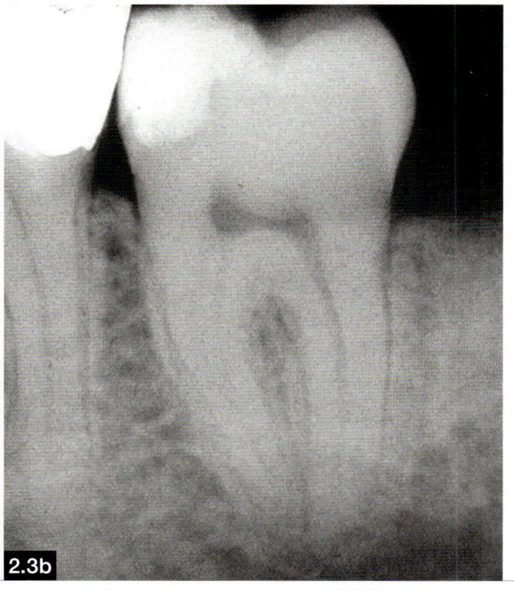

2.3b

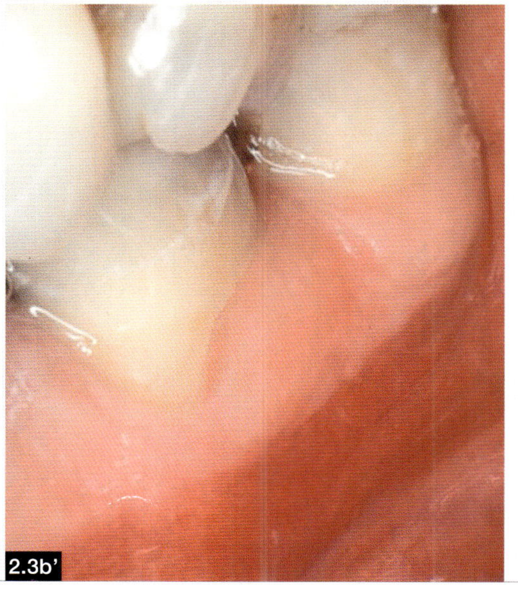

2.3b'

Fig. 2.3b-3b': The extraction of 38 leads to the resolution of the septic process and the implication of the distal mandibular alveolar bone at 37.

Skin fistulas

Skin fistulas are rare in modern times. This condition was more frequent in the past, probably because people less frequently underwent dental treatment. They are often mistaken for dermatological manifestations and usually persist over time, generating significant bone lesions.

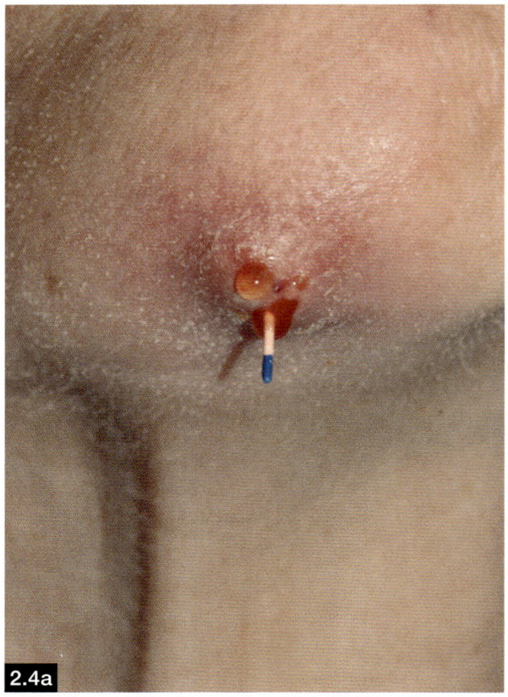

Fig. 2.4a: Suppurative skin fistula in a patient over 70 years old, with a gutta-percha cone inserted.

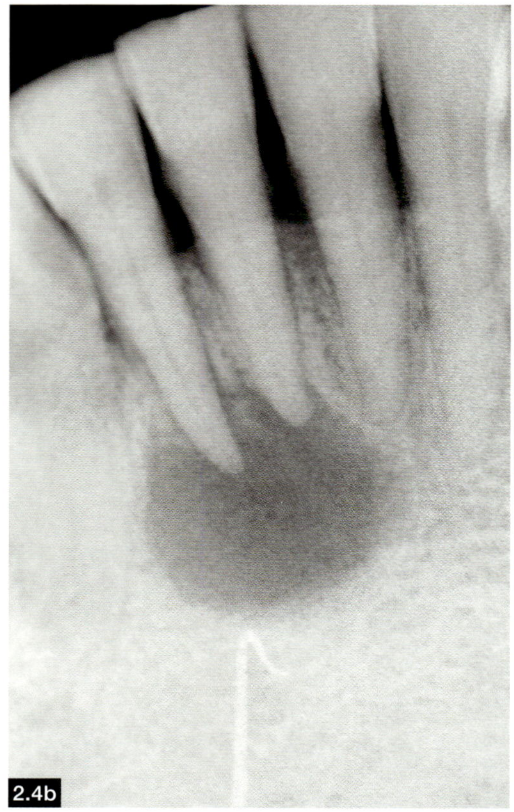

Fig. 2.4b: Two-dimensional radiographic image of a large rarefying lesion at the load of 31, having had them withdrawn the vitality with thermal tests.

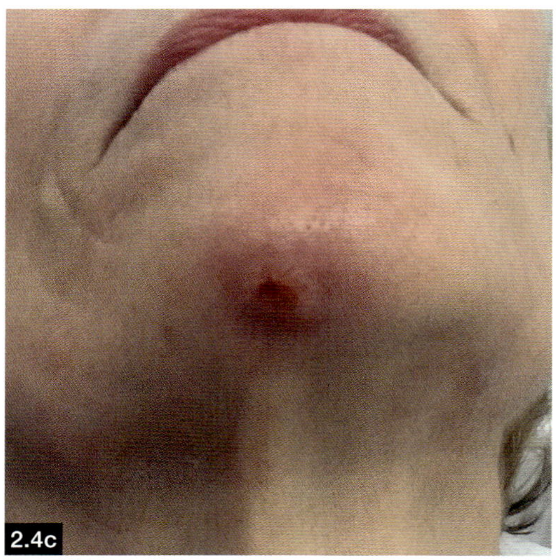

Fig. 2.4c: Same injury after 6 months.

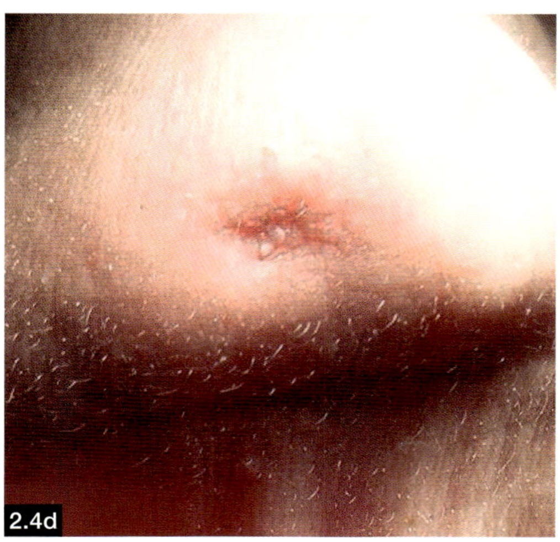

Fig. 2.4d: The therapeutic choice was that of the extraction because of lingual probing exceeding 10 mm. The fistula is regressing, but a large skin lesion is still present.

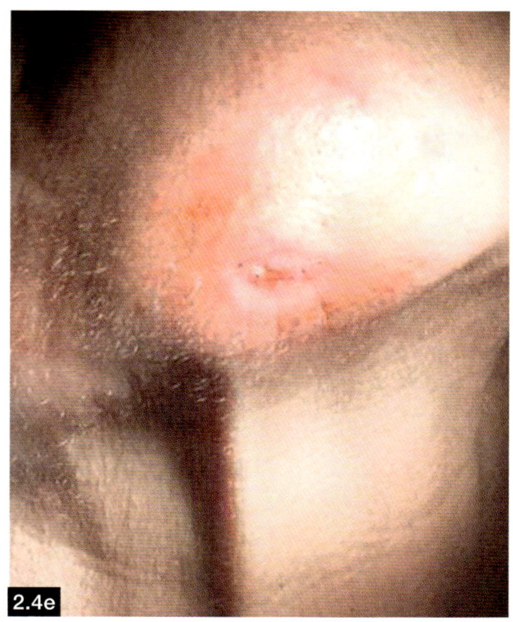

Fig. 2.4e: Skin lesion after 2 months.

Intra-oral inspection

Observation of deficient restorations

The finding of inadequately sealed restorations can be considered a warning. Several studies have documented the extent to which an inadequate restoration can be conducive to bacterial contamination of the root canal and periapical tissues.
In this sense, clinical analysis through a scrupulous systematic review of the literature is necessary[13].

Observation of missing restorations

The lack of restorations can also be predictive of endodontic periapical lesions.
Ricucci et al.[14, 15] highlighted that the gutta-percha seal, although exposed to oral fluids, is sufficient for preventing bacterial aggression; however, periradicular lesions of endodontic origin are common in teeth without complete restorations.

Fistulas

Fistulas can have varying characteristics: from a simple orifice of the vestibular mucosa, more rarely in the palatine area in the upper teeth and lingual area in the lower, to a hypertrophic evagination.
Pus often comes out of the fistula, either spontaneously or after vestibular acupressure. A fistula that drains spontaneously or otherwise is often prognostically unfavorable because this sign is linked to periapical infections sustained by bacteria that have colonized the root surface and therefore can only be eliminated with surgical procedures.

Swelling

Less frequently than with a fistula, a tooth with periradicular disease may present with visible swelling.
The observation can be supported by the subsequent periapical palpatory examination. After making an exploratory flap, tooth extraction due to a fracture is performed to determine the quality and position of the lesion.

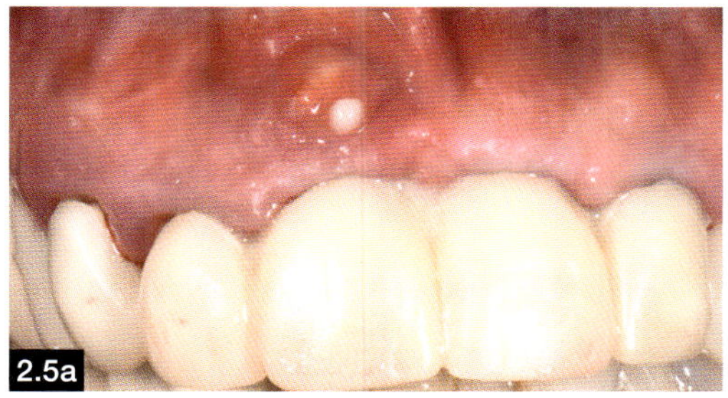

Fig. 2.5a: Supporting vestibular fistula: a low location suggests periodontal involvement.

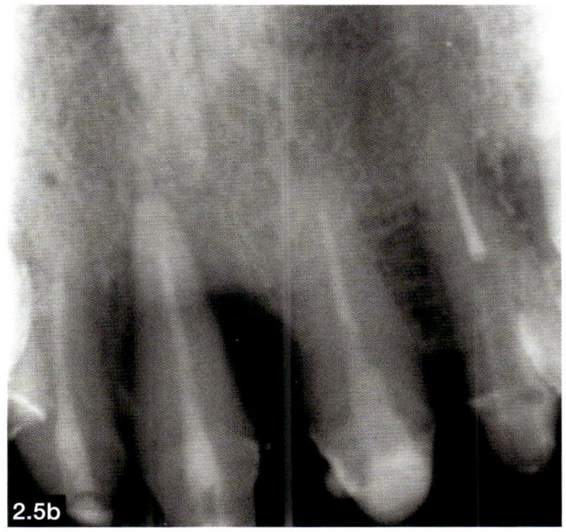

Fig. 2.5b: X-ray image showing deep bone resorption.

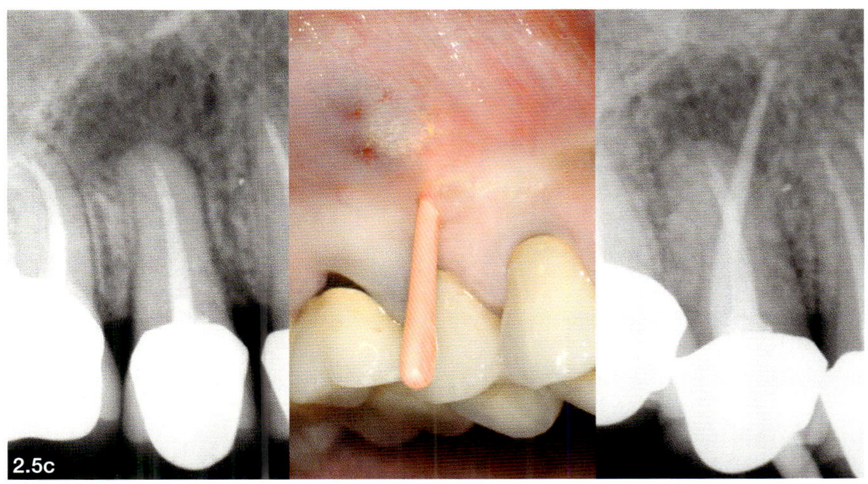

Fig. 2.5c: Examination with endodontic radiography followed by the examination of the fistula to precisely analyze the cause of the disease; in this case, doubt remains.

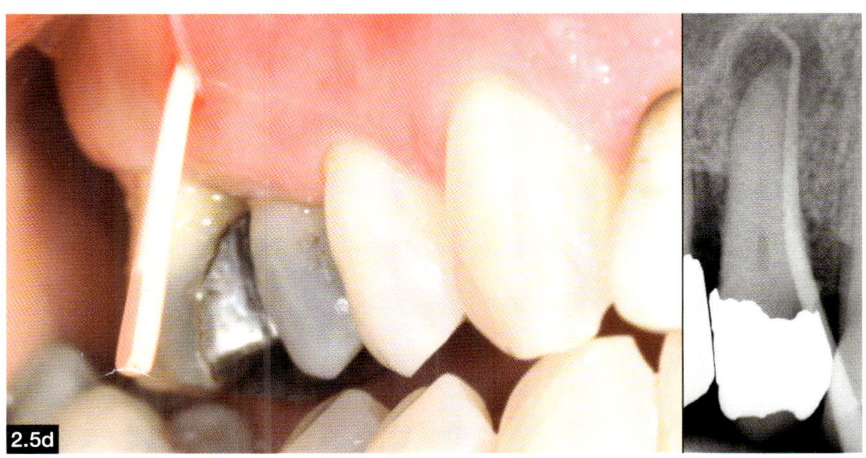

Fig. 2.5d: Image identical to the previous one but in which an obvious indication is given by the gutta-percha cone.

▶ *continue to page 84*

CASE REPORT 1

Abnormal closure of upper premolar

As mentioned repeatedly, the teeth should be carefully examined during the intraoral inspection; in this specific case, the patient reported severe pain when chewing on tooth no. 24. Visually, the tooth had a composite reconstruction with two strange pins that were difficult to consider root canal posts.

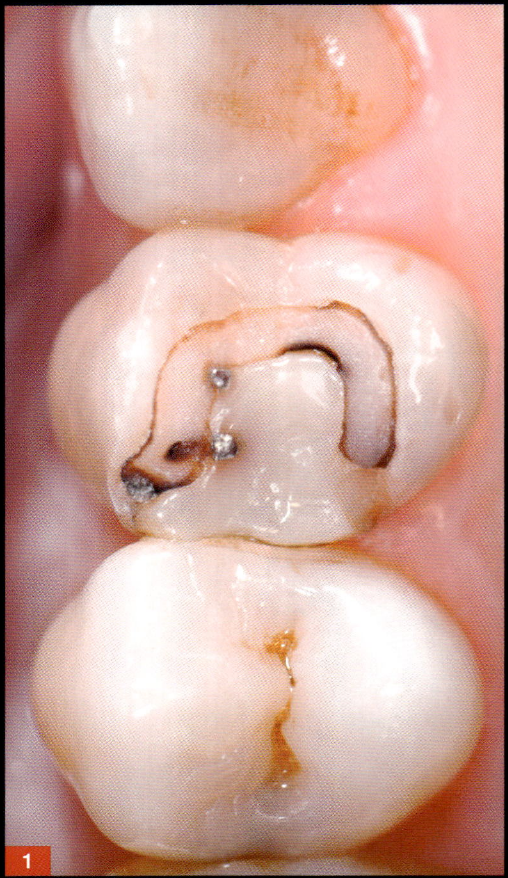

Figure 1: Visual inspection of teeth no. 23, 24, and 25; in no. 24 note the two small metal marks in the composite material.

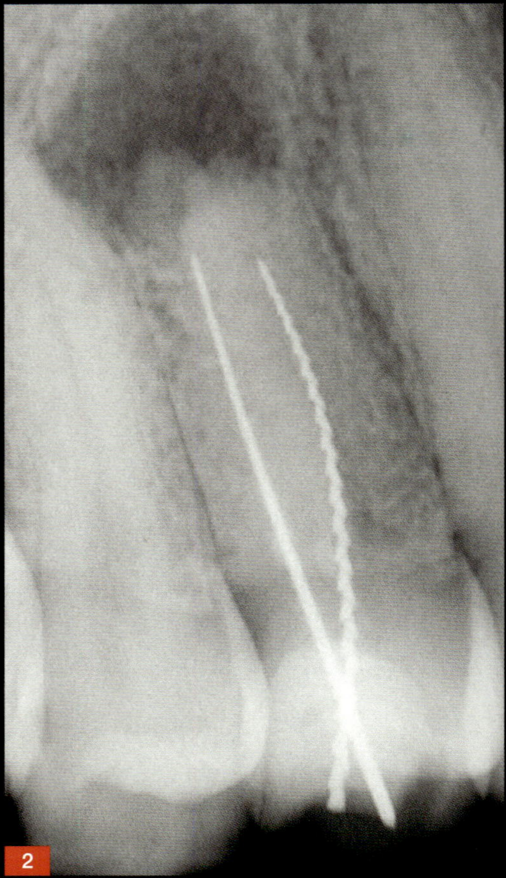

Figure 2: Radiographic examination certifying the presence of two endodontic instruments (Hedström file) intentionally broken at the entrance to the access cavity. The radiolucent periapical lesion is larger than 7 mm.

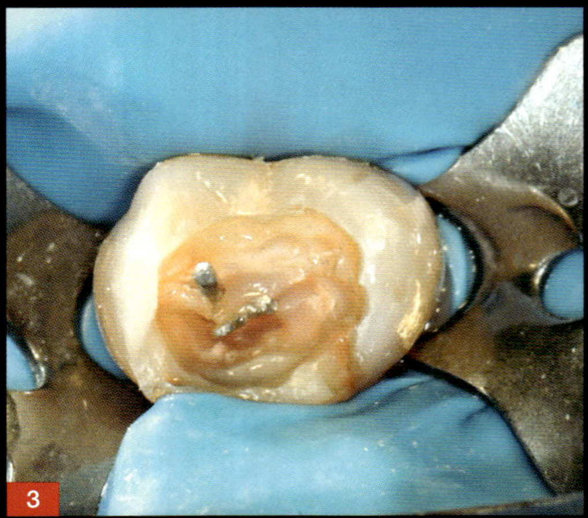

Figure 3: The first phase of opening the coronal access exposes the head of the instruments.

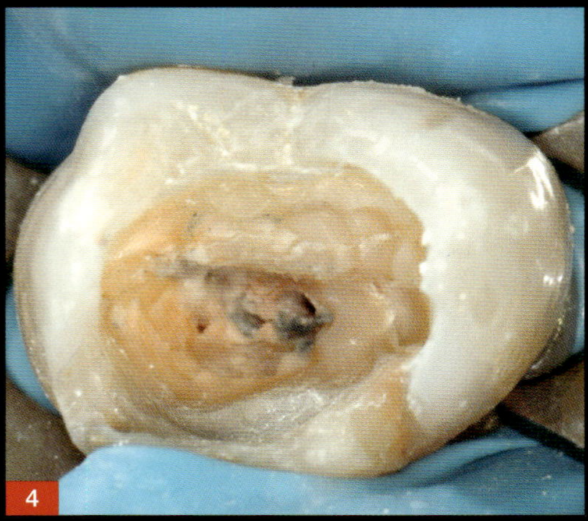

Figure 4: The bottom of the pulp chamber is severely calcified.

The X-ray examination revealed two root canal instruments, deliberately used as endodontium closure systems. A clear, radiolucent lesion was seen at the apex of the tooth.
The procedures for freeing the endodontium of the obstructions were not easy,
and the filling of the root canals also involved a slight extrusion of the material. The longitudinal controls have defined the success of the treatment about 6 years after the intervention.

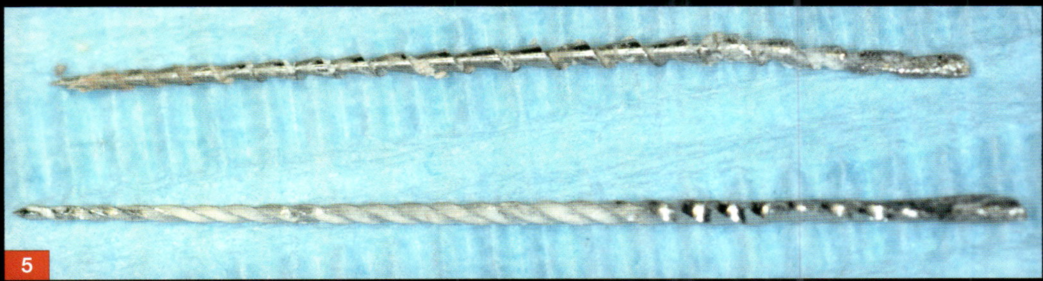

Figure 5: The two instruments (Hedström file and a k-file) extracted from the canals without fractures.

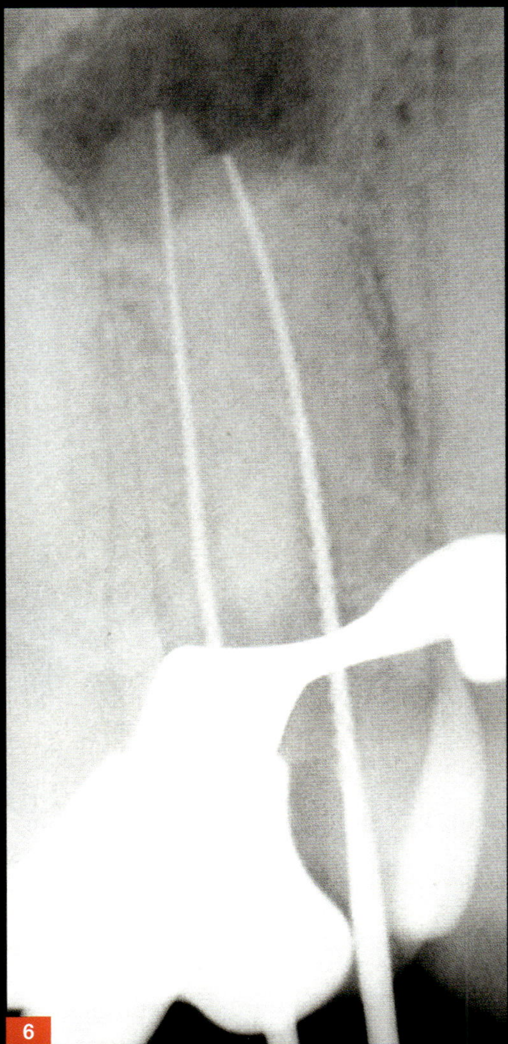

Figure 6: The X-ray of the working length.

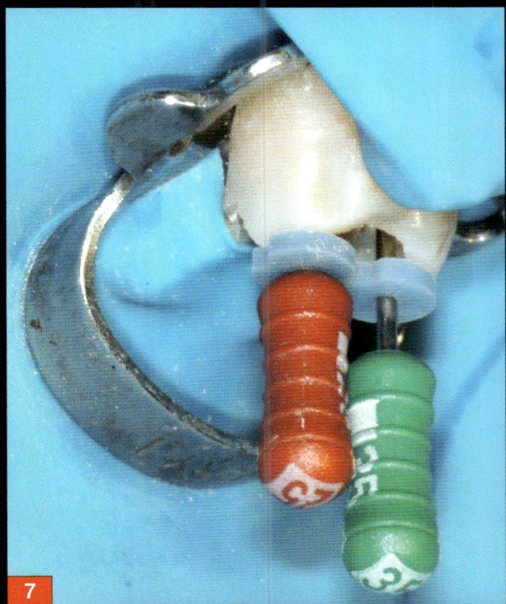

Figure 7: The two instruments inserted in the root canals certify different dimensions at apical level.

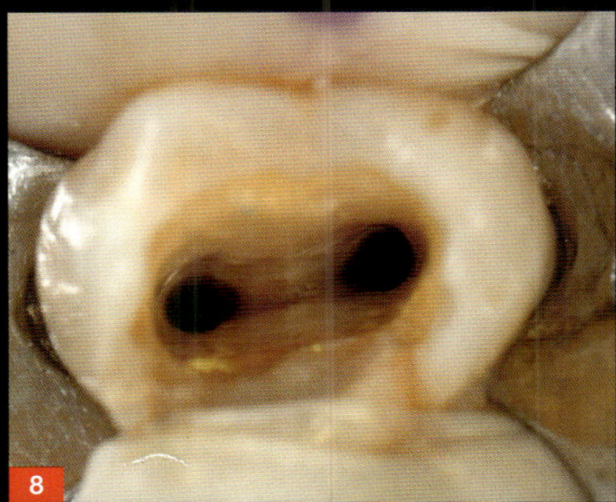

Figure 8: The canals are perfectly shaped; note the difference to image 4.

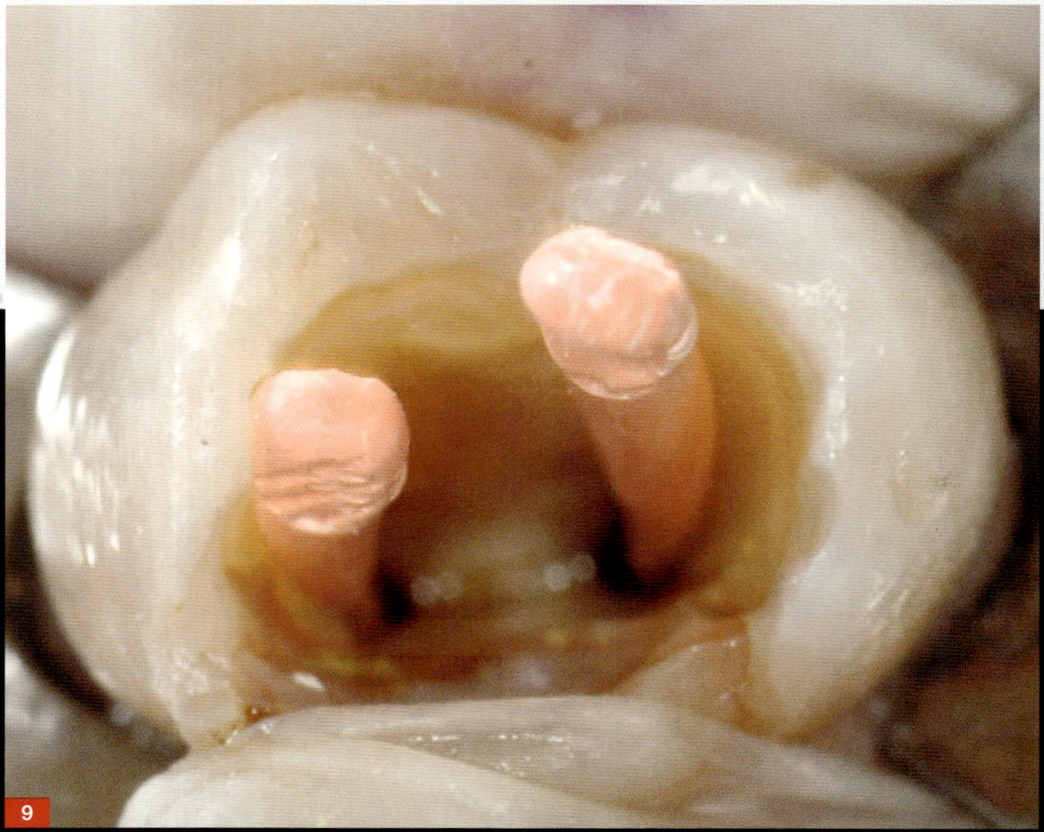

Figure 9: The two gutta-percha cones adapted inside the root canals.

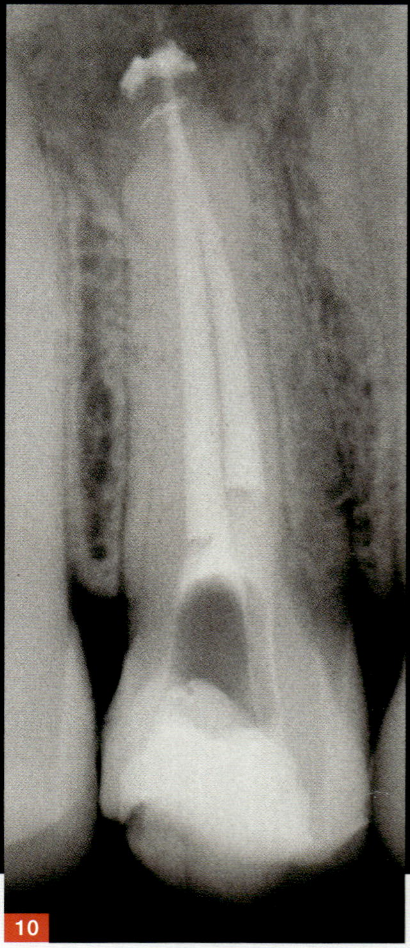

Figure 10: Closure of the endodontic space; note the slight overfill.

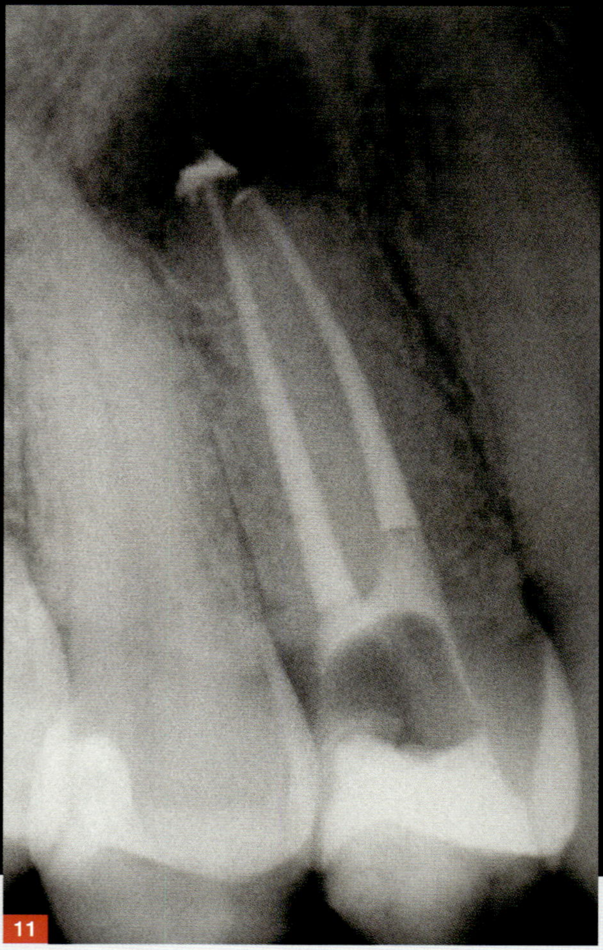

Figure 11: The same closure from another angle highlighting the two different apical outlets.

The various stages of healing. As shown, about six years have elapsed between 12 and image 16. The time required for a lesion of this magnitude to regress completely is very variable and each radiograph, if considered individually, could be considered a failure.
In actual fact, the clinical situation and the patient's symptoms always reassured the dentist and, at the end of the process, the bony structure was reorganized around the root apexes, once again enclosing them, as if it were an intact tooth.

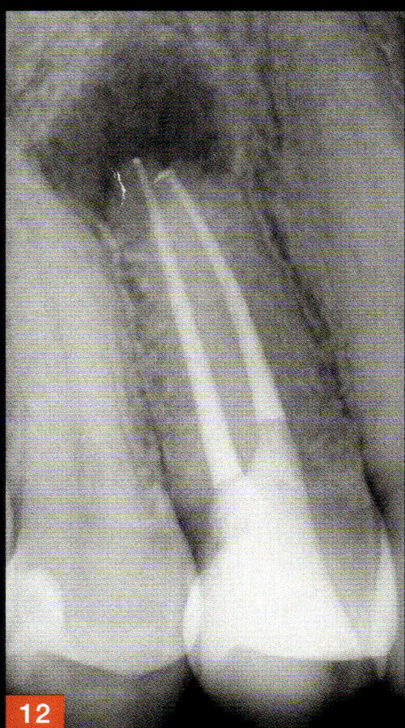

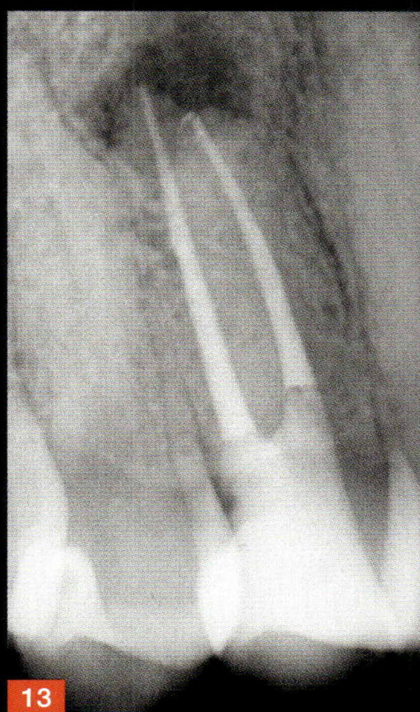

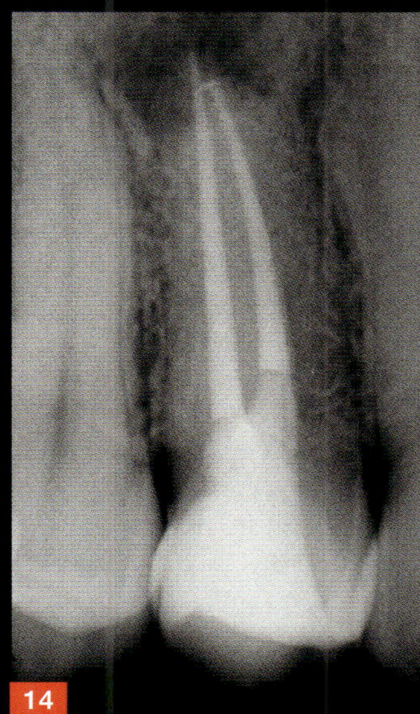

Figure 12: Follow-up x-ray 1 month after treatment.

Figure 13: Follow-up x-ray 6 months after treatment.

Figure 14: Follow-up x-ray 6 months after treatment with different projections to the x-ray in Figure 13.

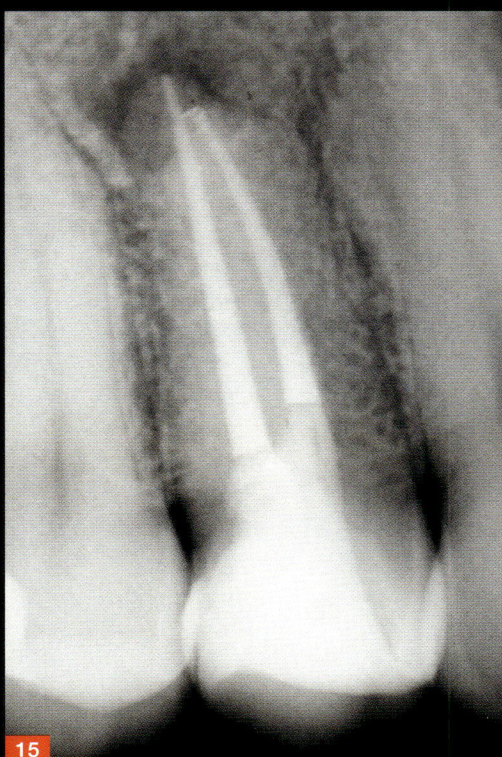

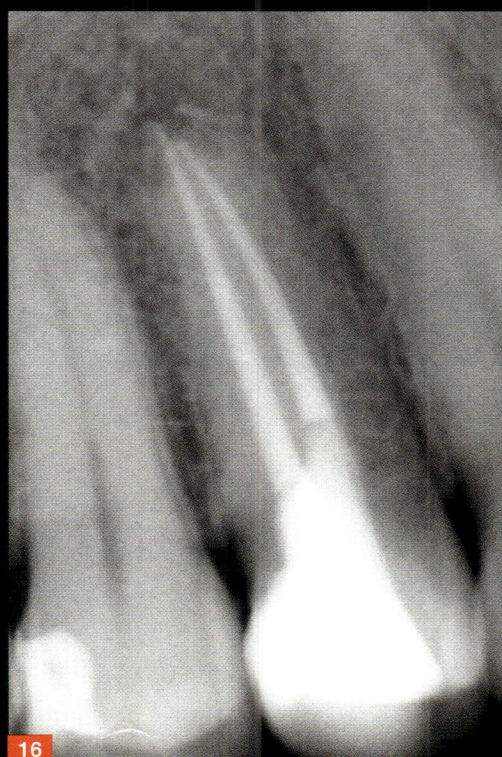

Figure 15: Follow-up x-ray 1 year after treatment.

Figure 16: Follow-up x-ray 6 years after treatment.

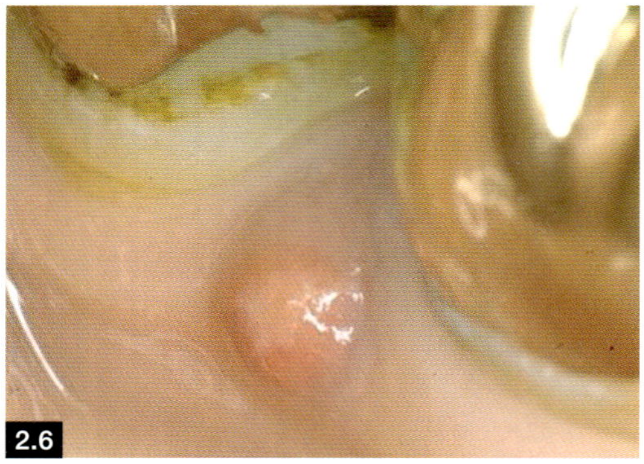

Fig. 2.6: Example of a fistula with an interdental position; as the location is often misleading, this type of fistula must be investigated with the insertion of a gutta-percha cone that gives an idea of the origin of the infection.

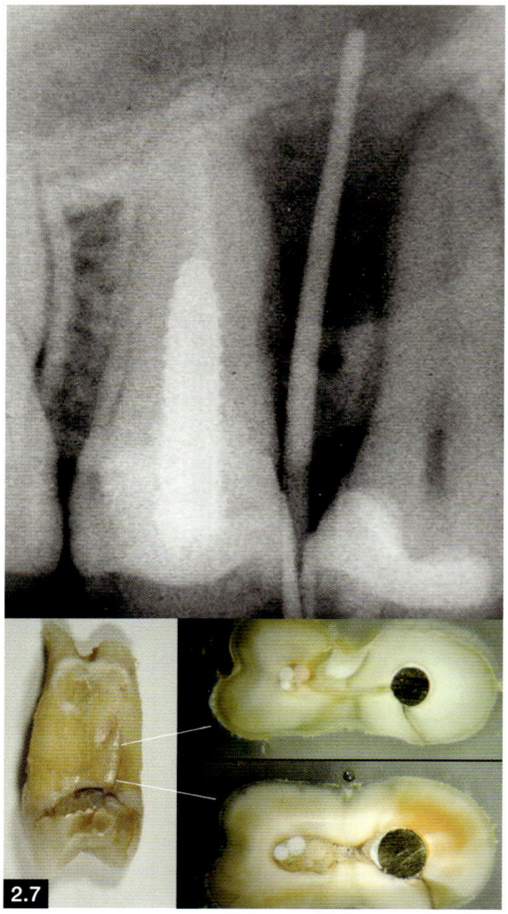

Fig. 2.7: Example of a fistulograph, i.e., a radiograph with a gutta-percha cone inserted, which should identify to the lesion site. The picture remains uncertain.

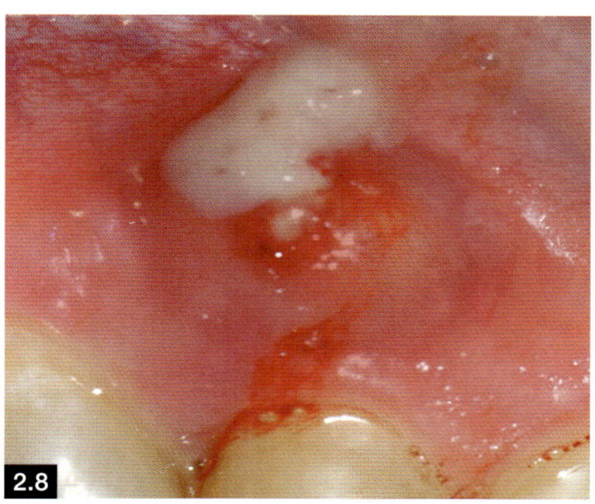

Fig. 2.8: Suppurative periapical fistula; this uncommon situation is often connected to and fed by a periapical lesion full of bacteria proliferating on the root surfaces, and therefore refractory to endodontic treatment.

A high risk of fracture should be considered in teeth with root canal posts, particularly of the screwed metal type.

Intra-oral instrumental examination

This second phase, which is not always separated from the previous one, is important for outlining the most relevant prognostic factors from a clinical point of view.

Pulp vitality tests

In the absence of an X-ray examination to evaluate pulp vitality, it must be determined whether the target tooth or teeth have undergone alterations to the endodontic tissue, especially when these teeth have already been treated. A detailed description of the vitality tests, whether thermal, hot or cold, electrical, or with other more sophisticated systems, will not be given in this text. These tests must be carried out when periapical disease of endodontic origin is suspected.

Palpation

Passing a finger over the alveolar area of the teeth affected by periapical disease can cause pain. As mentioned previously, swelling can be observed, and is almost always the expression of chronic inflammatory events of the tissues surrounding the dental root. The palpation of the periradicular vestibular regions often reveals provoked pain, which can be a crucial element in the diagnosis of periapical disease after endodontic treatment.

Circumferential probing

Beyond the periodontal considerations mentioned above, testing the periodontal tissue is an important clinical diagnostic maneuver. A "tubular" probing, that is, a single part of the circumference of the gingival collar, is a negative prognostic sign. Indeed, it is frequently associated with vertical fractures of the root, conditions that are currently unsolvable, and not always easy to diagnose, but fatal for the affected tooth. These conditions must be intercepted in time because they often lead to significant bone loss, making a subsequent implant solution impracticable.

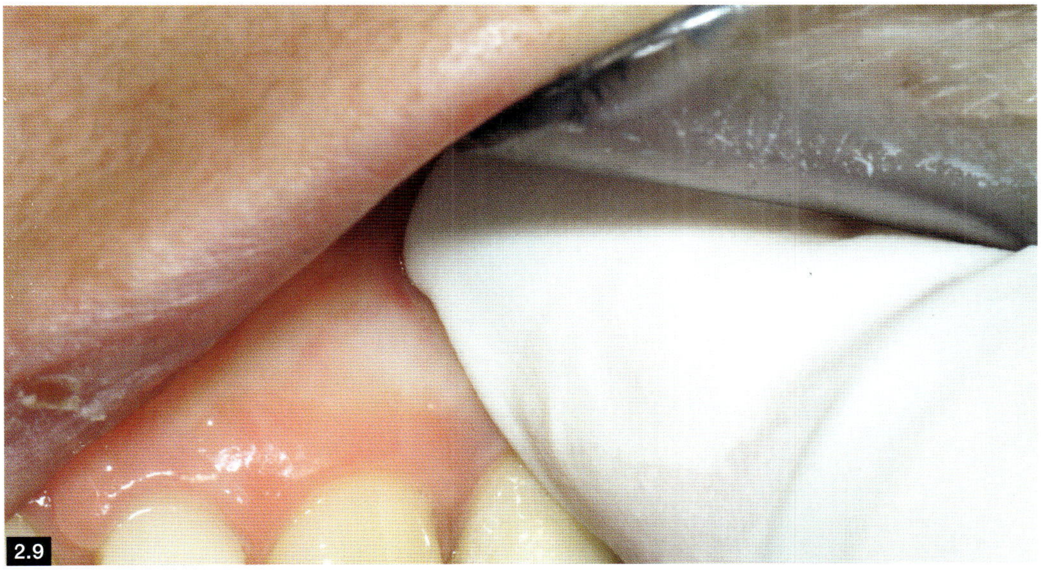

2.9

Fig. 2.9: Palpation of the apex; this maneuver shows the periradicular contour of the teeth; a bump, which may be painful, may be observed near the apex of the tooth concerned.

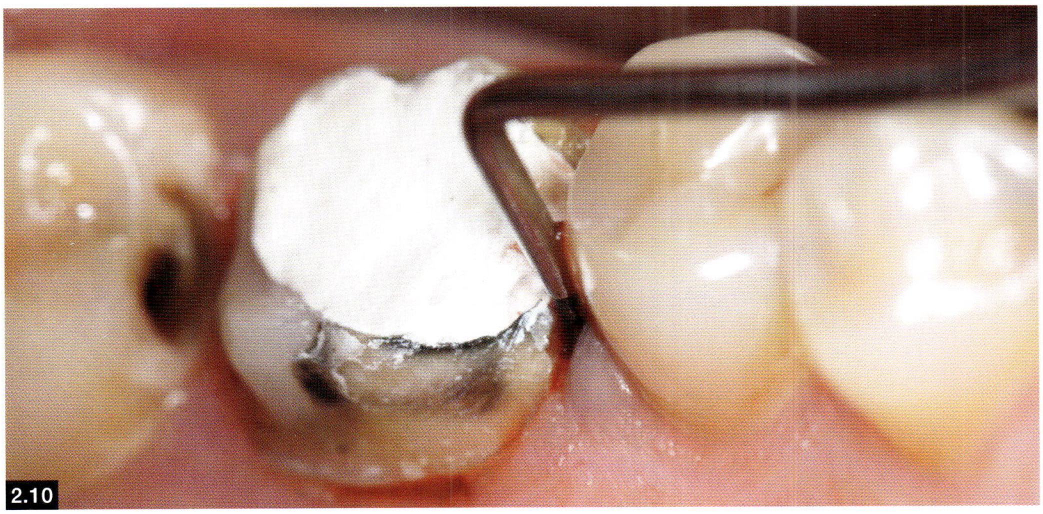

2.10

Fig. 2.10: Circumferential probing is fundamental in the diagnostic phase; spot probing.
Deep probing that is radically different to that observed along the entire circumference of the tooth is often suggestive of longitudinal root fracture.

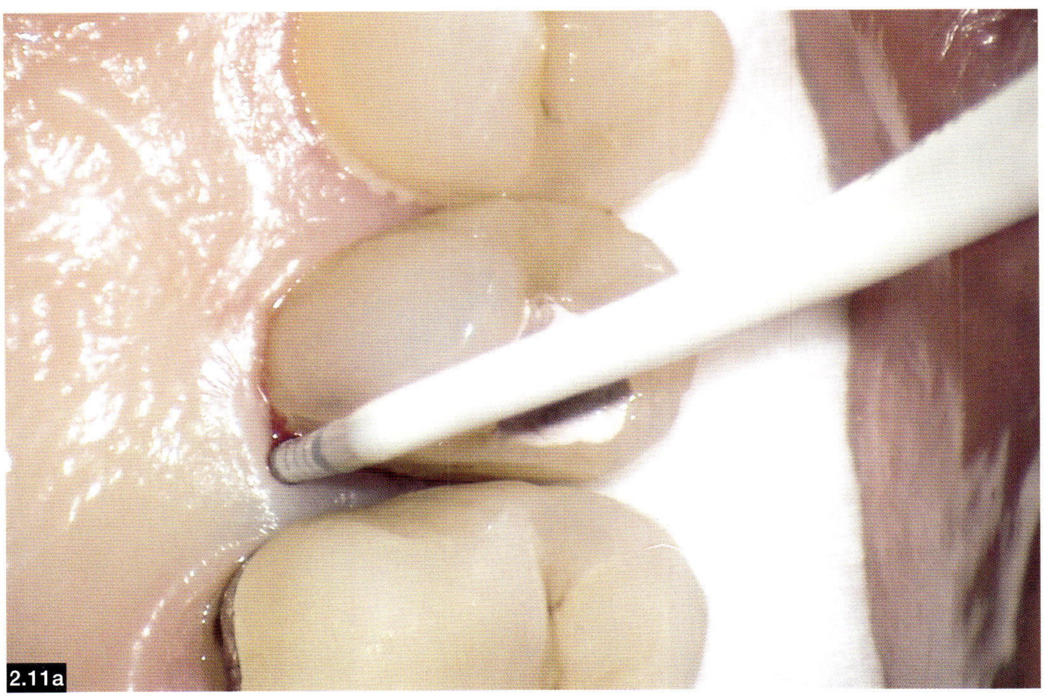

2.11a

Fig. 2.11a: The clinical examination reveals the presence of distal deep probing, which was confirmed on the radiographic examination by distal bone loss.

Fig. 2.11b: Inspection of the root surface under microscopic magnification excludes the presence of a vertical fracture. An intrasulcular fistula was diagnosed, and it was decided to proceed with retreatment.

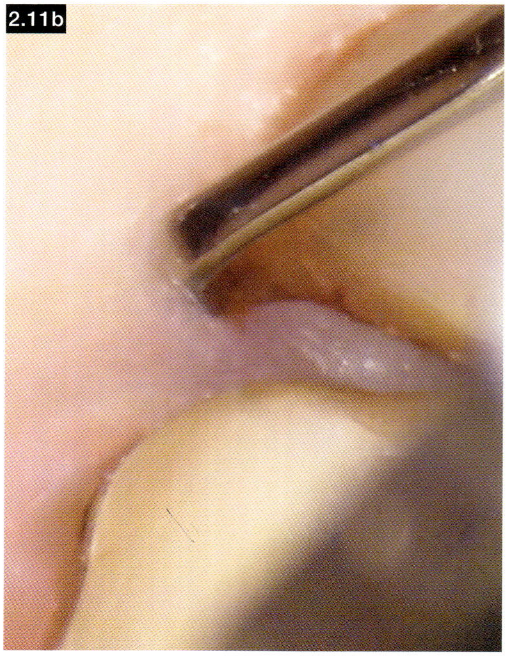

Fig. 2.11c: Canal closure shows the presence of a lateral canal (in the area left empty by the previous treatment; see Fig. 1.11a) communicating with the area of bone thinning.

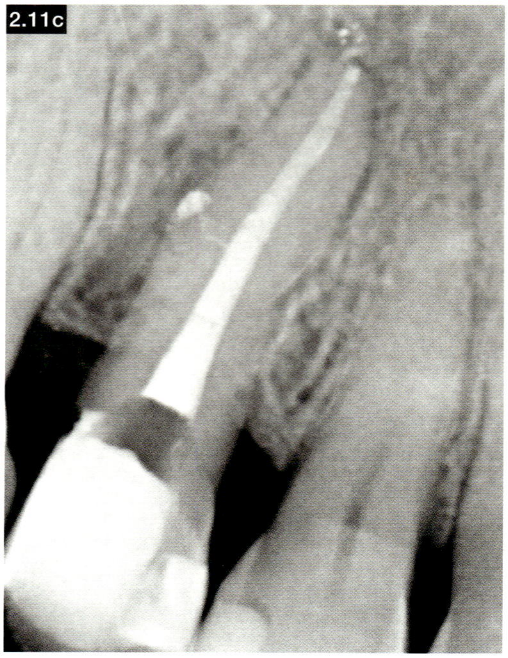

Fig. 2.11d: Airtight closure of the endodontium and disappearance of the symptoms as well as a tangible improvement in the radiographic situation allow us to consider treatment a success and confirm the correctness of the diagnostic and therapeutic procedures.

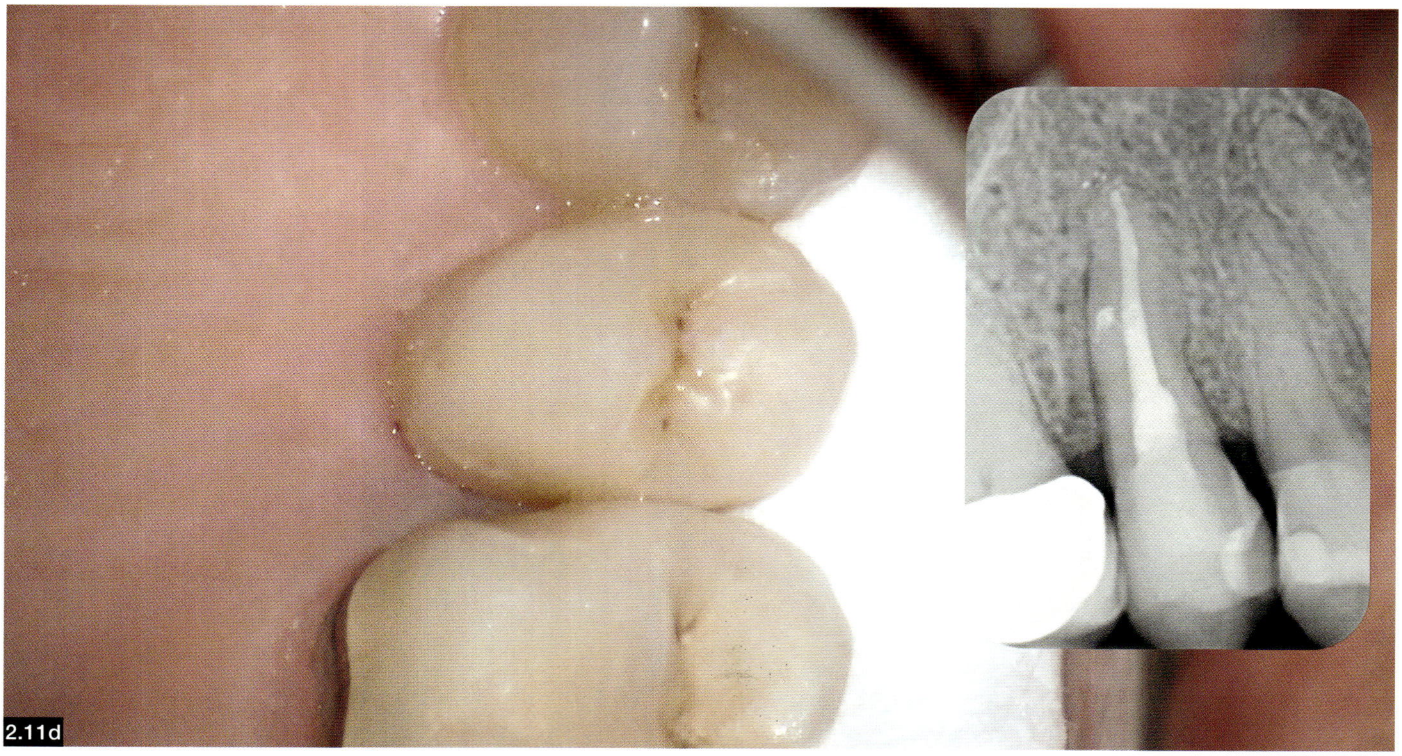

CASE REPORT 2

Upper lateral incisor with periapical lesion and fistula

A fistula at the distal apical area of tooth no. 22 immediately gives rise to the suspicion of a periapical lesion of endodontic origin in a tooth with a prosthetic crown. The endodontic reconstruction treatment was performed in a single appointment, because the tooth is in an area with a high esthetic value.

▶ *continues on page 88*

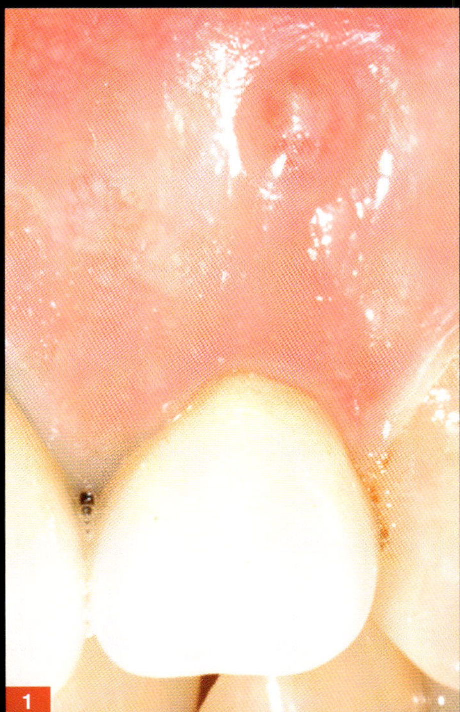

Figure 1: Frontal view of tooth no. 22 with an overt fistula in the periapical area.

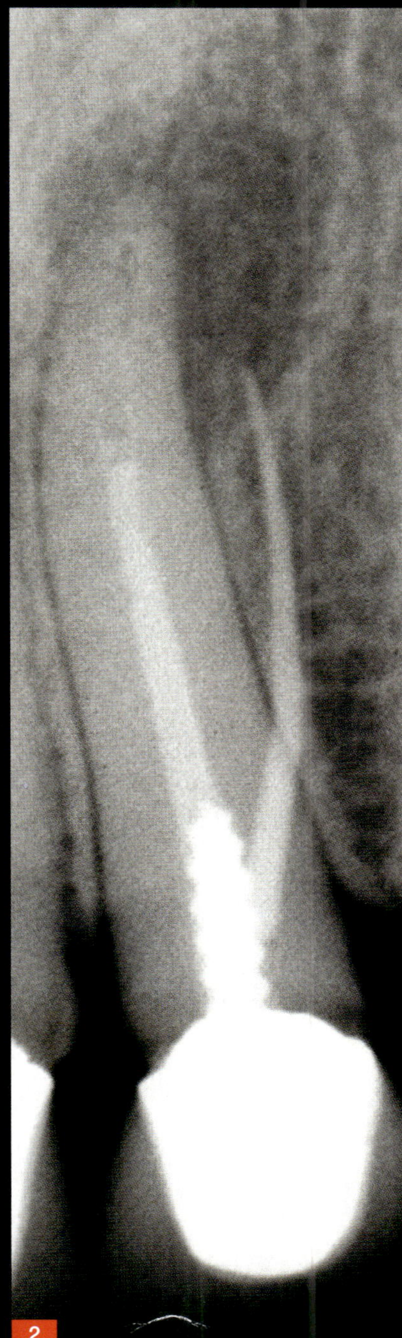

Figure 2: Radiograph with the inserted cone; the radiolucent lesion leaves no doubt about the endodontic origin of the lesion. It is interesting to note that a screw-retained root canal post complicates the endodontic access.

Figure 3: The gutta-percha cone inserted into the fistula to observe the origin of the lesion.

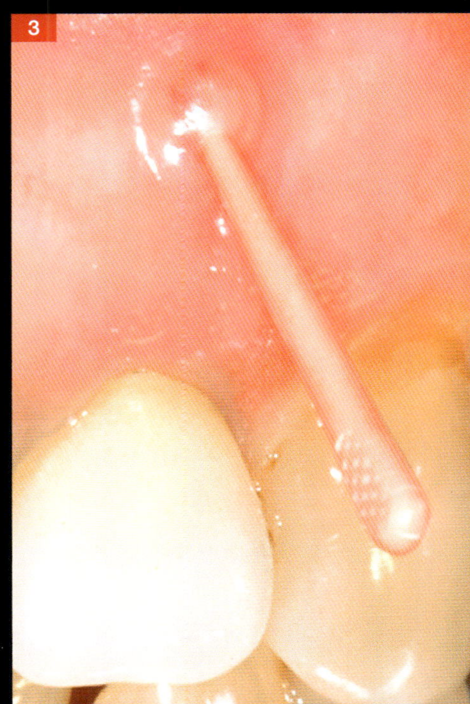

Figures 4 and 5: The post became visible once the crown had been removed and was subsequently unscrewed.

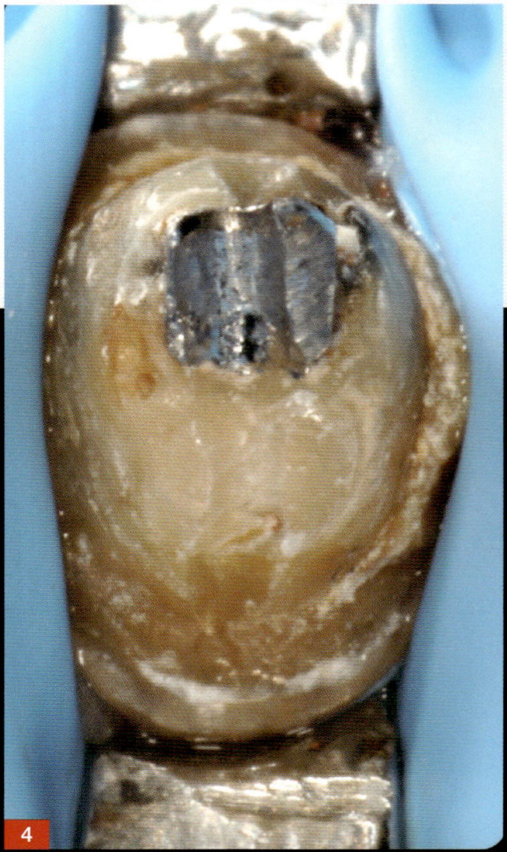

4

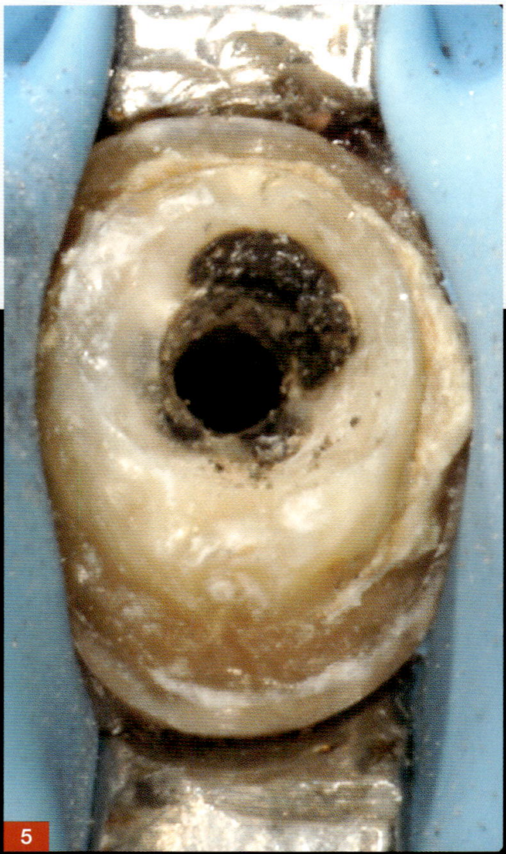

5

Figure 6: The new path inside the root canal that, as often happens in the upper lateral, has a distal curvature that will slightly complicate the shaping maneuvers.

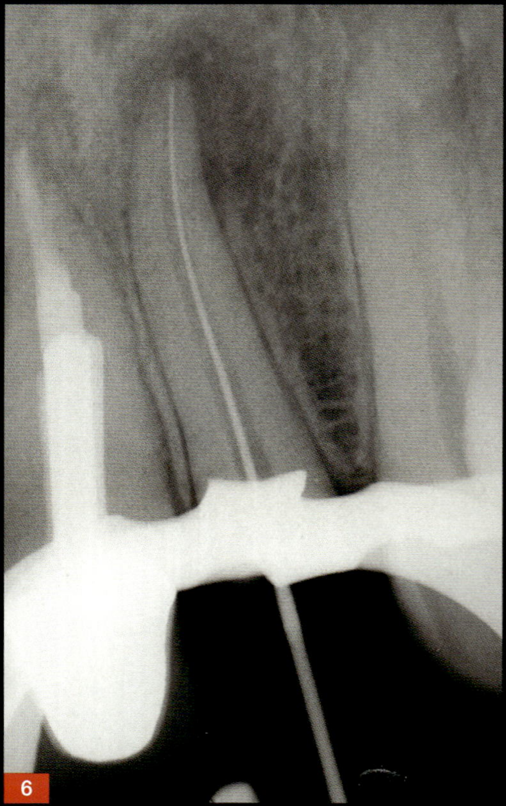

6

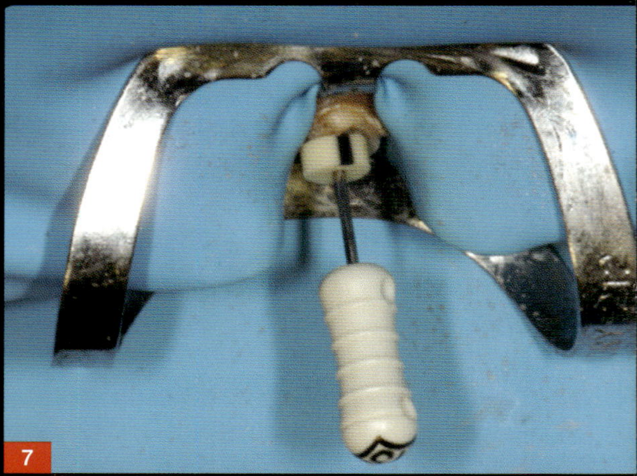

7

Figure 7: The tool inserted to validate, through the electronic apex detector, the path of the new instruments.

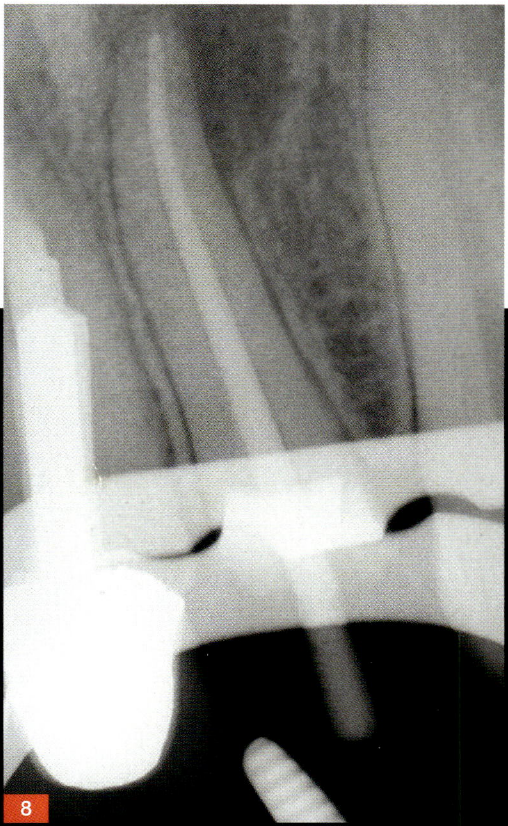

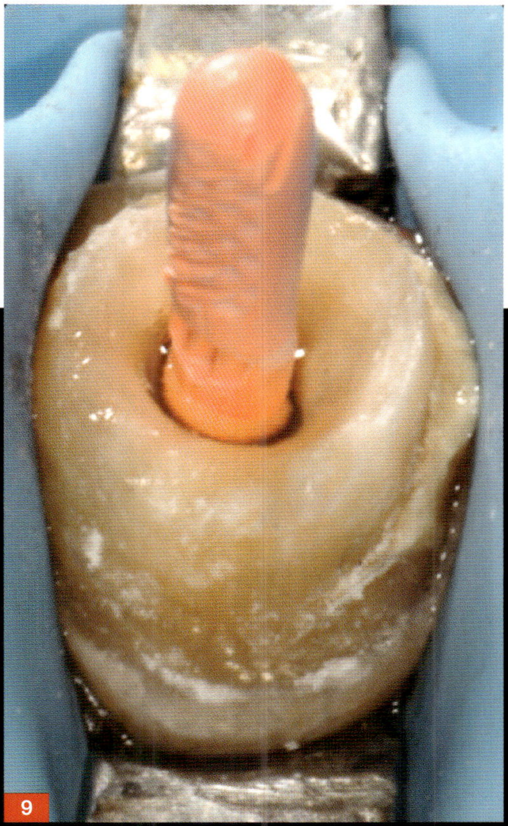

Figure 8: The gutta-percha cone test.

Figure 9: The cone fits snugly against the walls; respecting the working length and the length of the truncated cone system will be fundamental for obtaining a perfect filling of the endodontium.

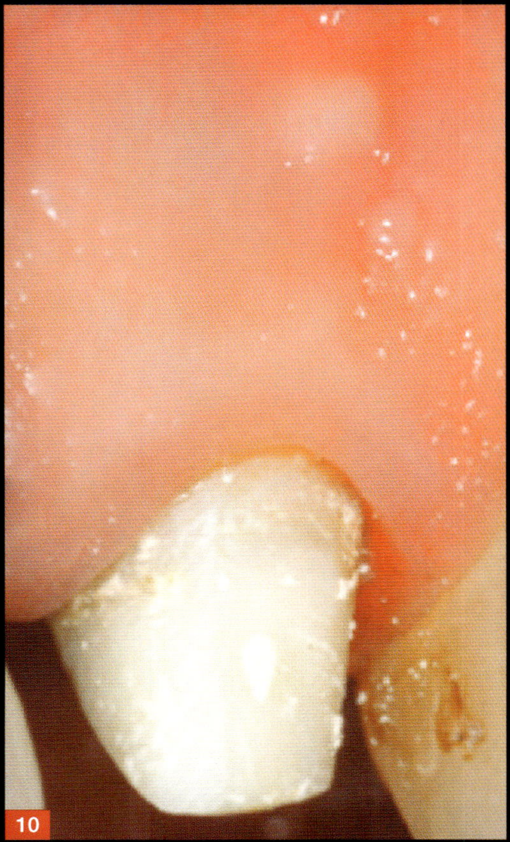

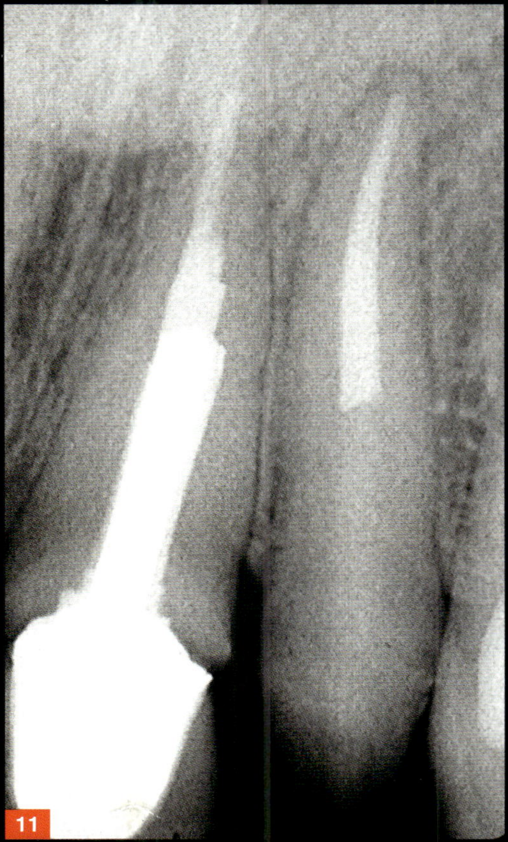

Figure 10: The shrunken fistula leaves a fibrous scar.

Figure 11: The success of the treatment and the disappearance of the radiolucent lesion, a sign of a reaction of the surrounding bone tissue, which is desirable in all cases of treatment but not always achieved in cases like these.

Percussion

The vertical percussion of the tooth suspected of having a periapical lesion reveals – although it was not reported by the patient in the medical history collection phase – pain that can be moderate or severe, when compared with that the same maneuver causes on a nearby or contralateral tooth not affected by this disease.

Clinical tests can also be performed, such chewing on a cotton roll that, not infrequently, can reveal non-remediable dental fractures (Figs. 2.12 and 2.13).

Mobility

Testing dental mobility always presupposes a suspicion of involvement of the periodontal structure, whether it is direct due to a condition specific to the periodontium or mediated by a strongly destructive evolution of the periodontium by the residual intraradicular infection.

Mobility patterns are always associated, except for the acute phases, with serious pathological situations that would advise against complex endodontic retreatment.

Fig. 2.12: The percussion test is often conclusive if neighboring teeth are affected by the same disease; pain on percussion is a characteristic sign of the involvement of periapical tissue.

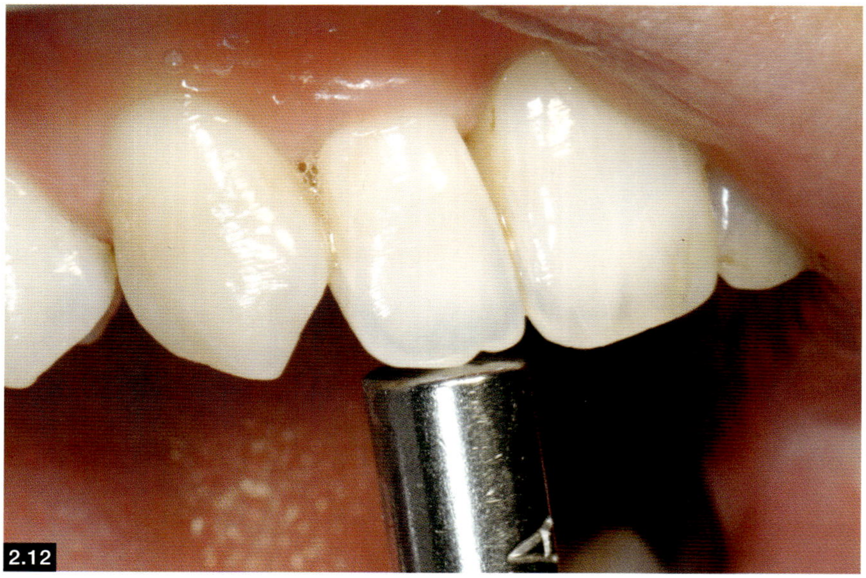

Clinical examination

Clinical examination remains important in the diagnostic phase because it makes it possible to consider the tooth affected by periapical disease in a broader context; in these cases, the radiological diagnosis, which will be discussed below, is decisive. The information collected during the anamnestic phase and the clinical tests, as well as the observation of the clinical status, is essential for formulating the diagnosis and defining a prognosis that, as reported by many data from literature[11], is strongly mediated by the patient's status, the location of the tooth in the arch the type of restoration, and its future functional destination, among others.

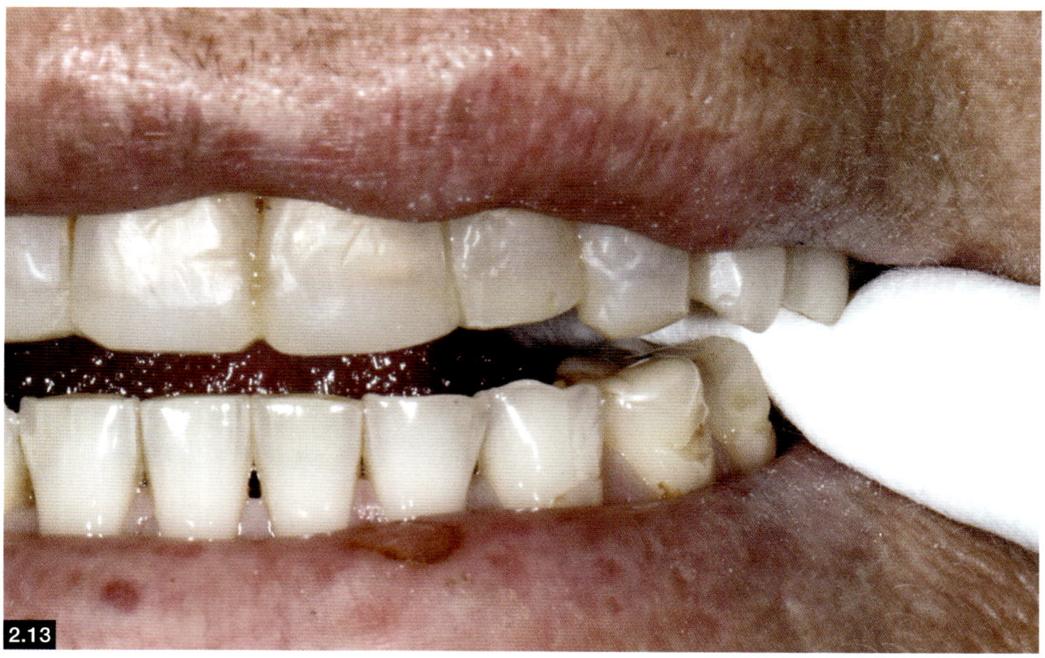

Fig. 2.13: Inserting a cotton roll between the dental arches and clenching the teeth is recommended for a patient suspected of having a more or less extensive root lesion, often a fracture.

Radiology

Radiographic examination is essential in the diagnosis of endodontic periapical diseases. The careful observation of a two-dimensional radiogram is fundamental for an infinite series of elements that can be deduced from the black-and-white image.

Endodontic X-ray

The easiest way to identify a periapical disease is radiographic examination (Fig. 2.14a-b). It is conducted electively through the use of endodontic radiographs with several projections that are rigorously centered by dedicated plate holders.
In a multiradicular tooth, the use of multiple images aims to accurately discern which of the roots is responsible for the periapical pain. However, the identification of disease with this type of examination is not always precise. Indeed, as was well described over fifty years ago by Bender and Seltzer[16], an absence of involvement of the cortical bone in the destructive process caused by the periapical granulomatous reaction makes the lesion "invisible" radiographically, and it can only be supposed through a detailed examination of the periradicular contour, where the lack of the periradicular radiotransparency continuity would provide a first sign of a disruption of the periodontal ligament, a fundamental clinical indication for establishing the onset of an inflammatory disease of the tissues that support the tooth that originates from the endodontum.
When the cortical bone is also involved, the radiotransparency will be evident. Thus, it must be considered to be larger than shown on the radiographic image.
The size of the lesion has significant diagnostic and prognostic values, providing the dentist with the information needed to identify the type of treatment to be carried out, as we will see later.

2.14a

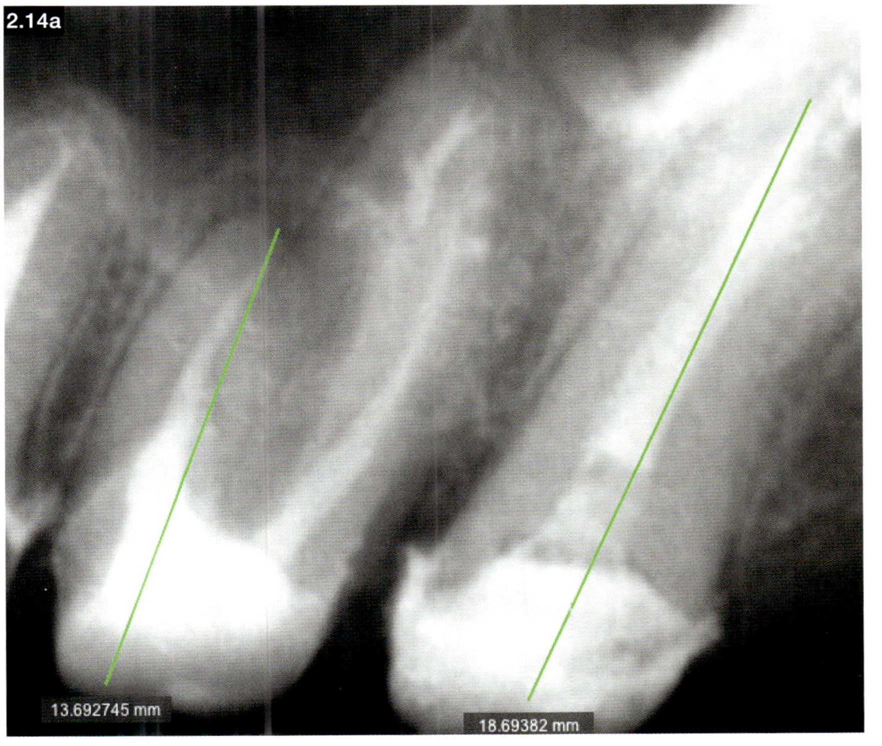

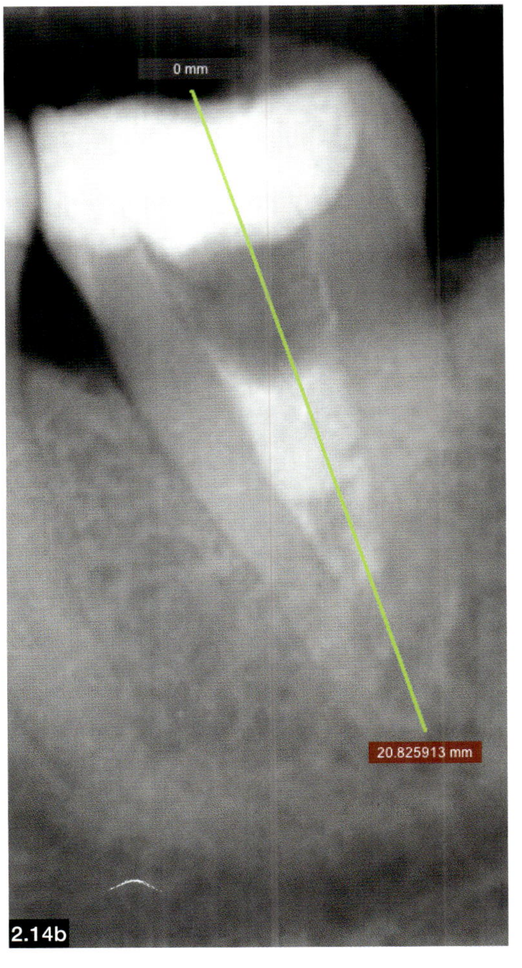

2.14b

Fig. 2.14a-b: The two-dimensional x-ray examination can be digital; as such, it can be enhanced by further information, such as the measurement of canal lengths.

Box 2.2 **RADIOLOGICAL TECHNIQUES**

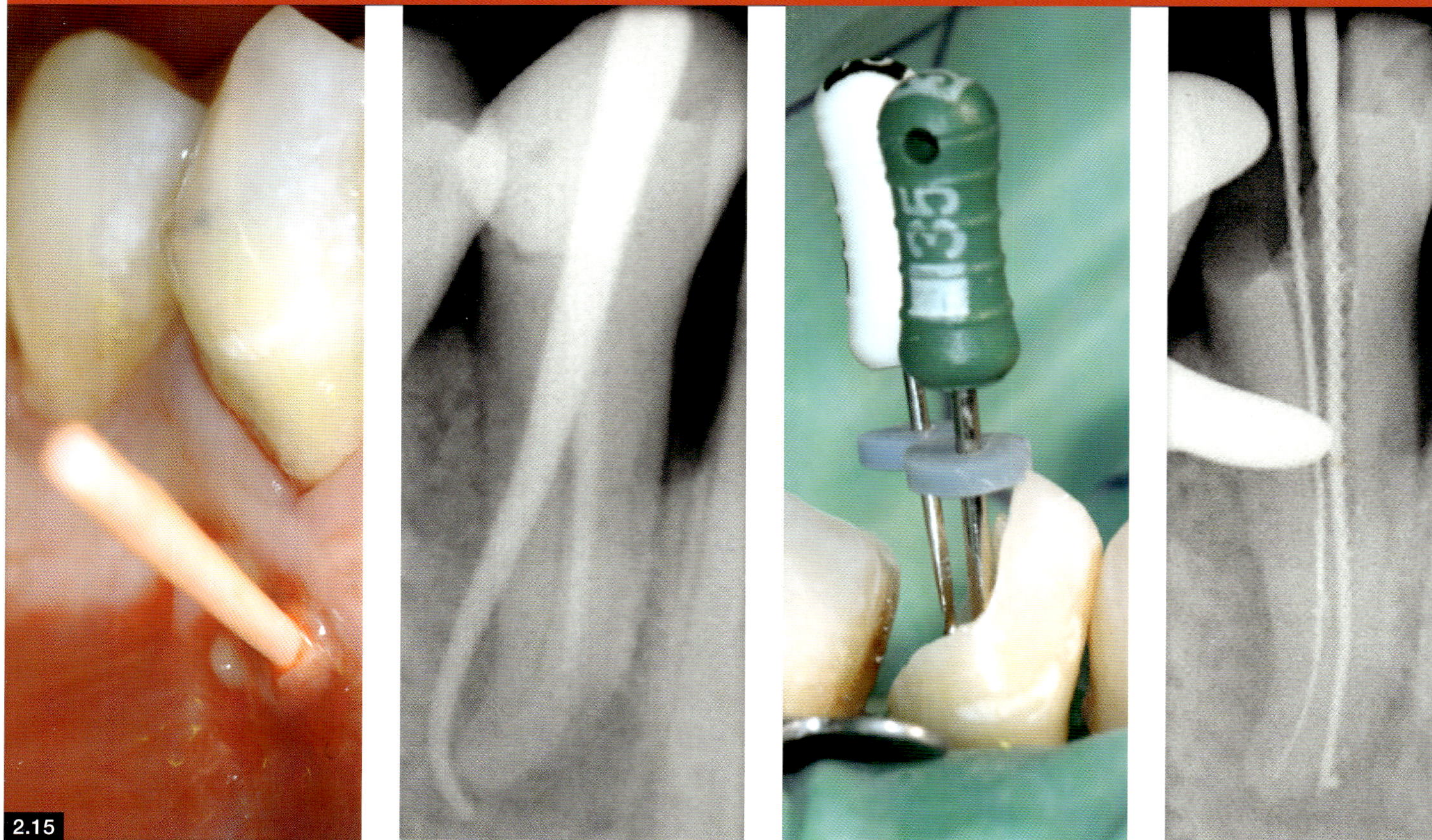

2.15

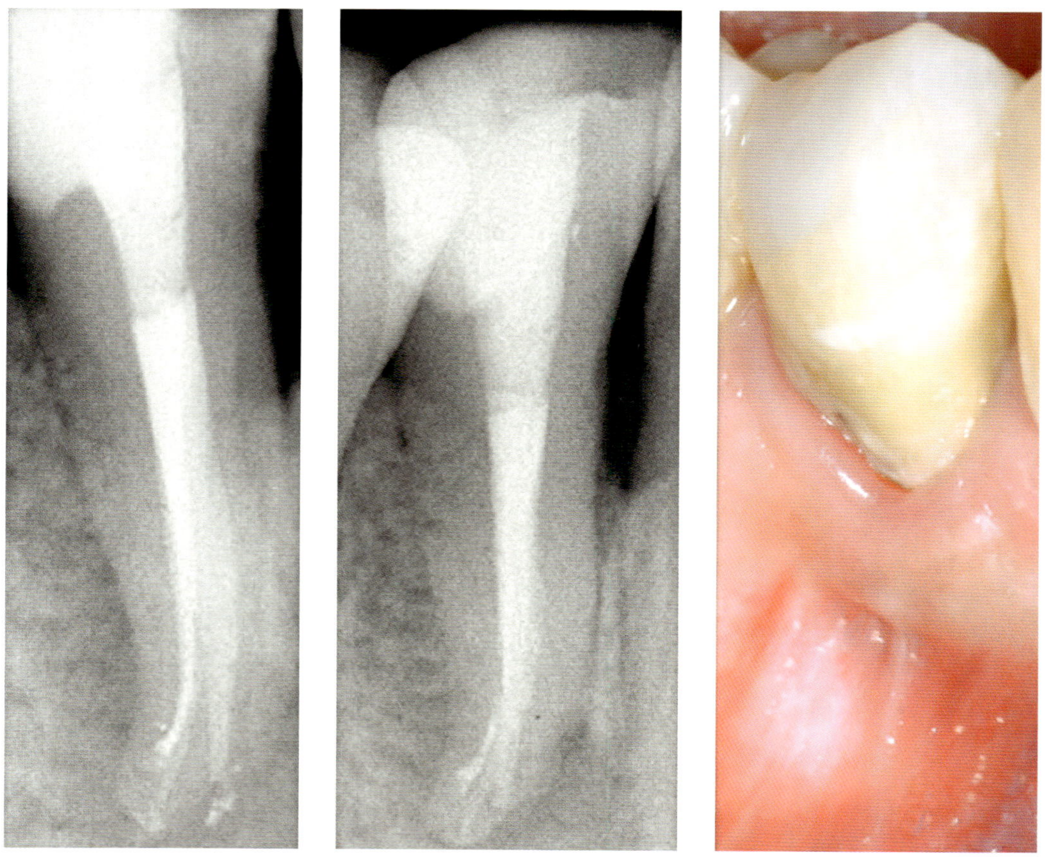

Fig. 2.15: In this case, the insertion of a gutta-percha cone in a fistulous path shows an evident periapical lesion of endodontic origin; the suspicion that the tooth has an endodontic involvement on two canals can be corroborated by the overprojected x-ray images that provide this information.

Hoen MM, Pink FE. *Contemporary Endodontic Retreatment: an Analysis Based on Clinical Treatment.* J Endod 2002;28(12):834-836.

As is well described by the drawings, the so-called projection of the vestibular object can be understood by examining the images and corresponding drawings.

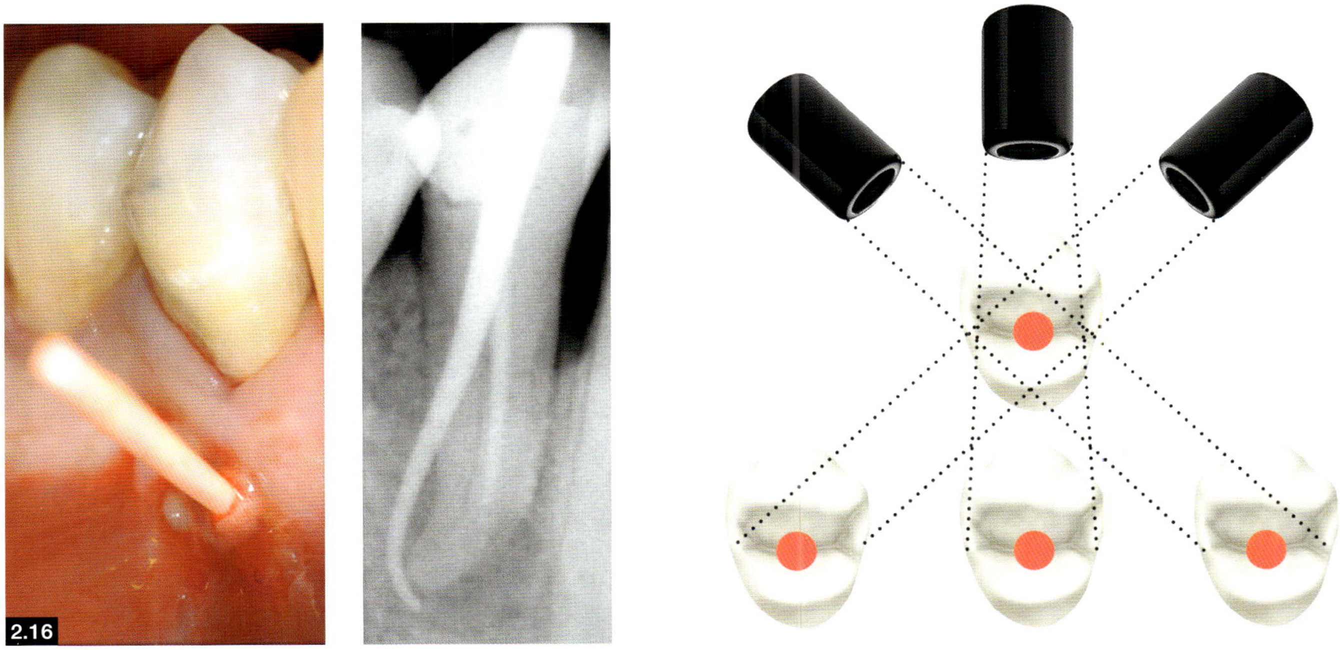

Fig. 2.16: When the root only has one canal, will be at the center of the root and will always appear centered on the film regardless of the x-ray projection.

The clinician is aware that, in accordance with "the buccal object rule", in a mesial or distal angled x-ray, the internal markers in the vestibular position (such as files or cones during the intraoperative x-rays or canal fills of the previous endodontic treatment) "move away" from the radiogenic source: therefore, if the tube is angled mesially, the vestibular findings will appear in a distal position on the x-ray, whereas if the tube is angled distally, the vestibular findings will appear in a mesial position. In this case, the mesial positioning allows the visualization of the vestibular canal.

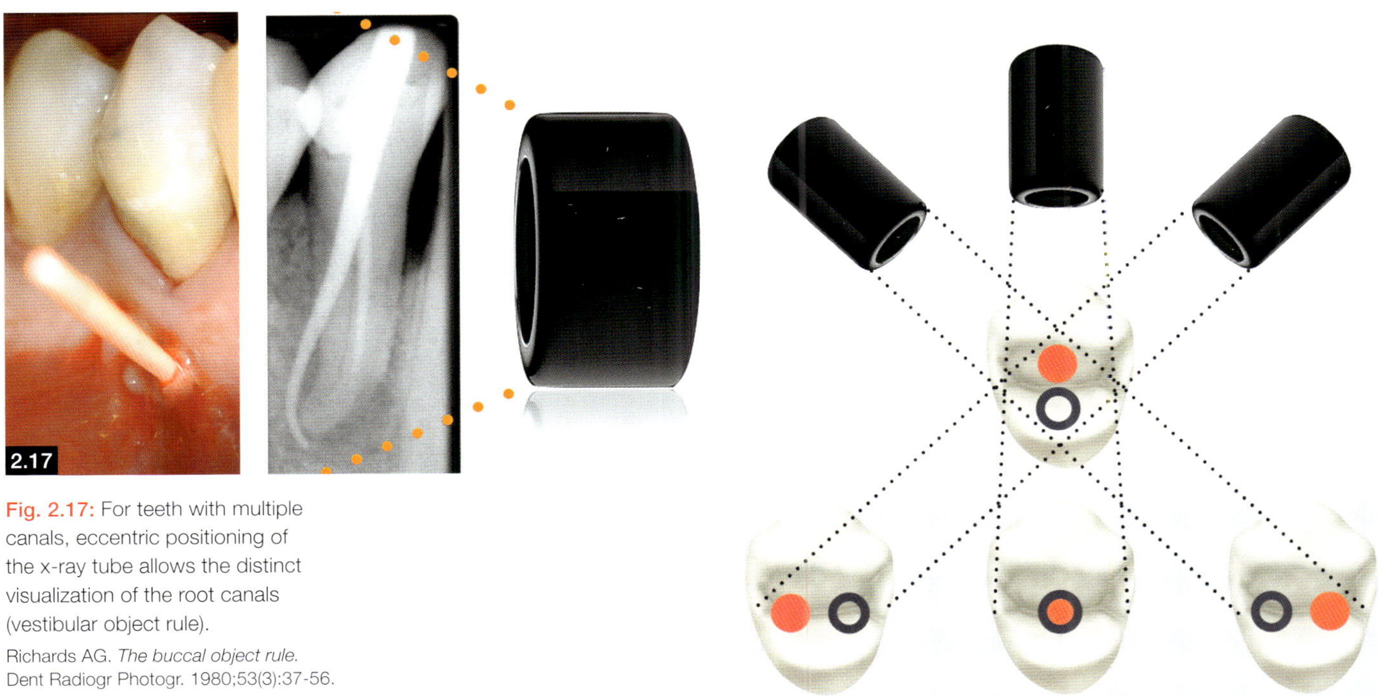

Fig. 2.17: For teeth with multiple canals, eccentric positioning of the x-ray tube allows the distinct visualization of the root canals (vestibular object rule).

Richards AG. *The buccal object rule.* Dent Radiogr Photogr. 1980;53(3):37-56.

ELEMENTS TO BE EXAMINED IN TWO-DIMENSIONAL RADIOLOGY

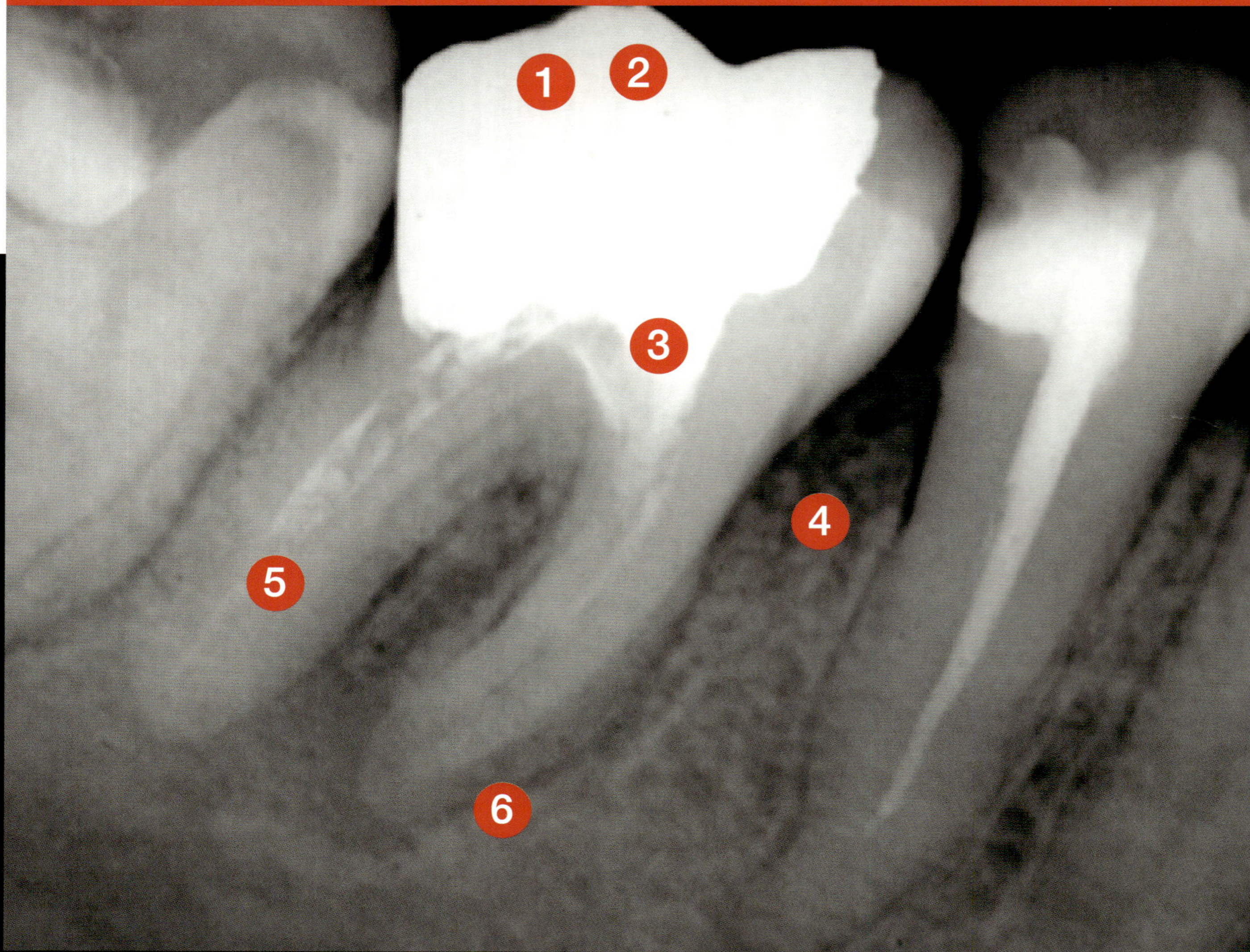

1 The appearance of the retreating material must be carefully evaluated because the choice of cutters will be fundamental for proper access to the endodontium.

2 The endodontic radiograph should be performed with a centering device.
If it is not, as in the case shown here, incorrect projections alter the picture and do not allow reproducible subsequent follow-up.

3 The bottom of the pulp chamber and the canal inlets must be well represented; the morphology will provide indications on the method to be employed for opening. Often, mistakes in the opening of the endodontium lead to errors that compromise the entire therapy.

4 The pericoronal contour should not show areas of radiotransparency that could lead to a suspicion of concomitant periodontal lesions, root fractures, or high perforations.

5 The canal content must be examined with great care: an uneven appearance is a sign of an incomplete condensation of the filling material. It is often associated with the use of gutta-percha-free cements.

6 The periradicular contour must be evaluated by examining the entire perimeter of the root. Each discontinuity is a sign of the inflammatory reaction of the bone tissue.

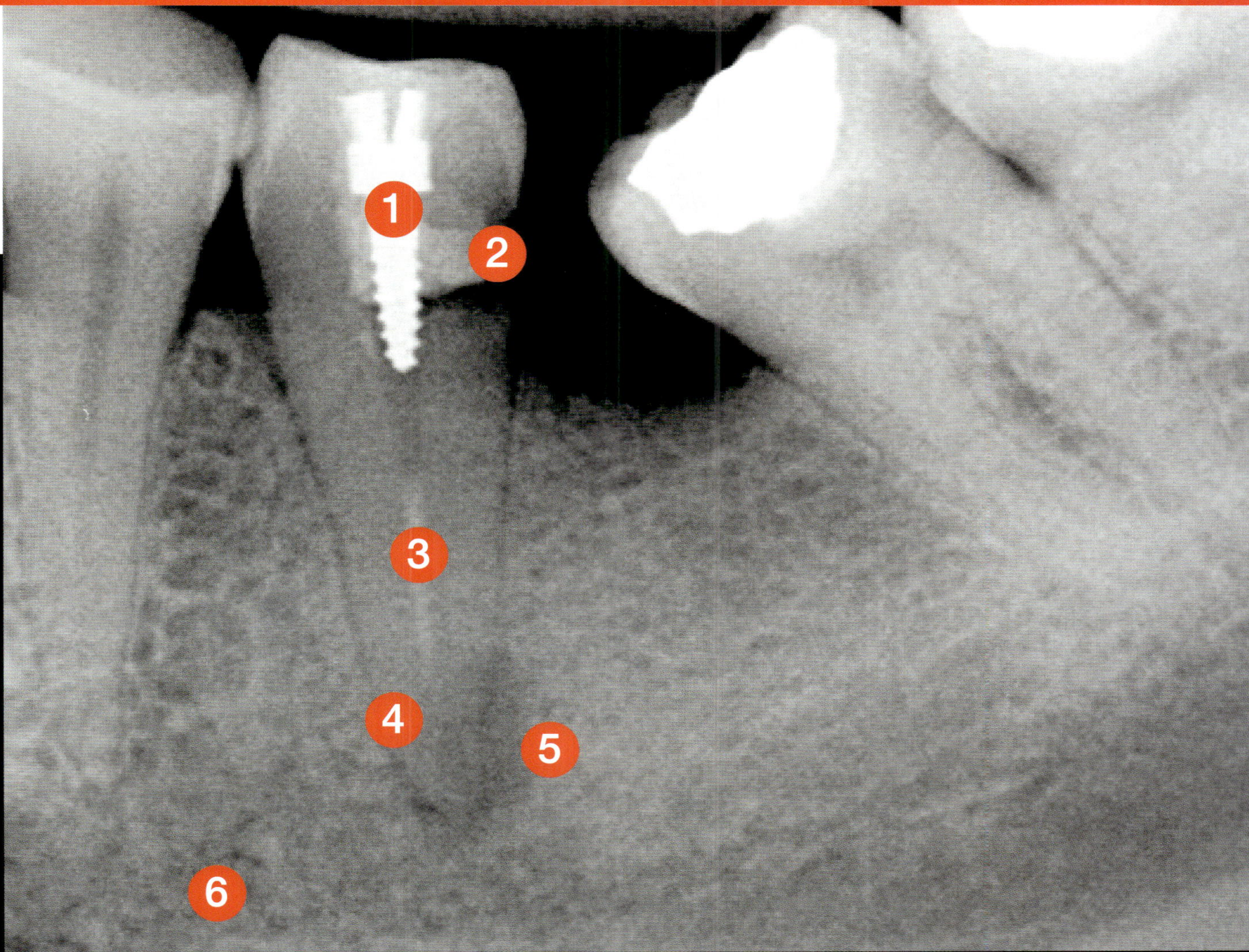

1 The presence of radiopaque root canal posts must be noted: the further they are inserted in the canals, the more difficult it will be to remove them.

2 The coronal seal must be continuous and uniform; otherwise, coronal infiltration might be suspected.

3 The filling level is an important element in assessing the quality of endodontic treatment; closures that are more than 2 mm from the radiological apex must be considered unsatisfactory.

4 The radiographically visible presence of an insufficiently filled canal lumen is a favorable prognostic element for retreatment.

5 A change in the radiotransparency of the bone is the unequivocal indicator of an inflammatory reaction associated with the presence of bacteria inside the root canal.

6 In the lower quadrants, the mental foramen must always be identified when visible.

Three-dimensional radiology

Cone Beam Computed Tomography (CBCT)

Cone beam computed tomography (CBCT) is a radiological examination that is similar to computerized axial tomography (CT) but is characterized by some relevant peculiarities.
The latest generation CBCT systems are compact appliances (similar to orthopantomographic equipment) that use an X-ray source that, making a single turn with synchronous movement of the radiogenic source and the detector around the patient to be examined (the amplitude of rotation can vary from 180° to 360°), emits a conical or pyramidal beam (hence the name "cone beam").
The detector thus acquires an entire volume with a cylindrical or spherical shape (FOV) and, thanks to the reduction of the performance times, the exposure times and dose of radiation absorbed by the patient are limited.

Fig. 2.18a: Tangential section of volumetric examination: you can appreciate the false road with its perforation (red arrow). The clinician who reported the case reported profuse bleeding to the canal probe. The electronic locator provides an apical length of many millimeters shorter than the root length.

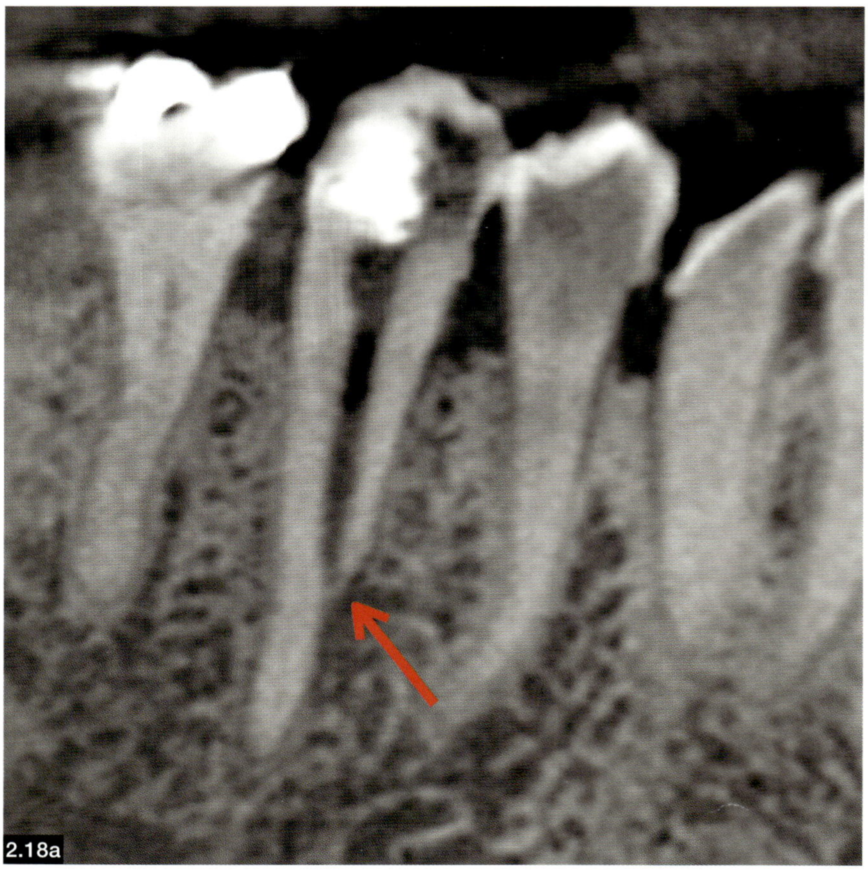

The acquired volume is then processed using appropriate software to obtain a set of two-dimensional images that are diagnostically valid in the three planes of space (tangential, transversal, and axial). Compared with modern multi-slice computed tomography (MSCT), CBCT is more precise and detailed in detecting small high-contrast structures; CBCT also entails considerably lower radiogenic exposure than MSCT[17, 18].

An Italian study conducted in 2003[19] proposed the use of CBCT for preoperative diagnostic analysis in cases of endodontic surgery on the palatine roots of the upper molars; its extensive use was then validated scientifically in 2007, when some studies compared the sensitivity and specificity of these radiographic examinations with the traditional two-dimensional ones[20].
In subsequent studies, the authors highlighted a specificity 25% higher than that of traditional X-rays in the diagnosis of periapical disease[21-29].
An effective review[30] was recently published, and a number of indications for the clinical use of this review have been proposed by the European Society of Endodontics[31].

In addition to scientific data in the strict sense of the term, three-dimensional diagnostics in endodontics has applications in the following areas:

- the identification, localization, and extent of periapical disease; the possible involvement of one or more roots; and the involvement of neighboring noble structures, such as the maxillary sinus and the lower alveolar nerve and the mental foramen;
- in cases of internal and external resorption;
- in traumas of the lower third of the facial bones;
- in traumas of doubtful cases and in the failure of endodontically treated teeth.

The advantages of a rational use of CBCT are therefore obvious; however, the greater radiogenic exposure to which the patient is subject, compared to two-dimensional endodontic radiographs, must be considered.

Therefore, CBCT can be considered an excellent diagnostic solution in ambiguous cases.

In diagnostic evaluations in endodontically treated teeth, we must consider how CBCT can have a reduced diagnostic/decisional impact as a result of artifacts (beam hardening) due to the presence of radiopaque materials (metal intracanal retention, gutta-percha, radiopaque cements, prosthetic artifacts, etc.) that can reduce the specificity of CBCT scans. Indeed, artifacts can induce an incorrect diagnosis: for example, some types of artifacts (streaks) can be mistaken for fractures or perforations.

In recent times, special software has been used to partially remedy these disturbances. Precisely for this reason, the massive use of CBCT for endodontics diagnostics is to be considered with due caution; nevertheless, ignoring its existence would be extremely limiting.

For this reason, the clinician's decision to use this type of examination must always consider two fundamental parameters: the justification parameter (based on guidelines, the clinician must always limit patient exposure by collecting all the necessary diagnostic information first) and the optimization parameter (when the clinician decides that the examination is necessary, the optimal settings must be adopted and patient exposure must be kept to a minimum).

However, the examination allows access to areas of the periodontium that cannot be identified with normal x-rays, with a percentage 38% higher than the traditional two-dimensional radiographs[32, 33]. In this regard, the cortical bone of the maxilla can act as an X-ray screen to allow the identification of large periapical lesions[16].

The diagnostic opportunities in teeth affected by irreversible pulp disease should also be considered, but they go beyond this treatment in the strict sense; in a study on corresponding roots, the identification of periapical rarefactions associated with these clinical pictures was 20% in X-rays and 48% in CBCT exams[34].

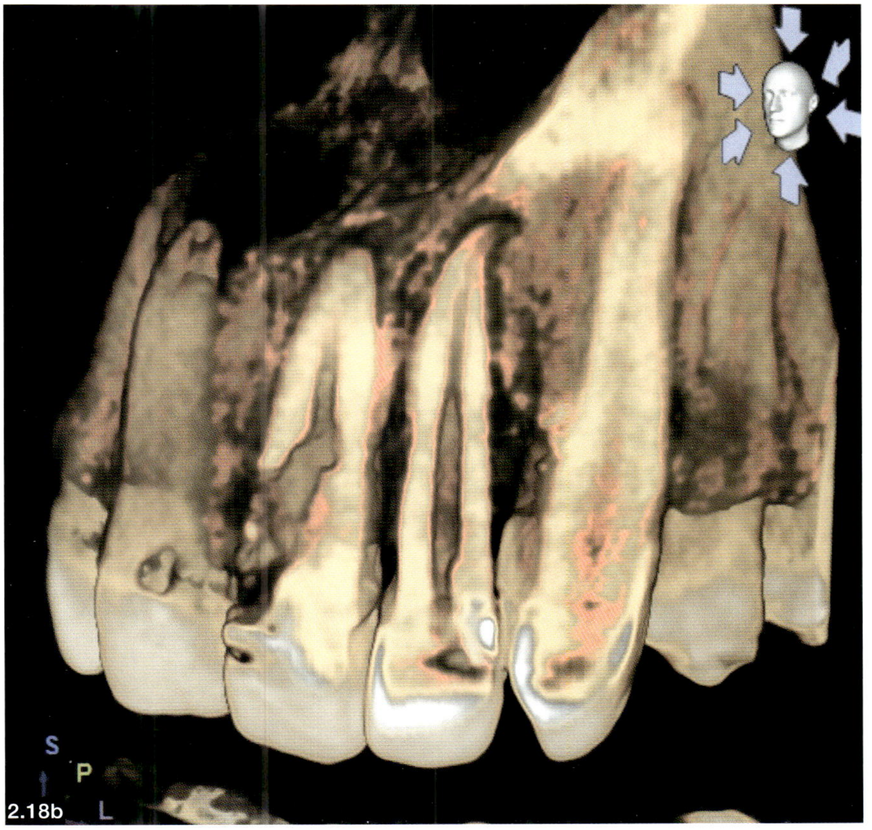

Fig. 2.18b: Rendering of small FCV frontal area upper arch where DOV is obvious:

- arge periapical lesion with a consequent apical reshaping of 1.1;
- nitial cervical resorption of 1.1;
- extensive pathological external corono-radicular resorption of 2.1: the tooth can no longer be recovered.

The peculiar curvature of the apical third of the lateral incisor often causes endodontic failure of these teeth.

These data confirm that many dental diseases characterized by irreversible pulpitis patterns have already developed an inflammatory periradicular reaction that will condition their future prognosis.

These findings were emphasized by Cheung et al.[28] to confirm the inaccuracy of traditional endodontic radiographs. The clinically evaluable results were then further corroborated by experimental findings, confirming that the two-dimensional radiographic image must be interpreted with caution. These results indicate that CBCT is far more sensitive than traditional endodontic radiographs, whether analog or digital, in diagnosing periapical disease of endodontic origin.

Further points in favor of the three-dimensional examination remain: the possibility of identifying the disease and determining its real extent, particularly in the case of multiradicular teeth, as well as the detection of areas of the endodontium not reached by the previous canal treatment.

The identification of root fractures, especially those deep in the periodontal tissues, is fundamental for sparing patients retreatments, which are often labor-intensive, with an unfavorable prognosis. We will devote a separate paragraph to this subject.
Returning to the analysis of the endodontic space, the images in different projections provide information regarding the anatomy of the tooth and the filling of the root canals. The congruence between the length of the canal filling and the estimate of the canal size in the two-dimensional picture can already be evaluated. However, the degree of filling, the compactness of the gutta-percha, and the occupation of all the spaces of the endodontium represent a set of elements of judgment that cannot be neglected, especially when talking about retreatment. These last elements will be easier to examine and evaluate in the three-dimensional examination.

Under-instrumented canals are extremely common in endodontic treatments, as reported by studies that have highlighted how much endodontic space is not touched by endodontic instruments during the shaping phase[35, 36].
Beyond these important considerations, identifying voids within root canals or uninstrumented root canals is much simpler with the use of a three-dimensional system than with a two-dimensional system[34]. Identifying possible contaminated areas of the root canal will help to create the conditions for the new treatment to be more effective. In conclusion, CBCT can play a leading role in the decision-making process for endodontic failures.
In these cases where the collection of information, the clinical examination, and the two-dimensional radiology techniques do not allow a certain diagnosis, the three-dimensional examination is indispensable.

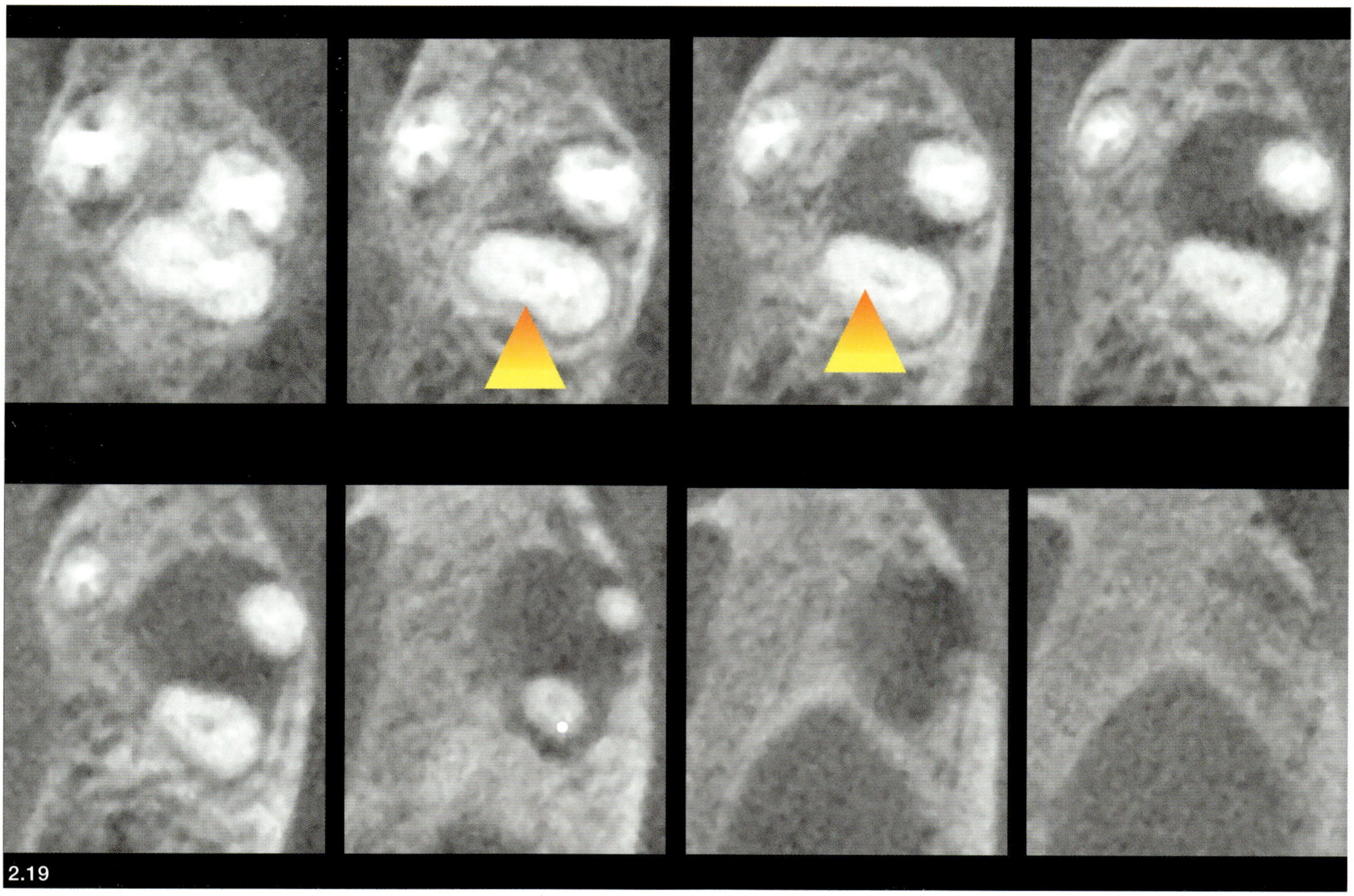

2.19

Fig. 2.19: Upper left molar sections. The images show incomplete filling of the mesial canal, a good filling of the other canals, and a substantial injury in no. 27. In a two-dimensional framework, all sections would not have been possible to examine everything in such detail. In addition, the various sections avoid being contiguous with the upper maxillary sinus, which simplifies the treatment plan.

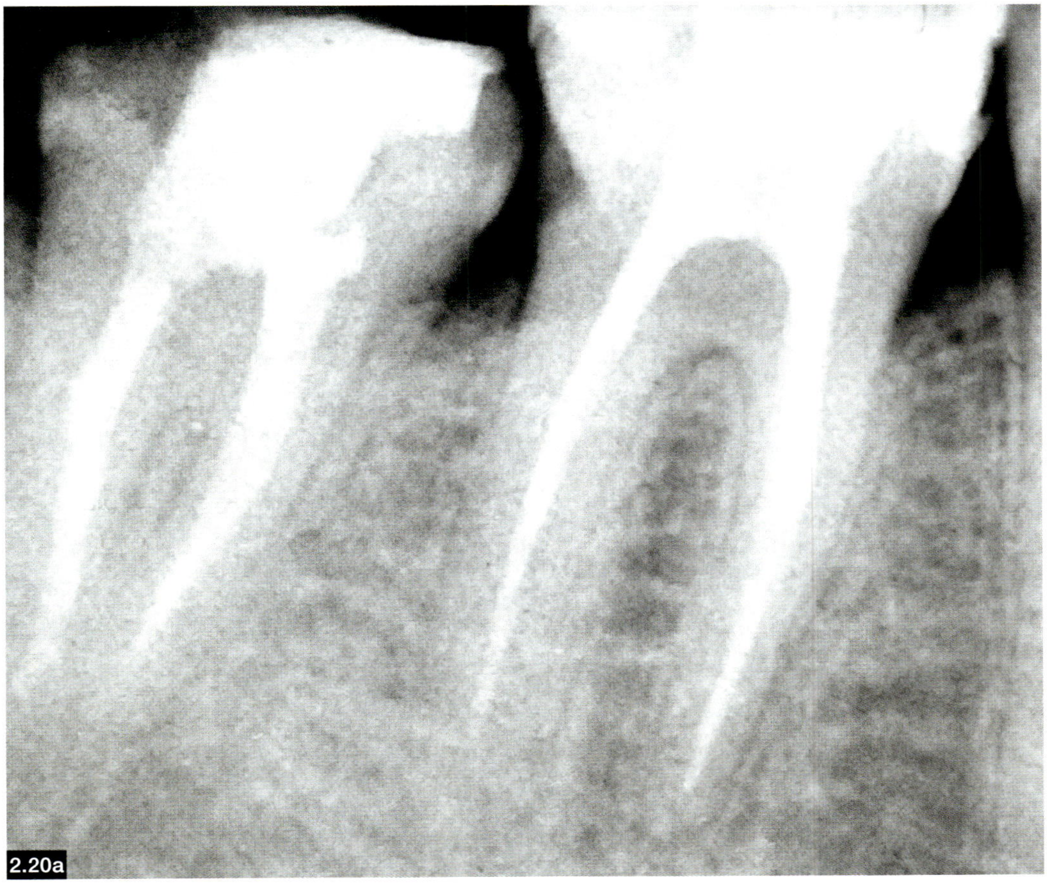

Fig. 2.20a: Lower molars with endodontic treatments performed; the patient still complains of the pain in the presence of heat and with changes in pressure (at high altitudes).

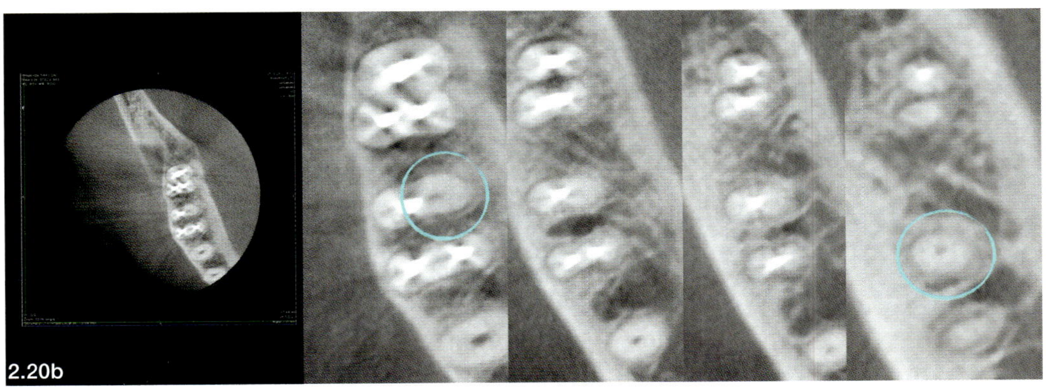

Fig. 2.20b: Examination using three-dimensional x-rays highlighting a canal of the untreated distal root (blue circle) that ends separately but converges towards the apex.

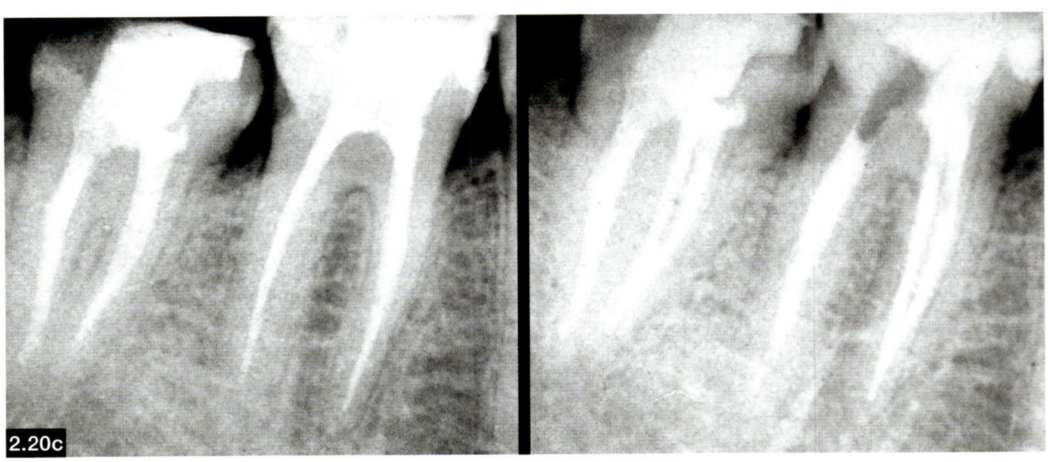

Fig. 2.20c: Retreatment has had the desired effect. Note the difference in tapering at the distal root of tooth 46.

▶ *continue to page 127*

CASE REPORT 3

Adjacent periapical lesions in the molar and premolar area

Radiographic examinations often underestimate the extent of periradicular lesions in previously treated teeth and, in addition, do not provide correct information on the content and filling of the root canal.

Figure 1: Preoperative x-ray. Note the small medial root size of no. 16 and the slightly radiolucent area around the medial root of no. 16 and the periapical area of no. 15.

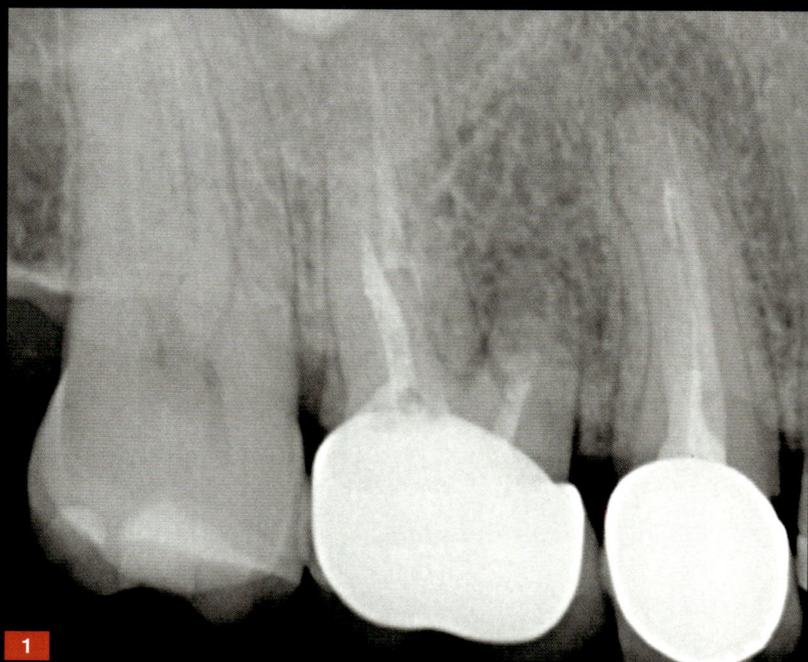

1

Figure 2: 3D CBCT reconstruction showing a bone lesion in teeth 16-15 and the need for the surgical resection of the medial root of tooth 16.

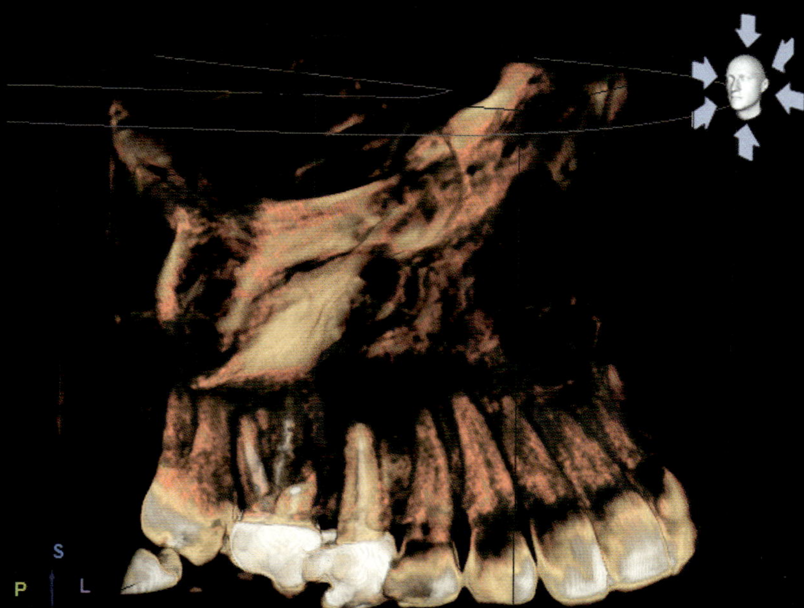

2

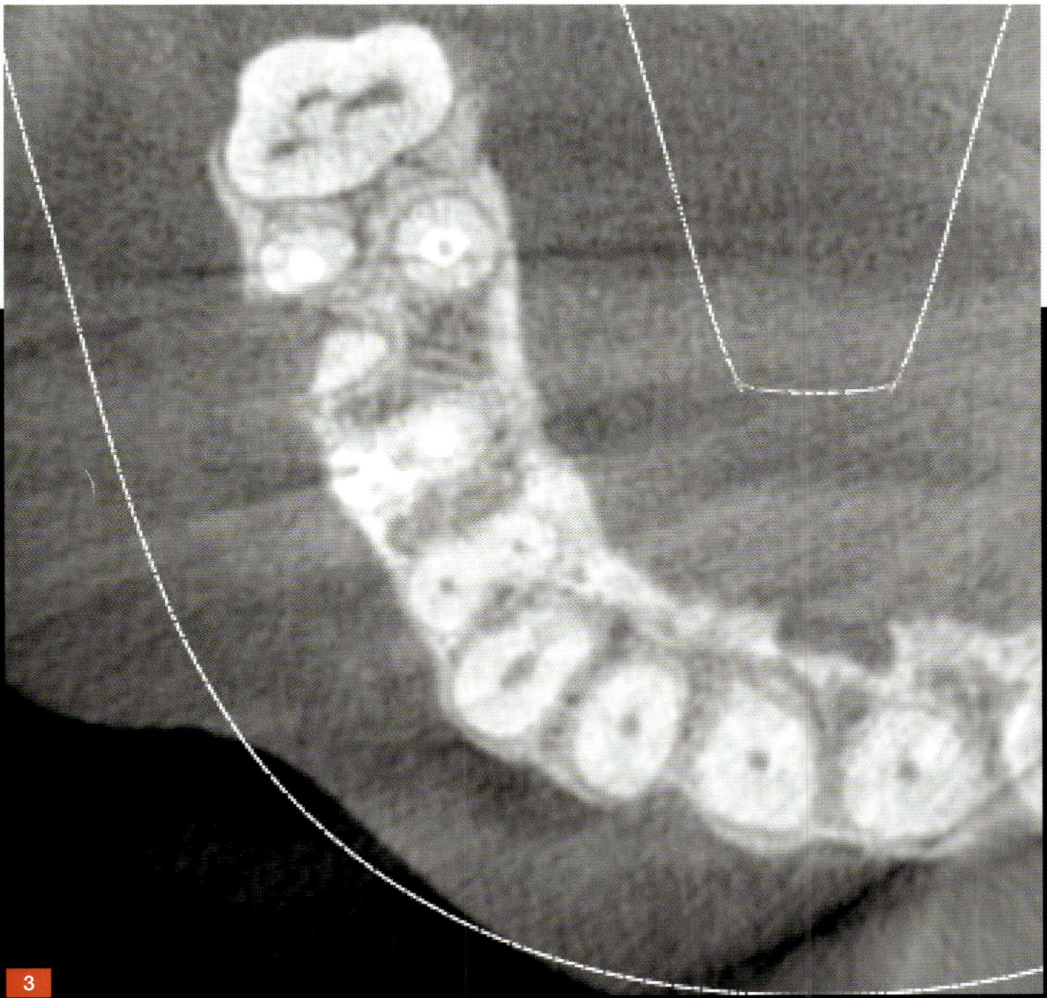

3

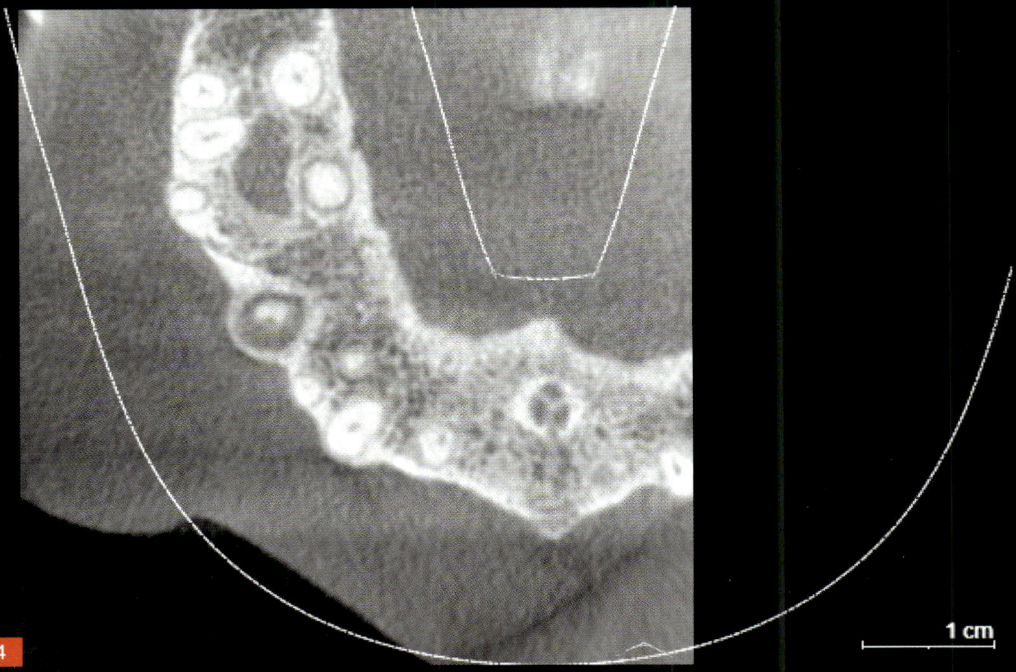

4

Figures 3 and 4: Axial section obtained by CBCT, at coronal level (Figure 3). The resection of the medial root of tooth 16 and the erosion of the cortical vestibular bone are visible. At a more apical level (Figure 4), the periapical radiolucent lesion at tooth no. 15 is evident, together with the widening of the periodontal space of the palatine and distal roots of tooth 16.

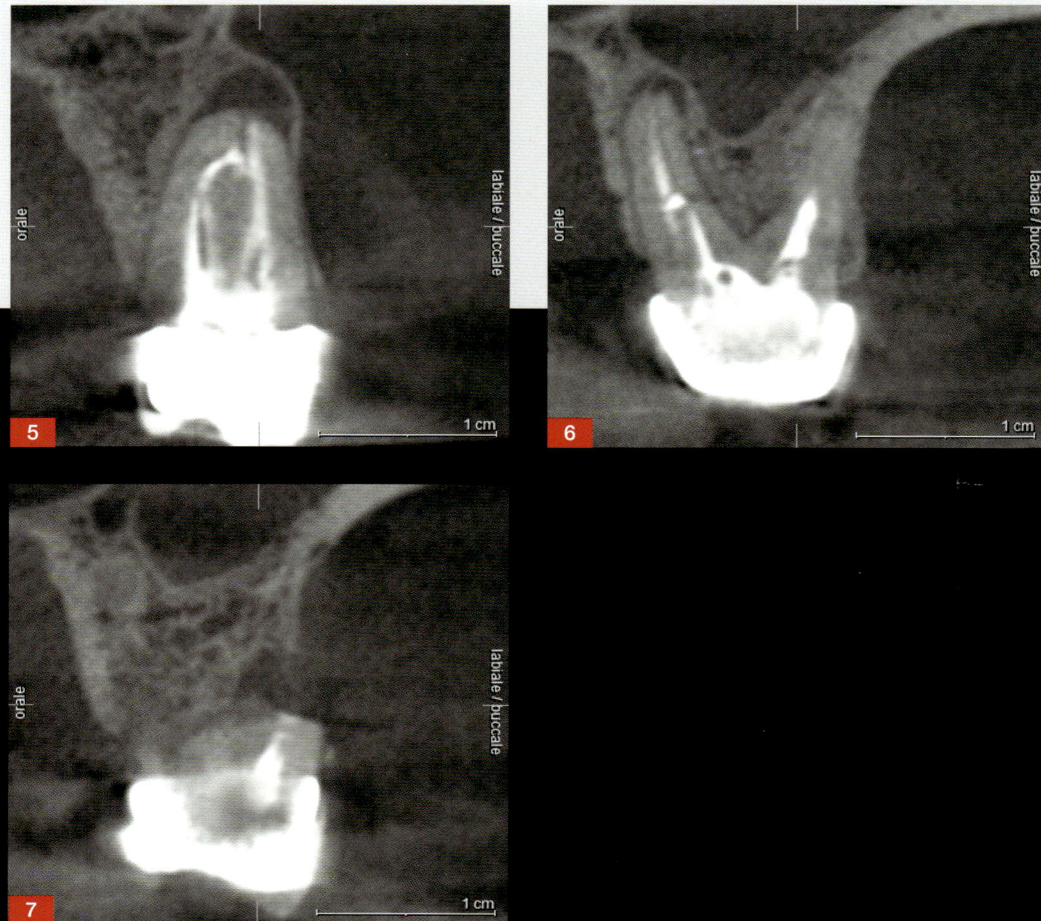

Figures 5-7: Coronal CBCT slices showing a periapical lesion in tooth 15 and the curvature of the palatine canal in the vestibular direction (Figure 5). The lesion can be detected on the palatine root (Figure 6) and the medial root resection of no. 16 (Figure 7).

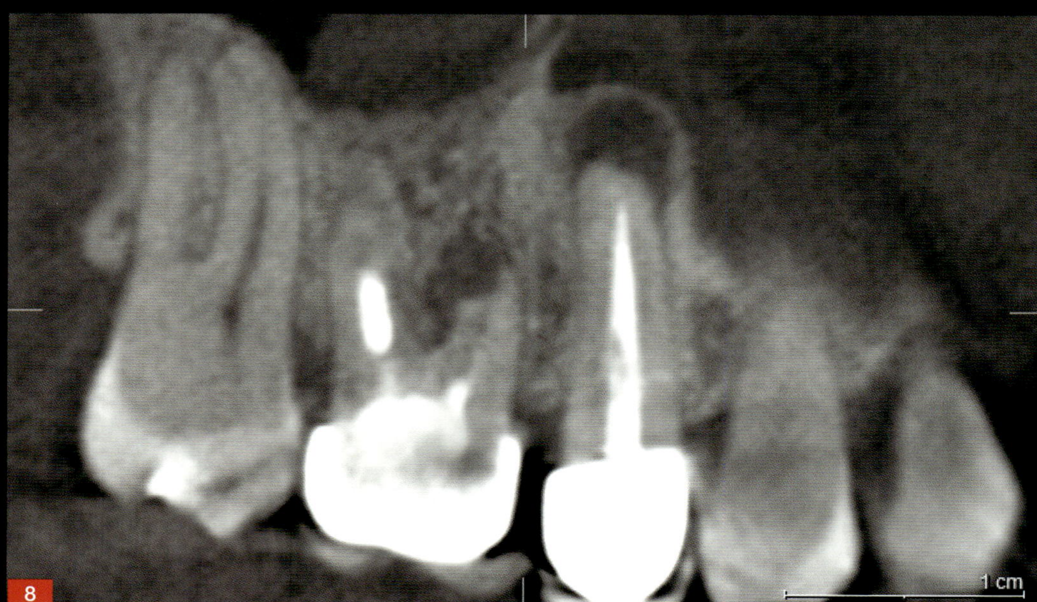

Figure 8: Sagittal CBCT slice showing the periapical region of no. 15, the lesion and resection of the medial root of no. 16.

9

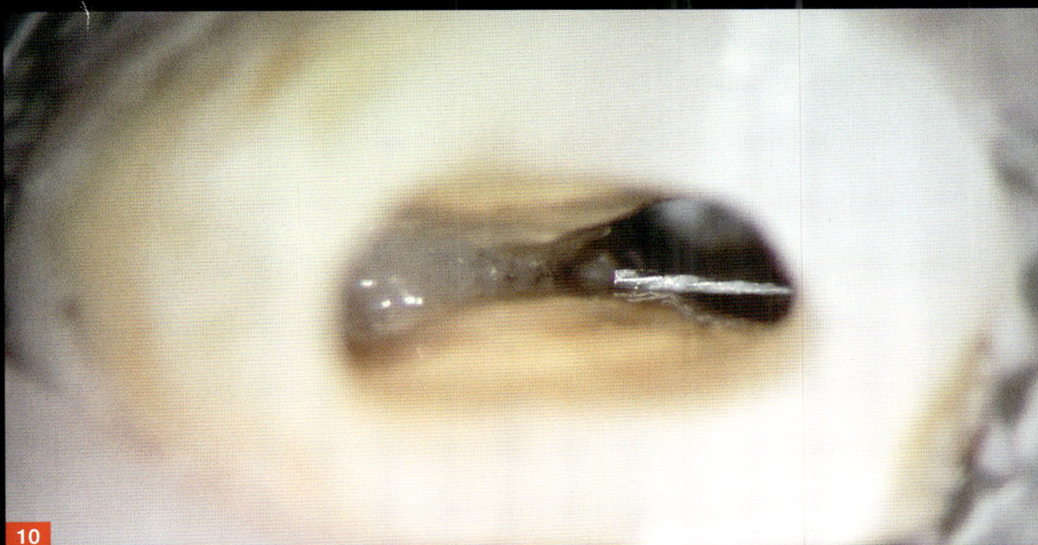

10

Figures 9 and 10: Intraoperative images showing the broken instrument in the palatine canal (Figure 9) and its subsequent removal (Figure 10).

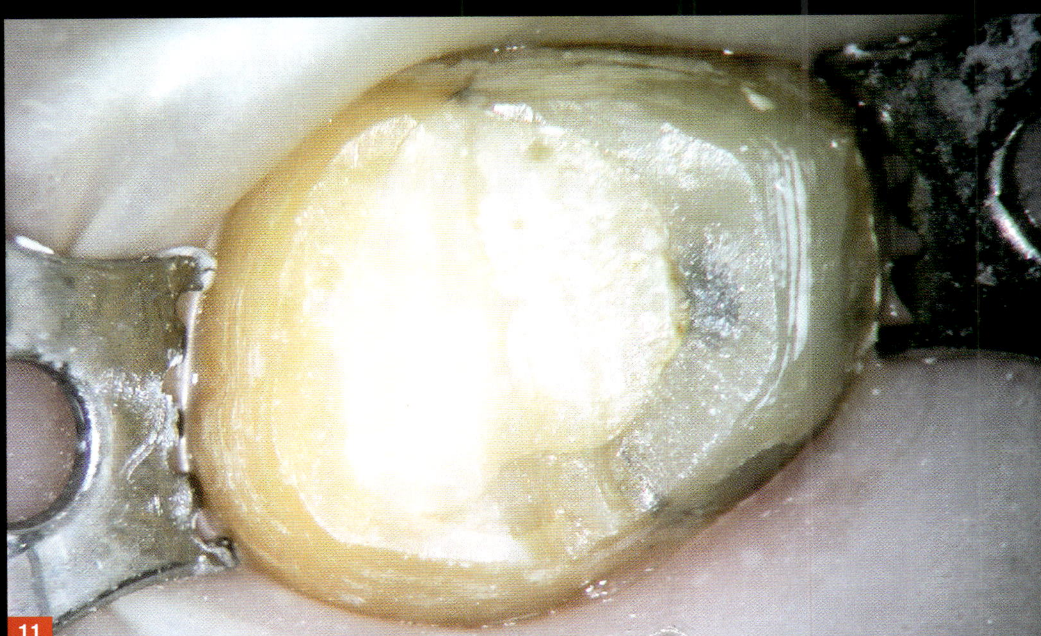

11

Figure 11: Intraoperative image of the abutment of no. 16 after isolation with rubber dam.

Figure 12: Note the old canal filling material inside the palatine canal. Note the lack of a snug fit between the filling material and the canal walls.

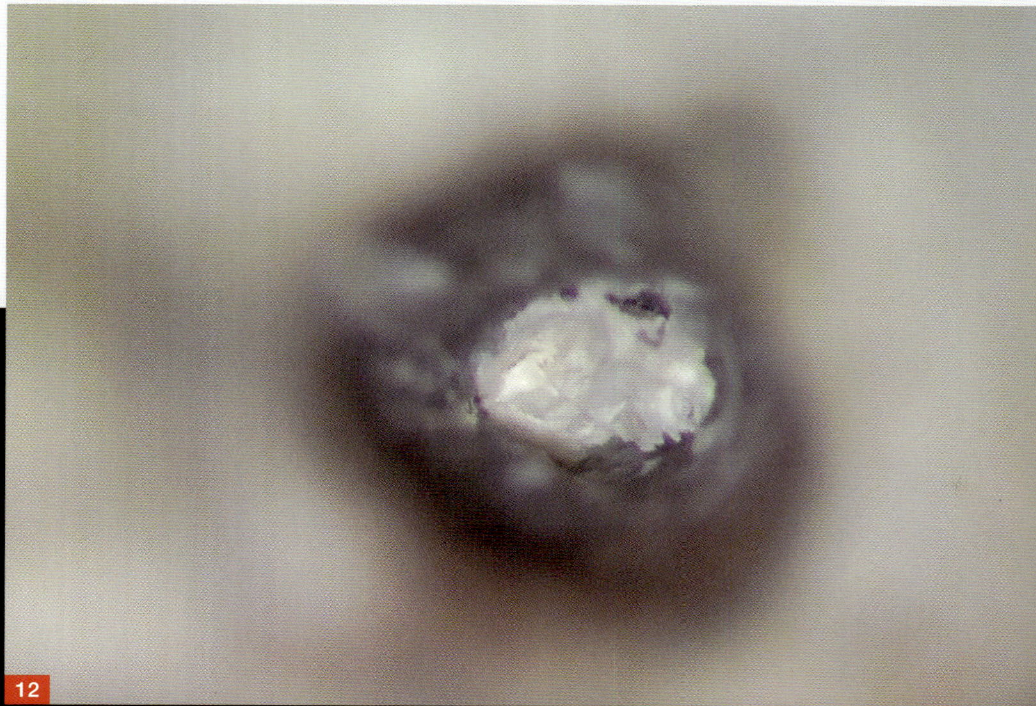

Figure 13: Intraoperative view showing the very wide MB1 canal reshaped after endodontic surgery and the MB2 canal, which was not found and has an independent outlet.

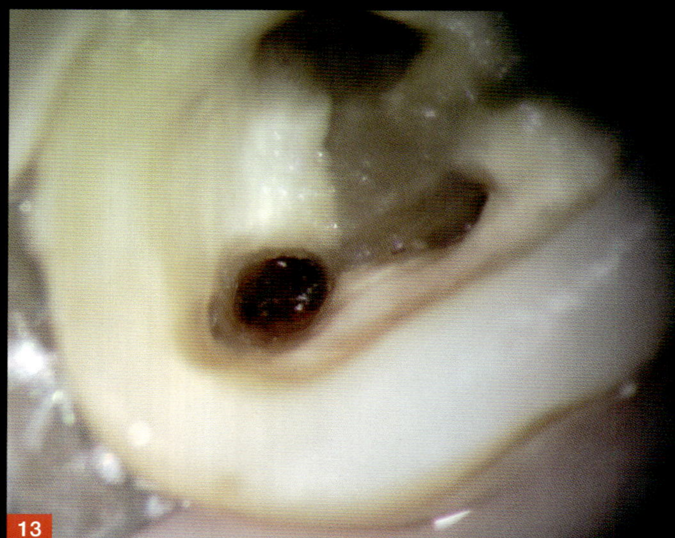

Figures 14 and 15: Details of the access cavity before (Figure 14) and after root canal filling (Figure 15).

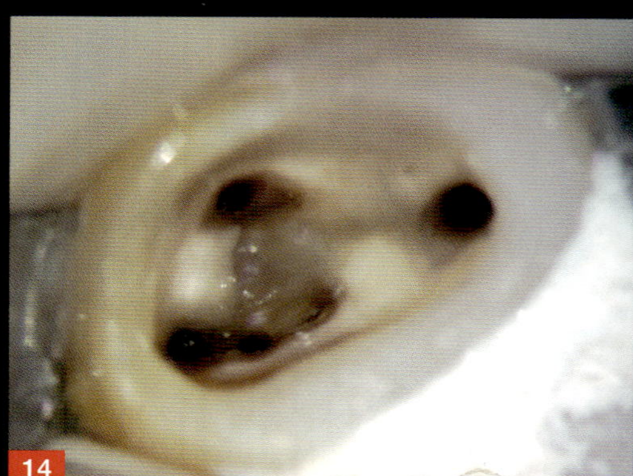

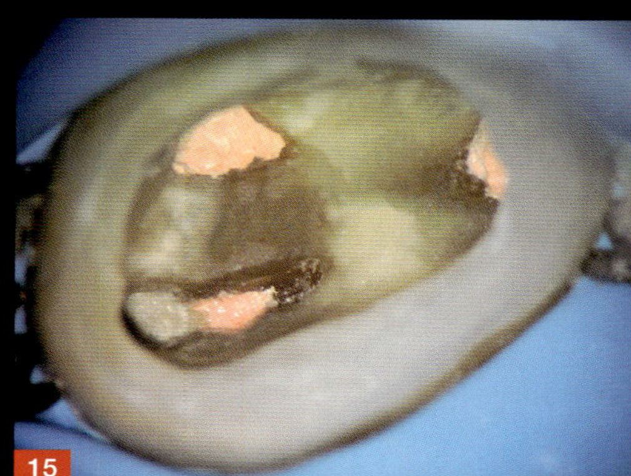

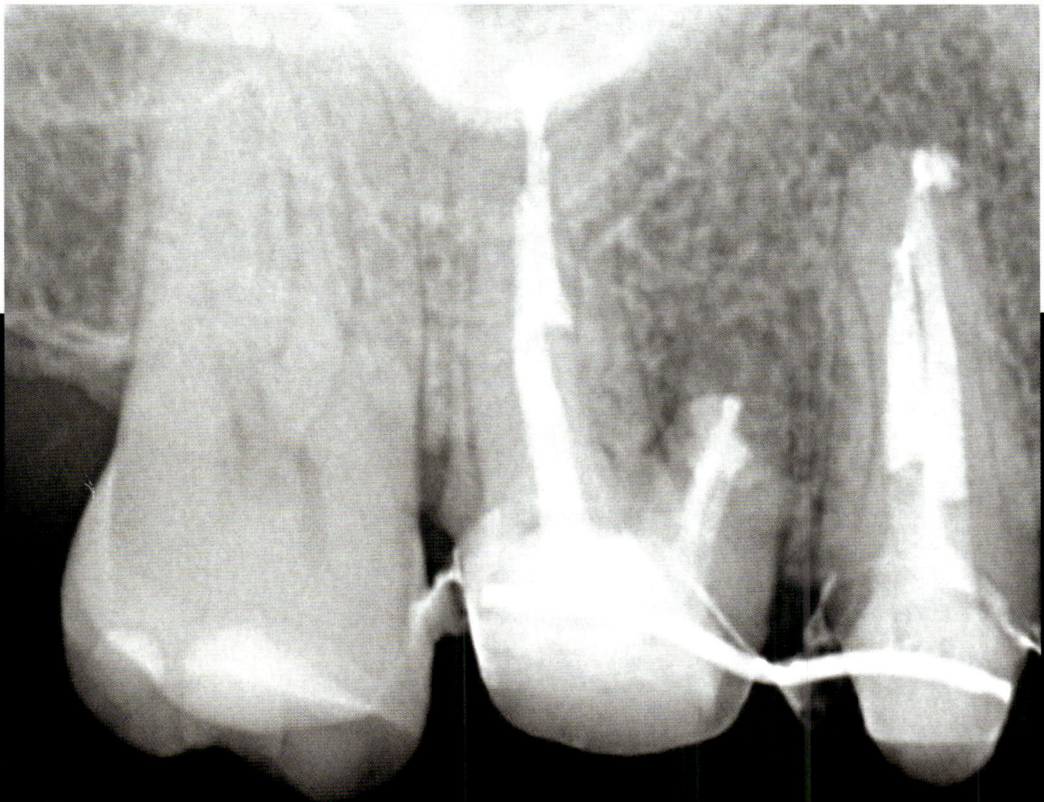

16

Figure 16: Final X-ray. Note the confluence of the canals in tooth no. 15 and independence of the medial canals of no. 16.

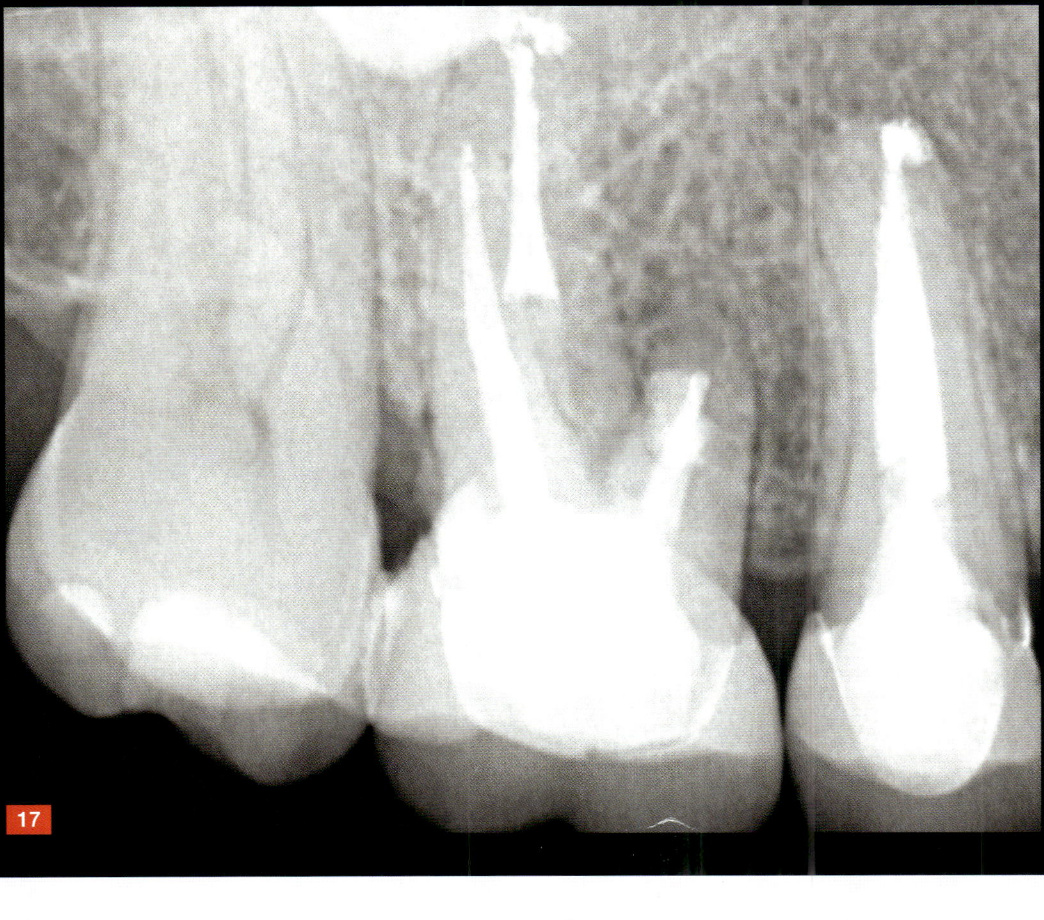

17

Figure 17: 3-month follow-up x-ray showing well-defined bone around tooth no. 15 and the medial root of no. 16.

CASE REPORT 4

Diagnosis of perforation/radical fracture of premolars

In cases such as that presented, establishing the clinical and radiological situation, through a three-dimensional view, is essential for guiding the treatment plan. Relying on two-dimensional X-rays would have led to the design of an incorrect treatment plan.

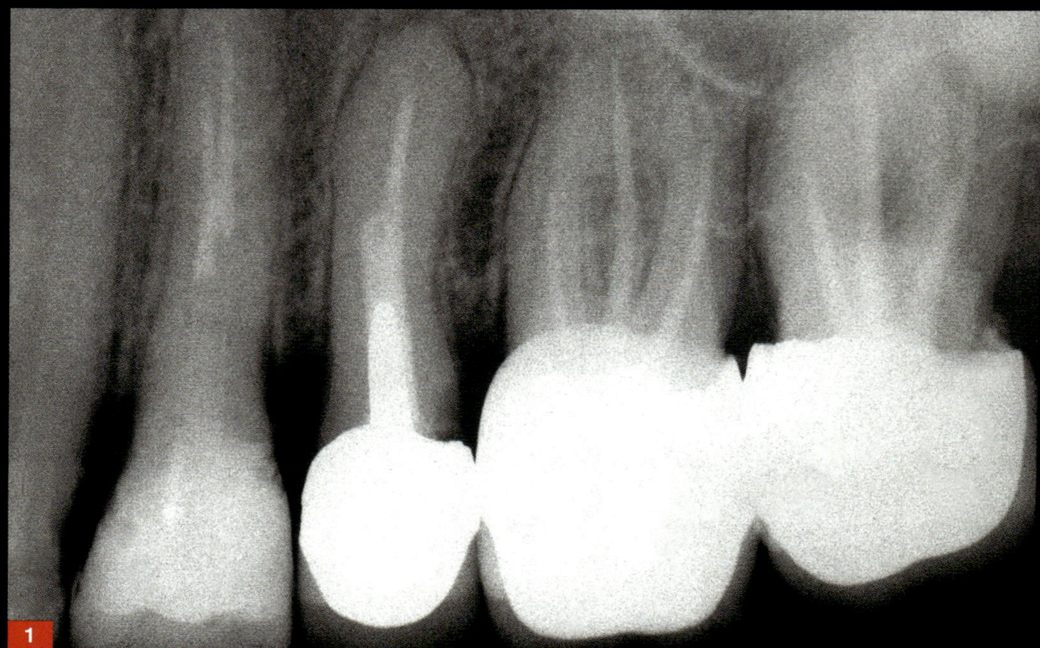

Figure 1: Initial x-ray showing a distal carious lesion, a large intracanal retention and a slight enlargement of the periapical space at tooth no. 25.

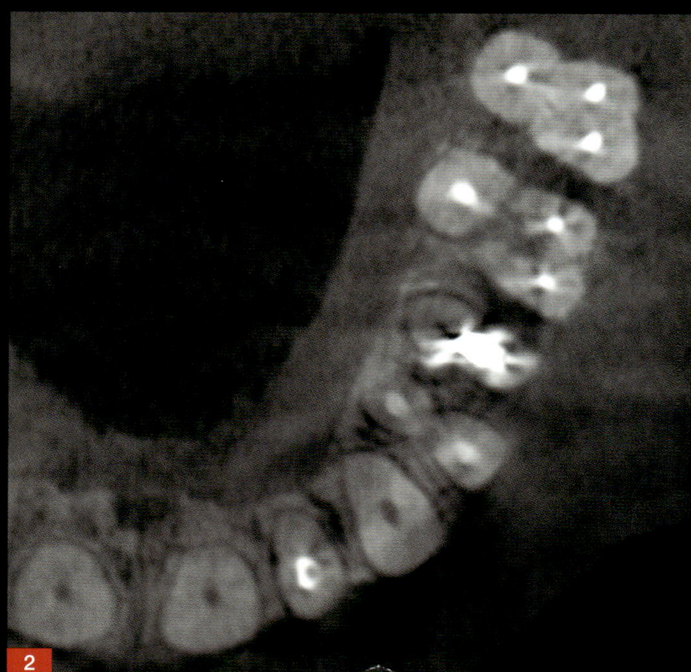

Figure 2: Axial CBCT slice showing incorrect positioning of intracanal retention with probable root fracture.

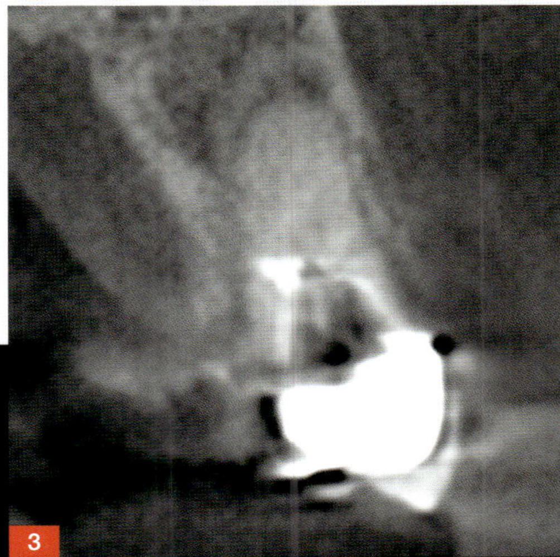

3

Figure 3: Coronal CBCT slice showing significant loss of tissue at tooth 25.

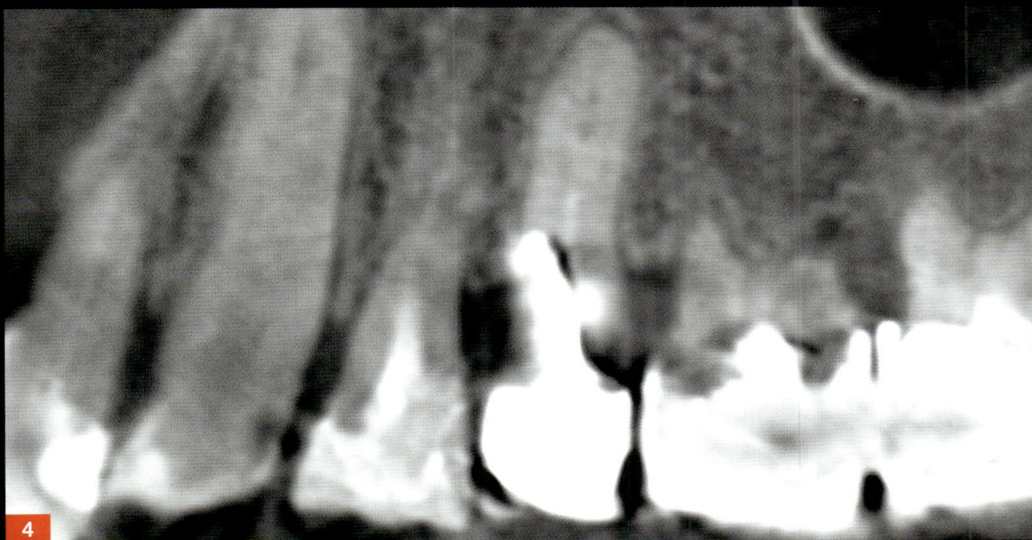

4

Figure 4: Sagittal slice showing the mesial perforation of the intracanal retention of tooth 25 and a slight enlargement of the periapical space.

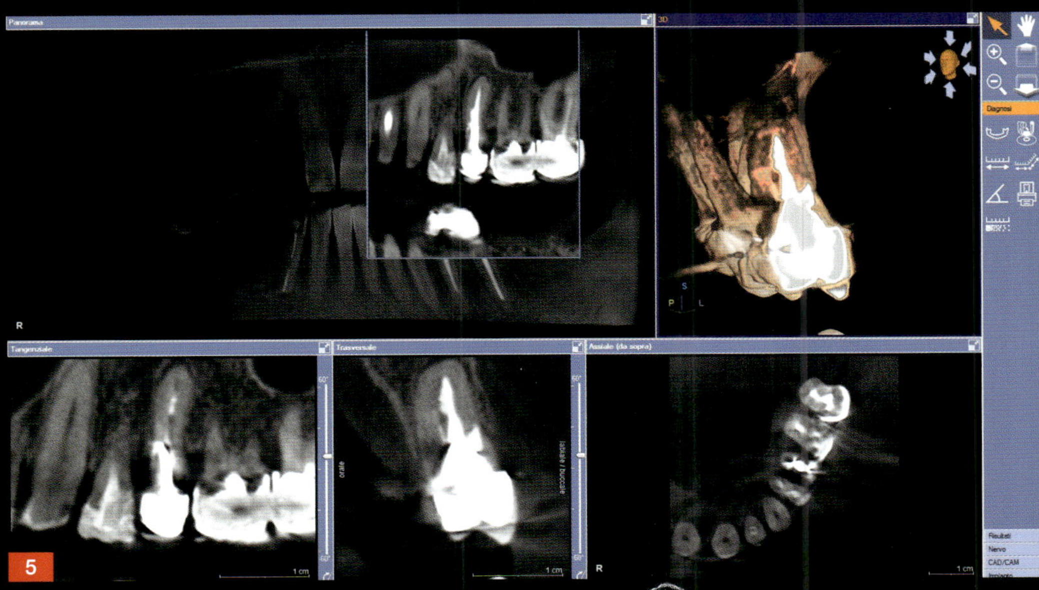

5

Figure 5: CBCT reconstruction software working window, making it possible to simultaneously navigate between the axial, coronal and sagittal slices and the 3D reconstruction.

CASE REPORT 5

Identification of a broken instrument in the distal root of the upper molar

Although the broken instrument in the distal root of the upper molar is evident even with two-dimensional analysis alone, the execution of radiographs that provide a three-dimensional picture helps to formulate a proper operational strategy.

Figure 1: Preoperative intraoral radiograph showing a tapered root profile of tooth 26 and a broken instrument inside the distal canal.

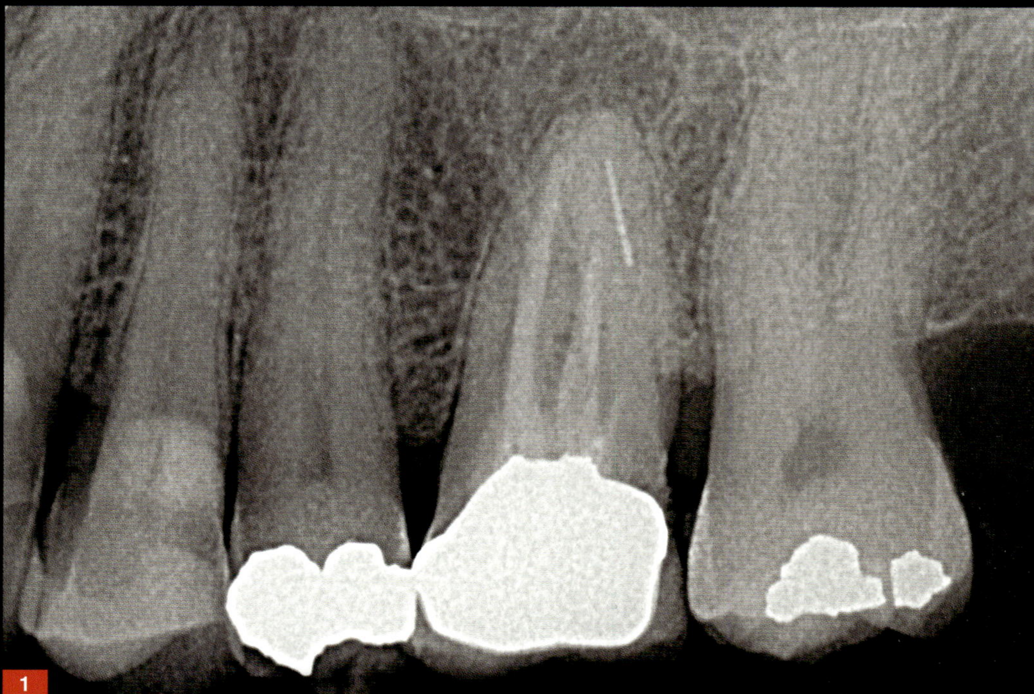

1

Figure 2: 3D CBCT reconstruction showing the broken instrument and periapical lesion of tooth no. 26.

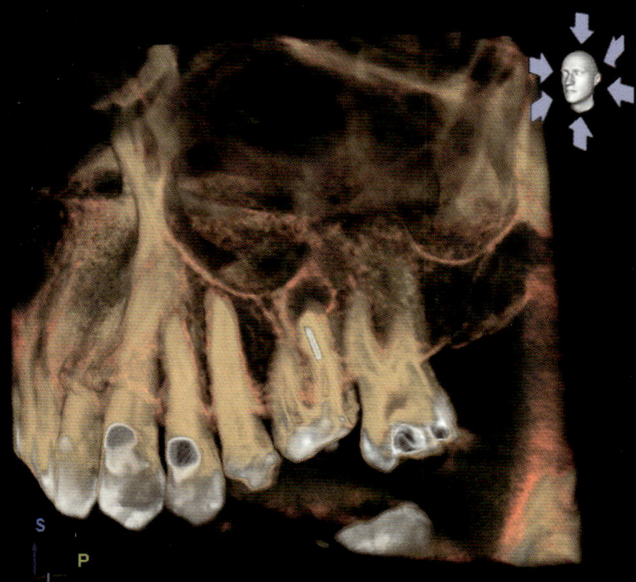

2

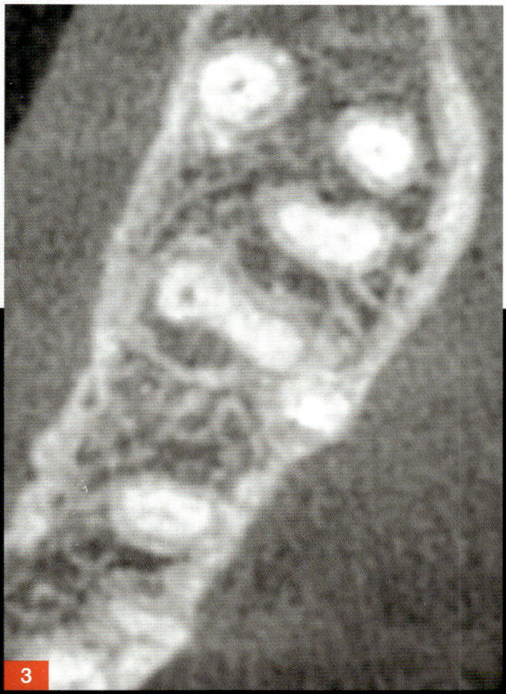

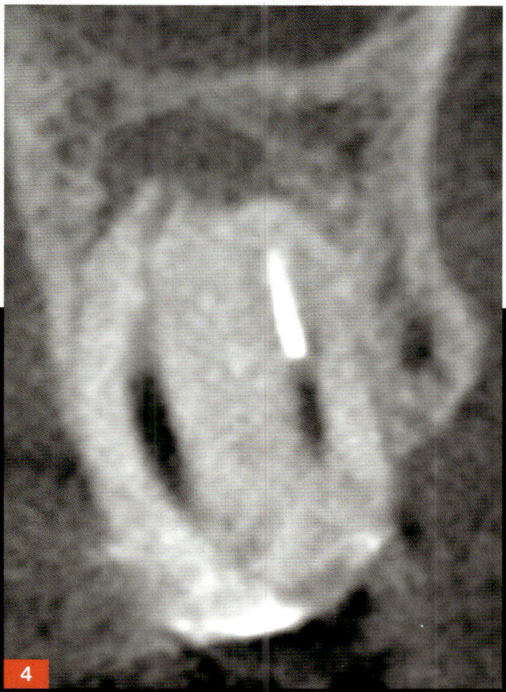

Figure 3: Axial CBCT slice showing non-converging canals and periapical lesion of the palatine root.

Figure 4: Coronal section showing the broken instrument in the distal canal and the periapical lesion involving the palatine and distal canals.

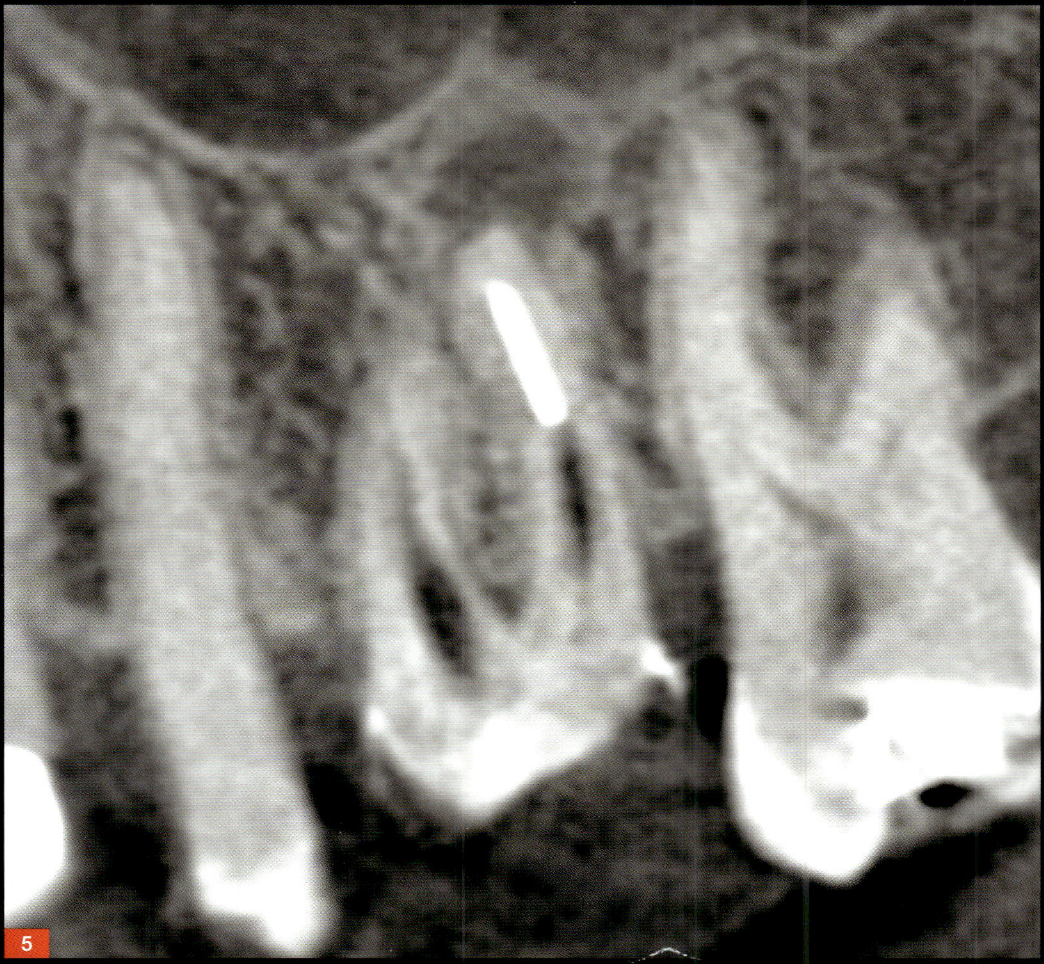

Figure 5: Sagittal section showing the broken instrument in the distal canal and the periapical lesion.

Figures 6 and 7: Preoperative clinical images (Figure 6) and after removal of the gold-ceramic crown of no. 26.

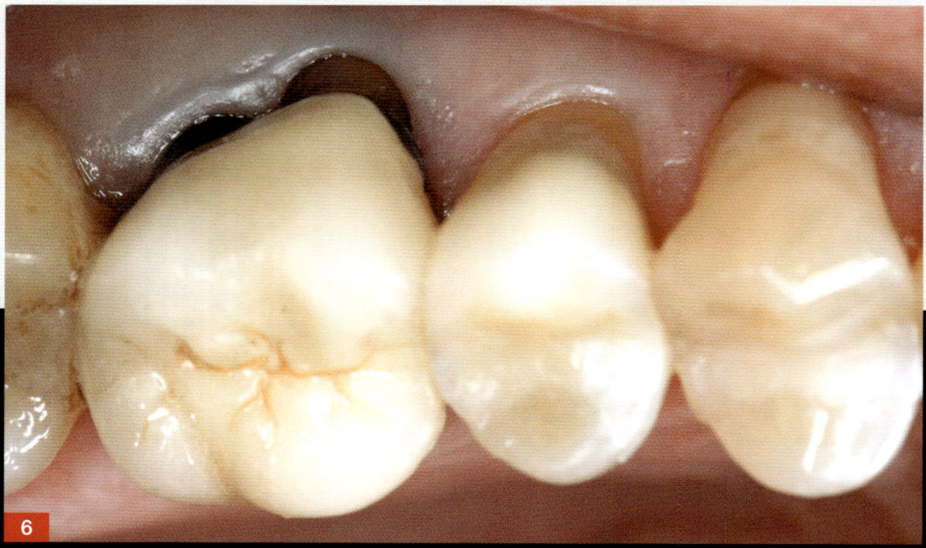

6

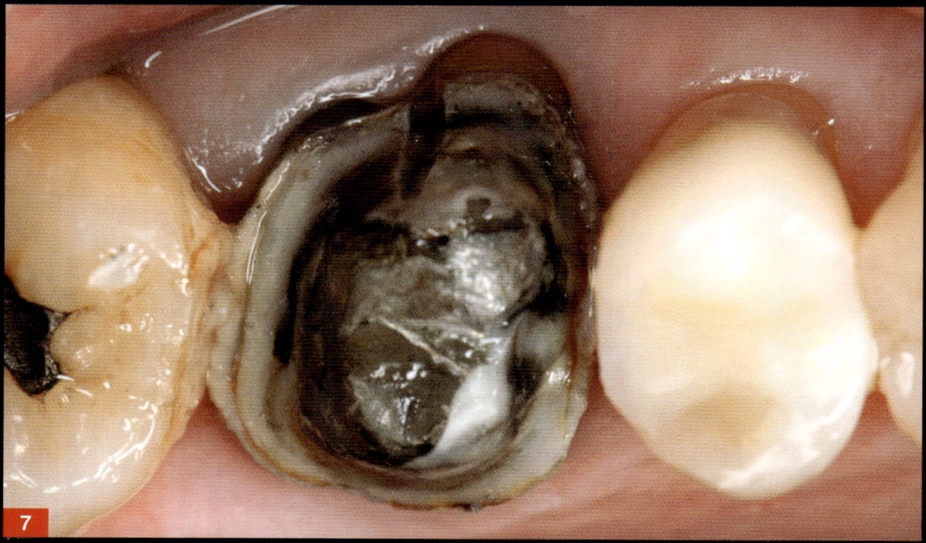

7

Figure 8: Manual probing of canal MB2.

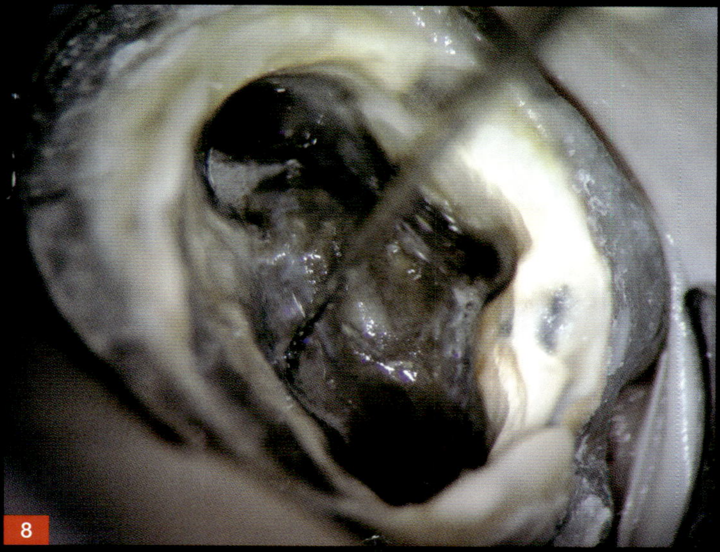

8

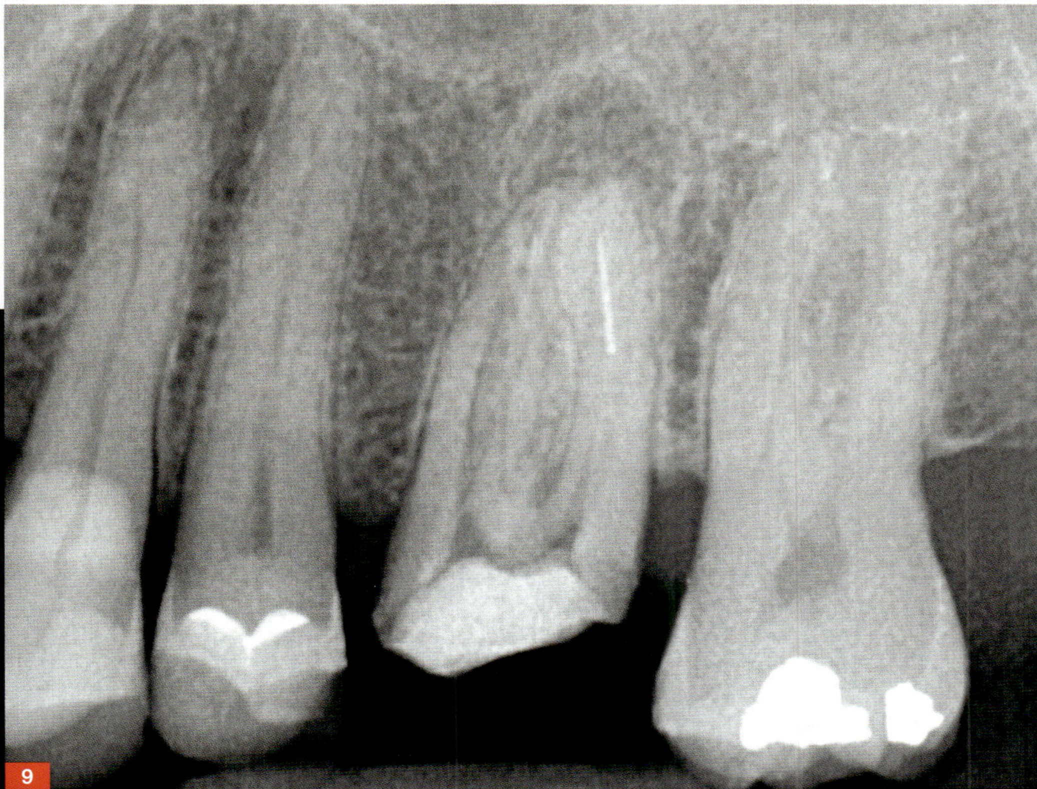

Figure 9: X-ray showing the emptying of the filling from the root canals.

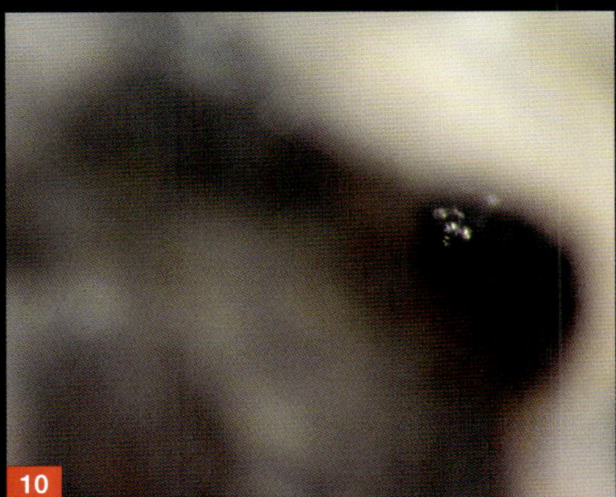

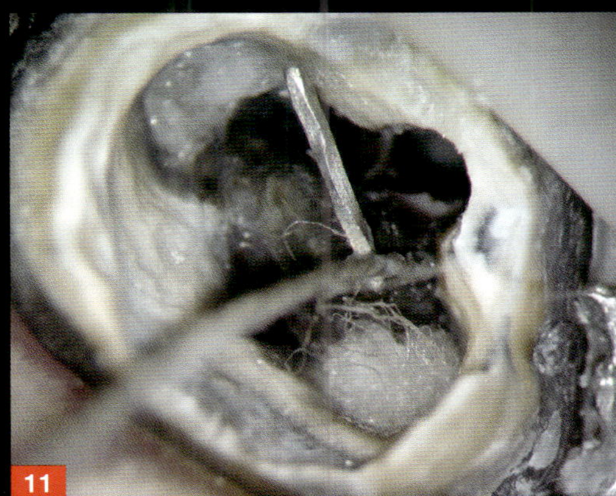

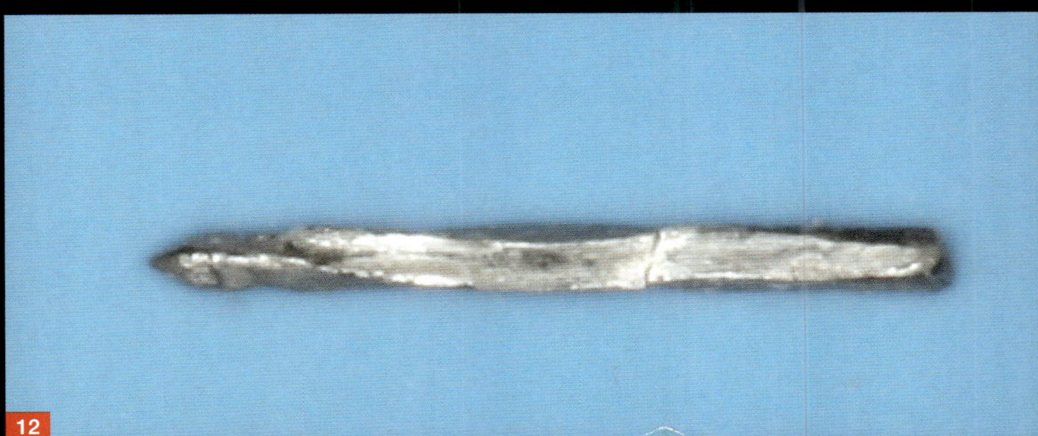

Figures 10-12: Isolation of the broken instrument from the distal canal (Figure 10); removal (Figure 11) of the broken instrument; situation after removal (Figure 12).

Figure 13: X-ray showing complete removal of the broken instrument from the distal canal of tooth 26.

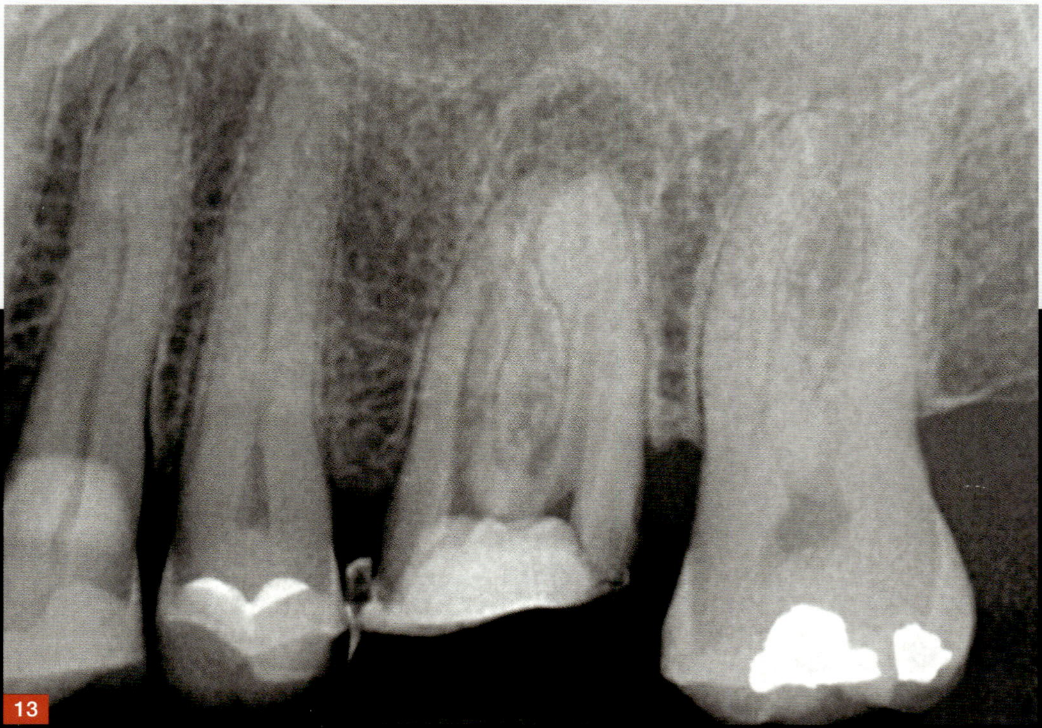

13

Figures 14 and 15: Intraoperative images of the completed access cavity.

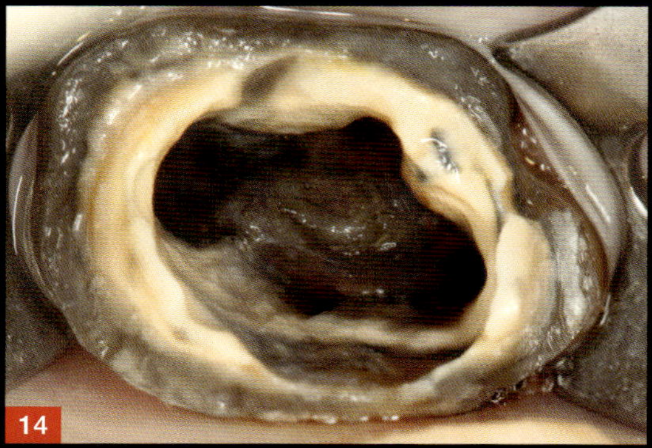

14

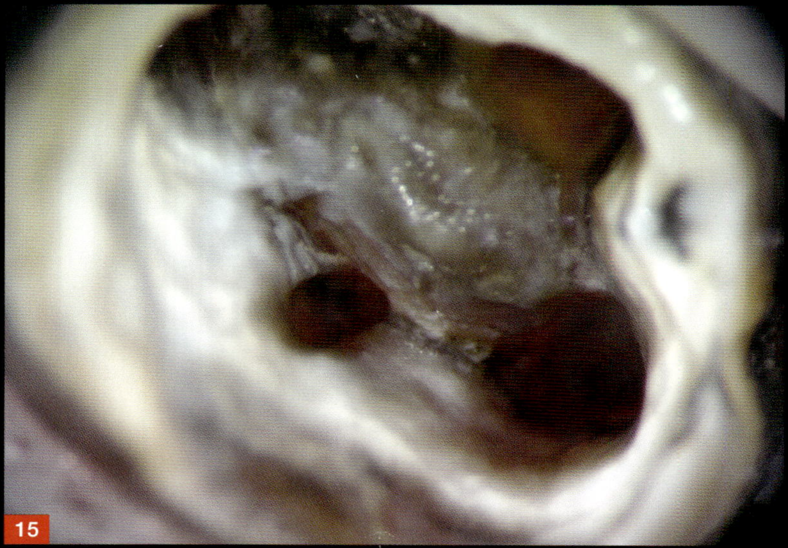

15

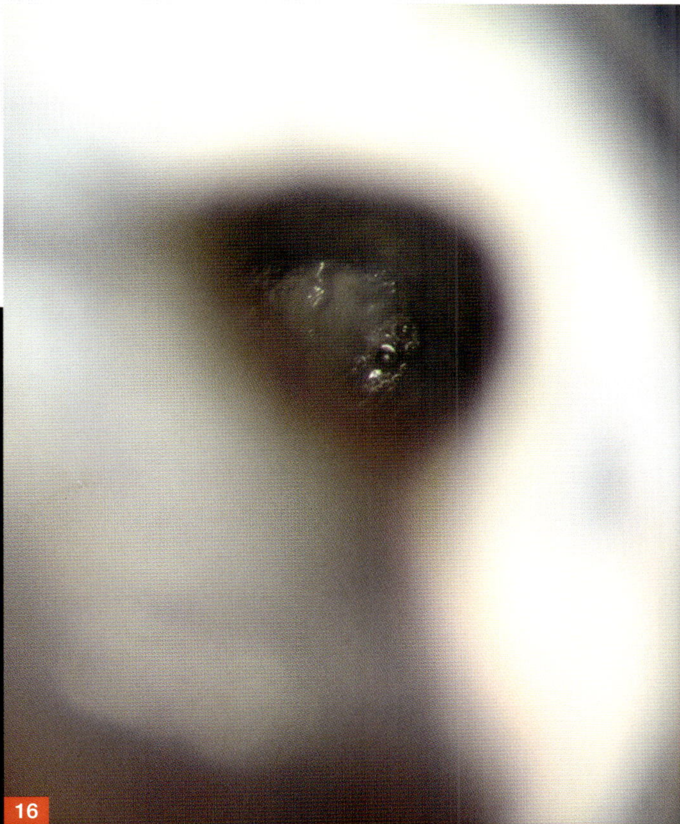

16

Figure 16: Detail of hypochlorite activity inside the distal canal. In such cases, it is mandatory to clean for a long time.

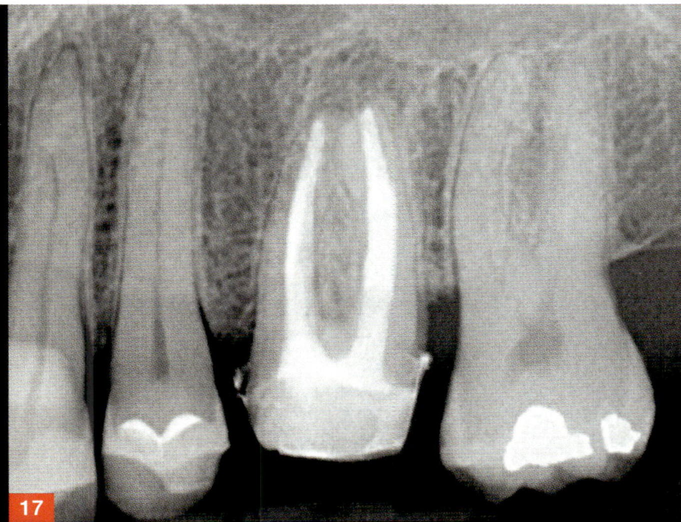

17

Figure 17: Final radiograph showing a good degree of compaction of the root canal filling material ending at the level of the radiographic length.

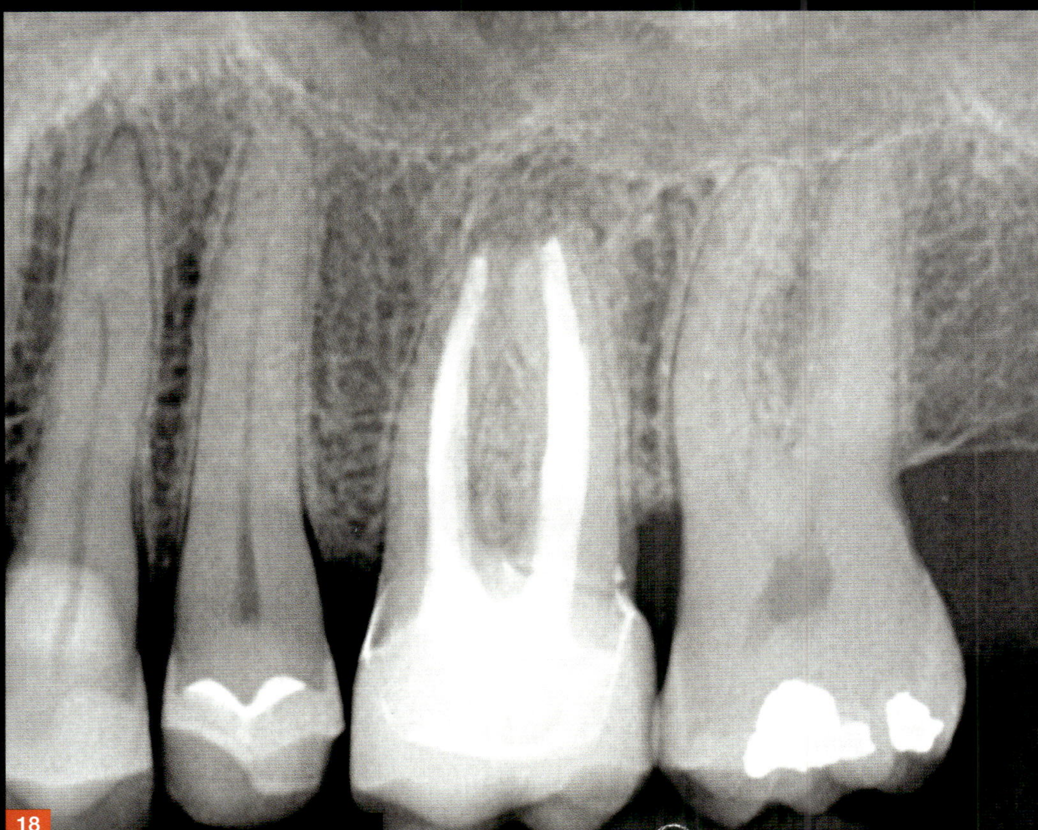

18

Figure 18: A 4-month follow-up showing an improvement in the periapical lesion of tooth 26.

CASE REPORT 6

Diagnosis of periradicular rarefaction in a lower cuspid

A radiolucent lesion of a flawlessly-filled cuspid with a peculiar canal morphology way, raises the suspicion that the lesion may be fed by the adjacent teeth and the CBCT examination confirms the diagnostic hypothesis.

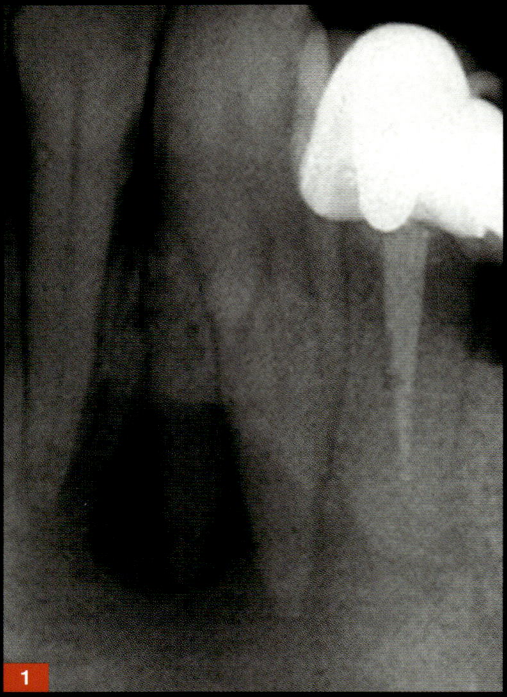

Figure 1: Preoperative radiograph, note the apical radiolucent lesion at tooth 33.

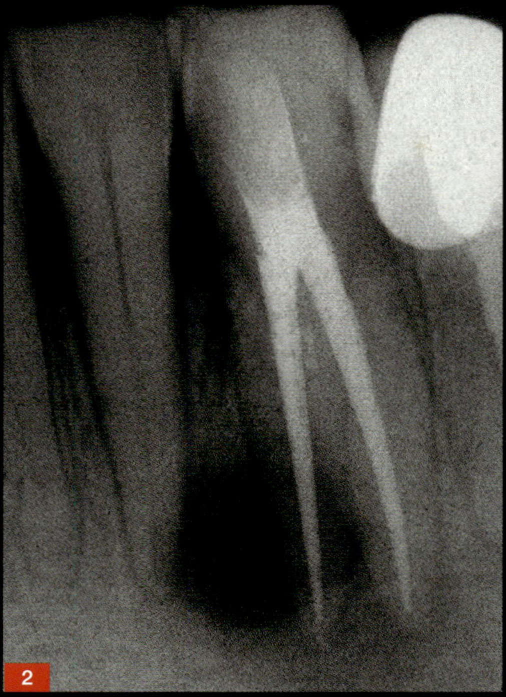

Figure 2: 4-month follow-up x-ray showing tooth no. 33 with two distinct roots, root canal filling to measure radiographic work and persistence of the periapical lesion.

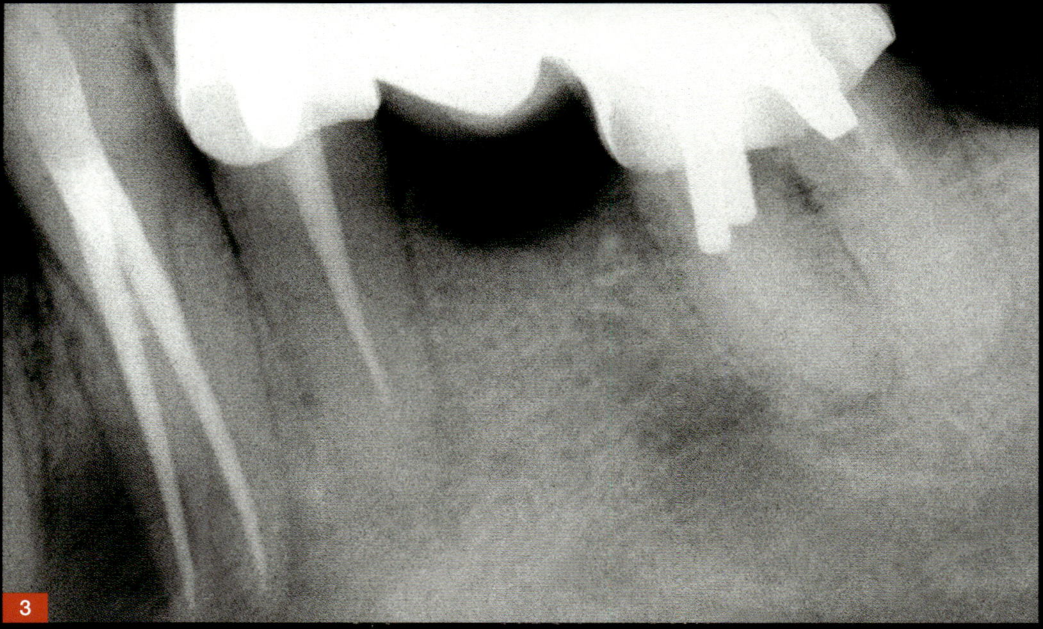

Figure 3: Follow-up x-ray at 6 months showing the persistence of the periapical lesion at tooth 33.

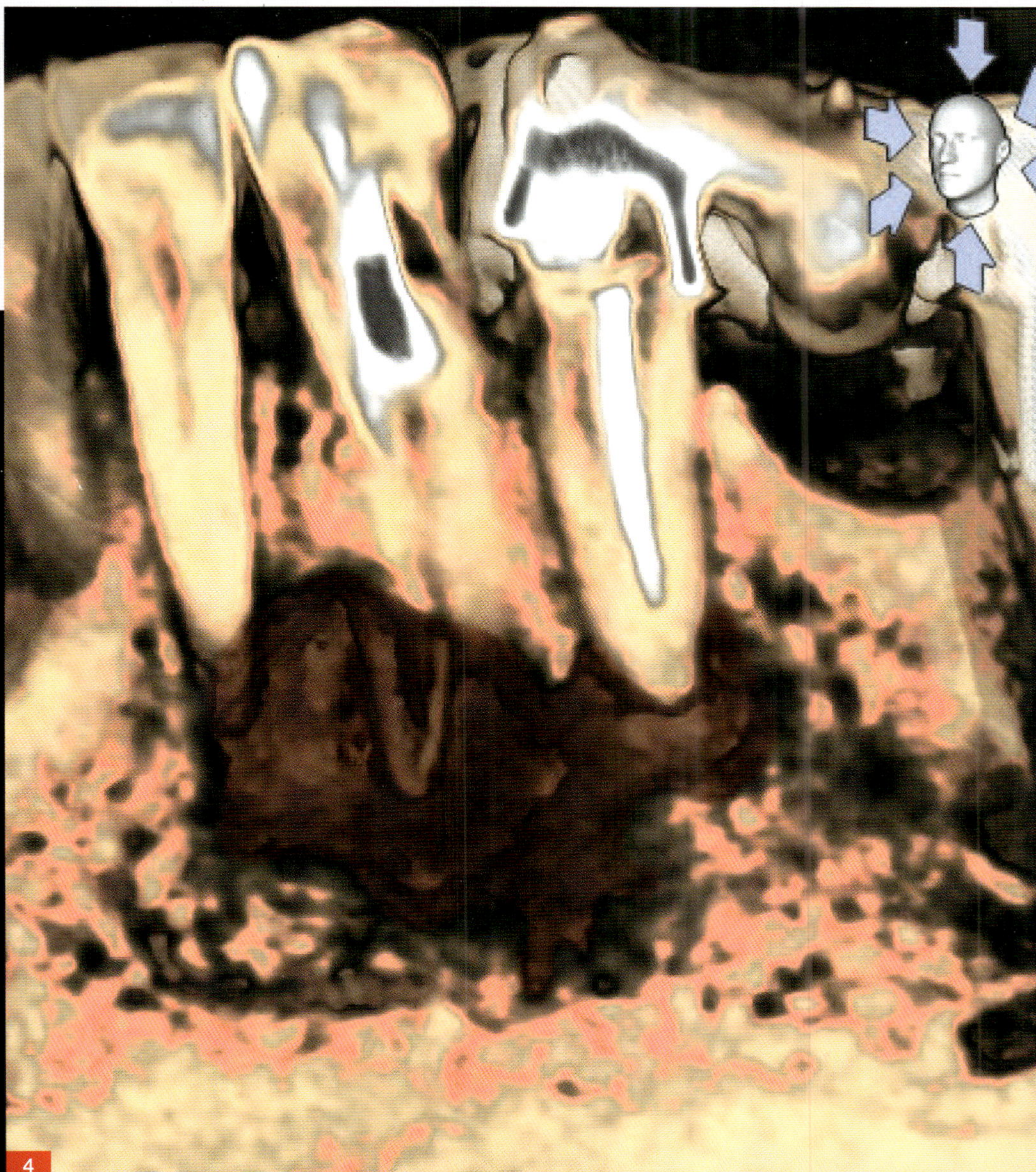

Figure 4: 3D CBCT reconstruction showing the extent of the periapical lesion; note the involvement of teeth 32, 33, and 34.

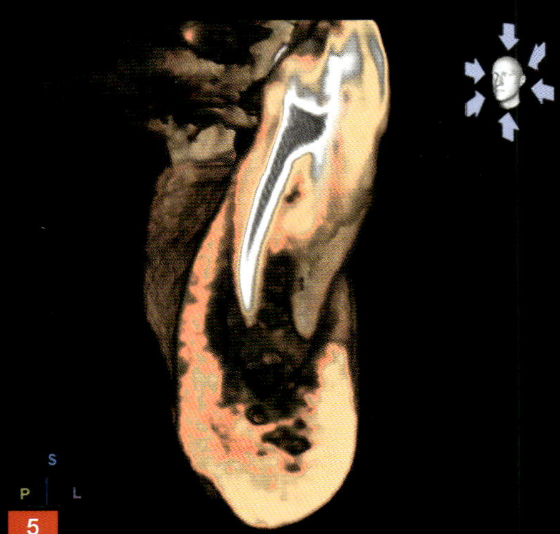

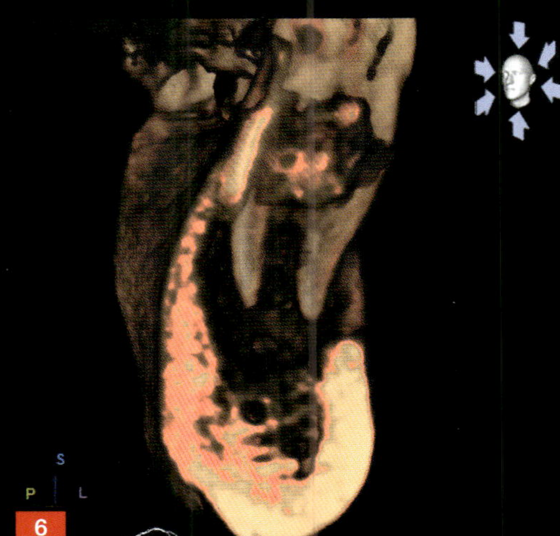

Figures 5 and 6: 3D reconstruction of the CBCT coronal slice showing the two roots of tooth no. 33 and the bone lesion.

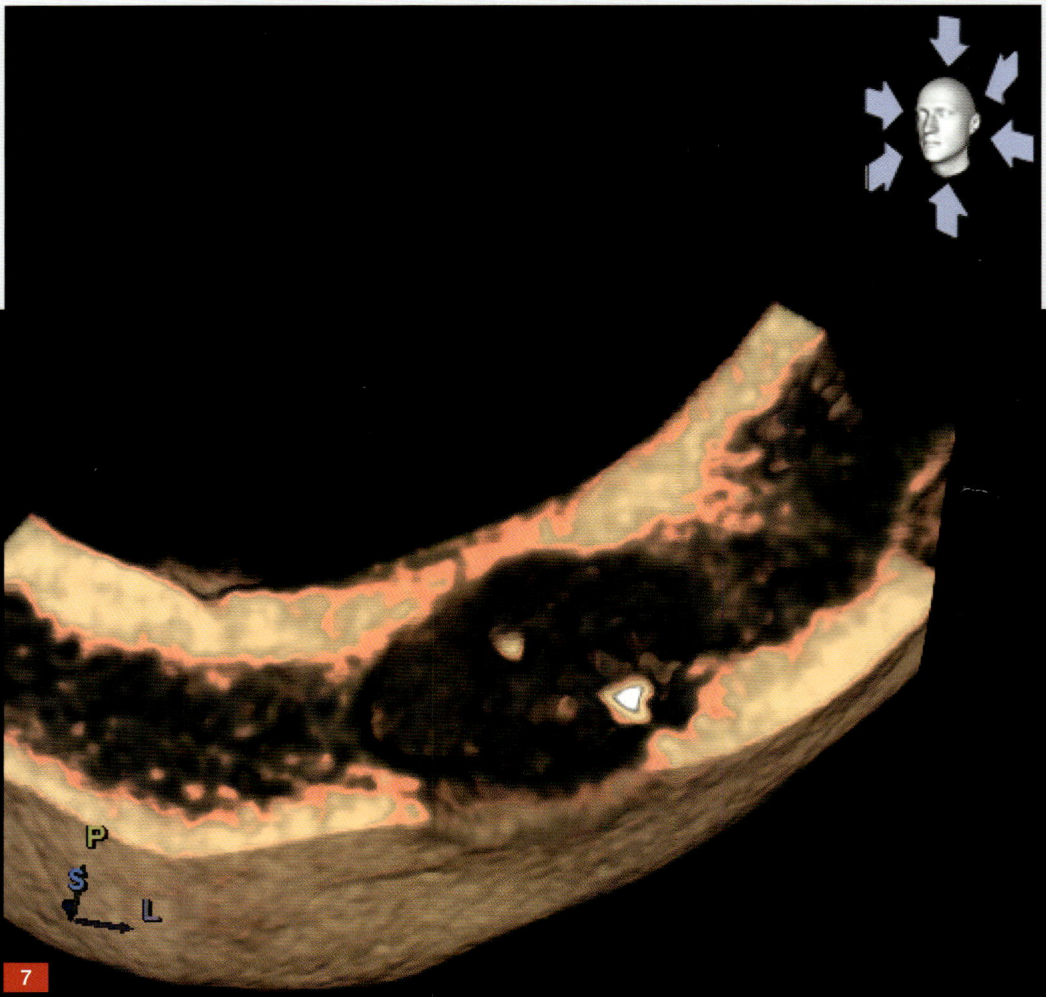

Figure 7: 3D reconstruction of the CBCT axial slice showing the bone lesion and the involvement of root apexes.

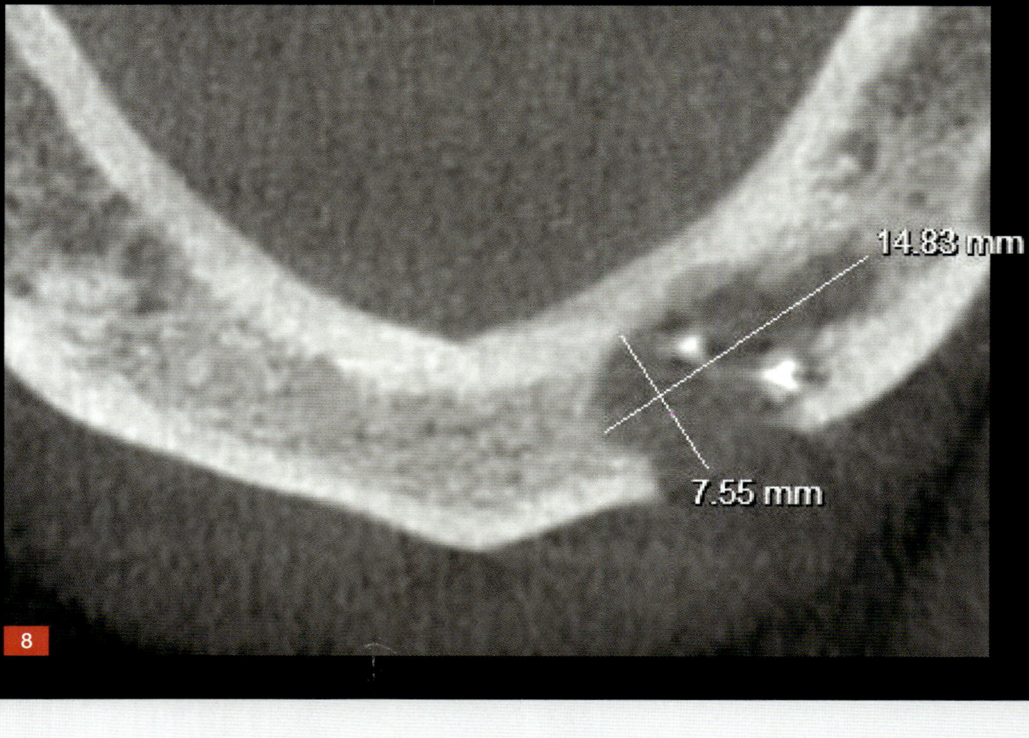

Figure 8: CBCT axial slice showing the actual size of the lesion.

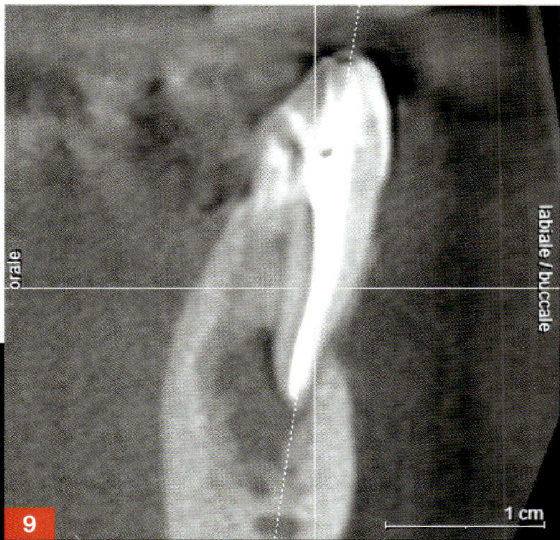

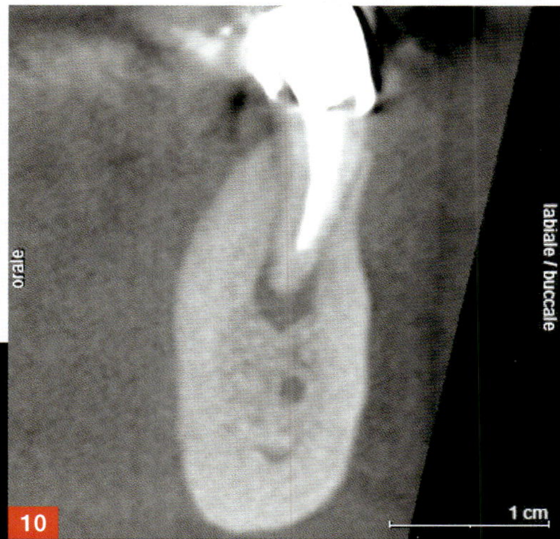

Figures 9 and 10: Coronal CBCT slice showing involvement of tooth no. 33 within the lesion.

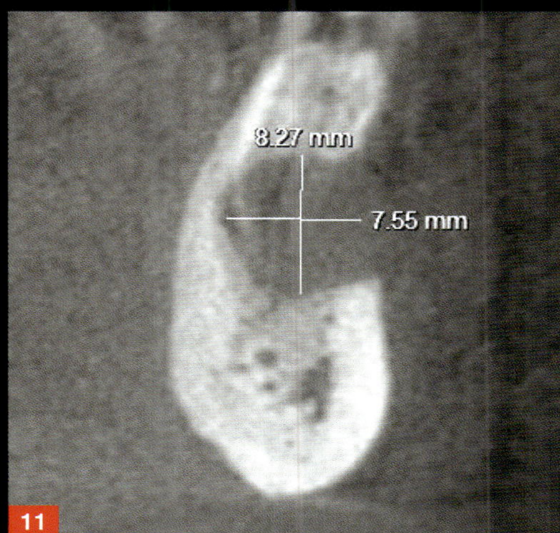

Figure 11: Coronal CBCT slice showing the actual vestibulo-lingual extension of the lesion.

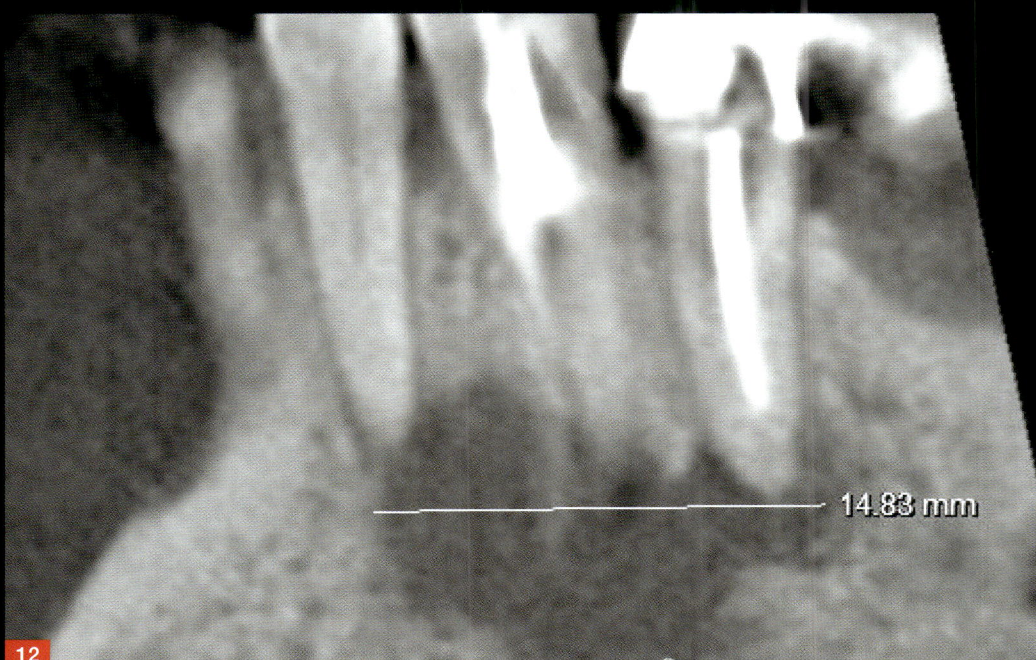

Figure 12: Sagittal CBCT slice showing the mesio-distal extension of the bone lesion.

CASE REPORT 7

Diagnosis of root perforation in a lower molar

In cases like this, the two-dimensional view leaves no diagnostic doubt; once again, however, the CBCT evaluation becomes essential for establishing where to perform access to the mesial endodontium not explored or shaped during the previous intervention.

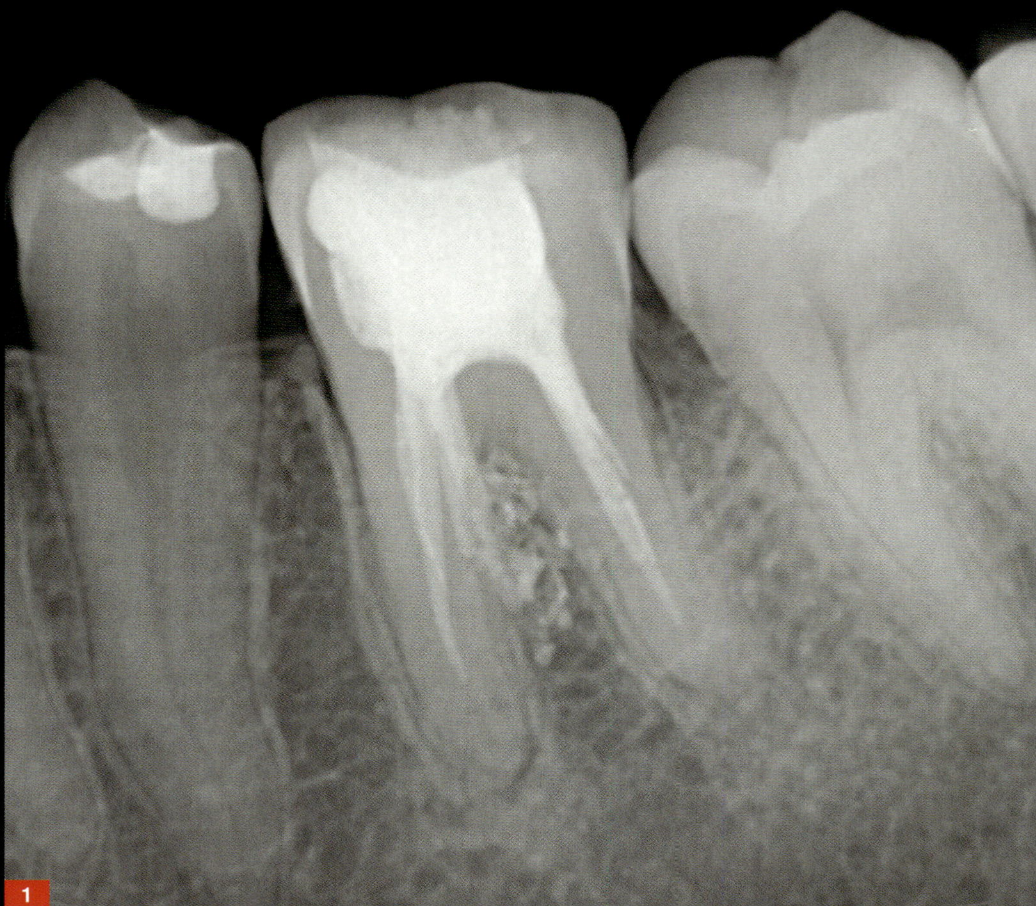

Figure 1: Preoperative x-ray: tooth no. 36 has an incorrect endodontic treatment with "short" canal filling and a suspicion of false canal with the presence of material in the inter-radicular space.

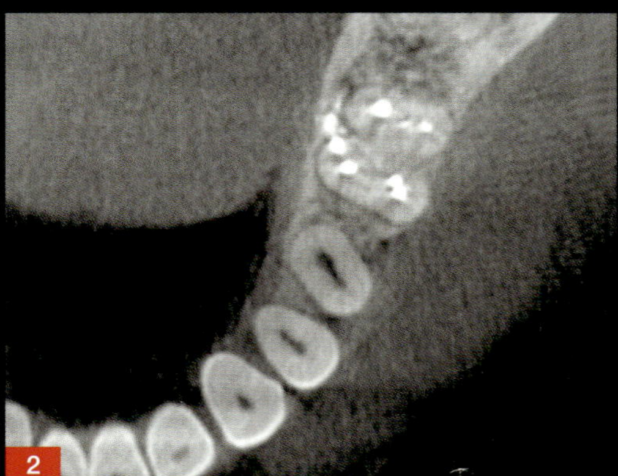

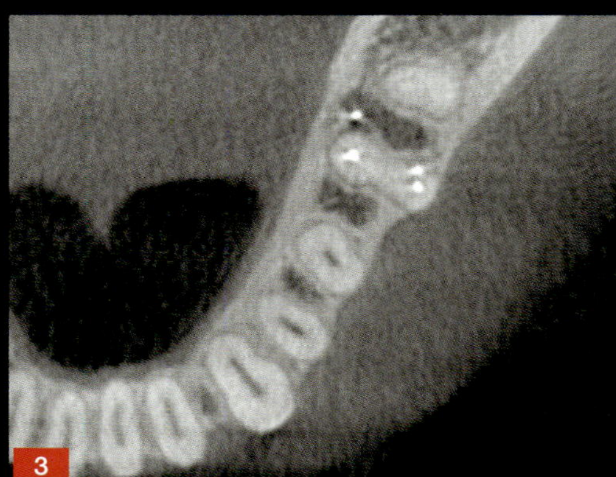

Figures 2 and 3: The definition of the axial sections of the CBCT evaluation makes it possible to highlight very clearly a false lingual canal with perforation and presence of endodontic material outside the endodontic space as well as a false canal in the mesio-vestibular canal.

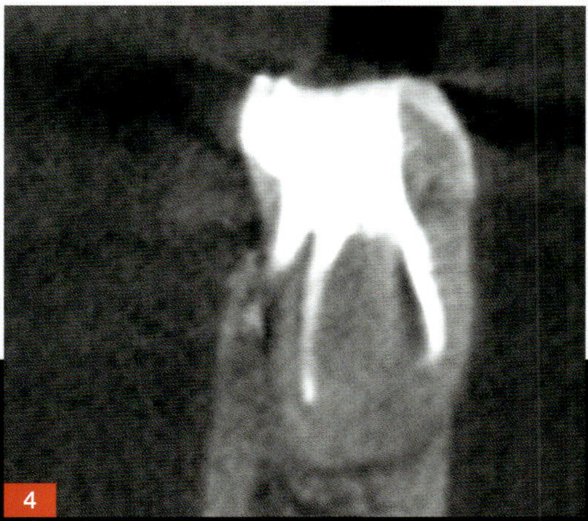

4

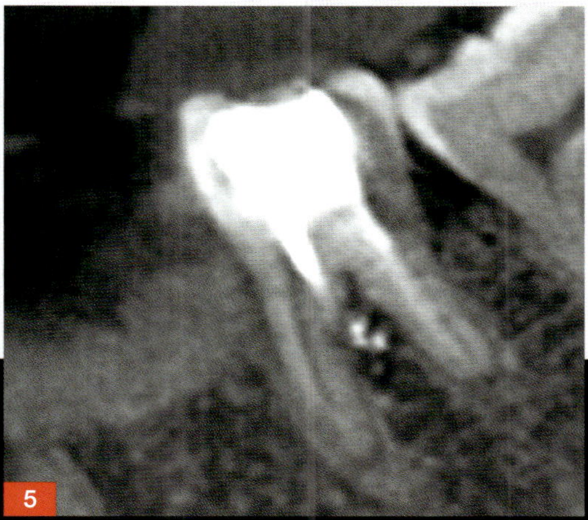

5

Figure 4: Coronal CBCT slice showing the lingual perforation of tooth no. 36.

Figure 5: Sagittal CBCT slice another view of the perforation with the presence of root canal filling material in the periodontal tissues.

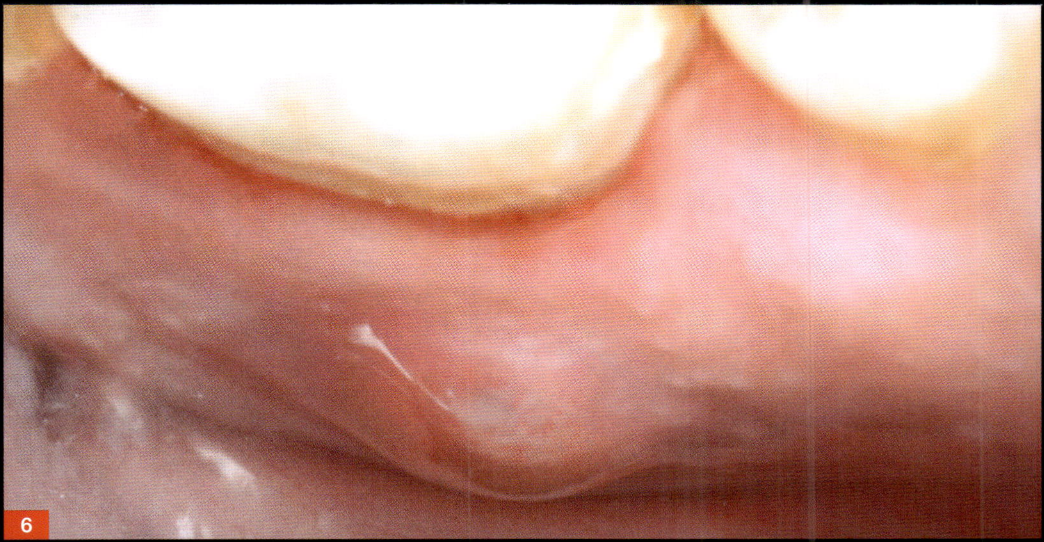

6

Figure 6: Preoperative clinical picture showing the presence of lingual swelling at tooth 36.

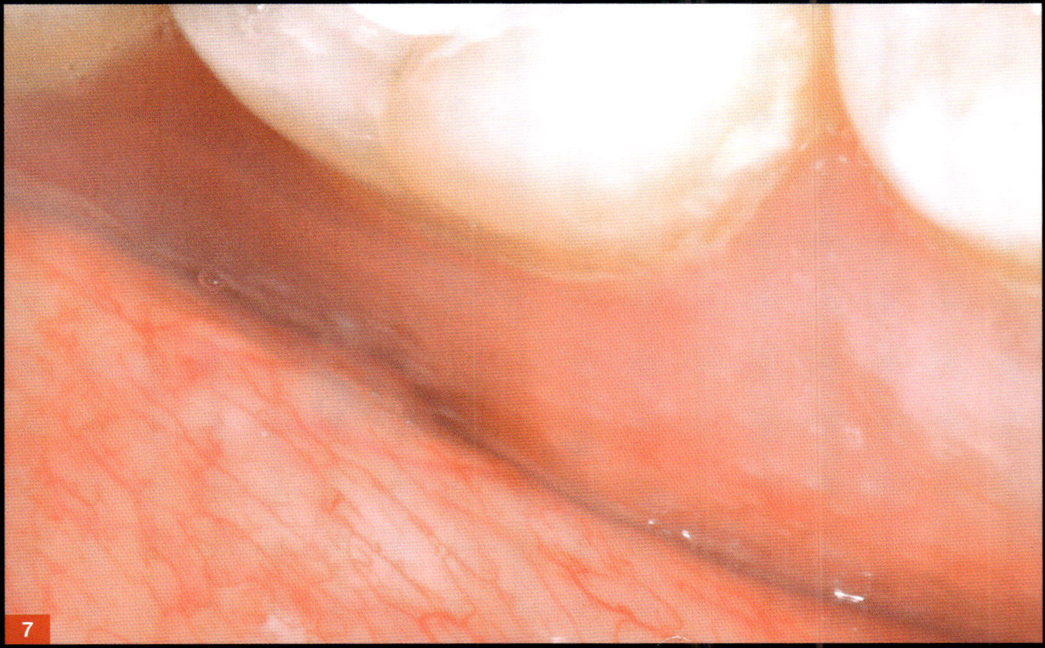

7

Figure 7: Photograph taken 7 days after medication showing the disappearance of the swelling and the return to normal of soft tissue color.

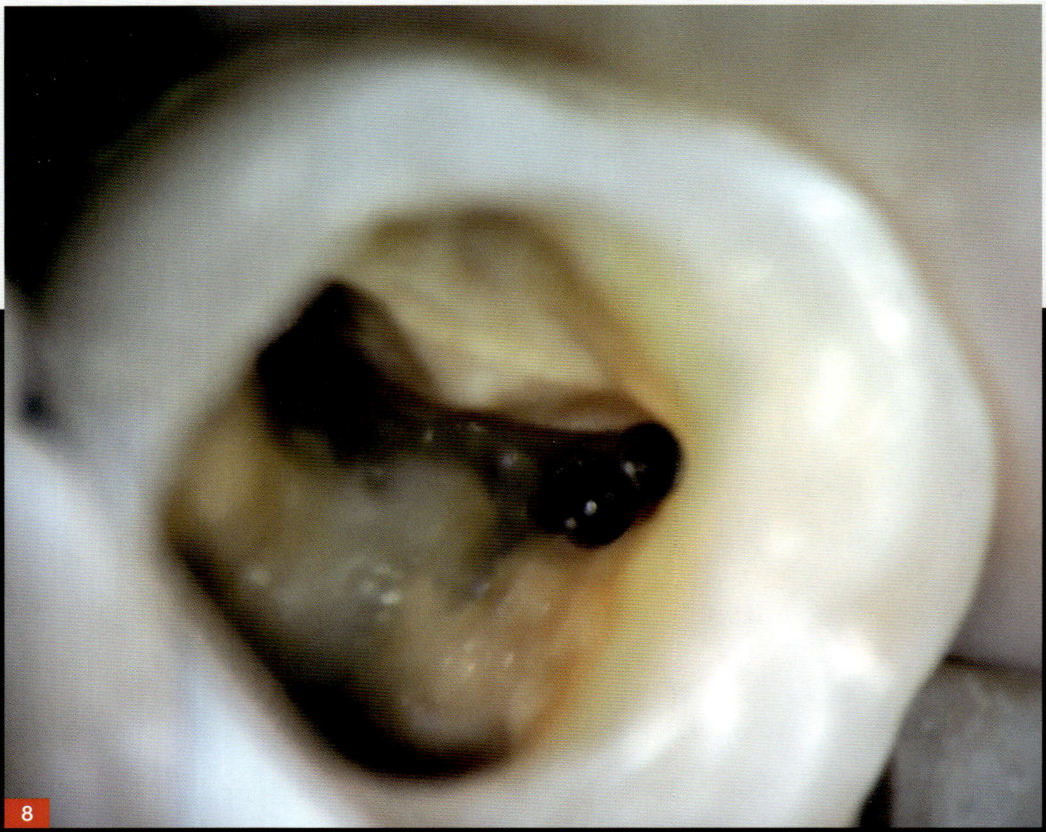

Figure 8: Intraoperative picture of the mesial canals under the microscope showing the presence of a false canal just mesially to the entrance of the mesio-vestibular canal.

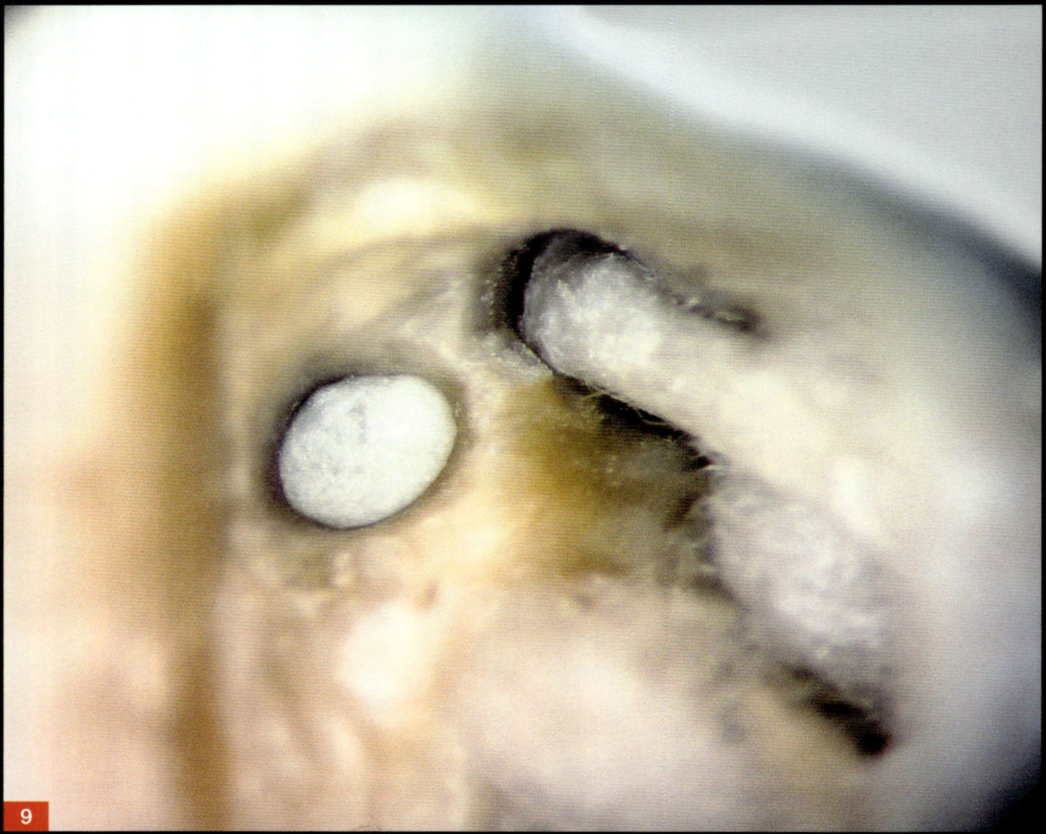

Figure 9: Intraoperative microscopic photo of MTA placement in lingual perforation after the protection of the canal openings by means of paper and cotton cones.

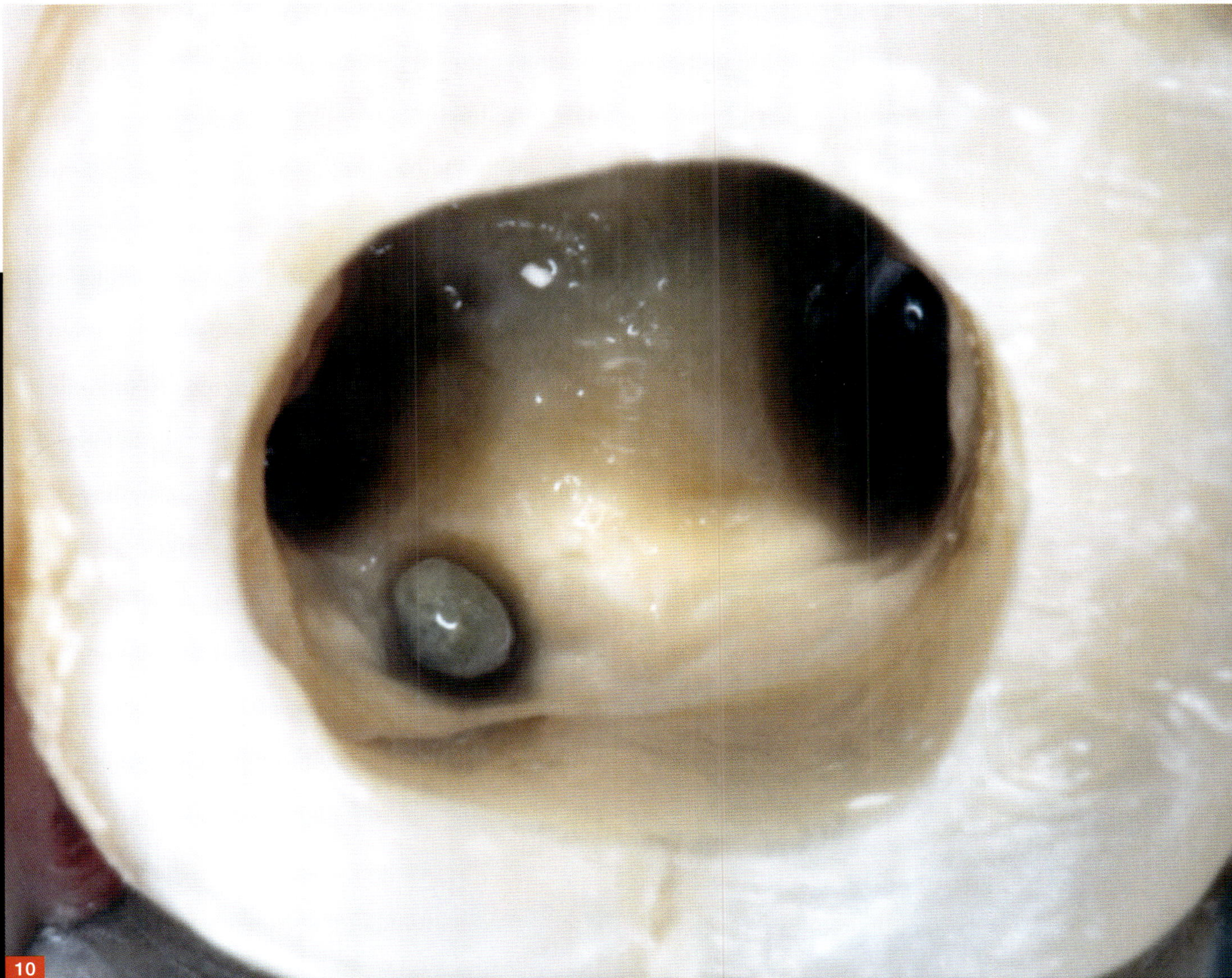

10

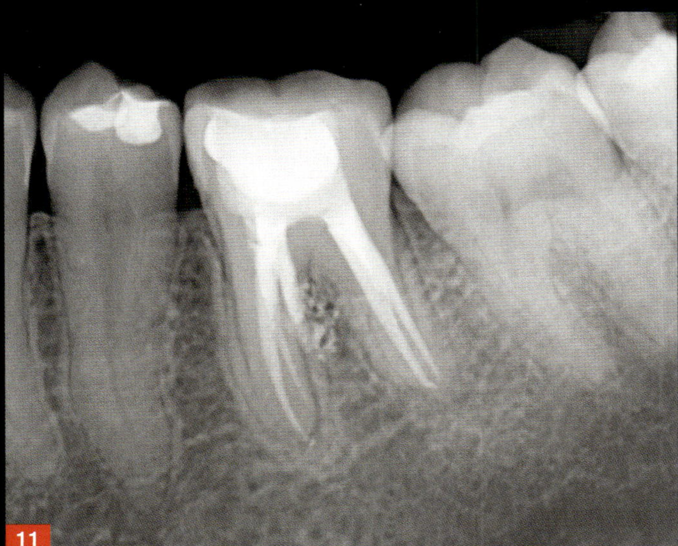

11

Figure 10: Intraoperative photo of access cavity and repaired lingual perforation.

Figure 11: 3-month follow-up periapical x-ray: note the independence of the 4 root canals and the repair of the perforation.

CASE REPORT 8

Diagnosis and therapeutic evaluations of cervical resorption in an upper canine

The presence of swelling in teeth without previous treatment should always be part of the differential diagnosis, as it is distinctive of inflammatory lesions of endodontic origin.

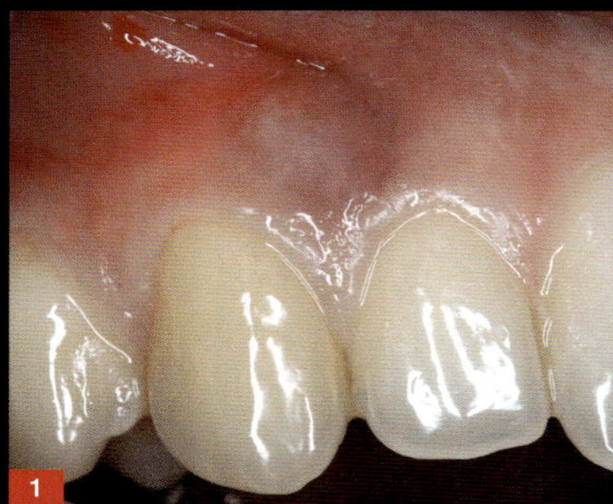

1

Figure 1: Clinical picture showing gingival swelling at tooth no. 13.

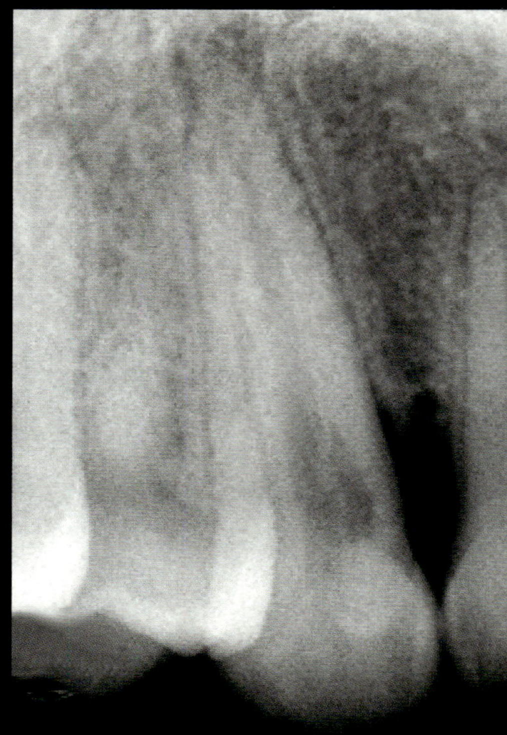

2

Figure 2: Preoperative radiograph showing a periapical radiolucent lesion at tooth 13 and a large resorption gap in the same tooth.

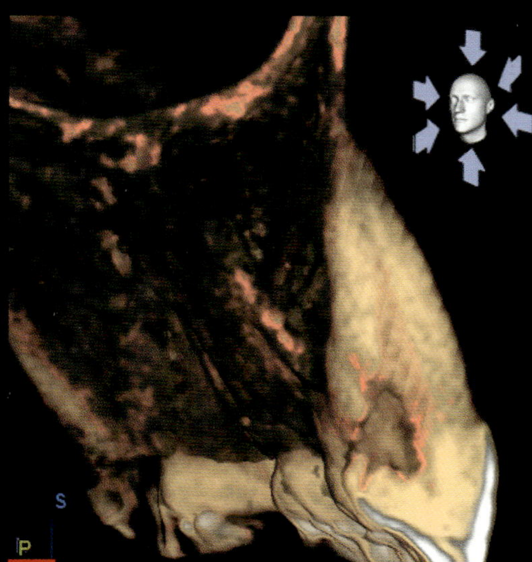

3

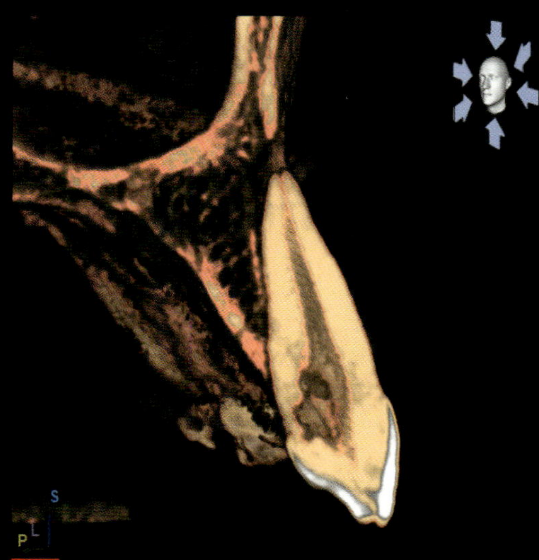

4

Figures 3 and 4: 3D rendering using CBCT showing the resorption gaps (Figure 3) and the presence of periodontal communications.

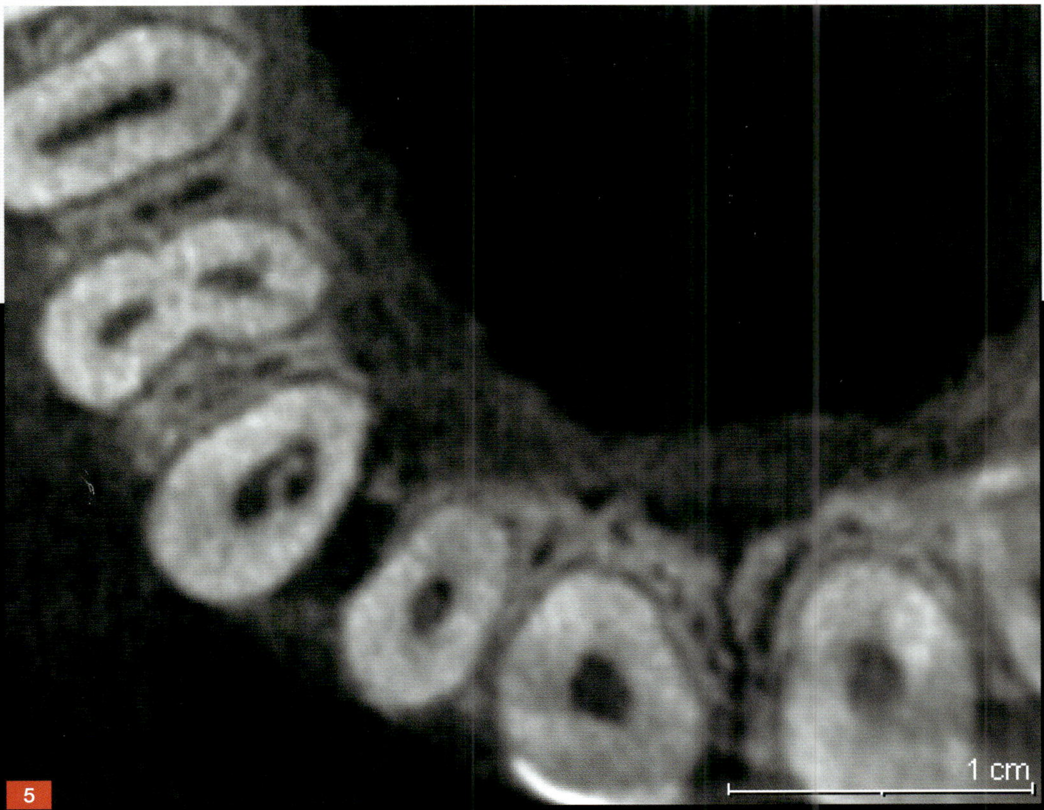

5

Figure 5: Axial CBCT slice showing resorption gap at tooth 13.

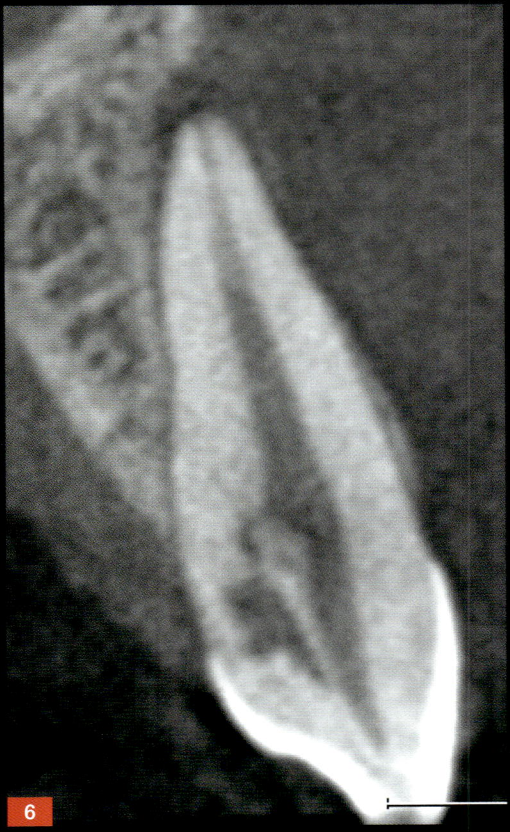

6

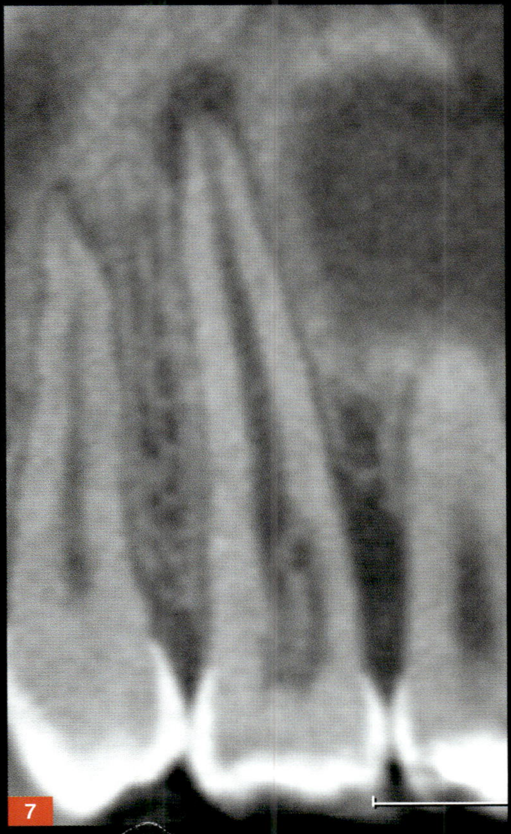

7

Figure 6: Coronal CBCT slice showing the periapical lesion in tooth 13 and the resorption gap.

Figure 7: Sagittal CBCT slice showing the periapical lesion in tooth 13 and the resorption gap.

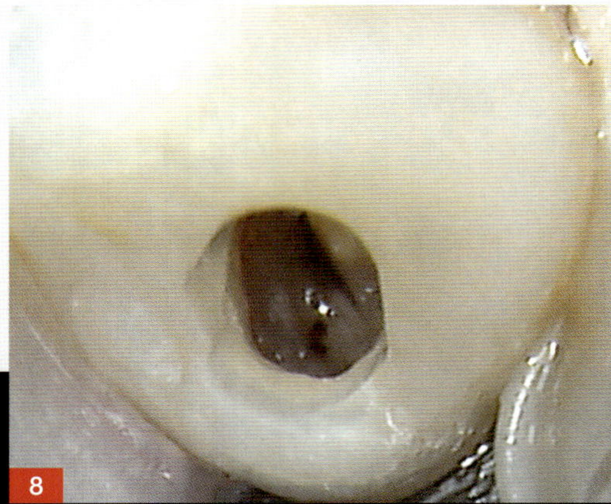

Figure 8: Access cavity in which the blood from the perforation is visible.

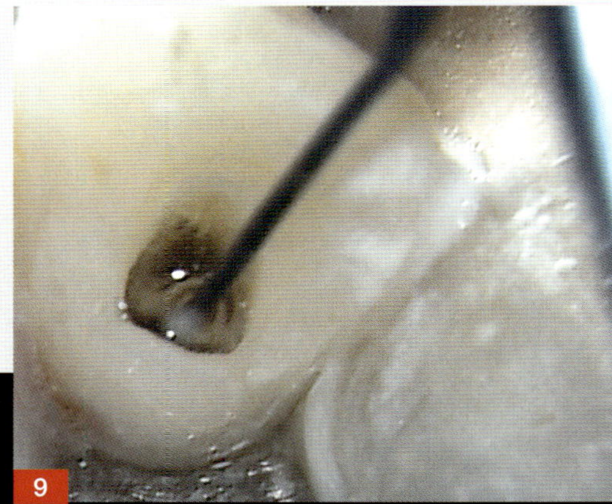

Figure 9: Activation of the irrigants by ultrasound.

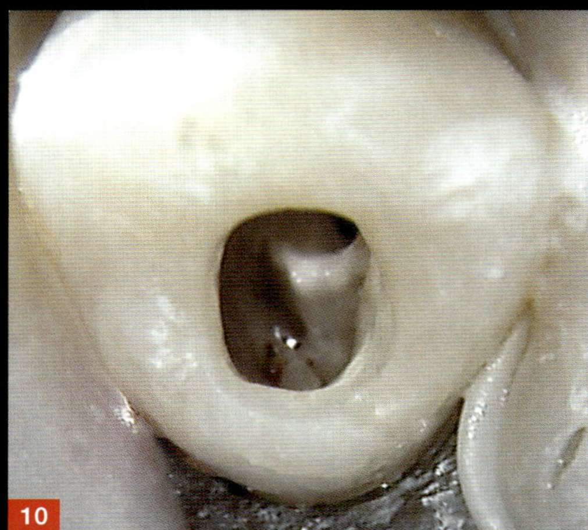

Figure 10: Resorption after cleansing.

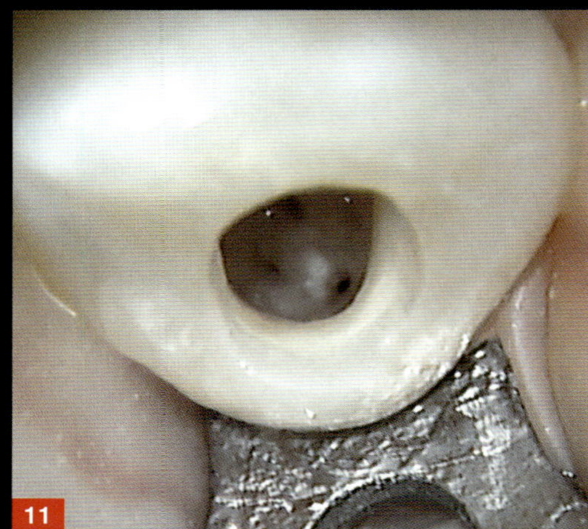

Figure 11: The root canal and the two perforations.

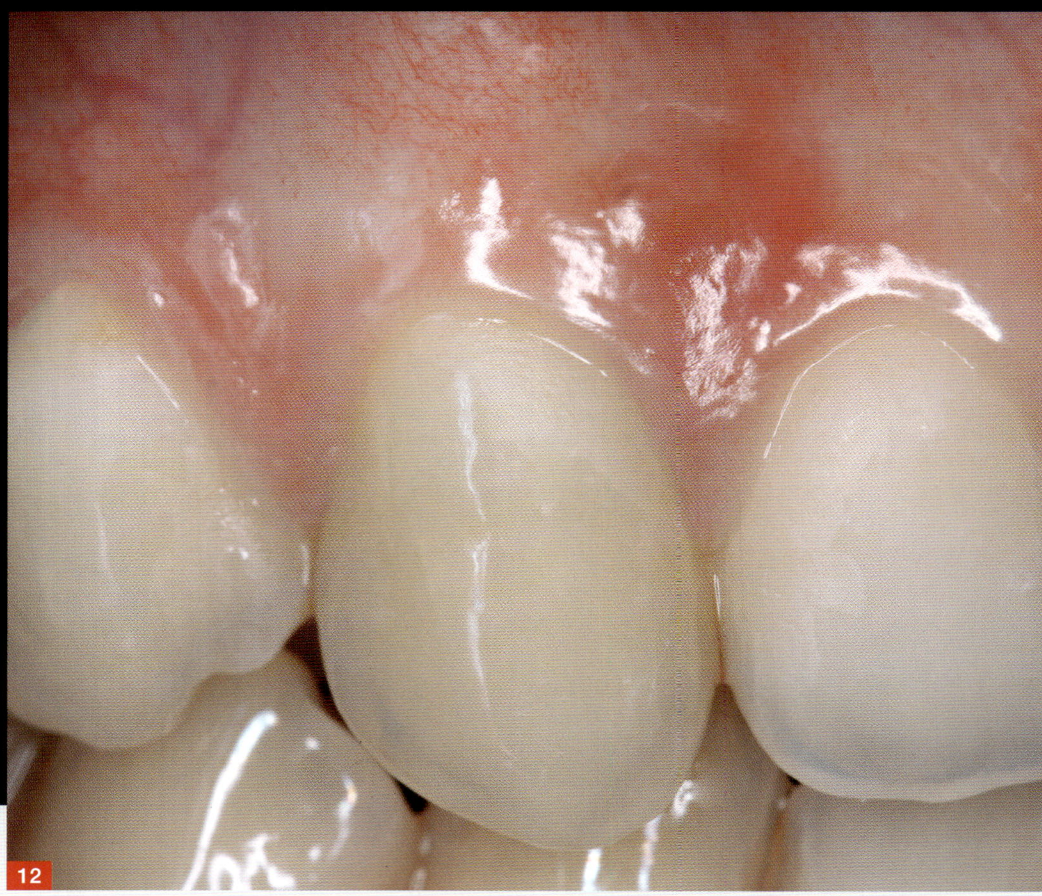

Figure 12: Clinical image showing soft tissue healing after 10 days.

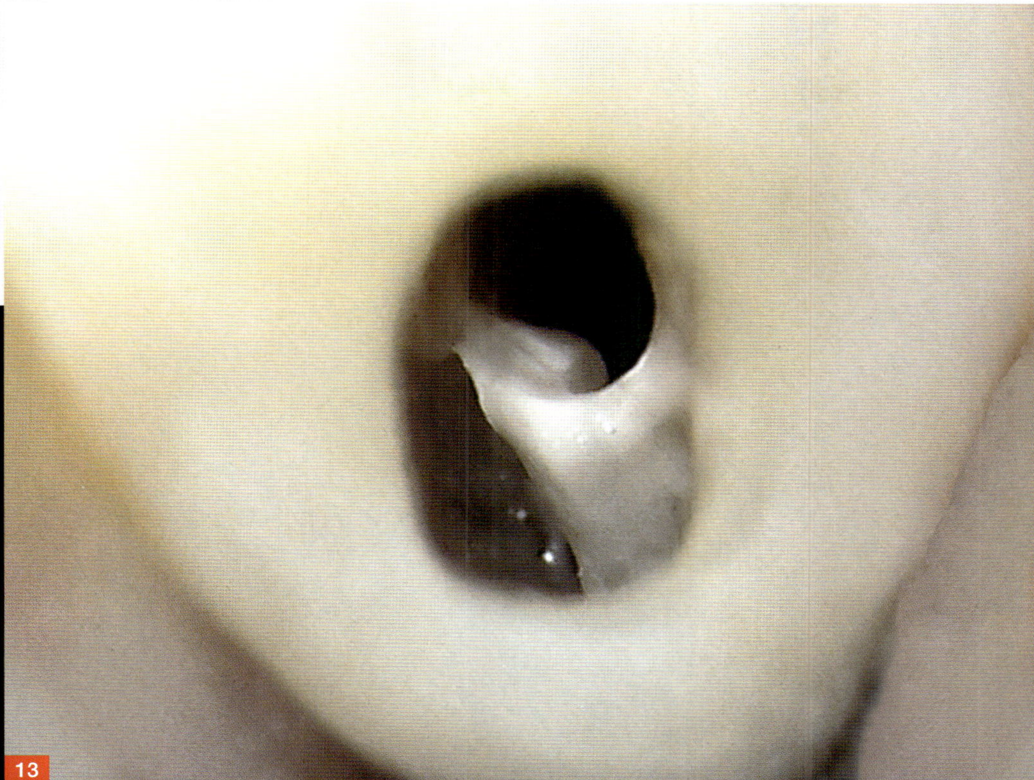

Figure 13: Resorption after cleansing and instrumentation using ultrasonic tips.

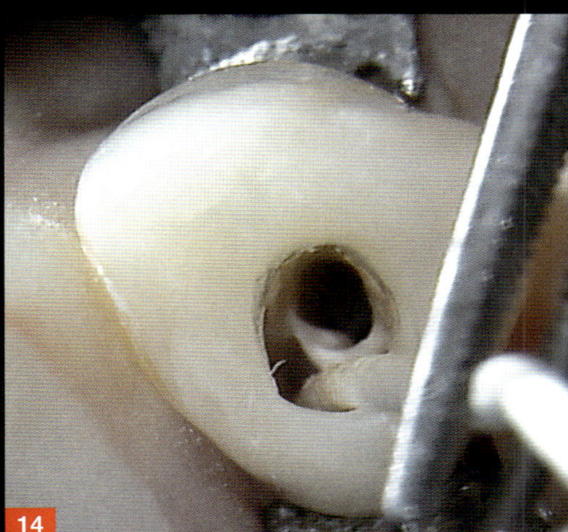

Figure 14: Drying of the perforation by means of well-calibrated cones of sterile absorbent paper.

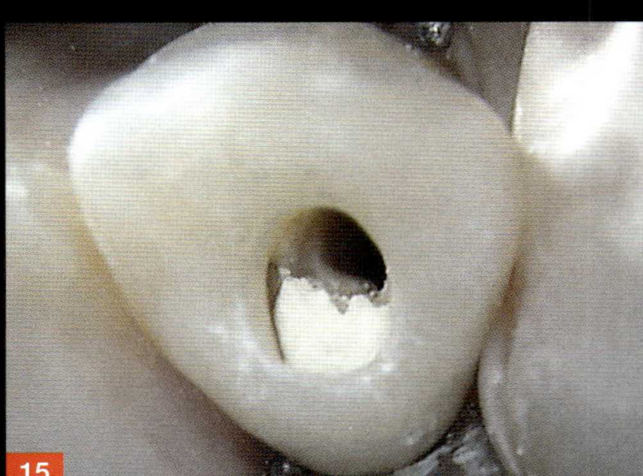

Figure 15: Perforation repaired with MTA.

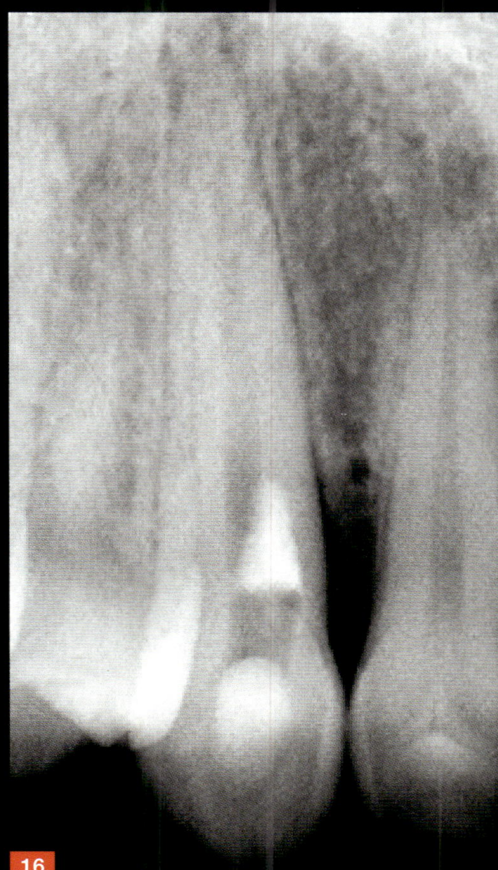

Figure 16: X-ray showing closure of the perforation with MTA.

Figure 17: Hardening of the MTA. In the past this process took 48 to 72 hours; the new formulations have far shorter hardening times.

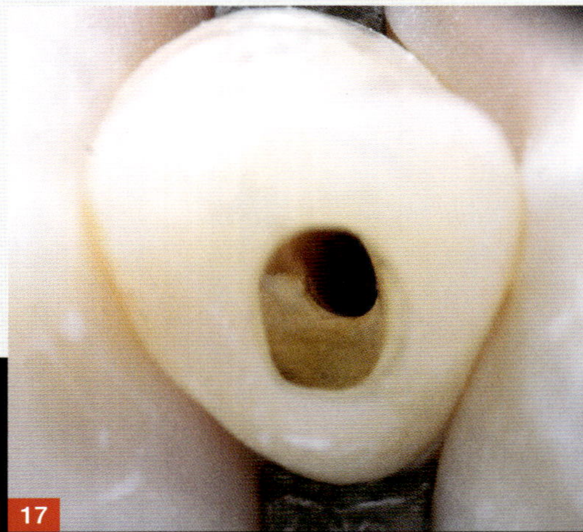

17

Figure 19: Clinical image of the follow-up after 3 years showing absence of soft tissue swelling.

Figure 18: 3-month follow-up x-ray showing initial healing of the periapical lesion of tooth 13 and the absence of periodontal problems.

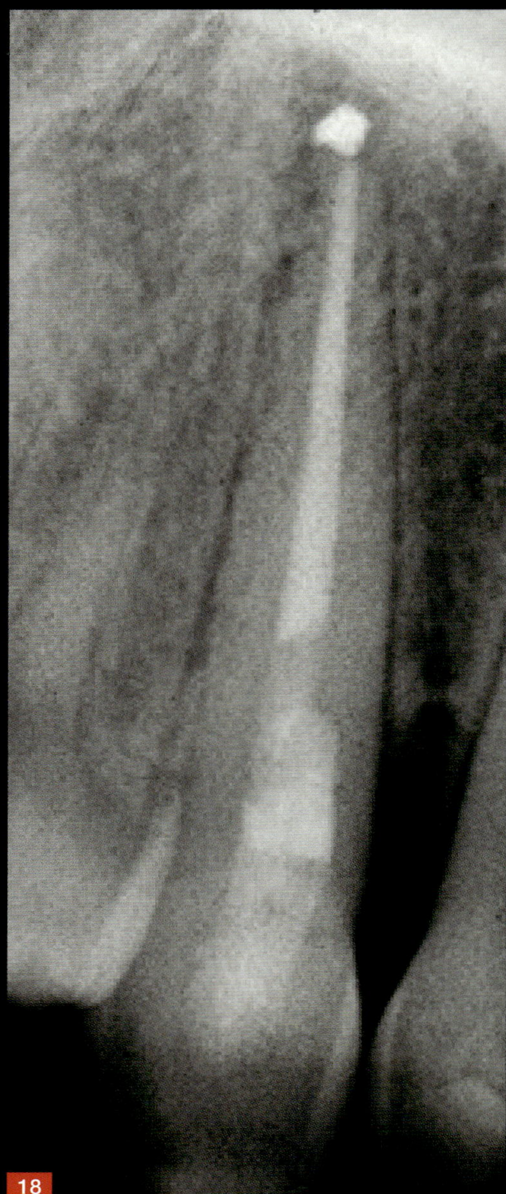

18

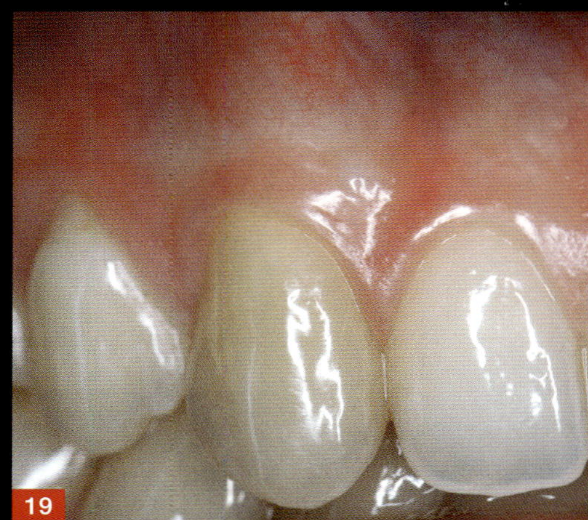

19

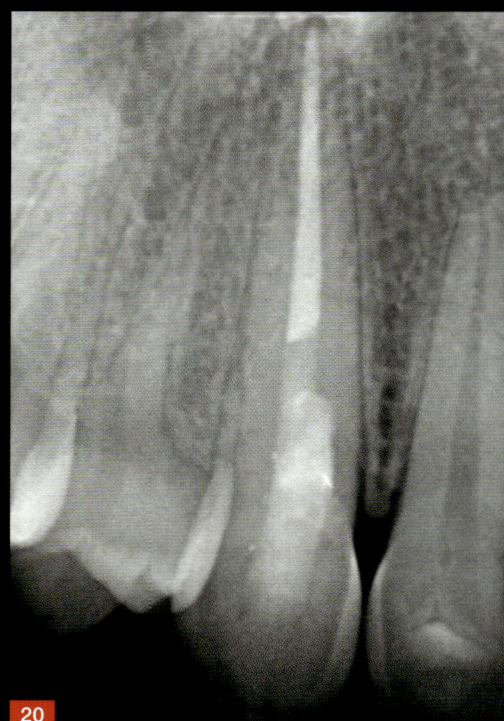

20

Figure 20: 3-year follow-up x-ray showing complete cement resorption beyond area of apex and apical healing.
A very small area of apical radiotransparency remains, which can be attributed to a small scar tissue.

Some studies have been carried out, most of which in vitro, and have not yielded encouraging evidence: as already mentioned, the "disturbance" caused to the radiopaque materials present inside the root canal complicates the success of this type of radiographic examination[37, 38].
The association between the presence of root canal posts, particularly metal ones, and the vertical root fracture has already been reported in the literature many years ago[39-41]. Suspicion of irreparable injury can be supported by clinical examinations and traditional radiographic findings without the need for a CBCT examination.
However, in uncertain cases, additional support, if only for the location of the lesion, can be obtained from the CBCT examination.
As the radiograph can be scrolled in a corono-radicular direction, the presence of a root fracture can be hypothesized if, as illustrated in Chapter 1 on page 35, bone rarefaction is already present in the first slices of radiograms immediately below the pulp chamber floor.

Box 2.3 **ROOT FRACTURES**

Root fractures deserve a separate chapter; they are increasingly found in previously treated teeth. Recent studies have pointed out that indications for retreatment or retrograde surgical therapy are misinterpreted because the signs of periradicular disease are unclear and not easily interpreted[42,43].
The teeth in which a vertical root fracture should be suspected are those in which one or more of the factors listed in Table 2.2 are present upon clinical or radiographic examination.

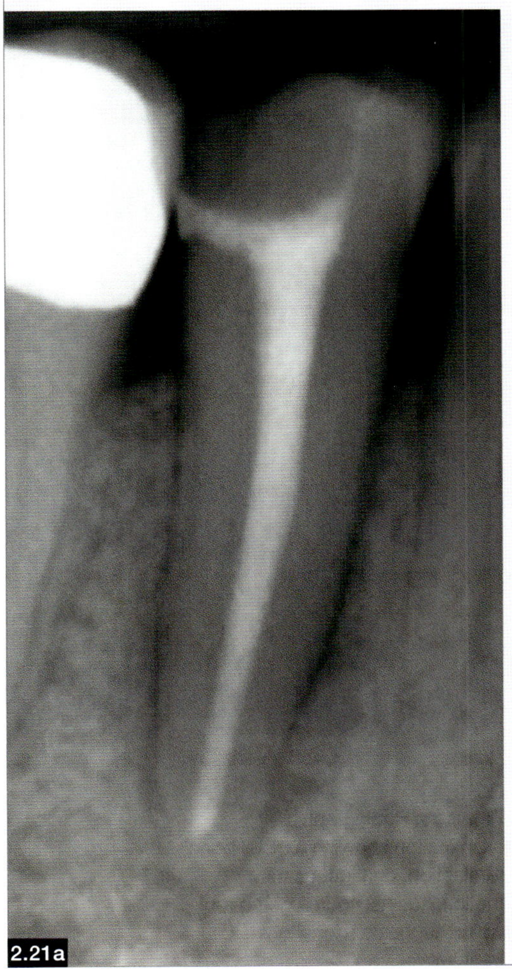
2.21a

Fig. 2.21a: Apparently well-performed endodontic treatment has a barely noticeable rarefaction along the entire length of the root contour.

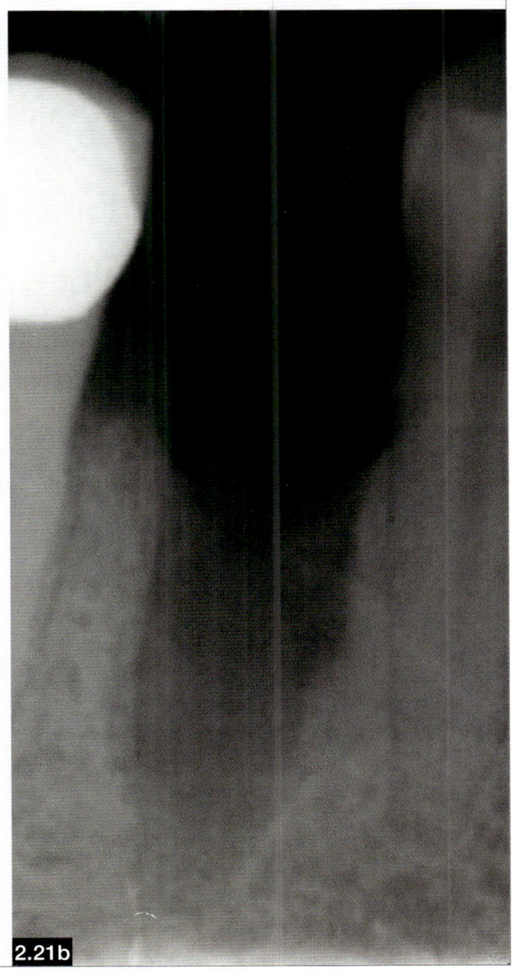
2.21b

Fig. 2.21b: Outcome of the extraction for a vertical root fracture; note the great impairment of the bone compartment.

Fig. 2.22: Clinical image of upper premolars showing a healthy tooth and a treated tooth, specifically nos. 25 and 24. Chewing pain was attributed to a periapical lesion on 24.

Fig. 2.23: Radiographic examination highlights an idiopathic periapical lesion at tooth 25, lacking all the elements known to cause pulp injury.

Fig. 2.24: High-magnification examination shows a fracture line path incompatible with the presence of the tooth in the patient's mouth.

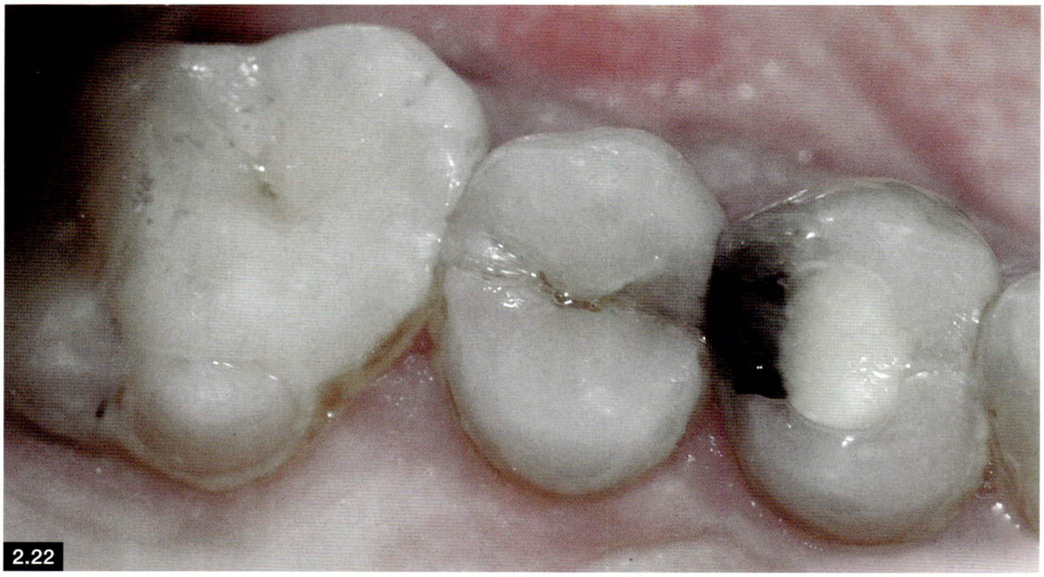

2.22

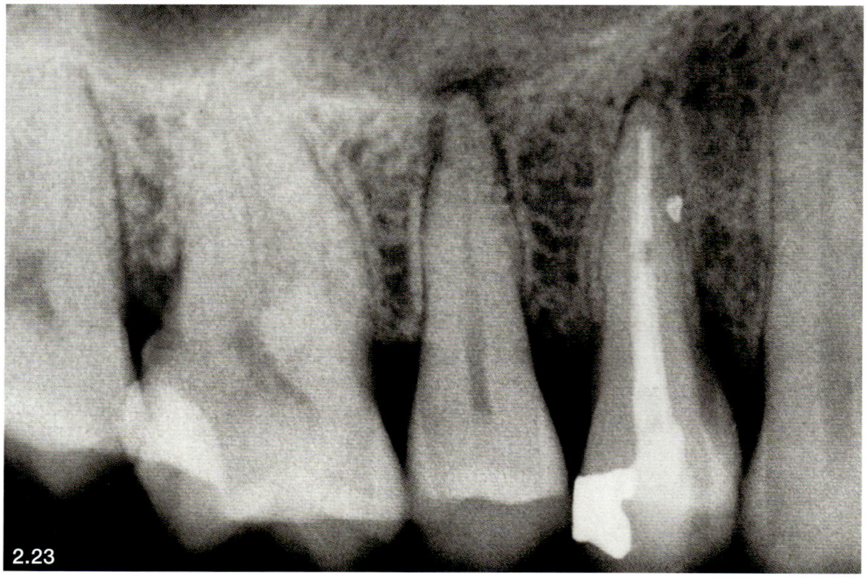

2.23

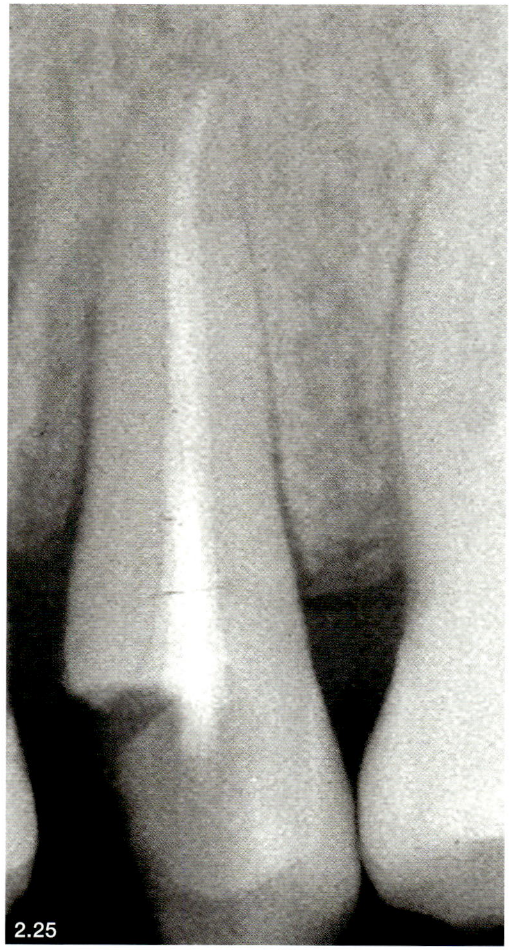

2.25

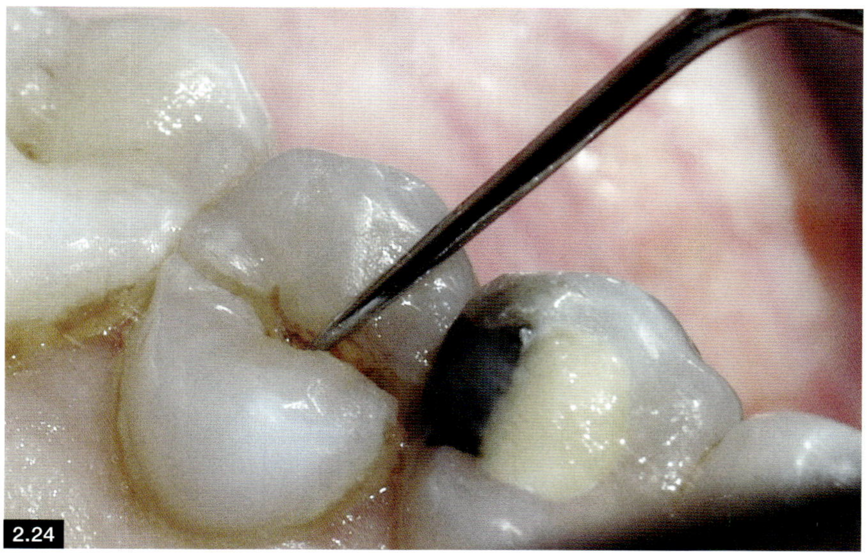

2.24

Fig. 2.25: Radiographic examination showing a distal bone rarefaction, contiguous to the longitudinal course of the root, which suggests a longitudinal fracture.

Table 2.2 **RISK FACTORS**

• BRIDGE PILLARS, ESPECIALLY IF TERMINAL	• FISTULAS AND SWELLINGS THAT TEND TO NOT TO REGRESS DESPITE TREATMENT
• RECONSTRUCTIONS WITHOUT CUSP COVER	• X-RAY EXAMINATION REVEALING WIDE RAREFACTION UNRELATED TO INCONGRUOUS ROOT CANAL TREATMENT
• ROOT CANAL POSTS	
• SCREW-RETAINED (THREADED)	
• ICONIC CROWNS ROOT CANAL POSTS	
• PERIRADICULAR TUBULAR PROBING	• MOBILITY

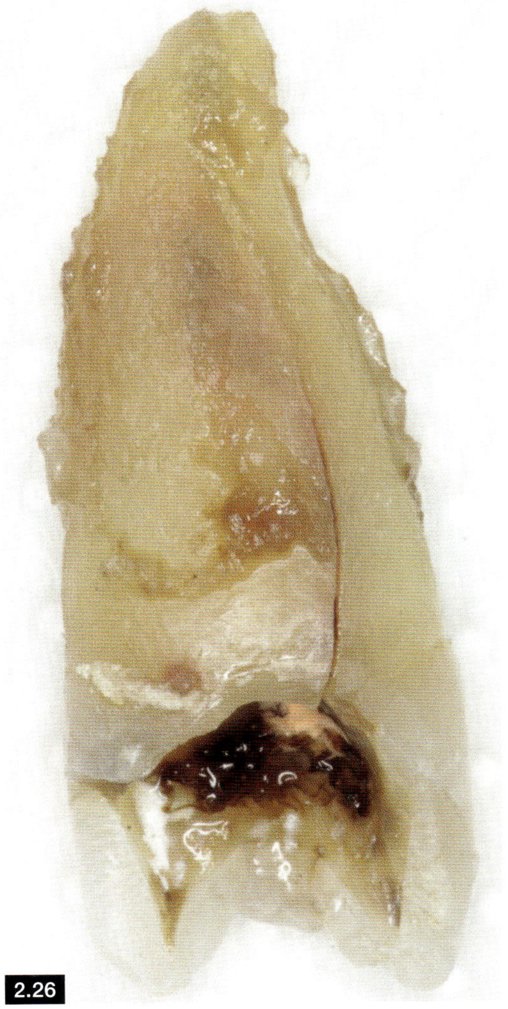

2.26

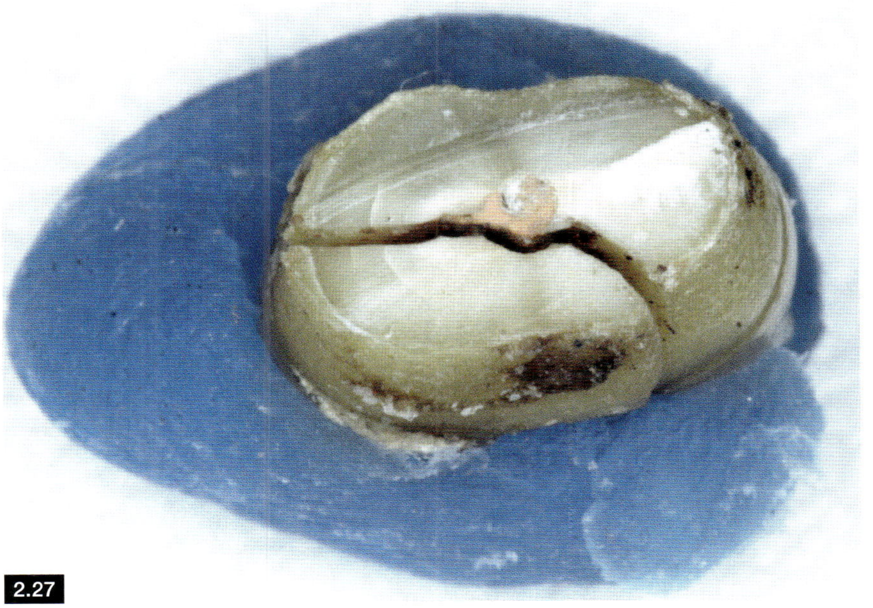

2.27

Fig. 2.26: Vision of the lesion in longitudinal cut.

Fig. 2.27: Same clinical picture as in the previous case with evidence of axial cut fracture.

The elements that need attention are those listed in Table 2.2, but those most commonly present are represented by the disproportion between the size of the radiographic image and the inadequacy of the corresponding canal treatment and the periodontal tubular probing, i.e., in a single precise area of the coronal perimeter[44, 45].

In other words, root canals with good-to-medium-quality treatments show very large areas of radiotransparency, not limited to the apical area, in periradicular space.
Although some studies have described the treatment of root fractures with various methods [46, 47], there is a lack of evidence on the effectiveness of these treatments with adhesive procedures, with or without dental banding by means of prosthetic artifacts. In addition, the root fracture often starts from the periapical area and, once it is visible in the coronal area, it has already caused a significant inflammatory reaction, which consistently destroys the bone structure.
This destruction subsequently leads to a technical inability to insert osseointegrated implants and sometimes requires regenerative procedures; vertical root fractures must therefore be diagnosed early to avoid major bone lesions.

References

1. Nair PN *Pathogenesis of apical periodontitis and the causes of endodontic failures.* Crit Rev Oral Biol Med. 2004;15(6):348-381.
2. Haapasalo MS Y; Ricucci D *Reasons for persistent and emerging post-treatment endodontic disease.* Endodontic Topics, 2011;18(1):31-50.
3. Sjogren U et al. *Factors affecting the long-term results of endodontic treatment.* J Endod, 1990. 16(10): p. 498-504.
4. Ricucci DG, D *The compromised tooth: conservative treatment or extraction?* Endodontic Topics, 2006. 13(1): p. 108-122.
5. Abbott P, *Diagnosis and management planning for root-filled teeth with persisting or new apical pathosis.* Endodontic Topics, 2008. 19(1): p. 1-21.
6. *Success and failure in endodontics: an online study guide.* J Endod, 2008. 34(5 Suppl): p. e1-6.
7. Hamedy R et al. *Patient-centered endodontic outcomes: a narrative review.* Iran Endod J, 2013. 8(4): p. 197-204.
8. Friedman S, *Considerations and concepts of case selection in the management of post-treatment endodontic disease (treatment failure).* Endodontic Topics, 2002. 5(1): p. 54-78.
9. Kirkevang L, *Root canal treatment and apical periodontitis: What can be learned from observational studies?* Endodontic Topics, 2011. 18(1): p. 51-61.
10. Friedman S, S. Abitbol, and H.P. Lawrence, *Treatment outcome in endodontics: the Toronto Study. Phase 1: initial treatment.* J Endod, 2003. 29(12): p. 787-793.
11. Ng YL et al. *Outcome of primary root canal treatment: systematic review of the literature -- Part 2. Influence of clinical factors.* Int Endod J, 2008. 41(1): p. 6-31.
12. Pirani C et al. *Long-term outcome of non-surgical root canal treatment: a retrospective analysis.* Odontology, 2015. 103(2): p. 185-193.
13. Gillen BM et al. *Impact of the quality of coronal restoration versus the quality of root canal fillings on success of root canal treatment: a systematic review and meta-analysis.* J Endod, 2011. 37(7): p. 895-902.
14. Ricucci D et al. *A prospective cohort study of endodontic treatments of 1,369 root canals: results after 5 years.* Oral Surg Oral Med Oral Pathol Oral Radiol Endod, 2011. 112(6): p. 825-842.
15. Ricucci D and JF Siqueira Jr, *Recurrent apical periodontitis and late endodontic treatment failure related to coronal leakage: a case report.* J Endod, 2011. 37(8): p. 1171-1175.
16. Bender IB and S Seltzer, *Roentgenographic and direct observation of experimental lesions in bone: II. 1961.* J Endod, 2003. 29(11): p. 707-12; discussion 701.
17. Hofmann E et al. *Cone beam computed tomography and low-dose multislice computed tomography in orthodontics and dentistry: a comparative evaluation on image quality and radiation exposure.* J Orofac Orthop, 2014. 75(5): p. 384-398.
18. Hofmann E et al. *Comparative study of image quality and radiation dose of cone beam and low-dose multislice computed tomography--an in-vitro investigation.* Clin Oral Investig, 2014. 18(1): p. 301-311.
19. Rigolone M et al. *Vestibular surgical access to the palatine root of the superior first molar: "low-dose cone-beam" CT analysis of the pathway and its anatomic variations.* J Endod, 2003. 29(11): p. 773-775.
20. Estrela C et al. *Accuracy of cone beam computed tomography and panoramic and periapical radiography for detection of apical periodontitis.* J Endod, 2008. 34(3): p. 273-279.
21. Patel S *New dimensions in endodontic imaging: Part 2. Cone beam computed tomography.* Int Endod J, 2009. 42(6): p. 463-475.
22. Patel S et al. *The detection and management of root resorption lesions using intraoral radiography and cone beam computed tomography - an in vivo investigation.* Int Endod J, 2009. 42(9): p. 831-838.
23. Scarfe WC et al. *Use of cone beam computed tomography in endodontics.* Int J Dent, 2009;2009:634567.
24. Cheng L et al. *A comparative analysis of periapical radiography and cone-beam computerized tomography for the evaluation of endodontic obturation length.* Oral Surg Oral Med Oral Pathol Oral Radiol Endod, 2011. 112(3): p. 383-389.
25. Patel S et al. *Radiographs and CBCT--time for a reassessment?* Int Endod J, 2011. 44(10): p. 887-888.
26. Patel S et al. *The detection of periapical pathosis using digital periapical radiography and cone beam computed tomography - part 2: a 1-year post-treatment follow-up.* Int Endod J, 2012. 45(8): p. 711-723.
27. Ahlowalia MS et al., *Accuracy of CBCT for volumetric measurement of simulated periapical lesions.* Int Endod J, 2013. 46(6): p. 538-546.
28. Cheung GS WL Wei and C McGrath *Agreement between periapical radiographs and cone-beam computed tomography for assessment of periapical status of root filled molar teeth.* Int Endod J, 2013. 46(10): p. 889-895.
29. Moller L et al. *Comparison of images from digital intraoral receptors and cone beam computed tomography scanning for detection of voids in root canal fillings: an in vitro study using micro-computed tomography as validation.* Oral Surg Oral Med Oral Pathol Oral Radiol, 2013. 115(6): p. 810-818.
30. Patel S et al. *Cone Beam Computed Tomography in Endodontics- A review.* Int Endod J, 2014.

31. Patel S et al. *European Society of Endodontology position statement: The use of CBCT in Endodontics.* Int Endod J, 2014. 47(6): p. 502-504.
32. Pope O, C Sathorn and P Parashos, *A comparative investigation of cone-beam computed tomography and periapical radiography in the diagnosis of a healthy periapex.* J Endod, 2014. 40(3): p. 360-365.
33. Davies A et al. *The detection of periapical pathoses in root filled teeth using single and parallax periapical radiographs versus cone beam computed tomography - a clinical study.* Int Endod J, 2015. 48(6): p. 582-592.
34. Karabucak B et al. *Prevalence of Apical Periodontitis in Endodontically Treated Premolars and Molars with Untreated Canal: A Cone-beam Computed Tomography Study.* J Endod, 2016. 42(4): p. 538-541.
35. Paque F and OA Peters, *Micro-computed tomography evaluation of the preparation of long oval root canals in mandibular molars with the self-adjusting file.* J Endod, 2011. 37(4): p. 517-521.
36. Paque F, M Zehnder and G De-Deus, *Microtomography-based comparison of reciprocating single-file F2 ProTaper technique versus rotary full sequence.* J Endod, 2011. 37(10): p. 1394-1397.
37. Ozer SY, *Detection of vertical root fractures of different thicknesses in endodontically enlarged teeth by cone beam computed tomography versus digital radiography.* J Endod, 2010. 36(7): p. 1245-1249.
38. Ozer SY, *Detection of vertical root fractures by using cone beam computed tomography with variable voxel sizes in an in vitro model.* J Endod, 2011. 37(1): p. 75-79.
39. Dutra KL et al. *Influence of Intracanal Materials in Vertical Root Fracture Pathway Detection with Cone-beam Computed Tomography.* J Endod, 2017. 43(7): p. 1170-1175.
40. Elsaltani MH, MM Farid and MS Eldin Ashmawy, *Detection of Simulated Vertical Root Fractures: Which Cone-beam Computed Tomographic System Is the Most Accurate?* J Endod, 2016. 42(6): p. 972-977.
41. Hassan B et al. *Comparison of five cone beam computed tomography systems for the detection of vertical root fractures.* J Endod, 2010. 36(1): p. 126-129.
42. Maddalone M et al *Prevalence of vertical root fractures in teeth planned for apical surgery. A retrospective cohort study.* Int Endod J, 2018. 51(9): p. 969-974.
43. von Arx T, E Roux and W. Burgin, *Treatment decisions in 330 cases referred for apical surgery.* J Endod, 2014. 40(2): p. 187-191.
44. Metska ME et al. *Detection of vertical root fractures in vivo in endodontically treated teeth by cone-beam computed tomography scans.* J Endod, 2012. 38(10): p. 1344-1347.
45. Patel S et al. *The detection of vertical root fractures in root filled teeth with periapical radiographs and CBCT scans.* Int Endod J, 2013. 46(12): p. 1140-1152.
46. Floratos SG and SI Kratchman, *Surgical management of vertical root fractures for posterior teeth: report of four cases.* J Endod, 2012. 38(4): p. 550-555.
47. Uzunoglu E et al. *Effect of ethylenediaminetetraacetic acid on root fracture with respect to concentration at different time exposures.* J Endod, 2012. 38(8): p. 1110-1113.

- Describe **endodontic access strategies** for retreating previously instrumented and filled canals.
- Describe the **techniques for removing** coronal obstacles and **posts**.
- Provide solutions to problems that arise in inappropriately previously instrumented and filled root canals.

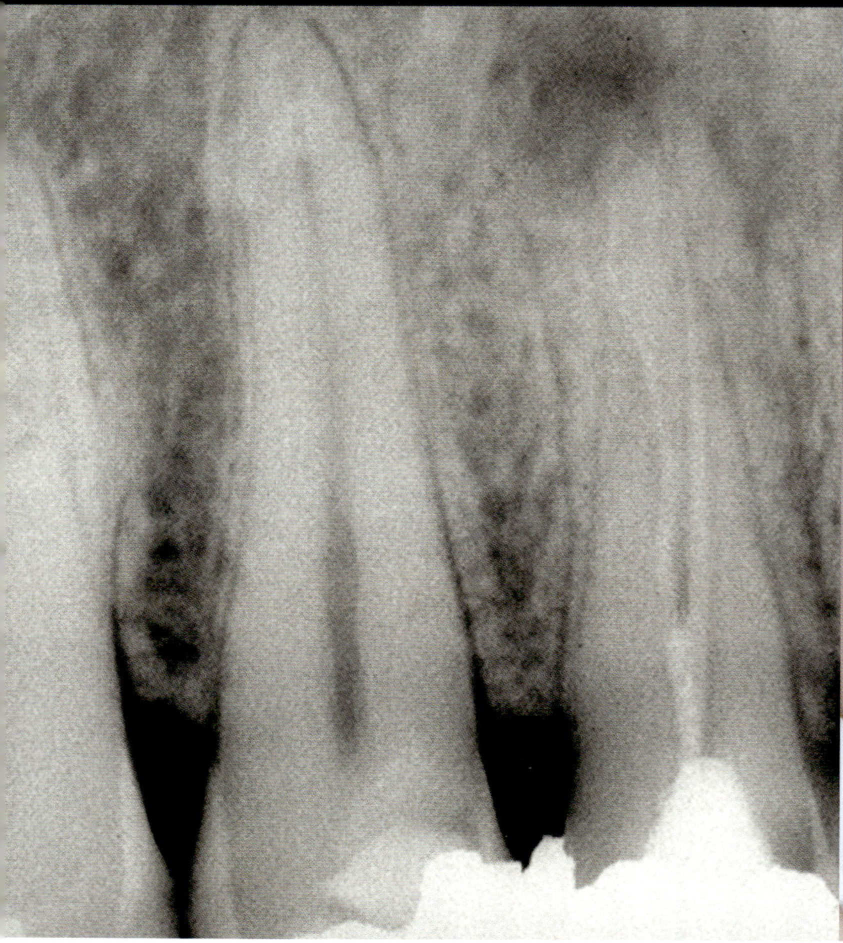

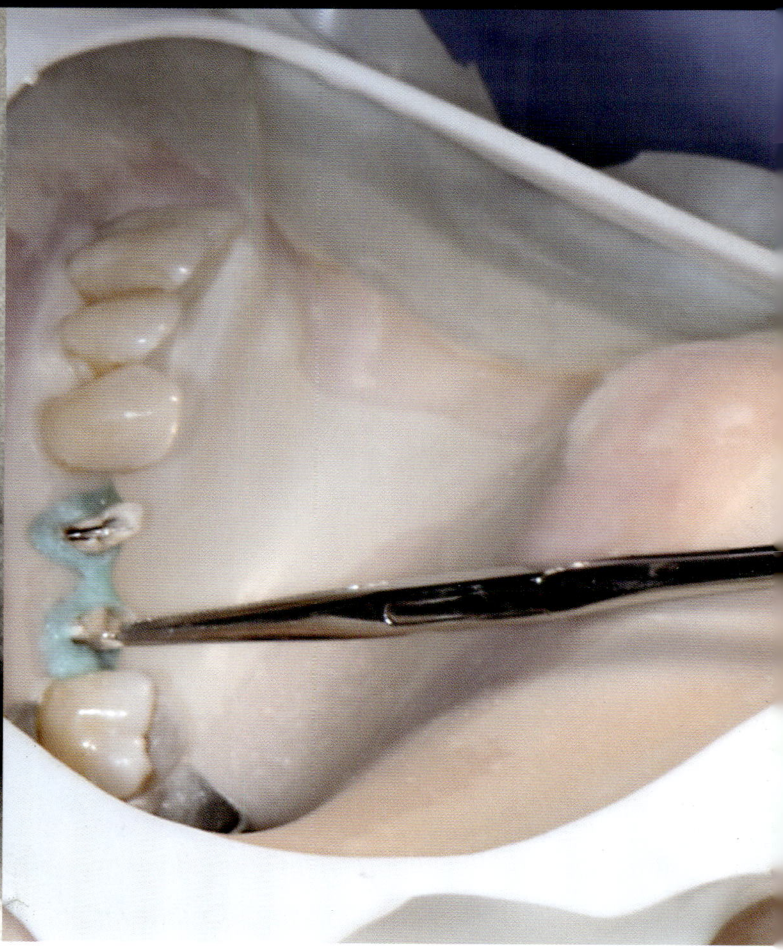

Enrico Cassai, Massimo Giovarruscio,
Francesca Cerutti

03

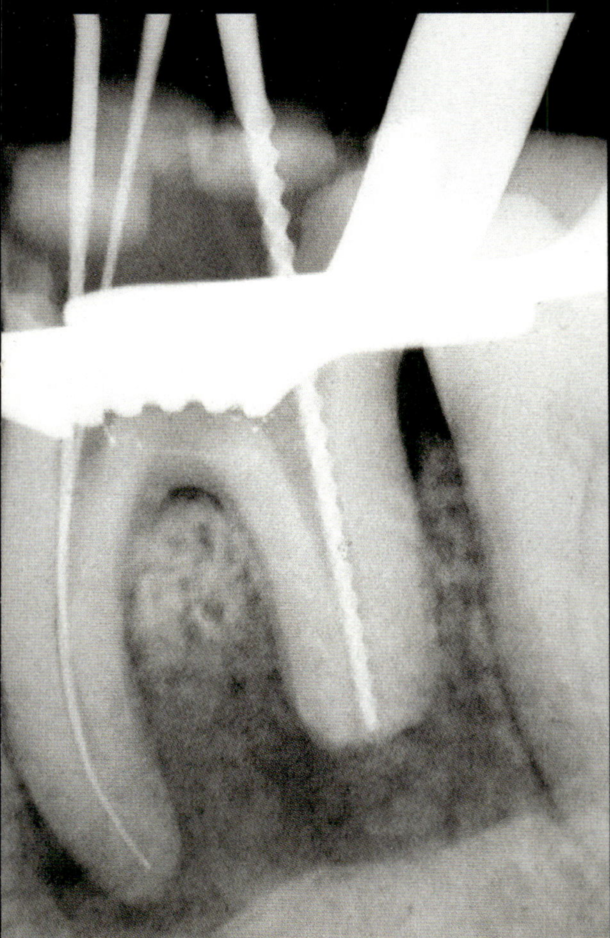

Clinical procedures for accessing the endodontic space

Techniques for removing all kinds of coronal and intracanal obstructions in the retreatment process

ELEMENTS TO BE ANALYSED BEFORE RETREATMENT IS PERFORMED

ANTERIOR TEETH

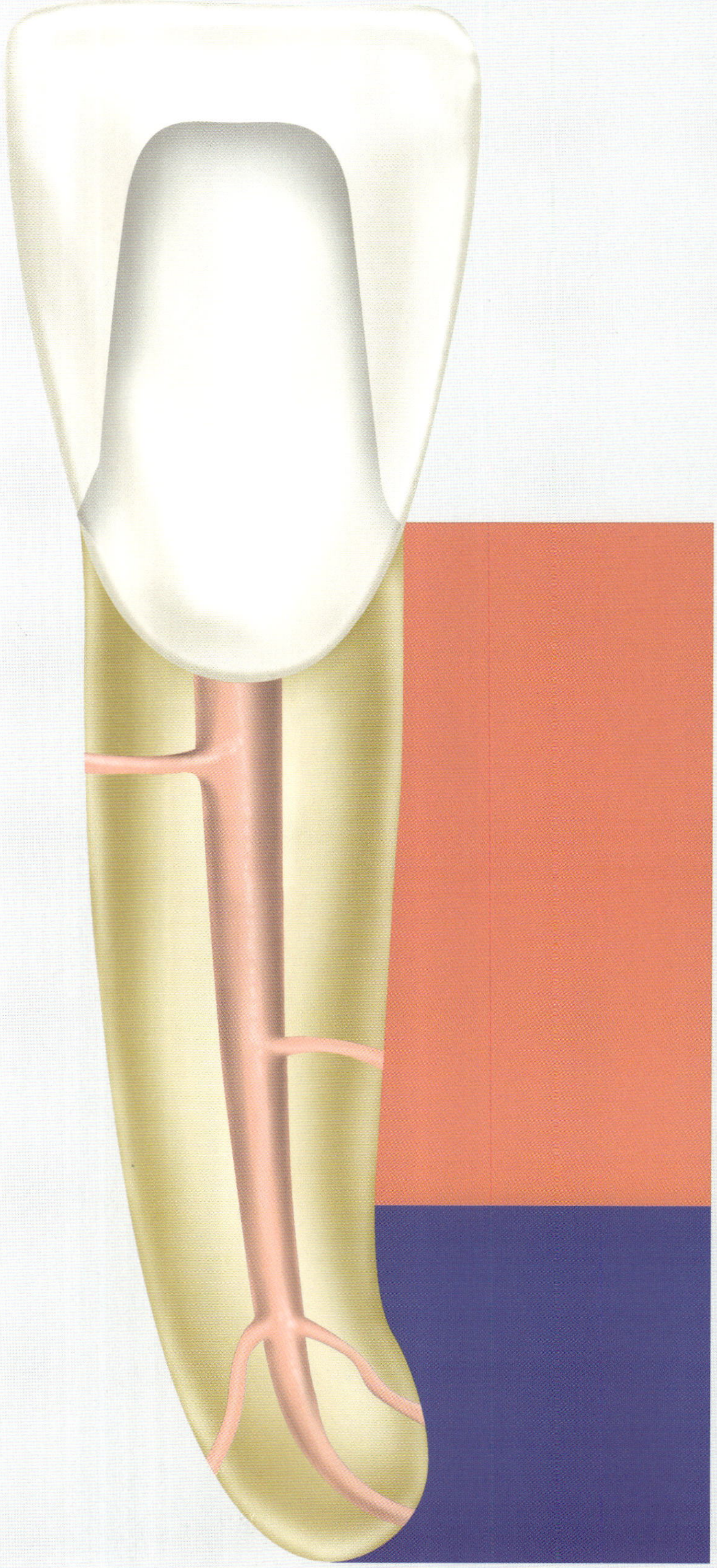

1. Coronal access becomes essential in the anterior teeth given their high aesthetic value; during retreatments the correct opening of the pulp chamber is a fundamental initial requirement.

2. Evaluation of the existing coronal restoration: should it be preserved or replaced?

3. The level of filling of the root canal lumen should be assessed by a preoperative radiographic examination.

4. A correct apical seal is of paramount importance to the success of endodontic therapy. In certain cases, in the anterior teeth, large diameters make this procedure complex.

POSTERIOR TEETH

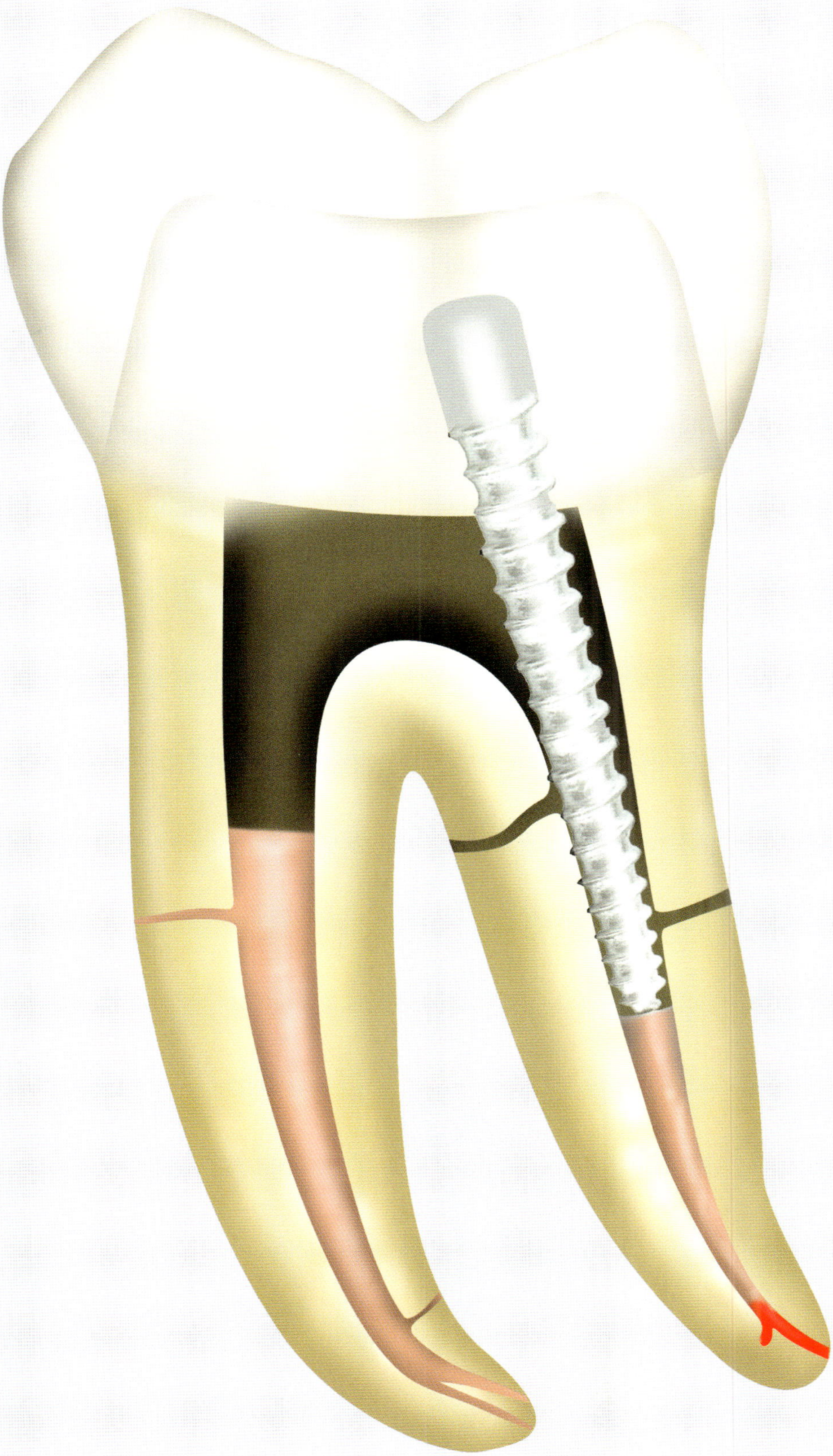

1. Coronal access through the removal of existing restorations is not greatly affected by the aesthetic aspect.

2. Root canal posts come in a range of different shapes and types and many techniques and tools can be used to remove them. A proper pre-operative evaluation will enable the clinician to make the most appropriate choice.

3. Perforation is an iatrogenic mistake that, when correctly diagnosed, can be successfully managed thanks to the methods and dedicated instruments currently available.

4. Due to the anatomical complexity of the root canals, one of the main causes of failure in posterior teeth is the failure to treat the entire endodontium.

5. Broken instruments represent an obstacle that can be removed or bypassed depending on the canal anatomy and the location of the instrument.

6. Due to the complexity of the apical anatomy, it is very common to find blocks and ledges in posterior teeth requiring retreatment.

Preliminary considerations on endodontic access

When commencing a retreatment procedure, it is appropriate to make a distinction between the anterior and posterior teeth. In addition to the potential surgical difficulties in recovering a tooth that has already been treated, the aesthetic nature of this intervention suggests that not all patients will be happy with the end result: the use of osseointegrated implants in the anterior area (with a high aesthetic value). The substantial complexity of managing this area with implant therapy will urge the clinician to make every effort to preserve teeth with a reasonable prognosis[1-3]. Most of the difficulties of retreating teeth in this area are associated with:

- the anatomy of the area (apexes of considerable size/immature/ mature, wide canals)
- the presence of intracanal retention (cast posts, metal or fiber posts)
- the material inside the canal to be removed
- any iatrogenic mistakes.

In addition to these conditions, we must also underline the great importance of the aesthetic factor: this can lead clinicians to adopt a multidisciplinary approach aimed at preserving the natural tooth.

When it comes to function, the primary advantage of treating teeth in the anterior area lies in the limited occlusal load that must be borne by the teeth: it is, therefore, possible to maintain teeth in the arch even in cases of unfavorable crown-root ratios.

In cases where retreatment is not the most suitable clinical option, endodontic surgery is a therapeutic alternative that guarantees very high success rates.

Conversely, the retreatment of a posterior tooth is relatively unaffected by aesthetic considerations. In certain circumstances in which the tooth is severely compromised and its recovery is difficult, clinicians may consider replacing the tooth with an osseointegrated implant[4, 5] (an issue that we will review in greater detail in Chapter 10). Clinicians must, therefore, carefully assess the operational difficulties associated with the removal of all obstacles that prevent proper disinfection and the introduction of a new effective apical seal. The reconstruction-related considerations in the preoperative phase are also different for the anterior and posterior sectors.

It is useful for clinicians to be able to accurately assess the stages of therapy. This is because it is essential to maintain aesthetic results in the anterior sector that are acceptable to the patients throughout the entire duration of treatment, i.e. until the resolution of the periapical disease.

If the use of a temporary crown is considered necessary, it may be helpful to prepare an alternative prosthetic restoration before proceeding with the removal of the existing one.

In this regard, the adaptation the existing restoration, rather than its elimination, may be considered.

Furthermore, it is essential to ensure easy access to the root canal system when retreating: if the reconstruction limits the appropriate and necessary access, there is an indication for the root canal system to be removed.

Fig. 3.1a-b: Correct case management in terms of cleaning, shaping and filling, combined with an appropriate restoration that collectively lead to case resolution (at 10 years).

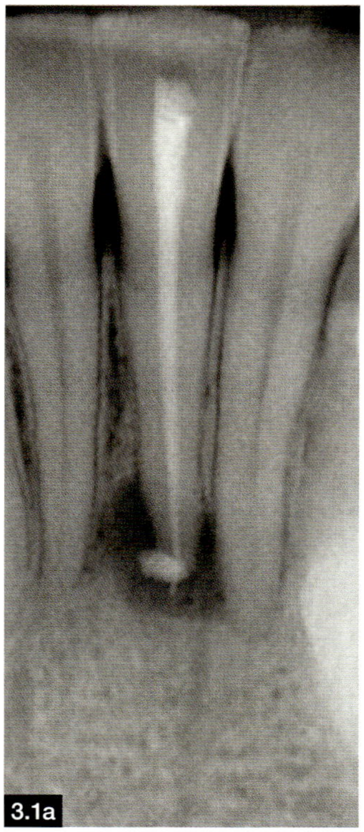

3.1a

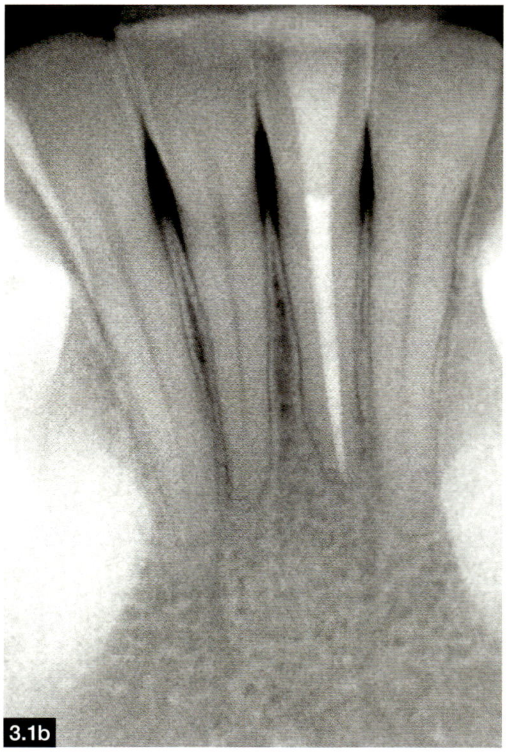

3.1b

Lower molar with complicated anatomy and inappropriate treatment

CASE REPORT 1

After a careful preoperative radiographic analysis, the case presents a large coronal amalgam restoration, a post screwed into the mesial canal, inadequate canal filling in terms of length and the probable presence of a broken instrument in the mesial root, together with an anatomical conformation that is difficult to manage in the apical third of both roots.

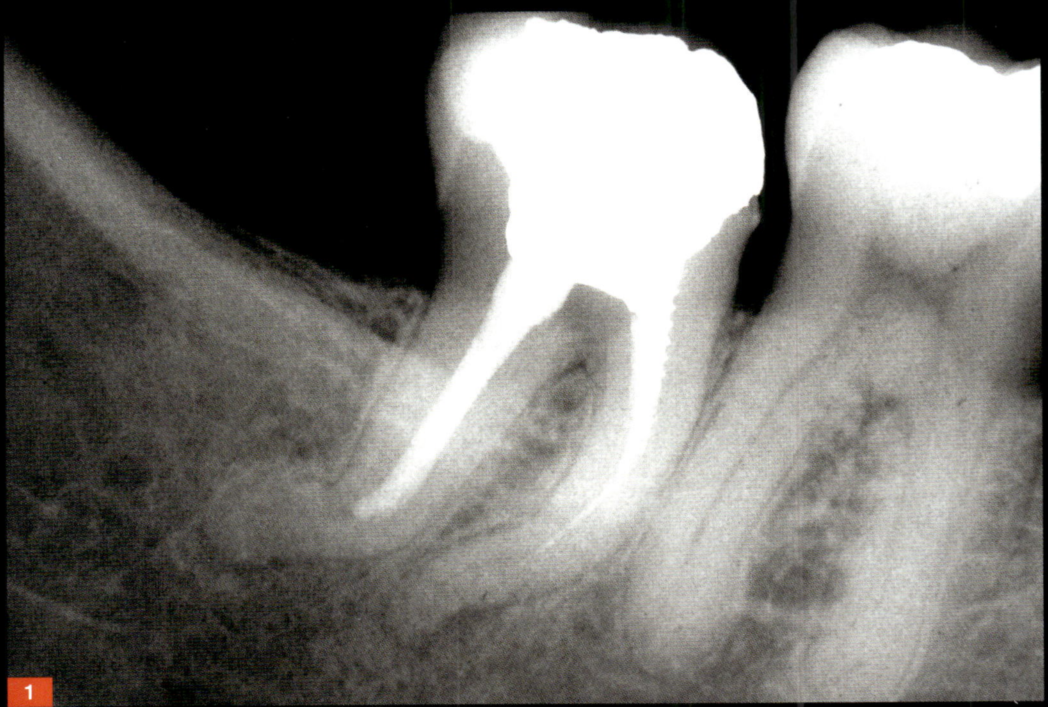

1

Figure 1: The initial case which, as described, presents a series of elements that could urge the clinician to consider whether or not to perform retreatment.

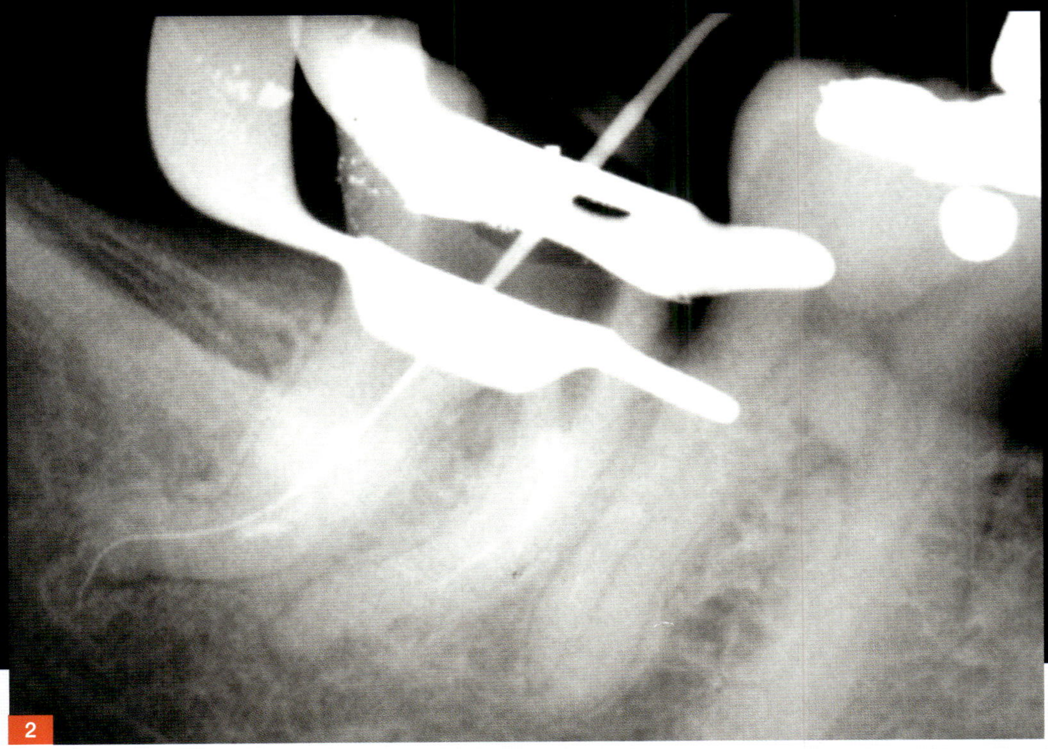

2

Figure 2: Once the coronal obstacles have been removed, the distal canal, which is scarcely visible in the preoperative x-ray is instrumented.

The case was treated in the correct sequence by removing the broken instrument, cleaning, shaping and filling the root canal system. The therapy was completed with adequate coronal restoration. Seven years later, the clinical and radiographic success is maintained.

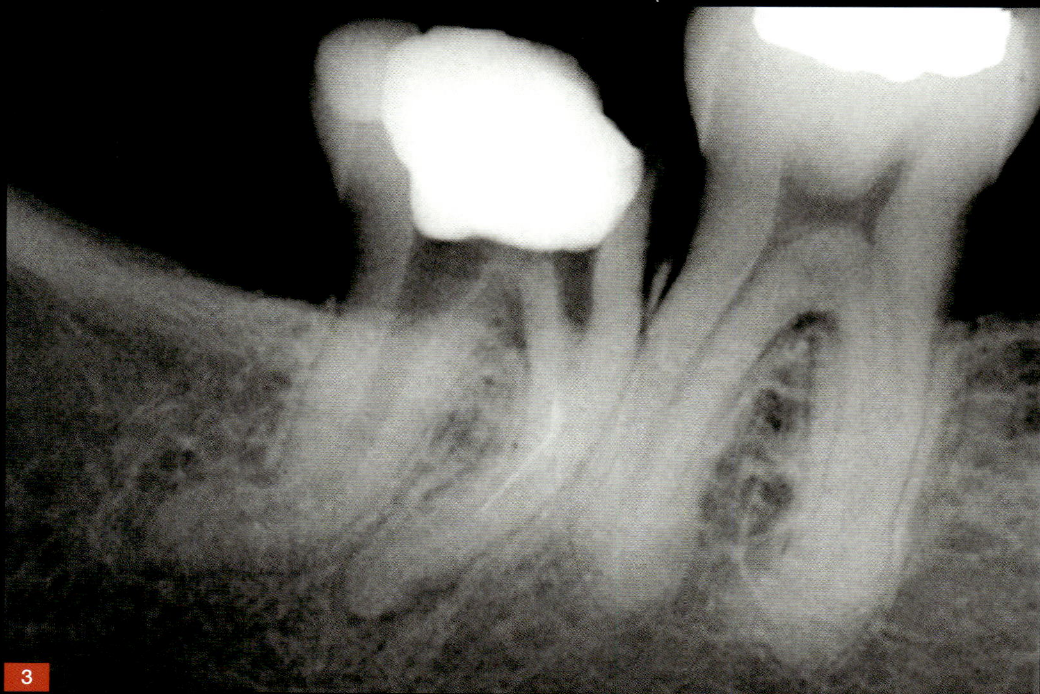

Figure 3: Once most of the canal content has been removed, the broken instrument has to be extracted.

3

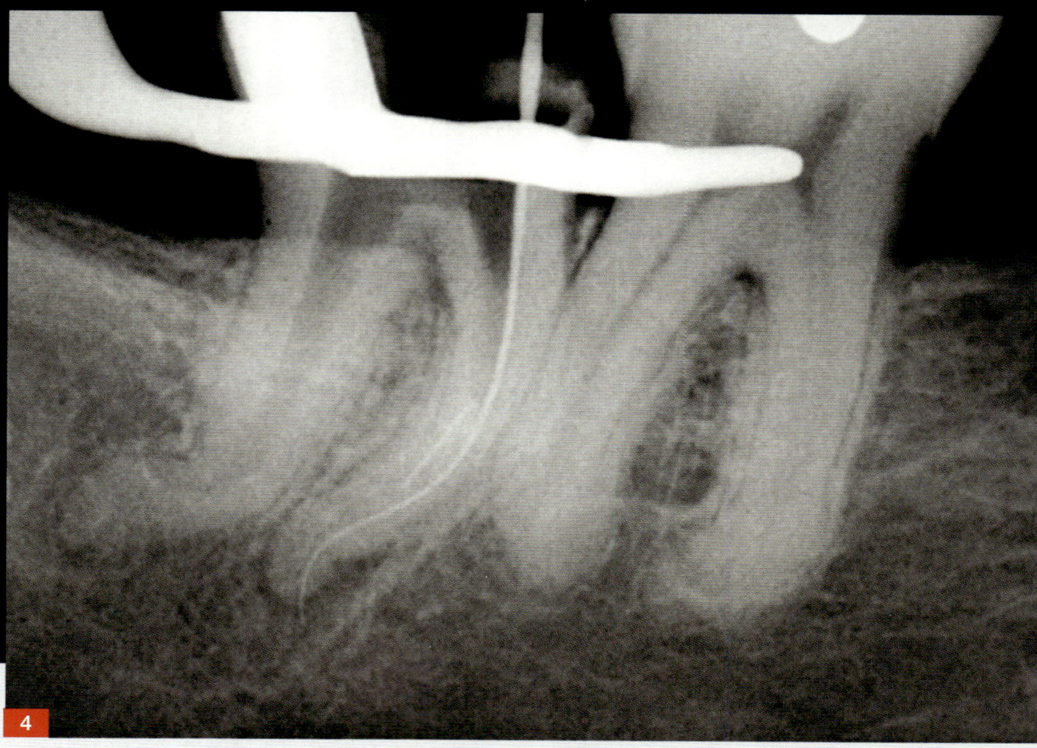

Figure 4: In a first step, it is possible to pass alongside it, creating space for the subsequent extraction.

4

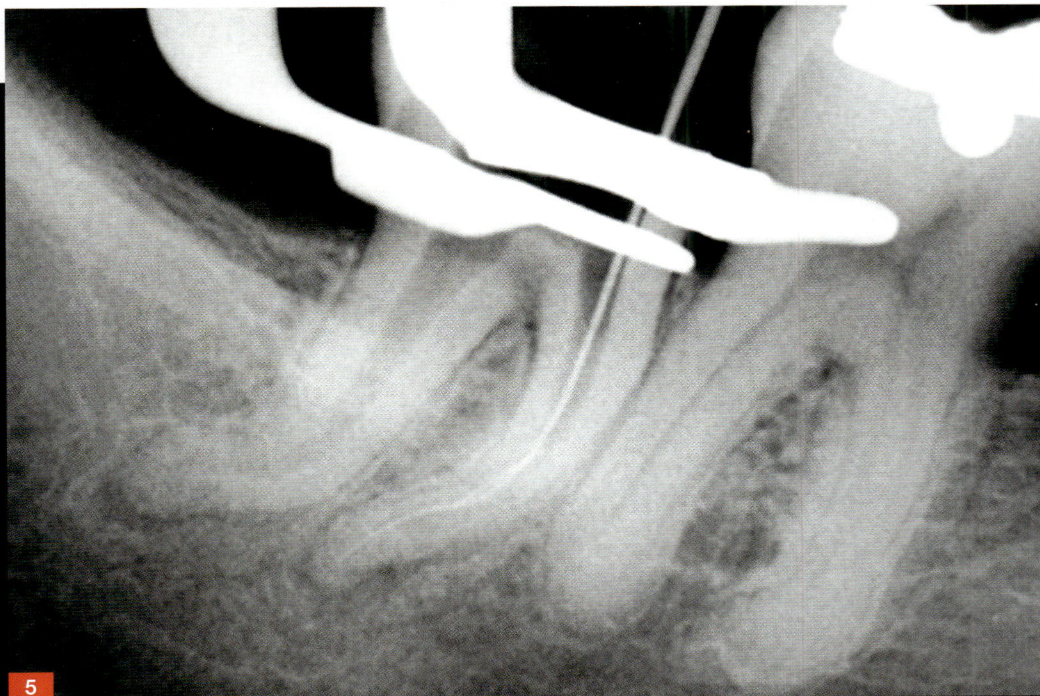

Figure 5: The space of the mesial canals is now greater in order to extract the instrument.

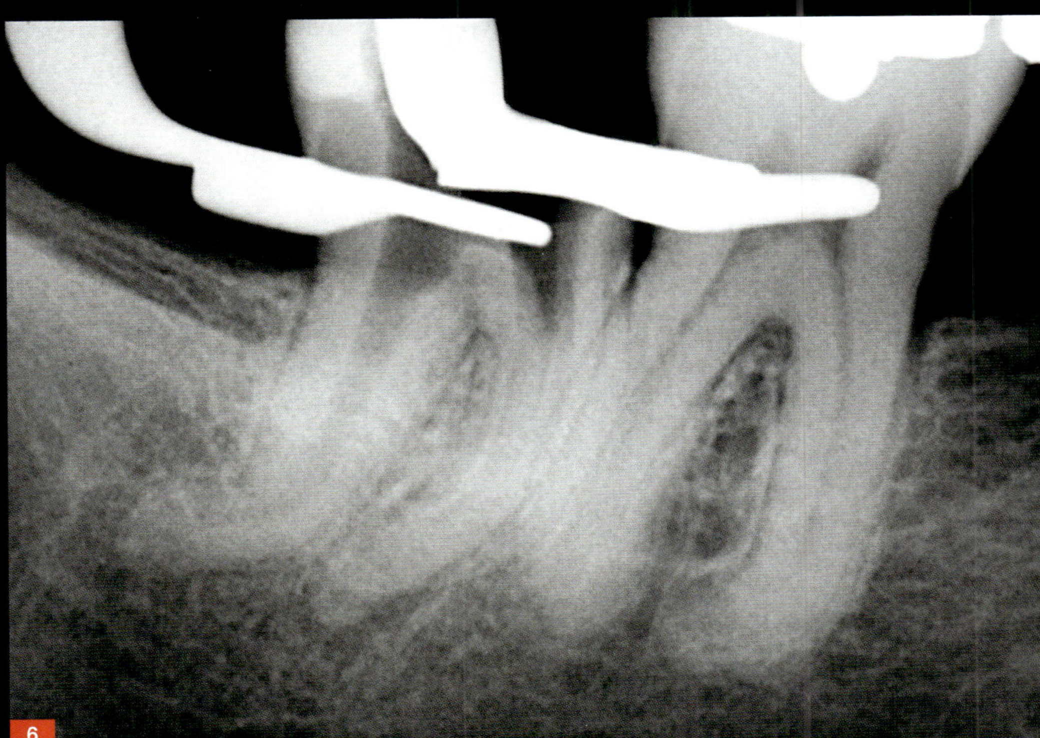

Figure 6: The instrument is pulled out and the canals can be shaped correctly.

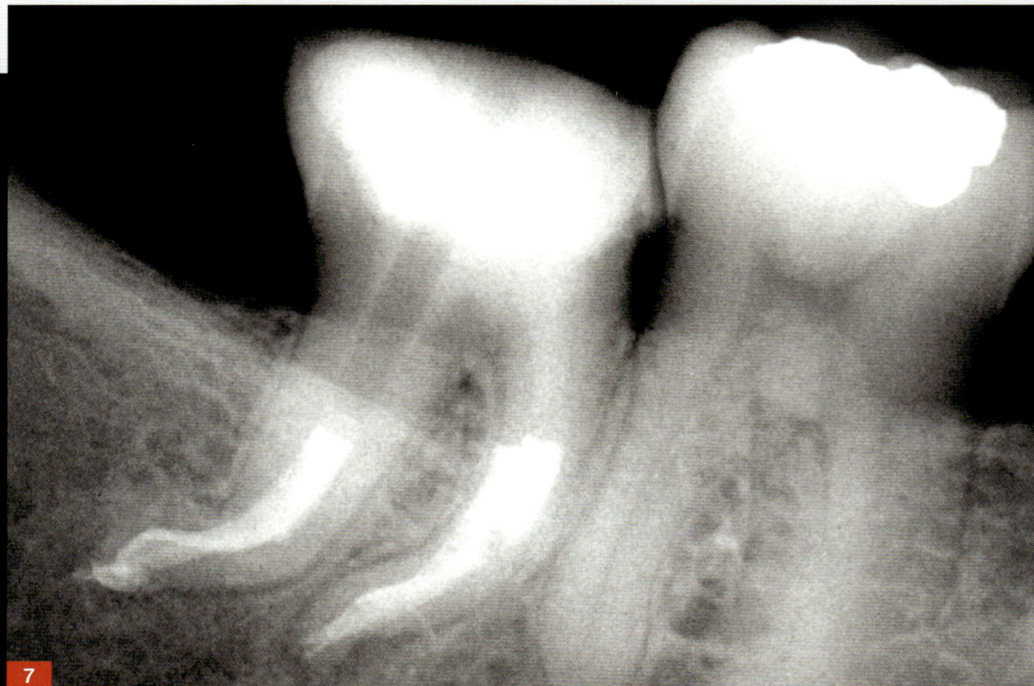

Figure 7: Root canal filling and coronal restoration with fiber post and composite material.

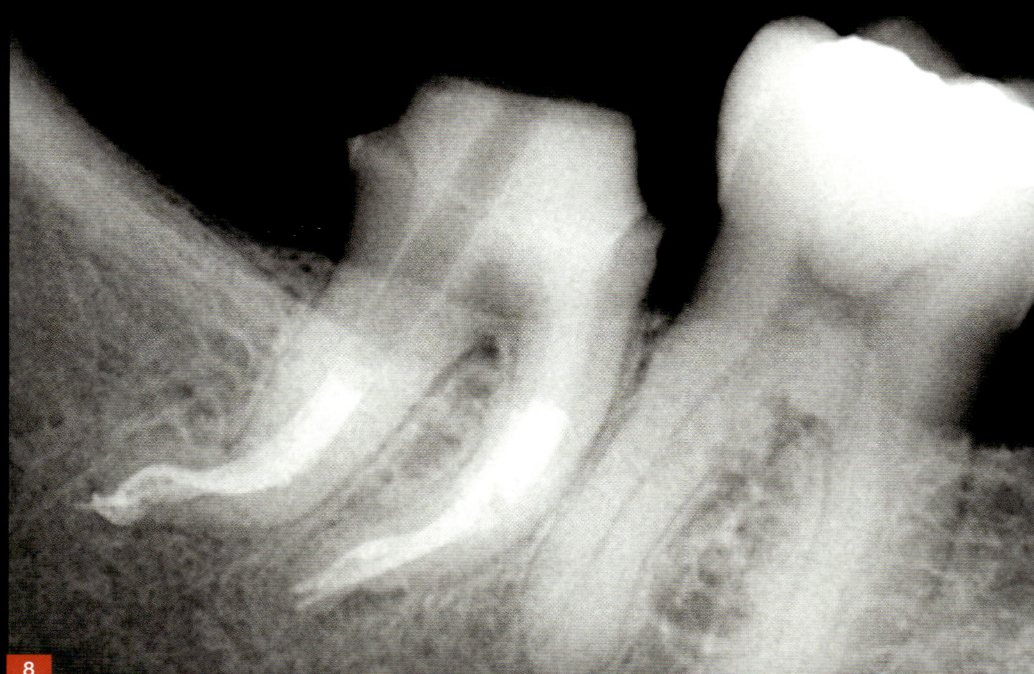

Figure 8: Chamfer preparation for a restoration with complete cuspal covering.

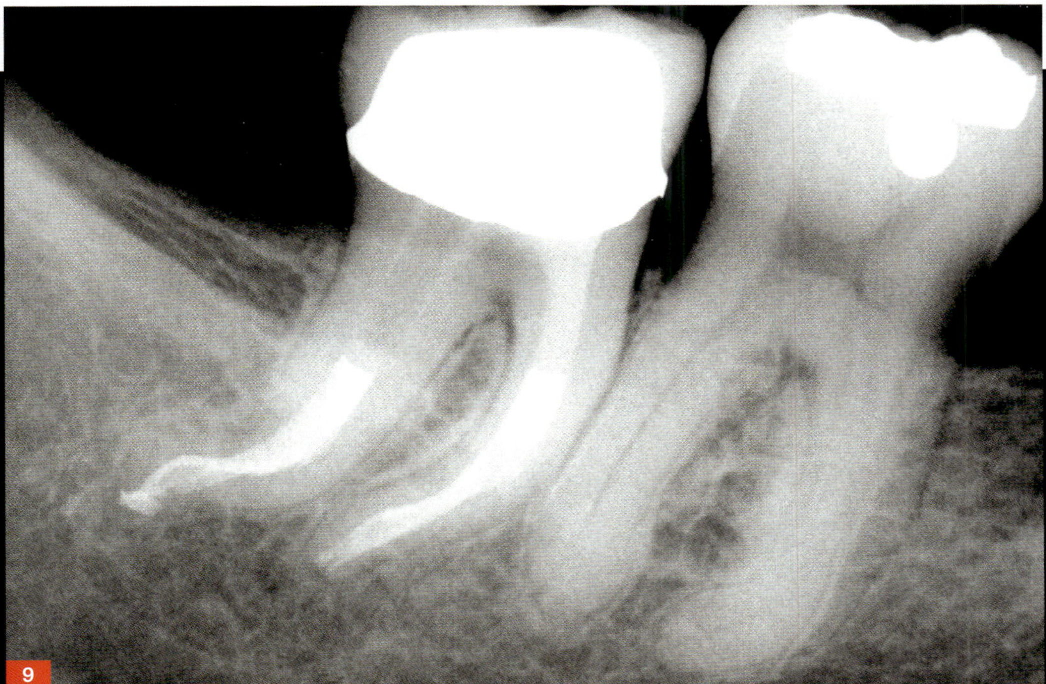

9

Figure 9: A metal-ceramic crown ensures a perfect coronal seal.

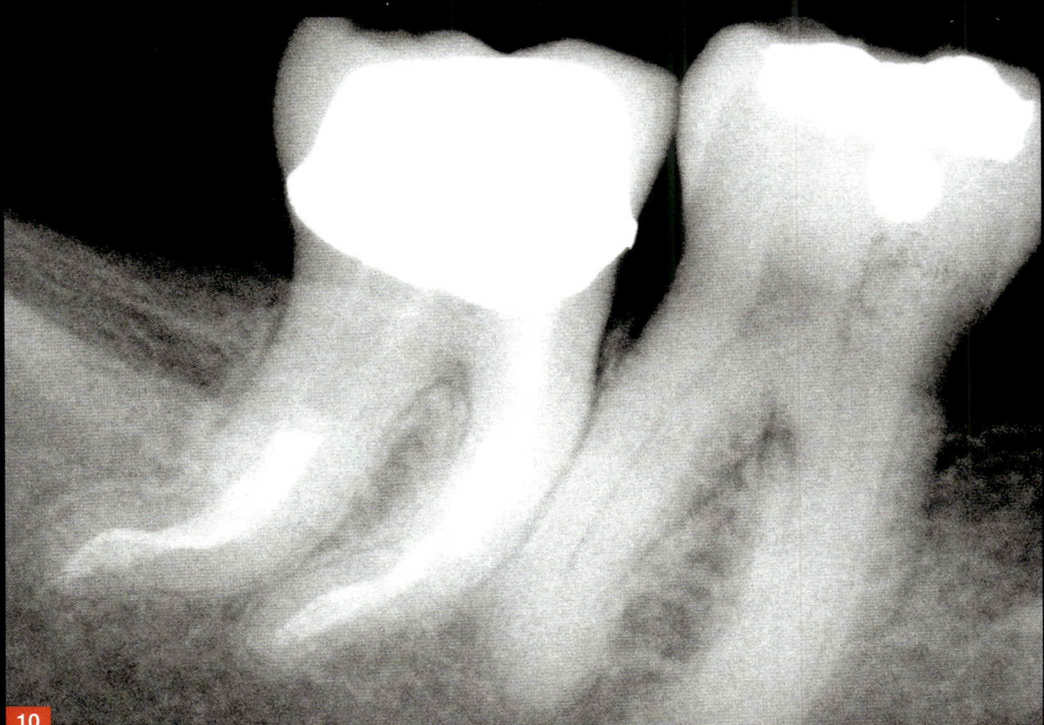

10

Figure 10: X-ray examination after 7 years.

CORONAL ACCESS TYPE OF RESTORATION

- **Direct**: **Amalgam**, **Composite** → **Demolition**; **Partial conservation**
- **Indirect**: **Gold**, **Gold-ceramic**, **Integral ceramics**, **Composite** → **Removal**; **Removal and temporary restoration**; **Conservation**

However, a fundamental question still remains: which operative sequence should be followed to ensure good access to the endodontium?[6]
In short, the operational pathway consists of two phases:

1. First, it is necessary to remove everything that limits access to the root canal system at coronal level;
2. Second, the canals should be emptied, by removing the filling material placed during primary endodontic therapy and, if necessary, overcoming obstacles that prevent the apical limit from being reached.

Passing through or removing the existing coronal restoration, with the indispensable elimination of any decay tissue, is essential for acquiring proper access to the canal system. However, it is also necessary to exploit coronal infiltrations to prevent bacteria from returning and colonizing the root canal system[7, 8].
Therefore, the removal of coronal obstacles is a clinical step that makes it possible to:

- obtain correct access to the duct system
- remove the supposedly contaminated material from the coronal part of the tooth
- obtain correct visibility of the deep endodontium to better understand the extent of the present obstructions.

Only after having carefully completed this first phase should intra-canal obstacles be considered, and will be removed as follows:

- The intracanal posts in the various forms, if present
- The filling material placed in the canal
- Any broken instruments (which can be by-passed instead, if possible)
- Steps and/or calcifications, if possible.

Particular attention should be given to forgotten and, therefore, not instrumented, disinfected, and filled canals. A separate role is intended for root perforations, whether associated or not with the situations described above. However, we will focus on this issue in greater detail in chapter 7. An extensive examination of the types of clinical behavior that can be used during retreatment processes is presented in a systematic review by Del Fabbro et al.[9].

Coronal obstacles: how to remove them

There are many coronal reconstructions that need to be performed in retreating teeth. The fate of the existing restoration is closely related to the initial status of the tooth, the sector to which it belongs, and the difficulties and risks associated with its removal. However, one thing remains certain: the passage through an old coronal reconstruction must facilitate and not hinder retreatment. In addition, we need to ensure the structural integrity of the coronal seal during both retreatment and in the immediately subsequent phases.

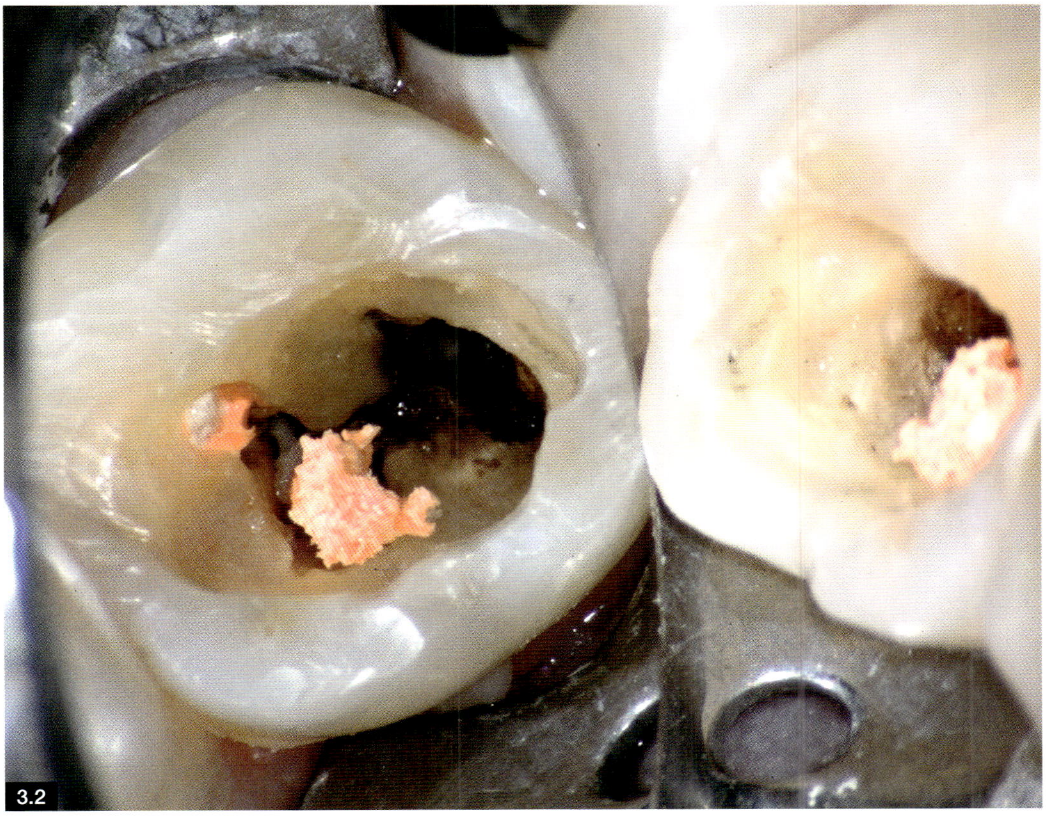

Fig. 3.2: The pulp chamber is often incorrectly cleaned when ret eating.

Direct restorations

Accessing the endodontic space in natural teeth with direct restorations may not be relevant; of course, any further secondary carious processes must be eliminated with great care.
Small periodontal interventions are sometimes also required at this stage to allow a proper sealing of the future coronal access and the efficient positioning of the rubber dam, an essential isolation material during the operational phase.
If treatment requires several work sessions, this preliminary restoration phase would be invaluable for restricting any temporary dressings. However, we should not remove all previously placed restoration material. Indeed, in some cases, having established a good seal will provide a good basis for accomplishing proper coronal access.
Discolored dental crowns are often found in anterior tooth retreatment due to the pigmenting effect of the sealers and gutta-percha used in previous canal therapies. Therefore, the complete elimination of these elements from the inside of the clinical

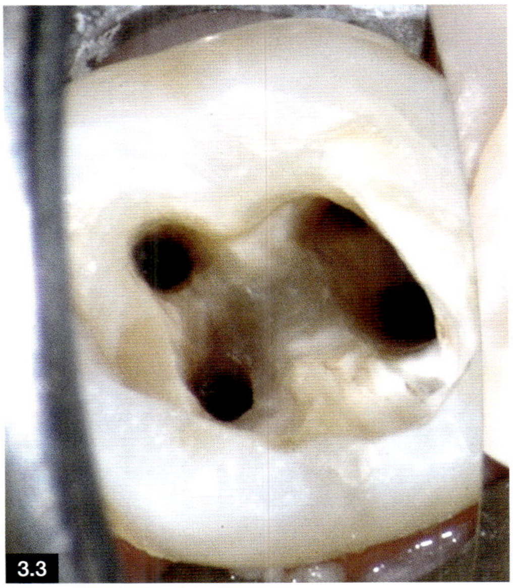

Fig. 3.3: The access has been changed and completely cleaned.

crown or canal entrance is crucial not only for ensuring good access to the endodontic root space but also for attenuating and/or eliminating dyschromic processes in the clinical crown[10].
A set of suitable instruments, summarized in Table 3.1, must always be present when accessing the endodontic space in order to be able to deal with any situation,

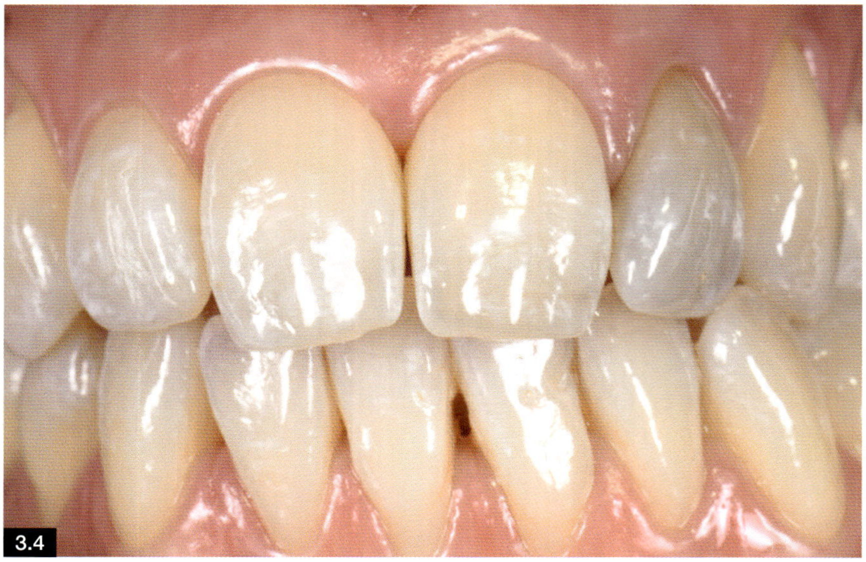
3.4

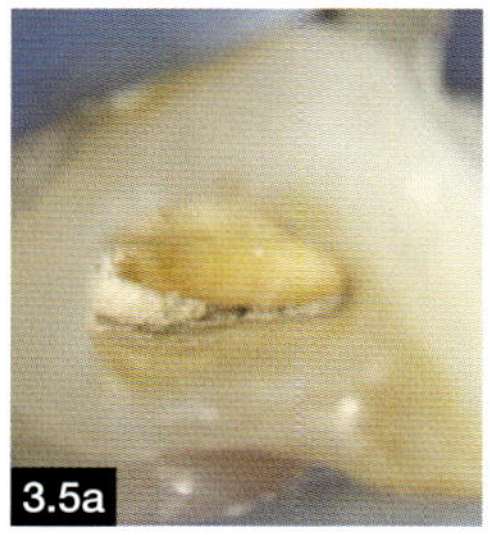
3.5a

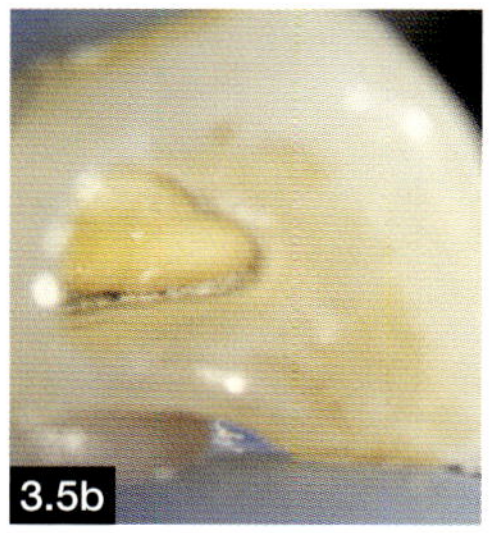
3.5b

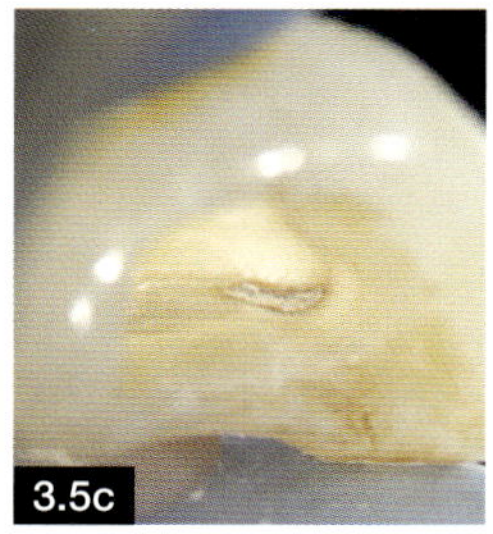
3.5c

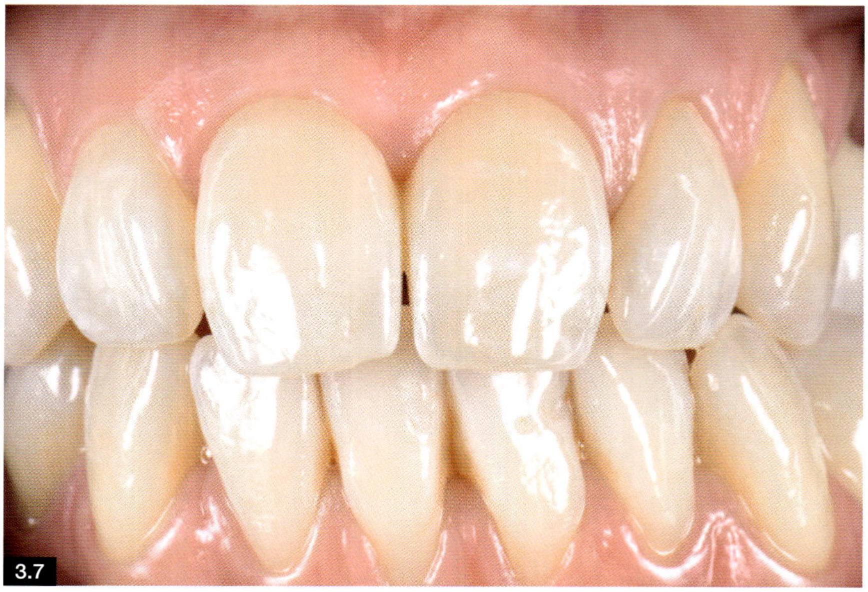
3.7

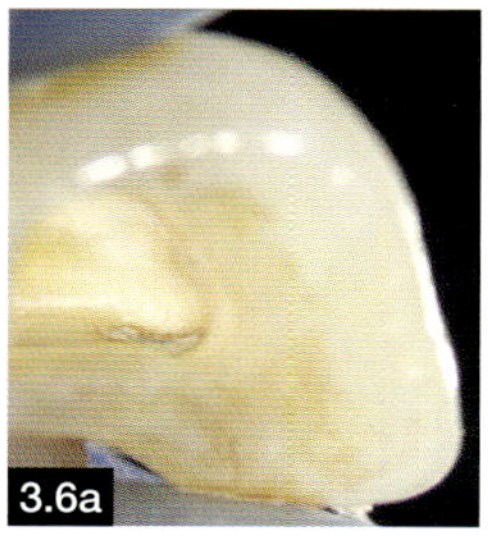
3.6a

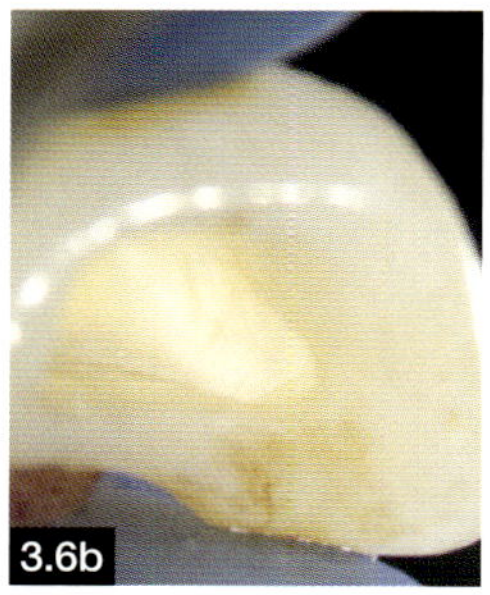
3.6b

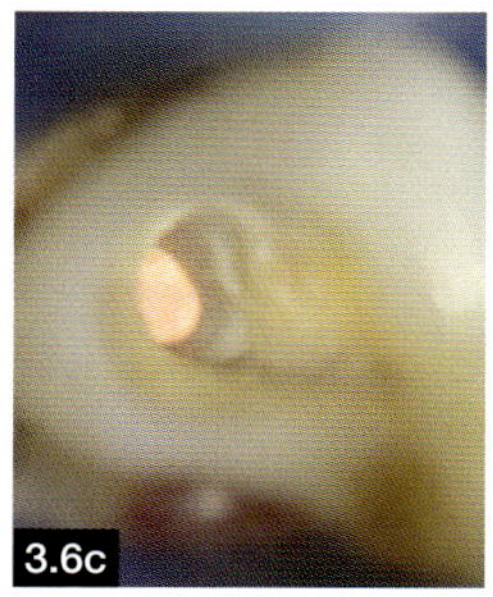
3.6c

Fig. 3.4: The frontal photograph shows a discolored lateral incisor.

Fig. 3.5a-c: The opening of the pulp chamber reveals an excessive amount of root canal sealer that has not been removed.

Fig. 3.6a-c: A thorough cleaning of the crown and a filling level below the sealer-enamel junction lead to the elimination of the discoloration.

Fig. 3.7: Frontal view at the end of the treatment. A substantial change in tooth color is notable.

whether related to the material or reconstruction to be removed, or to the supporting tissues of the tooth. Other tools may also be useful, such as a burr or scaler to discard any tartar residues or overfills.
Amalgam removal is common in the posterior sectors (Fig. 3.8 and 3.9) and it must be performed under a rubber dam, with high speed suction[9], thus providing all the necessary protection for patients, caregivers, and operators[11].
A multi-blade tungsten carbide bur (see Table 3.1), possibly new, mounted on a turbine or a red ring contra-angle with an abundant jet of water is used; when placing it between the dental walls and the restoration, the removal is easy and does not damage the residual dental tissue excessively.
If the amalgam extends into the root canals, then it is not recommended to use high-speed milling burrs because the procedure could prove difficult and dangerous (because of the risk of creating furrows or false paths).
It is suggested that clinicians should use ultrasound with strong metal tips combined with abundant irrigation to remove undercuts that prevent mobilization of the reconstruction (see Table 3.1).
The removal of composite or resinous

Table 3.1 **INSTRUMENTS FOR ENDODONTIC RETREATMENTS**

Rotary instruments	Ultrasonic instruments	Hand-tools
Blue ring/red ring contra-angle	Piezoelectric hand-pieces (subsonic or ultrasonic)	Excavators
Long-stemmed, diamond and tungsten carbide FG/CA burrs	Diamond and non-diamond handpiece burs	Probe DG 16 (7)

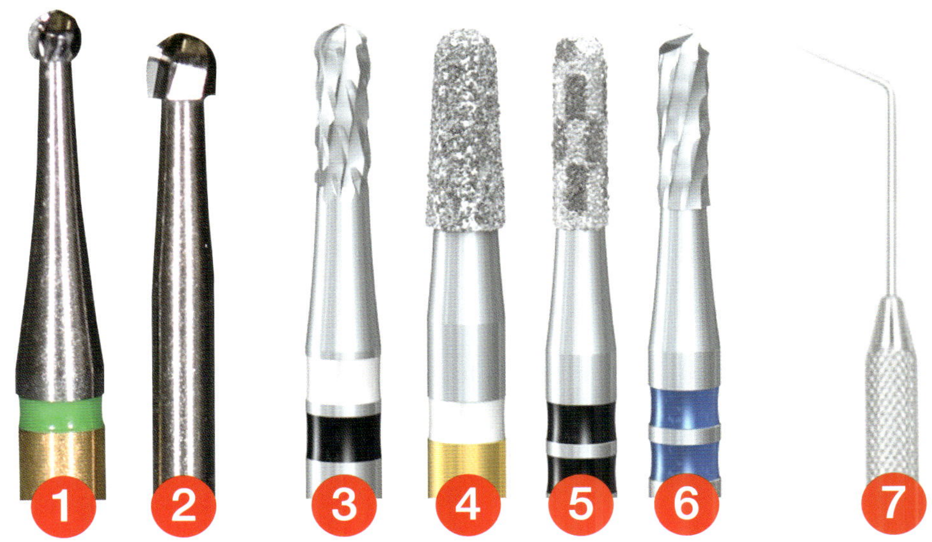

Description of the burrs

It is advisable to use a sequence of specific instruments to optimize time and reduce the overall treatment steps. Depending on the material to be removed, different milling burrs can be used, e.g. rosette milling burrs for micromotors (**1**) or contra-angle milling burrs with red rings (**2**) for dental tissues. Diamond burs are also available that have been specifically designed for rapid composite removal (**4**) (Komet 5985) or to remove hard all-ceramic zirconium dioxide (**5**) (Komet 4ZRS).
The rapid removal of silver amalgam can be easily performed with cross-blade burrs (Komet H32) (**3**) (Komet H4MCL) (**6**).

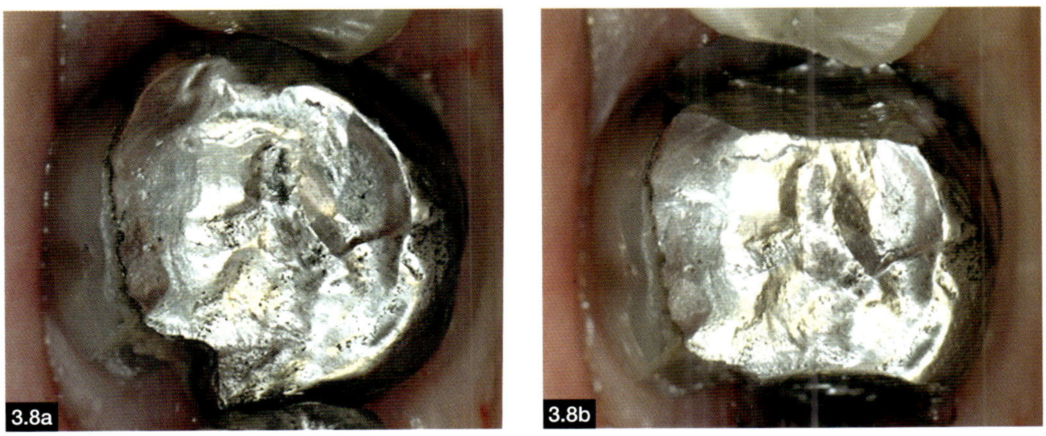

Fig. 3.8a: A block of silver amalgam that must be removed.

Fig. 3.8b: Mesial separation and distal view allows the efficient positioning of the dam.

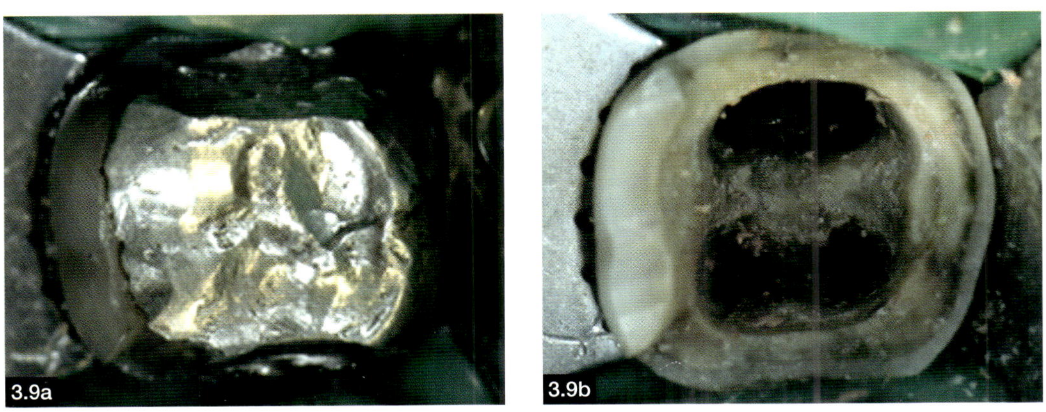

Fig. 3.9a: The dam is in place.

Fig. 3.9b: Complete removal of the amalgam.

Fig. 3.10: It is possible to numerically analyze the length and the size of root canals with modern radiographic systems.

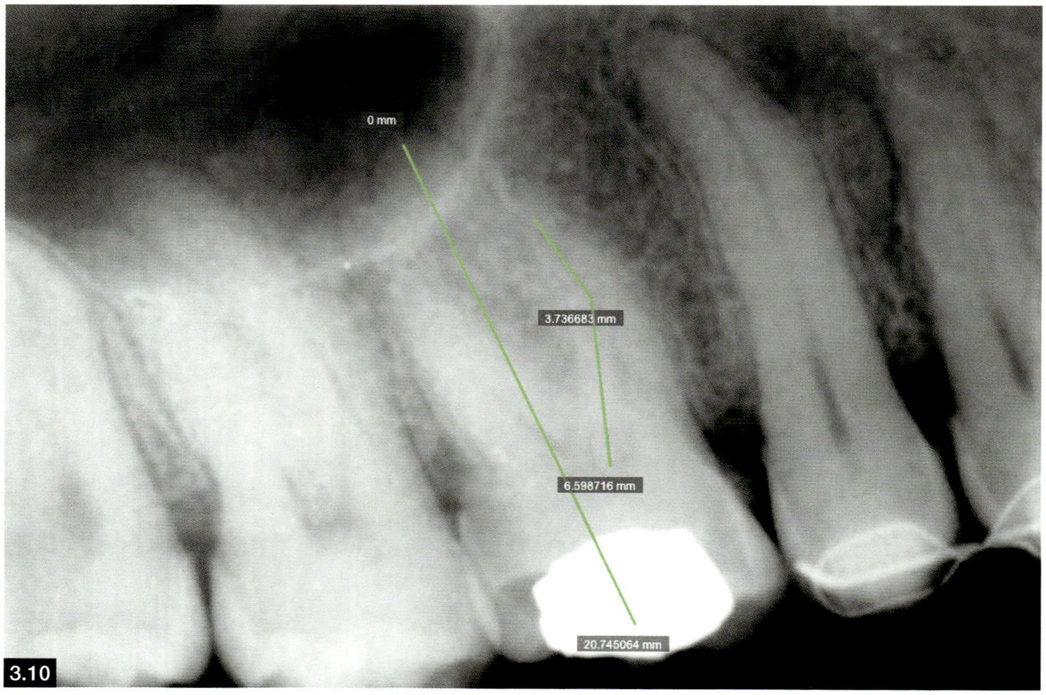

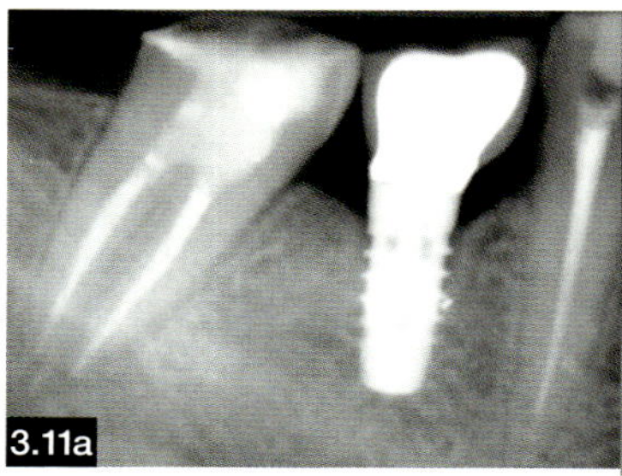

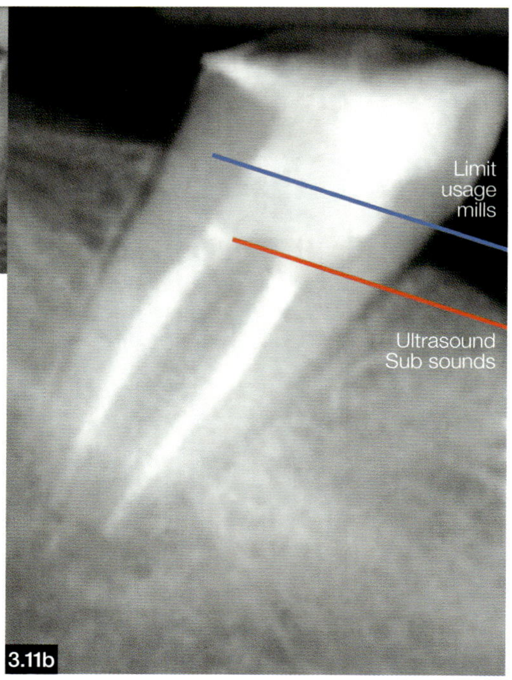

Fig. 3.11a-b: A thorough radiographic analysis may suggest the use of dedicated ultrasonic drills to safely reconfigure the cavity access.

materials requires a separate mention because these materials tend to blend in with dental tissues very efficiently, and hence their identification can be very challenging. Indeed, the prominent risk associated with this issue involves the involuntarily elimination of healthy dental tissue: for this reason, it is advisable to use dedicated ultrasonic tips that are dry so as to provide better visibility of the operating field (Fig. 3.11).

The tip acting on the material must be carefully assessed under sufficient optical magnification (magnifying glasses or surgical microscope) and with the help of a suitable light source. Furthermore, the operating field should be cleaned using the air spray of the chair syringe, directed alternately towards the operating field and the clinician's mirror.
Rinsing the cavity with water will help to enhance the color differences between the resin and the moistened dentin.
For this purpose, a wash with pure alcohol is useful. If this process does not allow the clinician to distinguish dentin from composite, the DG 16 probe can be used to scratch the cavity walls: composites and all resin materials can then be identified by the presence of a distinct black scratch.
In the posterior areas, and to avoid excessive aggressiveness that may facilitate iatrogenic damage (perforations) or the loss of important information regarding the correct position of the canal openings, it would be useful to remove most of the pre-existing restoration with a coarse-grained bur mounted on a turbine to a distance of 1 mm from the floor. Consequently, the clinician should use ultrasonic inserts to release the latter part. This is a very essential process in cases

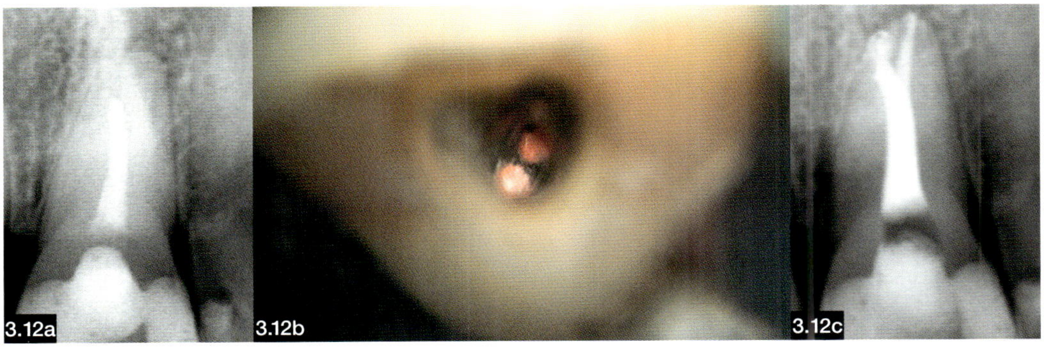

3.12a 3.12b 3.12c

Fig. 3.12a: Improper endodontic treatment of an upper central incisor with an unusual anatomical configuration.

Fig. 3.12b: Access through the existing composite restoration.

Fig. 3.12c: The treatment performed shows a doubling of the apex.

where the restoration material is in direct contact with the floor of the pulp chamber Once unsuitable dental tissues and old restorations have been removed, the clinician should then consider whether or not the cavity needs to be pre-built to regain lost coronal walls and recreate adequate coronal morphology. This process, which is significantly more important in the posterior sectors, will facilitate the creation of a new pulp chamber with four walls (Figs. 3.13-3.17).
When considering significantly extensive composite restorations, it is prudent, but not compulsory, to carry out the cleaning

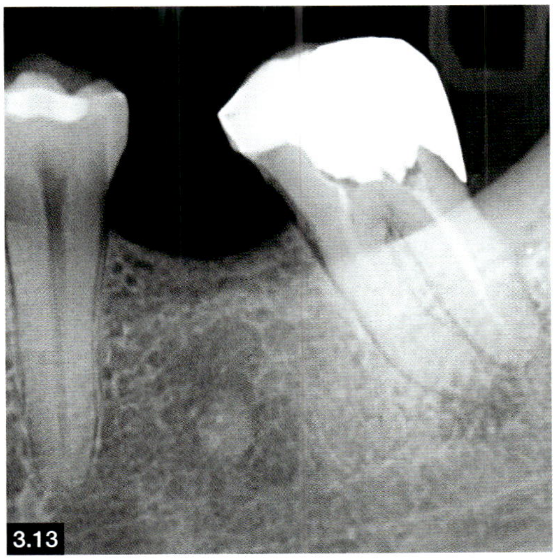

3.13

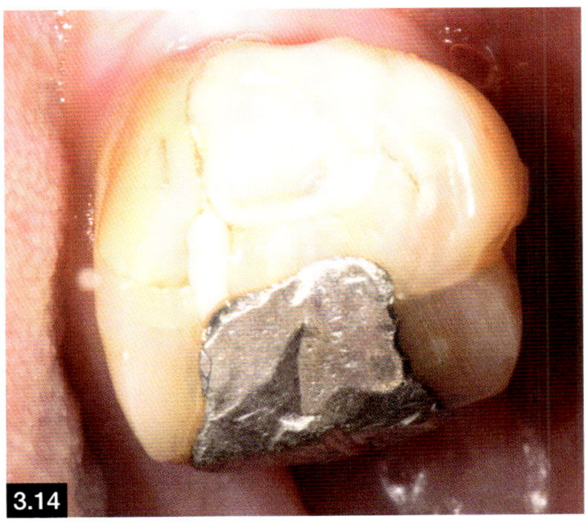

3.14

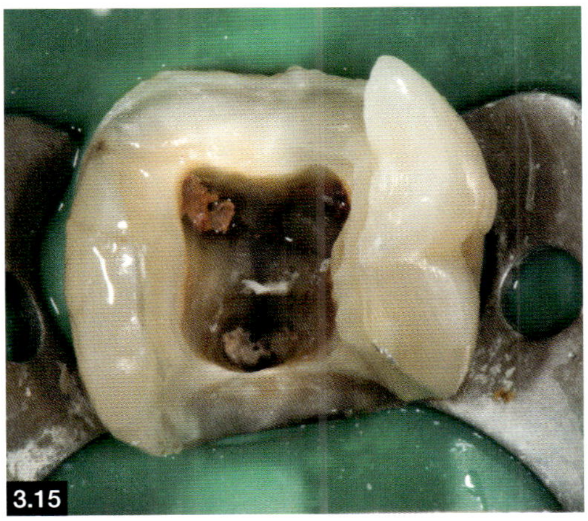

3.15

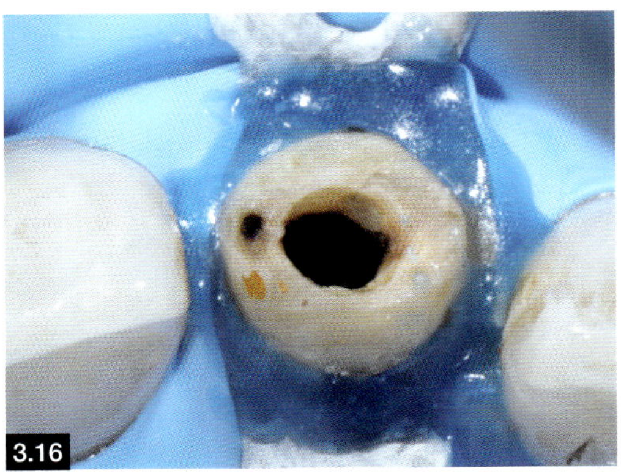

3.16

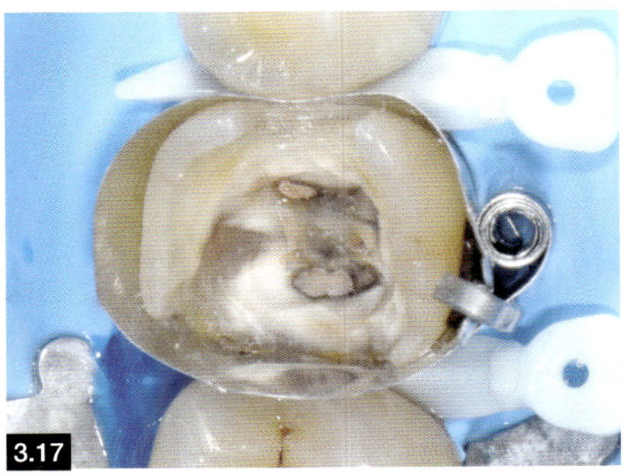

3.17

Fig. 3.13: A lower molar needs to be retreated, as illustrated in the x-ray image.

Fig. 3.14: The clinical picture shows a wide filling (Composite) in the mesial portion and amalgam in the distal portion.

Fig. 3.15: Removal of the restoration reveals a significant loss of dental tissue.

Fig. 3.16: The positioning of the "liquid dam" allows temporary field isolation.

Fig. 3.17: The subsequent reconstruction of the distal wall; the composite cavity makes the endodontic cavity perfectly isolated even in the case of intermediate dressing and treatment over several sessions.

CASE REPORT 2

A retreatment in a discolored central incisor

Retreatment situations often involve the aesthetic aspect of the teeth; not infrequently it is precisely the discoloration of teeth, such as that represented in this case, that leads the patient go to the dentist.
The request therefore becomes twofold: to resolve the aesthetic situation and restore health

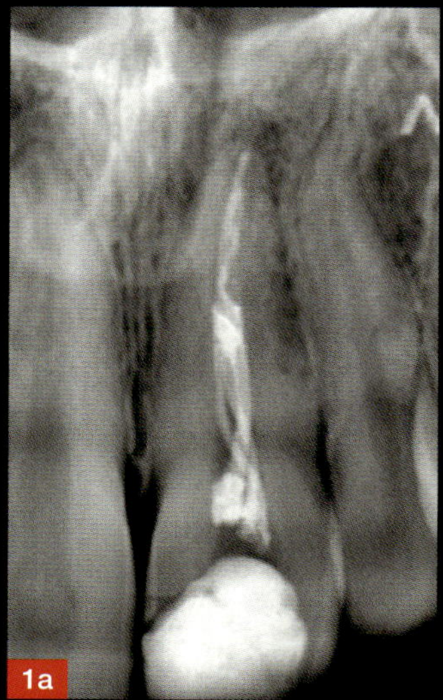

1a

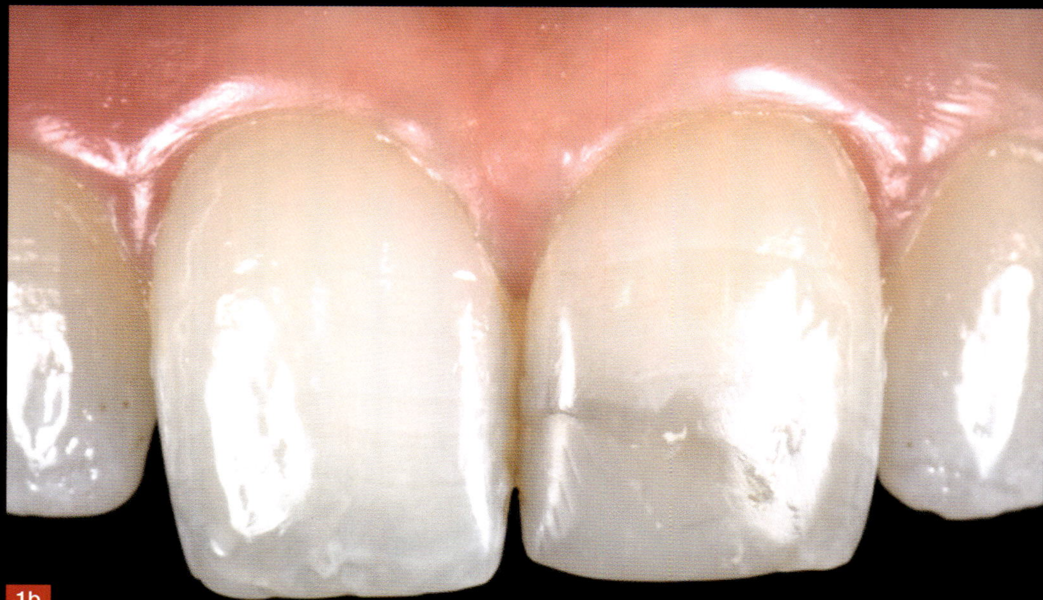

1b

Figure 1a: The x-ray image shows an inappropriate canal therapy.

Figure 1b: The slight discoloration of tooth no. 21 is associated with an infiltrated and inappropriate composite reconstruction.

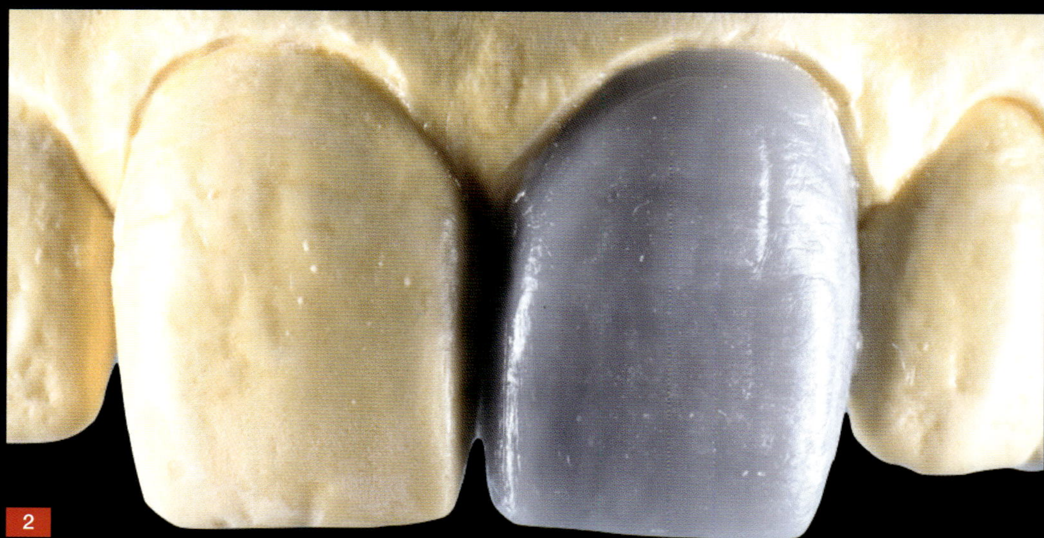

2

Figure 2: In order to obtain an anatomically sound restoration, waxing is performed.

to the apical dental and periodontal tissues. In this case, the discoloration is very evident and is often caused both by the incorrect opening and cleaning of the pulp chamber and by the incorrect use of root canal sealers during the treatment phases.
Thorough cleaning of the coronal compartment will eliminate aesthetic problems and the correct disinfection and sealing of the endodontium will lend new health to the dental and periodontal system.

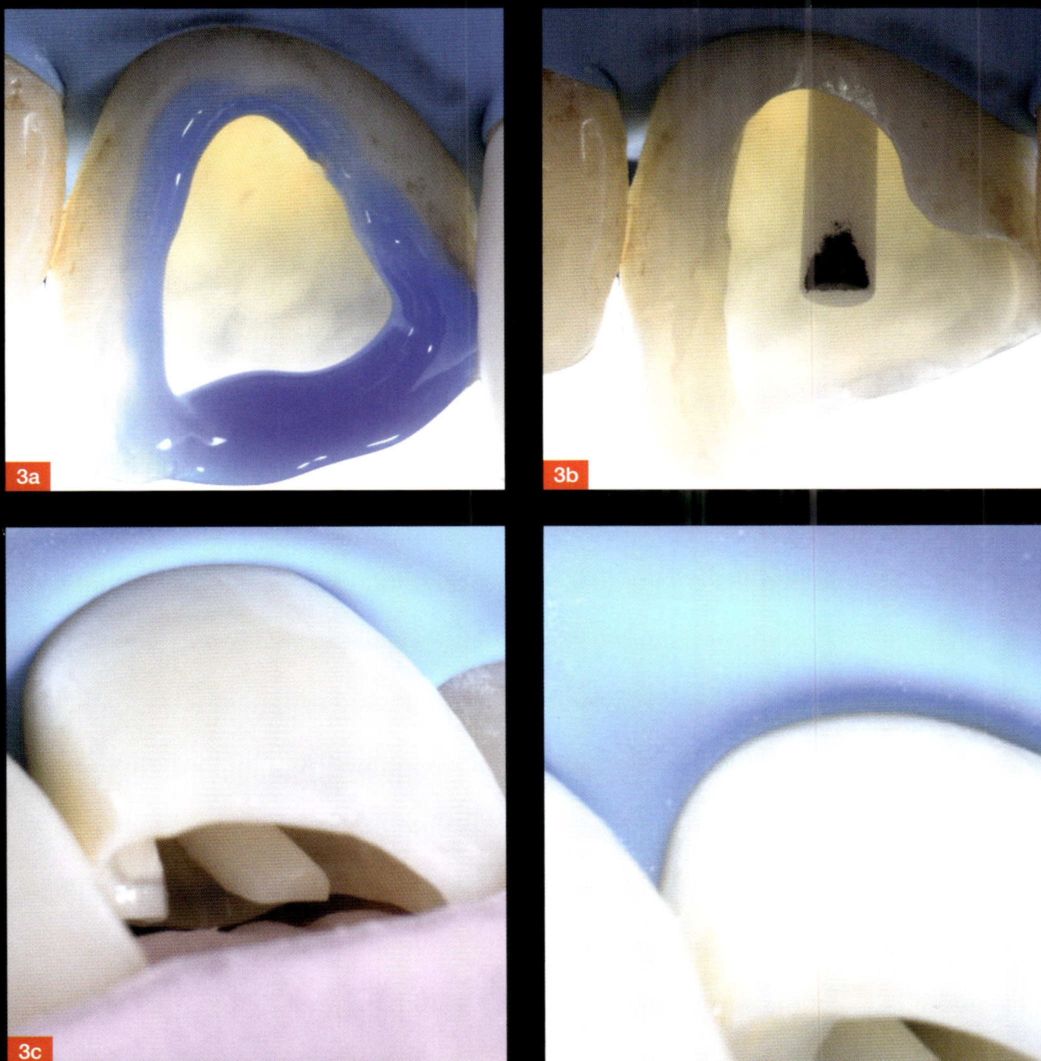

Figure 3a-c: Once the endodontic treatment is complete, we proceed with fiber pin-retained restoration to support the large amount of restoration material placed, by virtue of the residual walls predominantly in enamel.

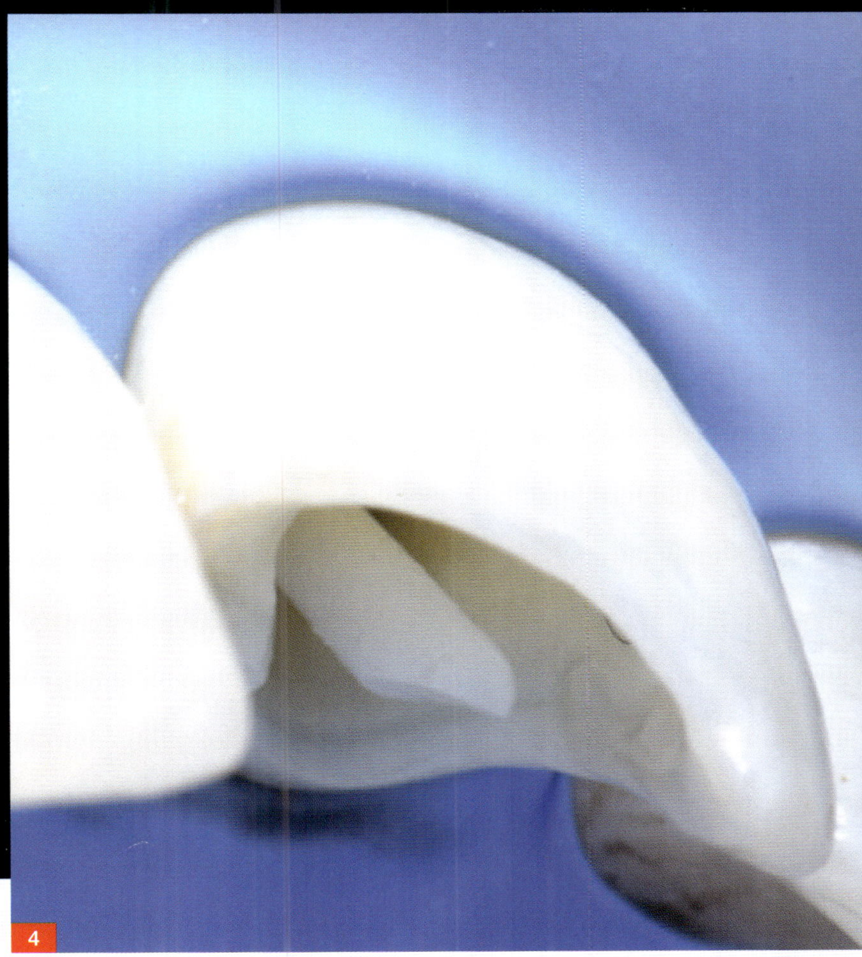

Figure 4: The silicone guide, obtained from the waxing, provides an excellent basis for the definitive composite reconstruction and for the correct management of the space between the post and the composite.

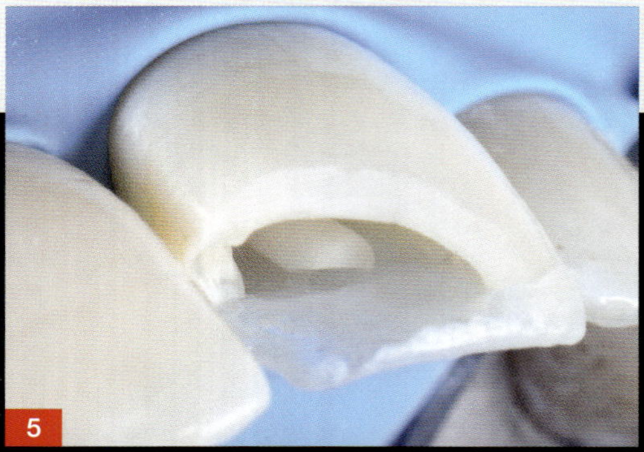

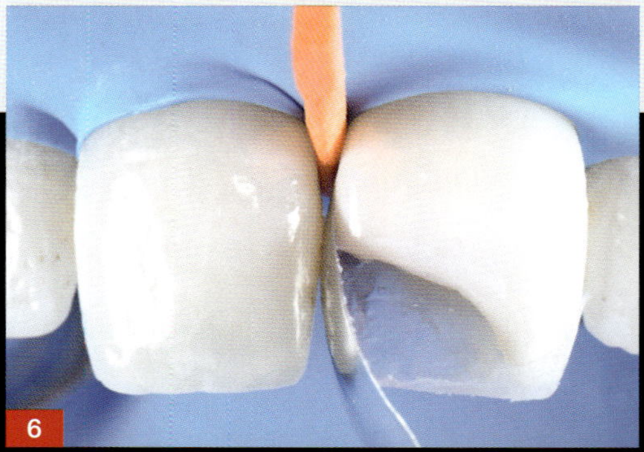

Figure 5: The fiber pin has been suitably modified to maintain the correct space between the pivot and the palatal composite wall.

Figure 6: Correct adaptation of a posterior matrix for a better anatomical configuration of the fourth class.

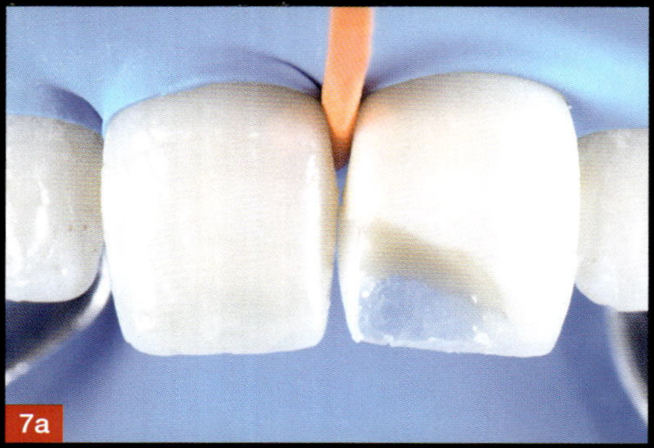

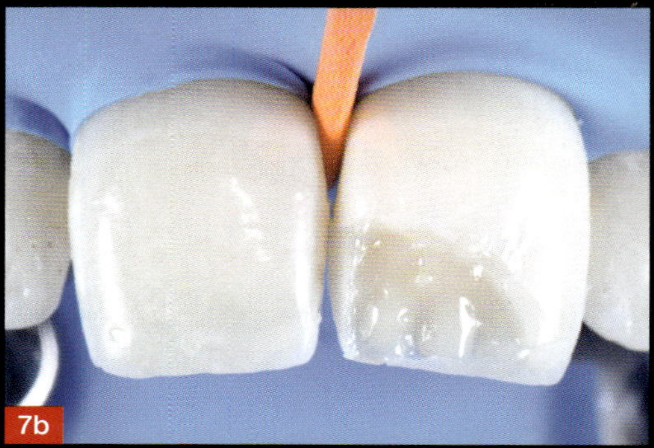

Figure 7a-b: Different phases of the layering of the composite mass, with realization of the dentinal mamelons.

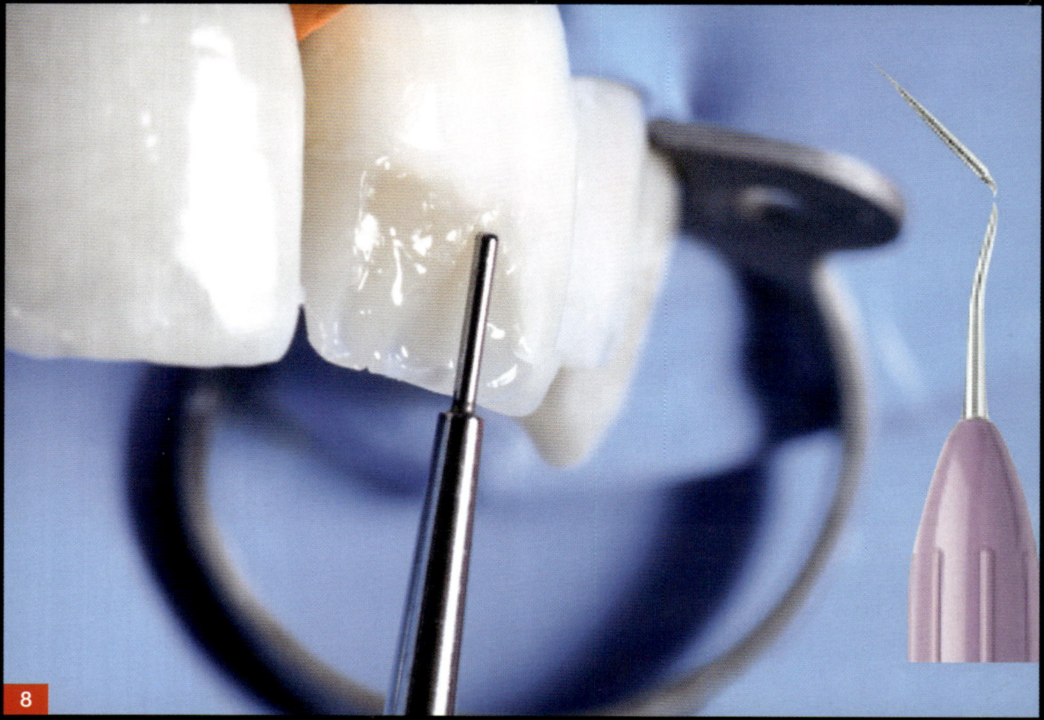

Figure 8: Use of the dedicated tool (LM Dental Measurement) to check the correct thickness of the enamel.

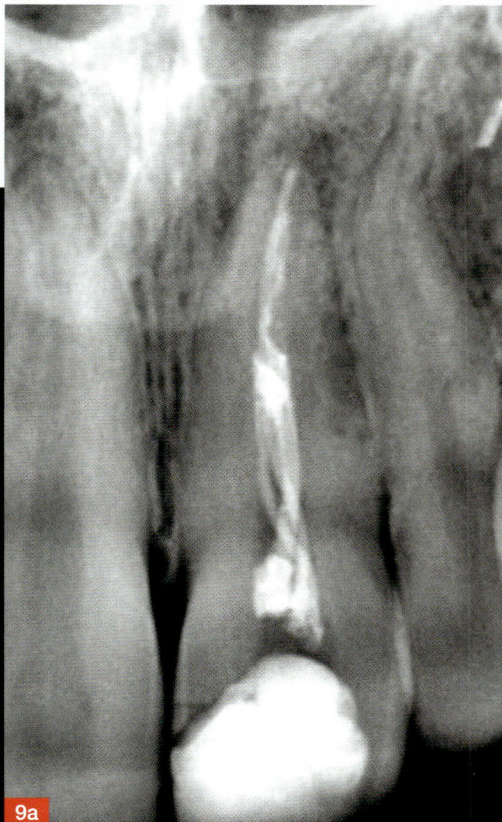

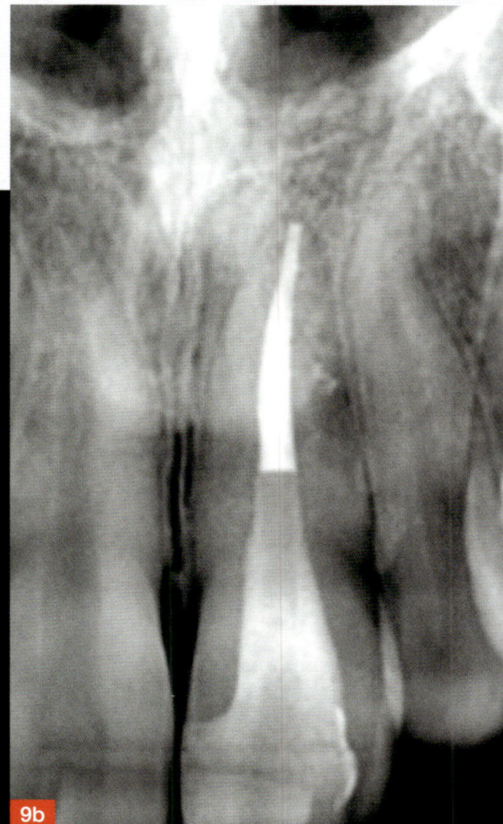

Figure 9a: The initial situation in the x-ray view: note the poor canal filling. In such cases, retreatment can have great opportunities for success.

Figure 9b: Postoperative x-ray showing the perfect performance of endodontic-reconstructive therapy.

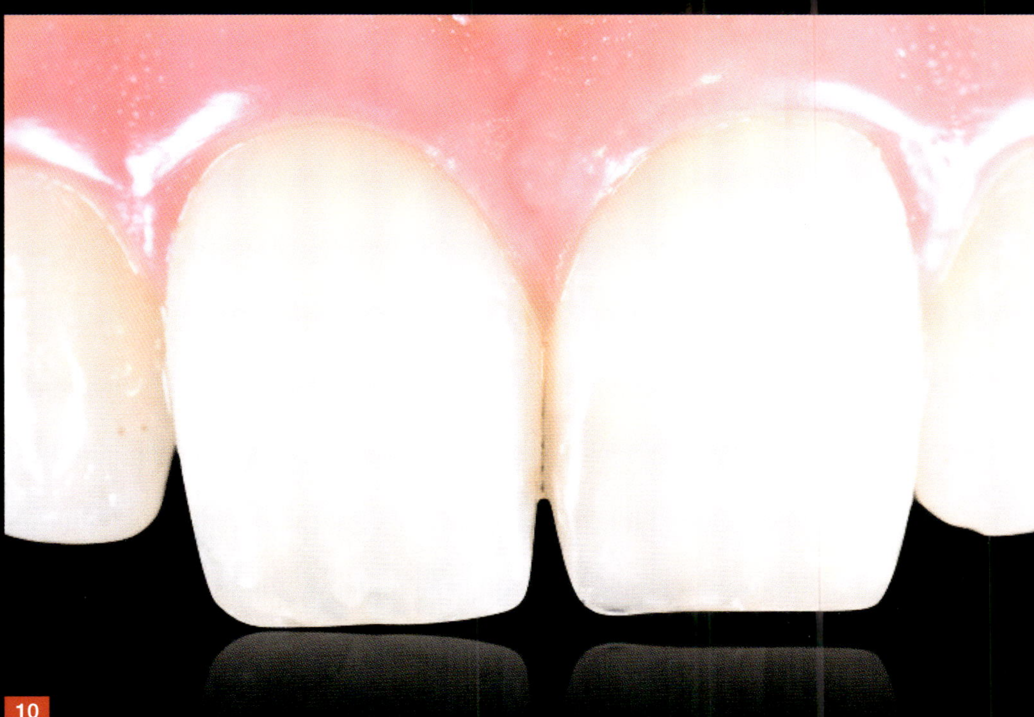

Figure 10: The final case showing perfect aesthetic integration, very different from the initial situation.

CASE REPORT 3

Retreatment of maxillary left first molar

This patient's main complaint was of pain on his upper left molar, which was very tender under pressure. At the clinical examination, there was a splint crown on teeth 26 and 27, and tooth 26 was very tender on percussion, an abscess was located on the buccal side of tooth 26 (Fig. 1). A radiographic examination was performed with periapical radiograph: tooth 26

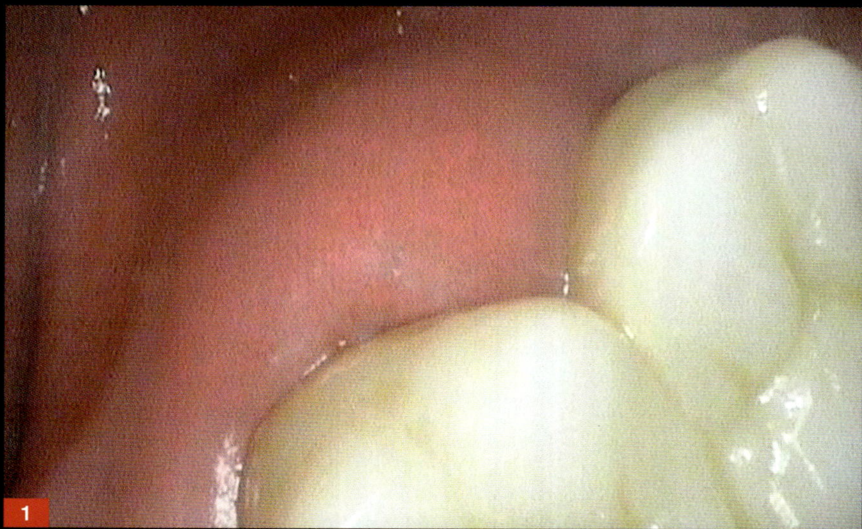

1

Figure 1: Clinical examination of the buccal part of the upper molar.

Figure 2: Periapical radiograph showing three canals and an apical lesion on the mesial root of tooth 26.

2

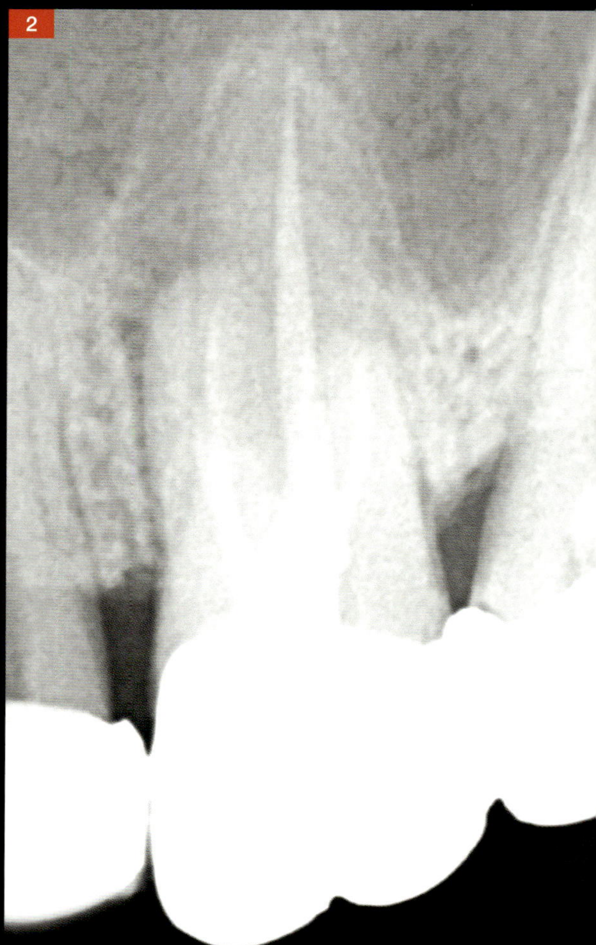

Figure 3: An endodontic ultrasonic tip such as BUC 1A (Obtura Spartan) or StartX #3 (Dentsply Sirona Endodontic) is needed to remove residual material from the pulp chamber area. This is important since we cannot use highspeed burs to clean the material in the pulp chamber due to the risk of perforating the furcation. It is also necessary to refine and explore the mesial area to search for any extra and overlooked canals.

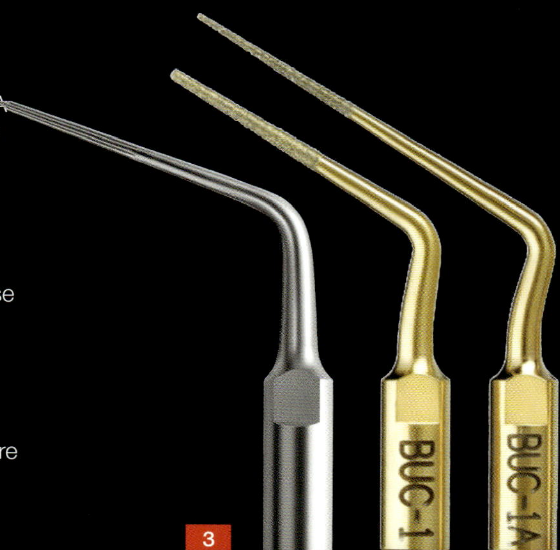

3

was endodontically treated and showed three canals; there was an apical lesion on the mesial root of tooth 26 and the crown margin still looked acceptable (Fig. 2). Retreatment was then planned for this tooth due to the possibility of intra-radicular infection with a possible overlooked canal on the mesial root. The cavity access was made through the crown using a diamond high speed bur as far as the pulp chamber area. A week after treatment, when the patient came for follow-up, the pain had already disappeared, the tooth was functional and asymptomatic, and the abscess had healed. Filling was then performed to complete the retreatment and seal the canal.

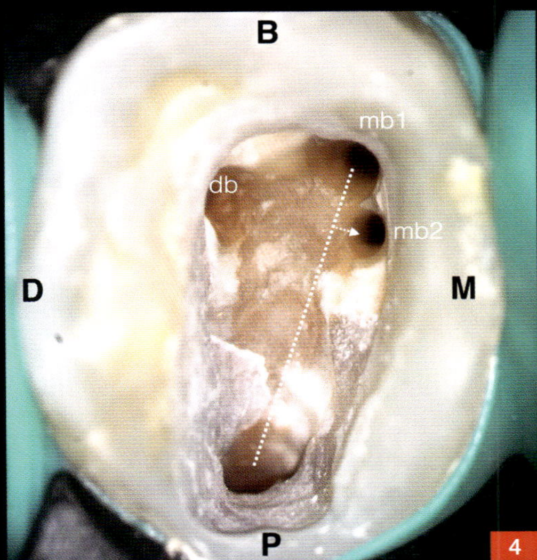

Figure 4: The area requiring exploration for a potential missed MB2 canal is usually palatal to MB1 and slightly mesial to a line drawn between MB1 and the palatal canal.

Figure 5: After refining and exploring the possible extra ME canals, lastly, missed canals were found. There were three mesial canals (MB1, MB2 and MB3), one distal canal (DB) and one palatal canal. After root canal preparation for all five canals (shaping and cleaning) the tooth was temporarily closed for further observation.

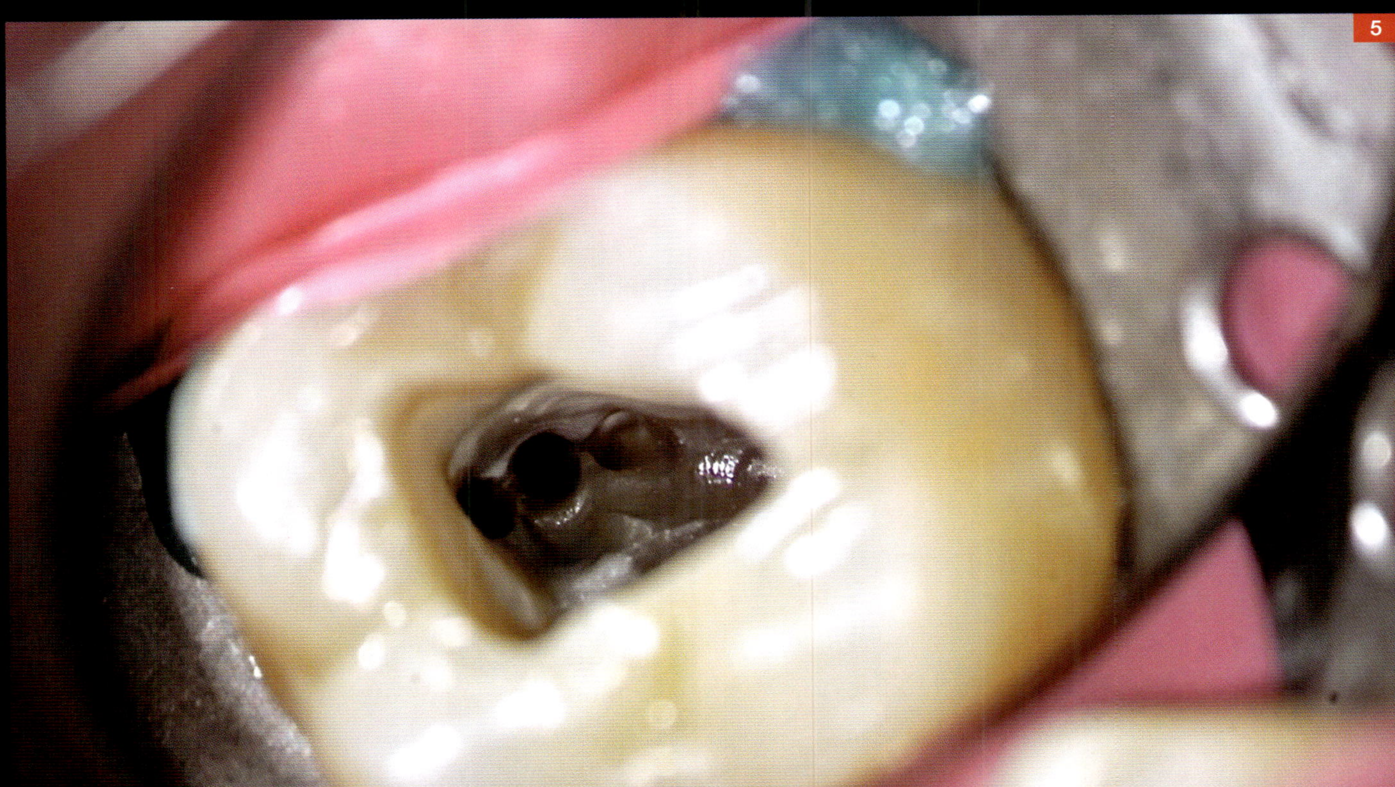

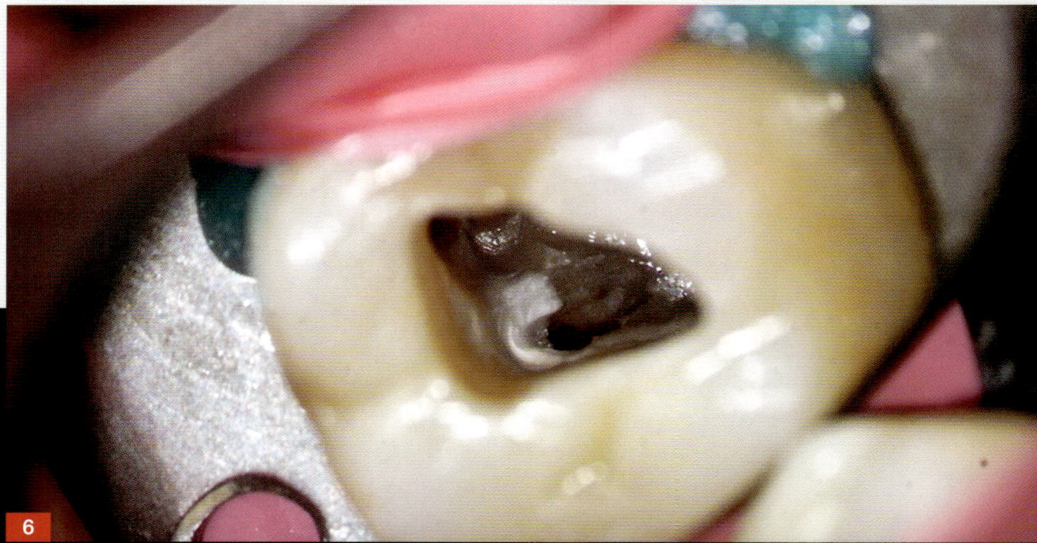

Figure 6: The mesio-buccal aspect of the tooth; an enlargement of the canal orifice made by ultrasonic tips reveal the MB2 canal.

6

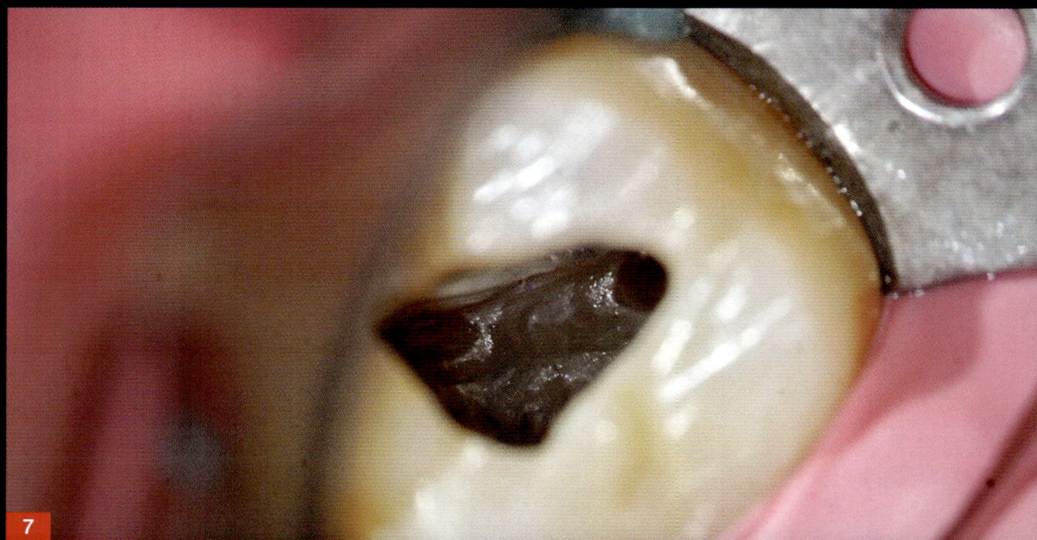

Figure 7: The palatal and disto-buccal canals were only refined using diamond coated ultrasonic tips to favor better root canal instrumentation.

7

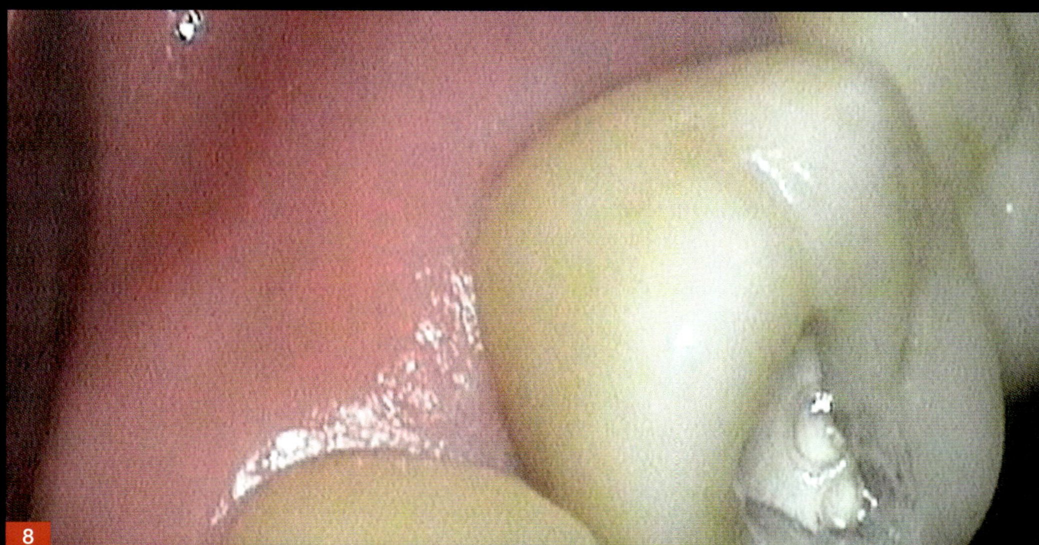

Figure 8: The swallowing deceased after proper decontamination of the whole root canal system by intermediate medication with calcium hydroxide.

8

9

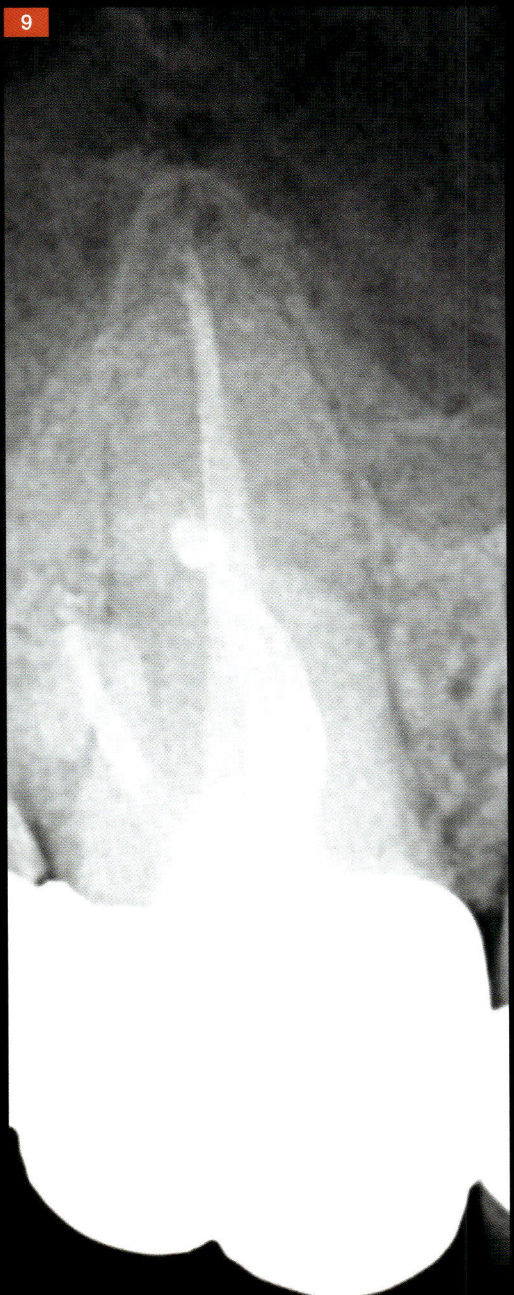

10

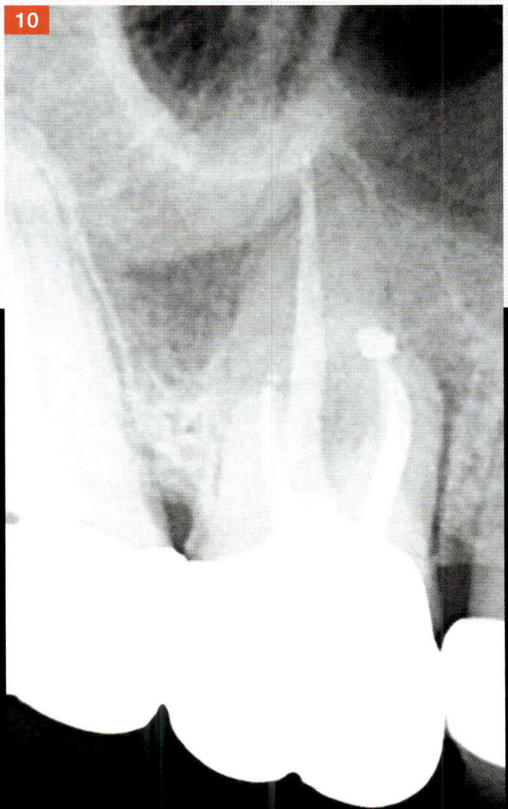

Figure 9: The final x-ray; a slight apical enlargement is still present at the apex of the palatal root. Satisfactory sealing was achieved on both the mesial and distal root canals.

Figure 10: The x-ray after 6 months, partial recovery of the apical transparency can be noted, no other symptoms were reported at that time.

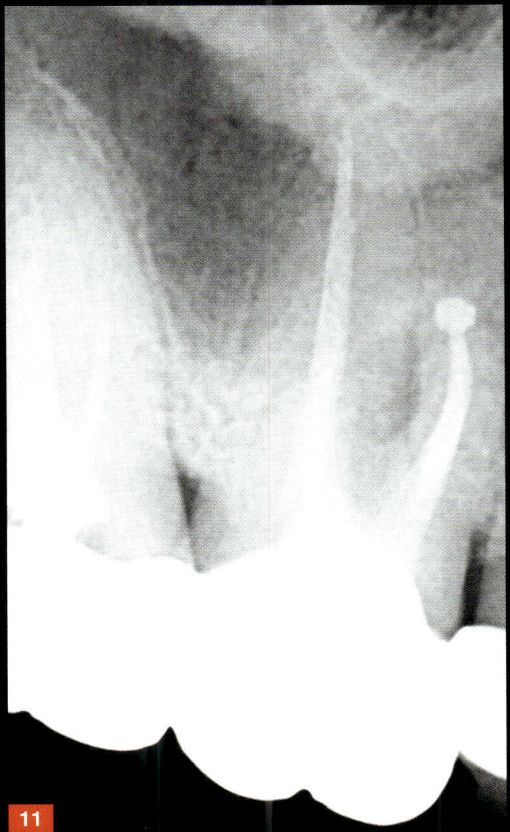

11

Figure 11: One year after the retreatment, a complete recovery of the apical transparency can be seen, no other signs or symptoms were reported at that date.

ADHESION

Restricting access to the endodontium **with adhesive and composite systems** makes the process more effective because the dentin has not been contaminated by chemicals.

phases of the coronal part prior to inserting the rubber dam. In this way, access to endodontic space will be highlighted in the best possible way, especially in cases where previous fillings, following an X-ray investigation, are very deep and may confuse the clinician when attempting to access the root canal.
Once the entire coronal aspect has been isolated in the best possible way, the operating field will also be efficiently isolated because the missing parts of the dental crown will have been reconstructed using composite materials. If the dentin surfaces are efficiently cleaned, a necessary condition for obtaining bacteria-free root access as far as possible, the *adhesion* that can be achieved at this stage will be significantly greater, in terms of both quality and quantity, since the dentin has not yet been contaminated by canal irrigation. Therefore, adhesives, particularly the so-called "self-etch" (or "etch and dry") type – be it single- or two-component – can be used to condition the dentin substrate and bond it to the composite. The latter can be a conventional composite or a fluid composite with low viscosity, thus providing a useful basis for future reconstruction which, in most of these cases, is of the indirect type. The latest generation composite materials, otherwise known as "bulk-fills" that seem to be indicative of this procedure[12] as well as glassinomer sealers modified or not with resin[13] can also be taken into consideration.

Indirect restorations

Often, an indirect restoration, such as a single restoration or a bridge element, has to be performed during the coronal access phase in cases of retreatment. We will primarily consider the following individual elements.

Preservation of an indirect restoration

When coronal restoration appears to be adequate, it may be decided to perform the retreatment process by creating the access cavity through the restoration itself[14] or, where possible, to attempt to decement the prosthetic artifact without damaging it, and then reconstruct it at the end of the therapy.

Access while maintaining the existing crown

The ability for cavity access through an existing crown presents a number of difficulties:

- Modification of the occlusal morphology, which, in some cases, may not be usable as a guide for creating a correct access cavity
- Risk of misfire if the abutment is not aligned with the coronal restoration
- Possibility of causing irreparable ceramic chipping
- Excessive weakening of the crown and abutment structure
- Aesthetic damage that is difficult to repair using a composite material.

In aesthetic areas, however, this type of solution can be advantageous when the intention is to preserve the appearance of the patient's smile, obviously taking care to practice access to the endodontium in the palatal or lingual area of the restoration, before placing the rubber dam.
It is advisable to postpone the use of a dam because an appropriate and effective view of the crown and of the orientation of the bur in three dimensions can protect against eccentric accesses that often result in perforations.

Metal-ceramic crown

Clinicians must be very careful in the initial drilling phase, which is usually performed with a coarse-grained diamond bur to remove the ceramic component of the crown, and facilitate a slightly oversized access, compared to that of a natural tooth, and then insert a tungsten carbide bur suitable for drilling metals. Care should also be taken not to touch the ceramic interface to avoid chipping. Once the access has been established, the tapered drills normally used in conventional coronal access procedures, whether diamond or un-machined

tungsten carbide, can be extremely valuable in defining access to the endodontium and in removing debris – such as sealer or gutta-percha – from previous therapies. Moreover, it is very important to use the milling burrs at low speed using a multiplier hand piece or a blue ring contra-angle hand piece.
It is also advisable to use new burrs to achieve a more effective cut. This will limit vibrations during the cutting process and the risk of crack development in the ceramic material.
Even at this point, ultrasound seems an indispensable modality for cleansing and eliminating the above materials, as demonstrated in the related imaging material. It is important to avoid placing the shaft of the ultrasound tip against the prosthetic crown, as this may cause cracks in the ceramic that can lead to the uncovering of the underlying metal.
It is also essential to warn the patient of the risk of fracturing the ceramic during the coronal access phase, especially if the tooth in question is located in an aesthetically relevant area: to prevent this from happening, it is recommended that clinicians take an impression and develop a temporary replacement crown, provided the original crown is irreparably damaged during the chamber access phase. In this process, it is important to remember the assistance that magnifiers (glasses or surgical microscope) with accessory light sources can provide.

Once this phase has been completed, there are three possible situations:

1. The emptying of the coronal component does not affect the seal of the crown.
2. The coronal seal is partially compromised, but the stability of the crown remains sound.
3. The coronal seal is highly compromised and the stability of the crown is dubious.

In the first two cases, the use of glass ionomer composites or sealers – either self-curing or light-curing – appears to be the best way to guarantee a good seal when trying to access the deep endodontium. It should be remembered that, in certain cases, it may be necessary to perform endodontic retreatment over several sessions, and hence the intermediate dressing must be contained in this space. Otherwise, the infiltration of salivary fluids would cause new bacterial contaminations in root canals already largely emptied, thus favoring the onset of septic postoperative reactions.
If certain instability in the crown is detected, it is important to find an immediate alternative solution using resin or polycarbonate temporary coverage to replace the crown.

Crown or veneer in feldspar, glass or zirconia ceramics

The above selection criteria also apply to the latest generation of aesthetic ceramic materials.
The risks are often linked to the possibility that the ceramics may fracture and, therefore, can no longer be used during the treatment phase and in the subsequent period.
The role that these restorations play in the healing phase is far from negligible.
Therefore, designing a new restoration in teeth that have a good, but not entirely certain, prognosis needs to be considered.
On the basis of these considerations, the maintenance of the previous *restoration* – which meets the necessary waterproofing requirements – may represent a valid alternative even to temporary resin materials and new restorations. This is especially true in cases of teeth that were reconstructed with highly aesthetic materials in the anterior areas.
If an access cavity is to be made on a lithium disilicate or zirconia crown, it is advisable to use a dedicated burr for cutting these materials mounted on a turbine, considering that the exact thickness can vary from 0.5 to 2 mm.
If the procedures for removing the material used in the previous treatment do not compromise the stability of the crown, and do not visibly affect the surfaces on which micro-cracks and lamellar detachments can be seen, simple repair of the endodontic access using composite materials could ensure sufficient longevity to the old reconstruction. Consequently, reagrdless of the medium chosen, the possibility that the restoration will remain intact following removal, or will be damaged, remains high.

RESTORATION

The maintenance of the **old restoration** can be an important element of the retreatment phase.

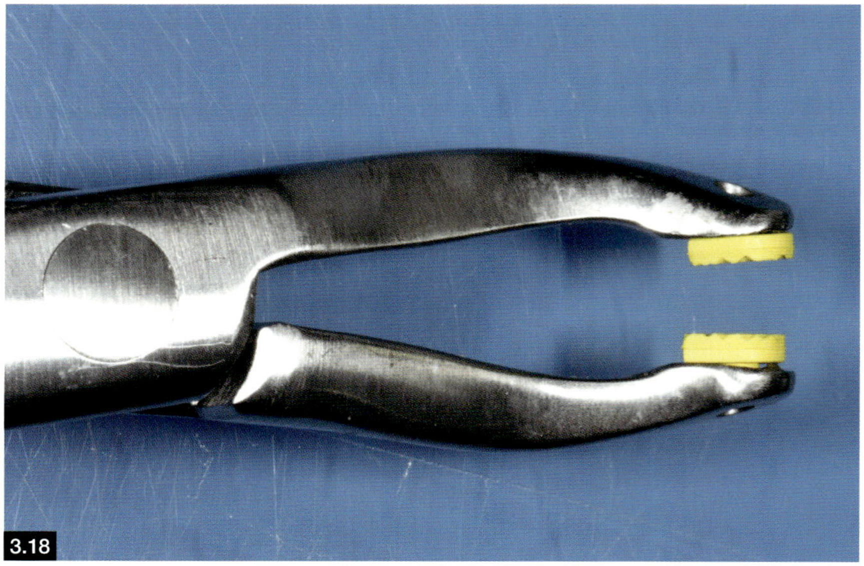

3.18

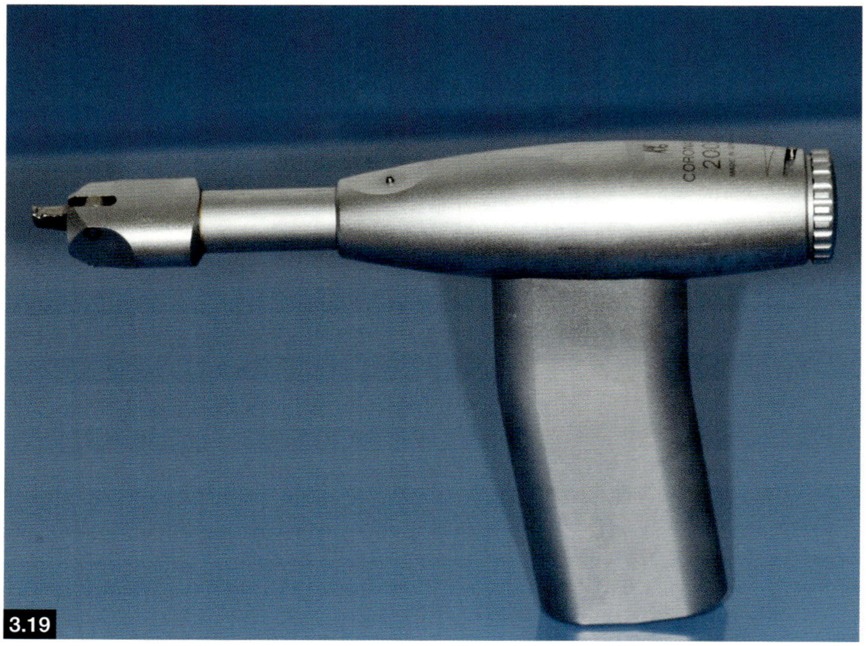

3.19

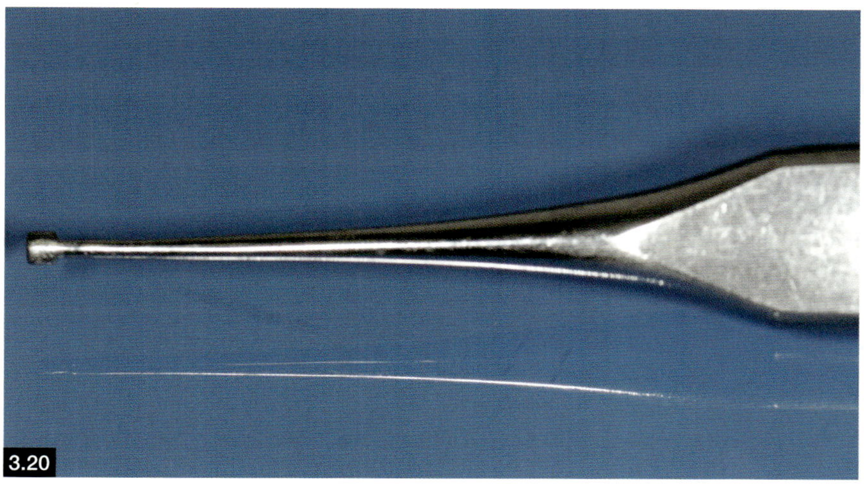

3.20

Elimination of indirect restorations

If the existing coronal restoration is not reliable or stable, literature suggests that clinicians should begin by removing the existing crown, the abutment (connecting element), and finally, any structures that limit access to the root canal system (e.g., posts, retention).
In this way, and by eliminating coronal interferences, it will be possible to treat the endodontium with better visibility and with compact instruments, thus minimizing the difficulty of the operation[15].
This technique involves the complete sacrifice of the existing crown in favor of the possibility of preserving as much of the dental structure of the underlying prosthetic abutment as possible.
It is also the option that allows the best immediate evaluation of the condition of the underlying abutment.
Crown removal can be difficult.
The crown's retention depends on many factors such as the type of preparation, the design of the underlying restoration, and the sealer used for fixation.
There are many tools that simplify this procedure, and they can be broken down into three categories (tool folders):

1. Grasping tools (silicon grip pliers; Fig. 3.18)
2. Percussion instruments (CORONAflex™, KaVo) and/or hand hammers (Fig. 3.19)
3. Passive or lever instruments (Metalift™ or WAMKey; Fig. 3.20).

Evidently, the clinician must be aware of the risks or/and benefits of these tools before proceeding with the removal of an intact crown or of an existing restoration[16].

A summary of crown removal methods and corresponding pros and cons can be found in Table 3.2.
Regardless of the medium chosen, the possibility that the restoration will remain intact, or minimally altered, following removal remains high. Hence it is essential to efficiently plan all related processes and prevent the unnecessary removal of prosthetic restorations.

Table 3.2 **TOOLS AND OPERATIONS FOR ELIMINATING CORONAL OBSTACLES**

Method		Operational phases	Notes
Cutting the crown		Use a dedicated drill to create a groove from the gingival surface to the incisal surface. In the cut created, insert a flat-headed tool and spread the two edges appropriately so as to lose the connection with the abutment below.	Destroys restoration and saves dental tissue.
Leverage movement		Insert an instrument (e.g. chisel or excavator or avulsion lever) to lever in uneven spaces between the tooth and restoration that undermine the stability and quality of the crown.	Risk of tooth fracture, especially when the restoration is not perfectly consistent with the abutment.
Pliers		Dedicated pliers with rubber-coated tips able to 'grasp' the crown.	Risk of restoration fracture due to a lack of force control. If a core post is present, the risk of root fractures increases considerably because of the applied displacement forces.
Decementation systems	Richwil Crown and Bridge Remover	A water-soluble resin – softened in water – can be easily inserted into the anatomical undercuts (apically to the tooth equator). Patients should close their mouths and compress the block of resin for about two thirds of the thickness. When the resin cools down, patients are then asked to quickly open their mouths.	The risk involves possible decementation of any prosthetic restoration present in the antagonist arch.
	Crown removal systems (manual and mechanical extractors)	The extractors used can be manual or mechanical. Manual extractors are characterized by inserts that are placed under the edge of the restoration to be removed (e.g. drop hammer). When a force is applied to the end of the system, this force is transmitted to the insert and, consequently, to the restoration, thus generating a sudden pulling force on the material with which it is sealed. In well-integrated restorations, it can be difficult to place the insert below a margin. Mechanized systems (e.g. CORONA flex™, KaVo) are very effective and use pneumatic force to break the sealing material. These systems are usually more comfortable for the patient, despite a greater risk of chipping the ceramic coating of the crowns.	Minimal damage to the restoration which may, in many cases, be reused. It is also possible for ceramic coating to chip. They are contraindicated when indirect all-ceramic restorations sealed with adhesive techniques are to be removed.
	WAMKey	After drilling a small hole in the vestibular or lingual surface of the crown and creating a space between the abutment and the restoration, the key is then inserted into the hole. It is turned until the crown is lifted. It is particularly effective if the reconstructed core is solid. Removed crowns can be reused as temporary restorations.	Effective system for reusing the crown as a temporary restoration. The abutment below must be intact.
	Metalift™	This is a self-tapping screw that is inserted through a hole in the occlusal surface of the restoration. Then turned, it applies a force to the core, thereby favouring the detachment of the crown.	Effective system for reusing the crown as a temporary restoration. The abutment below must be intact.
Ultrasound		Ultrasound used at high power and with abundant irrigation - either with a simple tip for hygiene and prophylaxis or with dedicated tips - can generate micro-fractures in the sealer structure, and hence decrease the degree of crown fixation.	They are often insufficient for removing the restoration by themselves. By contrast, they are useful for reducing the force needed to remove the restoration by other means.

(Modified from[16])

Bridge elements

The possibility of treating teeth that act as bridge pillars (anchors), in a similar way to the teeth discussed earlier, is secondary to numerous diagnostic and prognostic considerations.

When this opportunity arises, the clinician has two distinct choices:

1. The bridge can be removed, stored, and refreshed;
2. The bridge cannot be safely removed and must, therefore, be broken to ensure access to the endodontium.

In the latter case, the above rule applies to single crowns, whereas in the former case, the use of instruments such as air hammers (CORONAflex™, KaVo) can be useful for the atraumatic removal of the bridge (Fig. 3.21a-d).

It goes without say that this operation involves several risks. However, and in order to prevent a poorly performed endodontic retreatment due to access difficulties, clinicians should consider the compromise of using an abutment for its supporting tissues.

When faced with very uncertain situations, the use of the retrograde seal apicecdomy surgical technique can be the choice of election even in cases of an endodontic space that was poorly sealed during previous therapy[17].

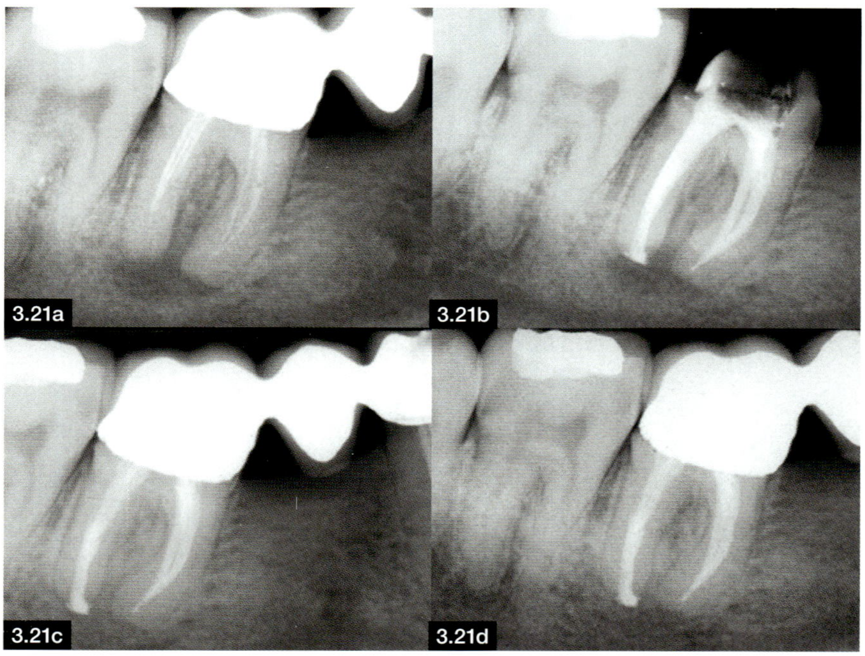

Fig. 3.21a-d: a) The preoperative X-ray shows an apical lesion of the distal bridge abutment (tooth 4.6);

b) Bridge removal makes access easier;

c) The bridge can be reused at the end of treatment;

d) Subsequent control exhibits that the bridge is still functional and the periapical endodontic lesion is resolved.

The importance of using the appropriate instrumentation in endodontics is strategic to achieving excellent results that are a prerequisite for preserving teeth and, in this specific case, improving the quality of ultrasonic sources.

New tips, which come in a great variety of shapes and sizes, allow an efficient combination of power and precision of cut in order to reach the deepest parts of the endodontium without compromising its integrity. The use of magnification systems (magnifying glasses and/or surgical microscope) together with the use of ultrasound sources

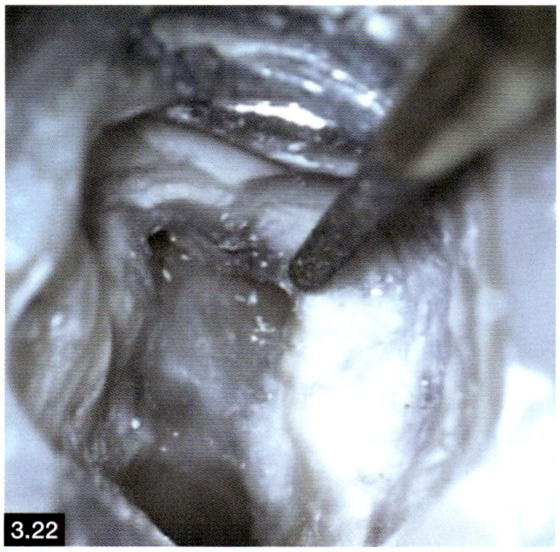

3.22

with dedicated tips, has facilitated an profound increase in the precision of the dentist's work, with a considerable saving of dentinal tissue and greater predictability of the final clinical result. The synergy of the microscope-ultrasound combination represents the best clinical combination for safety and control of the operational phase. Martin[18] was the first to introduce ultrasonic sources in the endodontic field, and more specifically, in the field of canal therapy and root resection. In the 1980s, Martin and Cunningham[19] introduced the term "endosonics" that was defined as the ultrasonic synergistic system of root canal instrumentation and disinfection.

Properties of ultrasound

Ultrasound pulses contain the oscillations induced on objects with a frequency above the audible limit (20 kHz). The energy required to induce these oscillations can be generated by two different methods: the magnetostrictive and the piezoelectric principle[20].

The magnetostrictive method converts electromagnetic energy into mechanical energy

Box 3.1 **ULTRASONIC SYSTEMS USED TO PERFORM AN ENDODONTIC RETREATMENT**

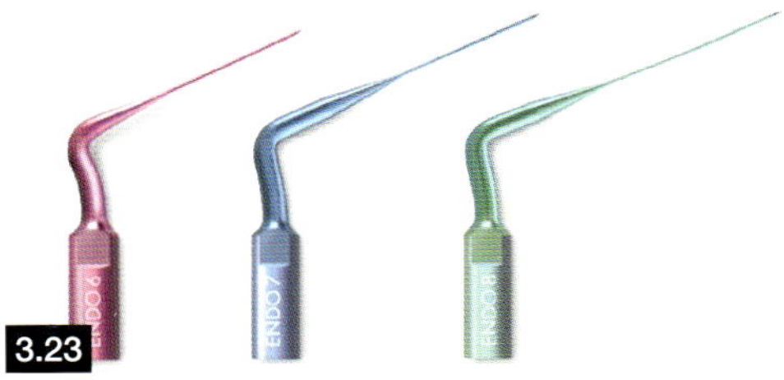

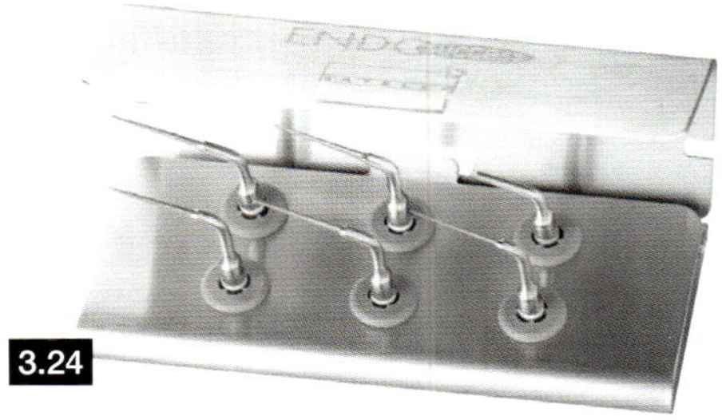

Fig. 3.22: A diamond ultrasonic tip in action.

Fig. 3.23: Useful ultrasonic tips for removing deep intracanal obstacles (ProUltra, Dentsply Maillefer, Switzerland).

Fig. 3.24: Useful Ultrasonic tips for removing deep intracanal obstacles (Endoset, Acteon, France).

through a pack of metal strips, where alternating magnetic fields produce approximately 25 kHz vibrations on average. With the piezoelectric principle, a crystal that changes its size under the effect of an electric charge, causes a mechanical oscillation, without the corresponding development of heat that is instead present in the magnetostrictive method, and a higher frequency of 40 kHz. The frequency range used in the original ultrasonic units was between 25-40 kHz; "low frequency" solutions operating at between 1 and 8 kHz (sub-audible) were proposed, thus resulting in lower levels of shear stress and reduced alterations of the tooth surfaces[21].

Modern piezoelectric units, which are used in endodontics as well as in surgical applications, can benefit from these distinct advantages in terms of cutting efficiency. The tips of these units, in fact, move with a linear "piston-like" motion as opposed to the "elliptical-oscillatory" motion of the magnetostrictive units. The position of the nodes and antinodes of a free endosonic file activated by a 30 kHz piezoelectric generator develops along the length of the file: the variation in amplitude of the vibration of the file does not increase progressively as the power generated increases[22]. The less invasive and more conservative characteristics of piezoelectric units find specific applications – when used with dedicated inserts – in orthograde endodontics during the pulp chamber access phase (search for hidden canals, removal of intra-canal obstacles, and calcifications), in the activation of irrigation solutions, and in surgical endodontics for the preparation of the retrograde cavity.

Clinical applications of ultrasound

As mentioned earlier, the combination of ultrasound and magnification is of fundamental importance for addressing cases of retreatment in both anterior and posterior segments. The first clinical situation in which the use of ultrasound tips presents with enormous advantages involves the review of the access cavity for identifying canal orifices to retreat. During the retreatment process, it is very common to find incorrectly prepared access cavities where clinician can find the pulp horns, typically in the front teeth, or the chamber roof of the premolars.

We are well aware of how difficult it is to regrind an access cavity, in such cases, because it is necessary to respect the original anatomy of the tooth without altering the chamber floor and, in particular, how complex it is to modify and restore proper access to all canal entrances.

The high cutting accuracy and the excellent visibility of the operating field are the main advantages of using ultrasonic drills in these cases[23].

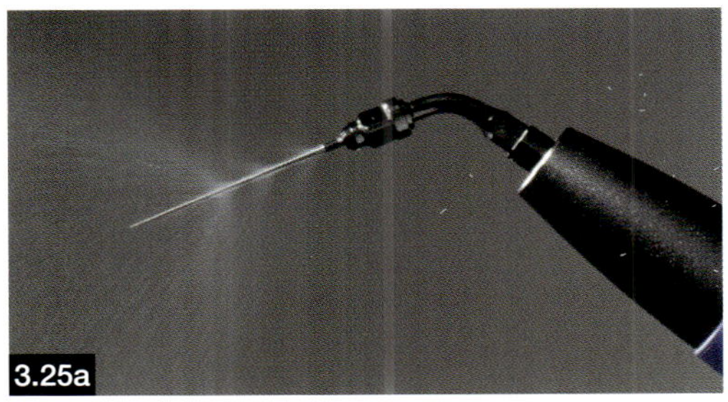

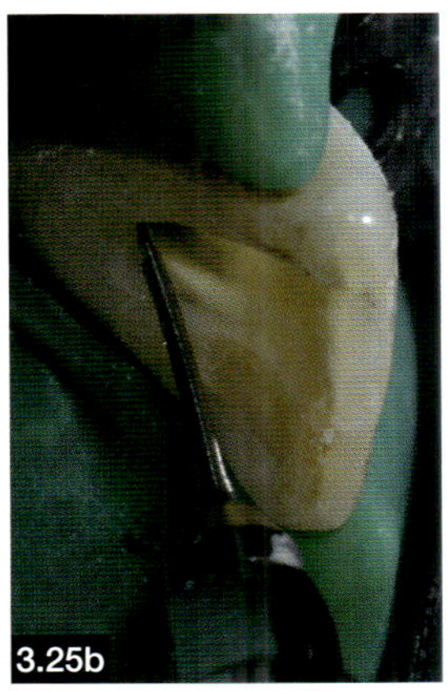

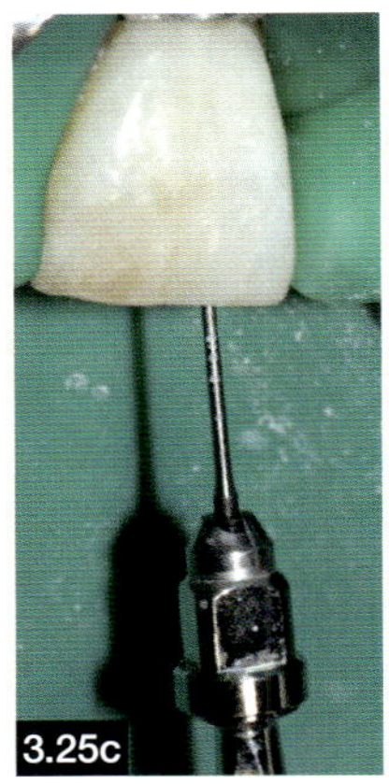

Fig. 3.25a-c: Action of the K-File ultrasonic tip (EMS, Switzerland).

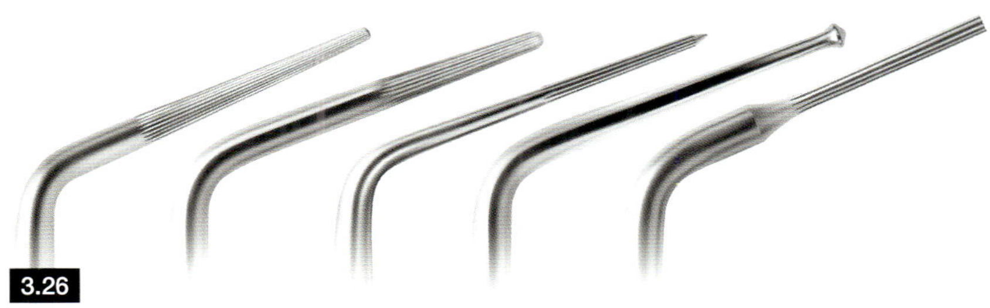

Fig. 3.26: Ultrasonic tips for finishing the pulp chamber (Start-X, Dentsply Maillefer Switzerland).

CASE REPORT 4

Retreatment passing through a bridge

Endodontic lesions in bridge abutment elements often pose operational dilemmas. Removing the bridge, which may be recent, warrants the replacement of the prosthetic artifact with a temporary one. Passing through the bridge, i.e. creating an access route without removing the bridge, has the dual advantage of retreatment without exposing the patient and the operator to additional costs. Good resolution may be obtained with a simple repair. In this case, the latter route was followed.

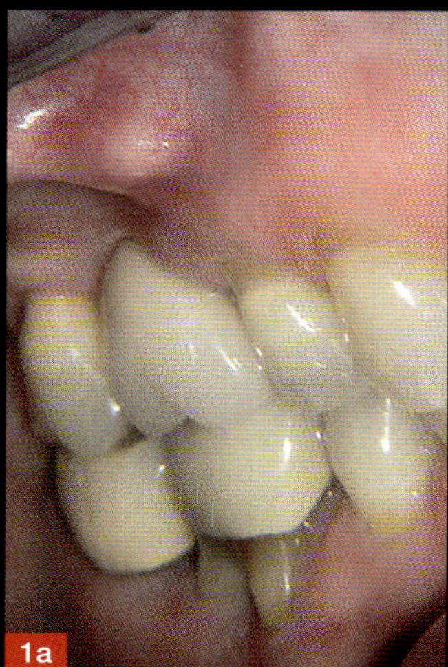

1a

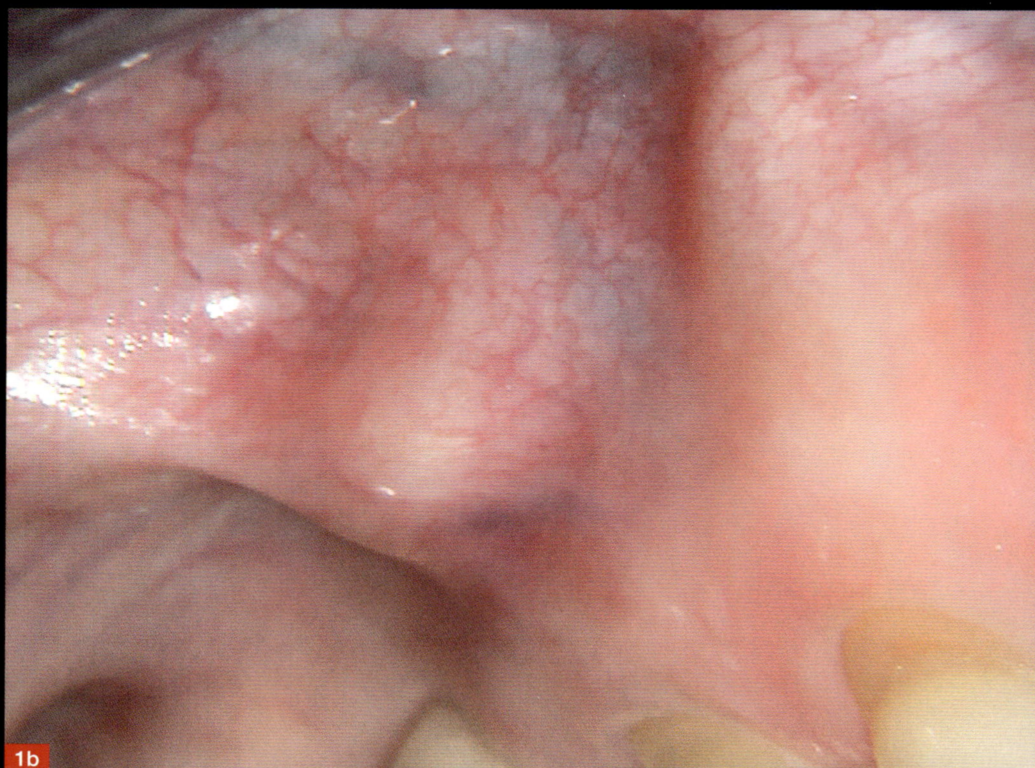

1b

Figure 1a: An obvious periapical reaction is appreciable at the mucous level of the first upper premolar.

Figure 1b: Mucosal examination at higher magnification.

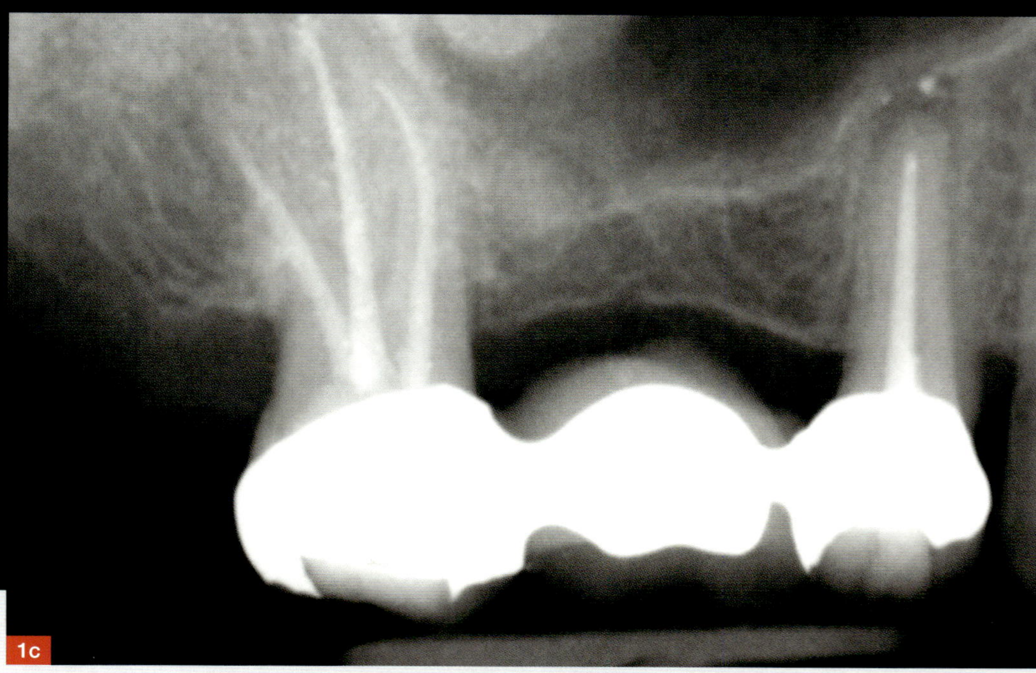

1c

Figure 1c: The x-ray image.

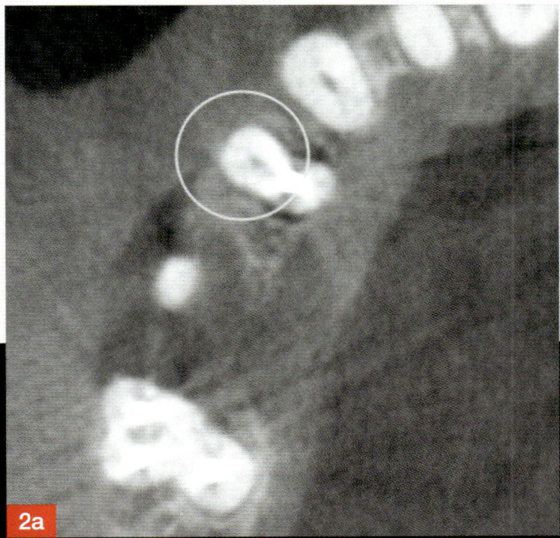

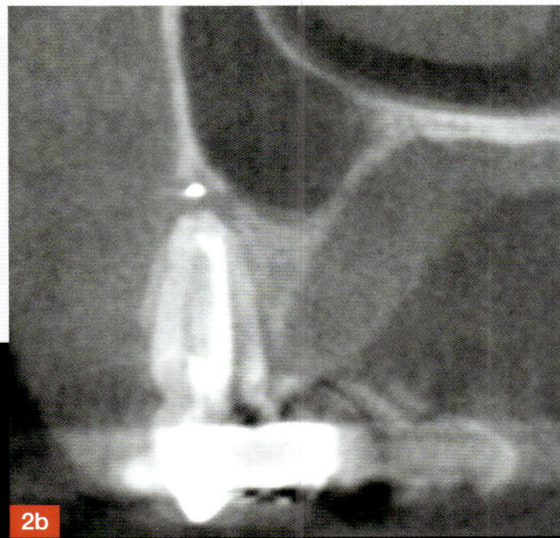

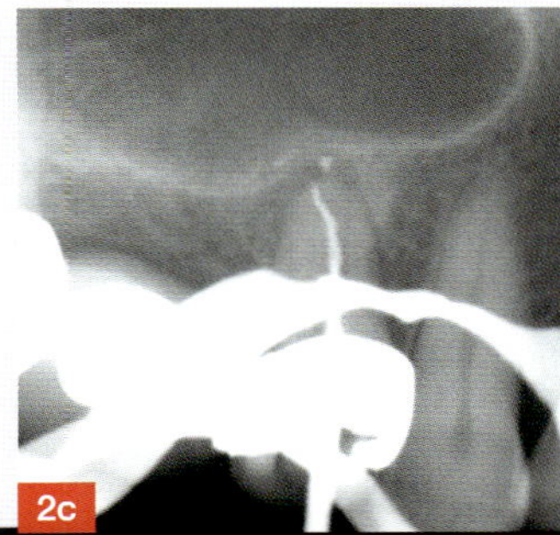

Figure 2a: CBCT examination showing an instrumented canal at the level of the first premolar (vestibular canal), the septic content of which is likely to be responsible for the periapical reaction.

Figure 2b: Another angle shows the presence of a step in the apical area.

Figure 2c: The instrument inserted in the root canal overcoming the step.

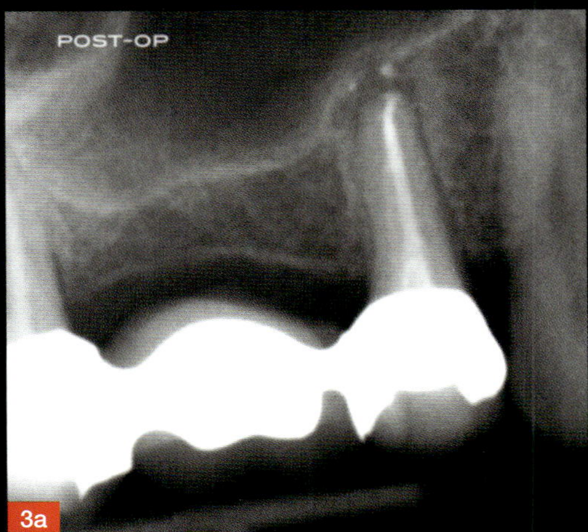

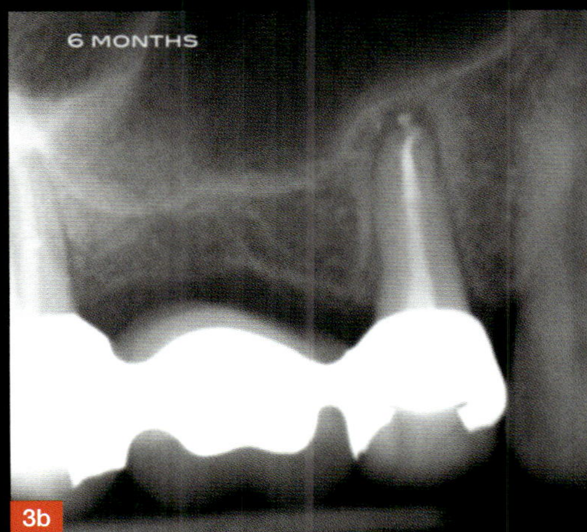

Figure 3a: The treatment is over.

Figure 3b: The clinical picture at six months.

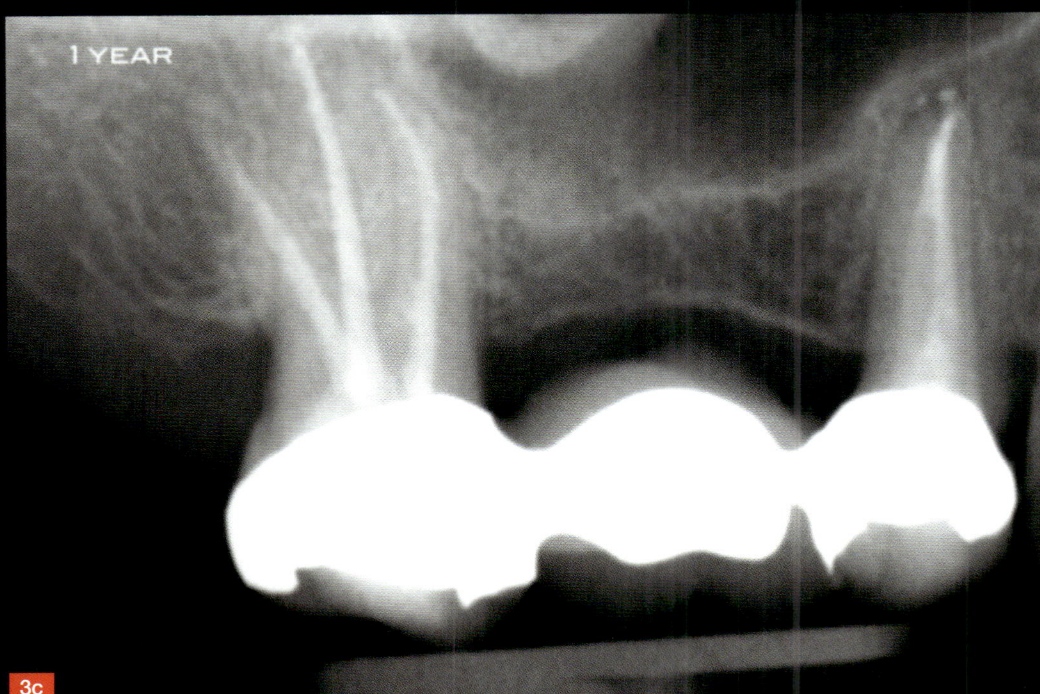

Figure 3c: Evolution at 1 year.

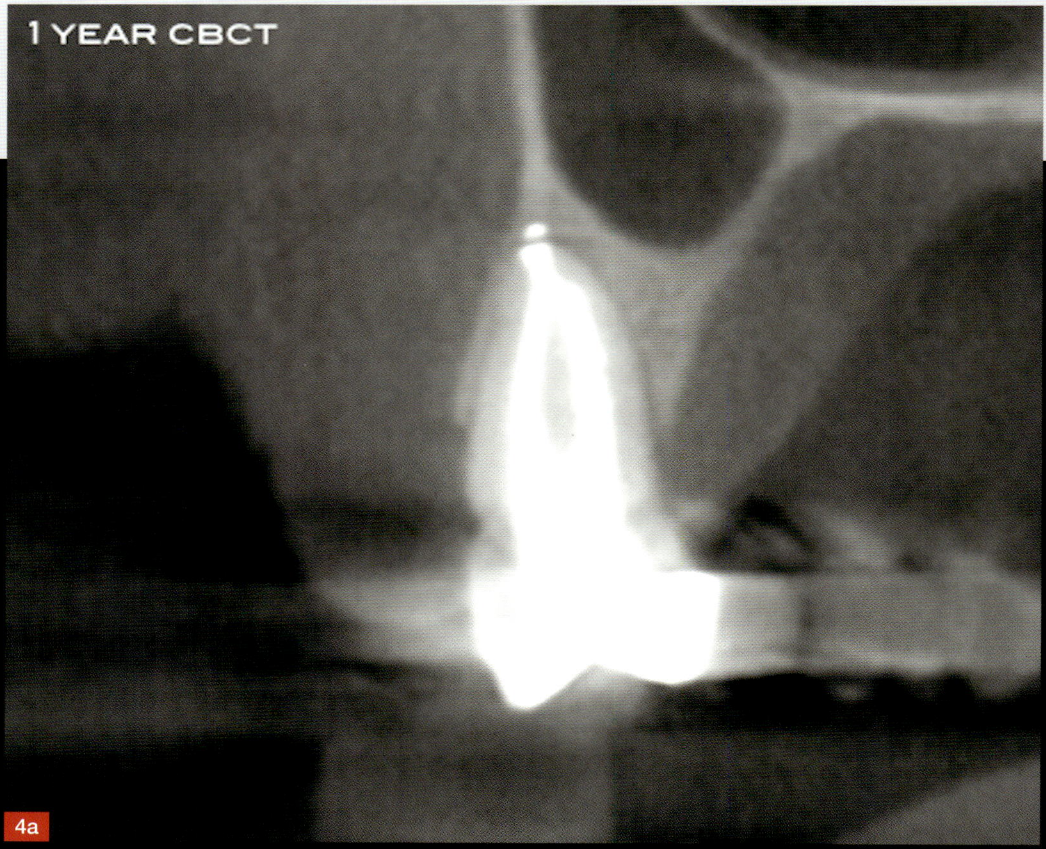

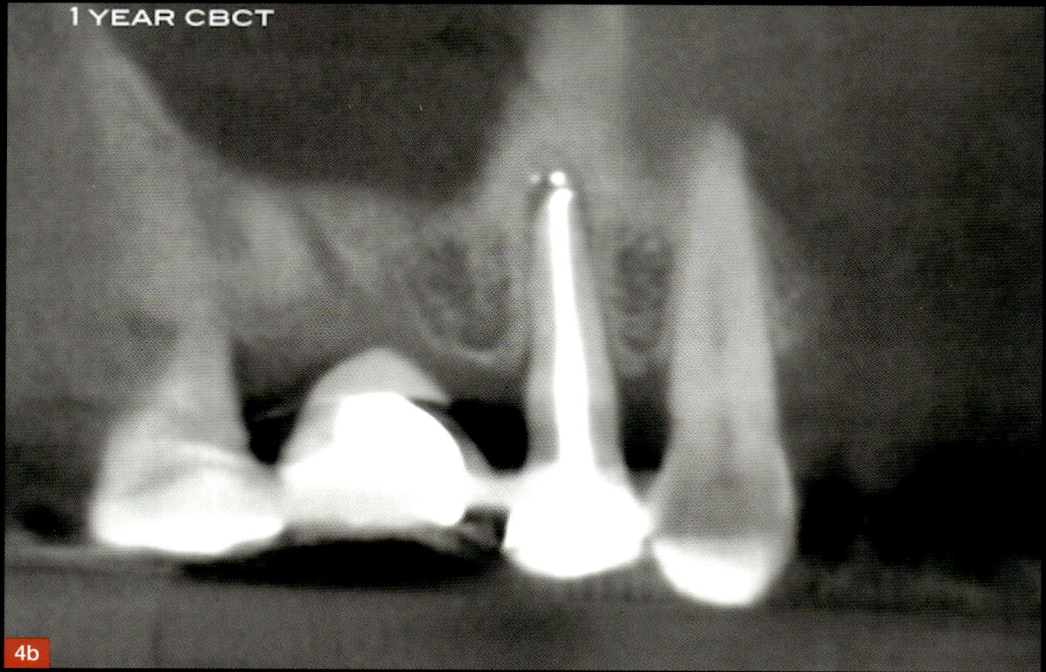

Figure 4a-b: The same image as in figure 3c in two different projections, the resolution of the apical lesion is almost complete.

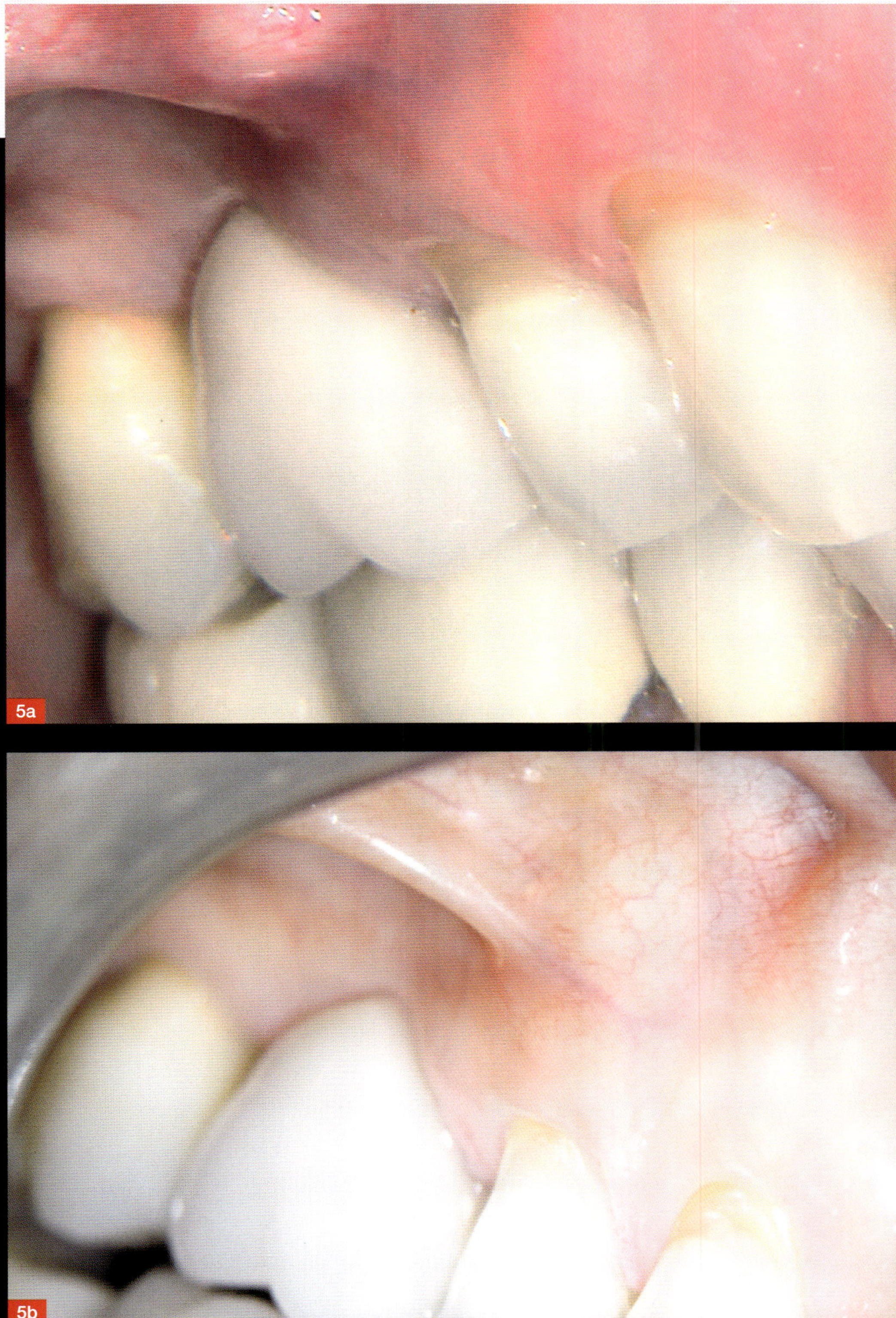

Figure 5a-b: The clinical appearance is comforting; the bridge still has a good functional prognosis.

Intra-canal obstacles: a preliminary analysis

In endodontically treated teeth with endodontic periapical lesions, the root canal content can vary.
The need to remove the infected root canal contents and the materials used previously is a prerequisite for accessing the root apex and performing proper shaping, cleaning, and filling of the root canal system.
A large number of techniques that assist the removal of intra-canal obstacles have been proposed since the end of the last century[24, 25]: burrs[26], specific pliers[27], ultrasonic instruments[28, 29], shaping in the presence of solvents, chelating agents, or sprinklers[30], as well as microtube systems using mechanical or adhesive techniques for the removal of fragments of endodontic instruments embedded in the canal lumen[31], and extractors[32-36].
These procedures are not always risk-free, so it is important for clinicians to consider the available treatment options and correctly inform the patient before beginning treatment.
The difficulty of removing intracanal obstructions is, of course, greater in the posterior areas of the mouth, where the root anatomy is less favorable, and its position compromises overall visibility, despite the fact that appropriate magnification and lighting instruments can be used.
A reasonable use of ultrasound-activated instruments can be useful for the removal of fractured instruments and cemented posts, as highlighted in literature since 1981, because ultrasonic tips or instruments mounted on special hand pieces (endosonic files) can reach greater depths in the root canal system[37].
When removing an obstacle from a root canal must always be considered the anatomical structure of the tooth involved and the surrounding tissues in mind.
Excessive removal of the dentin component when removing an obstacle will complicate the restorative aspect and will worsen the prognosis of the tooth.
It should be remembered that a straight access to the obstacle is essential in order to facilitate maximum visibility of the object: for this reason visibility is reduced when access is limited (for example, in curved and narrow canals).
The use of the surgical microscope is essential for obtaining a direct view and better illumination of the work area, and therefore certain cases will be unmanageable if this instrument is not available (Fig. 3.36). Obviously, the

Table 3.3 **CLINICAL REASONS THAT DETERMINE THE FORMATION OF INTRA-CANAL OBSTACLES**

CAUSE	CONSEQUENCES
Inadequate cavity access	Possible deviations in the path of the instruments inserted inside the root canal can result in the development of caps, false pathways, and fractures of the root canal instruments.
Insufficient preparation of the coronal portion of the canal	If the coronal portion of the canal is inadequately prepared, coronal interference can force mechanical instruments to work in a decentralized position, thus increasing the risk of fractures, canal obstruction, steps, and false pathways.
Insufficient use of irrigators	The mechanical tools currently used have excellent cutting capabilities and tend to displace the debris they produce. Insufficient irrigation can lead to the packing of organic material residues, gutta-percha, and sealer located inside the root canal. This will, in turn, facilitate the formation of caps and obstructions.
The use of instruments that are inflexible and too large in diameter for the canal lumen or instruments with incorrect mechanical properties	Steel and large diameter instruments tend not to adapt to the underlying morphology, thus increasing the risk of step formation. Excessive pressure in the apical direction exerted during the use of mechanical instruments can also facilitate the formation of steps when the tip of the instrument engages against the canal wall.

Box 3.2 **SILVER CONES**

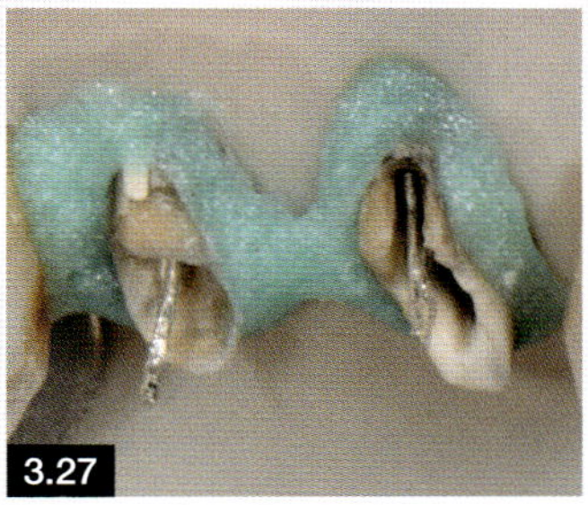
3.27

Although they have not been used for many years, silver cones are sometimes found inside root canals to be retreated are often eroded by electrolytic phenomena and are very fragile. However, and as demonstrated by clinicians who have documented the underlying methodology, great caution is needed when removing them. Ultrasonic sources are not always indicated, but they can be useful for releasing the silver cone from the surrounding filling material or endodontic sealer. When approached with caution, the process of removing a silver cone from a root canal is a fairly simple operation, and allows for subsequent effective endodontic shaping, as demonstrated by the case shown here. This is because the size of the cones rarely matches the actual size of the canal.

Fig. 3.27: Protruding silver cones in two premolars.

Fig. 3.28: Extracting the silver cones is the best solution.

Fig. 3.29: Detail of the plier tip.

Fig. 3.30: Utilizing the drop hammer may be advantageous.

Fig. 3.31: A detail of the grasp area.

Fig. 3.32a-b: The removed cones.

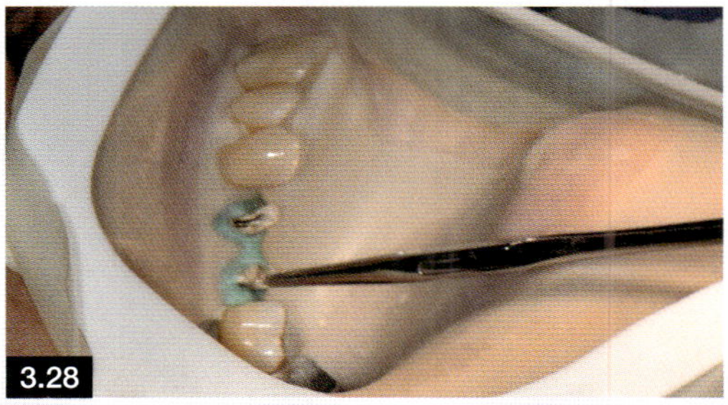
3.28

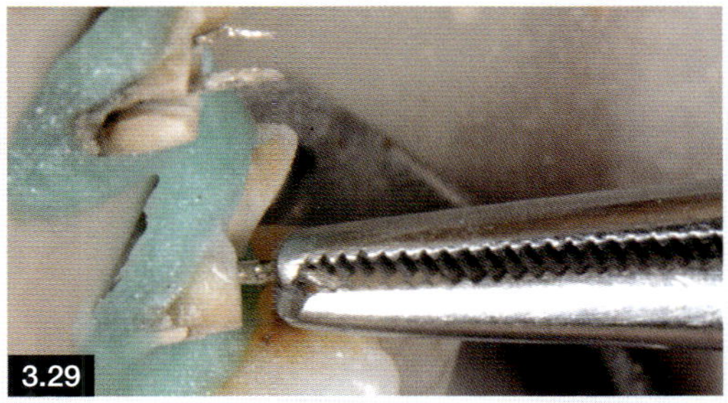
3.29

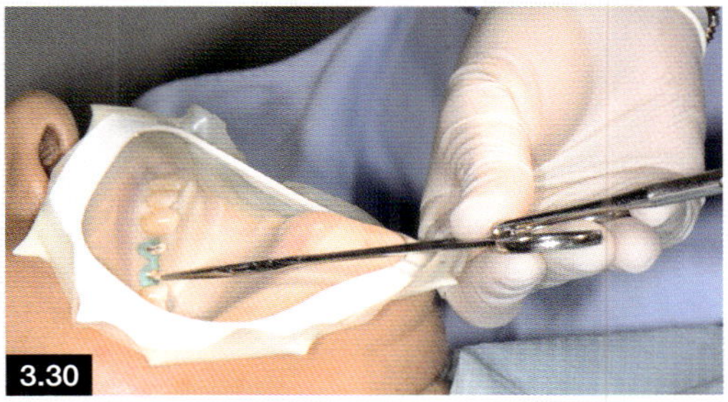
3.30

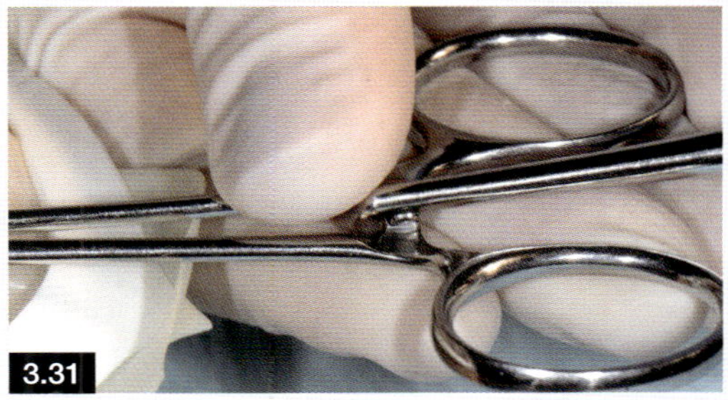
3.31

Fig. 3.33: The presence of a long silver cone and an apical lesion propends for retreatment.

Fig. 3.34: The empty canal.

Fig. 3.35: Endodontic space filling.

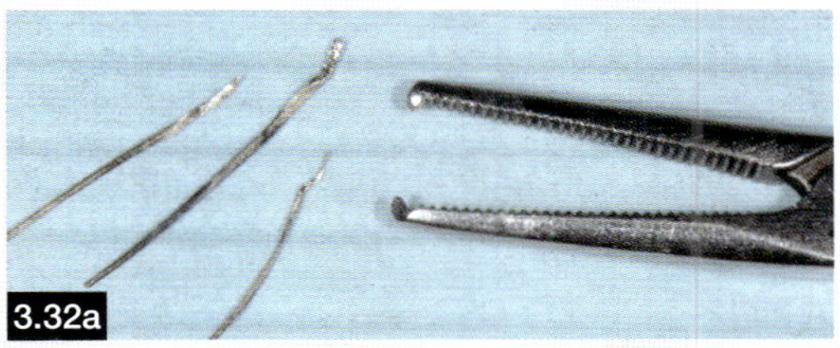
3.32a

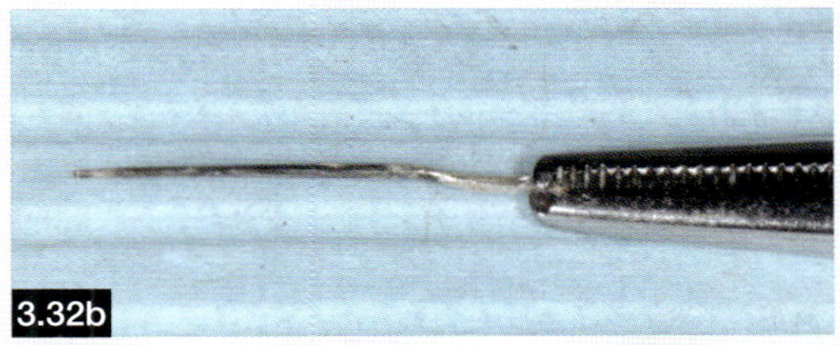
3.32b

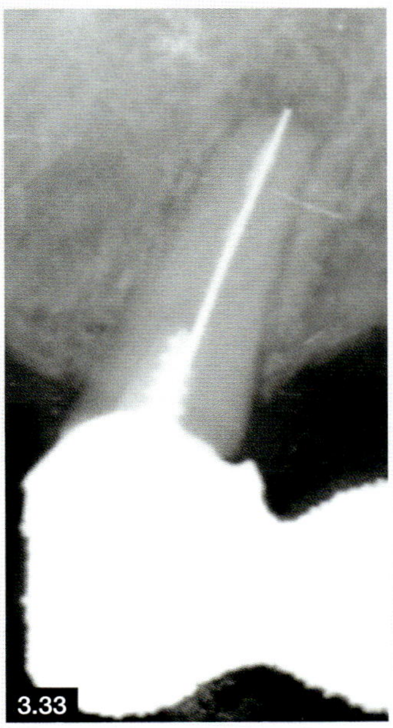
3.33

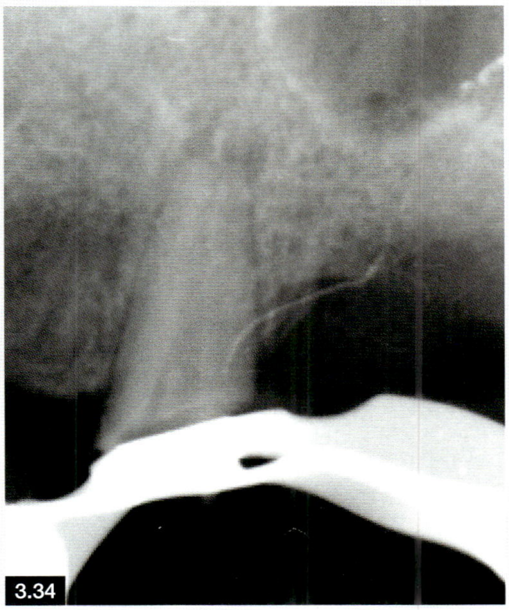
3.34

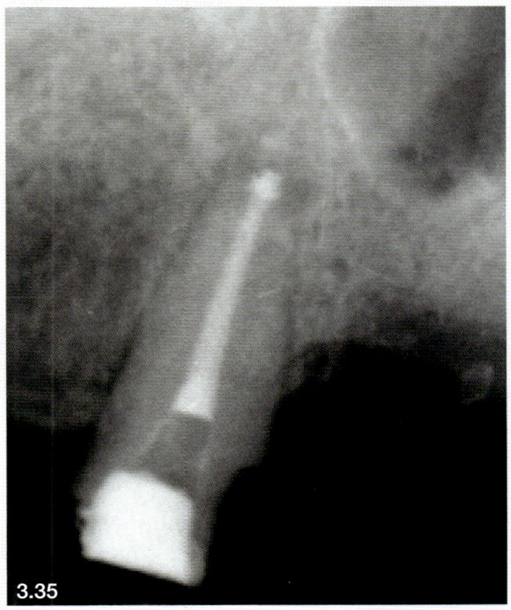
3.35

CASE REPORT 5

Silver cone removal: a challenge in retreatment procedures

Silver cone removal is a key point in retreatment cases; although less common than in the past, this type of filling material always represents a challenge and a concern for the endodontists. In this case, a patient with a lower molar, restored with amalgam filling build up under a crown was referred to the specialist for retreatment.

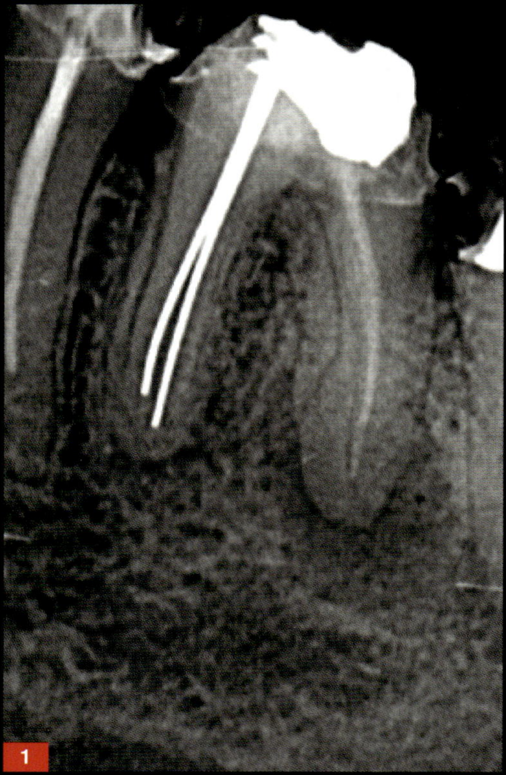

1

Fig. 1: Peri-apical x-ray showing root canal filling performed using silver cones, with chronic apical periodontitis on both the mesial and distal roots.

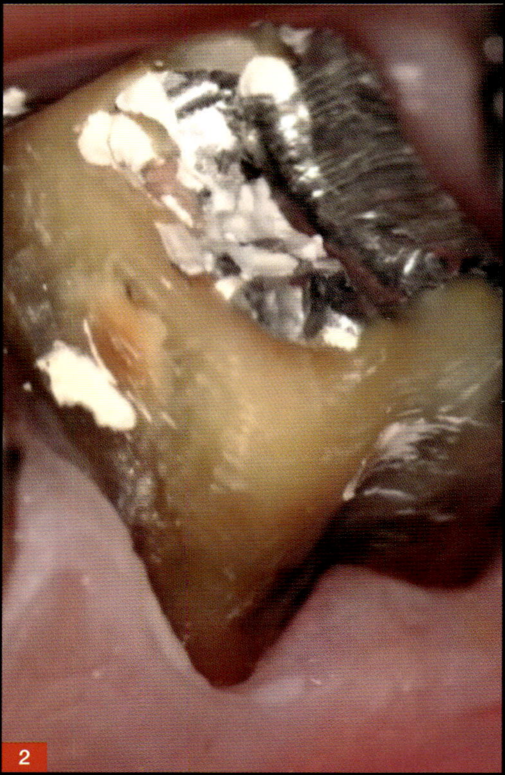

2

Figure 2: The tooth was asymptomatic to percussion. The mesial canals have been filled using silver cones embedded in the amalgam restoration with two silver cones reaching the amalgam in the access cavity.

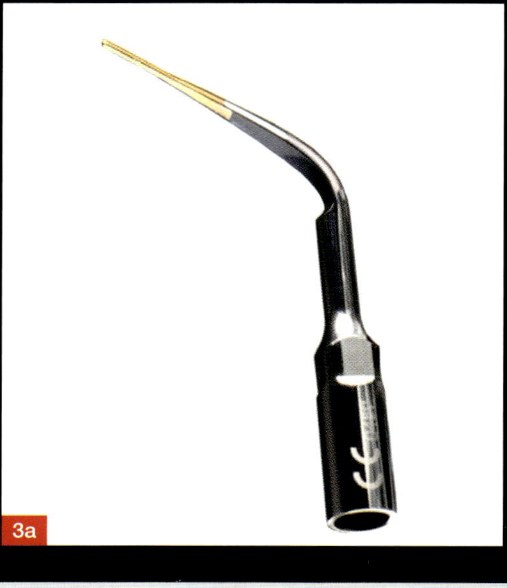

3a

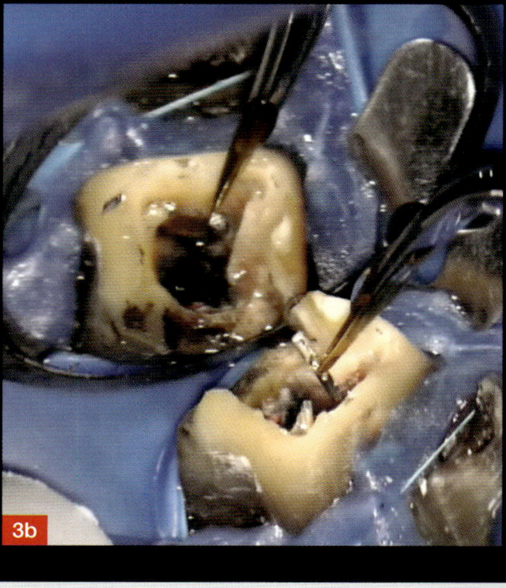

3b

Fig. 3a-b: After rubber dam placement on teeth 35-36, the amalgam was removed taking care not to touch the silver cones. The access cavity was cleaned to make space around the tip of the silver cones.
It is essential not to cut the protruding part of the cones as this would make it impossible to grasp them, making their removal more difficult.
An ultrasonic tip was used to remove the silver cones in the mesial root.

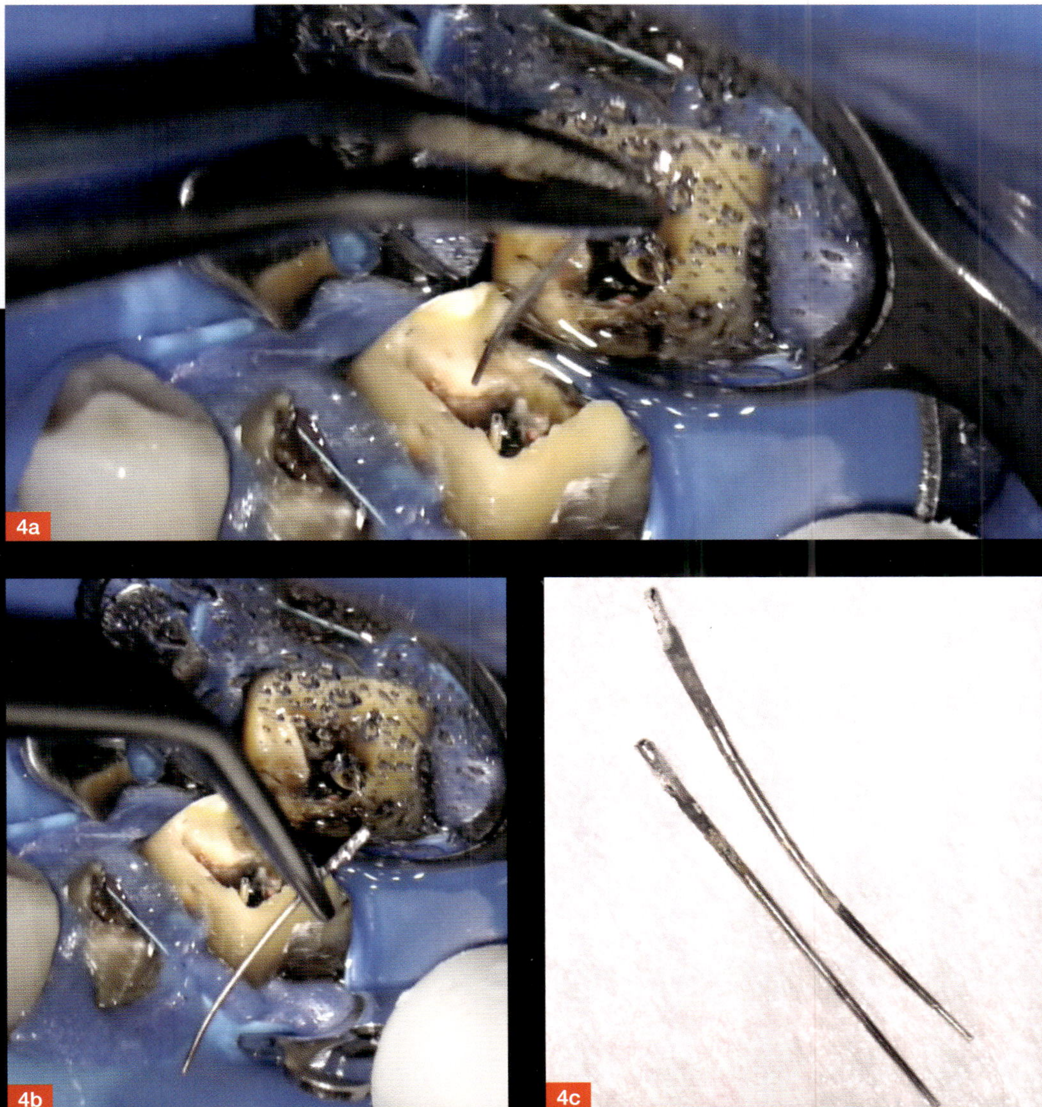

Fig. 4a-c: A series of lateral ultrasonic strokes were performed under water irrigation with correct occlusal direction, thus creating groves in the soft silver alloy. Each of the silver ones was gradually removed from the canal.

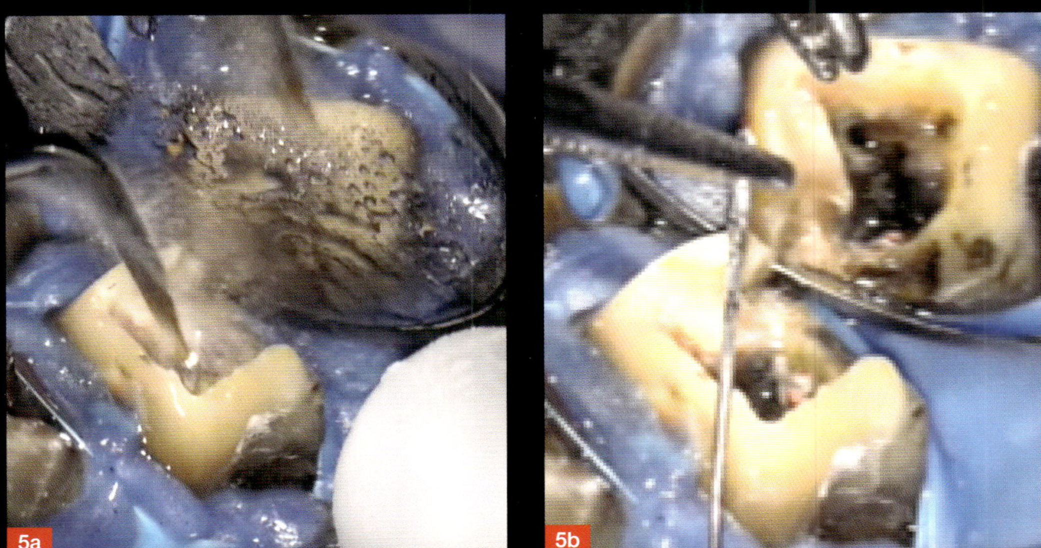

Fig 5a-b: The previously described operative sequence was utilized to remove the other silver cone.

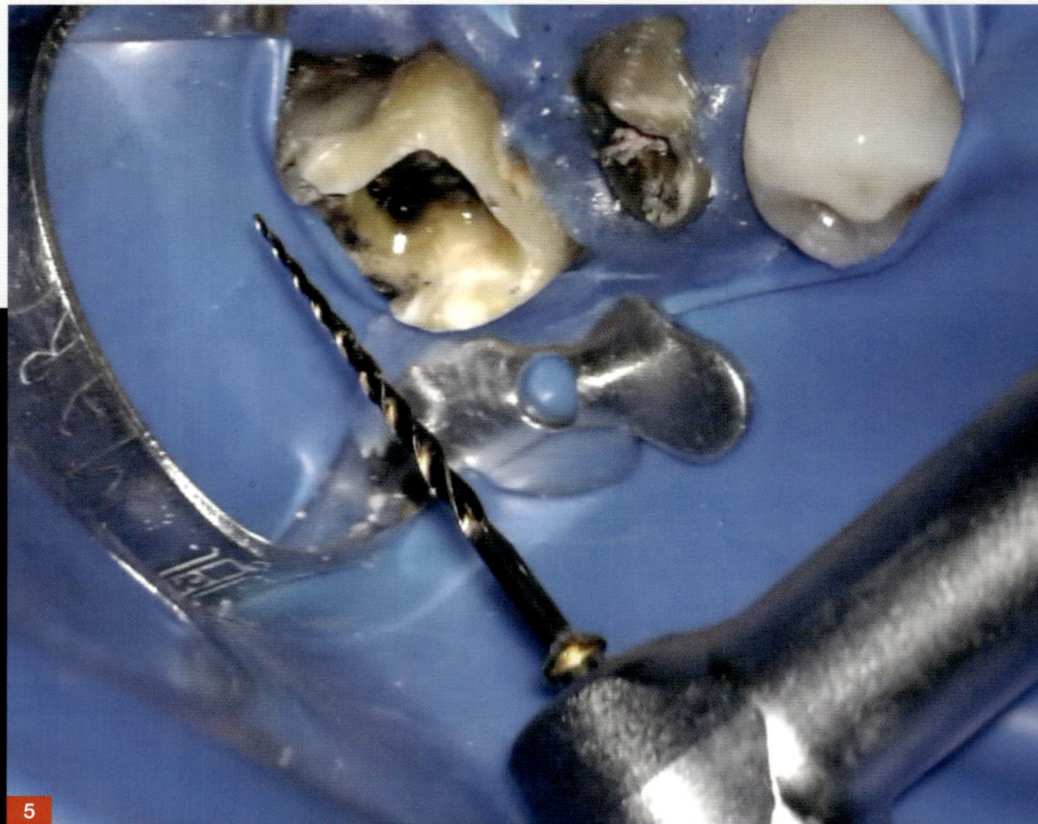

5

Fig. 5: To complete the root canal treatment, all three canals were pre-flared with appropriate NiTi rotating instruments (One Flare, Micro Mega), and retreated using xylol solvent to dissolve the old filling.

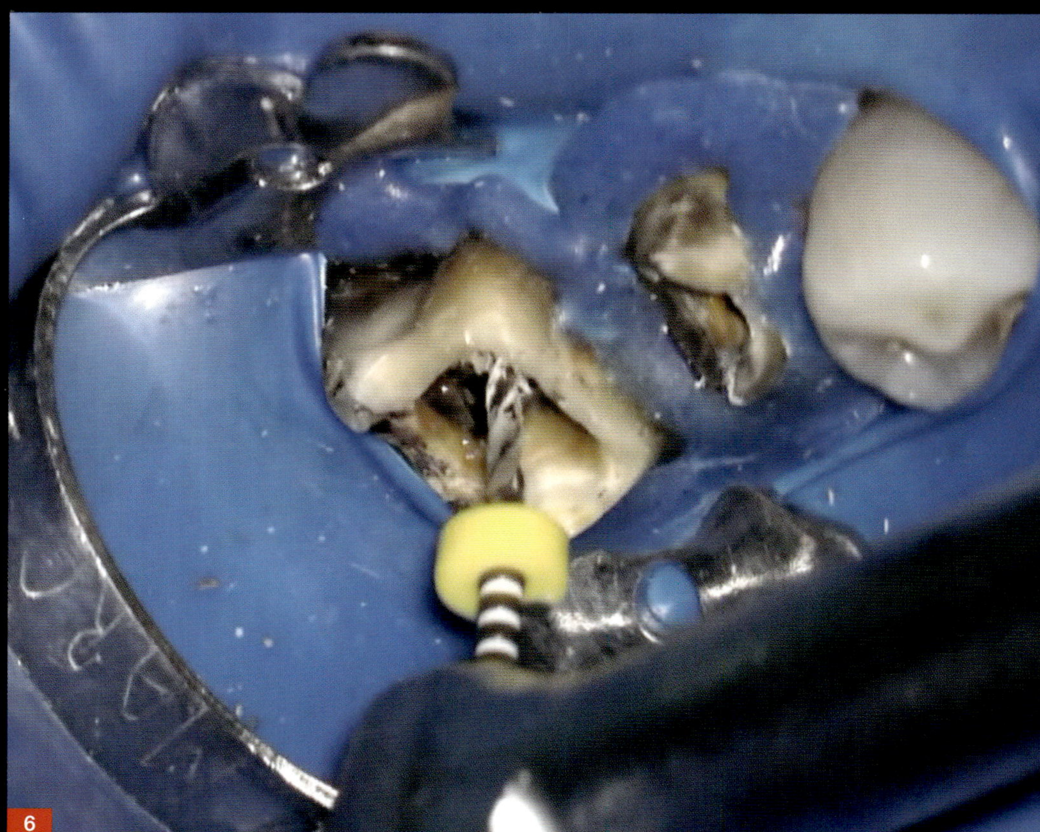

6

Fig. 6: After reaching the working length and achieving the glide path, the root canals were shaped with other NiTi instruments (Protaper Gold F1, Maileffer Dentsply, SUI).

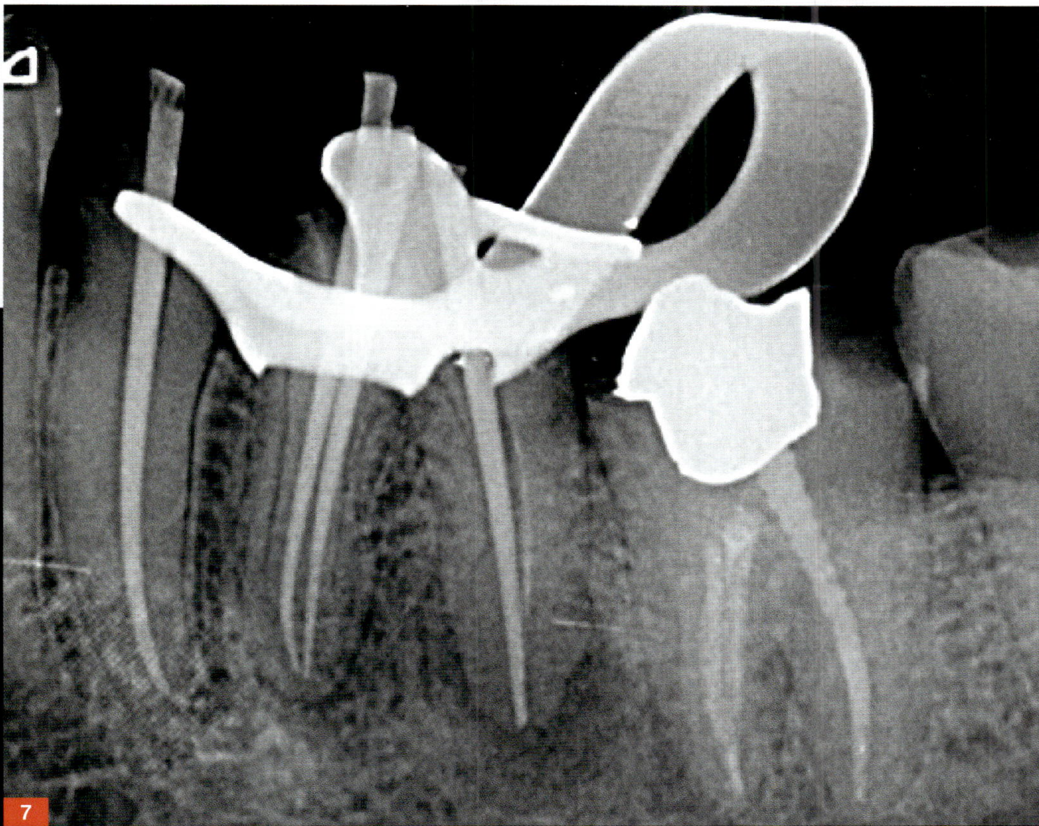

7

Figure 7: Copious sodium hypochlorite irrigation under sonic activation with dedicate device (EndoActivator, Dentsply) was performed to achieve optimal cleaning; the gutta-percha cone test.

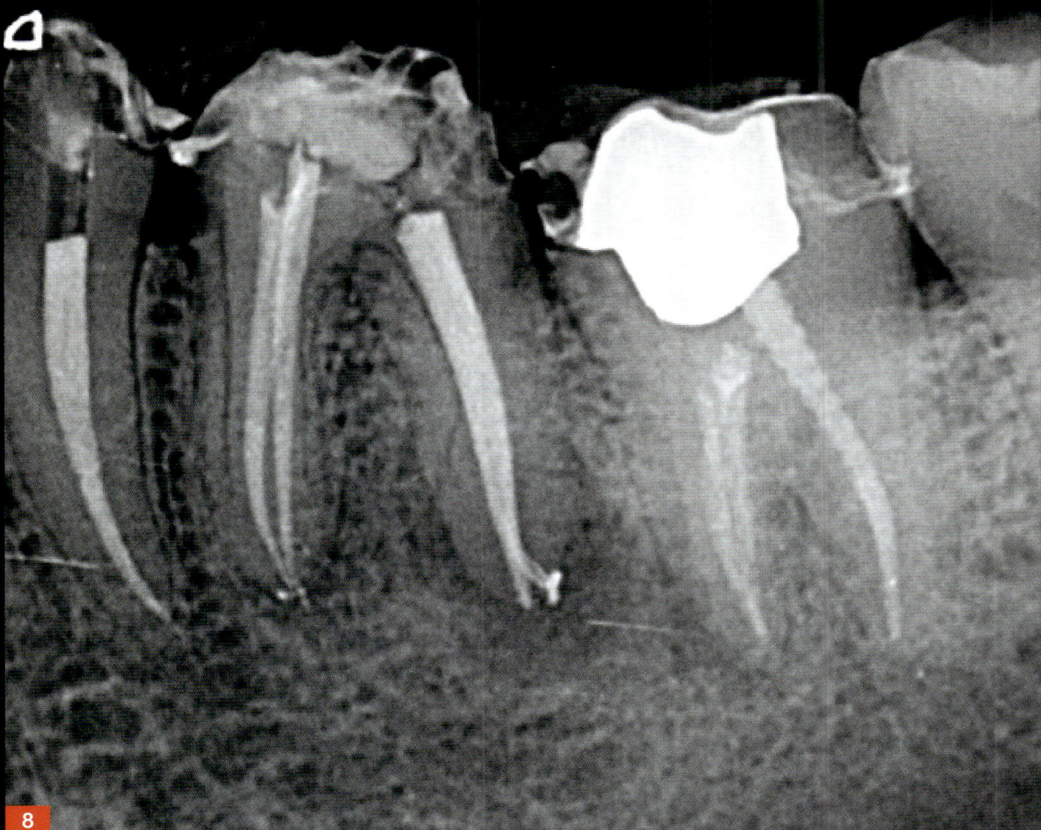

8

Figure 8: Warm vertical condensation was utilized to obtain a complete obturation of the whole root canal system.

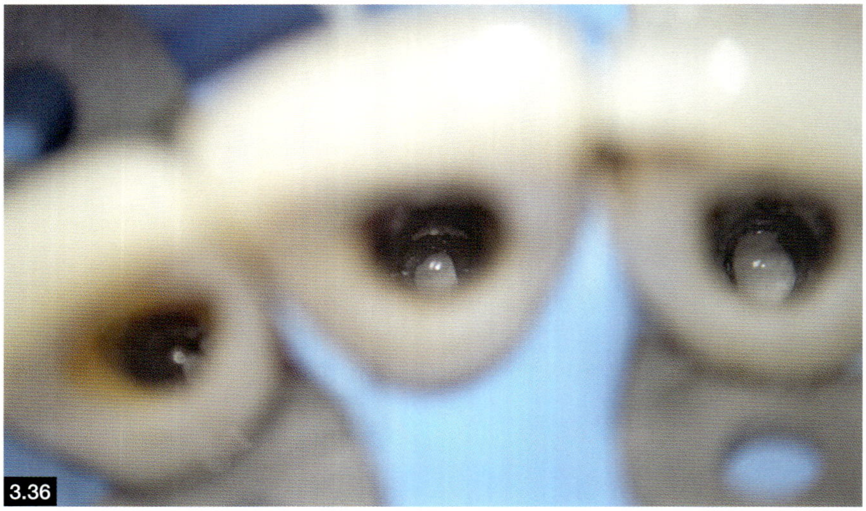

Fig. 3.36: The viewy with the operating microscope allows the best possible interpretation of the canal route.

Tab. 3.4 **LIST OF INTRACANAL MATERIALS FOR USE IN RETREATMENTS**
• FILLING MATERIALS
Gutta-percha
Sealers
Preheated gutta-percha carrier system
Silver cones
• ENDODONTIC POSTS
• FRACTURED INSTRUMENTS

operator's skills and experience play a critical role in the success and safety of removing these obstacles. A perfect use of these techniques must be acquired before clinical use[38], involving a sufficiently long, yet necessary, learning curve to cope with and resolve endodontics retreatment procedures in the best possible way.

Removal of endodontic posts

Teeth that have lost a significant amount of tissue are often reconstructed with the help of metal alloy or fiber posts, in order to improve the resistance of the tooth-restoration unit to mechanical loading. When dealing with a tooth retreatment, it is important to understand what type of endodontic retention is required for removal and its relationship with the residual tooth structure. This can be achieved by taking one or more endodontic radiographs and, if necessary, in order performing three-dimensional radiographic examinations such as CBCT, to define the nature, size, and structure of the post, as well as the proportions between the post and the root. According to Castrisos and Abbott,[39] the indispensable parameters to consider to successfully remove a post are the following:

- Type, diameter and length of the post[40]
- Root length and diameter
- Residual coronal and root structure
- Type of sealer used ("classic" sealers, such as zinc oxide-phosphate and epoxy resins, are easier to remove than composite sealers)[41]

Other factors to be considered in case assessment involve the type of reconstruction needed, the interocclusal space, and the position of the post in relation to the occlusal surface and the canal orifice.
Indeed, in the latter case, the more posterior a post is, the more complex its removal will be, especially in patients with reduced mouth opening.
Thanks to this initial analysis in the preoperative phase, it will be possible to understand whether it is advisable to proceed with the retreatment process and remove the coronal and intraradicular obstacles or whether it is preferable to choose a surgical approach, a subject that we will review in Chapter 8. If a retreatment process is preferable, it is then important to establish the most suitable strategies and tools to be used for the successful removal of the artifact, and the operative skills that are required. This will, in turn, allow for a greater understanding regarding whether and how the post can be removed and what risks are associated with the treatment (such as root fractures).
During the diagnostic phase, it is also important to observe the clinical signs of periodontal impairment or paramarginal fistulae in teeth restored with posts. In these cases, it is legitimate to suspect a root fracture rather than a true endodontic lesion.
Hence, it is imperative to develop a precise

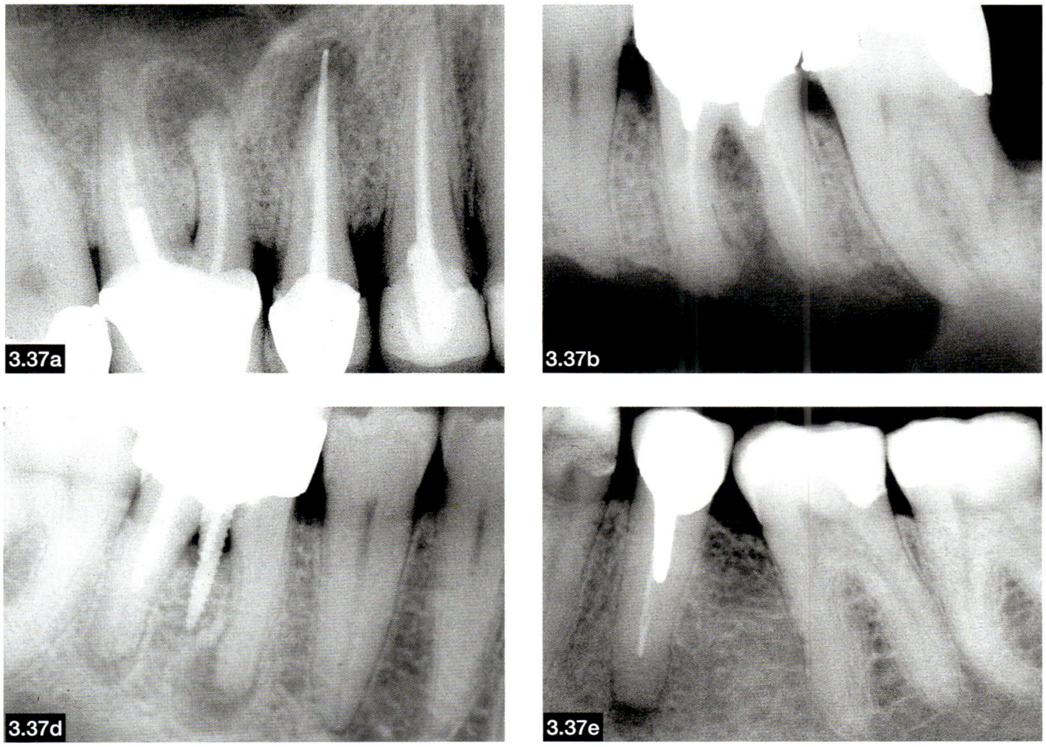

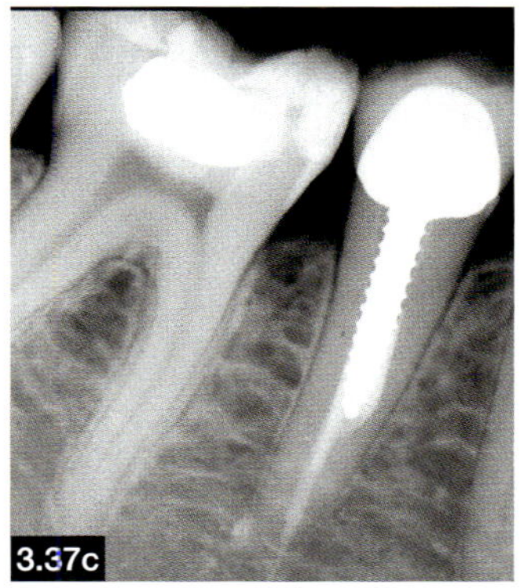

Fig. 3.37a-e: Various types of reconstructions can be identified with the aid of endodontic posts in teeth in which endodontic treatments have failed. However, failure does not depend on the presence of the post, but on its positioning, which can cause a perforation of the floor (Fig. 3.37d) or create a false path (Fig. 3.37c).

Table 3.5 **TYPES OF POSTS AND MEANS OF REMOVAL**

Post category	Post types	Shape	Tools to be used for removal	Procedures
Metallic screwed	Threaded in titanium, steel or alloy, not mobile	Cylindrical/ tapered	Ultrasound and pliers	Isolation of the post head from the retreatment material. Application of ultrasonic vibration. Unscrewing action that often exerts itself even during ultrasonic application.
	Cast artifacts (gold or other precious and non-precious alloys)	Anatomical	Ultrasound and/or specific post extraction tools	Isolation of the post head from the retreatment material. Application of ultrasonic vibration. Application of mechanical post-removal systems.
Cemented metal	Pre-formed (steel, titanium or other non-noble alloys)	Cylindrical/ tapered	Ultrasound and/ or dedicated post-extraction tools	Isolation of the post head from the reconstruction material. Application of ultrasonic vibration to the post head and between the posts and the sealer. Application of mechanical post-extraction systems. This process is usually simpler because of the poor congruence between the canal and the post.
Fiber	Glass fibers or carbon immersed in resinous matrices	Cylindrical/ tapered	Ultrasound and steel or tungsten carbide milling burs	The ultrasonic tips positioned in the center of the fiber post tend to disintegrate it. The only real difficulty regards the underlying visibility because fiber posts (except carbon posts, which are black) do not differ significantly in color from the resin and the surrounding dentin.
Ceramic		Tapered	Ultrasound and diamond burrs	Removal is very complicated. Diamond burrs can play a role in post erosion, whereas ultrasound can be used on the part attached to the resin sealer.

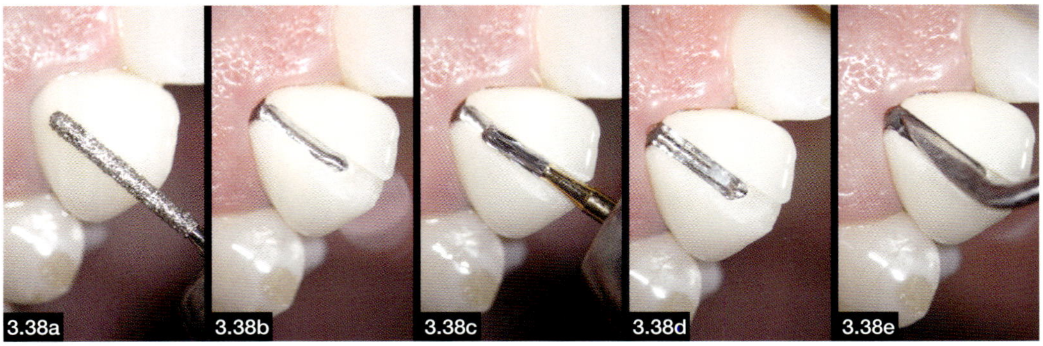

Fig. 3.38a-e: A crown anchored to the root by means of a post must be removed in order to perform a retreatment process. Consequently, the ceramic coating is removed with a diamond bur and the metal part with a tungsten carbide bur.
Once a vestibular groove has been created, a flat-headed instrument is inserted to displace the cemented crown.

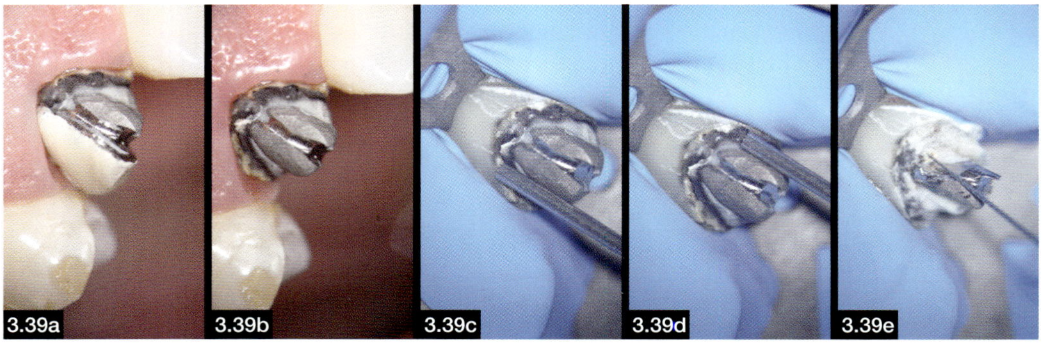

Fig. 3.39a-e: Once the post has been isolated, the dentin is treated with ultrasonic instruments.

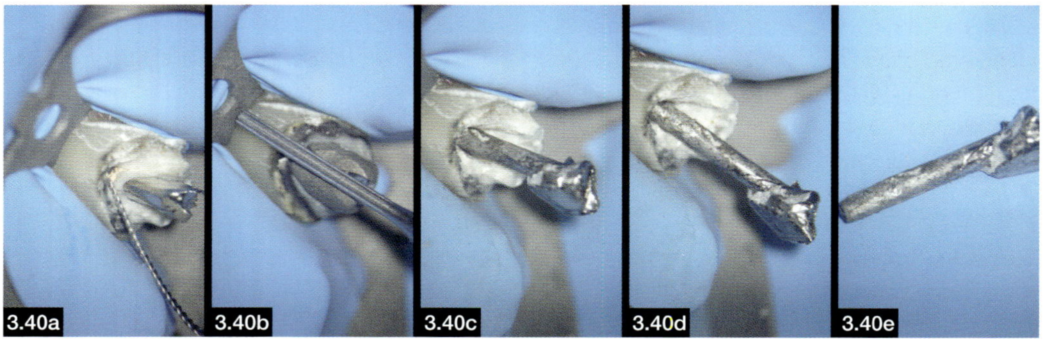

Fig. 3.40a-e: Further steps using ultrasound to mobilize the post. Note how ultrasonic files are used to remove the sealer and how ultrasonic tips mobilize the post.

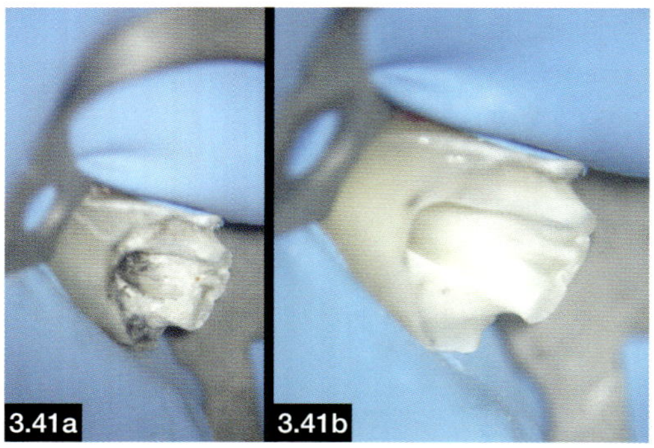

Fig. 3.41a-b: The post is removed.

and strategic plan that cannot be obtained with x-ray images alone, especially if two-dimensional.
The radiographic examination can provide us with a series of information regarding the type of post, its insertion depth, and the degree of contact with the canal walls, thus allowing clinicians to assess the relationship between the size of the post and the volume of the residual root.
This information can obtained with examinations such as CBCT[42-44].
It is fundamental for clinicians to have a knowledge and an understanding of the features of the various posts that are available on today's market, because the process of removing a post may vary according to the type of post to be removed. Table 3.5 summarizes the different types of post available. The sealer used to secure the post to the dentin structure may itself influence the post-extraction process.
In the past, the most widely used sealers were zinc oxide-phosphate, polycarboxylic sealer, glass ionomer sealers, and epoxy resins.
Today, with the growing popularity of adhesive composite materials, posts can get so close

to the root canal walls that their successful elimination can be challenging. The use of ultrasonic tips, whose vibration is useful for creating micro-cracks in the bonding material, can render post removal as a significantly easier process. Indeed, the force required to remove a cemented post once it has been treated with an ultrasonic tip, is about 25% lower than the force required in the absence of this kind of tip. The time required for this to occur can vary significantly, whereas cooling must be performed simultaneously, and must be consistent with the needs and the size of the post[45].

In other circumstances, the post may be poorly attached to the walls and, therefore, the vibration alone is able to remove it. Sometimes, it is useful to turn the ultrasonic tip around the head of the post so as to distribute the vibrations along all the attached surfaces.

In cases where the size of the post and the root allow, the mechanical action of the tip in the area of the interface between the post and the dentin facilitates the creation of an area of lower strength that can be exploited in the removal process.

Screwed metal posts

Screwed metal posts are very common and are often inserted a few millimeters into the endodontic space, making them easier to remove. Unscrewing them is the best choice. However, to perform this maneuver, the head must be freed from the restoration material retaining the post. When posts are screwed into the root canal, they should be removed counterclockwise. Ultrasound also favors the turning action; once most of the coronal part has been freed, it is possible to connect a suitable grasping tool to this portion to achieve the rotation required to remove the post from the endodontium. In these cases – given the poor congruence in the coronal areas between the post, which is usually narrower, and the canal lumen – the use of special ultrasonic inserts will be sufficient to remove the sealer from the dentin wall in the coronal area of the post space.

The most suitable instruments for this operating phase are endodontic files (K-File 15-20-25-30) mounted on special inserts that are, in turn, connected to ultrasonic handpieces. In addition, these tips can also allow clinicians to work deeper in the root canal between the post and the fixation sealer. This movement, when combined with the action exerted by ultrasonic vibrations, helps to fracture the sealer towards the apical part of the post[46].

The hardness of the sealers is the only constraint to complete the removal. However, extractors could be the first option, provided the head of the post allows their use.

It is recommended to cool the ultrasonic tip with water and spray, otherwise both the hand-piece and the ultrasonic tip may overheat the post, which could, subsequently, transfer this heat to the periodontal ligament.

If, on the other hand, the post is well-adapted to the canal, yet a considerable portion extends outside the canal opening, a hemostatic plier or similar device can be used to transfer ultrasonic energy indirectly to the canal space while simultaneously attempting to extract the post. The

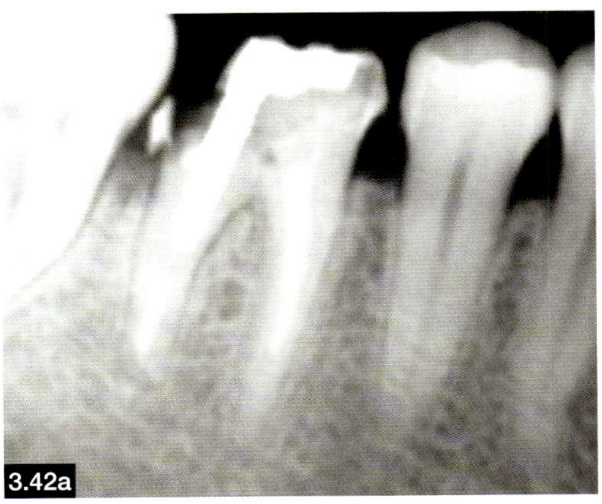

3.42a

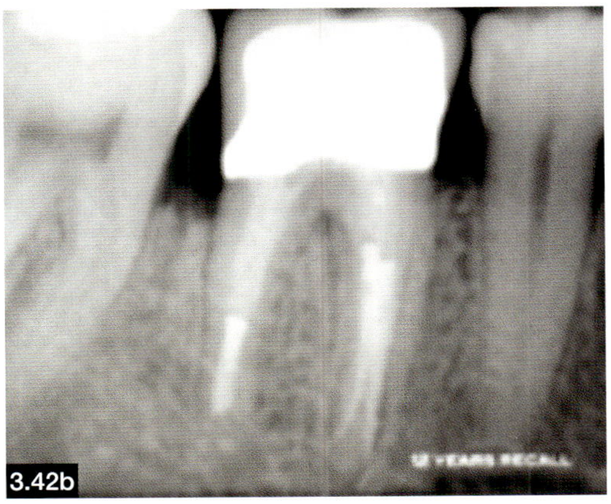

3.42b

Fig. 3.42a: An inferior molar with screwed post in the distal root.

Fig. 3.42b: The 12-year follow-up confirms the full resolution of the case.

clinician's assistant can use the ultrasonic tips directly on the hemostatic plier while the operator attempts to move and displace the post (four-handed technique) with small movements. However, when deciding to use this technique, the risk of dentinal crack formation on the root must be considered.
If the post its snugly in the the canal for an adequate length and diameter, and pliers are unable to grasp the (inaccessible) coronal part of the post, the effect of ultrasonic vibrations on the post alone may be limited. Consequently, the clinician should consider alternative treatments such as the use of extractors and dedicated burs to obtain post erosion. Tungsten carbide burs are particularly well suited to separating part of the post, as outlined at the beginning of the chapter.

Metal abutment posts

Cast metal posts usually fit snugly against the canal walls, and extend deep into the canal. In these cases, the clinician must assess the appropriateness and applicability of orthograde retreatment over the surgical option, because the root may be fractured or become very fragile while attempting to remove a cast post. In cases where the removal of the metal cast posts is straightforward, dedicated US-activated tips or extractors seem to be the most suitable tools for the task. The post removal kit (PRS/Post Removal System or Gonon) contains a plier, a bur for preparing the head of the post, five core burs of various internal diameters, five mandrels with an internal diameter of between 0.6 and 1.60 mm, a bar for exerting a higher torque, and an assortment of rubber shock-absorber discs of various diameters, to protect the tooth against the load generated by the extraction forces. Before using these mechanical extraction systems, it is necessary to completely isolate the head of the post inside the pulp chamber, and have direct access to and perfect visibility of the occlusal portion of the canal access. Once the appropriate core bur tool is applied to the head of the post, the clinician can commence the removal operation. A rubber disc is fitted on the mandrel to reduce traction so that the occlusal loads are evenly distributed over the tooth's contact surface.
By pushing the mandrel firmly against the post, the clinician can then start screwing it inwards by turning it counterclockwise. The strong apical thrust and the small counterclockwise rotation of a quarter turn will cause the mandrel to descend onto the head of the post, where it will tighten firmly and securely. The mandrel must be screwed into the head of the post by at least 1 mm, and if possible by 2-3 mm, taking care not to strip the thread.
Once the mandrel is firmly screwed onto the post, it is possible to place the plier correctly on the mandrel.
Holding the tool firmly with one hand, the other hand tightens the screw at the other end of the plier.

Fig. 3.43: a) Detail of a post extracted using a dedicated system; (b) an example of an instrument for endodontic post extraction (Gonon).

Fig. 3.44: a) Post in the root canal suitably cored for tapping with the Gonon system; b) the canal once the post has been removed.

Fig. 3.45: a) The x-ray view at the start of the case;
b) the x-ray of the free canal (note the non-effective amalgam seal);
c) root canal filling;
d) functional outcome some time later.

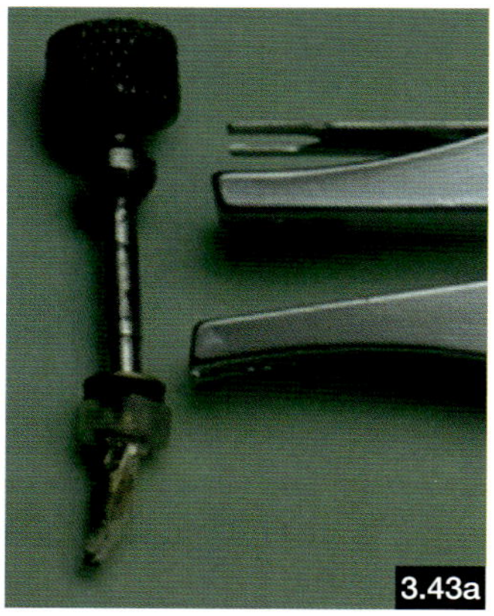
3.43a

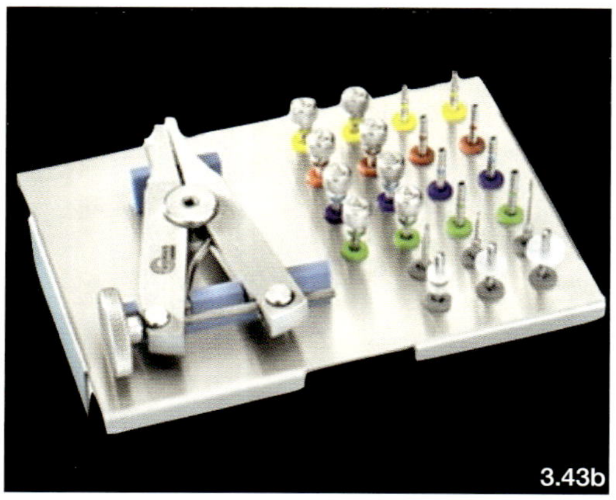
3.43b

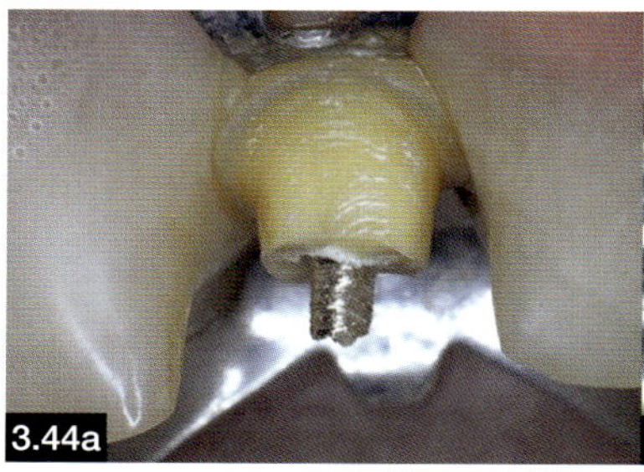
3.44a

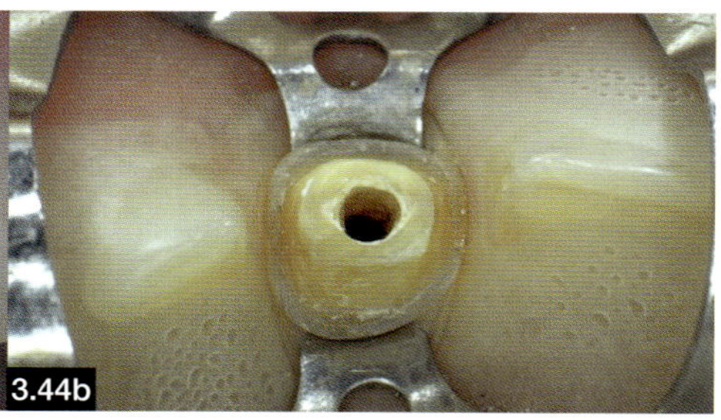
3.44b

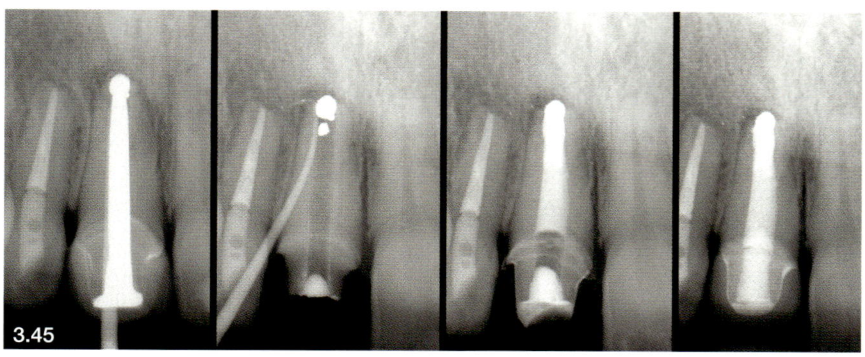
3.45

In this way, as the plier beaks begin to open, the pressure on the other end increases. At this stage, the clinician must make sure that the rubber disc is protecting the tooth correctly. If difficulties are encountered turning the screw at the end of the plier, the clinician should wait for a few seconds before continuing and, if necessary, place the ultrasonic-activated CPR 1 on the mandrel as close as possible to the post. On the one hand, this will decrease the post retention in the root and, on the other hand, it will further turn the nut and the screw at the end of the plier.
This combination is an excellent way to remove cast posts from roots. Subsequently, ultrasonic tips can be used to disintegrate the sealer or the fixing composite of the post until the gutta-percha is visible. If the post persists and still remains in the dentin compartment, the pivot bar can be inserted in the mandrel head to increase the leverage, and, at the same time, use the vibrations of the ultrasounds which, by disintegrating the sealer, would make the extraction process easier.

Fiber post

The retreatment of adhesively luted fiber posts in the root canal is one of the major difficulties encountered in endodontic treatment failure that requires the use of ultrasonic tips and adequate magnification[47]. The use of ultrasound to destroy the composite structure of the fiber posts seems to be the optimal method in these cases. The action of the ultrasound breaks down the longitudinal fibers and the resin matrix of the post, so as to entirely scrape it. Aesthetic white posts are more difficult to remove than carbon ones because their color often makes them hard to distinguish from dentin. This can lead to root canal axis loss and iatrogenic errors. During this procedure, it is important to operate in a dry place to ensure a direct view of the ultrasonic tip and the coronal portion of the post. It is also essential to remember to cool the tooth with air and water spray in order to remove the damaged post and dentin residues, and to facilitate a better view. To achieve therapeutic success, it is important to remove all composite materials used in the

Fig. 3.46: The X-ray shows the presence of an abutment post in a central incisor with coronal infiltration.

Fig. 3.47: New apical seal with MTA following removal of the post.

Fig. 3.48a: The coronal seal.

Fig. 3.48b: The functional outcome two years later.

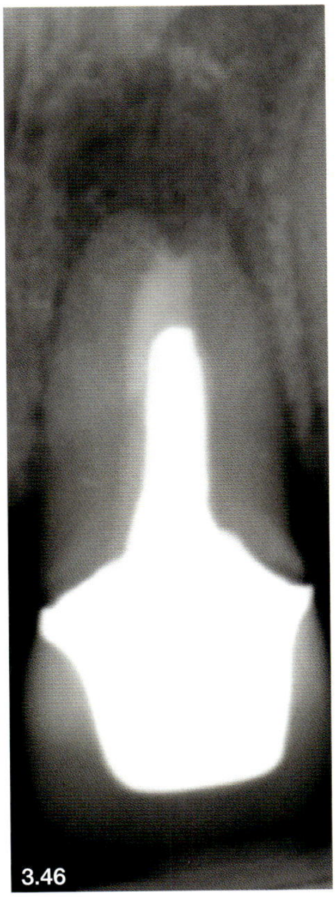
3.46

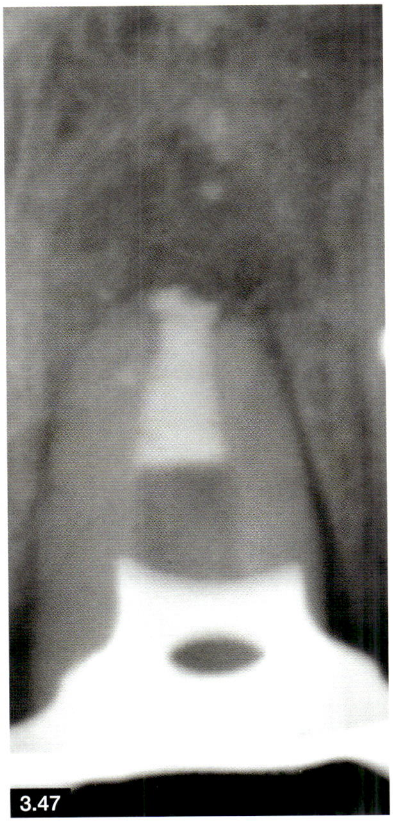
3.47

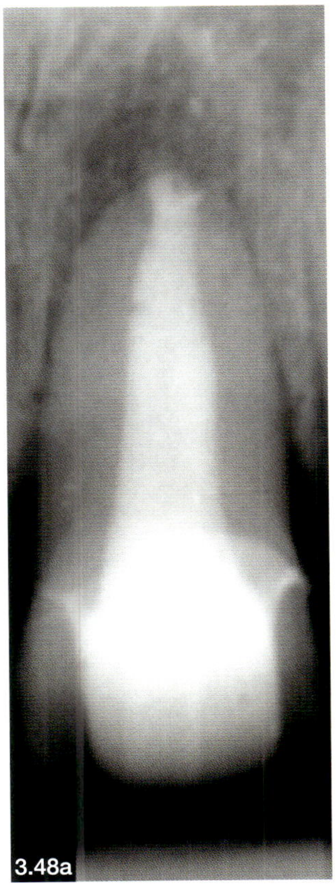
3.48a

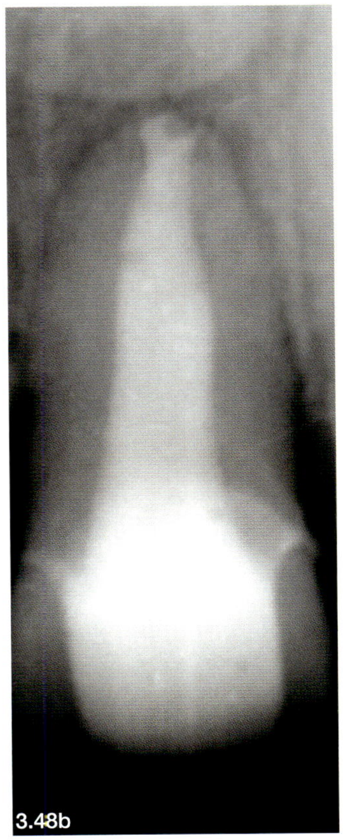
3.48b

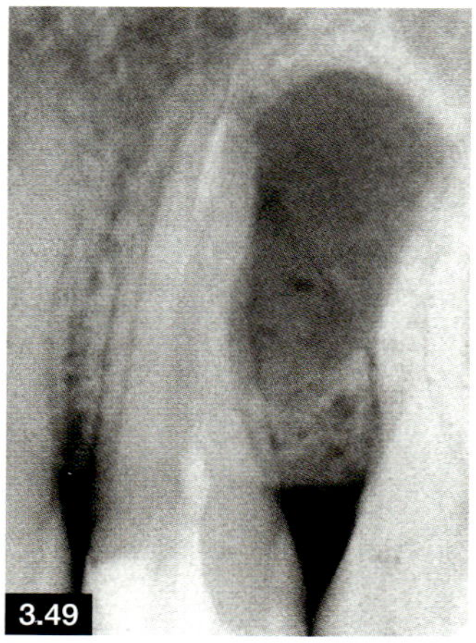
3.49

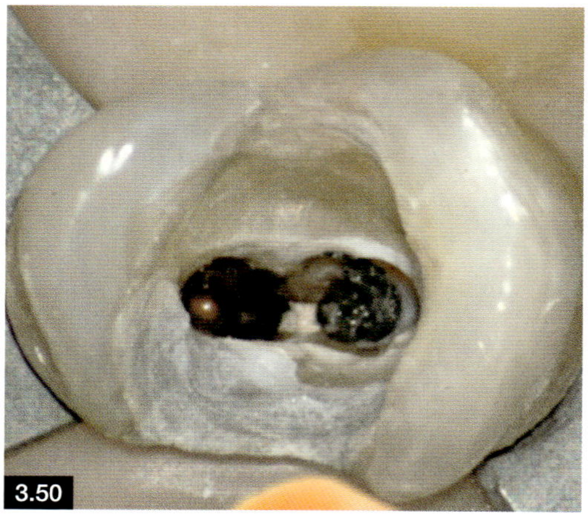
3.50

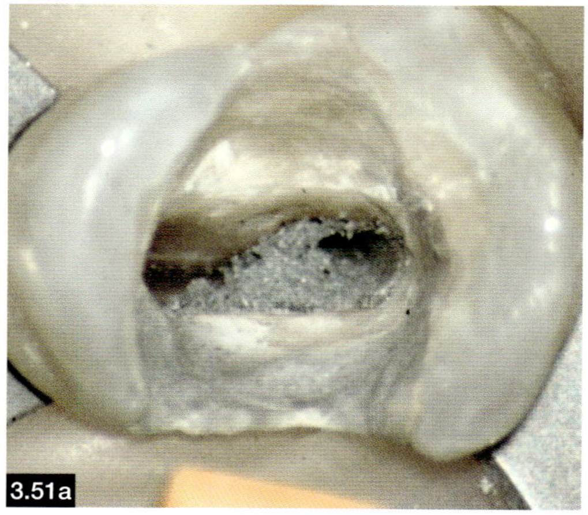
3.51a

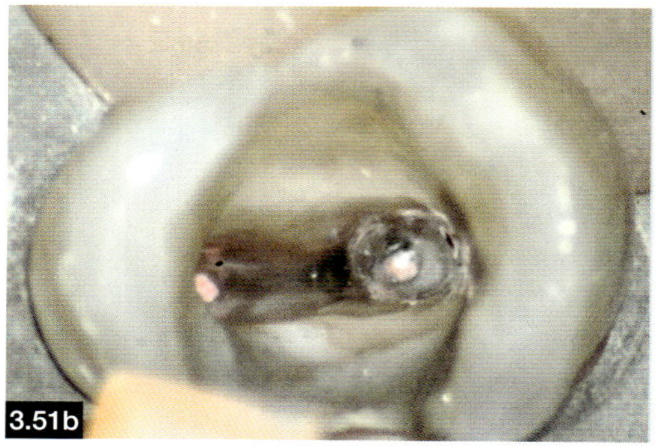
3.51b

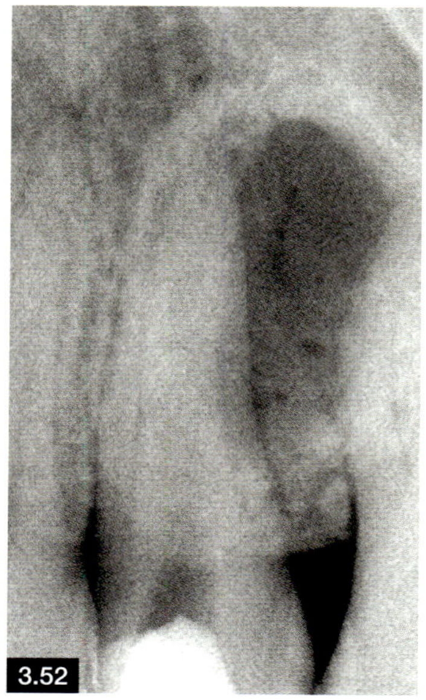
3.52

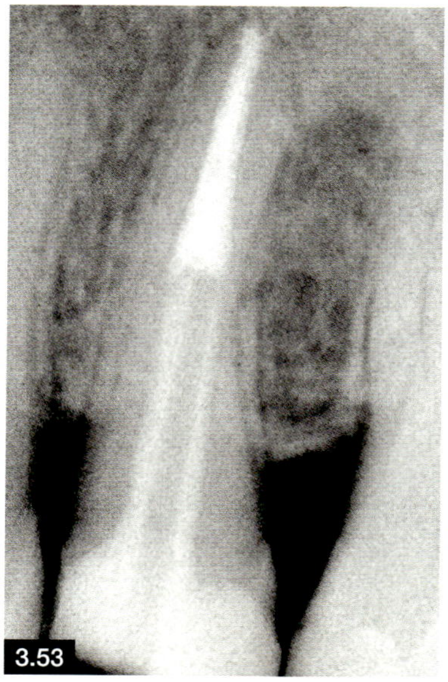
3.53

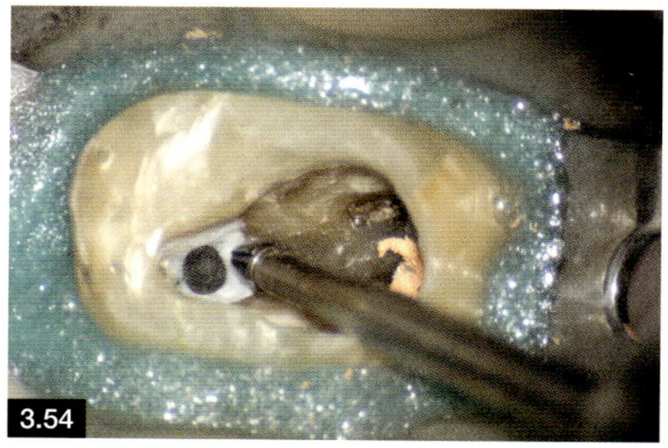
3.54

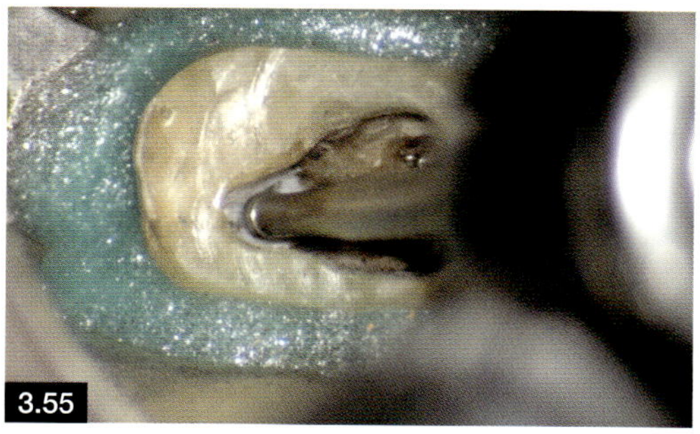
3.55

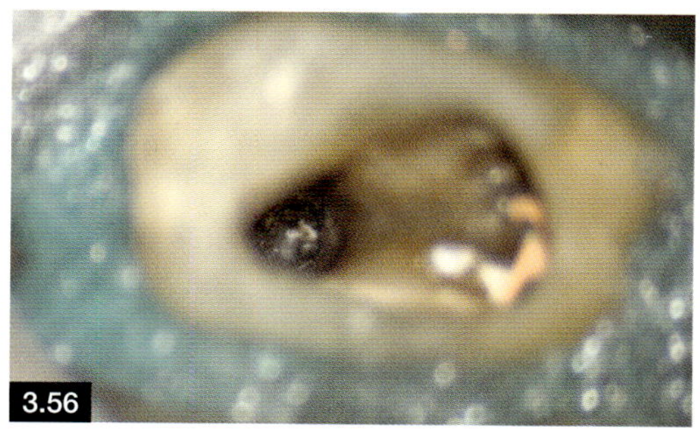
3.56

Fig. 3.49: This premolar presents a lateral lesion, the filling does not appear adequate, and the root canal is also sealed by a fiber post.

Fig. 3.50: The fiber post occludes the vestibular canal, whereas the other post has yet to be shaped.

Fig. 3.51a: The milling burs are used to break the post down to a gray powder that can be easily removed.

Fig. 3.51b: The canal can be easily retreated.

Fig. 3.52: The radiographic image of the canals free from endodontic obstructions.

Fig. 3.53: Follow-up of the case some time later shows the complete resolution of the lateral lesion.

Fig. 3.54: Another case of a fiber endodontic post cemented in the palatal canal.

Fig. 3.55: The triangular bur is ideal for use in cases like this.

Fig. 3.56: The free canal.

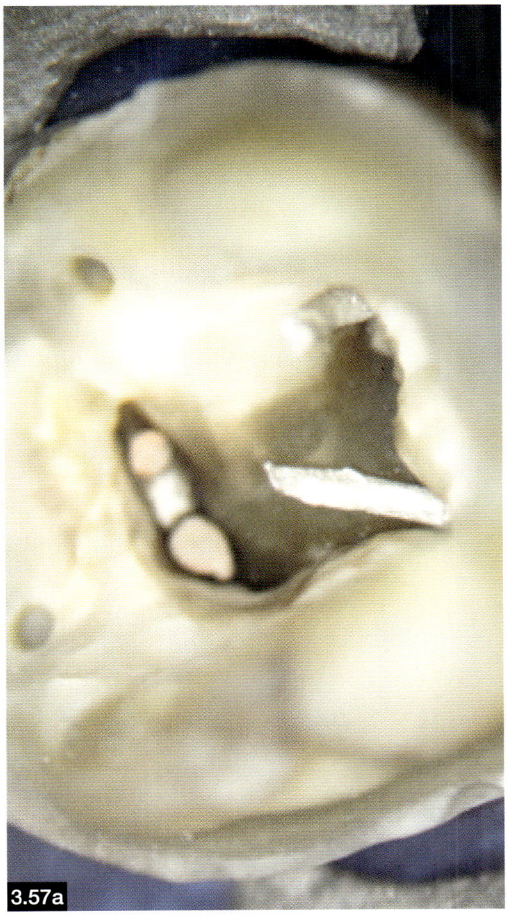
3.57a

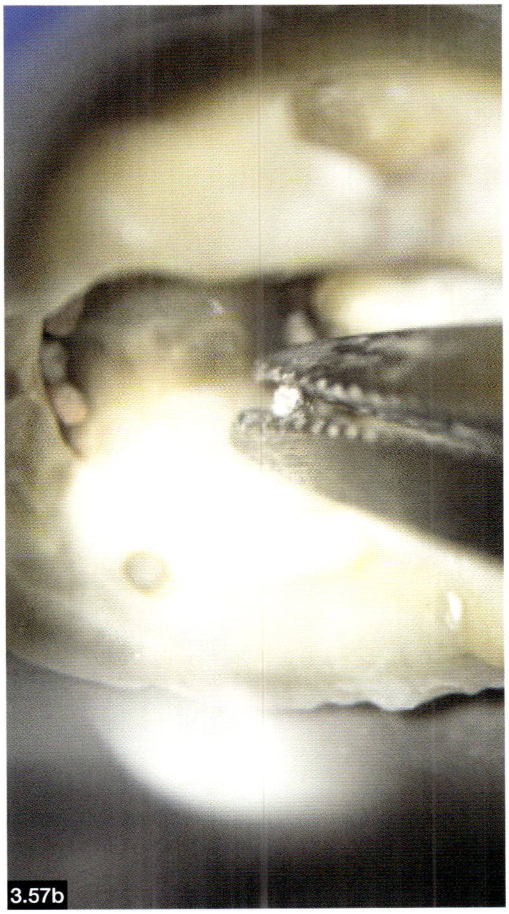
3.57b

Fig. 3.57a-b: Once it has been mobilized and is free in the cavity, a silver cone can be removed simply with pliers.

cementation process. If the adhesive process is performed perfectly, then it is often difficult to distinguish between the composite and the dentin walls. Hence, to remove this material, a magnification system should be used to guide the ultrasonic tip selectively over the remaining composite attached to the dentin. Selective removal of the composite is facilitated by the dark marks left by the tip of the drill or probe on the material, making it possible to distinguish it from the dentin.

Removal of the filling material

Once the access cavity has been reshaped and any endodontic post has been removed, it is necessary to identify the filling material that is present inside the root canals. Certainly, the evaluation of which material is present in the endodontium must have already been performed pre-operatively (Table 3.6) so that the choice

Table 3.6 **REMOVAL OF THE FILLING MATERIALS**

Type of filling	Tools	Level of difficulty
Endodontic pastes or sealers (Eugenol zinc oxide/Eugenol-based/ paraformaldehyde)	Solvents Ultrasound	Simple, but particularly difficult with some sealers.
Gutta-percha	Solvents Rotary instruments NiTi Alloy	Simple
Gutta-percha with plastic carrier	Solvents/Manual steel files Heat carriers Rotary instruments NiTi Alloy	Simple in wide, medium-length and curved canals, difficult in narrow canals.
Silver cones	Specific pliers	Complex because of the risk of separating the apical portion of the cone.
Resin-based filling materials	Ultrasound	Simple or medium, depending on canal volume and the visibility of the material.
Mineral-based sealers	Ultrasound	Complex

Table 3.7 **SOLVENTS**

Product or active substance	**Composition**	**Function**
Resosolv (Pierre Rolland, Acteon, France)	95% dimethylformamide and 1%-2% Cinnamomum cassia	Solvent for resinous sealers.
Endosolv E (Septodont, Paris, France)	50%-90% tetra-chloroethylene, 2.5%-10% isopentyl acetate, and 1% thymol	Solvent for zinc oxide eugenol cements.
Guttasolv (Septodont, Paris, France)	Eucalyptol-based gutta-percha softener	Active on gutta-percha and less active on eugenate-based sealers.
Chloroform	Triclomethane ($CHCl_3$)	Gutta-percha solvent, toxic, can be substituted with dichloro methane-methylene chloride.
Xylene or Xylol	Mixture of three benzene-derived isomers (C_8H_{10})	Useful in the dissolution of gutta-percha and sealer, as it is neutralized with ethanol.
Halothane (halothane)	Bromochlorotrifluoroethane	Active on gutta-percha.
Turpentine oil	Essential oil, extracted from coniferous resins	Solvent for both eugenol cements and gutta-percha.
Orange oil	Essential oil obtained from orange	Particularly active on eugenates, and therefore useful in the dissolution of sealers.
Eucalyptol Eucalyptus oil	Essential oil obtained from eucalyptus	Active on gutta-percha and less active on eugenate-based sealers.

of the technique and of any solvents used (Table 3.7) for faster removal can be confirmed by a subsequent intraoperative evaluation.

To confirm the diagnostic impressions with respect to the type of material present in the root canals, a DG16 endodontic probe must be inserted to test the hardness of the material. If necessary, a small amount of solvent can be added to the pulp chamber, to understand its direct effects on the material at the root canal openings. Based on these considerations, the clinician will then be able to understand which material needs to be removed from the root canals.

Removing pastes or endodontic sealers

Endodontic sealers or pastes are still used as filling materials.

Pastes can be classified into soft (easily removable) and hard, often impenetrable and, as such, non-removable. In general, and due to the method with which they are conveyed inside the root canals, the density of these pastes is higher in the coronal portion and lower in the apical portion.

Removal can be accomplished:

- Dedicated mechanical tools;
- Mechanical tools normally used for root canal shaping[48];
- Solvents (see Box 3.3);
- A combination of the above instruments and solvents.

However, the main problem in these cases is to verify the cleaning of the canal walls. Preoperative considerations when retreating a tooth filled exclusively with sealers, must also involve the presence of calcifications and resorptions.

It is also important to inform the patient that it is sometimes impossible to remove all the material in the root canals, and that episodes of postoperative septic

exacerbation may occur[49] (see Chapter 6). These sealers can promote a deterioration of dental aesthetics, especially in the anterior teeth, because the use of pastes combined with poor cleaning of the pulp chamber may generate tooth discoloration[50, 51].
In cases where the material is easily penetrated by the DG16 probe, tested at the level of the canal opening or in the coronal third of the canal lumen, the removal technique is based on the combined use of manual or rotating instruments with solvents.
However, special care should be taken to avoid excessive melting of the sealer so as to prevent it entering the dentin tubules, thus further complicating the overall treatment process.
The material should be softened so that the manual tools (initially) and the rotating tools (subsequently) can enter easily. If the material reaches the apex, the clinician should avoid exerting excessive pressure, in order to prevent it from leaking into the periodontium.
From a technical point of view, for soft sealers, removal is performed using:

- Dedicated mechanical tools (for example, Micro-Debrider, Dentsply Maillefer)
- Stainless steel or nickel-titanium mechanical tools for root canal shaping
- Ultrasonic k-files
- Solvents combined with mechanical instruments or paper cones.

Box 3.3 **USE OF SOLVENTS IN THE RETREATMENT PROCESSES**

A brief discussion on the role of solvents in the removal of canal content seems appropriate. Further information on this subject will also be provided in chapter 4. Although the possibility of softening the gutta-percha with heat or with the use of ultrasonic tips or dedicated endodontic instruments has greatly reduced the use of solvents, it is more suitable for eliminating the sealers and pastes that are often associated with the development of gutta-percha in the filling of root canals. The choice of one method over another may be questionable. However, and as well-demonstrated in various studies, some may be less suitable in certain circumstances. Chloroform, for example, seems to be more aggressive towards dentin tissues and, for this reason, eucalyptol or orange-oil extract should be preferred instead. Chloroform is also suspected of having a potential carcinogenic effect. It is certain that the use of solvents seems to be reducing the amount of debris expelled beyond the apex, and makes shaping more effective as the softened filling material is removed from the canal more quickly. According to some studies, xylene has proven to be the most effective solvent over other organic solvents. Essential oils (eucalyptus and orange) have proved to have similar dissolving capacities on some of the most frequently used endodontic sealers. The use of solvents does not seem to promote any adverse effects on the apical detectors during the shaping maneuvers. Last, but not least, solvents that have a real universal value, particularly with respect to methacrylate-based sealers.

Canakci BC, Er O, and Dincer A. *Do the Sealer Solvents Used Affect Apically Extruded Debris in Retreatment?* J Endod. 2015;41(9):1507-9.

Er O, et al. *Effect of solvents on the accuracy of the Mini Root ZX apex locator*. Int Endod J. 2013;46(11):1088-95.

Ferreira I, et al. *New Insight into the Dissolution of Epoxy Resin-based Sealers*. J Endod. 2017;43(9):1505-1510.

Karatas E, et al. *The effect of chloroform, orange oil and eucalyptol on root canal transportation in endodontic retreatment*. Aust Endod J. 2016;42(1):37-40.

Keskin C, Sariyilmaz E and Sariyilmaz O. *Effect of solvents on apically extruded debris and irrigant during root canal retreatment using reciprocating instruments*. Int Endod J. 2017;50(11):1084-1088.

Martos J, et al. *Dissolving efficacy of eucalyptus and orange oil, xylol and chloroform solvents on different root canal sealers*. Int Endod J. 2011;44(11):1024-8.

Saglam BC, et al. *Efficacy of different solvents in removing gutta-percha from curved root canals: a micro-computed tomography study*. Aust Endod J. 2014;40(2):76-80.

Solaiman M. & Al-Hadlaq. *Effect of chloroform, orange solvent and eucalyptol on the accuracy of four electronic apex locator*. Aust Endod J. 2013;39:112-115.

Yadav HK et al. *The effectiveness of eucalyptus oil, orange oil, and xylene in dissolving different endodontic sealers*. J Conserv Dent. 2016;19:332-7.

CASE REPORT 6

Fillings with endodontic pastes: strategies for removal

At first glance, the retreatment of teeth with endodontic pastes can appear very simple; once patency has been tested, the use of both ultrasound and solvents can be ideal.
In these cases, it is possible to make an "a priori" radiographic analysis, when it is possible to see the empty canal lumen inside or beyond its closing limit.

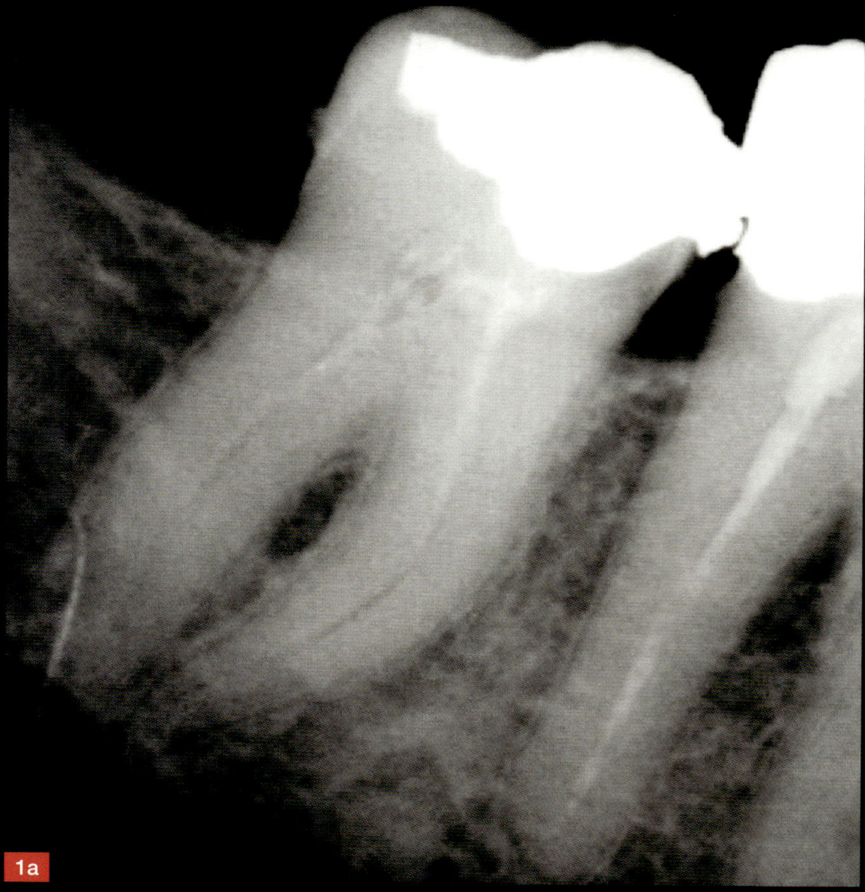

1a

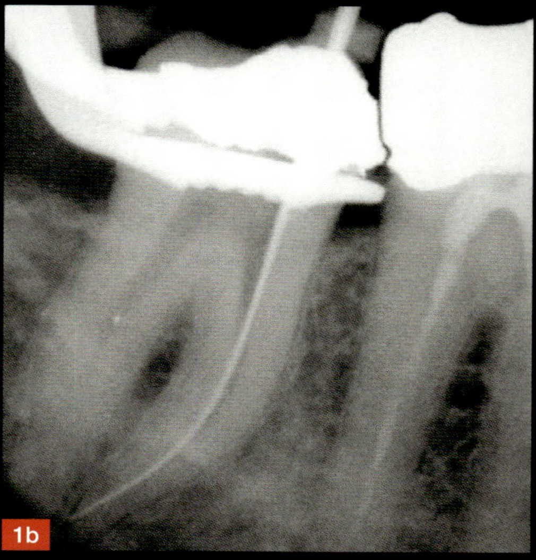

1b

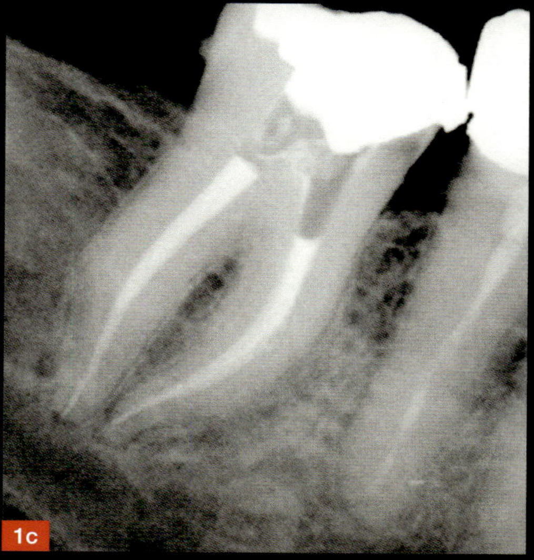

1c

Figure 1a: An emblematic example of canal closure using pastes; the molar is not instrumented and is only minimally filled.

Figure 1b: Working length confirmed by the endodontic file x-ray.

Figure 1c: Case with canal filling completed.

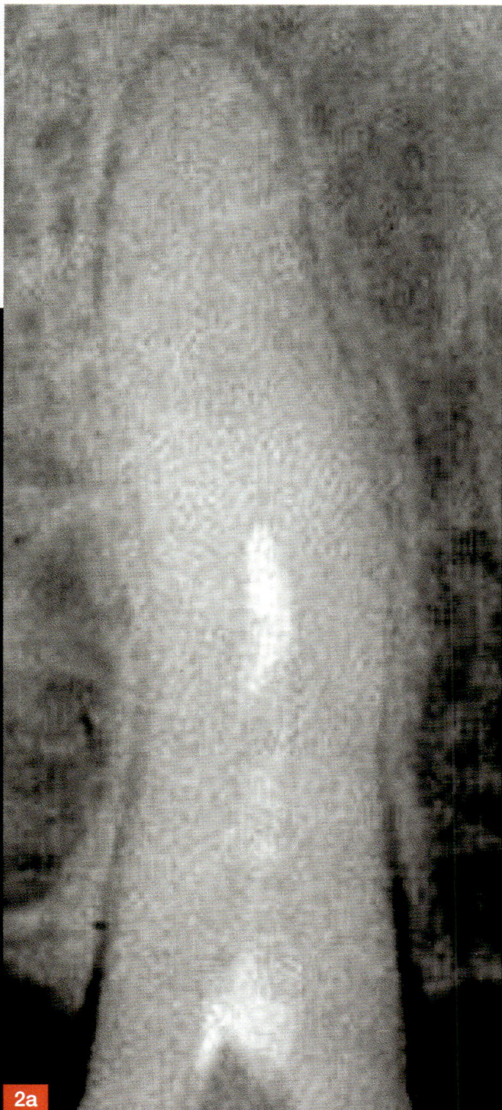

2a

Figure 2a: A premolar probably filled with iodoform paste.

Figure 2b: The retreatment is complete.

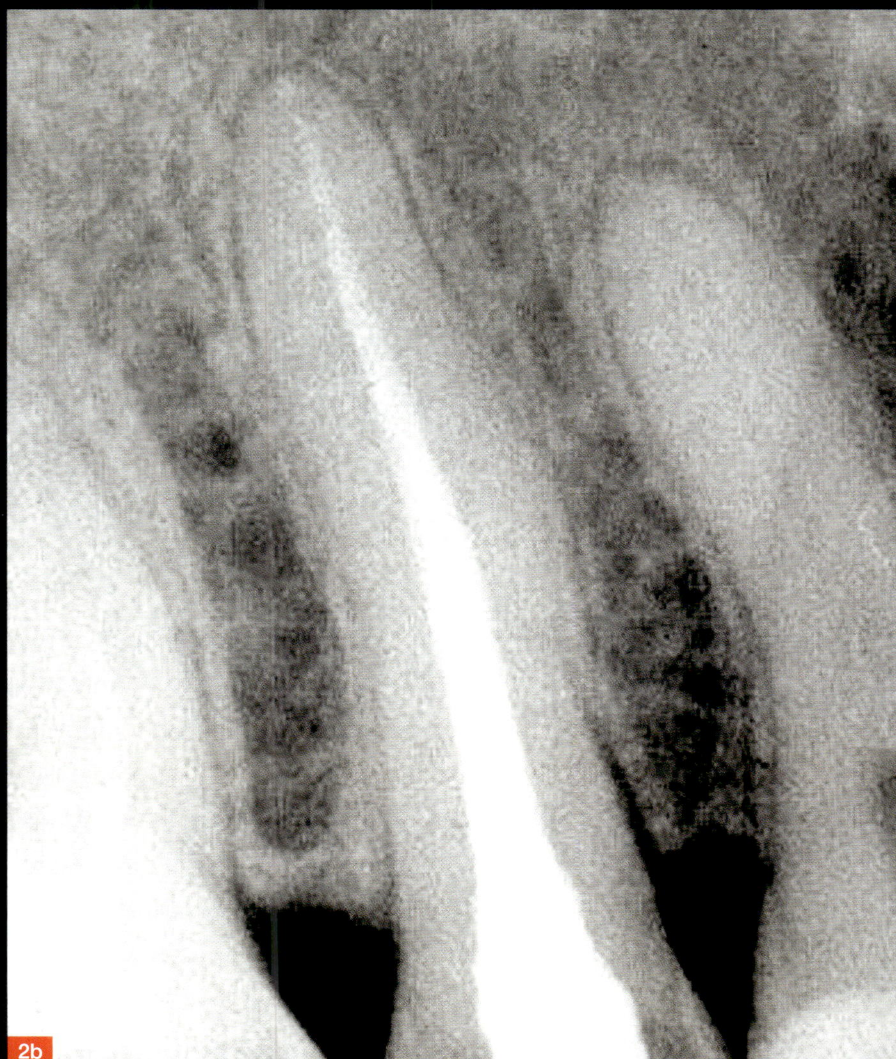

2b

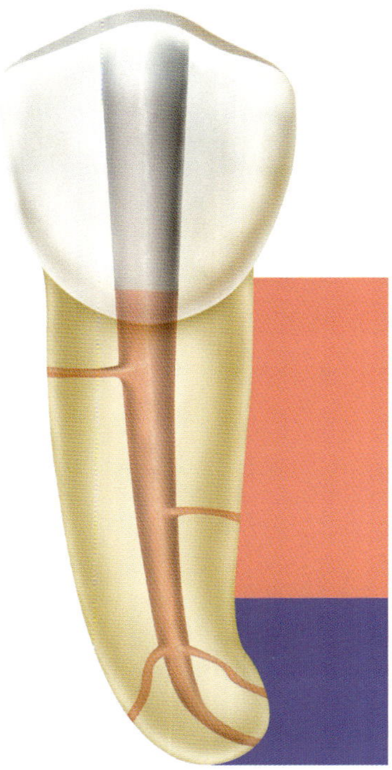

Figure 3.58: In the red zone you can always remove the gutta-percha with mechanical or ultrasonic instruments, whereas in the lower part (blue zone) it can be indicated to use solvents to soften the canal content.

Generally speaking, these sealers are softer than gutta-percha, and hence their removal is less questionable, even if a good level of cleanliness of the canal walls is obtained after a longer time[52, 53].

When dealing with a hard and impenetrable paste, however, it is advisable to proceed very slowly with ultrasonic diamond-coated burs to progressively wear down the filling material[49, 54].

More specifically, it can be stated that – if the material appears to be hard and not penetrable even once a particularly strong solvent has been introduced into the chamber (for example, Endosolv R, Septodont, France) – it can only be removed from the root canal mechanically. In this case, it is suggested to use ultrasonic tips (Start-X 3, Satelec ET 20-25, ProUltra 4 or 5) and ultrasonically activated k-files (ISO .20 or .25). Ultrasonic tips are designed to remove the coronal portion of the material, whereas the ultrasonically-activated k-files are used to remove the material when in the proximity of the apical area. It is clear that this approach requires high magnification and a well-lit field to safeguard the residual dental tissue. Therefore, the use of a surgical microscope is absolutely recommended.

Another aspect to consider is that this type of "forced removal" can only occur if the material to be removed is in a straight portion of the root canal or is easily accessible. If the material is located very apically or beyond a curvature, and it is impossible to achieve a straight access, then one of the greatest risks involves the selection of a wrong path and/or perforation.

Since the removal of hard pastes/sealers is time-consuming and particularly complicated, the recommendations are:

- Isolate several teeth, so that the axis of the teeth adjacent to the treated tooth can serve as a guide for the instruments used.
- Create a straight as possible access to the coronal portion of the material to be removed.
- Use ultrasound in combination with a magnifying medium and light source.
- During the apical penetration phases, perform intraoperative X-rays at different angles, using gutta-percha inserted at the level reached. This is to identify whether removal should be performed axially to the profile of the root (to avoid creating false paths) or not.

This should be performed with the aid of a magnifying glass and appropriate lighting. If it is necessary to remove sealer below a curvature, then it is advisable to proceed with pre-curved ultrasonic k-files.

Gutta-percha removal

Gutta-percha is the most frequently used filling material in endodontic treatments performed in recent decades with various techniques. Indeed, the filling technique used in primary treatment will reflect the difficulty of removing the filling material during retreatment[55, 56].

Other factors that can complicate the re-intervention are purely anatomical.

For example, the length, diameter, and configuration of the canal (e.g. curvatures, canal confluences, and isthmus)[57], also depend on how much of the original anatomy has been preserved (ledges, false paths, etc.)[55, 58].

Regardless of the filling technique used in primary therapy, the general indication is to proceed in a corono-apical direction, thus progressively freeing the canal from the gutta-percha, and minimizing the extrusion of irrigants[59-64].

The preoperative X-ray analysis allows the determination of the techniques that are most suitable for the clinical case in question.

It is, in actual fact, possible to act on gutta-percha with:

- Mechanical instruments;
- Ultrasonic instruments;
- Heat;
- Solvents;
- Manual or mechanical instruments combined with heat or solvents.

In general, and since the root canals are straight and wide in the anterior teeth,

▸ continue to page 188

Interradicular lesion in a lower molar

CASE REPORT 7

Injuries of the bone space of the lower molar furcation are often the subject of discussion by clinicians, who have to choose between endodontic treatment or retreatment and periodontal therapy (e.g., root section). In this case, a high fistula, which often associated with periodontal lesions, is visible.

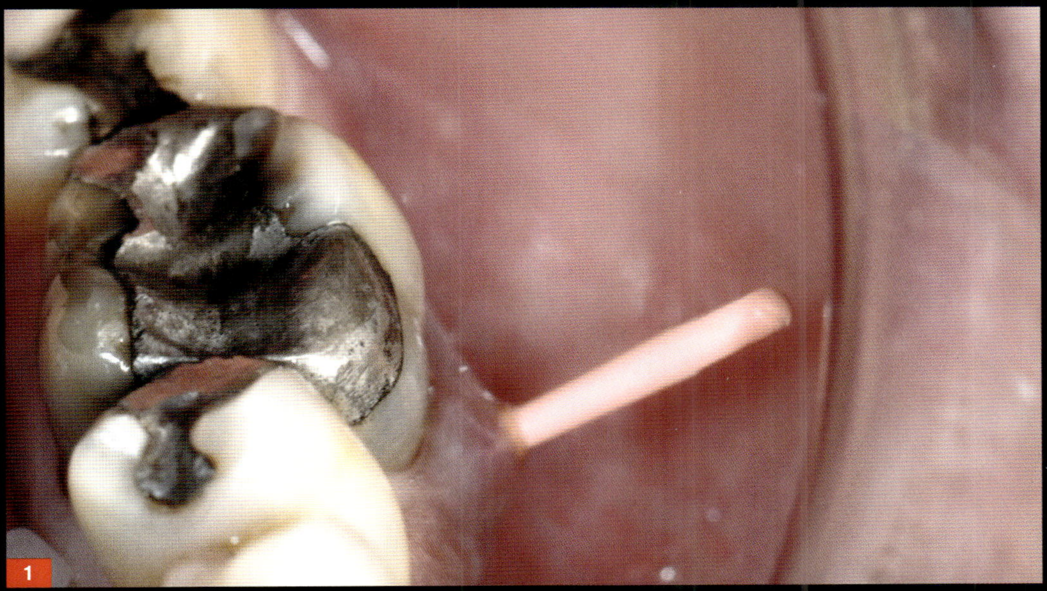

Figure 1: A fistula on a lower molar at the level of the furcation is highlighted by the insertion of a gutta-percha cone.

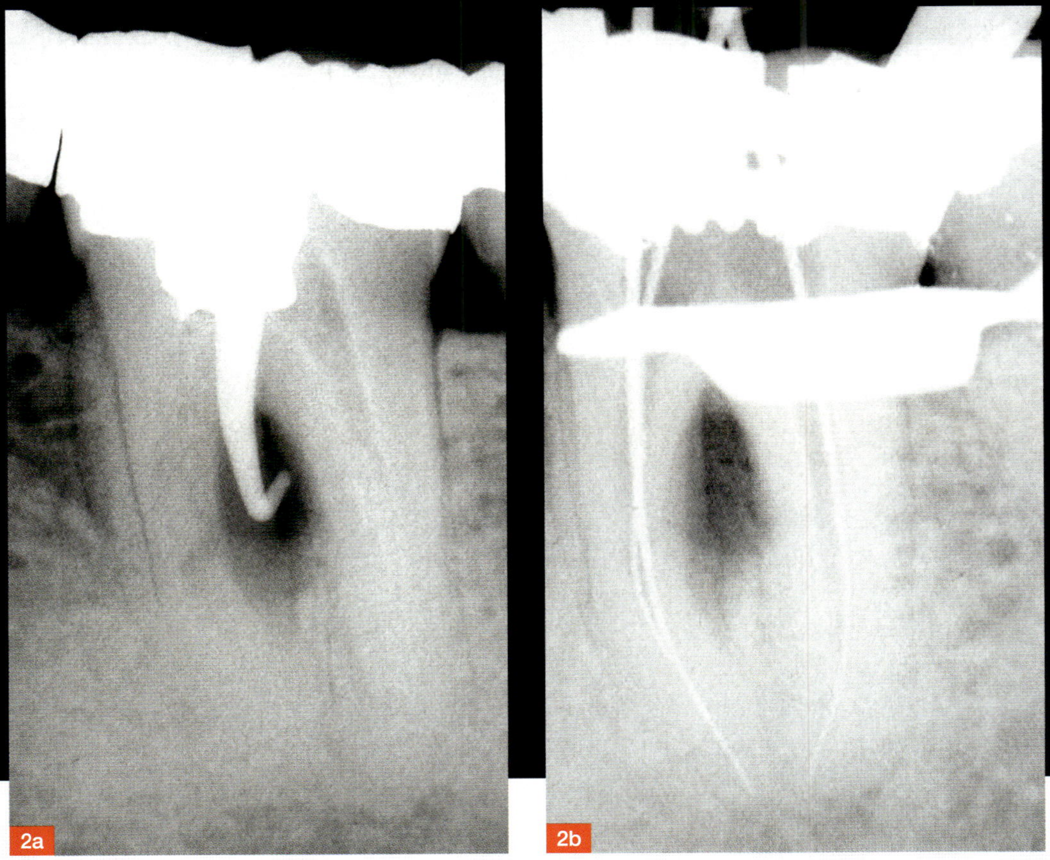

Figure 2a-b: The route of the cone, displayed radiographically, seems to lead to a diagnosis of forcible injury of periodontal origin; however, the canals do not appear have been treated correctly. We proceeded with the shaping and cleansing of the root canal system.

The radiographic examination does not make it possible to determine the nature of the lesion, but there is an indication for endodontic treatment if the tooth does not pass the pulp vitality tests or the previous therapy is clearly inappropriate or incomplete. If the endodontic anatomy has a communication with the periodontium at furcation level, a periodontal lesion may also develop.

Correct endodontic therapy leads to a complete resolution of the periodontal lesion.

Very often a lateral communication between the endodontium and the periodontal system

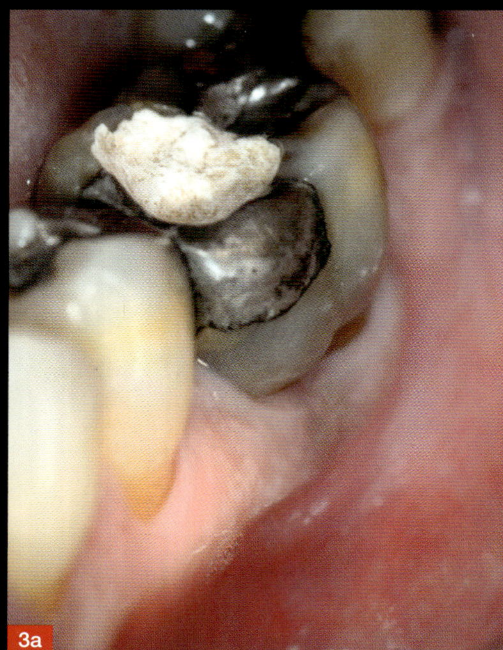

Figure 3a: At the check-up after one week, the fistula had disappeared, a clear sign of endodontic involvement in the interradicular lesion.

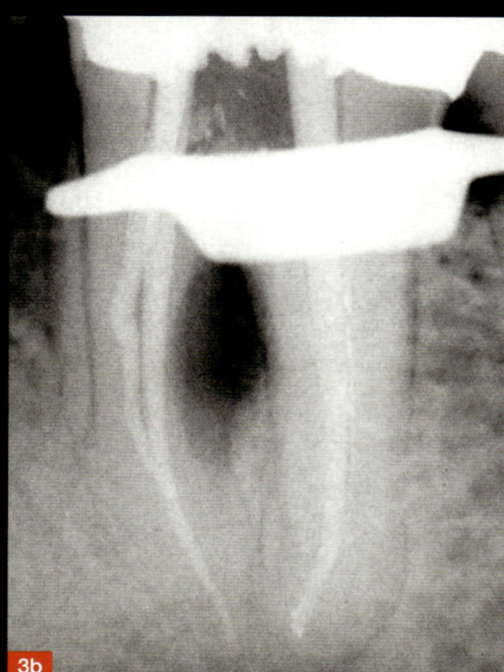

Figure 3b: The cone test shows a high confluence of the two mesial canals.

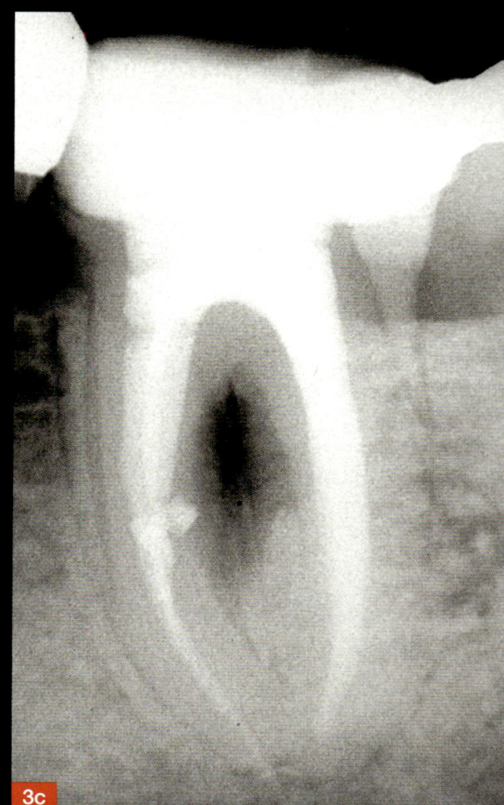

Figure 3c: The filling carried out shows a very wide endoparodontal communication, probably part of multiple side canals.

can be radiographically appreciated. In the early stages of retreatment, particularly if an intermediate filling with calcium hydroxide is used (see Ch. 4), the degree of reaction of the tissues surrounding the tooth can be observed between appointments. The disappearance of the fistula highlights the beginning of lesion resolution. The success of this case is due to the fact that the entire root canal system, including the accessory lateral canals, has been correctly shaped, cleaned and filled.

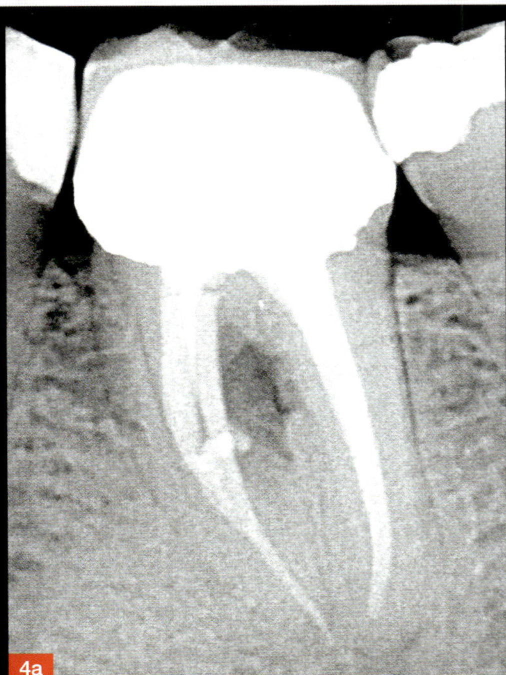

Figure 4a-c: The case observed after 1, 3 and 5 years: the excellent retreatment allowed the complete healing of the inter-radicular bone compartment, an evident sign that the compromise was only of endodontic relevance.

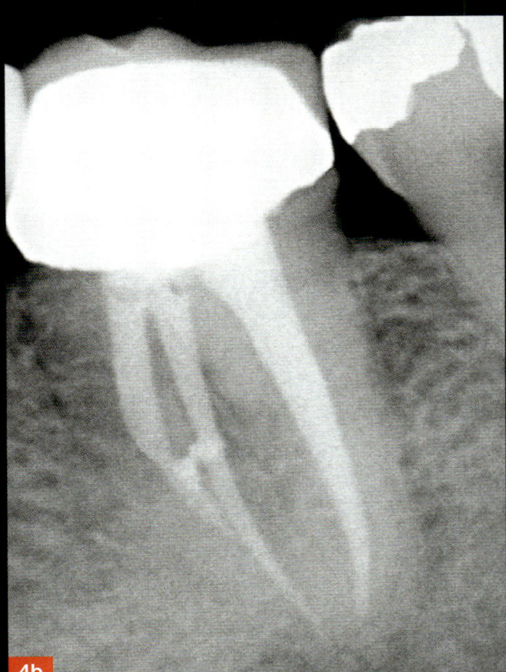

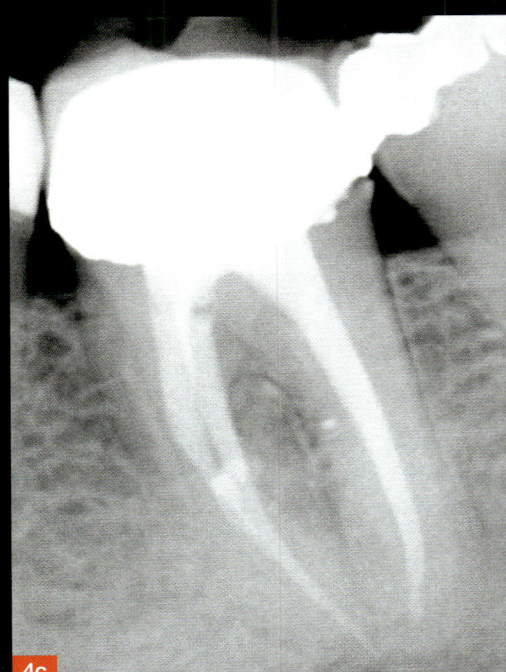

the best method for removing the gutta-percha is to use nickel-titanium rotary instruments mounted on dedicated hand-pieces[64]. This solution allows the elimination of large masses of gutta-percha without leaving residues on the canal walls[65-68]. For this purpose, instruments dedicated to canal retreatment or instruments normally used in primary endodontic treatment can be used[69-71]. The fundamental characteristics for an instrument to be effective are the following: good cutting capacity, an active tip that allows easy penetration into the gutta-percha, and a diameter (taper) that is large enough to remove a significant amount of material[72, 73]. The ultrasonic tips or ultrasonic k-files are very useful in root canals with irregular shape, particularly those that develop in the vestibular-palatal or vestibular-lingual sense where the simple use of rotary instruments does not guarantee complete contact with all canal walls.
The use of heat – conveyed by the same tip used by the gutta-percha heating systems during the condensation phases – increases the temperature, but also softens and partially removes the gutta-percha[74]. This system can be used on a stand-alone basis or combined with mechanical or manual instruments, and successfully facilitates penetration into the filling material. In cases gutta-percha is removed using mechanical action alone or combined with heat, specific solvents can be a valid alternative[75] because they can soften the gutta-percha and improve the efficiency of the mechanical instruments used – as they will now encounter a softer substrate on which to work.
Solvents can also be combined with manual instruments, with a significant increase in working time, and can be particularly useful for very large and oval root canals. The greatest disadvantage associated with the action of solvents is the fact that the dissolved gutta-percha tends to adhere to the canal walls, thus penetrating into the dentinal tubules and undermining the quality of cleaning[76].

In the preliminary investigation phase, in teeth that are considered filled with gutta-percha and, probably, sealer, it is possible to divide the radiological appearance of root canals into three broad categories, based on the quality of the filling:

1. Incomplete in length and width;
2. Incomplete in width but not in length;
3. Optimal.

All those canal fillings that appear at least three mm shorter than the radiologically evident apex on two-dimensional radiological analysis, will belong to category 1. Not infrequently, these images are also accompanied by obvious signs of radiolucency on the side of the filling (underfilling) and allow a glimpse of the canal lumen beyond the filling. This second characteristic is peculiar to category 2 whose primary difference compared to the category 1 is that the filling occupies the entire length of the radiologically visible endodontic space. Cases belonging to category 1 are most easily detectable with preoperative radiography. The presence of a single cone or cones placed without being heated can be identified when one observes that the root canal is filled with a material that has uniform radiopacity but low taper. In this clinical situation, it is advisable to limit the use of solvents to soften the coronal part of the gutta-percha and to use an H-file to screw in the endodontic portion of the gutta-percha cone, thus slowly extracting it from the canal in a single piece. When constant radiopacity is detected, with progressive tapering that may or may not reach the end of the root, gutta-percha removal can be effective using tools that are dedicated to canal retreatment such as those described on the next page.
Mechanical shaping tools can exert an effective action provided they are sharp and they have an active tip, which allows them to penetrate into the gutta-percha – if sufficiently large in diameter[78-80]. The mechanical removal

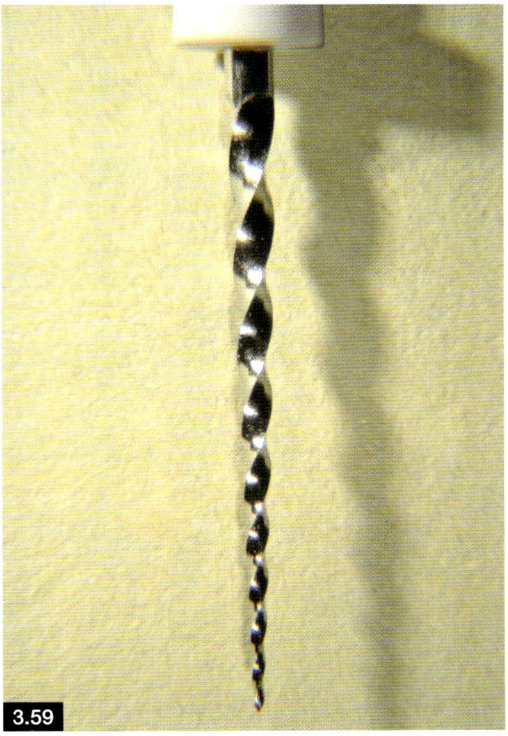

3.59

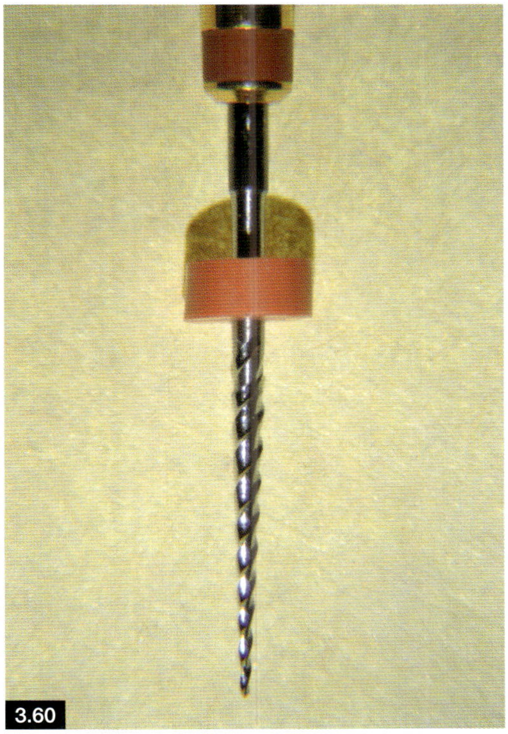

3.60

Fig. 3.59: Active cutting blade instrument that is ideal for removing gutta-percha (Maillefer, Switzerland).

Fig. 3.60: Similar instrument for removing gutta-percha (Micromega, France).

Fig. 3.61a-b: Two sections under a scanning microscope of instruments that are suitable for the mechanical removal of the gutta-percha. Note the active profile of the blades and the different thread designs.

Fig. 3.62a-b: Tools with different length and taper suitable for the mechanical removal of the gutta-percha (Komet, Germany).

action can also be performed using ultrasonic tips or ultrasonic k-files (very useful in root canals with irregular shape, where rotating instruments do not guarantee the complete emptying of the treated area)[81]. Where it is not possible to remove the gutta-percha using mechanical action alone, solvents may be used to dissolve the gutta-percha as follows:

1. Insert a dry instrument rotating at between 800 and 1000 rpm, without having introduced any solvent in the chamber, up to two thirds of the length of the filling material present.
2. Inject an active solvent into this material (see Table 3.7) and, with small K files, enter the mass of material (thus allowing the solvent to penetrate).
3. Absorb the amount of dissolved gutta-percha with paper cones.
4. Continue with k-file, solvent, and paper cones until the latter comes out clean when inserted into the root canal.

The action of the solvent softens the gutta-percha and favors the efficiency of mechanical instruments. The combination of solvents with the use of manual tools leads to a considerable increase in working time,

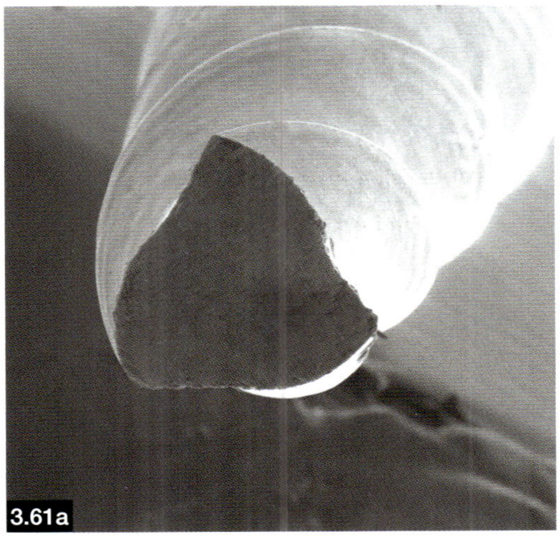

3.61a

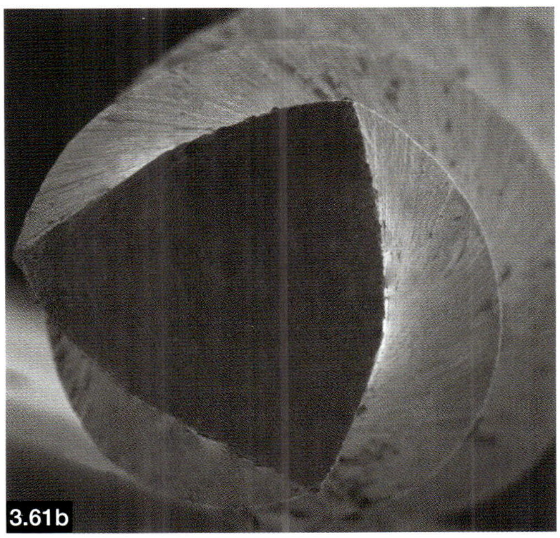

3.61b

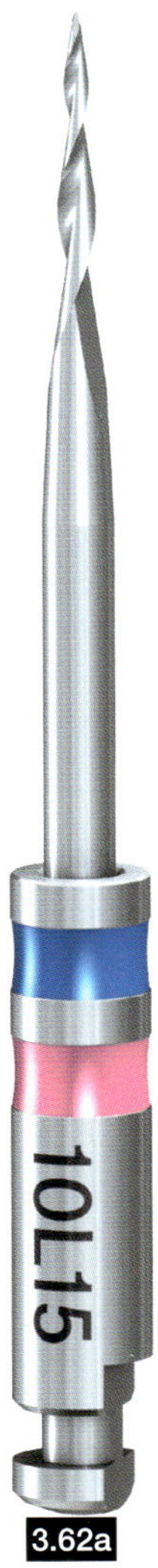

3.62a

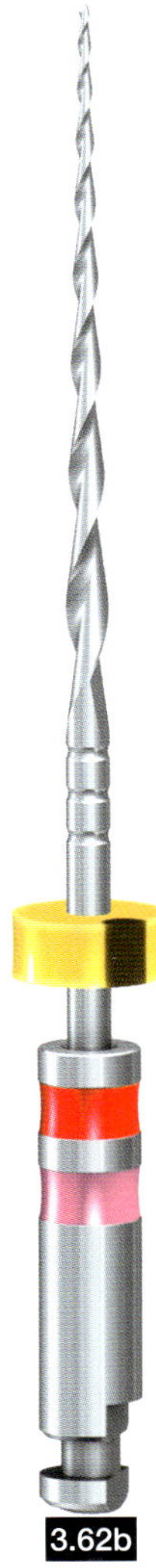

3.62b

greatly raising the risk of creating ledges and false paths. For this reason, the dissolution of the gutta-percha in the root canals using the heat generated by the “heat carriers” in the condensation phase of the gutta-percha, can be a very useful alternative.

Gutta-percha removal and the plastic carrier

When removing a filling with a gutta-percha system conveyed by a plastic carrier, the use of ultrasound is preferred to that of the drills because the heat and vibration will allow for an easier removal of the material without inadvertently sacrificing dentin.
Electronic heat carriers can be the instruments of election when ultrasound is not used.
Using solvents to isolate the plastic core and gripping it with a plier can be an effective alternative. There are several versions of these systems, with different cores and coatings. Thermafil (Dentsply Maillefer, Switzerland) is a gutta-percha coated plastic carrier, however, gutta-percha carriers with different chemical composition are also available (GuttaCore, Maillefer, Switzerland or Guttafusion, Dentsply Germany).
In addition, certain synthetic gutta-percha systems were widespread in the recent past (Resilon™, Kerr, USA). When considering removal, obturators with plastic carriers can create some additional problems over the gutta-percha ones, since the carrier cannot be affected by the solvents that we normally use. However, there is a groove along the carrier that, when engaged with a tool such as an H-file, facilitates its removal from the gutta-percha, thus rendering the process significantly easier.
In the preoperative phase, it is rather difficult to understand whether a carrier system has been used because the radiograph can only present a slightly more pronounced radiopacity than the characteristic radiopacity

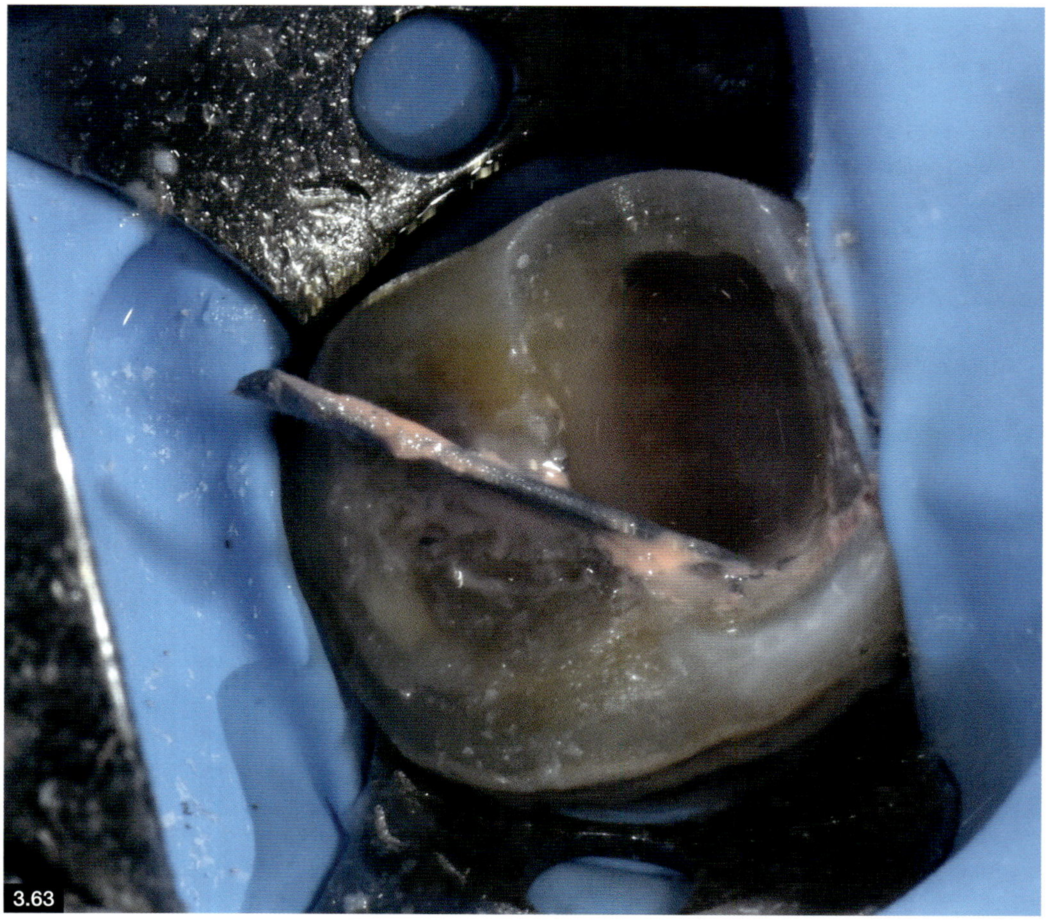

Fig. 3.63: The use of solvents has made it possible to dissolve the gutta-percha surrounding the carrier made of easily-removed plastic.

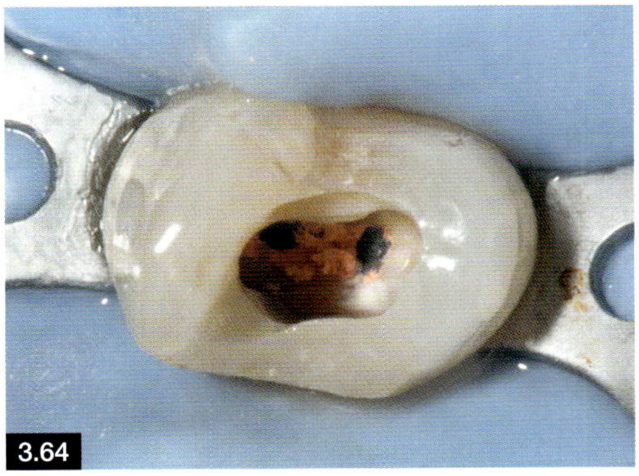

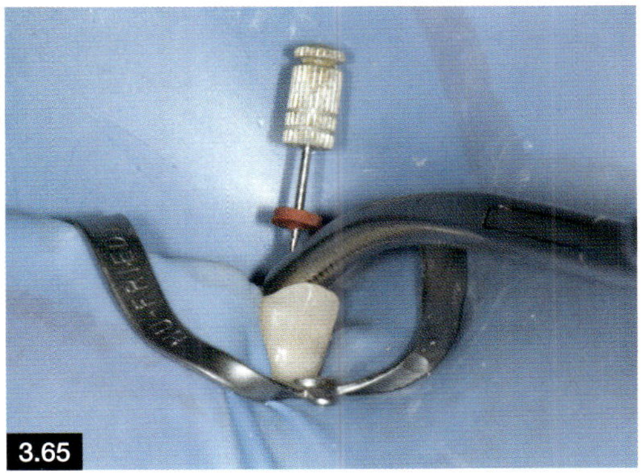

Fig. 3.64: An upper premolar has a root canal filling with a gutta-percha system and a plastic carrier.

Fig. 3.65: The insertion of a Hedström-type instrument is intended to engage the plastic carrier.

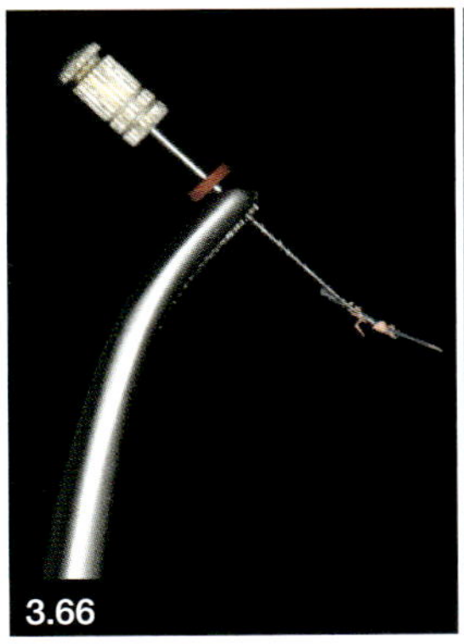

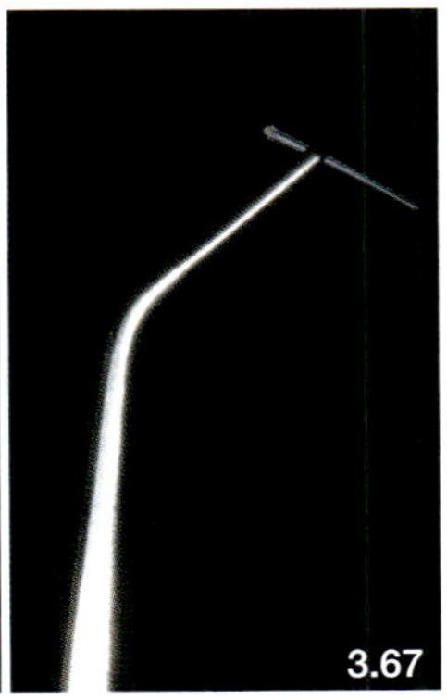

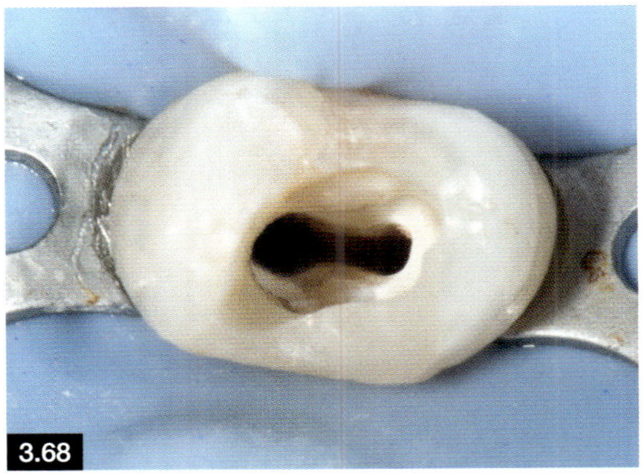

Fig. 3.66: The "mosquito" type clamp makes it possible to grasp the plastic carrier.

Fig. 3.67: Detail of a plastic carrier removed using college-style tweezers.

Fig. 3.68: The canals are completely clean and ready for the new seal.

of a filling performed using another hot system, with a constant taper.
Only in cases where the system has been inserted in a sub-instrumented root canal or where a correct taper has not been developed, is there a uniform radiopacity with a very limited taper.
The removal techniques classically described in literature include:

- introducing a gutta-percha solvent into the pulp chamber.
- moving the plastic core with a small DG16 or k-file probe inserted between the plastic core and the gutta-percha.
- pulling out the plastic core, inserting an H-file into the root canal so that the blades grip the plastic part of the core, and pulling gently in a coronal direction.

Another possibility is to insert the plugger an electronic heat carrier that is heated at 600 °C, for a few millimeters in the center of the plastic core in order to melt it, and then cool it down for 30 seconds with an air spray while pulling it gently in a coronal direction.
Some authors have also suggested using ultrasonic tips to perform the same method.
An alternative method, that is quite safe and fast, is to use a Ni-Ti rotating instrument (reciprocating or continuous movement) inserted in the gutta-percha and surrounding the carrier.
Proceeding in an apical direction, the instrument will remove the carrier – or pieces of the carrier – from the root canal[82]. It is important to use instruments with a good cutting capacity to allow the operator to work without exerting pressure in an apical direction, and to act quickly, thus reducing the risk of a fracture to the carrier[83]. In cases where the carrier is cut above the canal entrance, it can be removed using the systems used remove fractured instruments.
Removal of the gutta-percha surrounding the carrier, followed by the attachment of the carrier and its extraction, can be our final alternative[84].
Recently other obturators with a gutta-percha core have been introduced, and removal in these cases is significantly easier. Once most of the coronal portion appears more resistant has been softened, the remaining part of the filling system can be simply removed using the techniques described for the removal of the warm-compacted gutta-percha.

Unidentified and un-instrumented root canals

One of the major errors associated with failure in endodontics involves the incorrect assessment of the anatomy of the pulp chamber and root canals[85]. Failure to visualize, shape, clean, and fill one or more canals results in the development of an environment that is particularly favorable to colonization by bacteria, which can proliferate undisturbed within the tooth and generate considerable periapical reactions. In the case of radiolucent lesions that are larger than five mm, one should immediately suspect the presence of an endodontic space that has not been correctly explored. Therefore, the clinician must restart from this point, i.e. redesigning the access cavity correctly, in order to identify all canal openings. In these cases, better visibility and control are essential, hence it is advisable to use both dry and irrigated ultrasonic tips.

During this phase, the main purpose is to leave the pulp chamber floor intact, in order to better appreciate the respective lines present that help clinicians to identify the location of the canal openings. It may also be necessary to remove coronal calcifications, which can often obliterate the canal entrance.

The removal of calcifications is correctly performed through the use of ultrasonic tips that are always used with adequate magnification and suitable lighting. Intrapulpal calcifications (pulp stones) are often easy to remove, as they are not connected to the walls of the canal. However, the removal of dentin calcifications can be significantly more complex, and it is necessary to use the surgical microscope and organic dyes to examine the pulp tissue, thus preventing perforation[86].

These operations should not be random. A radiographic guide, preferably a three-dimensional one, will allow the operator to collect sufficient information to determine a suitable intervention strategy.

Therefore, the clinical findings of partial or entirely untreated canals is anything but random; reference is always made to the second canal of the mesial root in the upper molars (MB2)[87]. As repeatedly mentioned, this may be caused by an inadequacy, fin terms of the means used by the previous operator, by a distinct lack of knowledge related to the endodontic anatomy and its variables, by the presence of obstacles that prevent operators from reaching the canal entrance, or by the presence of calcifications that affect the entire root canals[88,89].

Proper treatment of these portions of the endodontium is often a prerequisite for clinical and radiographic success.

▶ continue to page 207

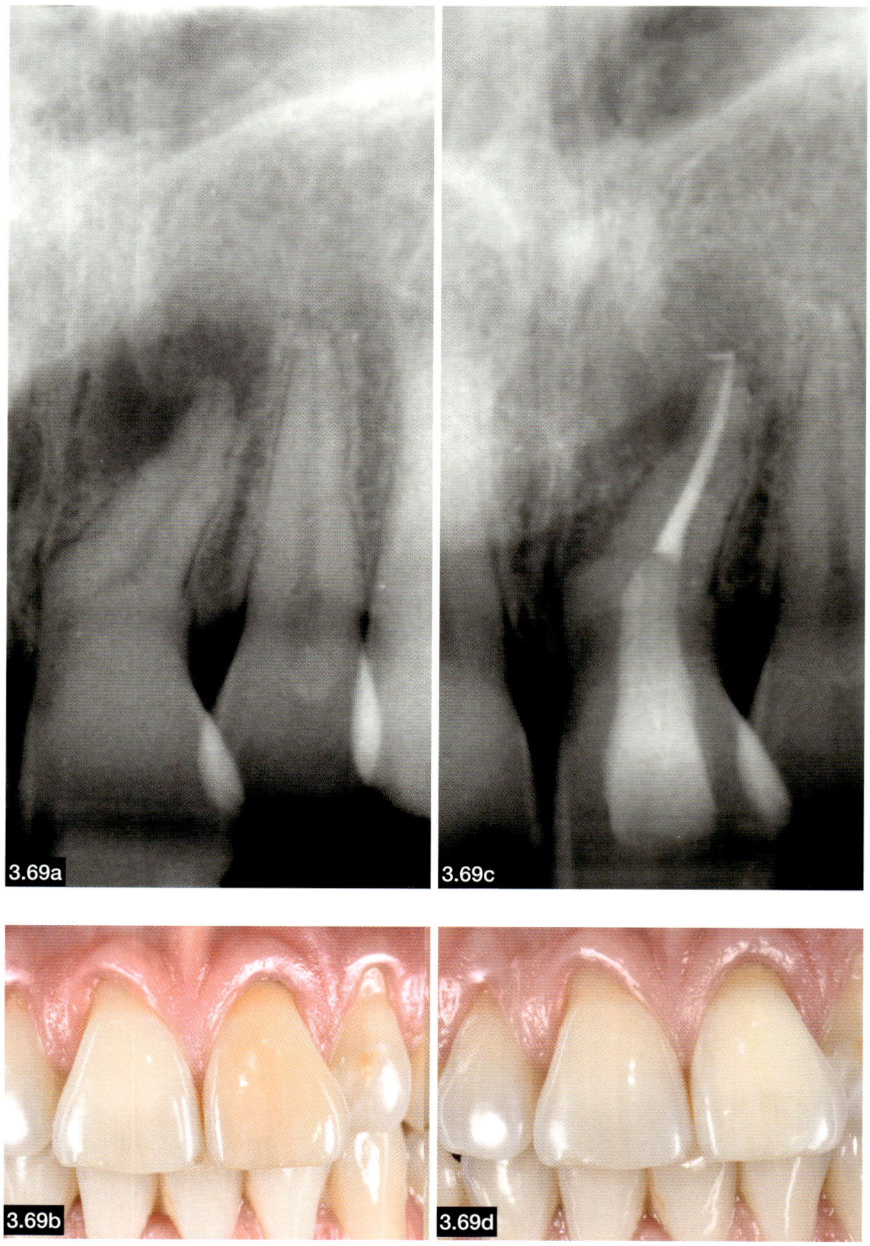

Fig. 3.69a-d: Calcified central incisor canal (a), the tooth appears discoloured (b); the canal is properly identified and instrumented (c) and it recovers its original ideal color following a whitening operation (d).

Uninstrumented canals, one of the main causes of periapical injury

CASE REPORT 8

Retreatment is necessary when closure and disinfection of the endodontic space is not possible; the causes are many but, as demonstrated by an interesting study by Karabucak et al.[85], the so-called forgotten canals, i.e. those not identified during the first treatment, are found in almost 45% of teeth with periapical lesions.

▸ continue to page 194

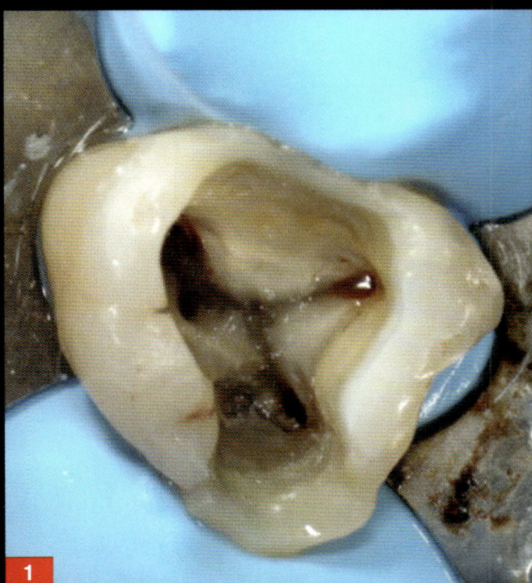

1

Figure 1: The reopening of a pulp chamber shows a singular geometry for an upper molar (two palatal canals).

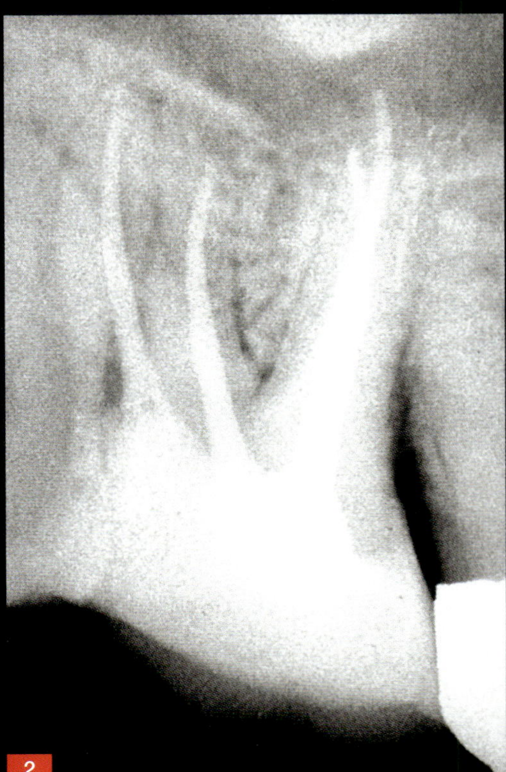

2

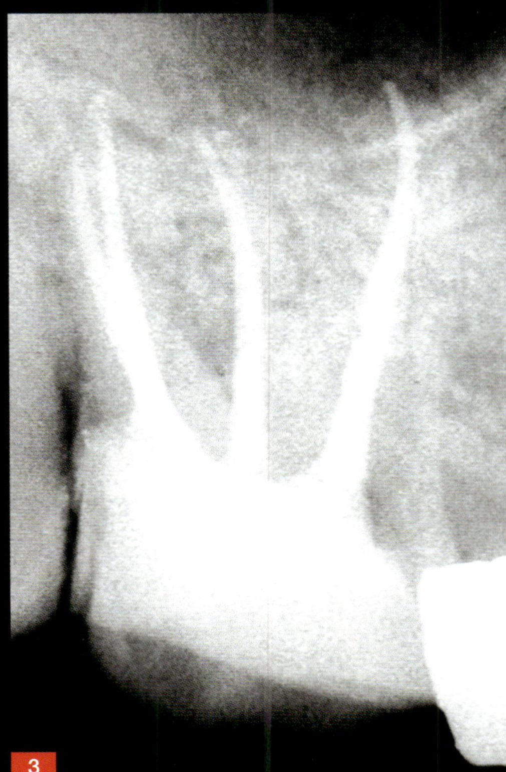

3

Figure 2: The x-ray does not show any apparent anatomical peculiarities.

Figure 3: A projection highlights a double palatine root that, if not sealed, could have generated a overt disease.

It is also clear that an uninstrumented root canal can provide an ideal biological niche for a very large quantity of bacteria which, in turn, can induce significant periapical reaction. Hence an interesting diagnostic hypothesis: in cases in which, faced with a satisfactory canal filling, a failure occurs, it is not uncommon to look for an uninstrumented canal within the endodontic compartment. CBCT is often useful in circumstances like these.

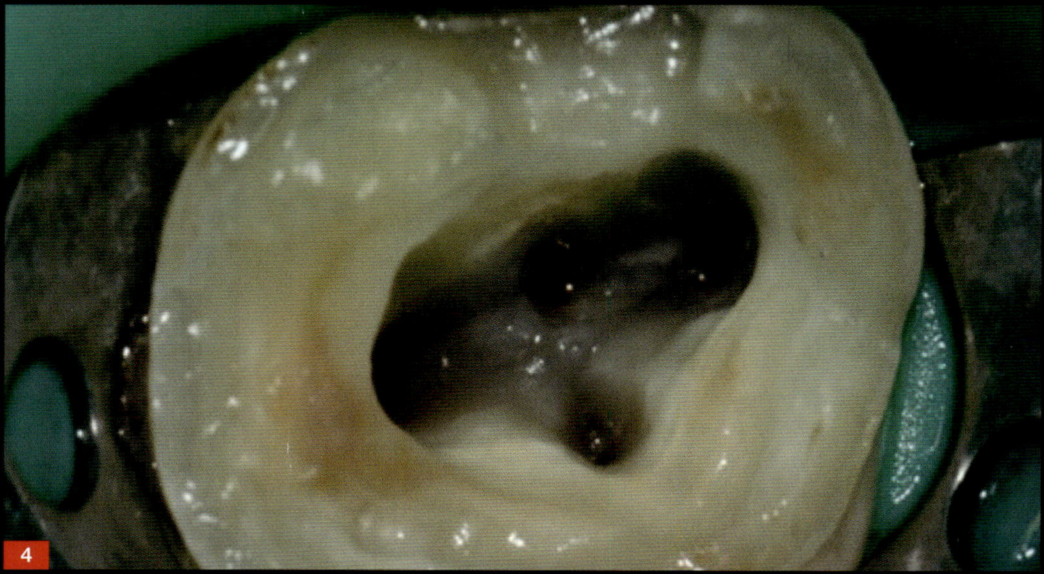

4

Figure 4: The examination of the pulp chamber of the upper molars must be performed bearing in mind that MB2 canals are common.

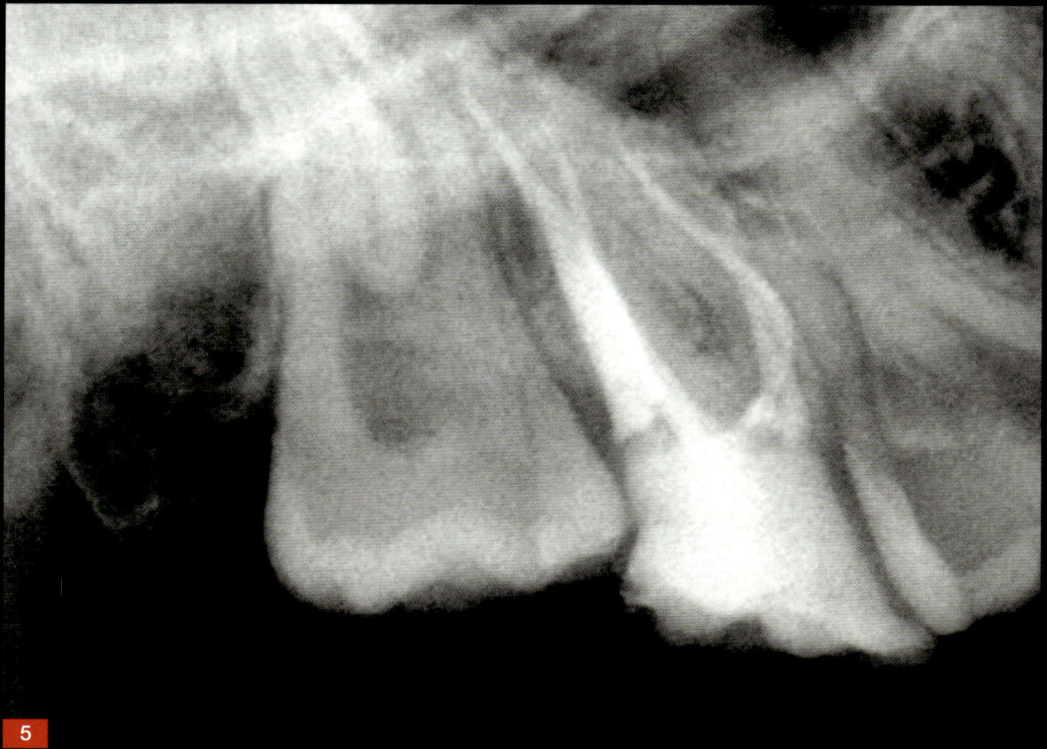

5

Figure 5: Endodontic filling highlights the complexity of the anatomy of the MB1 and MB2 canal.

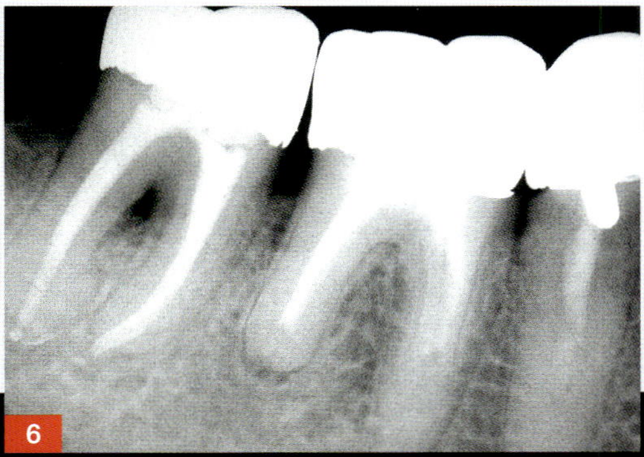

6

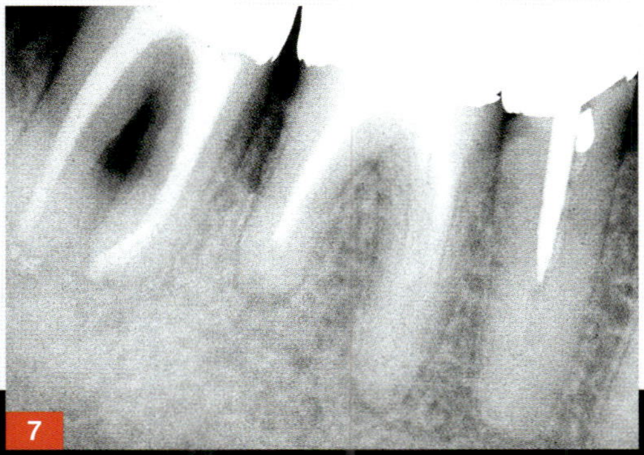

7

Figure 6: The X-ray picture of a second lower molar shows a frank radiotransparent inter-radicular lesion.

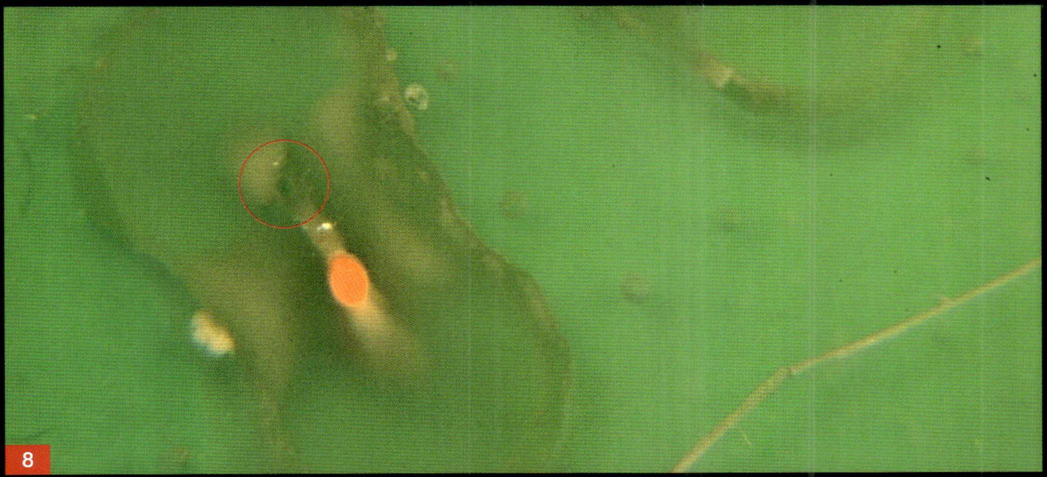

8

Figure 7: Monitoring after about 3 years, supported by lingual probing exceeding 7 mm, leads the clinician to conclude for an irreversible periodontal lesion and, given the pain symptoms, to extract the tooth.

Figure 8: A thorough examination of the images shows that the lingual canal had not been either identified or instrumented.

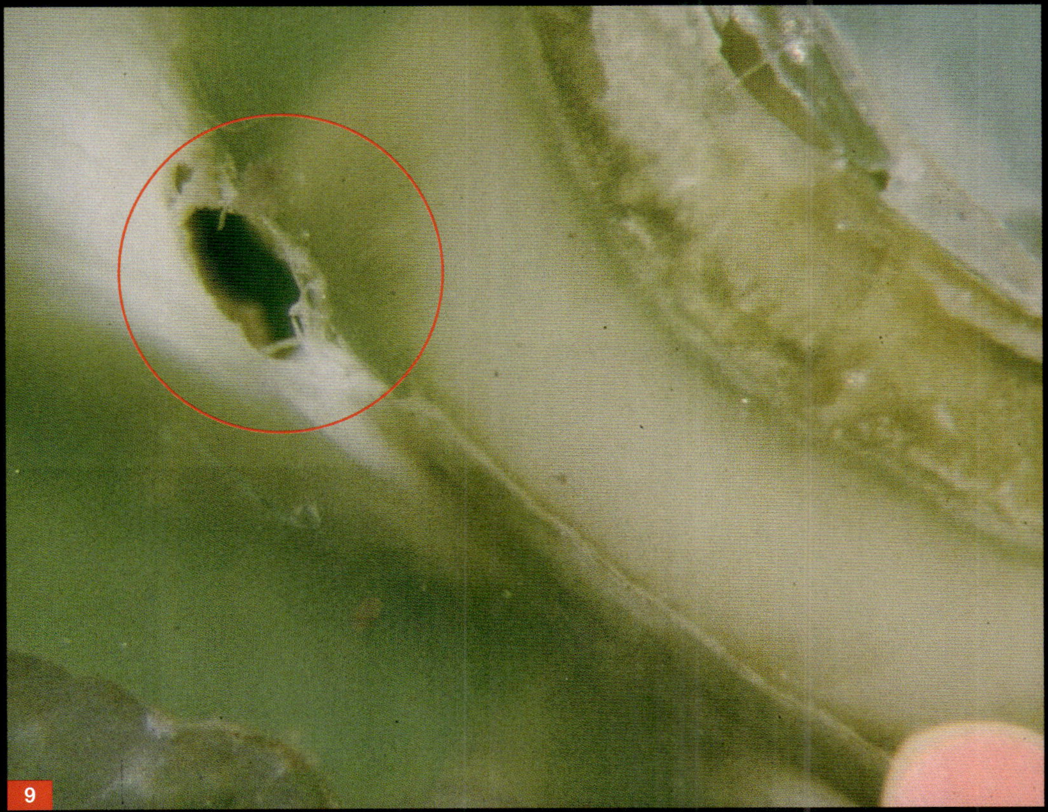

9

Figure 9: The same picture at higher magnification.

Figure 10a: An upper premolar in which an unconventional anatomy is suspected.

Figure 10b: Postoperative x-ray showing the complex anatomy of the tooth and the presence of three root canals and an accessory lateral canal.

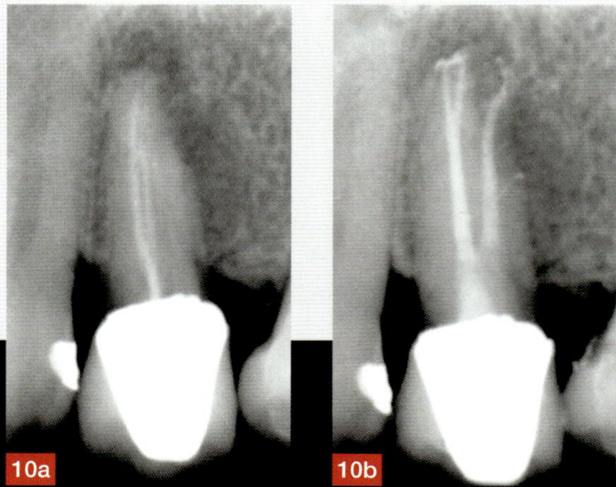

Figure 11a-c: A situation similar to the previous one, involving a premolar with a triradicular conformation that is clearly visible ony the CBCT examination.

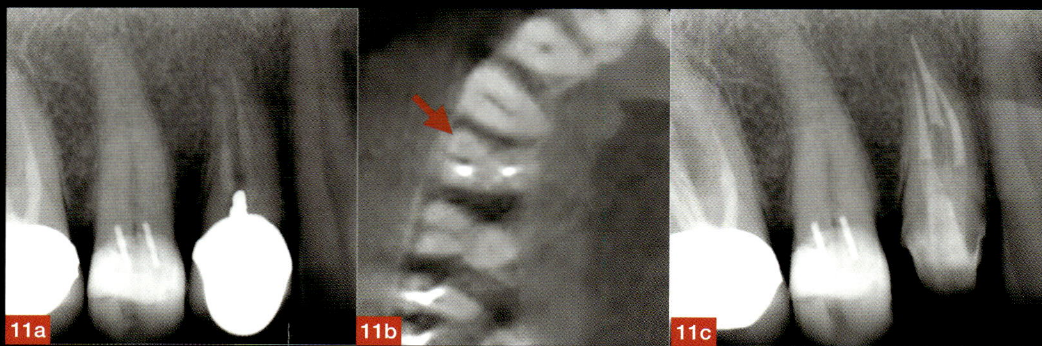

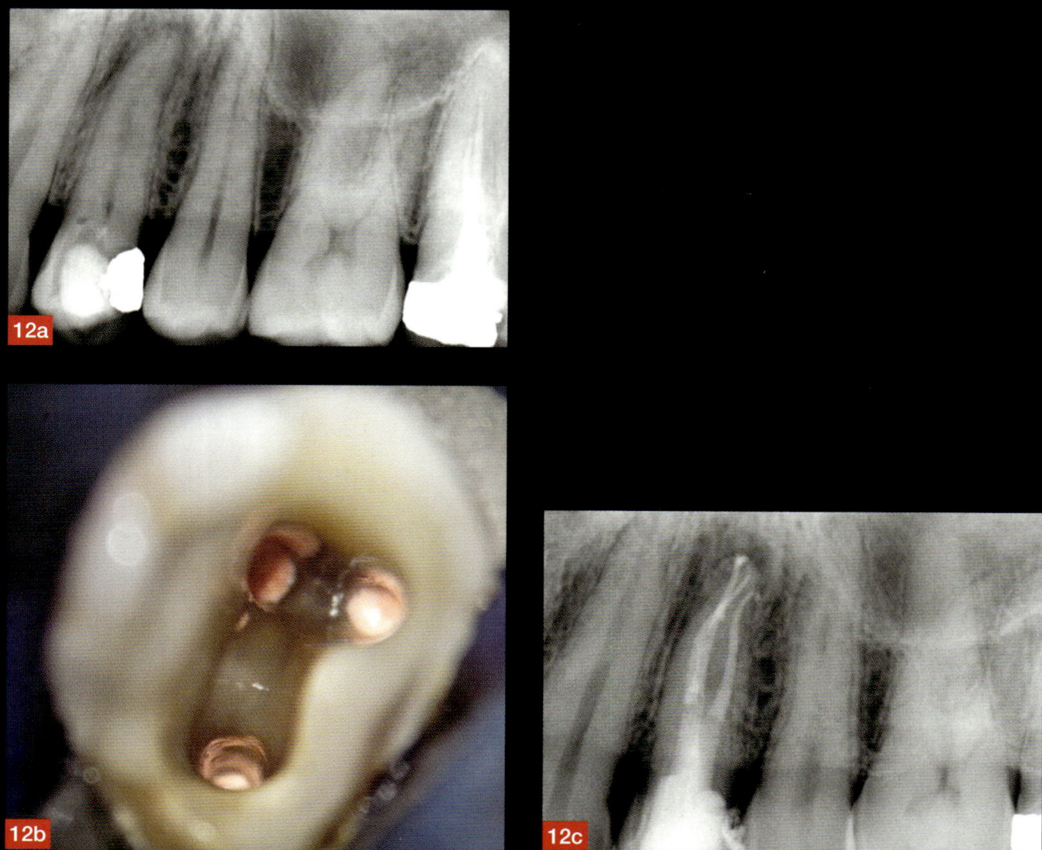

Figure 12a-c:
a) A premolar with three roots;
b) the intra-chamber appearance of the three canals;
c) the filling carried out according to the state of the art.

Complex anatomies in posterior teeth: a double challenge

CASE REPORT 9-18

Complex anatomies can present a challenge in routine root canal treatment; in cases of retreatment, the challenges are even greater due to the presence of further endodontic obstacles, such as a poor root canal filling or tenacious sealer, a ledge or a fractured instrument, a perforation or stripping; all these elements could be difficult to overcome individually and even more challenging when concomitant.

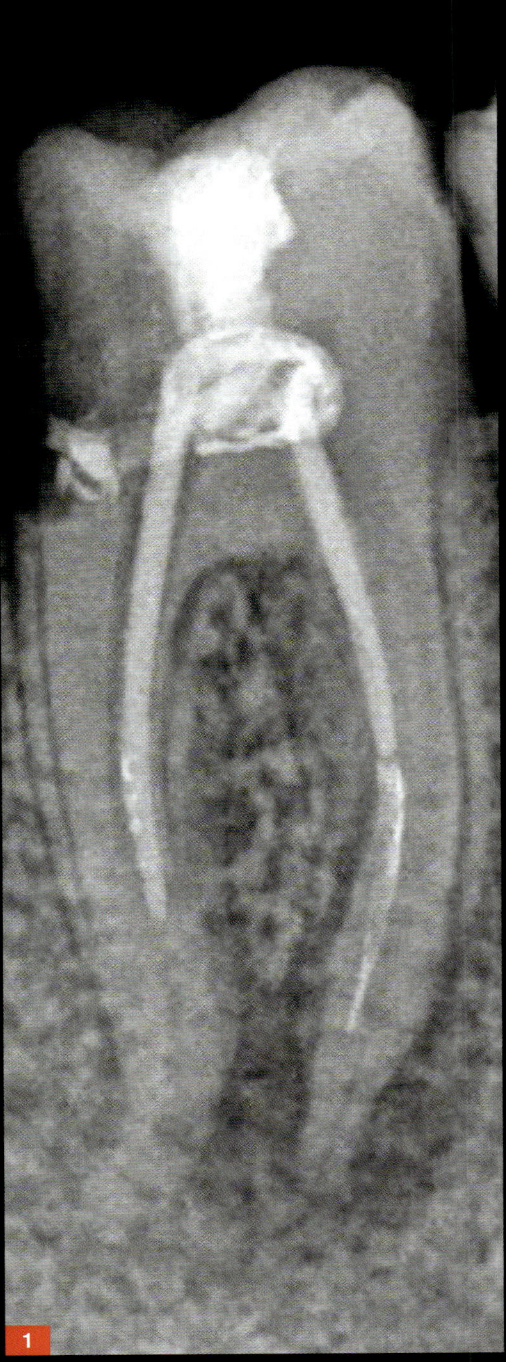

1

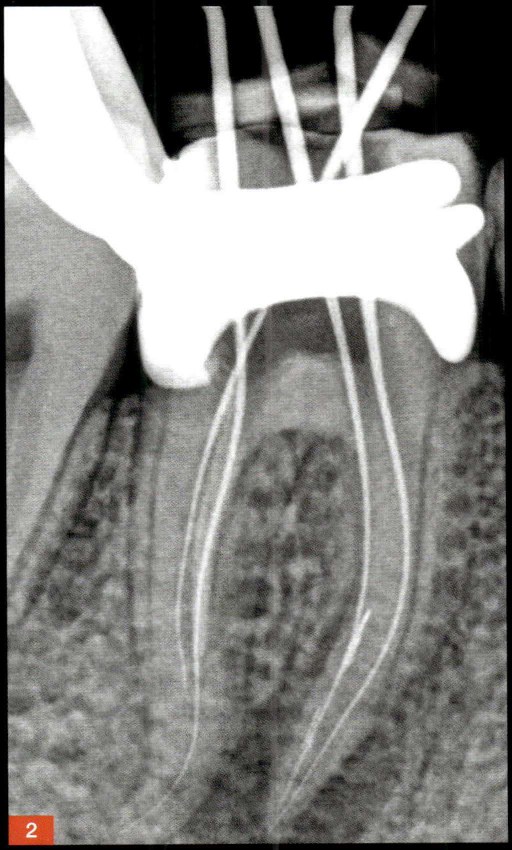

2

In this lower molar with a large carious lesion and a huge periapical inflammatory reaction a retreatment is advisable; the root canals have been poorly treated and the filling is inadequate, a broken instrument is observed in the mesial root. The strategy to adopt in cases like this should be properly planned before the clinical phase as the risk of canal blockages is particularly high. Disinfection protocols and ultrasonic devices are important tools in these clinical conditions.

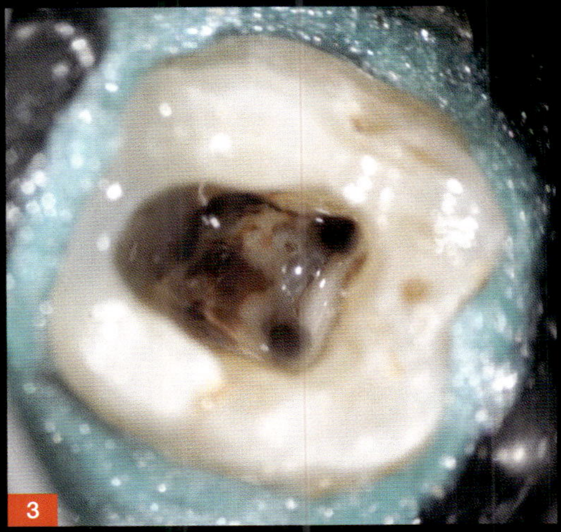

3

Figures 1-3: The endodontic access reveals an incomplete pulp chamber opening.

CASE REPORT 10

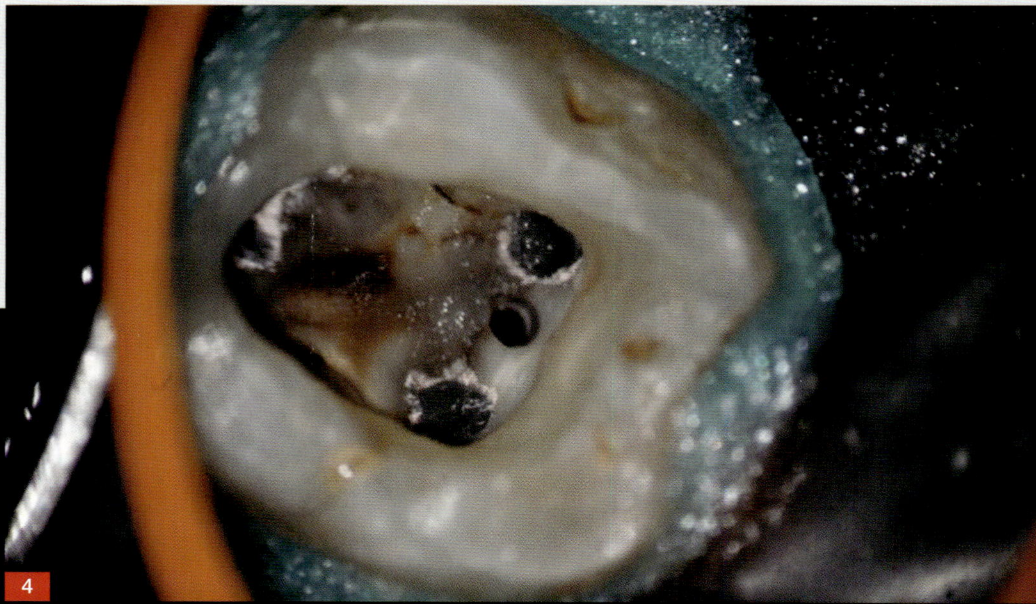

4

Figures 4-5: A median mesial canal was found, instrumented and sealed.

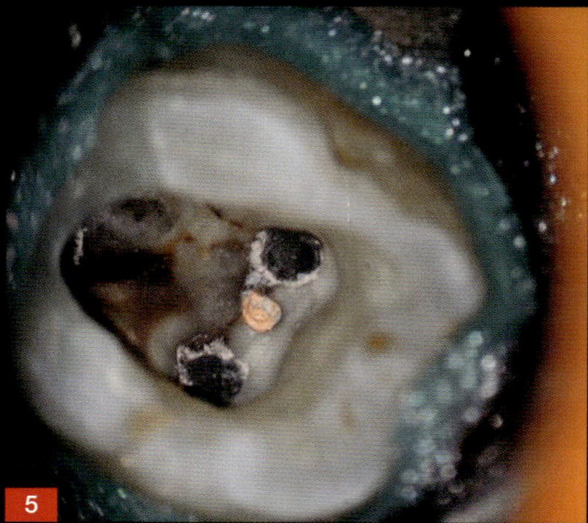

5

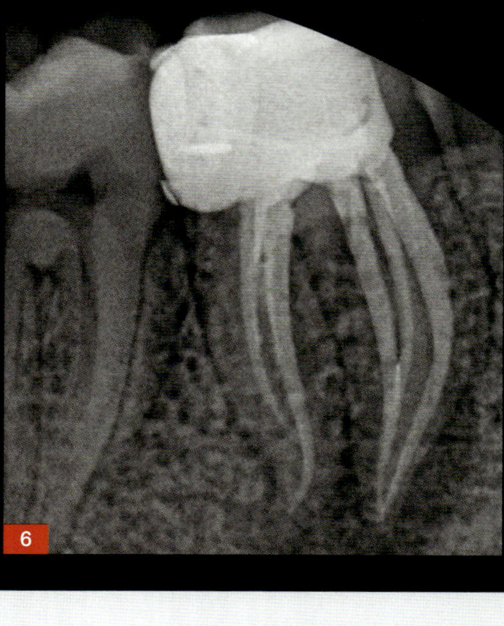

6

Figure 6: The final radiographic follow-up shows a correct filling of the whole endodontic space, the periapical lesion has a wide extension around the mesial root.

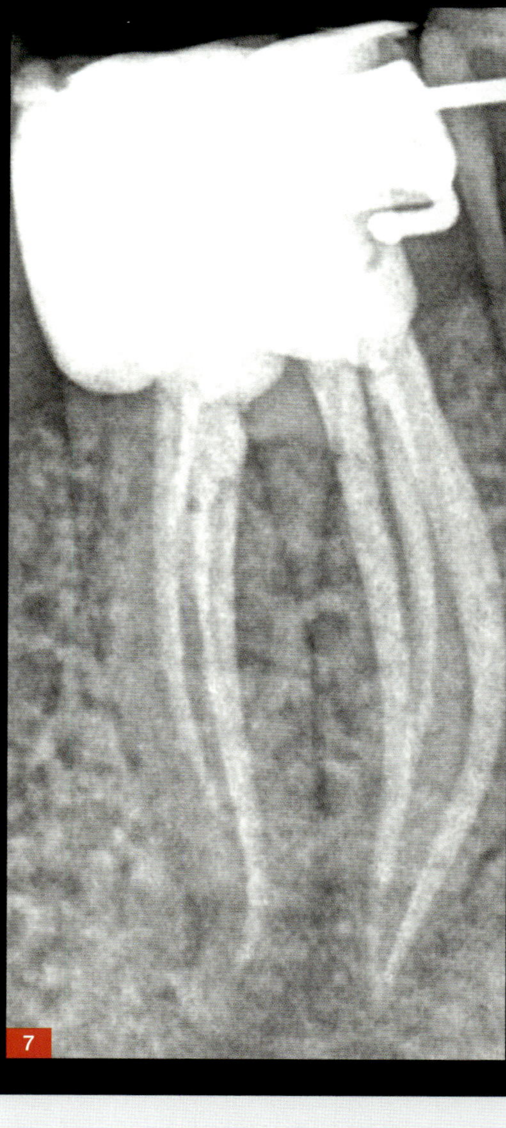

7

Figure 7: The one-year follow-up reveals a satisfactory healing process.

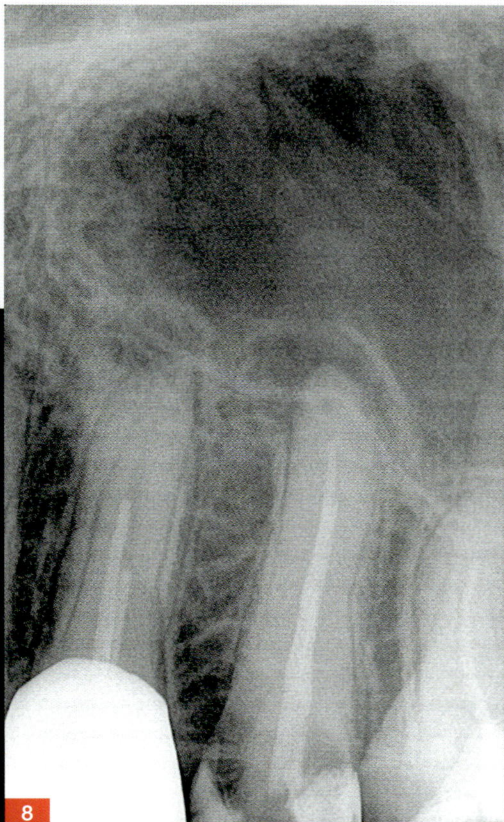

8

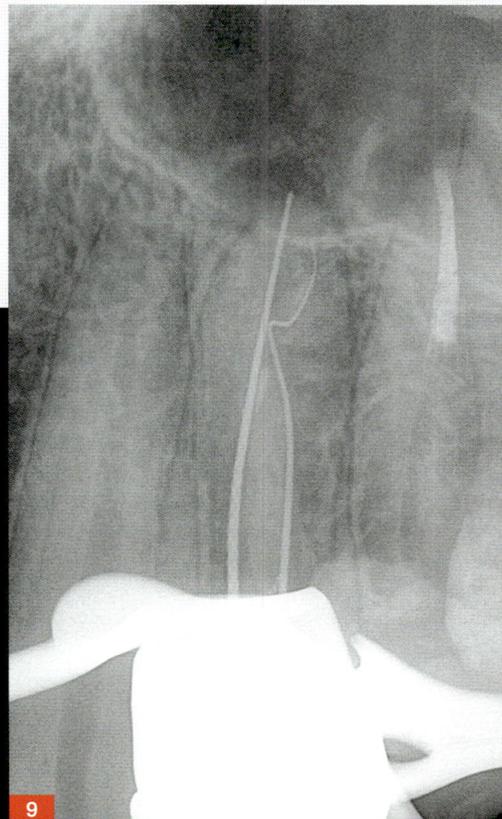

9

CASE REPORT 11

Figures 8-9: Upper premolars are always insidious teeth due to the huge number of possible anatomical variations; in the case presented the x-ray reveals a relatively simple root canal anatomy but the examination of the root canal reveals a confluence in the middle third.

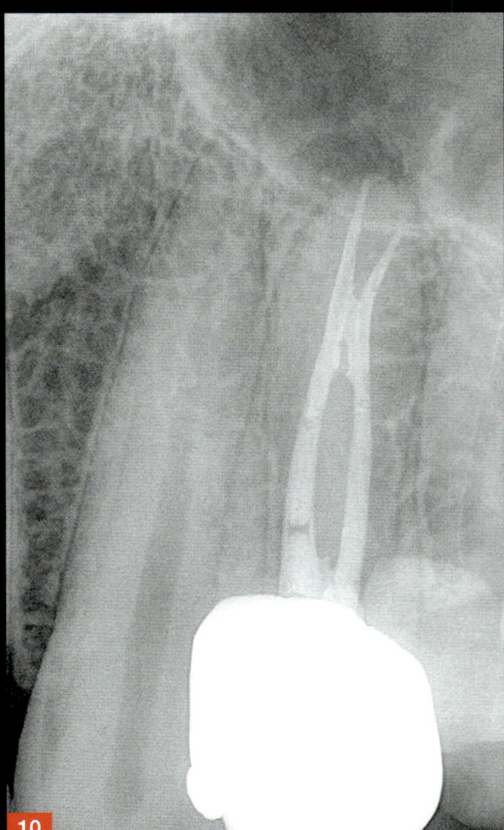

10

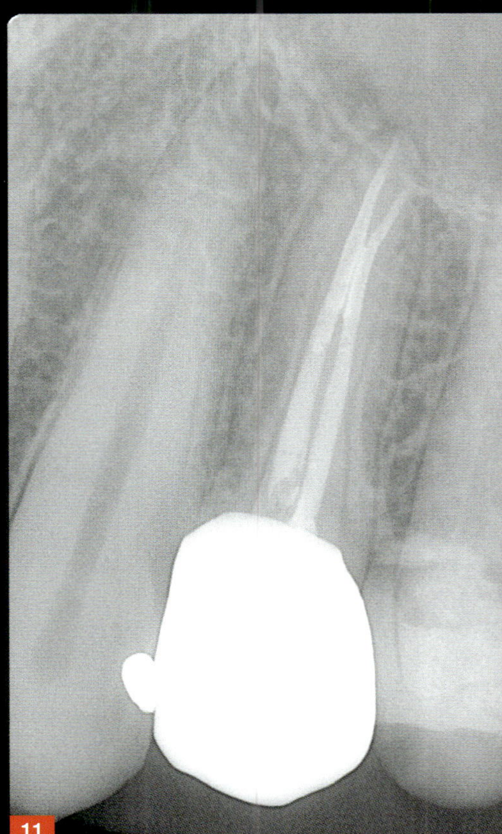

11

Figures 10-11: The sealing was optimal and the follow-up examination confirms a complete resolution of the periapical radiolucency.

CASE REPORT 12

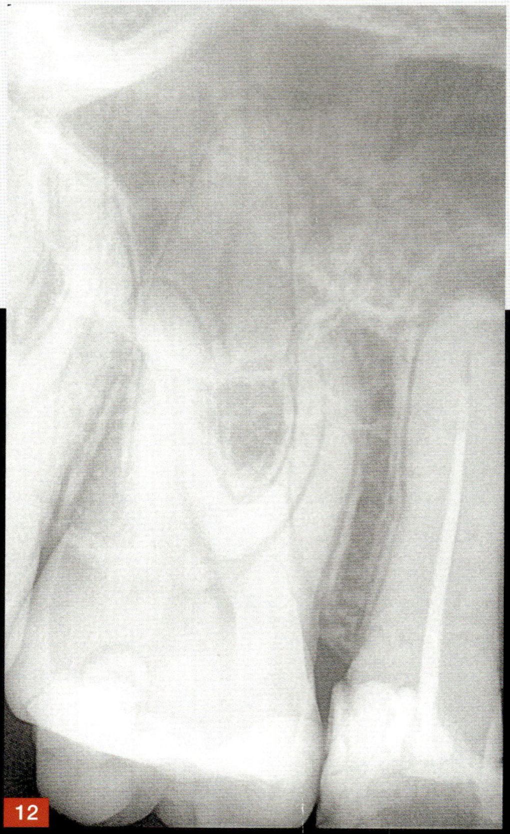

12

Figure 12: An incomplete root canal treatment should be retreated; an apical bifurcation was assessed and shaping was performed.

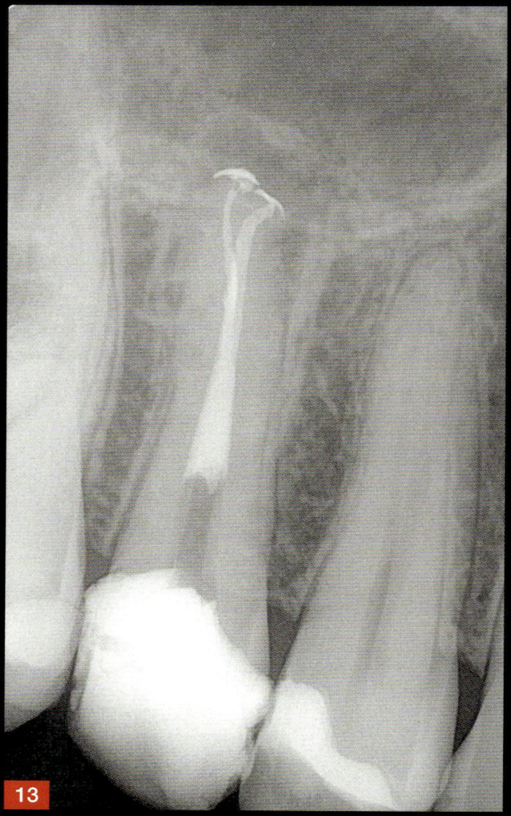

13

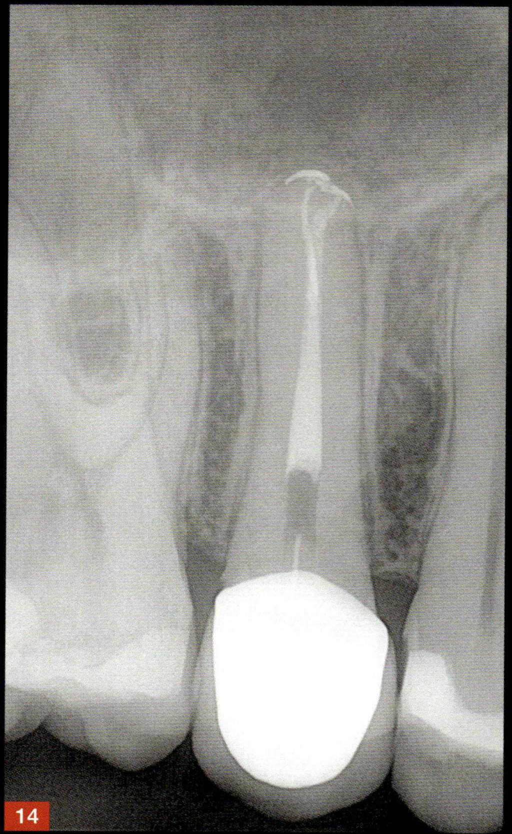

14

Figures 13-14: The final radiographical examination at the end of the treatment and the follow-up after one year (Fig. 14) confirm the success of retreatment.

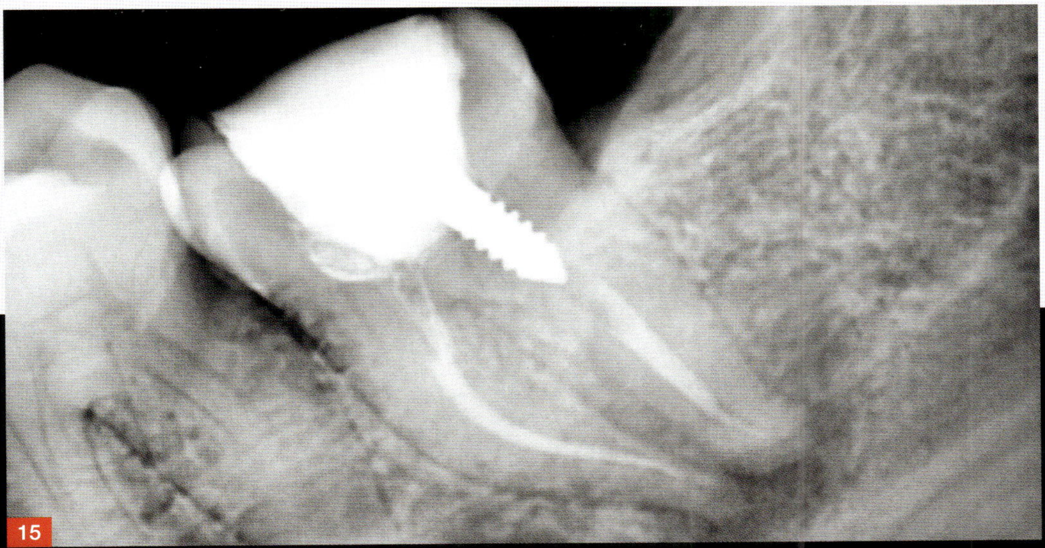

15

CASE REPORT 13

A thorough examination of the initial x-ray is a fundamental pre-requisite for planning a correct retreatment strategy; in this lower molar a vast periapical lesion surrounds the distal root.

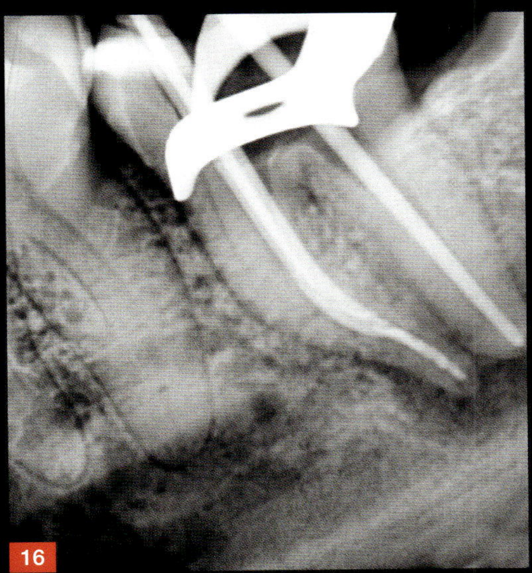

16

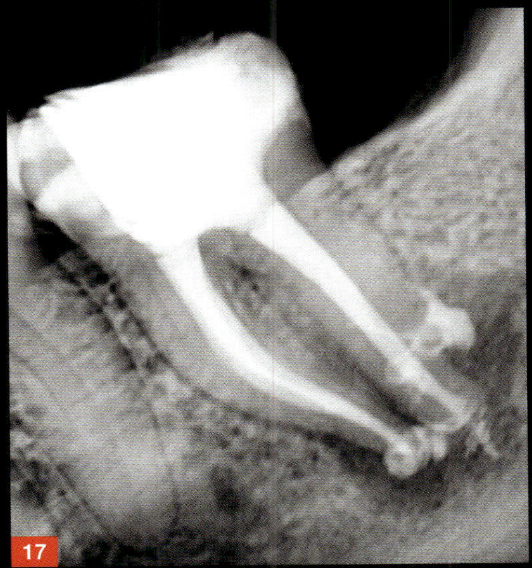

17

Figure 15: An apical delta should be suspected.

Figure 16: Careful irrigation procedures can clean the entire root canal system and lead to the sealing phase.

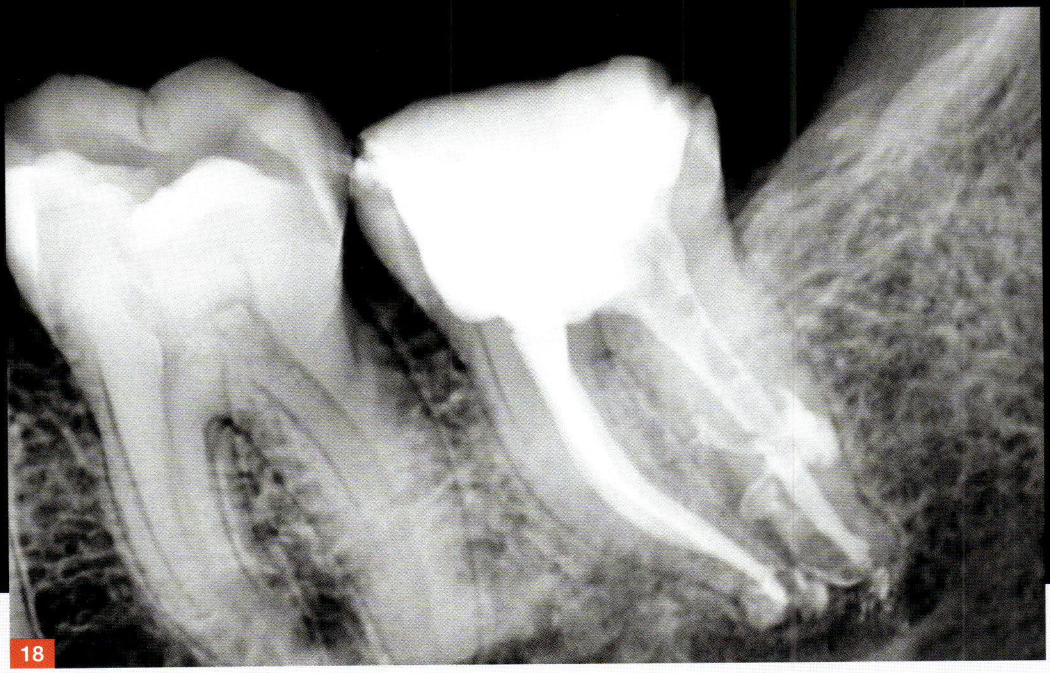

18

Figure 17: Several lateral canals were identified after vertical compaction of warm gutta-percha.

Figure 18: The extra-canalar excesses are seen to be depleted on the follow-up x-ray.

CASE REPORT 14

Figure 19: A relatively simple anatomy in an upper first molar is examined by pre-operative X-ray; although it might be considered an easy case, during instrumentation, particularly during the scouting phase a double apical curvature was identified. The shaping relatively dure might be conservative in order to preserve the morphology of the apical part.

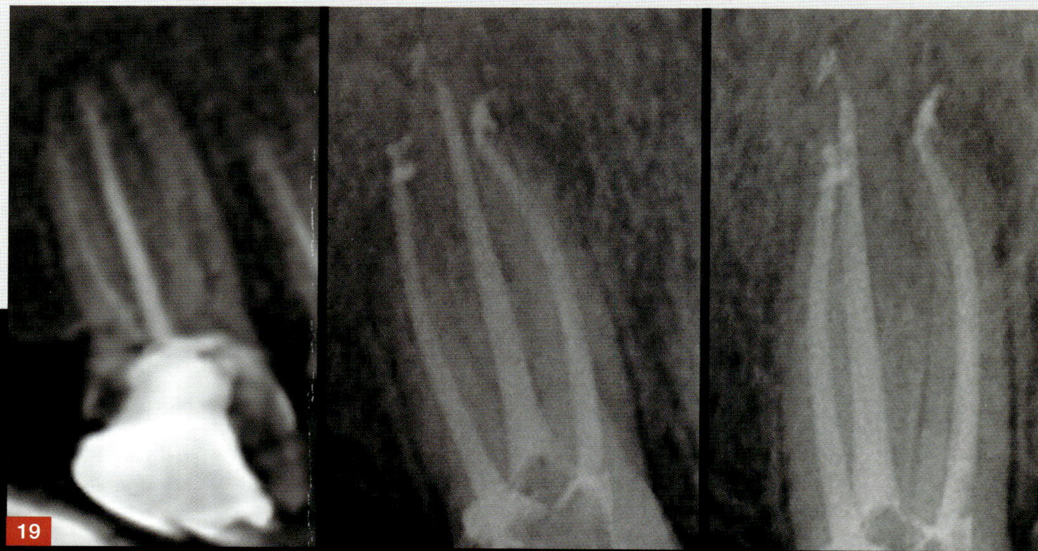

CASE REPORT 15

Figures 20a-c: Shaping procedures were accomplished focusing on dentine preservation and respect of the apical limit of the whole root canal system. The high point of confluence of the mesial root canals should be noted.

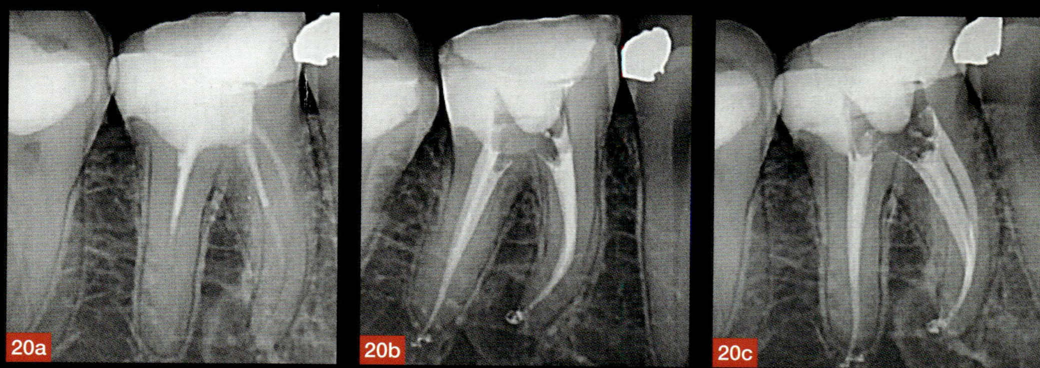

CASE CANALS 6

Figures 21a-c: A double convergence in the mesio-buccal and mesio-lingual canals were detected; a proper shaping of the endodontic space lead to a complete filling of both the root canals up to the apex.

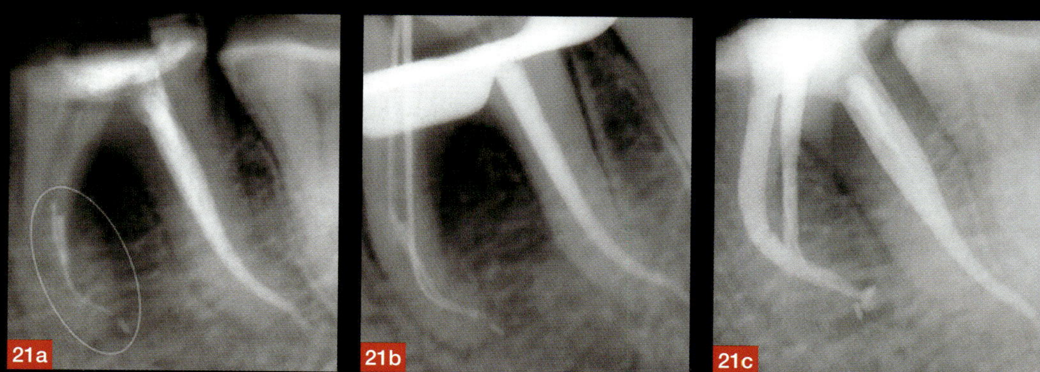

CASE REPORT 17

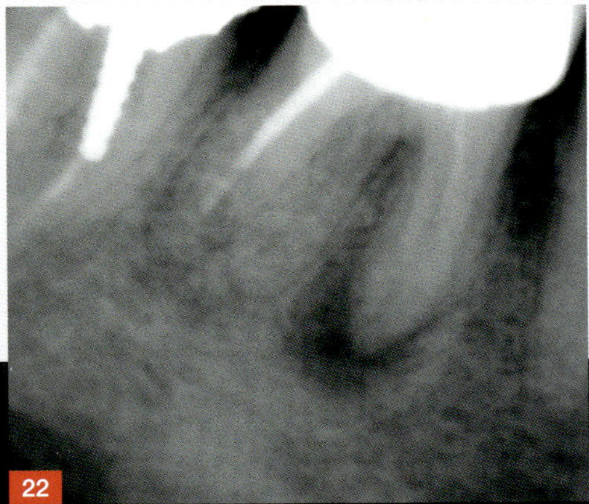

22

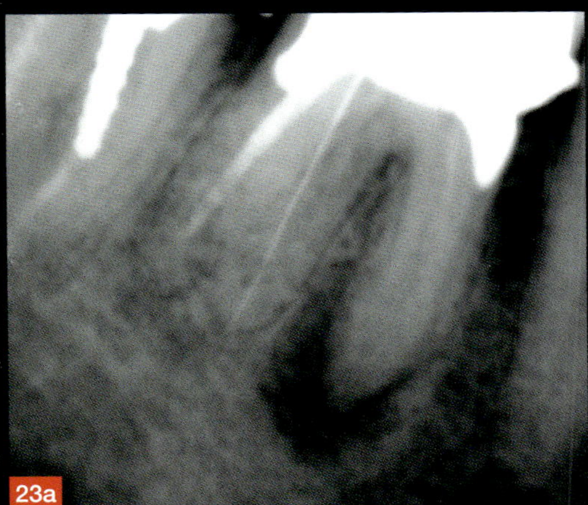

23a

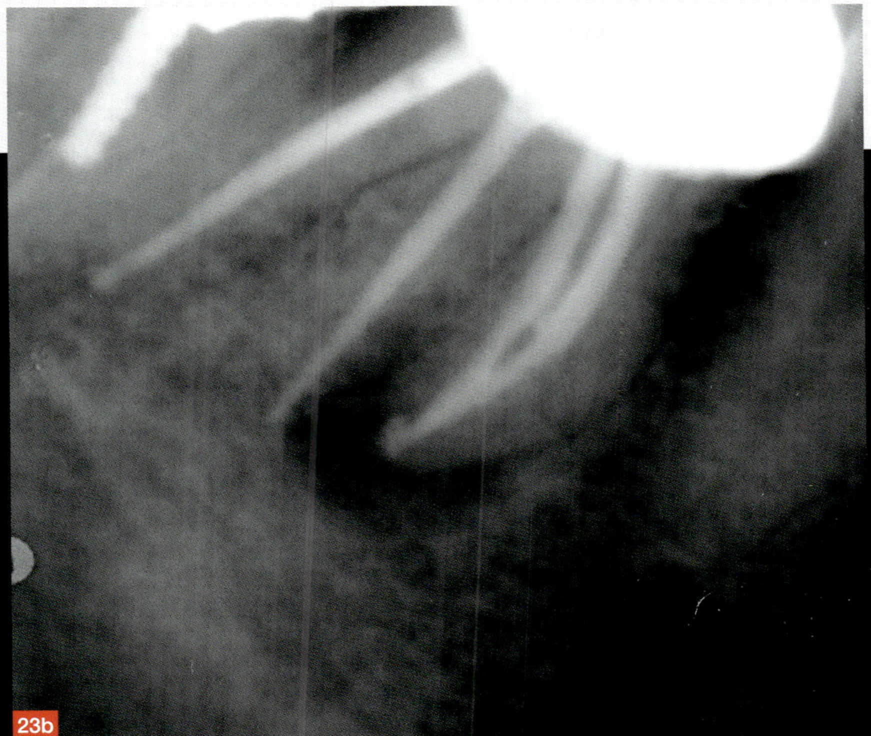

23b

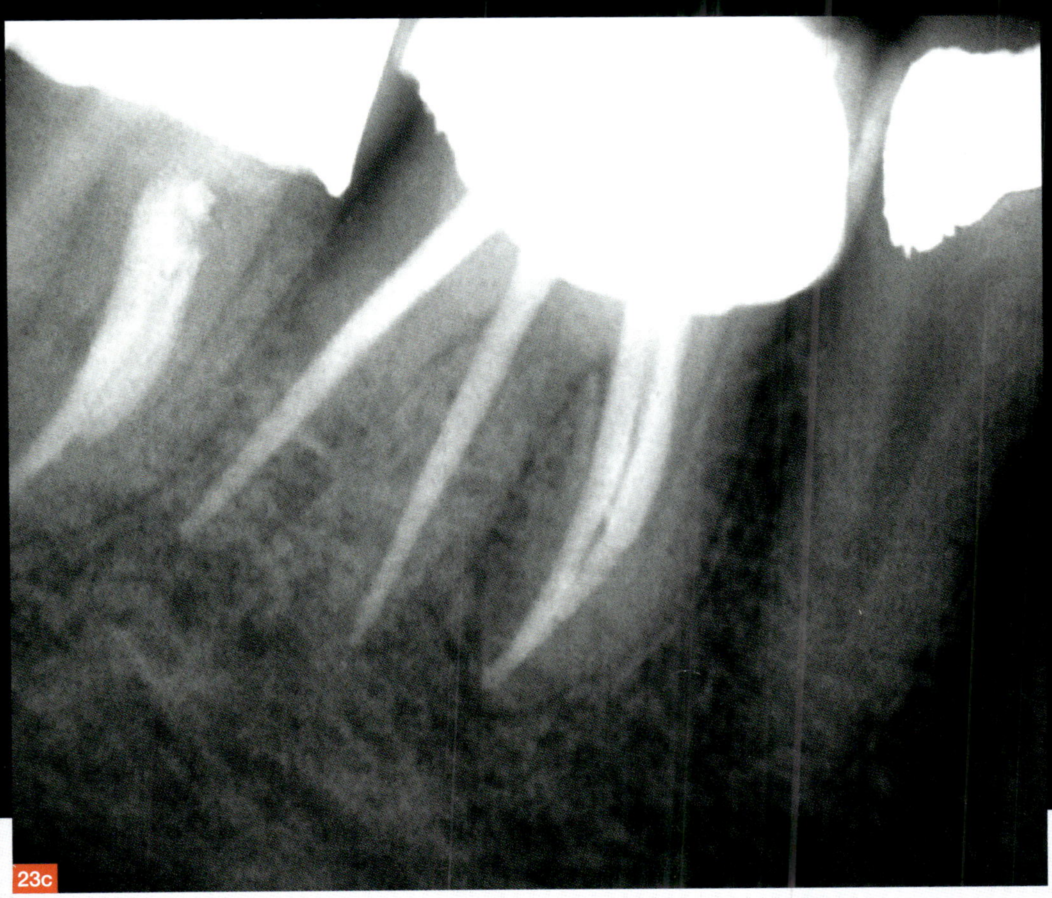

23c

Figure 22: A lower molar with large periapical lesion in mesial root and a double distal root, i.e. the so called "radix-enthomolaris".

Figures 23a-c: A radix enthomolaris case in lower first premolar, a different x-ray projection might be useful to identify these anatomical feature not uncommon in these teeth.

CASE REPORT 18

Root canal in the distal root of a lower molar is frequently neglected in shaping procedures; it is considered an easy root canal shape but, as shown in Figures 24-27, an abrupt curvature was identified and instrumented.

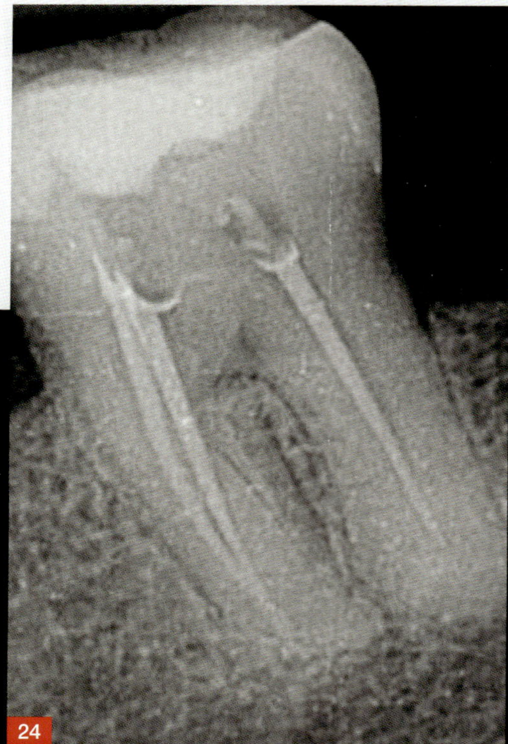

24

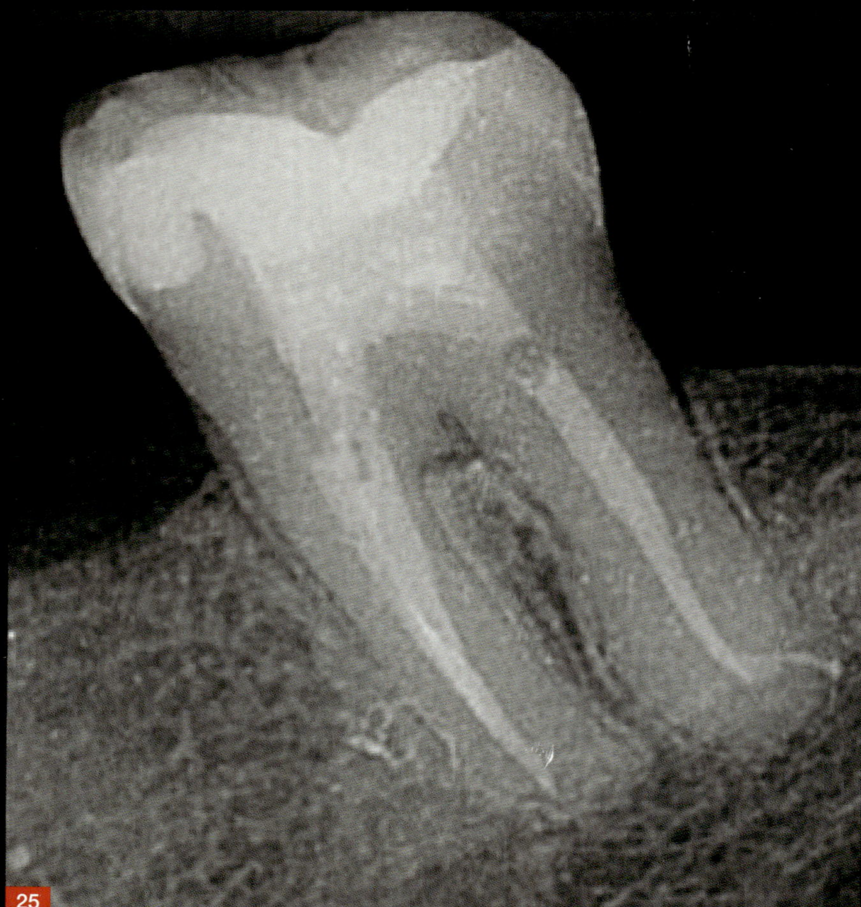

25

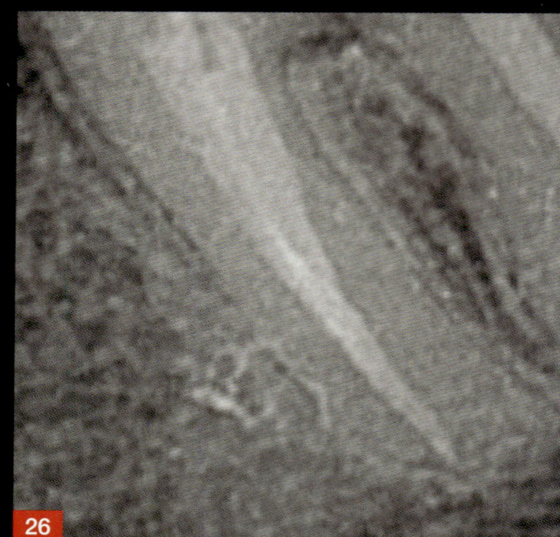

26

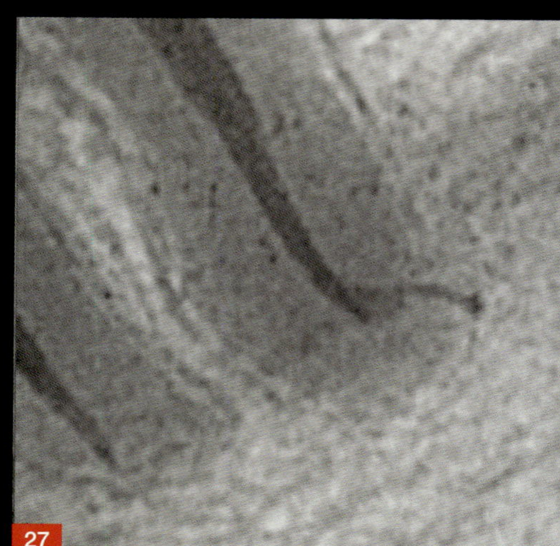

27

CASE REPORT 19

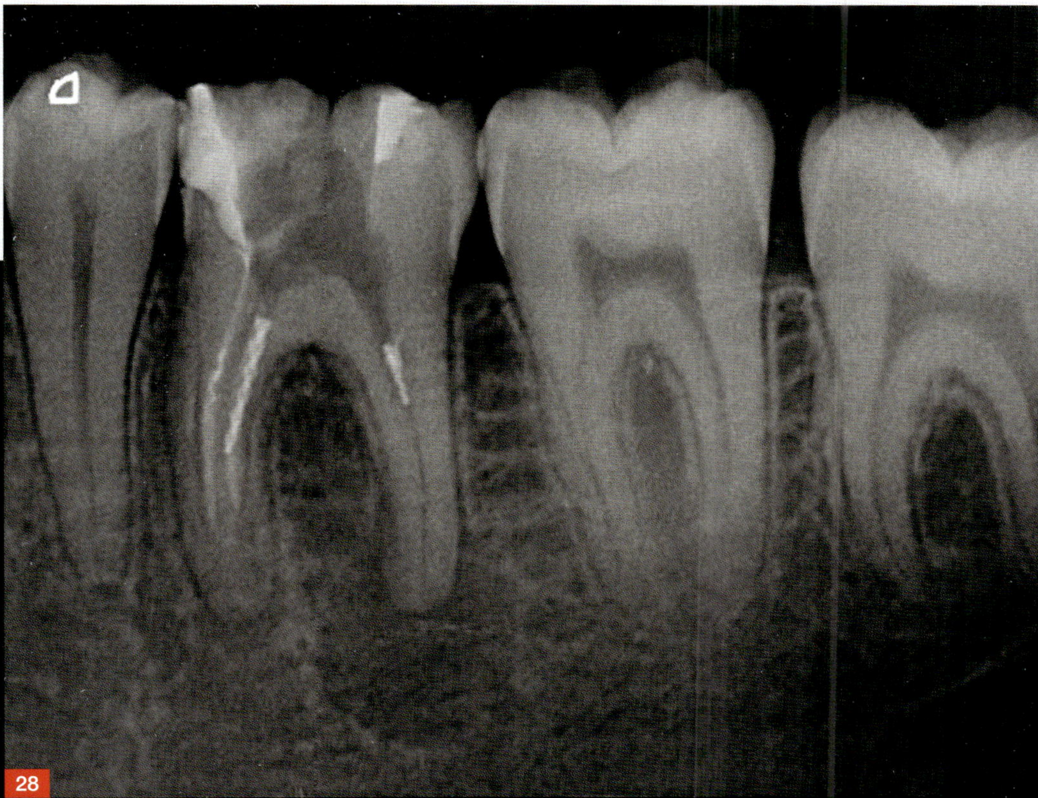

28

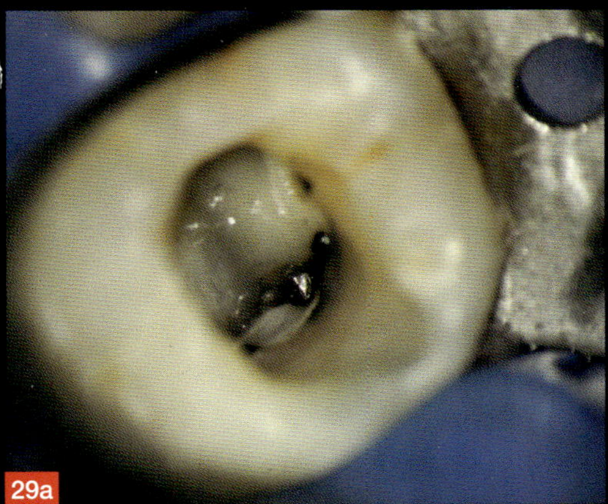

29a

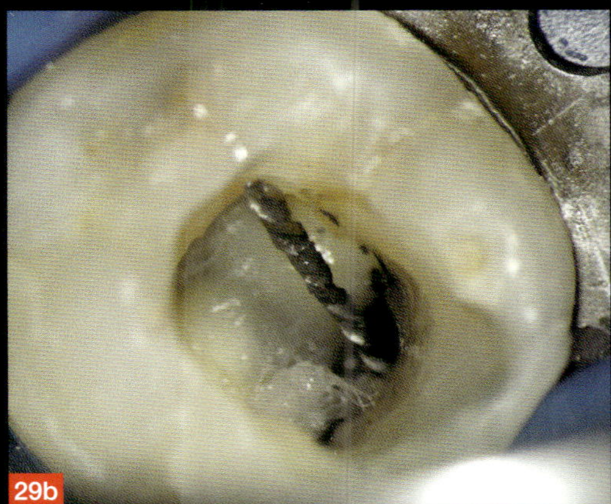

29b

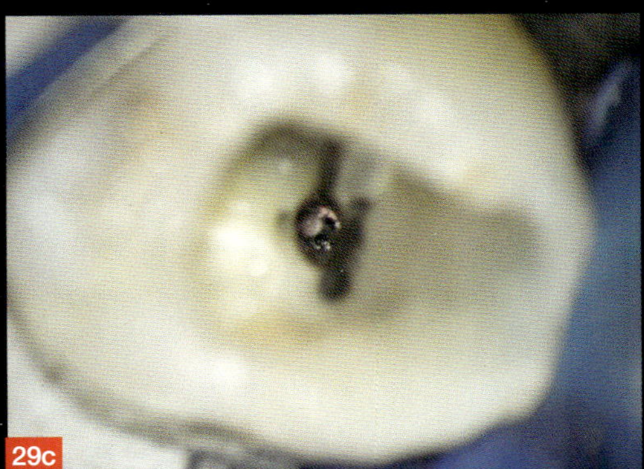

29c

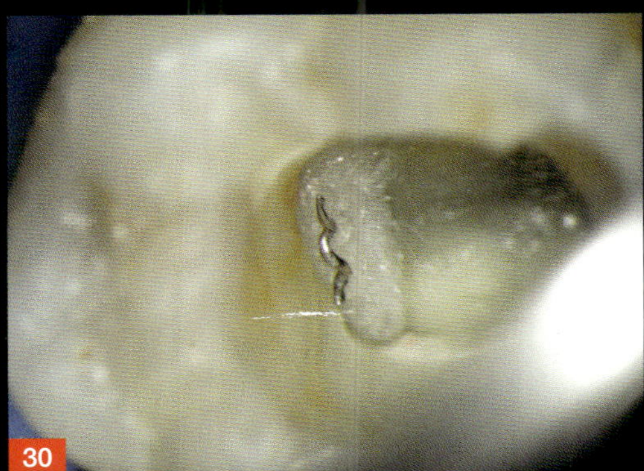

30

In Figure 28 a lower molar is to be retreated due to a large area of periapical radiolucency of endodontic origin; the removal of the three broken instruments could be the major challenge in this case, but a careful observation of the distal root reveals an abnormal extension of the periapical inflammatory reaction. A wider distal root canal should be suspected. Retrieving the instruments was the first step (Fig. 29 a-c)

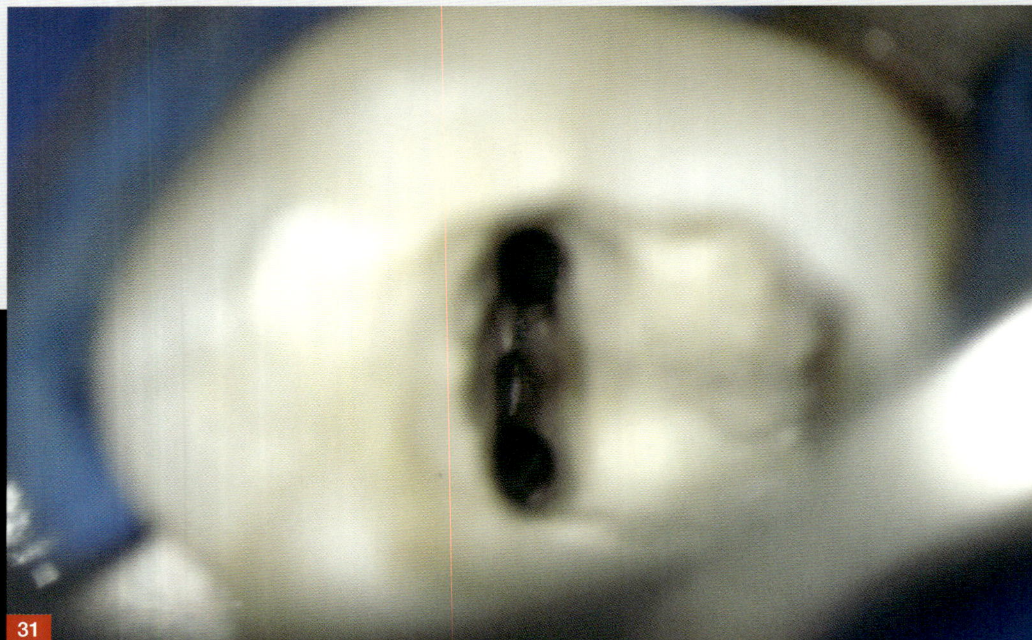
31

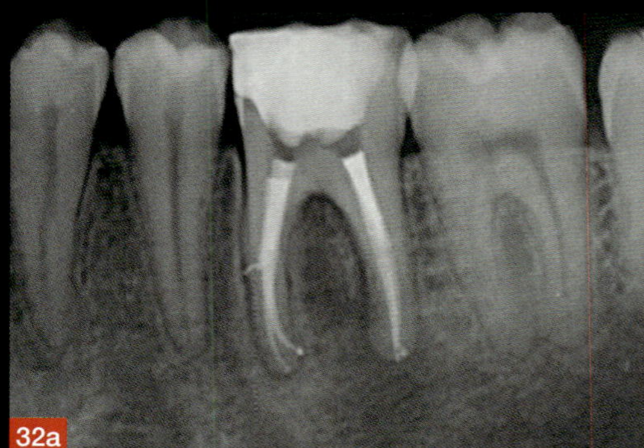
32a

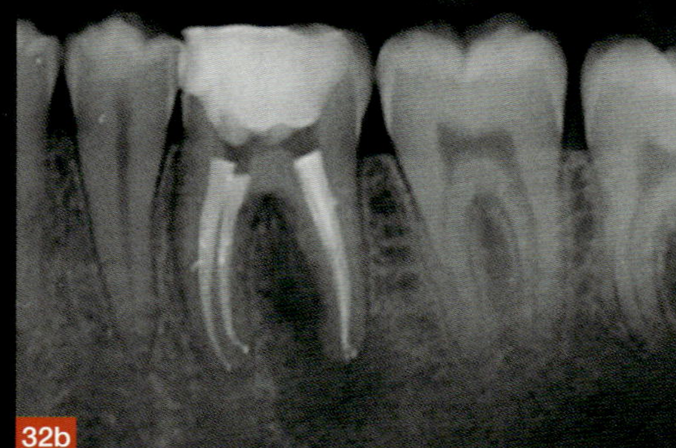
32b

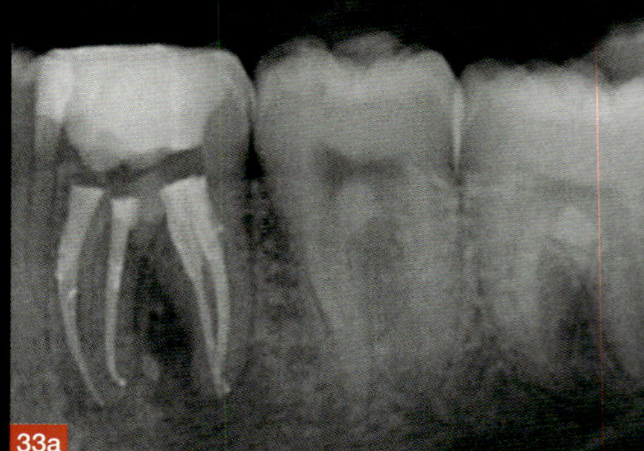
33a

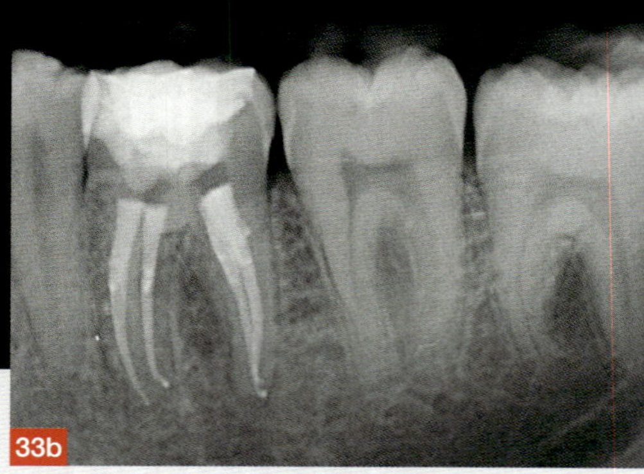
33b

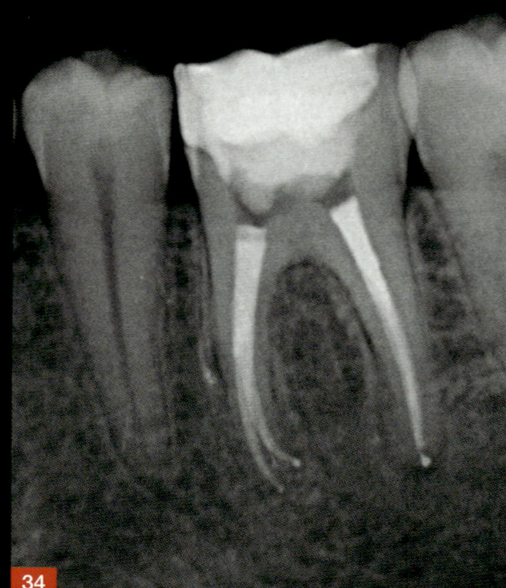
34

Figures 31-34: A wider opening of the distal root canal revealed a double-distal canal, converging at the apex; associated instrumentation with several checks of canal patency is the preferred shaping technique for obtaining a correct root canal morphology at the end of the retreatment.

Fractured instruments: therapeutic solutions

In the context of retreatment, the presence of one or more broken instruments inside the endodontium is not an uncommon occurrence[91-93] (Fig. 3.70).
The use of the surgical microscope, associated with devices such as ultrasound and extractors, allows the removal of most fragments. A correct preoperative evaluation[94], facilitated by the use of appropriate instruments and by practicing a correct access to the endodontium, can successfully allow the removal of broken instruments in more than 80% of all cases[95-97]. Furthermore, even in cases where the operator decides to bypass the use of instruments, the prognosis is still excellent[98].
However, during the preoperative phase, the clinician should evaluate the possibility of removing the fractured instrument or undergoing a new therapeutic solution, in relation to the endodontic and reconstructive prognosis[99, 100].
Before proceeding with the operative phase, the operator should thoroughly analyze the preoperative radiograph and the CBCT, if available, to determine the following:

- In which root canal the fractured instrument is located
- The size and the length of the fragment
- The type of instrument (try to understand, from the type of radiopacity of the fragment, what material it is made of)
- The position of the fragment in the root canal
- The anatomical characteristics of the root canal (length, curvatures, wall thickness)
- The possibility of obtaining a straight access to most of the coronal part of the fragment.

The type of instruments available to clinicians will allow them to choose whether to perform the operation personally or to refer the patient to a colleague who has the appropriate tools to effectuate this therapy (microscope, ultrasound, and extractors)[101]. More sophisticated techniques that involve the dissolution of instruments through galvanic processes[102-104] remain to be evaluated.
Nonetheless, if the tooth is to be preserved, there are three main therapeutic solutions:

1. Extracting the instrument
2. Incorporating it into the subsequent filling
3. Performing endodontic surgery.

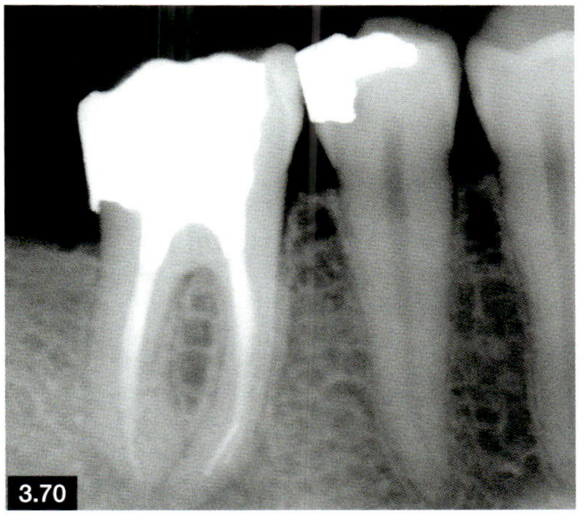

Fig. 3.70: Tooth with fractured instrument in the apical third of the mesial root.
This inconvenience is quite common when rotary instruments are used incorrectly [87, 88].

Box 3.4 CAUSES OF INSTRUMENT FAILURE

Understanding the main cause of instrument failure can help and guide the clinician in choosing the optimal technique for removing or by-passing the instrument (Table 3.8).
If the portion of the instrument is small and located in the apical region, a torsional stress fracture may be assumed. In this case, the rotating instrument may have encountered a narrower canal section compared to the tip, thus resulting in the tip being blocked, while the more coronal portion continues to rotate thereby causing instrument fractures. The same fracture mechanism is associated with obstructions due to the taper, which is generally accompanied by the fracture of a larger portion of the instrument that is not necessarily in the region of the apical third of the root[100, 101].
If, on the other hand, the broken instrument fracture is longer than 4-5 mm, and is located in the vicinity of or just beyond a curvature, especially in cases where its radius is large, one can assume a cyclic fatigue fracture mechanism[102]. In this case the instrument rotating in a curve, is subjected to two forces that simultaneously contract and stretch it. Consequently, the persistence of these forces induces a coronal fracture at the point where these forces are applied.

INSTRUMENT REMOVAL PROCEDURE

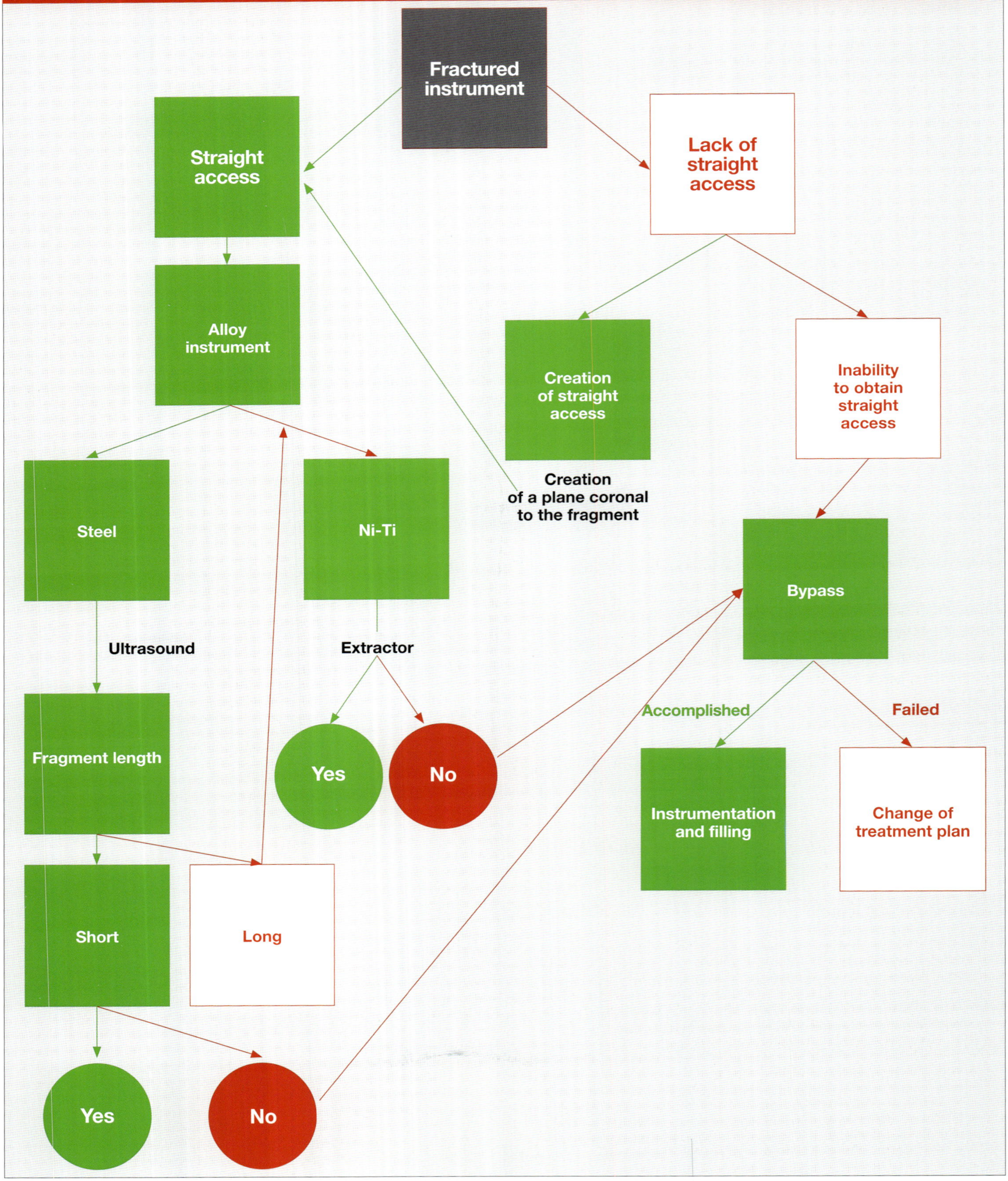

Several factors influence the possible removal of broken instruments from root canals:

1. The root canal anatomy
2. The location of the fragment
3. The type of instrument.

1. Canal anatomy (see diagram)

The possibility of removing or by-passing the fractured instrument depends on:

- The shape and diameter of the root canal
- The presence of curvatures or concavities
- The thickness of the dentin in the area where the fragment is located.

2. Location of the fragment (see diagram)

The position of the broken instrument inside the root canal influences the operator's choice. If the broken instrument is located in the coronal portion of the tooth, and provided there is a straight access, the chances of removal are high[103]. If the fractured instrument is located in the middle third of the root canal and before a curvature, the possibility of removal is associated with the likelihood of reaching the most coronal portion of the instrument. If this is not considered feasible, then the alternative option of bypassing the instrument would be a good strategy. On the other hand, if the instrument is beyond a curvature, the only option is to try and bypass it[104, 105].

The possibility of removing the fractured intracanal instrument also depends on the type of instrument. For instance, a steel file is generally easier to remove than a Ni-Ti file, which can be firmly inserted into the canal walls.The length of the fractured portion should also be considered, as this may affect the method of removal. It therefore goes without say that extraction techniques can vary according to the circumstances.

ELEMENTS OF CANAL ANATOMY: RISK FACTORS

Most coronal areas have greater dentin thicknesses. In the molars, as shown in the image, the dentin has a larger volume in the mesial areas and it is in these areas that it will be necessary to remove more material in order to free the fractured instrument inside the endodontium.

Area 1 - mesial: maximum security.
Area 1 - distal: maximum risk of perforations.

Area 2 - mesial: maximum security.
Area 2 - distal: high risk of erosion of the dentin wall.

Area 3 - mesial and distal: high-risk areas. Endodontic surgery could be the best choice.

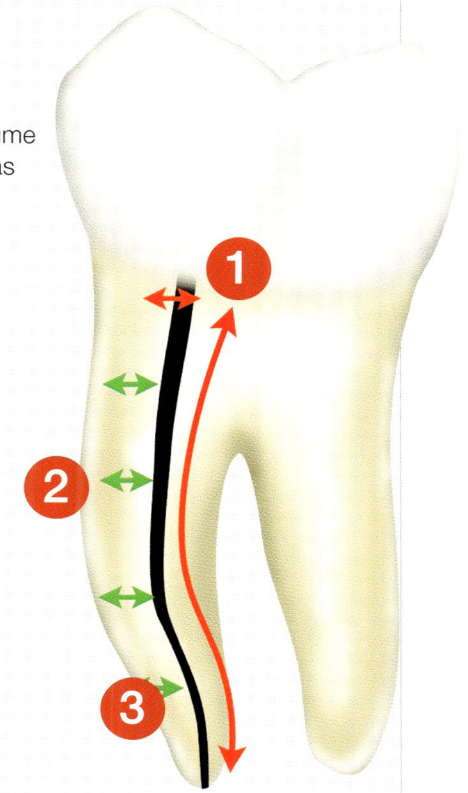

LOCATION OF THE FRAGMENT: RISK FACTORS

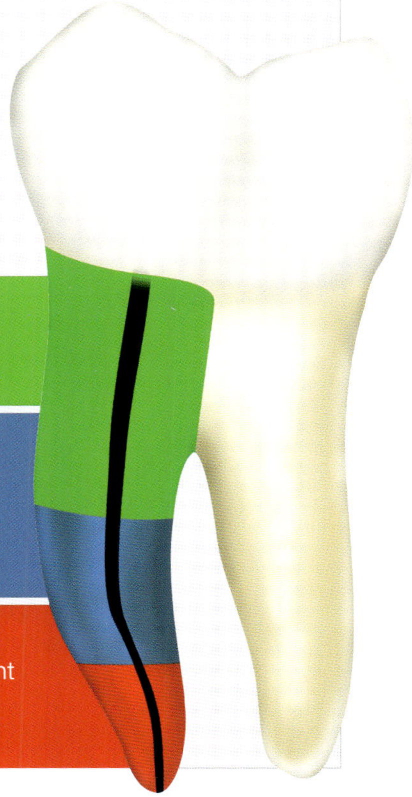

Fractured instruments in this area of the canal can be removed with a higher success rate.

The middle-apical third area poses a number of questions: the choice of either extracting the instrument or bypassing it, depends on the position of the fragment and the anatomy of this area.

Areas where removal appears to be very risky. In these areas, the instrument can be bypassed, otherwise endodontic surgery is required.

3. Type of instrument (see Table 3.8)

Table 3.8 **REMOVAL OF FRACTURED INSTRUMENTS BASED ON THEIR TYPE**

Type of fractured instruments	Means of removal	Clinical procedures
Hand-tools such as a k-file or reamer	Ultrasound Delicate tools	Difficulties vary according to the location, the length, and the anatomy of the tooth.
Hand-tools such as a Hedström file (H-file)	Ultrasound Delicate tools	The difficulties are similar to those indicated for k-files or reamers, but must take into account the particular morphology of the H-file.
Ni-Ti mechanical tools	Ultrasound Delicate tools	Removal can be more difficult because the instrument is flexible and always tends to rest against the root walls, making a grip difficult.
Lentulo spirals	Ultrasound	Removal can be very complex.
Ultrasonically-activated instrument parts (tips, k-files)	Ultrasound	The difficulties vary according to the location, the length, and the anatomy of the tooth.

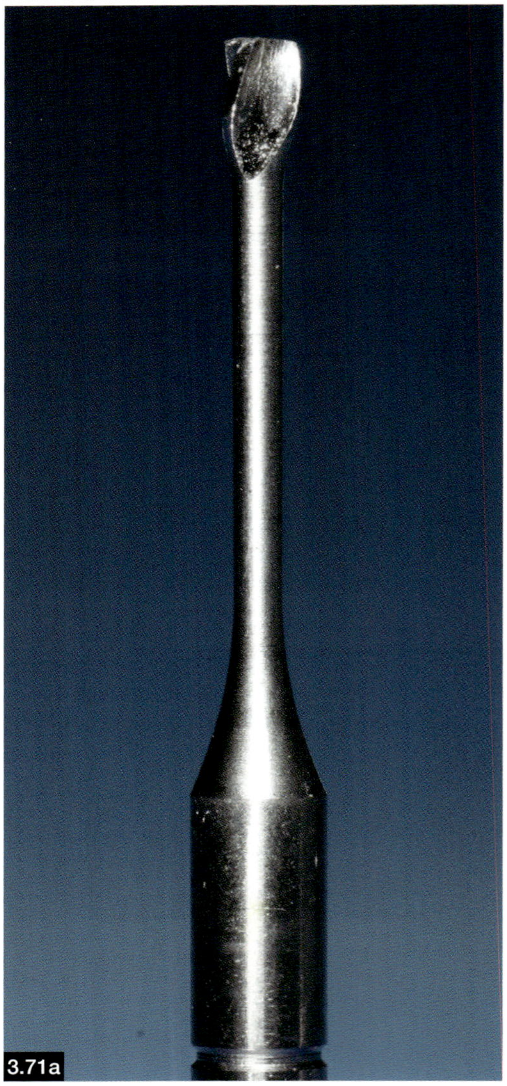

3.71a

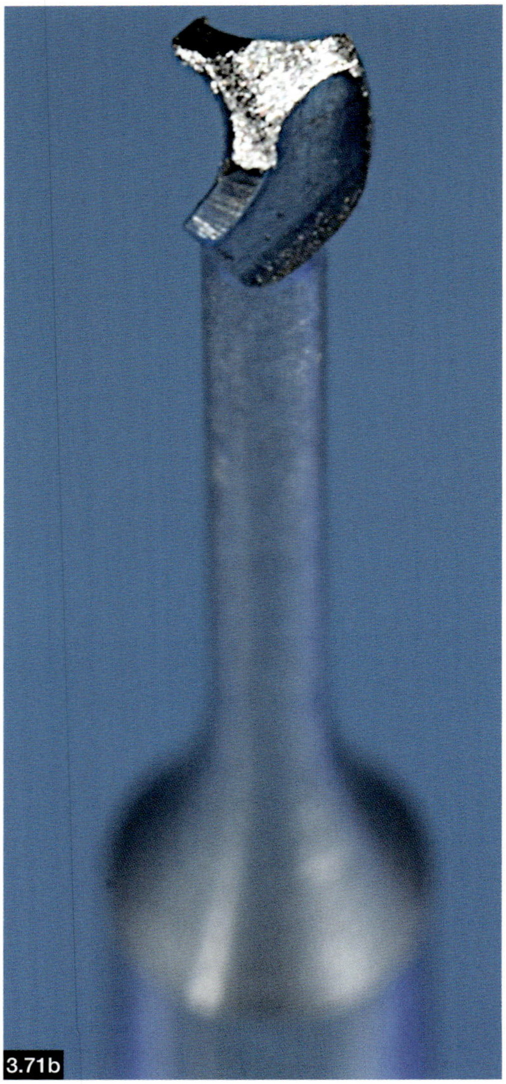

3.71b

Fig. 3.71a-b: a) Example of GG milling burr modified at the top to make deep cutting more effective (b) detail of the tip of the bur.

Clinical aids for the removal of fractured instruments

In addition to certain clinical competence and experience, the removal of a broken instrument from a root canal requires several instruments without which subsequent interventions can be ineffective or even detrimental to the long-term prognosis of the tooth. Some of these instruments are common to other retreatment techniques, and represent essential equipment for these types of clinical procedures.
The tools needed to extract a fractured instrument from a root canal are the following:

- **Gates Glidden burs.** The Gates Glidden (GG) (Maillefer; Switzerland) 1 to 6 burs have maximum diameters of 0.5, 0.7, 0.9, 1.1, 1.3 and 1.5 mm, respectively, and they are used to create an access to the root and a uniform funnel taper as far as the obstruction. They can also be used in a modified form, by cutting the tip horizontally in its distal part, thus accentuating cutting effectiveness, as shown in Figure 3.69b.
- **Dedicated ultrasonic tips.** These are stainless steel instruments, some of which are coated with zirconium nitride to improve their cutting life and efficiency. These tips are used in the coronal enlargement at the fragment, in order to create space for the use of additional ultrasonic tips or extractors. Titanium inserts with narrower diameters are also available; they are used at lower power, without a water supply and can move the fragment in deeper and apical spaces (see types on page 161).
- **The Stropko three-way adapter** (Vista Dental, Racine, Wisconsin) is used to generate an energetic but not exaggerated jet of compressed air, and allows, if well used, to collimate and direct air selectively in the areas of the operating field where they are necessary.
- **Magnification and lighting.** Microscopes provide variety of magnification options depending on the clinical circumstances, and the use of co-axial light can improve vision in a perfectly illuminated field without any irritating shadows.

Dedicated removal systems

This category includes all the accessories that can be effective in engaging the broken endodontic instrument and removing it from the canal.
Various systems are available.

- **iRS** (Dentsply Tulsa Dental, Tulsa, Oklahoma) is a two-component system designed for the mechanical engagement of broken instruments. It consists of a micro-tube, a small plastic handle to improve vision during positioning, a side window to improve mechanics, and a 45° beveled end to engage the coronal end of the broken instrument. Each screw wedge has a knurled metal handle (Fig. 3.72).
- Some **systems**, such as tips and hollow tubes in which cyanoacrylate is inserted to "glue" the instrument and extract it, can be useful (Fig. 3.73).
- **File Retrieval Kit** (Terauchi, Japan) (Fig. 3.74).

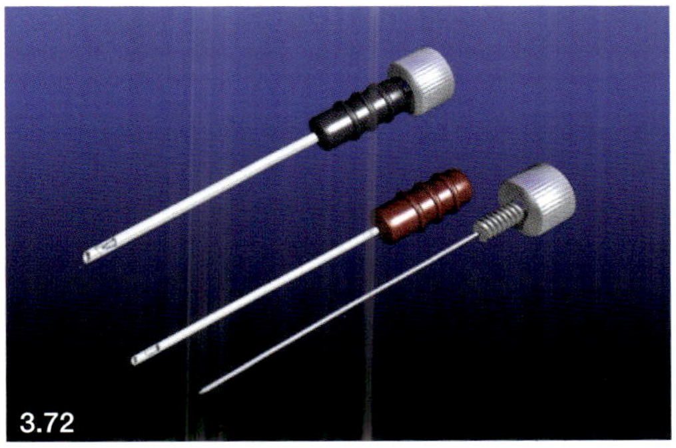

3.72

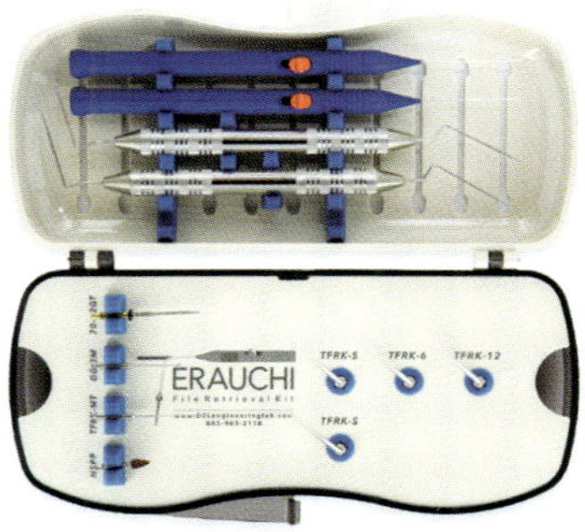

3.74

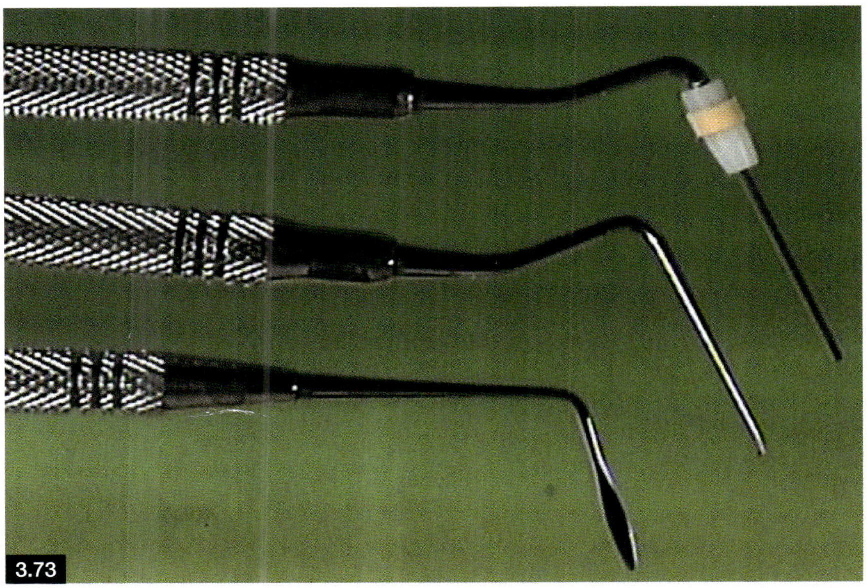

3.73

Fractured instrument removal techniques

The removal of the fragment can be divided into five distinct phases:

❶ Access to the coronal third of the fragment

The operator creates a straight access to the coronal portion of the fragment to obtain appropriate accessibility and vision. Gates Glidden burs or ultrasonic tips are used that very carefully avoid touching the fragment when creating the access.

❷ Partial mobilization of the fragment

Small ISO 08 or ISO 10 k-files can be used to by-pass the broken fragment. This maneuver can be simple provided the fragment is inside an oval canal or when there is adequate space between its coronal portion and the canal walls. Conversely, the maneuver can be extremely difficult to perform if the canal is round and the fragment is completely blocking the canal lumen.

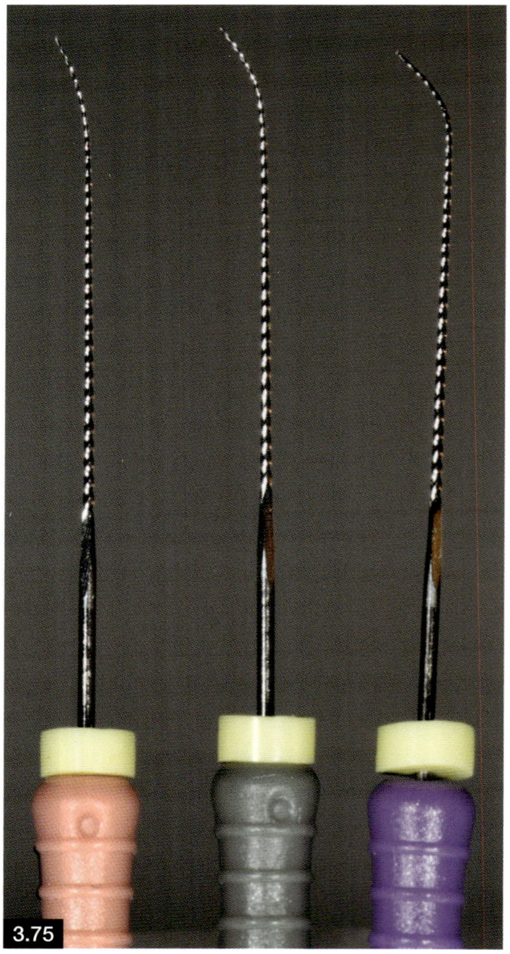

3.75

Fig. 3.75: Steel instruments with pre-curved tip of ISO 06, 08, and 10 dimensions, respectively, that are suitable for passing through narrow spaces such as those between fractured endodontic instruments and the canal wall.

❸ Removing the fragment with ultrasound

When space exists between the canal walls and the coronal part of the fragment, which no longer appears blocked, the ISO 15 k-file is introduced, mounted on ultrasound, thus enabling it to vibrate while alternating the jet of water, and eventually touching the coronal portion of the instrument. In most cases, the mobilized fragment comes out the canal. However, it is advisable – in the case of a multiradiculated tooth removal – to protect the openings of the other canals with a cotton or Teflon pellet so that the removed instrument does not fall into the other canals.

❹ Release of the coronal third of the instrument

If the coronal portion of the instrument cannot be by-passed and occupies the entire lumen of the canal, it is necessary to release at least a part of it in order to gain direct access. In this case, dedicated ultrasonic tips are used (ProUltra, ET20-ET25 Satelec) that must be applied to the dentinal walls to free the coronal region of the engaged fragment for height of at least 2 or 3 mm. Once the access to the released coronal part of the fragment has been obtained, it is possible to proceed according to phase 3.

❺ Use of the extractor

In the event that the instrument is not displaced from the root canal using an ultrasonically-activated k-file, although its coronal portion has been released, the operator should consider using an extractor. The majority of extractors consist of a tube with a plunger inside. Consequently, the operator allows the tube slide until it meets the head of the fractured

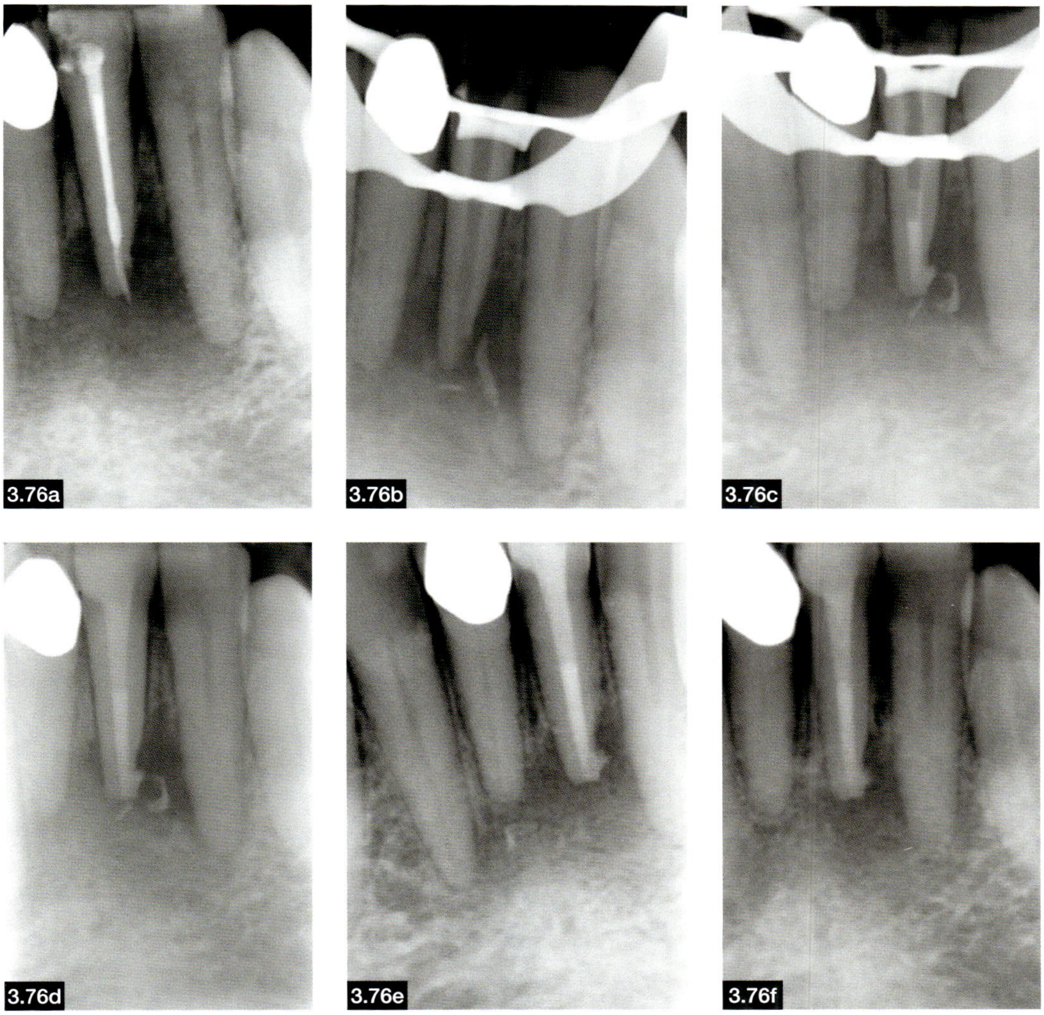

Fig. 3.76a-f: a) Retreatment of a lower lateral incisor inside which a Gates Glidden bur has been fractured; b) the bur is removed with difficulty using diamond ultrasonic tips and the canal appears to be patent; c) the filling of the third apical is accomplished with Mineral Trioxide Aggregate using an "apical plug" (see Chapter 5); (d) complete filling of the canal and reconstruction using a fiber and composite post; (e) evolution of the situation one year later; (f) evolution after three years demonstrating complete resorption of the inflammatory lesion.

instrument, and it is then gently extracted from the canal. The IRS system (Maillefer, Switzerland) consists of two tubes with different sizes (black 1 mm diameter, red 0.8). The final part of each of these tubes is rounded and has a window from which the fragment is extracted by screwing the plunger onto the head of the micro-tube. To use this type of extractor, the coronal portion of the fragment must be released by at least three mm.
The correctly selected micro-tube must be inserted passively into the canal until the coronal part of the fragment emerges from the lateral opening.
At this point, the plunger will be screwed counterclockwise to the microtube, which will, in turn, gradually descend until it locks the fragment in the side window. At this stage, the system will be extracted, together with the broken fragment. This system is particularly suitable for removing lentulo spirals or silver cones.

Technique for by-passing fractured instruments

In cases where the position of the fractured instrument or other factors do not allow its removal, the clinician will need to adopt different strategies aimed at by-passing the fractured instrument. Indeed, in these cases it is necessary to by-pass the fragment with small ISO 06, ISO 08, ISO 10 k-files (Fig. 3.72) – having pre-curved their tip – with a very gradual "watch-winding" motion, changing them very frequently to avoid fractures during this operation. Once the correct working length has been established, the root canal must be shaped entirely by hand using e.g. manual Ni-Ti instruments or stainless steel instruments with reduced taper.

Removal of a lentulo spiral

When the presence of a lentulo in a root canal observed at the preoperative radiographic examination is confirmed by clinical findings, it is imperative not to engage the visible portion to try to extract it. Indeed, although the coronal portion is free, the lentulo spiral could be more apically embedded. Once the access cavity has been modified according to operational requirements, it is therefore necessary to insert a chelator into the canal, shaking it with a small k-file in order to bypass the lentulo spiral laterally. At this point, you can use an extractor which, since the access is correct, can engage with the head of the instrument to remove it.

Canal obstructions and ledges: working sequences for by-passing them

One of the highest failure rates is found in cases where the root canal filling is a few millimeters shorter than the length of the root[111, 112]. In this type of retreatment, and following removal of the existing filling, the clinician has to re-establish canal patency and to overcome the deformations of the canal

Box 3.5 THE MEDICOLEGAL IMPLICATIONS OF LEAVING A FRACTURED INSTRUMENT INSIDE A ROOT CANAL *(Prof. Marco Scarpe*

In the professional "perception" of the Author, endodontics represents a category, within the super-specialized dentistry field, with a low risk of litigation.

If we look at the data from a large insurance sample (ANDI/Cattolica convention, approximately 13,000 members) and considering the long-term effect (~ 17 years), the endodontic field represents the 13.4% assigned to the "conservative/endodontic" group. Hence, if we extrapolate a value equal to 50% (in the case of endodontics in the "group" estimated for excess), we treat about 6.7% of these claims.

Out of the 5,040 claims for one period, we refer to claims that result in damage compensation amounting to 45% of those reported (6.7% of 5,040 claims over approximately 17 years), of which 45% are settled i.e. 9 claims/year on a national level.

It should also be considered, although certain information cannot be produced here, that the majority of accidents in endodontics relate to treatments or retreatments characterized by early prosthetic loading i.e. prior to the verification of the success/failure of the endodontic treatment. Here, the primary cause of the dispute is not necessarily the possible endodontic failure. Indeed, a prominent cause involves the need to re-enter after having finalized the intervention prosthetically.

We can, therefore, state that clinical endodontics is a "low-risk" field.

It is worth remembering, however, that some preventive measures, in our opinion, some simple but imperative preventative measures must be employed.

In the case of retreatment, and especially when retreating teeth containing fragments of fractured instruments, it is essential to explain to the patient (with the aid of images) the meaning of the intended "attempt" without guaranteeing certainty in terms of the result, i.e. indicating the alternatives in terms of the conclusion of the therapy (should we remove the instrument?, failure to remove, but good closure of the canal?). Consequently, the next step is to collect the patient's consent, which must also include one or two explanatory images.

If, on the other hand, endodontic colleagues notice that they have broken an instrument in the canal of their patients' teeth, should they tell their patients or not?

The answer is Yes, always. This is not based only on ethical considerations or those regarding equal opportunities and fairness, but also by virtue of that therapeutic alliance that has always been flaunted as an essential and fundamental element for the maintenance of good doctor/patient compliance. The patient has the right to be informed. Of course, the possibility of resolving the case through,

Claims data from Oris Broker
(ANDI/Cattolica Convention (1 January 2001 - 20 February 2018)

Claims reported in total:	5,040
Outstanding claims:	807
Claims settled:	4,233
Claims paid:	2,299 (55%)

Types of claims (%)	
ORTHODONTICS:	9.4
CONSERVATIVE DENTISTRY:	13.4
ORAL SURGERY:	17.5
IMPLANTOLOGY:	30.9
PROSTHETICS:	25.1
ANESTHESIA:	1
OTHER DAMAGES:	2.7

lumen caused by the previous treatment[113], whether they are blocks or ledges.
When analyzing the preoperative radiogram, it is necessary to try and understand the reason why the radicular apex was not reached. The most frequent causes are almost always pertaining to anatomical characteristics, such as canal curvatures or particularly narrow canals[114, 115].
Therefore, it is important to develop a therapeutic path using the right instruments: instruments that are very thin and pre-curved k-files, have adequate magnification, and consist of chelating solutions that favor the sliding of the instruments in the canal.

It may also be possible, in some cases, to pre-curve a Ni-Ti instrument brought manually up to the working length.
In this case, it is necessary to avoid reusing the instrument in subsequent therapies.
Generally speaking, when an obstacle is encountered in a straight portion of the canal, it is called block. If, on the other hand, the obstacle is close to a curve and a certain asymmetry between the existing filling material and the root profile is identified, then probably this is a ledge. The technique for accessing the root canal system when encountering these two types of obstacle is markedly different[116].

for example, the intervention of an experienced endodontist-microscopist should also be illustrated in these cases, which imply zero costs for the patient (in such a case, if properly handled, the claim provides for insurance settlement).
We also suggest clinicians record any potential adverse events in a specific folder confirming that they have already described it to the patient and that appropriate action will be taken to manage its consequences.
In the case presented in the endodontic x-rays, the colleague failed to notice a fractured instrument in the root canal of tooth 46. However, he chose to proceed with prosthetic treatment because of the pain the patient was experiencing. The patient was treated pharmacologically and it was not until the patient contacted another professional that an accurate diagnosis was performed.
Consequently, the patient was referred to an endodontic surgery specialist. Given the condition of the prosthetic treatment performed and the position of the instrument fragment, the specialist opted for retrograde surgery; in case of failure the dentist and the patient had agreed that the tooth would be extracted (prudent option). The case is ongoing but is well managed by the insurance company that indemnifies the colleague who performed the endodontic procedure with instrumental rupture.
With regards to the informed consent form, it should be noted that the use of this type of form requires its full completion. If the consent is not completely filled in then it is likely to facilitate further counter-productiveness. In the case of surgery on teeth containing fragments of fractured instruments, our advice is to attach to the x-ray showing the fractured instrument, specifying that attempts will be made to remove it and proposing alternative therapeutic solutions.

In short:

- The informed consent form should specify that instruments may fracture (see Chapter 2);
- Identify and record the fracture
- Perform operations to recover the instrument;
- If the instrument is left in place or by-passed, adequate follow-up is required.

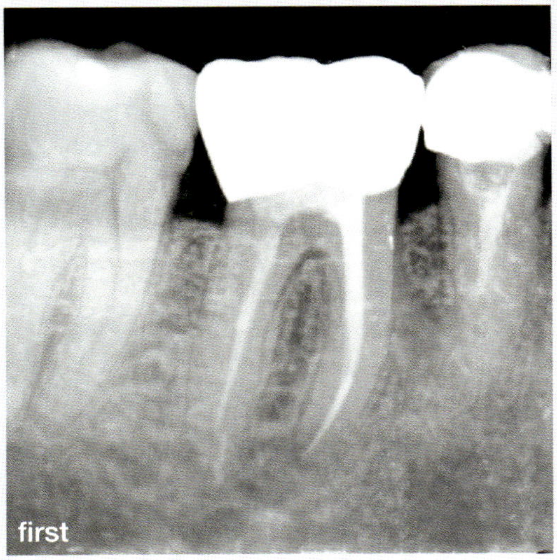

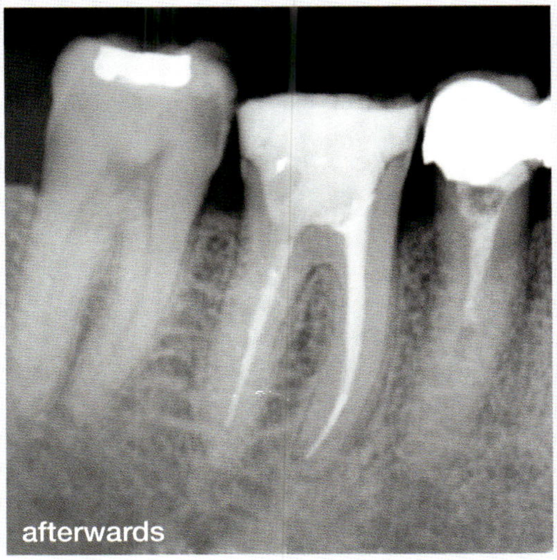

CASE REPORT 20

Fractured root canal instrument bypass at apical level

Fracture of endodontic instruments at the apical level can be a very complex event to deal with. Both the length of the root canal and its size can play an unfavorable role in removal. Therefore, clinicians should try to eliminate the problem by bypassing the instrument, shaping the surrounding spaces so as to incorporate the instrument into the

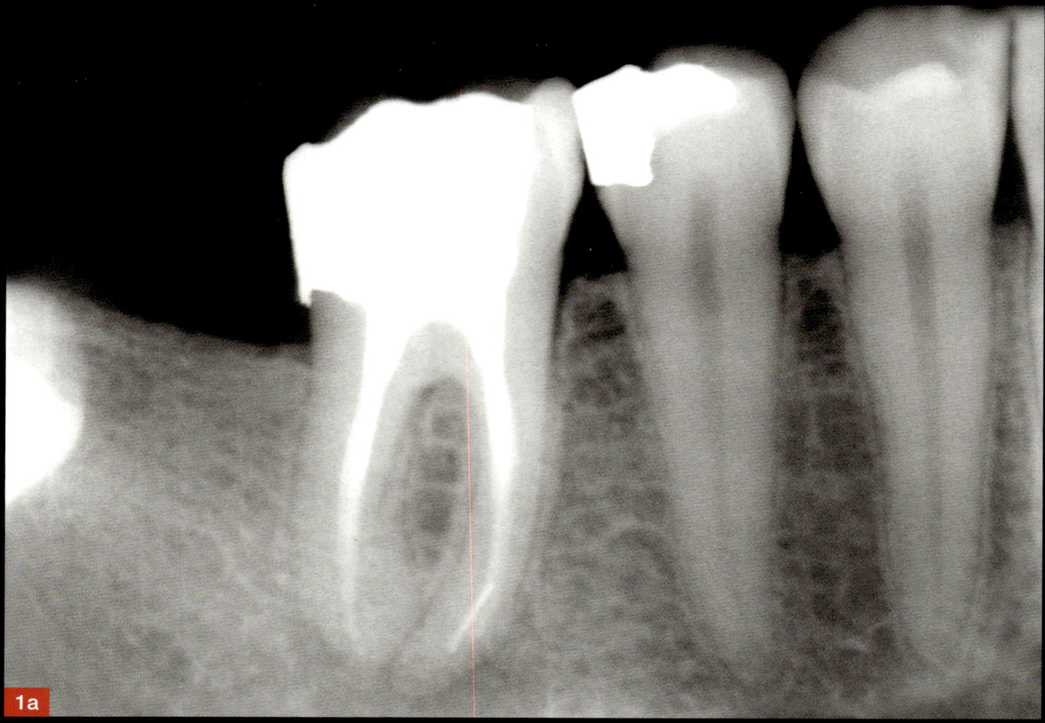

1a

Figure 1a: Molar with periapical lesion requiring retreatment.

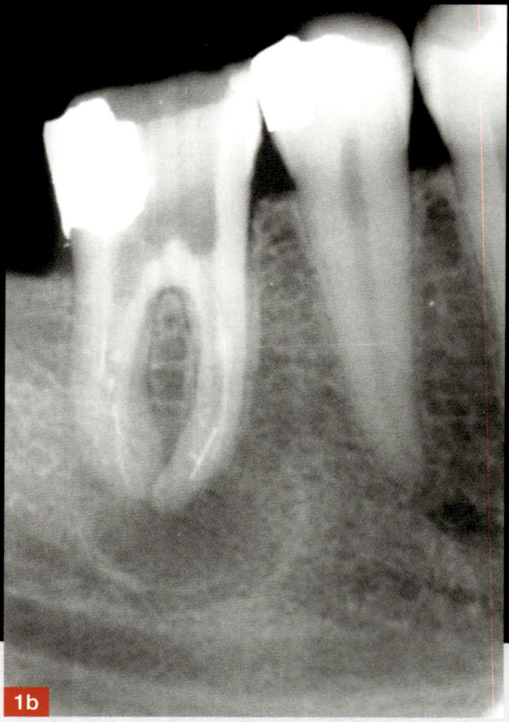

1b

Figure 1b: Note, once the endodontic space is emptied, the presence of an instrument that is difficult to remove.

subsequent filling. This operation is delicate and not without its risks. In this case, a lower molar, the key to success was the confluence of the root canals, which allowed adequate irrigation with powerful disinfectants in the apical area before correct filling was carried out.

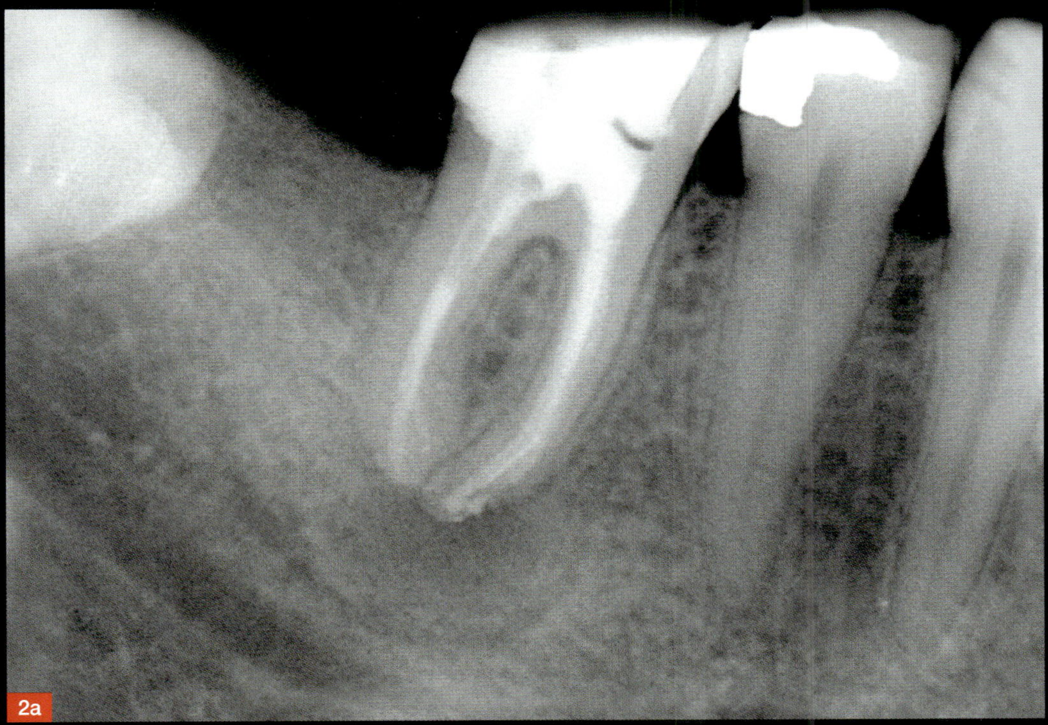

2a

Figure 2a: By-passing the instrument allowed for adequate disinfection and obturation of the root canals.

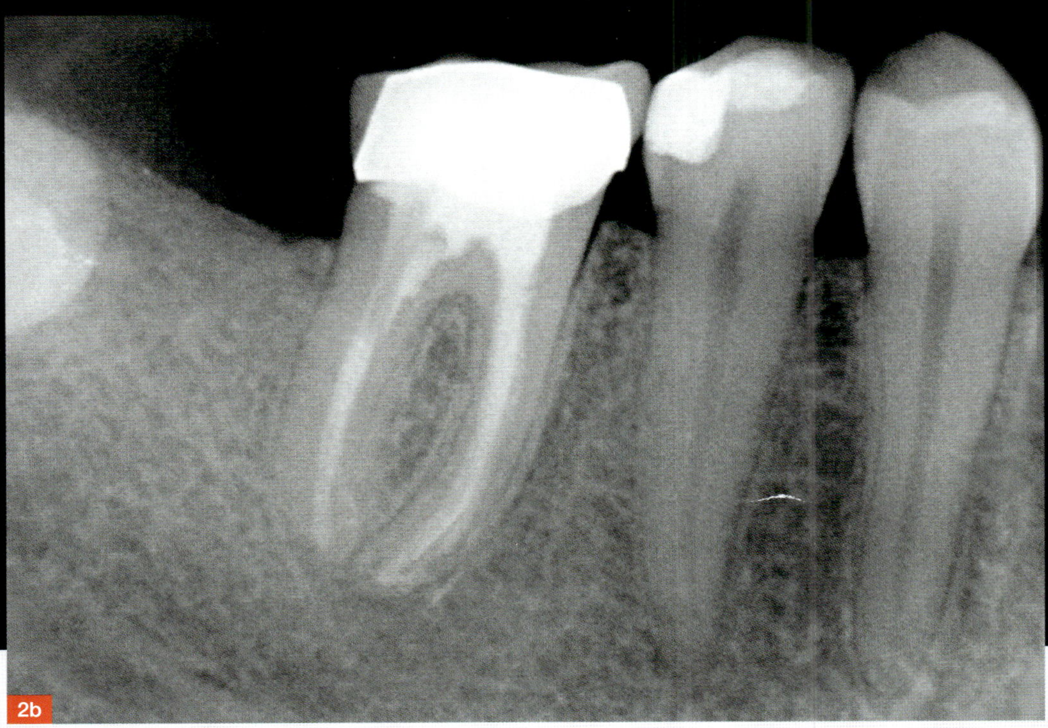

2b

Figure 2b: Follow-up six months later.

CASE REPORT 21

Removal of a broken instrument using the "super glue technique"

A 58-year-old female patient was referred by a colleague. In the radiographic examination, the second right upper pre-molar presented a fractured instrument located in the middle and upper third of the buccal canal. The treatment plan was to remove the fractured instrument to perform a correct root canal treatment. It was possible to remove the file

Figure 1: The initial x-ray examination reveals a fractured instrument in the mesio-buccal canal and an incomplete root canal filling in the palatal one.

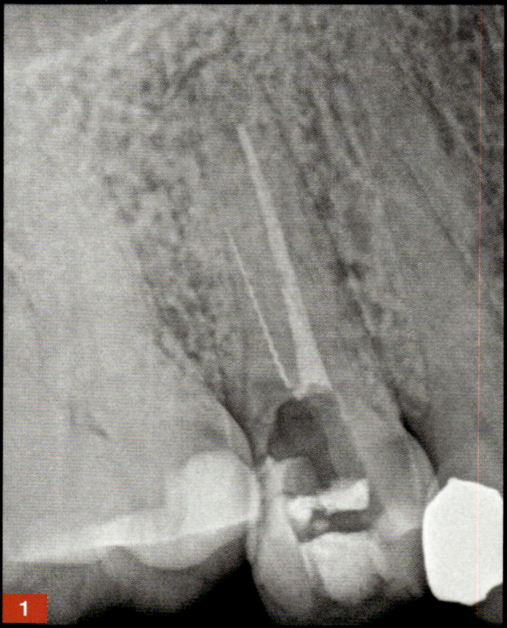

1

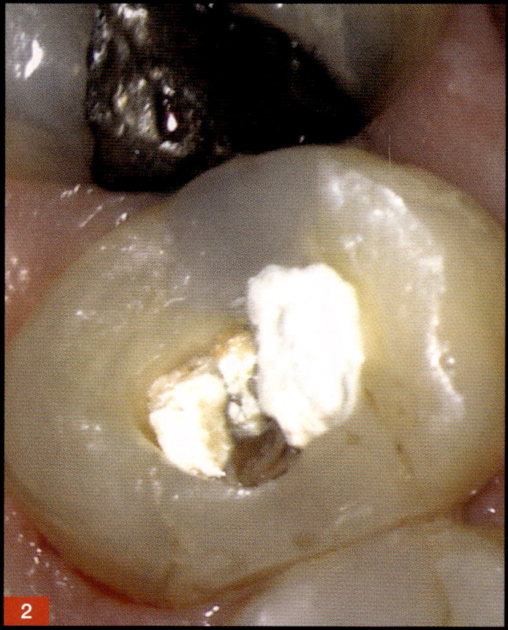

2

Figure 2: A poor provisional restoration was easily removed by ultrasonic devices.

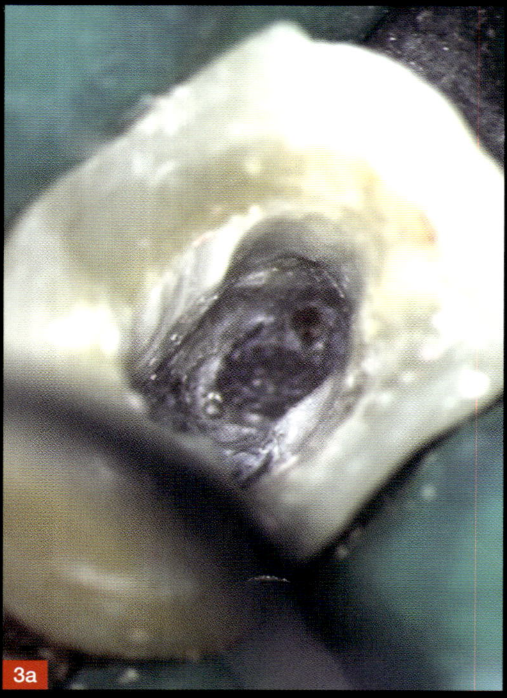

3a

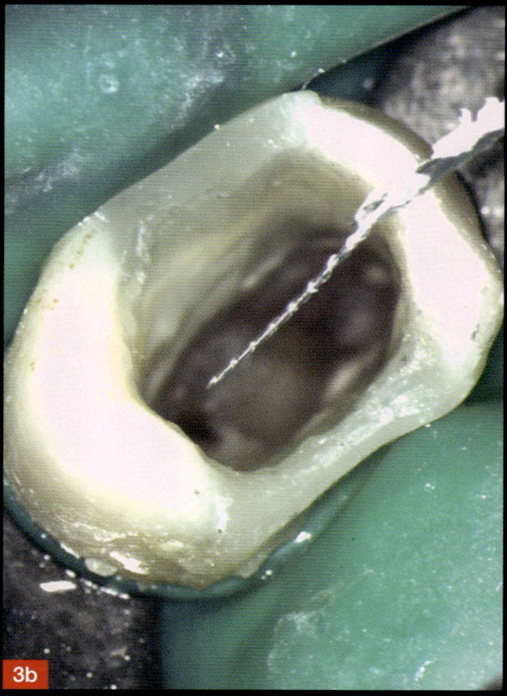

3b

Figure 3a-b: A better pulp-chamber opening was performed to identify the fractured instrument (Fig. 3) an appropriate needle with a dedicated glue was inserted to grasp the instrument.

by using several systems including a 27G (BD MicrolanceTM 3 Needles 27G × 3⁄4 "- 0.4 mm × 19 mm) irrigation needle and a cyanoacrylate glue (Cobra Pacific Super Glue).
The tooth was completely instrumented, disinfected, filled with gutta-percha and subsequently restored directly and definitively with composite resin.
This alternative method, involving the use of an irrigation needle and cyanoacrylate adhesive, might be considered in case like this as an economical and suitable alternative to other comparable methods.

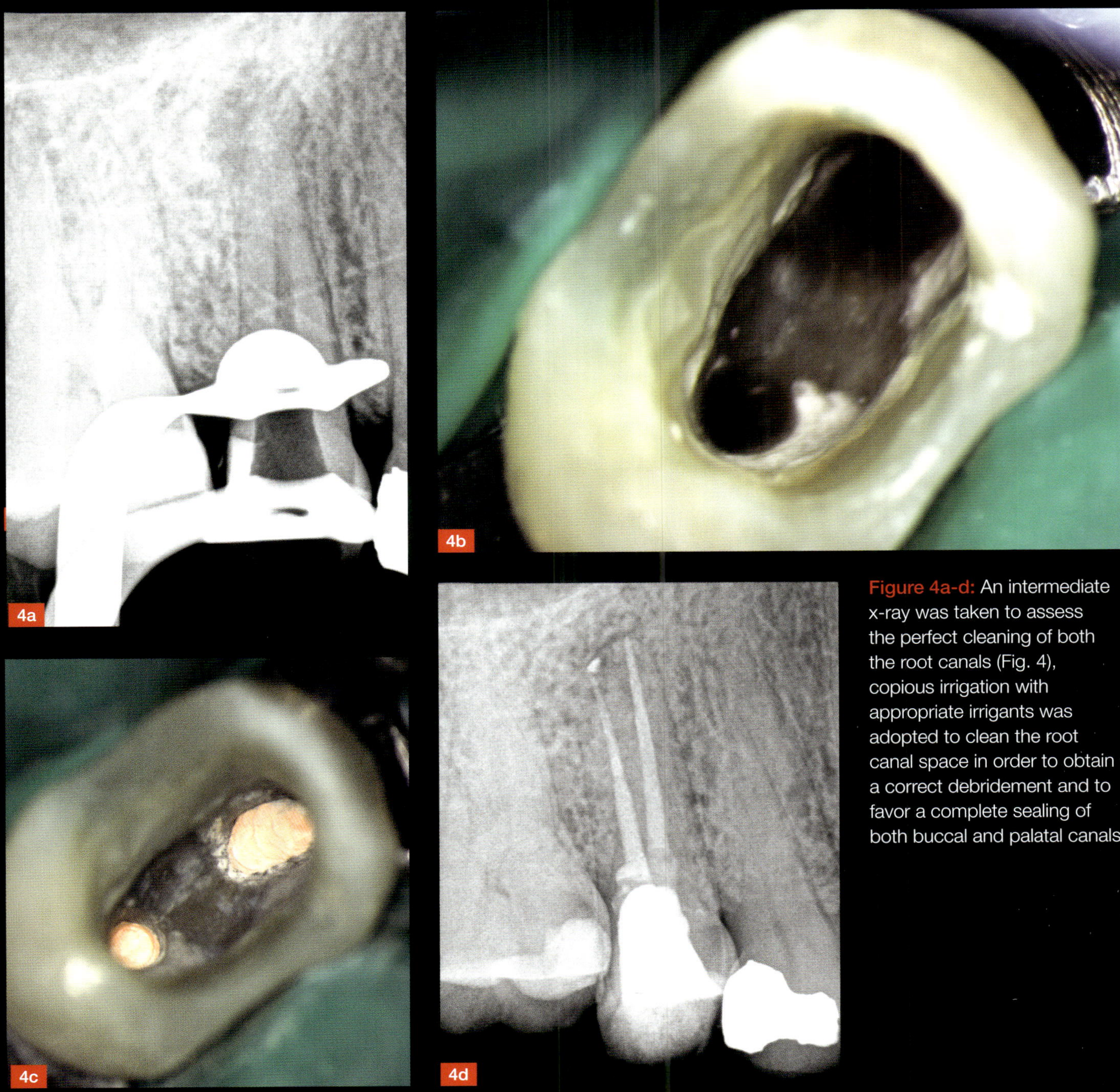

Figure 4a-d: An intermediate x-ray was taken to assess the perfect cleaning of both the root canals (Fig. 4), copious irrigation with appropriate irrigants was adopted to clean the root canal space in order to obtain a correct debridement and to favor a complete sealing of both buccal and palatal canals.

CASE REPORT 22

Fractured instruments: possible solutions

The fracture of an endodontic instrument in a root canal is an unlucky occurrence that may hinder the root canal procedure and negatively impact the endodontic treatment's outcome. A fractured instrument in itself may not cause treatment failure. However, fragments present in the root canal can interfere with appropriate root canal preparation. The overall endodontic

BY-PASS AND REMOVING PROCESS IN TWO DIFFERENT ROOT CANALS

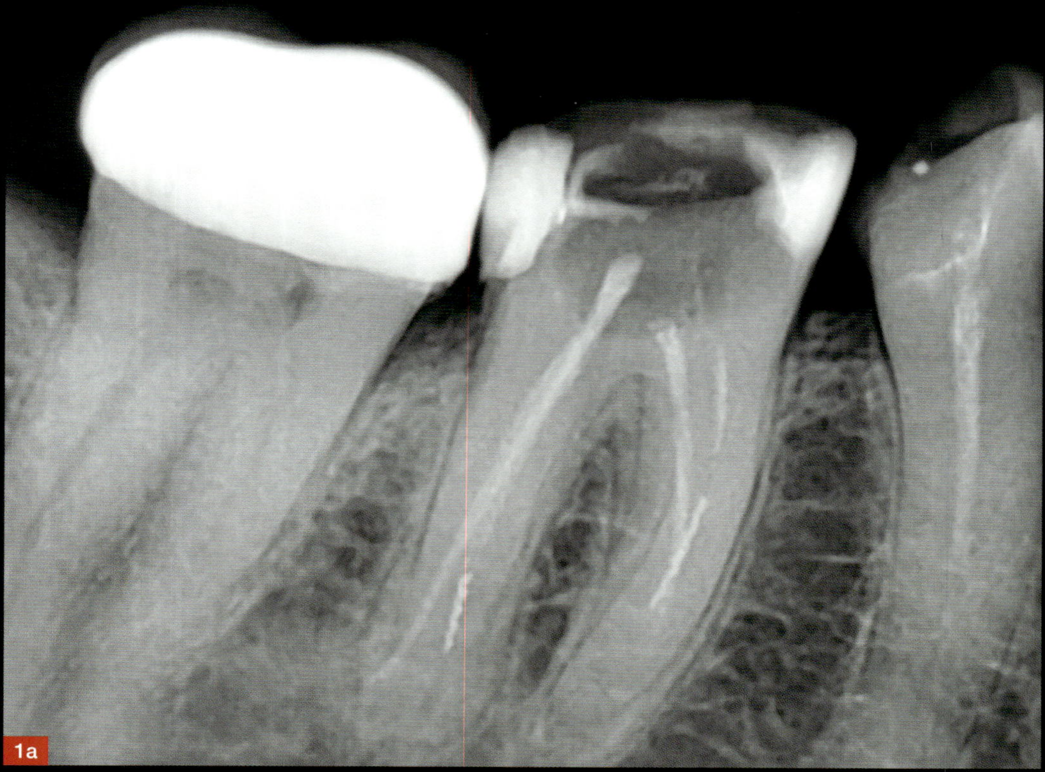

1a

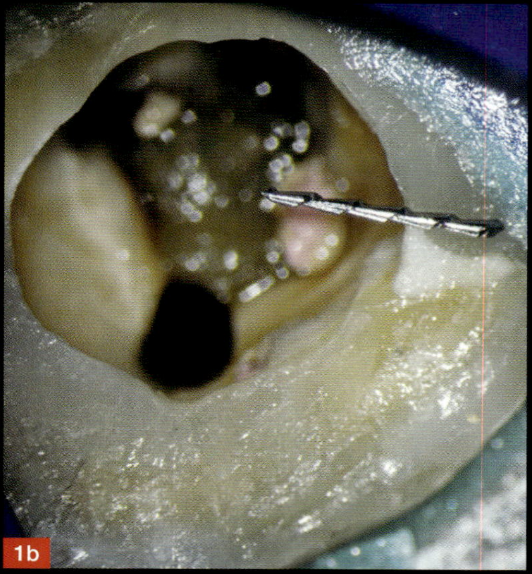

1b

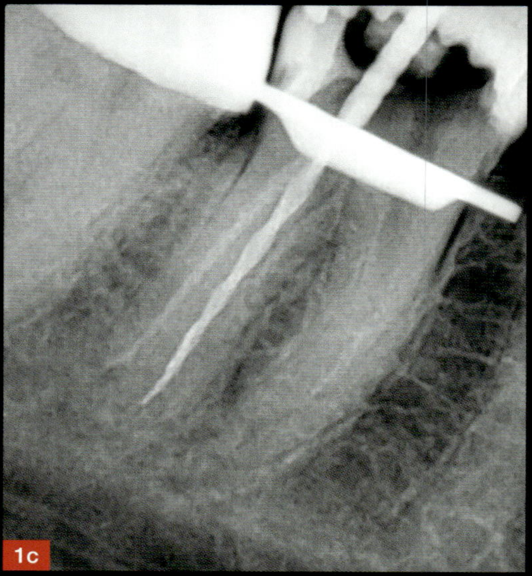

1c

Figure 1a-f: The by-passing technique is considered the more conservative approach, given the amount of dentin removal, compared to the retrieval techniques, especially if the fragment is located in the apical third.

prognosis, following instrument fracture, is likely to depend on the stage and degree of canal preparation and disinfection at the time of instrument fracture, the main prognostic factor, in such cases, is reported to be the preoperative periradicular status.
As reported in the main body of this text, with fractured instruments, there are two main options for accomplishing a correct root canal treatment: by-passing or removing it.

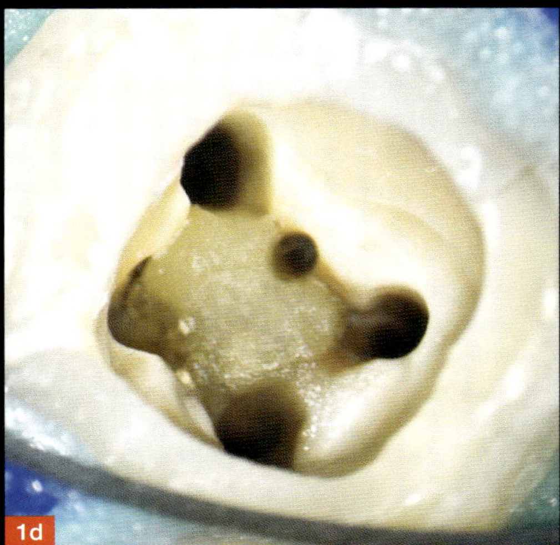
1d

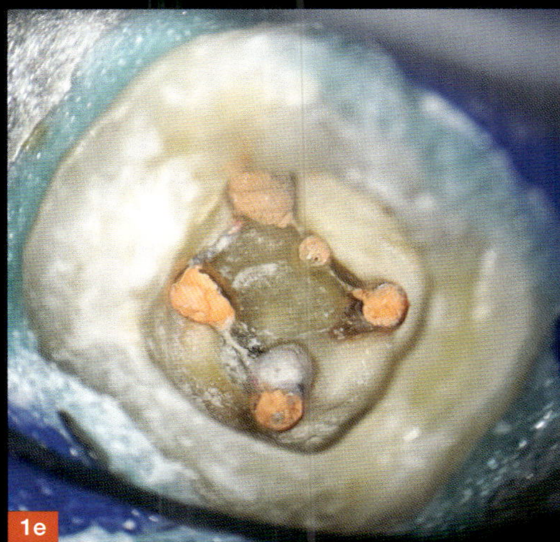
1e

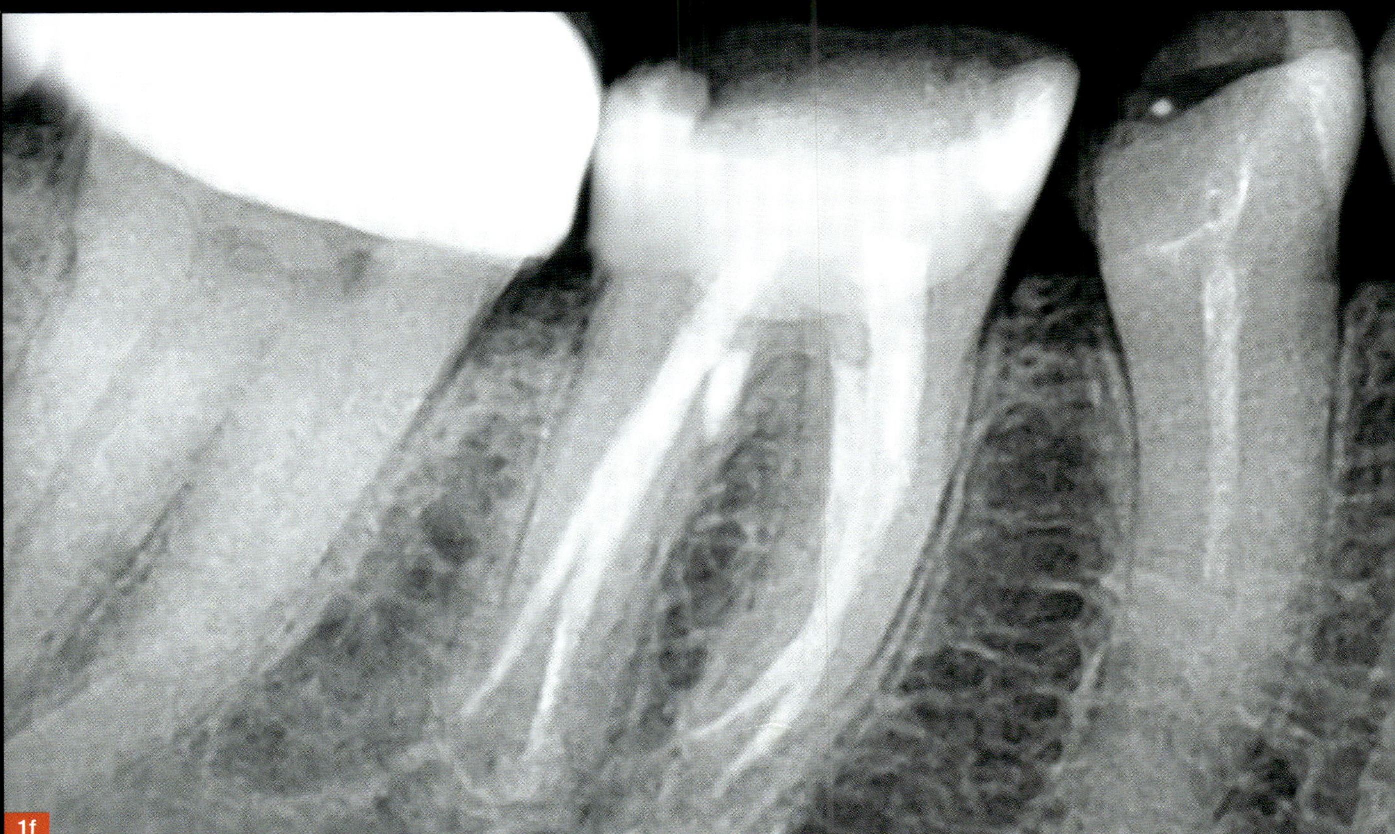
1f

REMOVAL OF A FRACTURED INSTRUMENT DEEP IN THE MESIAL ROOT OF AN UPPER MOLAR

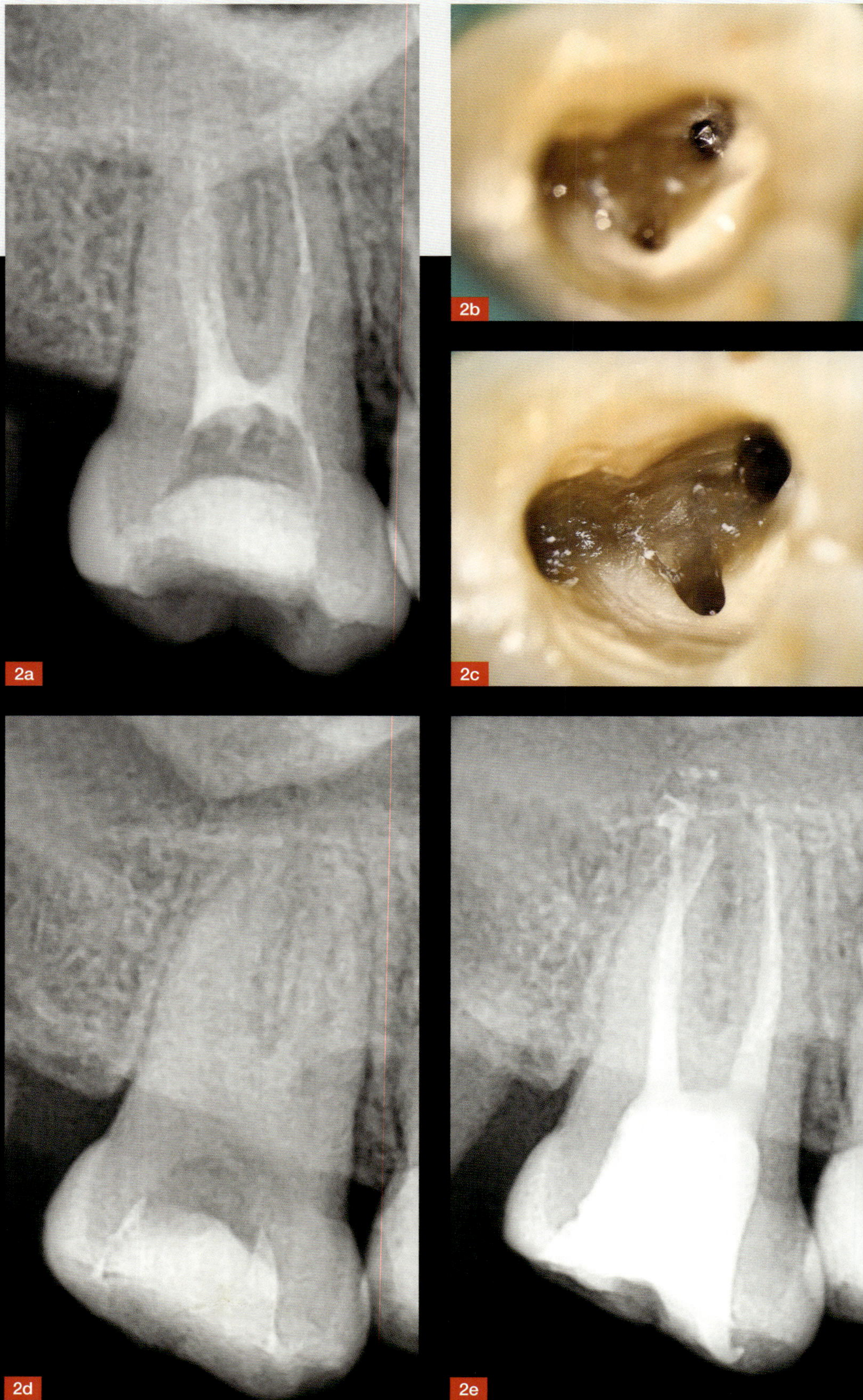

Figure 2a-e: The removal of fractured files is an effective technique and is the ideal solution for obtaining suitable obturation of the whole root canal system.

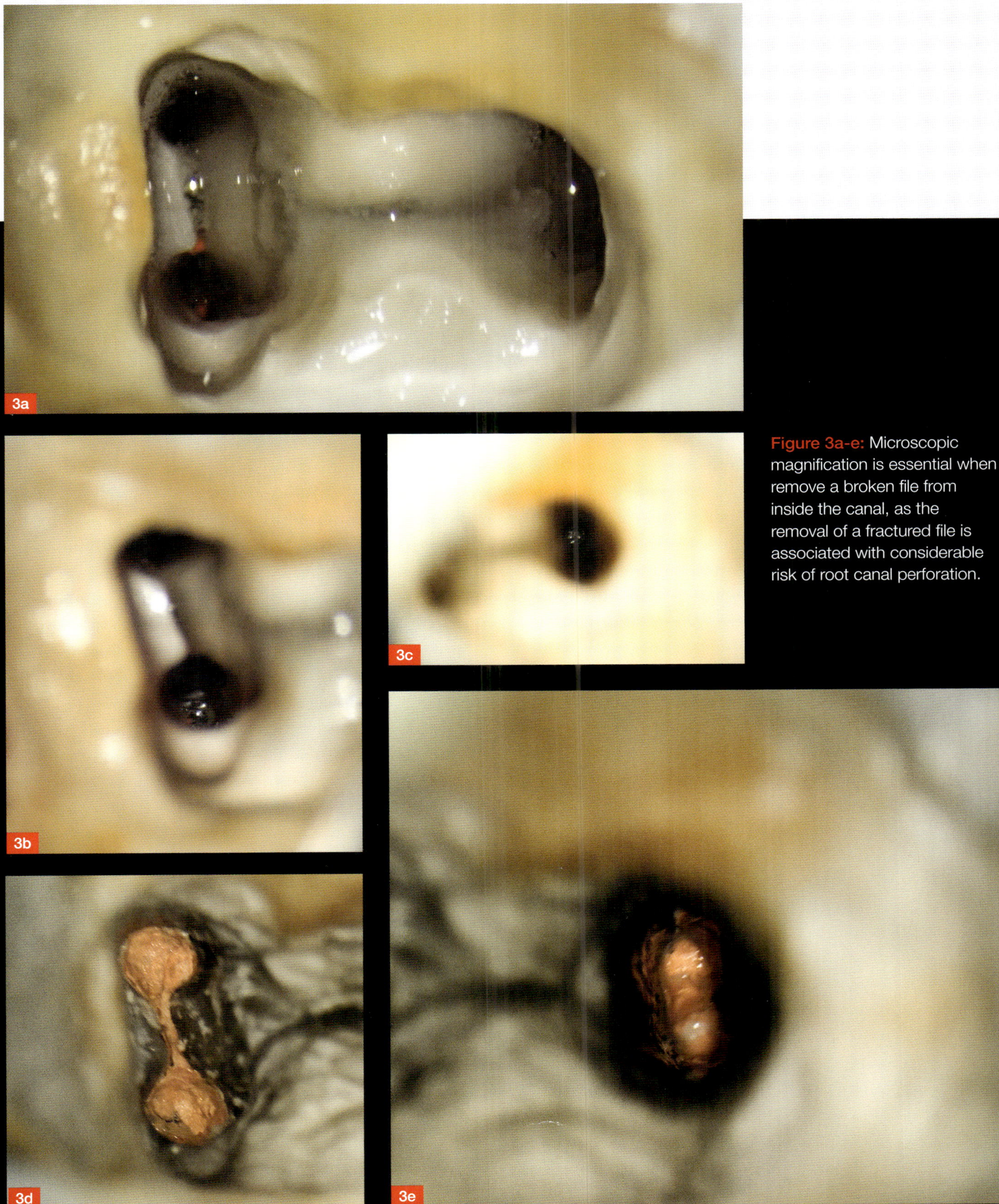

Figure 3a-e: Microscopic magnification is essential when remove a broken file from inside the canal, as the removal of a fractured file is associated with considerable risk of root canal perforation.

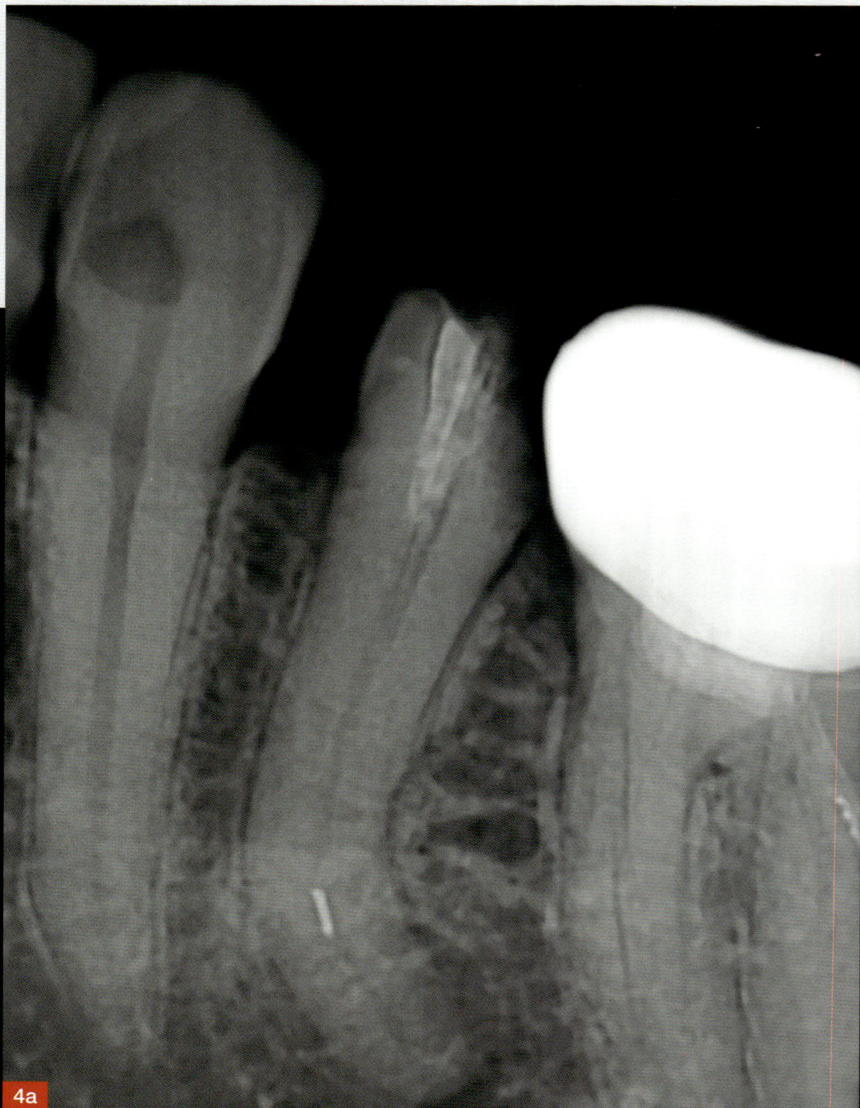

4a

CHALLENGING REMOVAL OF A BROKEN INSTRUMENT INSIDE A ROOT CANAL CURVATURE

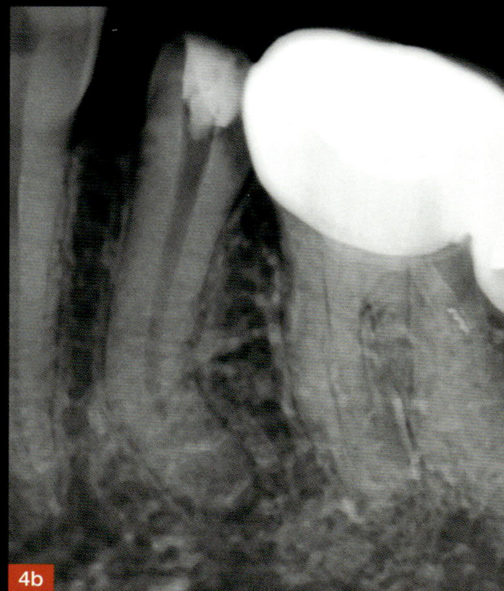

4b

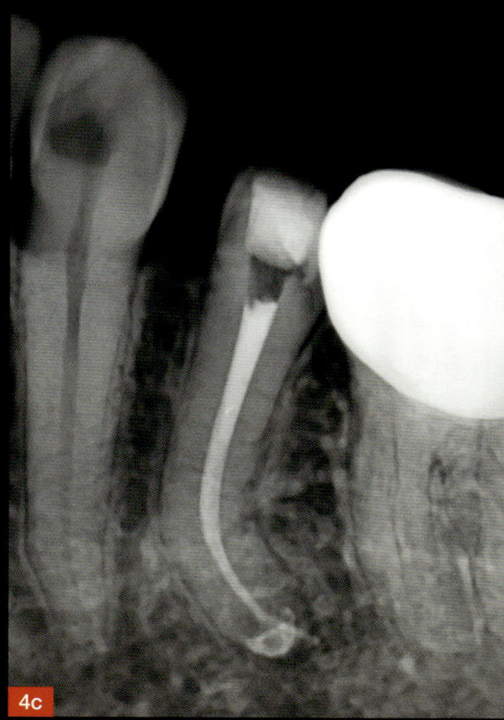

4c

Figure 4a-c: There are several methods for instrument removal: the use of ultrasonics techniques and devices being one of the most popular. In this case, a coronal enlargement was the pre-requisite for using the ultrasonic tip inside the curvature to dislodge the file fragment and extract it.

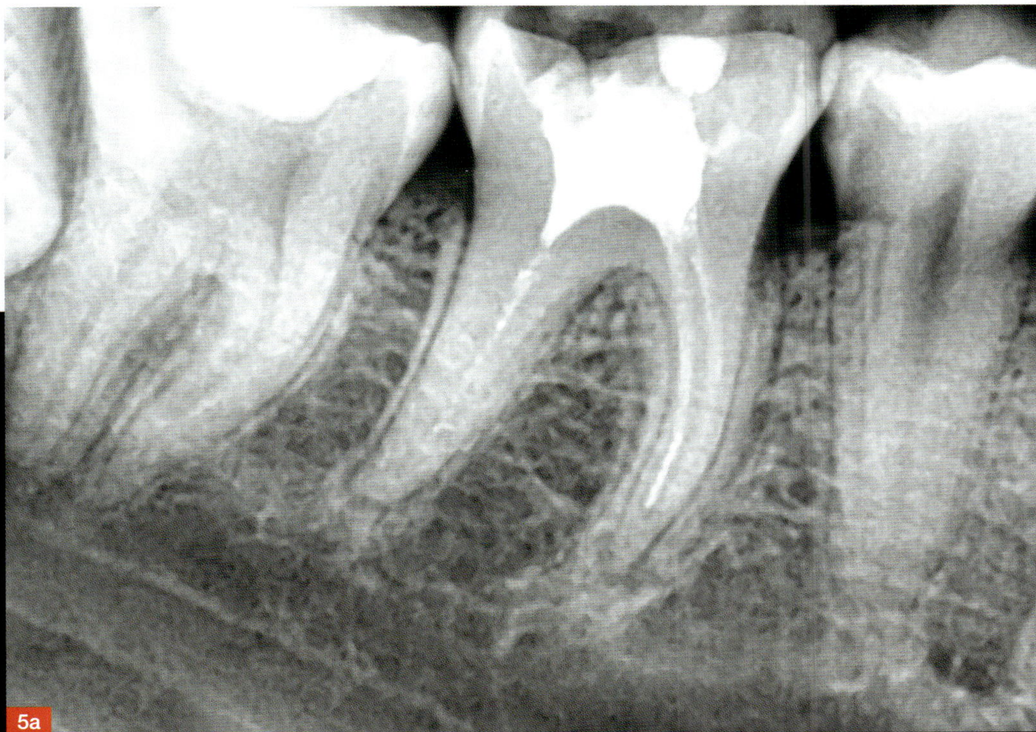

5a

GRASPING TECHNIQUES: A REAL ALTERNATIVE FOR REMOVING FRACTURED INSTRUMENTS (CASE REPORT 1)

Figure 5a-d: Loop, micro tweezers, pliers and/or forceps.

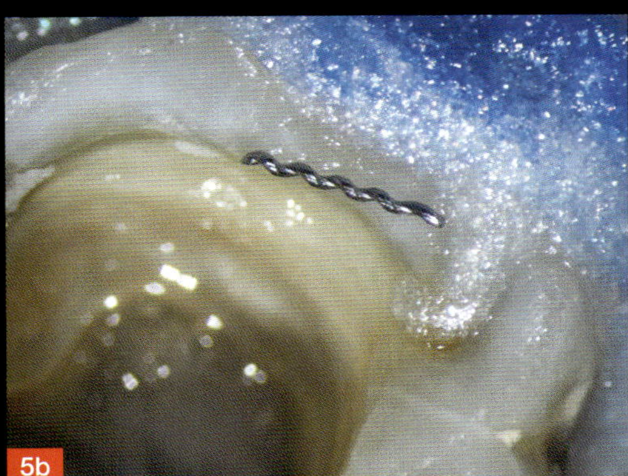

5b

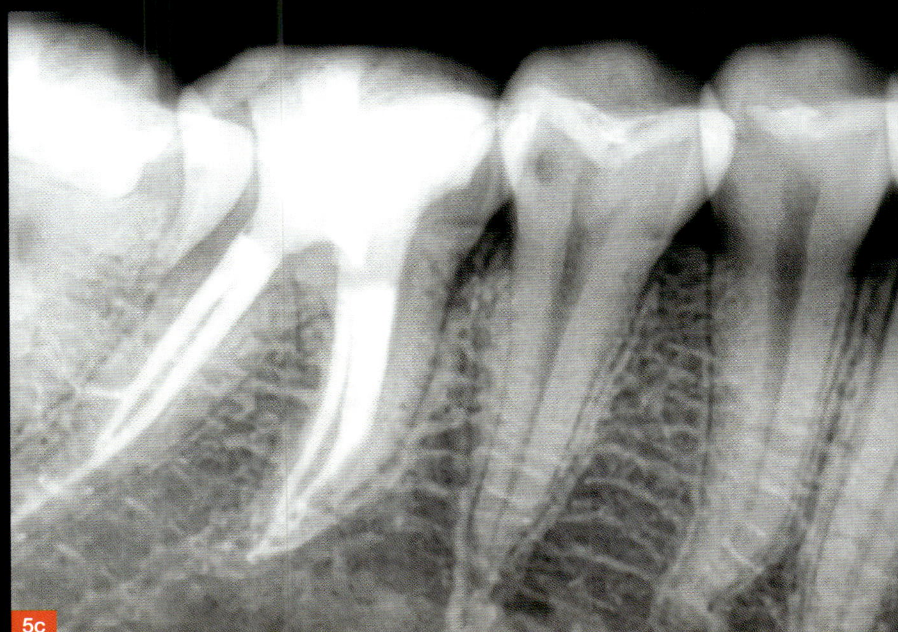

5c

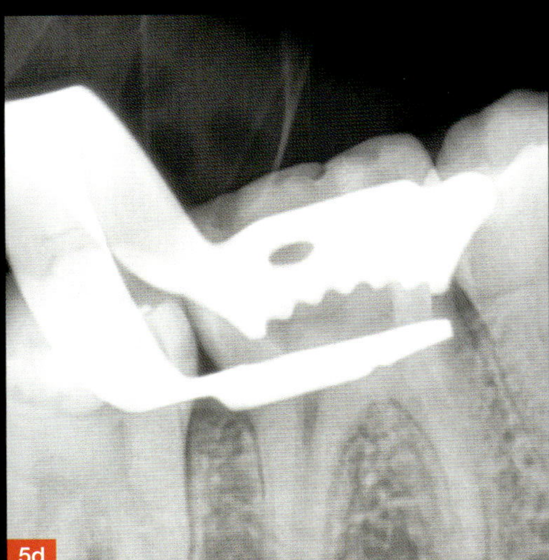

5d

GRASPING TECHNIQUES: A REAL ALTERNATIVE FOR REMOVING SEPARATED INSTRUMENTS (CASE REPORT 2)

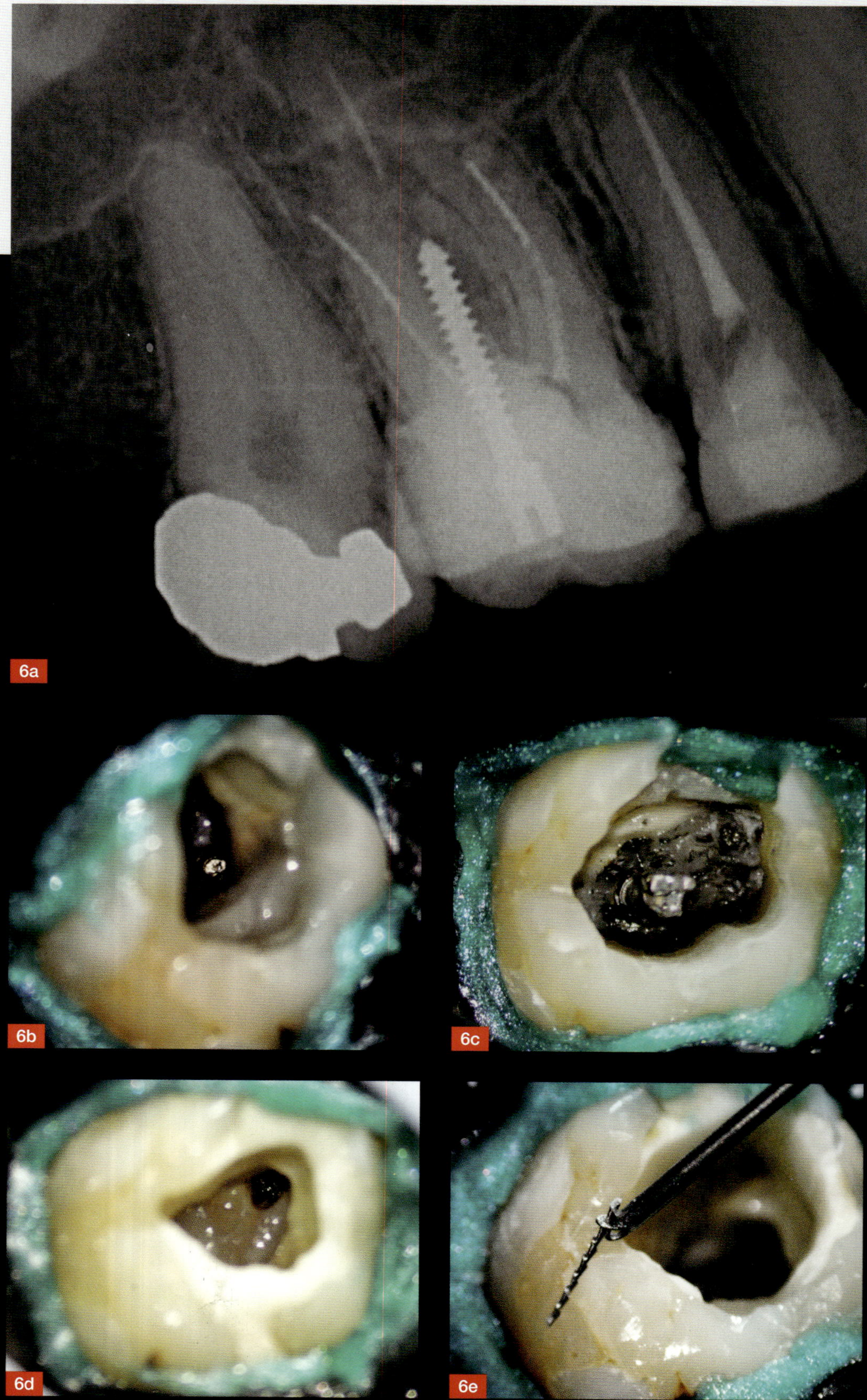

Figure 6a-i: Use of grasping tools such as microtube or wedging tube devices might be the only alternative suitable for removing fractured files such as H-files, deeply engaged in large canals.

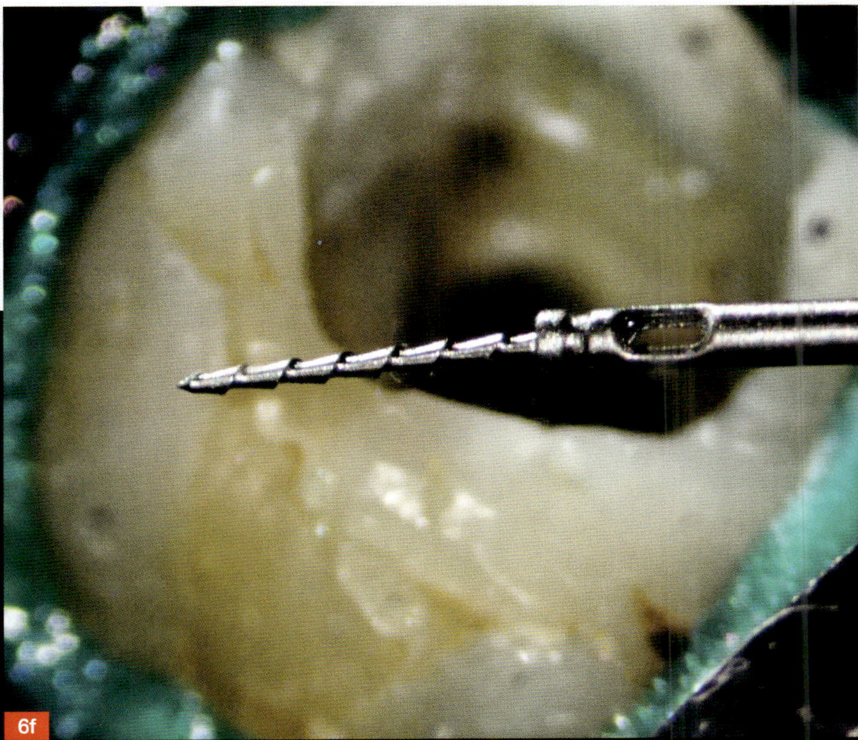
6f

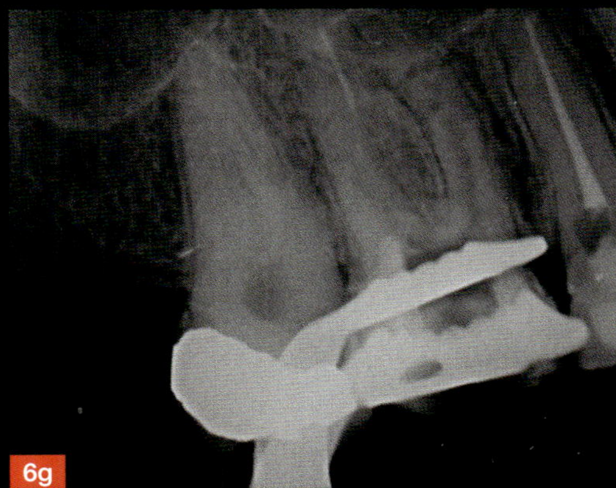
6g

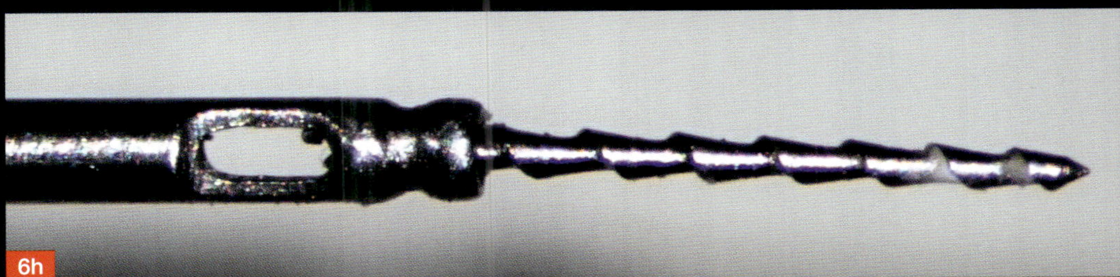
6h

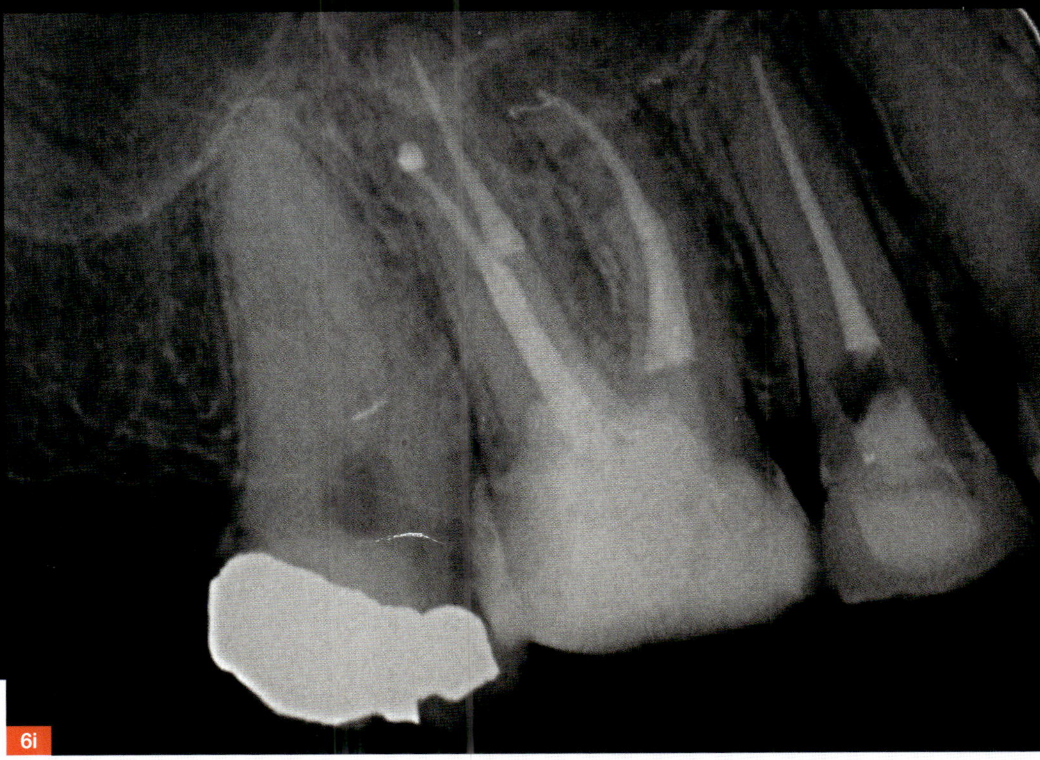
6i

CASE REPORT 23-26

Complex retreatment cases with ledges, perforation, fractured instruments and large periapical lesions

CASE REPORT 24

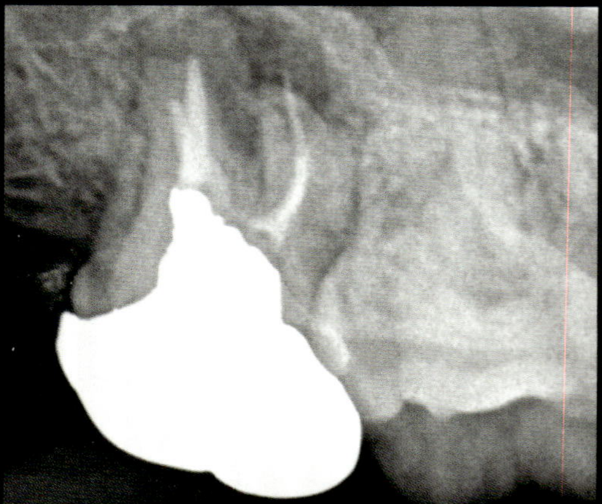

1

Fig. 1: Preoperative radiograph showing an extruded root filling cone (red arrow) on the mesialbuccal root with periapical lesions.

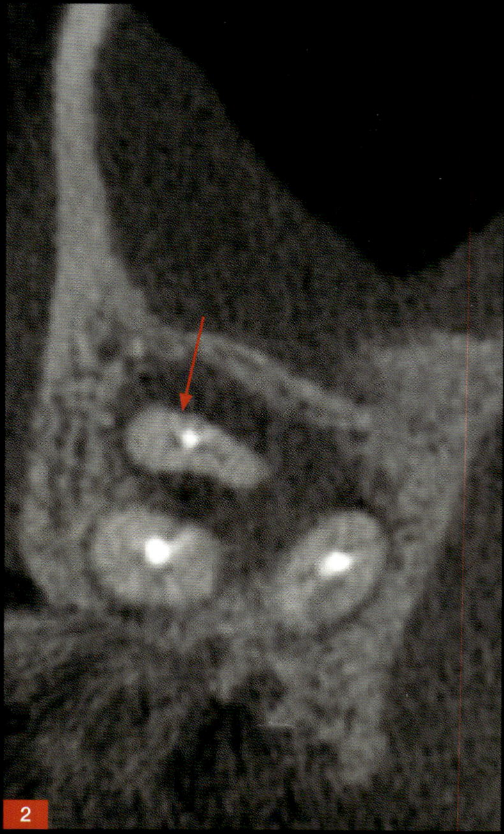

2

Fig. 2: Preoperative axial CBCT view in the middle third reveals an oval canal in the MB root with a large periapical lesion surrounding the root (red arrow).

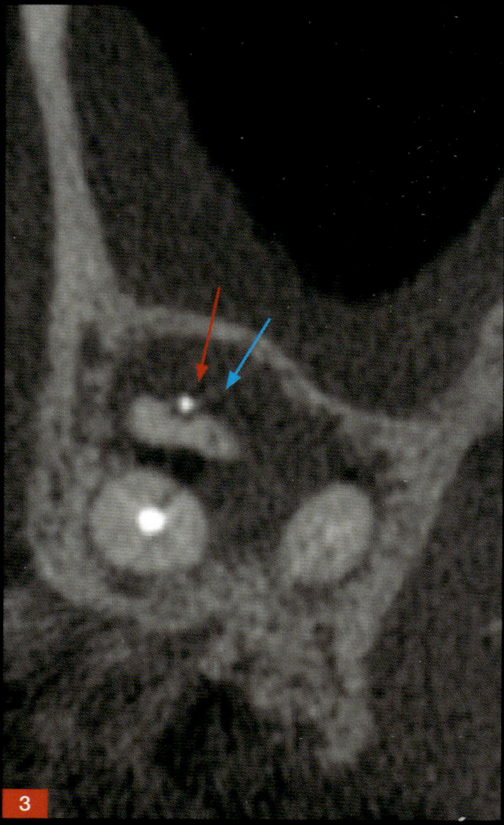

3

Fig. 3: Preoperative axial CBCT view in the apical third reveals the root filling deviating from the main canal in the MB root (red arrow) and the presence of another canal palatal to the root filling (blue arrow).

Complex retreatment can be roughly defined by the numbers of clinical challenges enclosed in each tooth; the CBCT scan is a fundamental starting point in the diagnostic process. Without the 3D X-ray examination several keys aspects would not be revealed, such as the presence of a fractured instrument, the volume of the periapical lesion, the root involved in the pathological process in multiradiculare teeth, fractures or perforations. Sometimes the radiopaque materials in the root may conceal a fracturedd instrument, making it difficult to measure the fractured instrument on the CBCT images. In some cases these materials are not confined inside the root canal and the part outside

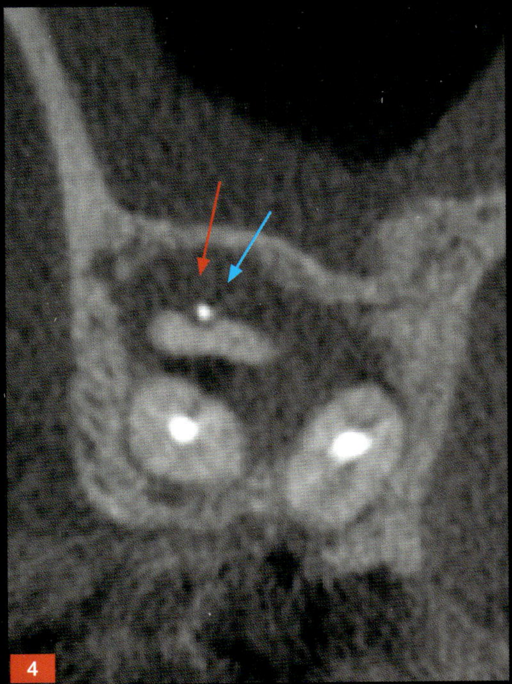

4

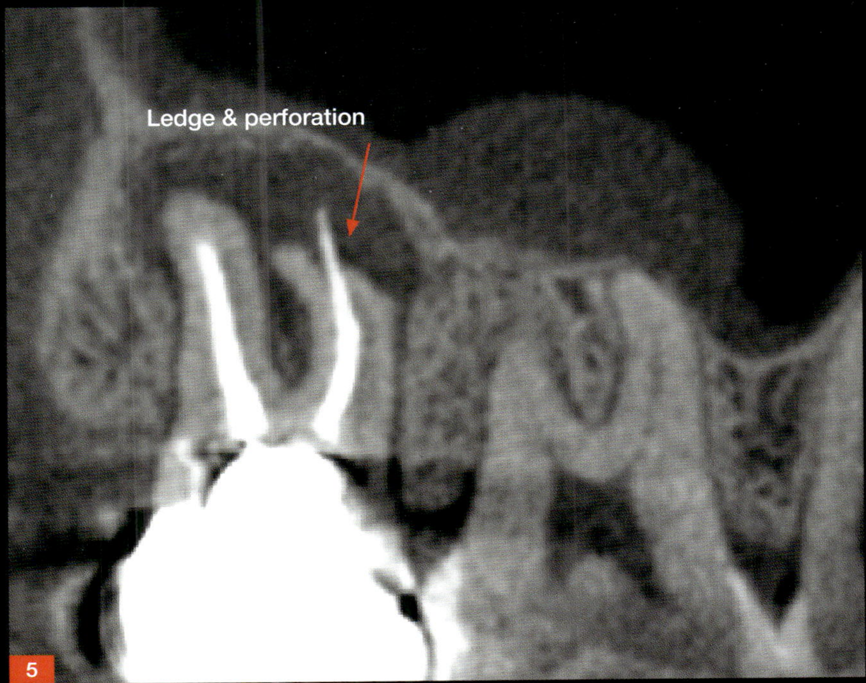

5

Fig. 4: Preoperative axial CBCT view just before the apical foramen reveals the root filling outside the MB root (red arrow) and the other canal remaining in the MB root (blue arrow).

Fig. 5: Preoperative sagittal CBCT view showing the root filling in the MB root extruded deviating from the apex (red arrow) with large lesions on the buccal roots.

Fig. 6: The preoperative sagittal CBCT view shows the original canal (MB2) in the center of the MB root (red arrow) with a large lesion on the MB root.

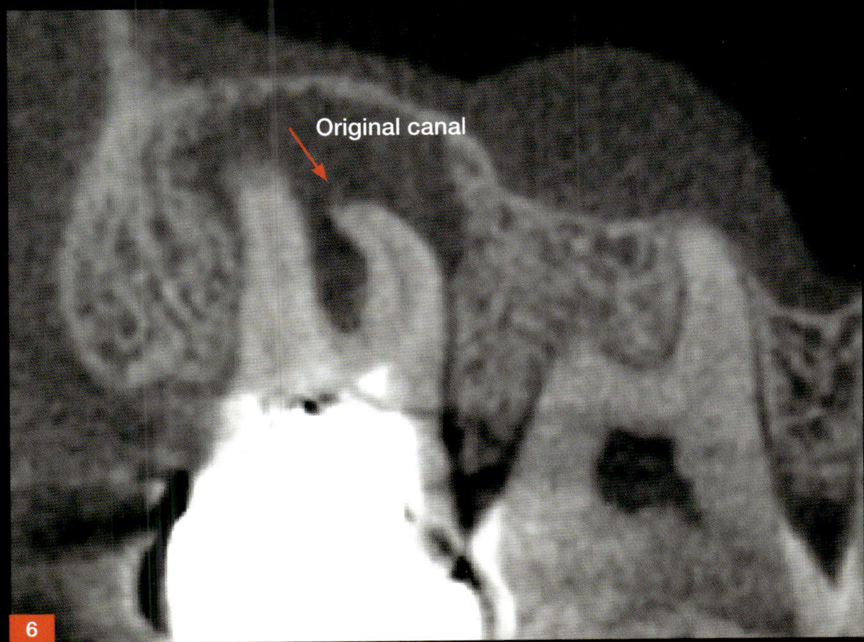

6

should be carefully removed using techniques and strategies carefully planned before the intervention. The patient should be examined not only from the endodontic point of view, as the periodontal probing depths on these teeth should be within normal limits. Symptoms often consist in mild sensitivity to percussion without spontaneous pain. From a clinical point of view the irrigating solutions for these root canal treatments was 5.25% NaOCl and 17% EDTA stirred using a TFRK-S ultrasonic tip. An alternative method could be to use irrigants with 5.25% Qmix 2in1 (Dentsply Sirona, USA). A Stropko device might be useful or drying and improving visibility in order to search for the fractured instrument

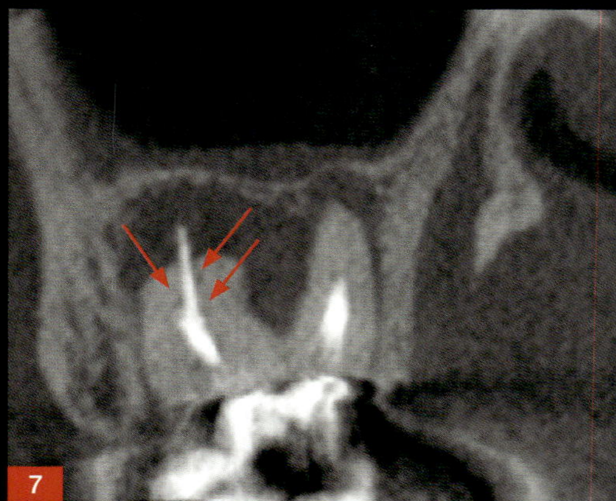

Fig. 7: Preoperative coronal view of CBCT reveals the root filling in the MB root extruded into periapical tissues and the presence of small voids between the root filling and the canal walls (red arrows).

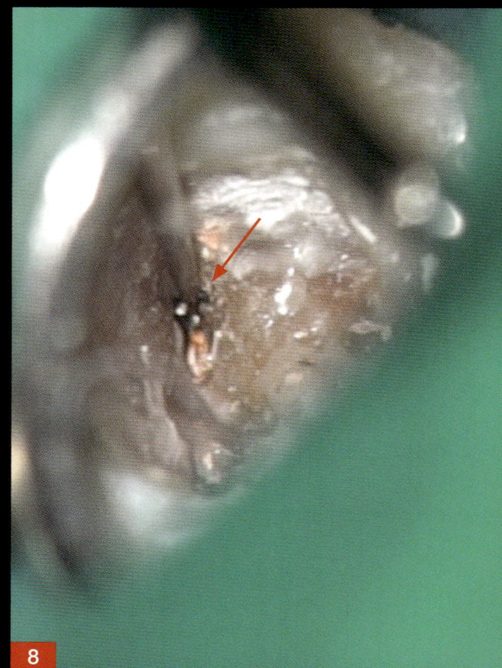

Fig. 8: Magnified image from the microscope shows the GPR hand instrument (red arrow) placed in the space between the gutta-percha cone and the buccal wall in the MB canal.

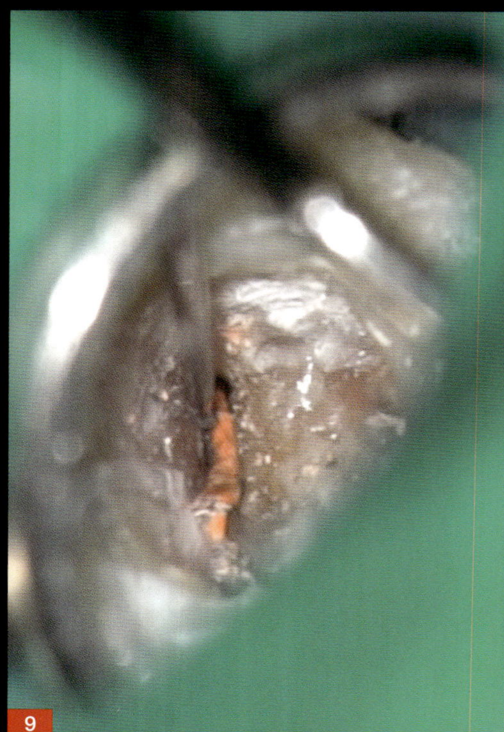

Fig. 9: Magnified image from the microscope shows the removal of the gutta-percha cone from the MB canal with the GPR hand instrument.

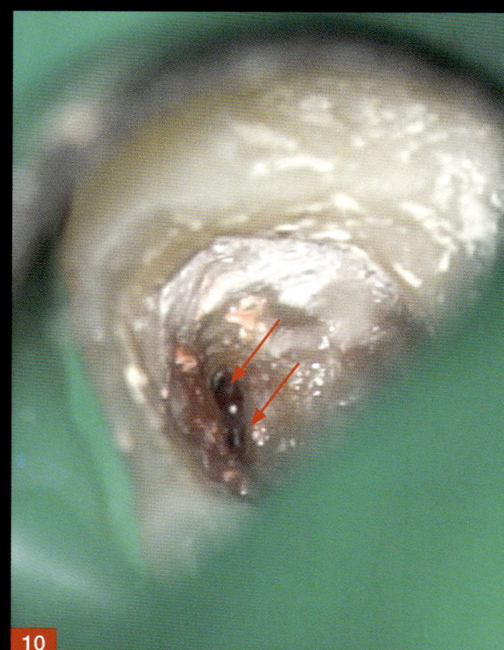

Fig. 10: Magnified image from the microscope reveals the MB canal with perforation (red arrow) and the original canal (blue arrow) palatal to it after the gutta-percha cone removal.

under the microscope. The ultrasonic tips must be sharpened with a brownie bur so that they can be placed in the narrow space between the fractured instrument and the inner wall. The sharpened TFRK-S ultrasonic tip was precurved to suit the canal curvature and it was placed in the space where a sticky feeling was obtained on the ultrasonic tip. During ultrasonic activation, the root canal was replenished with 17% EDTA and the ultrasonic tip was slid down along the inner wall into the space.
The ultrasonic tip was activated continuously in short up/down strokes at power 4 on a scale of 0 to 20.

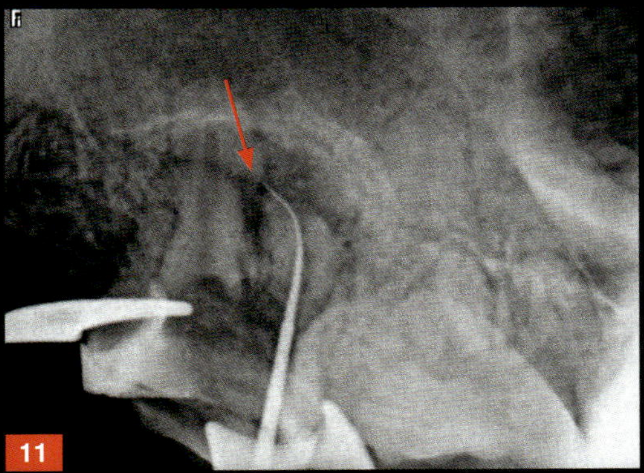

11

Fig. 11: The intraoperative radiograph shows successful negotiation of the original canal with a ProTaper S1 file (red arrow).

Fig. 12: The postoperative x-ray shows the MTA root fillings in the original canal (MB2) as well as the MB canal with perforation (blue arrows) including the DB and the palatal canals.

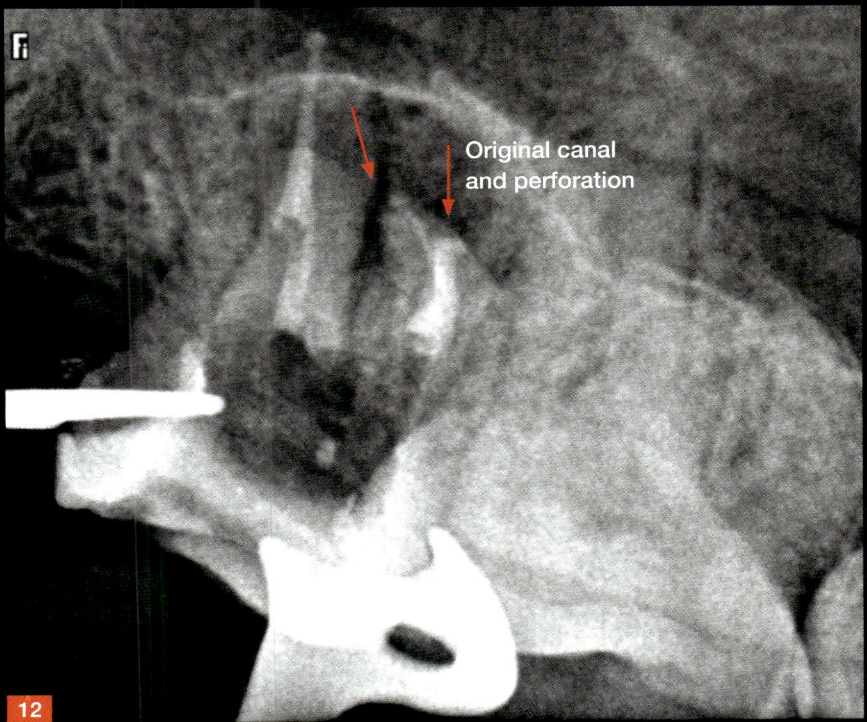

12

Fig. 13: Three month postoperative radiograph shows a reduction of the periapical lesions compared to those on the preoperative radiograph.

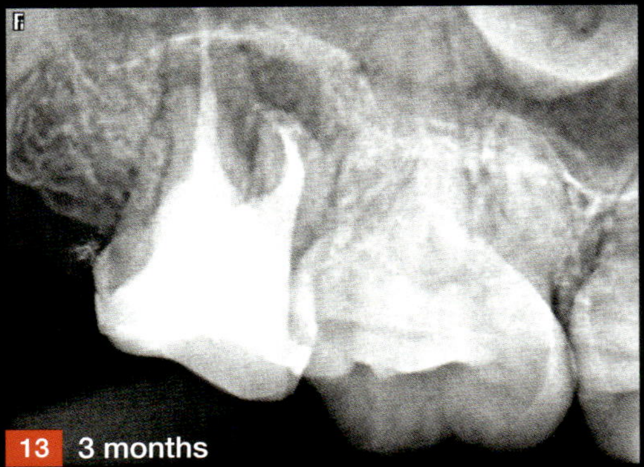

13 3 months

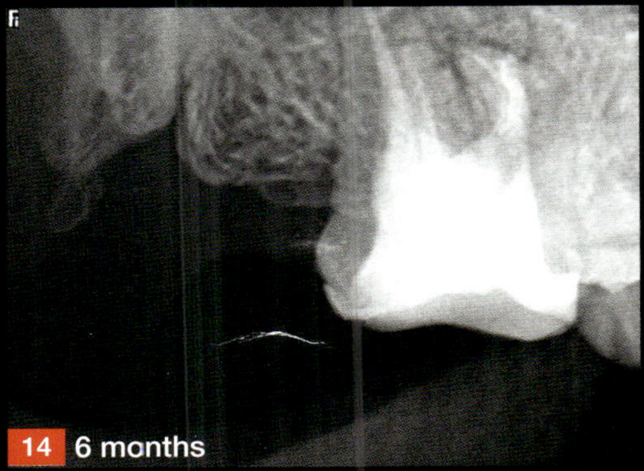

14 6 months

Fig. 14: The six month postoperative radiograph shows the periapical lesions had been significantly reduced compared to those on the preoperative radiograph.

Fig. 15: The six month postoperative sagittal CBCT view showing bone reformation (red arrow) in the defect on the buccal roots.

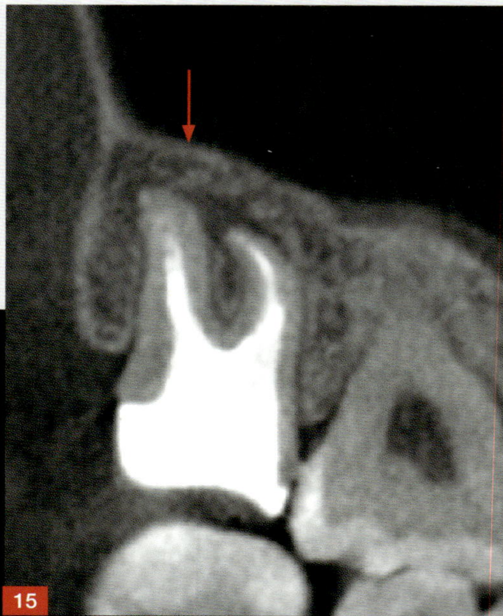

Fig. 16: Six-month postoperative sagittal CBCT view showing bone reformation (red arrow) in the defect around the perforation in the MB root.

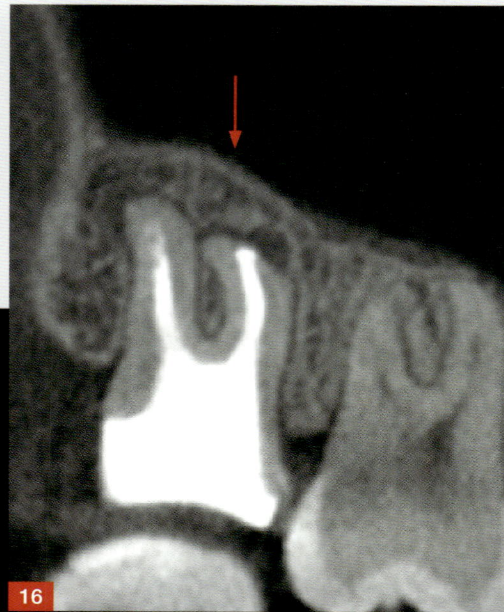

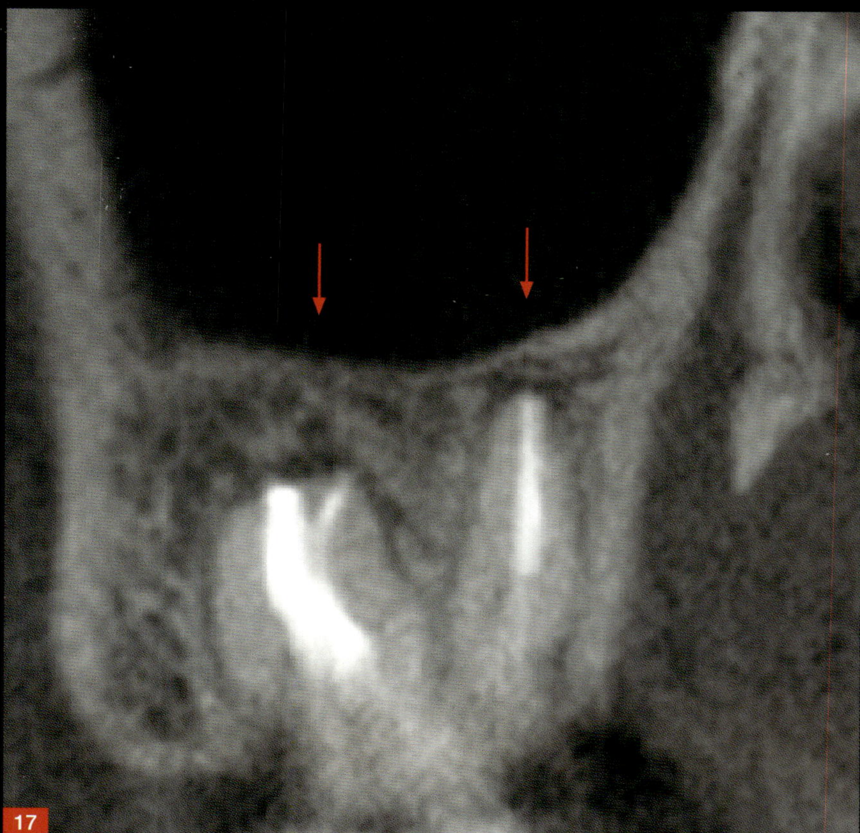

Fig. 17: Six-month postoperative coronal CBCT view showing bone reformation in the defect on the MB root and the palatal root (blue arrows).

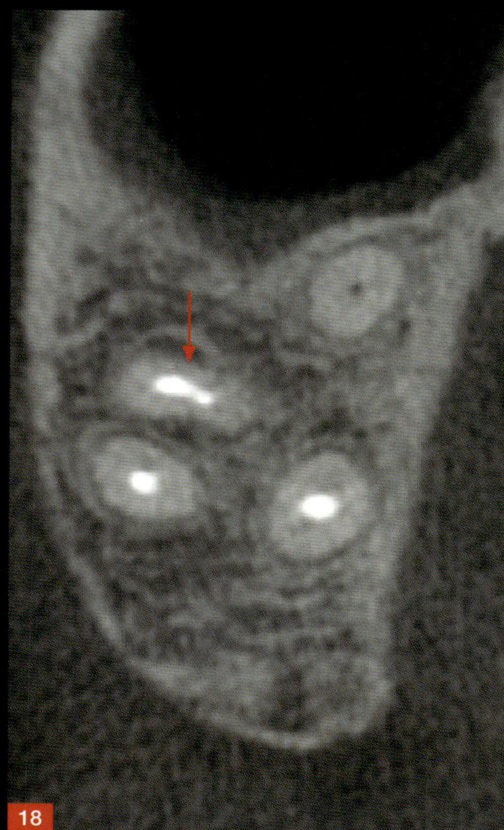

Fig. 18: Six-month postoperative axial CBCT view in the middle third showing MTA root fillings in the oval canal (blue arrow).

In some cases, the TFRK-S ultrasonic tip is used to both remove the root filling materials and create a small space between the canal wall and the root filling materials so that the manual gutta-percha removal (GPR) instrument (DELabs, Santa Barbara, CA) can be placed in it to remove the root filling materials. If this is done carefully, the root filling material extruded from the perforation, particularly in the mesio-buccal canal in upper molars, can be retrieved in one piece with the GPR instrument.
As these teeth present massive bacterial contamination it would be advisable to use further mechanical cleaning procedures, such as using an XP-Endo Finisher at 1,000 rpm in the

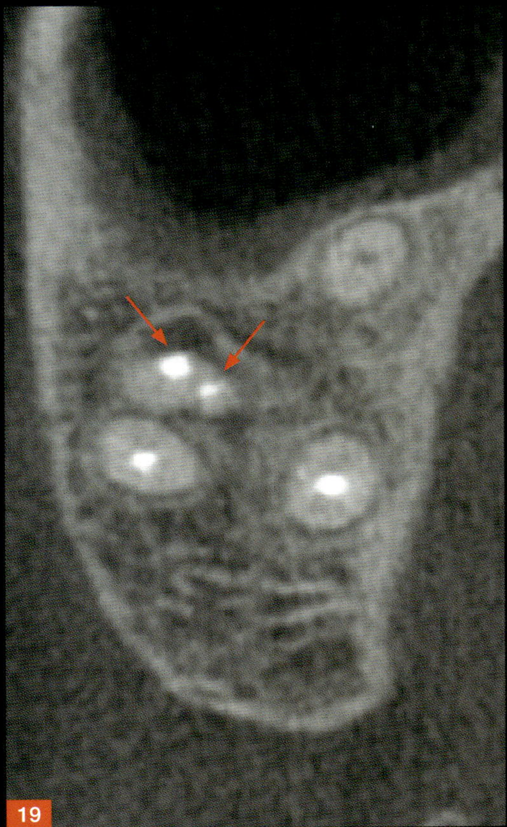

19

Fig. 19: The six-month postoperative axial CBCT view in the apical third shows MTA root fillings in the MB canal and the original canal (blue arrows).

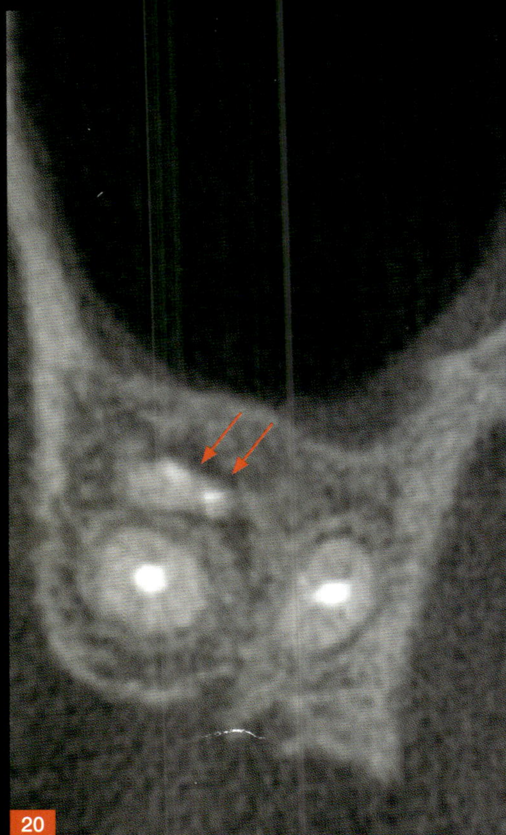

20

Fig. 20: Six-month postoperative axial CBCT view just before the apical foramen shows MTA root fillings in the MB canal with perforation and the original canal (blue arrows) with reforming bone surrounding the root.

presence of 5.25% NaOCl, followed by 17% EDTA for 30 seconds for each canal. In these canals, particularly those with perforation sites the filling material adopted should be ProRoot MTA (Dentsply, Tulsa, OK).

Postoperative x-rays should be taken to confirm the root fillings. Patients should have follow-up appointments 3 and 6 months after the non-surgical retreatment.

CASE REPORT 25

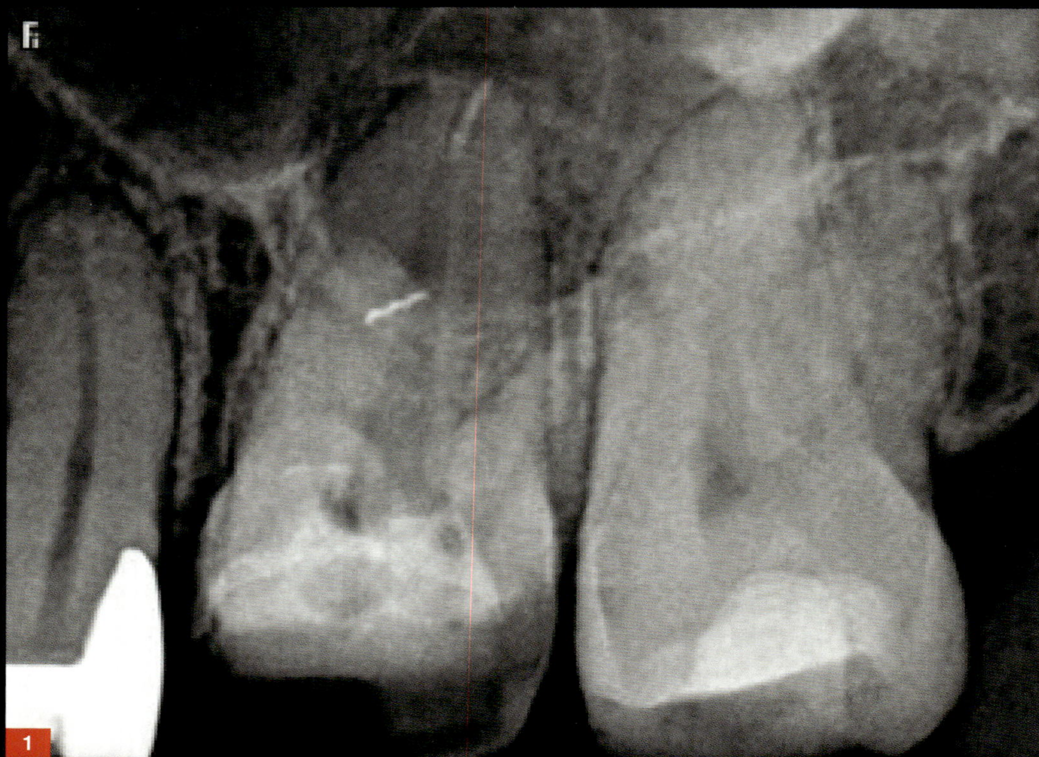

Fig. 1: Preoperative radiograph showing a fractured instrument in the MB canal around the curve (red arrow).

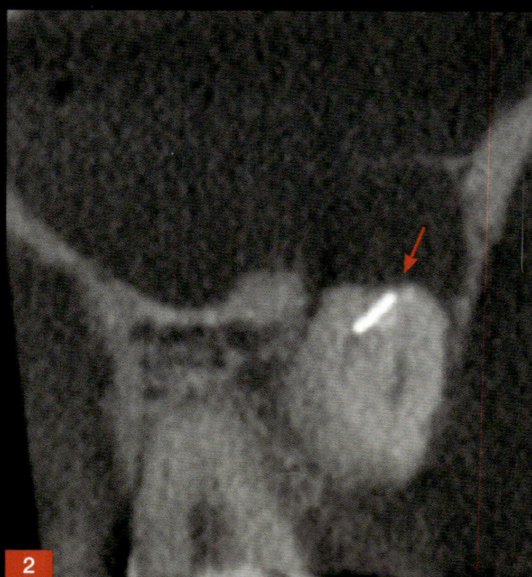

Fig. 2: Preoperative coronal CBCT view showing the separated instrument (red arrow) lying buccally in the MB2 canal with a large apical lesion elevating the sinus floor.

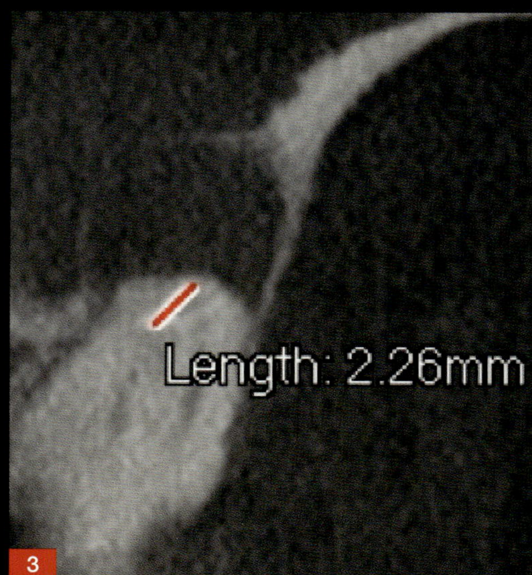

Fig. 3: The preoperative coronal CBCT view shows the fractured instrument measures 2.26 mm.

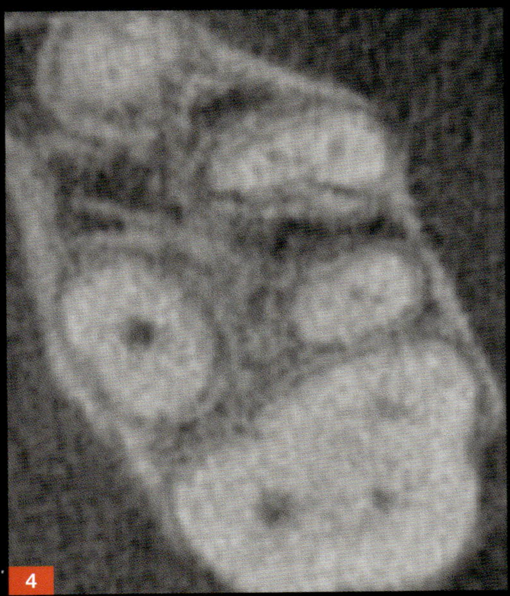

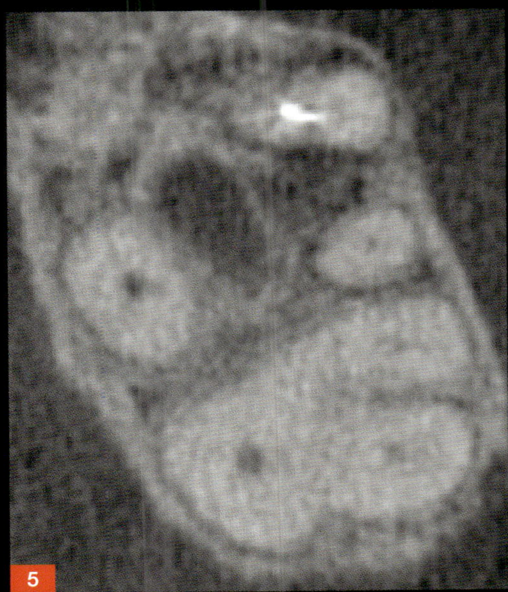

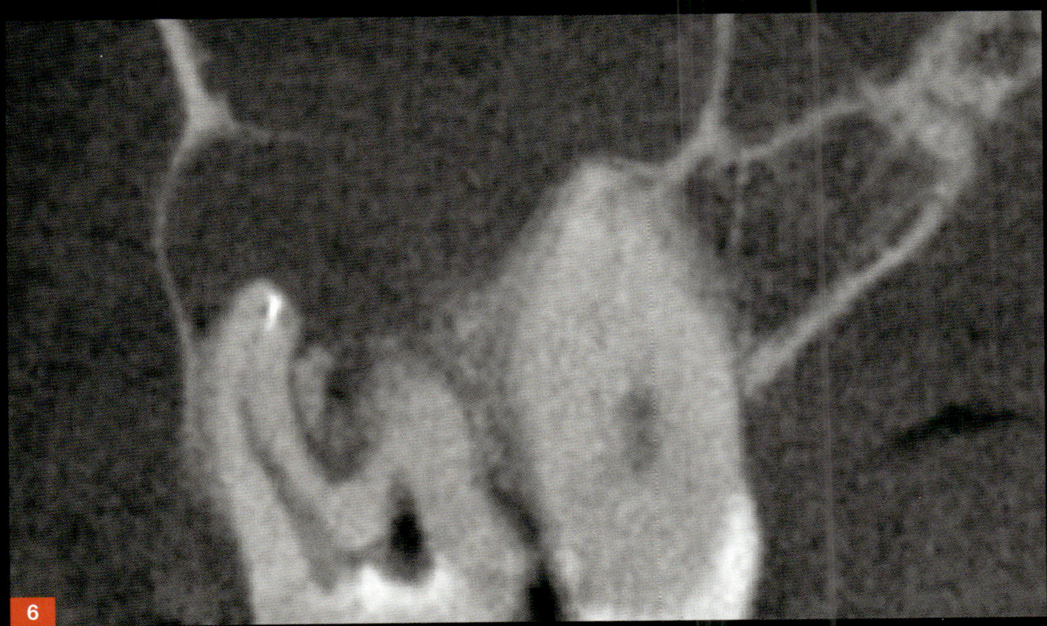

Fig. 4: Preoperative axial CBCT view in the middle third showing the presence of two canals (red arrows) in the MB root (MB1 and MB2).

Fig. 5: Preoperative axial CBCT view in the apical third showing the fractured instrument in the MB2 canal.

Fig. 6: The preoperative sagittal CBCT view in the apical third shows the separated instrument lying distally in the MB root with a large apical lesion developing in the sinus cavity (red arrow).

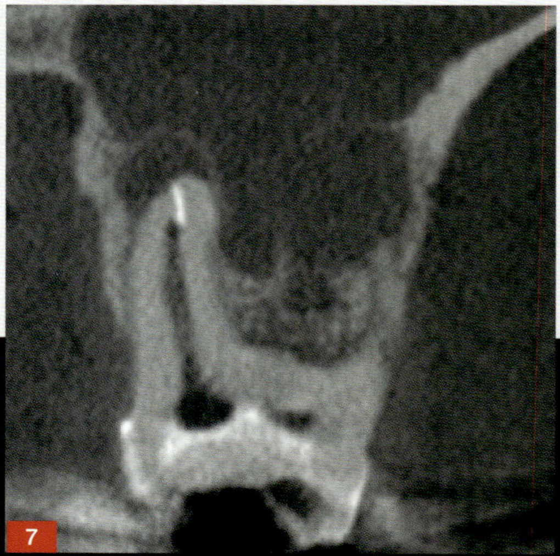

7

Fig. 7: Preoperative coronal CBCT view showing a periapical lesion on the palatal root elevating the sinus floor.

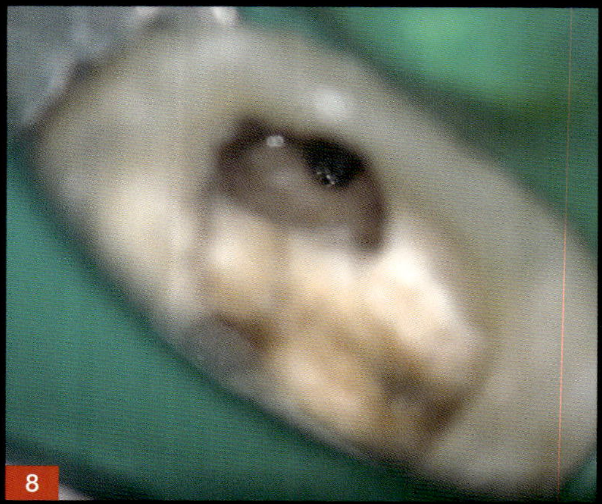

8

Fig. 8: Magnified image from the microscope showing the head of the fractured instrument in the MB2 canal (arrow).

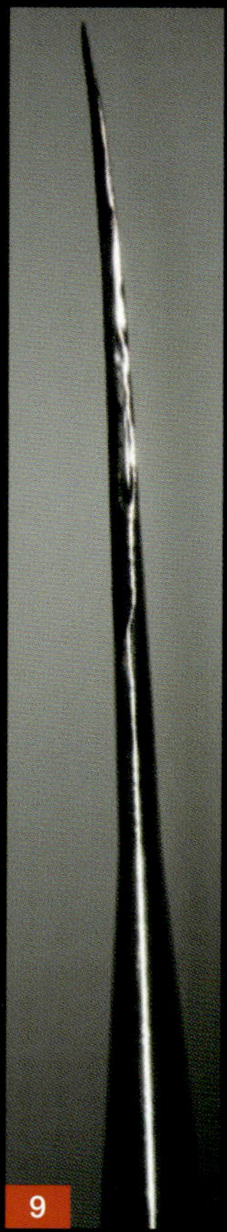

9

Fig. 9: TFRK-6 ultrasonic tip converted into a Katana shape to create a 90-degree semicircular space.

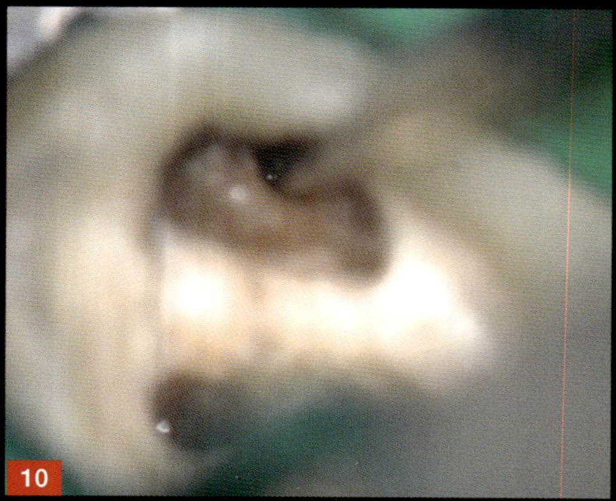

10

Fig. 10: Magnified image from the microscope showing canal preparation to create a semicircular space on the inner wall with a precurved TFRK-S in the MB2 canal (arrow).

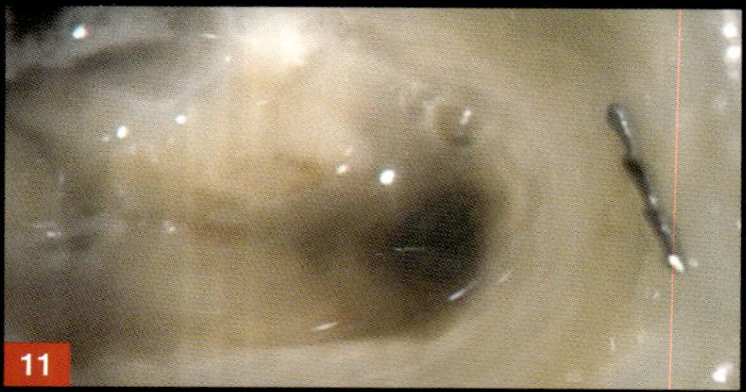

11

Fig. 11: Magnified image from the microscope showing the fractured instrument that was removed from the MB2 canal ultrasonically (arrow).

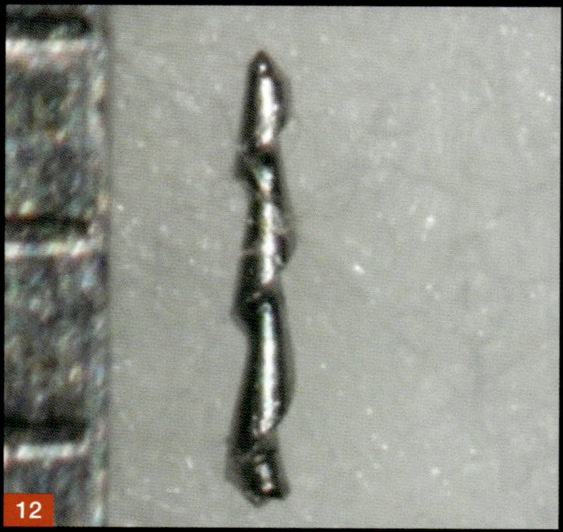

12

Fig. 12: Magnified image from the microscope showing the fractured instrument measuring 2.3 mm against a ruler.

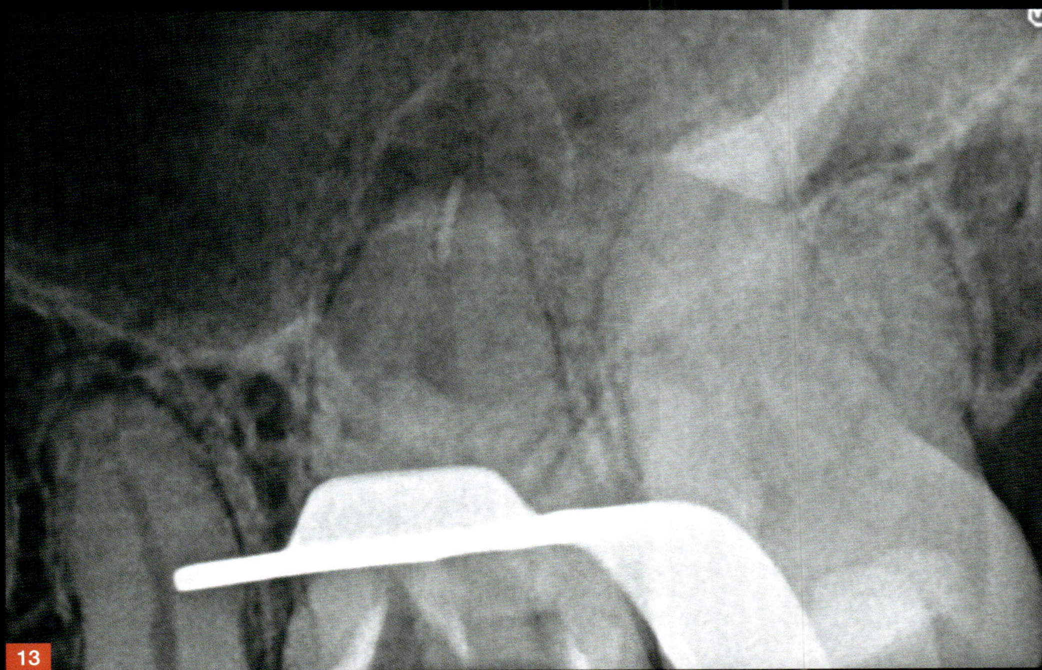

Fig. 13: The intraoperative radiograph confirmed the removal of the fractured instrument from the MB2 canal (blue arrow).

Fig. 14: Magnified image from the microscope showing a suctioning syringe (red arrow) was placed in the MB2 canal for drainage to remove the copious pus that was released upon instrument removal.

Fig. 15: The postoperative x-ray shows the minimally invasive preparation for instrument retrieval and MTA obturation in all the canals.

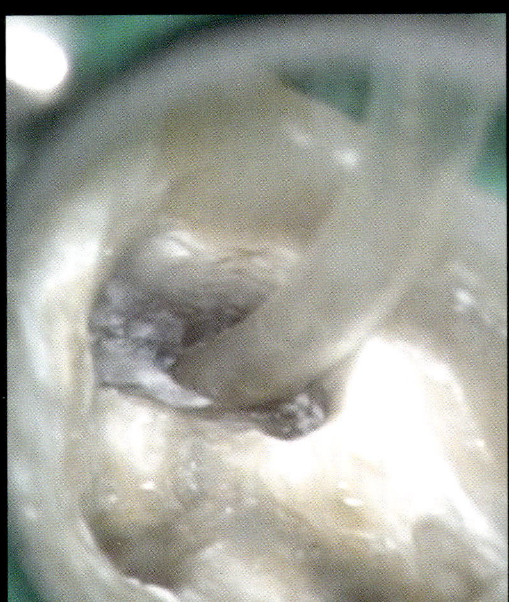

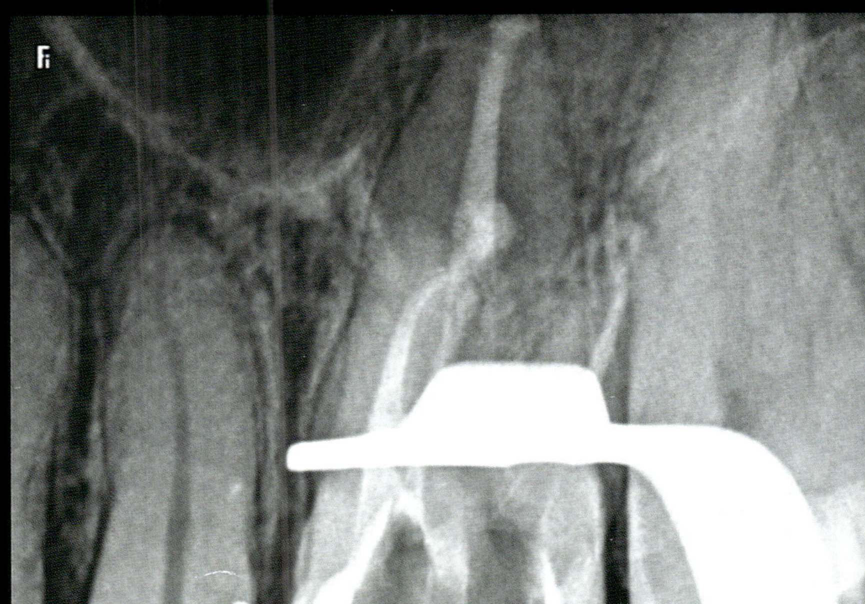

Fig. 16: Three month postoperative radiograph showing the minimally invasive preparation for instrument retrieval and MTA obturation in all the canals.

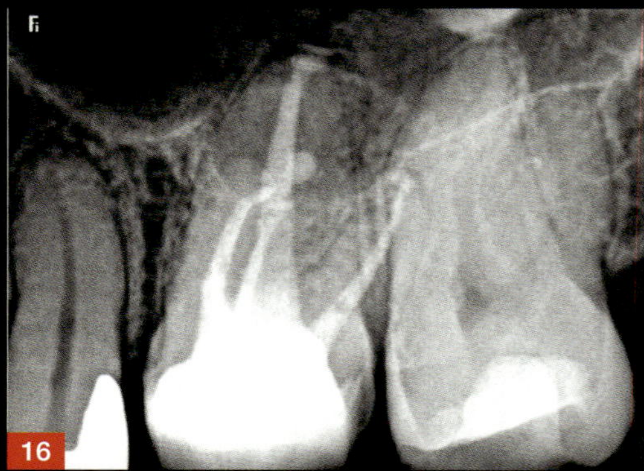

Fig. 17: Three month postoperative coronal CBCT view showing bone reformation in the defect on the MB root (blue arrow).

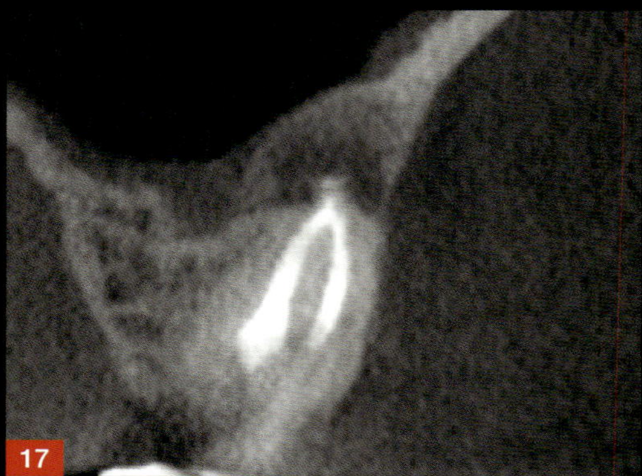

Fig. 18: Three month postoperative axial CBCT view showing MTA root fillings both in the MB1 canal and the MB2 canal (blue arrow).

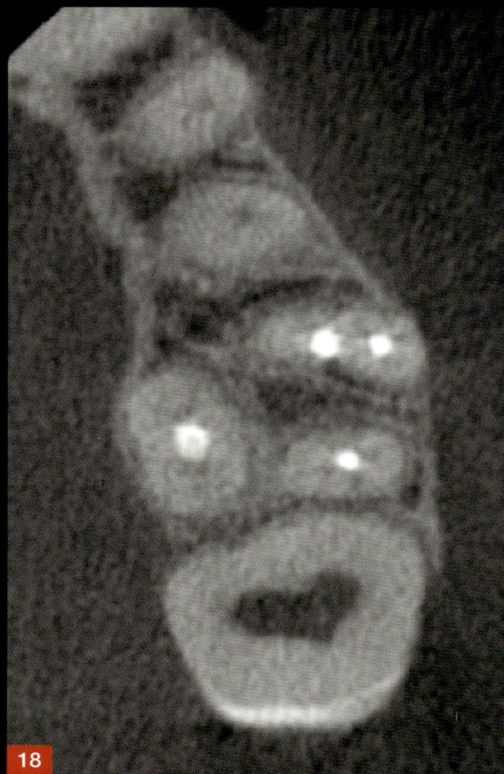

Fig. 19: Three month postoperative sagittal CBCT view showing bone reformation (blue arrow) in the defect on the MB root and the DB root.

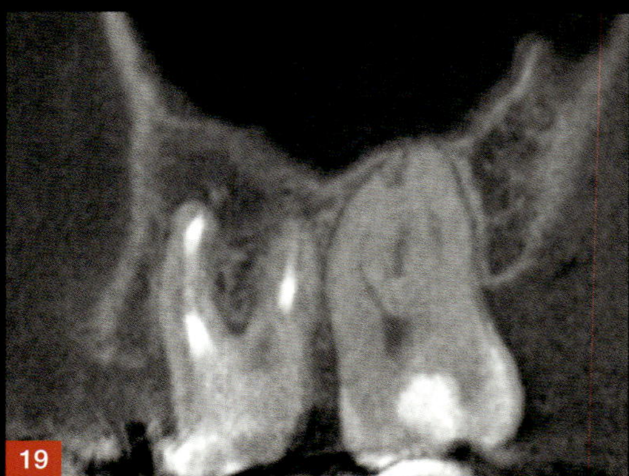

Fig. 20:Three month postoperative coronal CBCT view showing bone reformation in the defect on the palatal root (blue arrow).

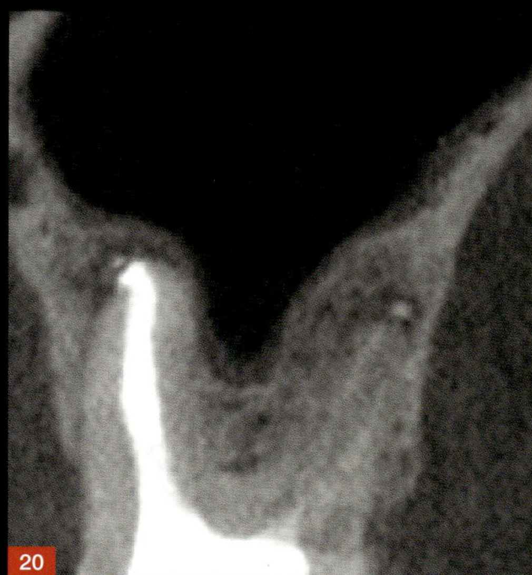

The patient was a 21-year-old female referred by a general dentist for removal of a fractured instrument and retreatment of the mandibular right first molar. The patient presented with mild sensitivity to percussion without spontaneous pain. The periodontal probing depths on this tooth were within normal limits. The 2D PA radiograph (Figs. 1 and 2) and the preoperative CBCT scan revealed the presence of a separated instrument in the mesial canal with a periapical lesion on the root. However, the radiopaque materials in the mesial root blurred the fractured instrument, making it difficult to measure it on the CBCT images. Upon removal of the temporary filling, calcium hydroxide was used as an endodontic dressing and it was

CASE REPORT 26

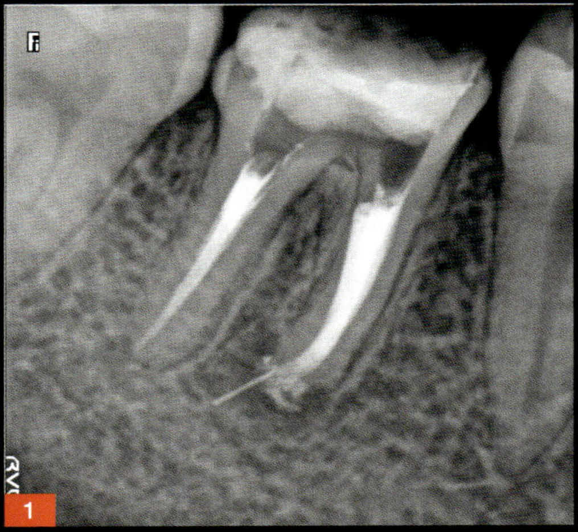

1

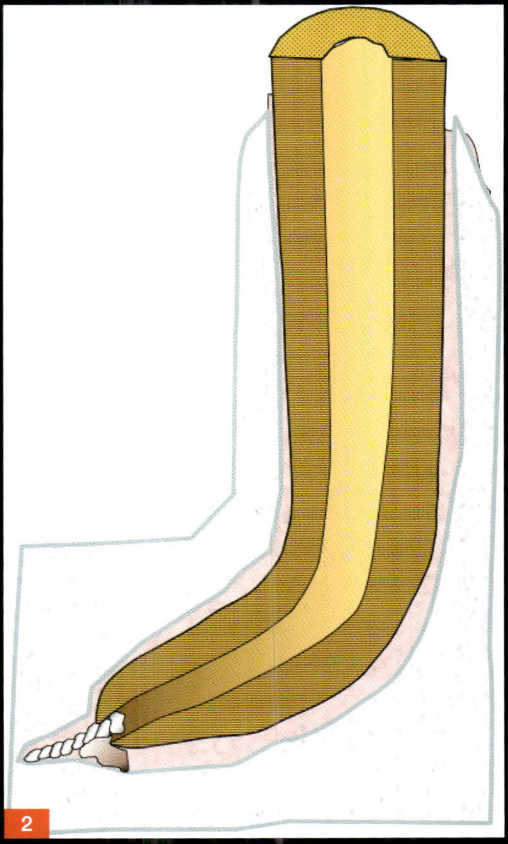

2

Fig. 1: Preoperative radiograph showing the fractured instrument (red arrow) beyond the curve in the mesial root.

Fig. 2: Schematic image of the mesial root showing that more than 90% of the instrument beyond the curve is outside the root.

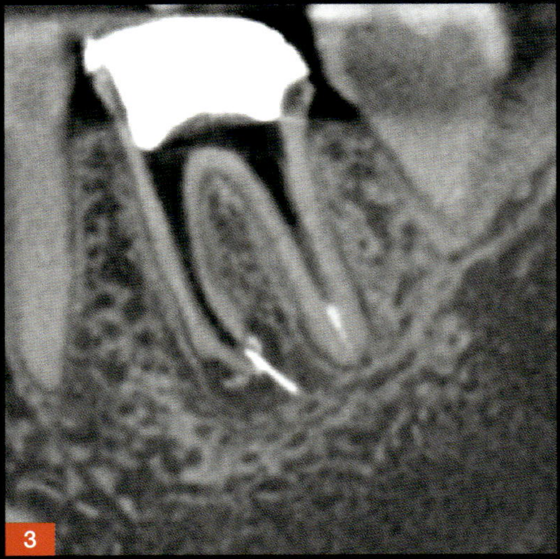

3

Fig. 3: Preoperative sagittal CBCT view showing the separated instrument (red arrow) lying distally in the mesial root with a small apical lesion and the majority of it extruded beyond the apical foramen.

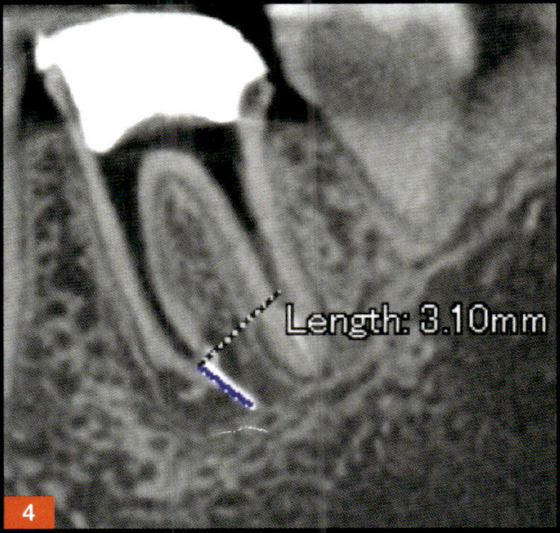

4

Fig. 4: Preoperative coronal CBCT view showing the fractured instrument measures 3.10 mm.

removed by irrigating the canal with 5.25 % NaOCl and 17% EDTA stirred using a TFRK-S ultrasonic tip. Subsequently, another CBCT scan (Figs. 3 to 7) and another radiograph (Fig. 8) were taken to clearly identify the fractured instrument. On the CBCT scan, 90% of the fractured instrument appears to be beyond the apical foramen with a periapical lesion. Apical periodontitis was diagnosed. The treatment plan was devised based on the findings from the CBCT images that showed the separated instrument measured 3.10 mm and the curvature of the canal measured 20 degrees against the line from the orifice to the fractured instrument, which made it possible to retrieve it with ultrasonics alone.

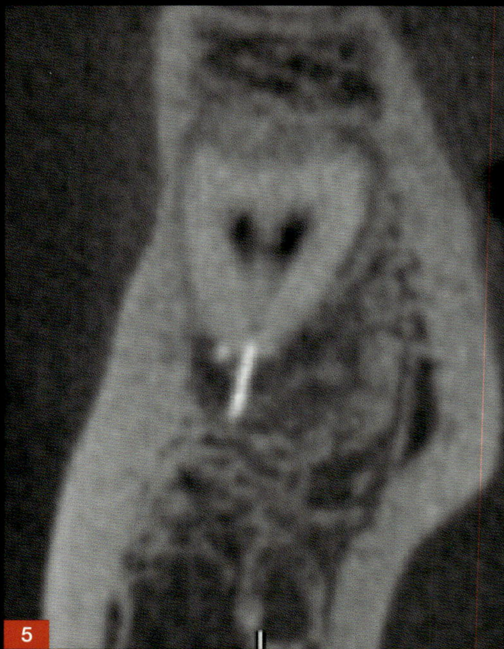

5

Fig. 5: Preoperative coronal CBCT scan showing that the MB canal and the ML canal merge into one canal in the apical third and the fractured instrument is beyond the join.

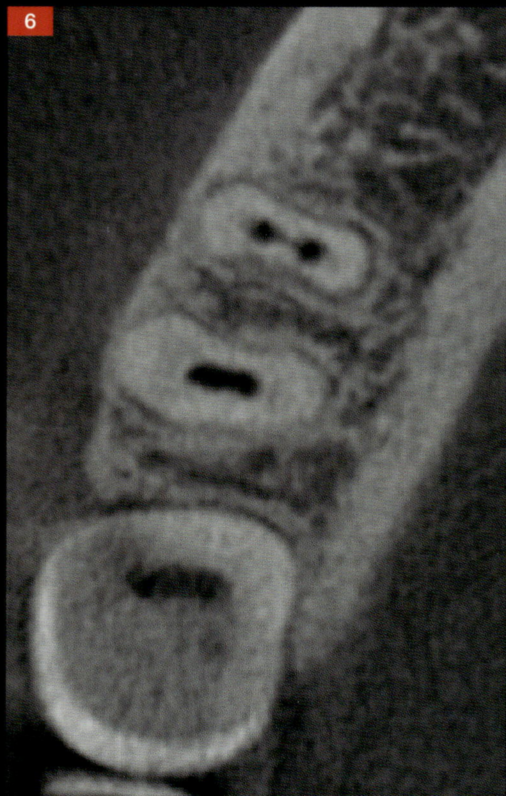

6

Fig. 6: Preoperative axial CBCT scan showing one canal in the distal root and two canals in the mesial root.

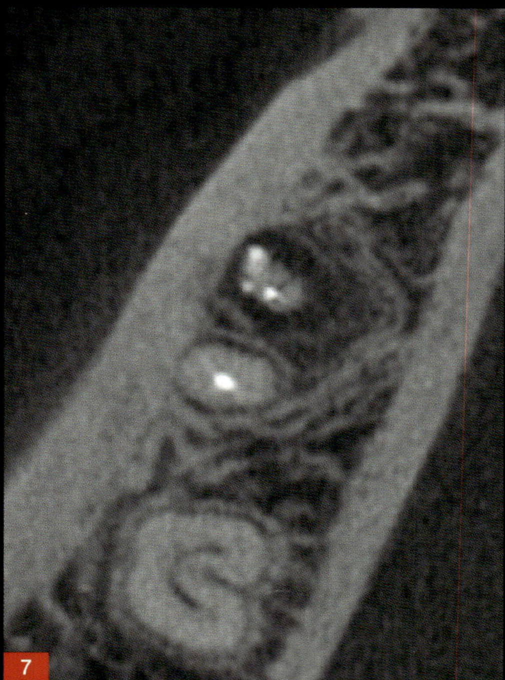

7

Fig. 7: Preoperative axial CBCT scan showing the fractured instrument (red arrow) in the mesial canal just before the apical foramen.

The inner wall for this instrument was found on the distal side of the mesial root. First the canal was irrigated with 5.25% Qmix 2in1 (Dentsply Sirona, USA) and dried with a Stropko irrigator and was examined to locate the fractured instrument under the microscope. However, it was not in a visible place and the coronal end of the fractured instrument seemed to be far beyond the curve (Fig. 9) as shown on the preoperative CBCT images. Therefore, the preparation for instrument retrieval started using the tactile sensation on the clinician's fingers in the presence of EDTA. The ultrasonic tip must be sharpened with a brownie bur so that it can be placed in the narrow space between the fractured instrument and the inner

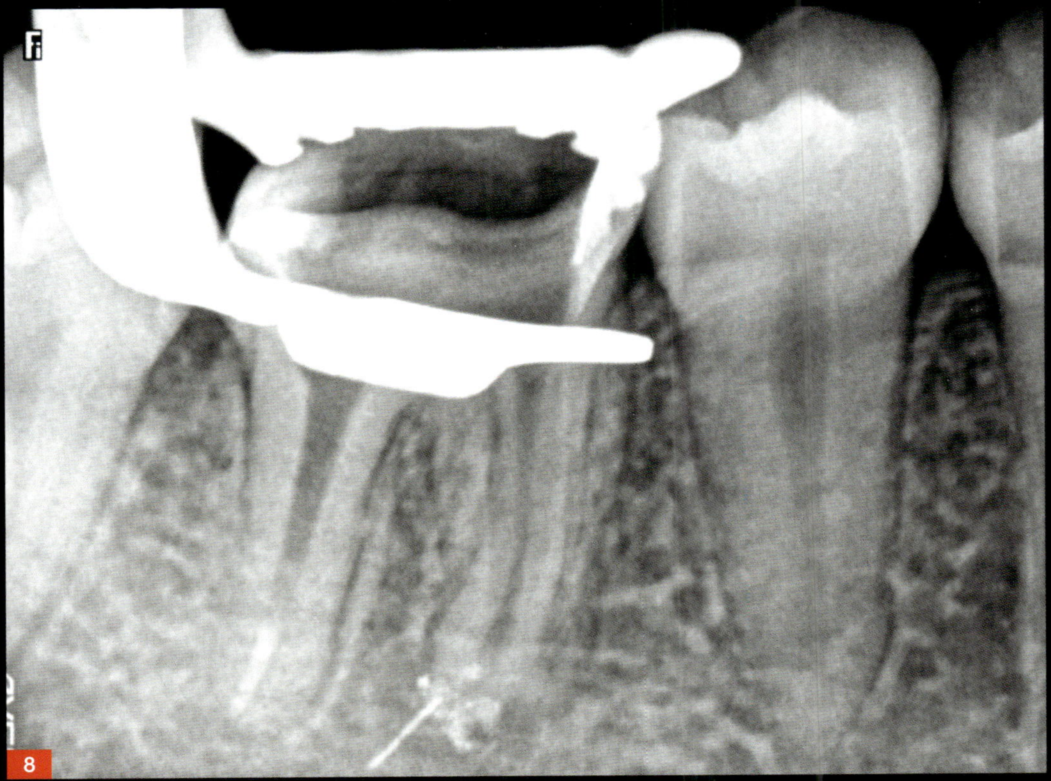

Fig. 8: The intraoperative radiograph taken after removal of calcium hydroxide medication reveals the separated instrument (red arrow) far beyond the curve and almost all of it extruded into the periapical tissues.

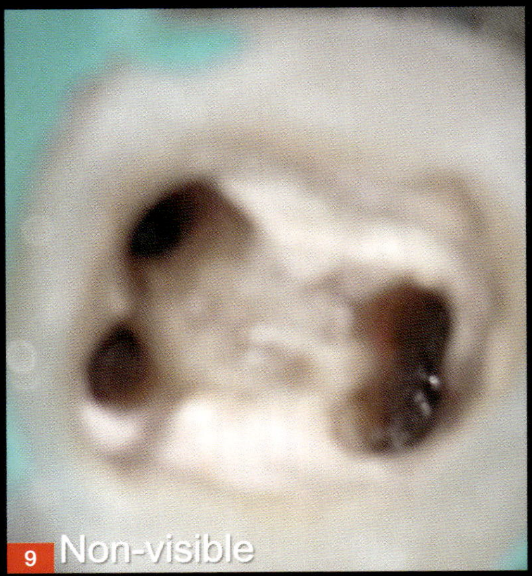

Fig. 9: Magnified image from the microscope showing that the fractured instrument is not visible in the mesial root under the microscope.

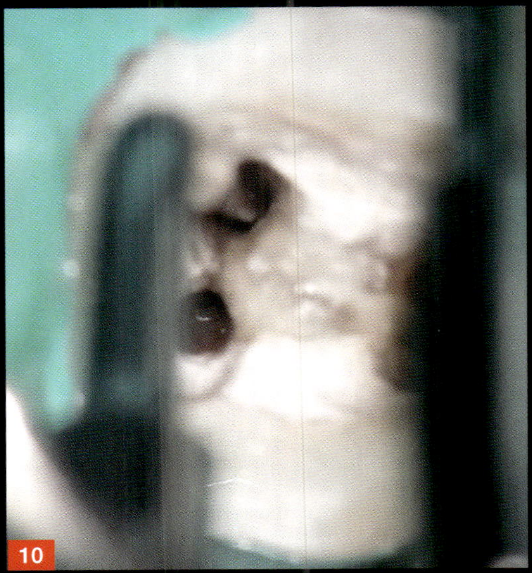

Fig. 10: Magnified image from the microscope shows the placement of the precurved TFRK-S in the space on the inner wall in the mesiolingual canal under the microscope.

wall. The sharpened TFRK-S ultrasonic tip was precurved suit the canal curvature and it was placed in the space where a sticky feeling was obtained on the ultrasonic tip (Fig. 10). Several radiographs were taken until one showed the ultrasonic tip placed in the space on the inner wall (Figs. 11 and 12). The root canal was replenished with 17% EDTA and the ultrasonic tip was slid down along the inner wall into the space. The ultrasonic tip was activated continuously in short up/down strokes at power 4 on a scale of 0 to 20. The fractured instrument came out of the canal a few seconds after the ultrasonic activation (Fig. 13).
The retrieved fractured instrument measured 3.1 mm on a ruler (Fig. 14), which matched the

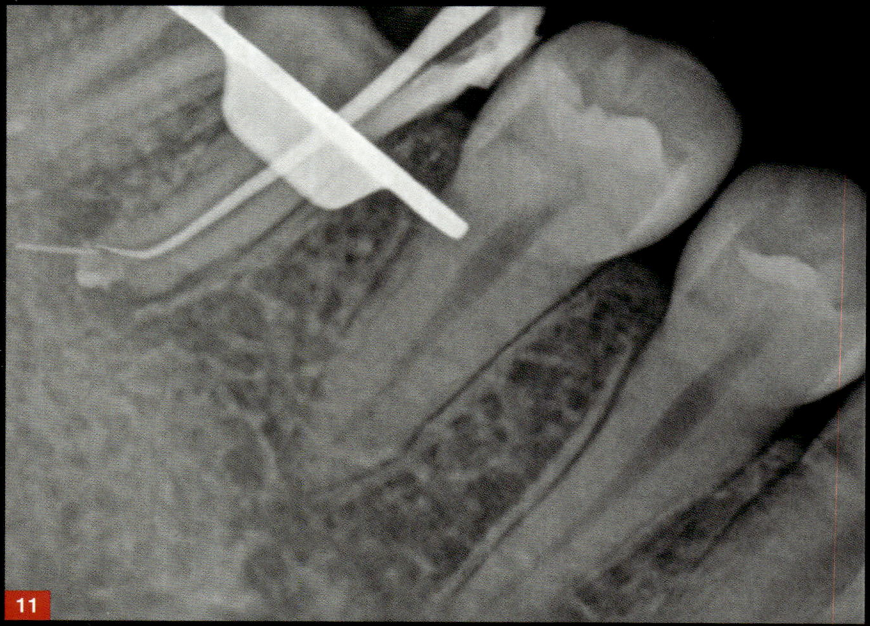

11

Fig. 11: The intraoperative radiograph taken after the placement of the ultrasonic tip (red arrow) shows it is in the space between the inner wall and the fractured instrument.

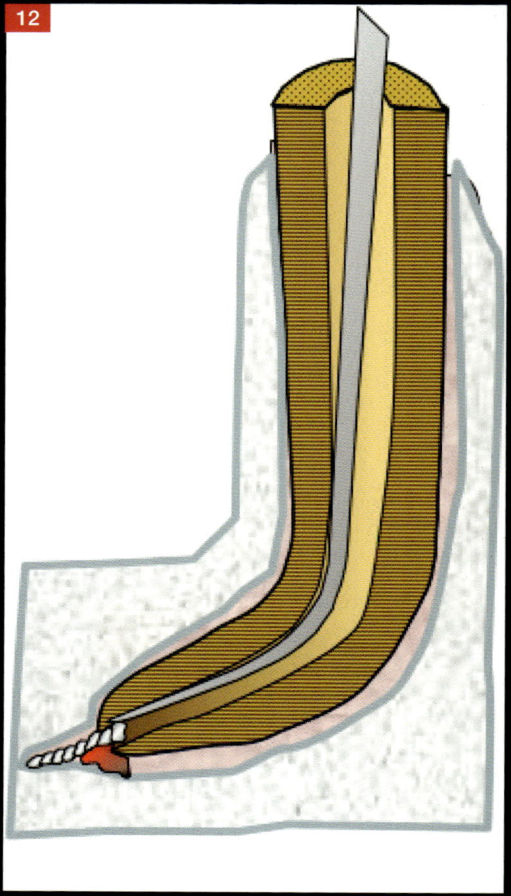

12

Fig. 12: Schematic image of the mesial root showing the ultrasonic tip placed on the inner side of the fractured instrument.

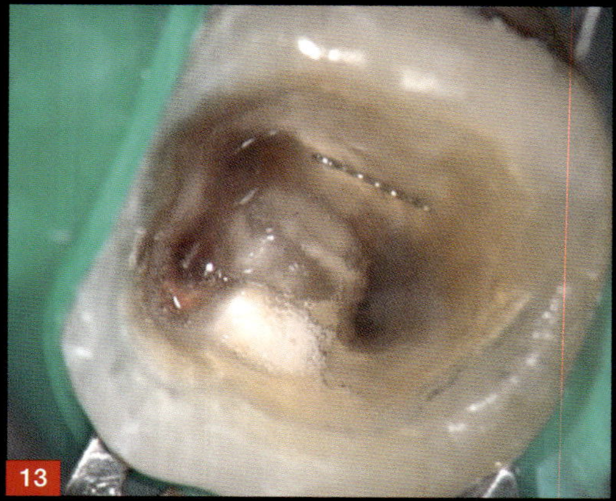

13

Fig. 13: Magnified image from the microscope shows the separated instrument that has just come out of the mesiolingual canal with ultrasonics

length of the fractured instrument measured on the CBCT images. A radiograph was taken to confirm the retrieval of the separated instrument (Fig. 15). All the canals were cleaned and shaped, followed by MTA obturation (Fig. 16). The postoperative radiograph shows that there was almost no dentin sacrifice during the preparation.
The three-month postoperative radiograh showed that good periapical healing was in progress compared to the preoperative radiograph (Fig. 17).

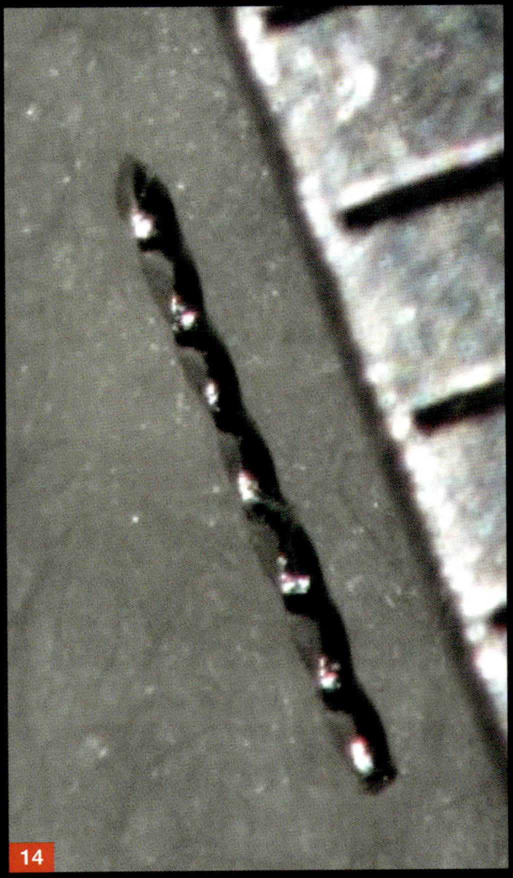

14

Fig. 14: The retrieved instrument measures 3.1 mm on a ruler.

Fig. 15: Intraoperative radiograph taken after removal of the separated instrument showing the successful removal of the fractured instrument (red arrow).

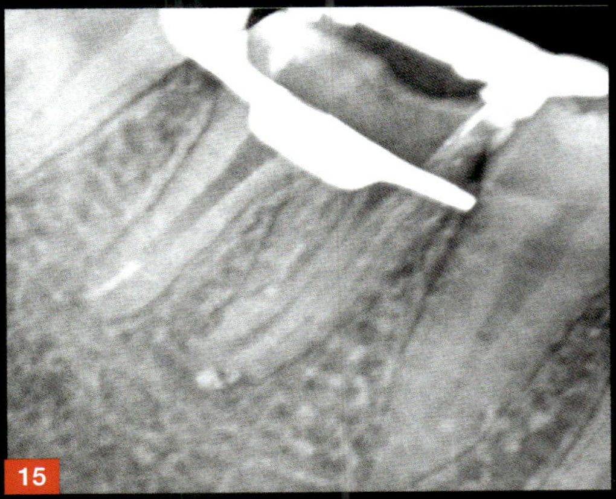

15

Fig. 16: Postoperative radiograph showing a minimally invasive preparation for the removal of the non-visible fractured instrument.

Fig. 17: Three month postoperative radiograph showing good periapical healing on the mesial root.

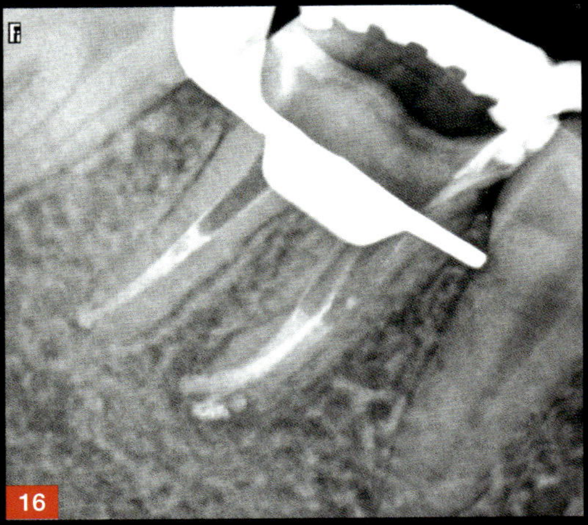

16

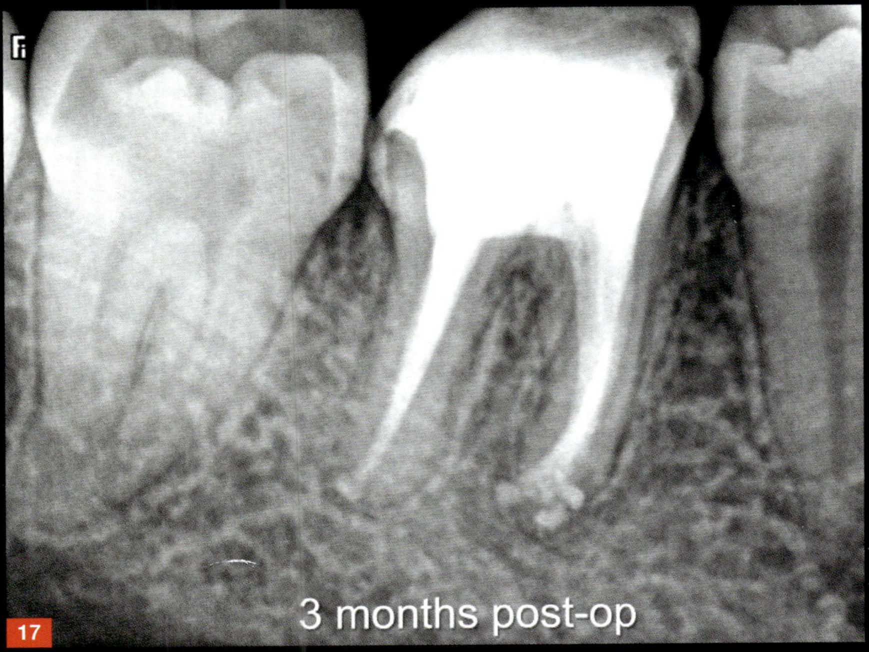

17

Bypassing a periapical ledge

When a ledge is identified the presents resistance to endodontic instruments by blocking them, it is necessary to evaluate its position in relation to the canal anatomy before attempting to overcome the obstacle. Indeed, it is often located at a curvature and the filling material appears in an asymmetrical position in relation to the center of the root[117].

In any case, the following steps must be carried out to bypass a ledge:

- Bear in mind that the actual canal is a few millimeters more coronal and on the opposite side to the bottom of the ledge, as shown by the drawing.
- Insert a pre-curved ISO08 or ISO10 k-file and make small clockwise movements in the apical direction. Then, insert a viscous chelator into the root canal until the tip of the instrument enters the original canal.
- Continue with the probing technique with watch-winding movements until you reach the presumed working length, perhaps with the help of an apex locator. Once the obstacle is bypassed, perform movements of half a millimeter beyond the apex with "to and fro" motions.
- Insert a k-file smaller than the one used to determine the working length, and bring it to the working length with "to and fro" movements until it easily reaches the apical third.
- Perform the same procedure with ISO 10 and ISO 15 k-file.

Bypassing apical blocks

The underlying causes for the formation of a block during the first phases of probing may be compaction in the apical third due to a part of the collagen in the pulp that was not completely removed, or dentin debris that was generated by the action of mechanical instruments (rotating or reciprocating) during the shaping phase and was, eventually, pushed apically.

The main reasons for the development of blocks inside the canal are attributable to:

- Inadequate cavity access
- Insufficient preparation of the coronal portion of the canal
- Insufficient use of irrigants
- Use of poorly flexible instruments that have a larger diameter than the canal lumen or mechanical instruments that were used incorrectly[117].

EXAMPLE OF A STEP

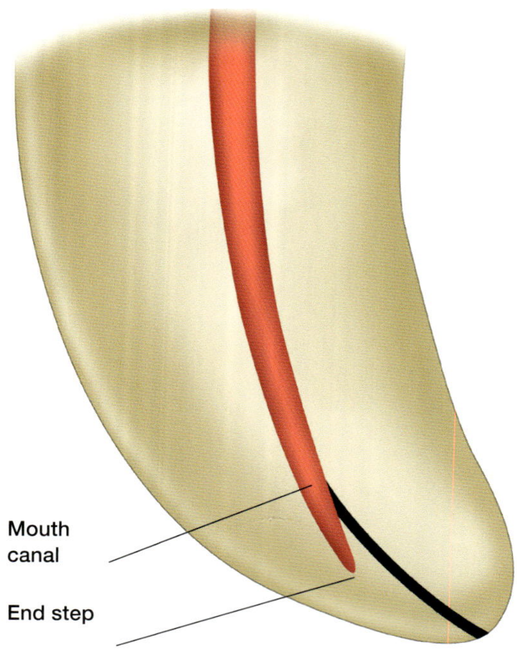

EXAMPLE OF BLOCK

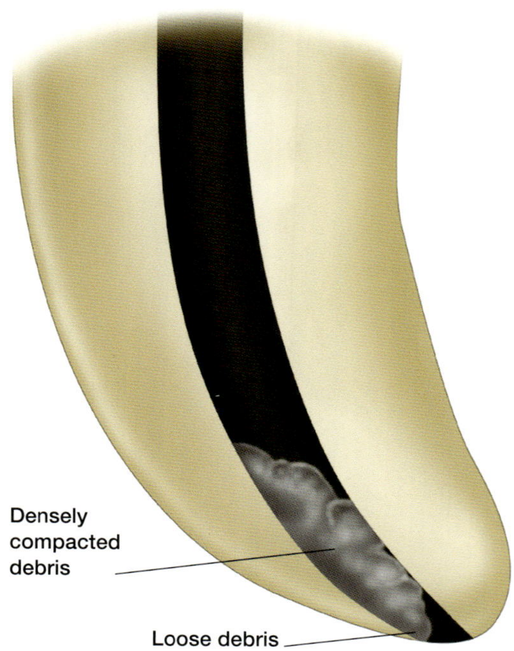

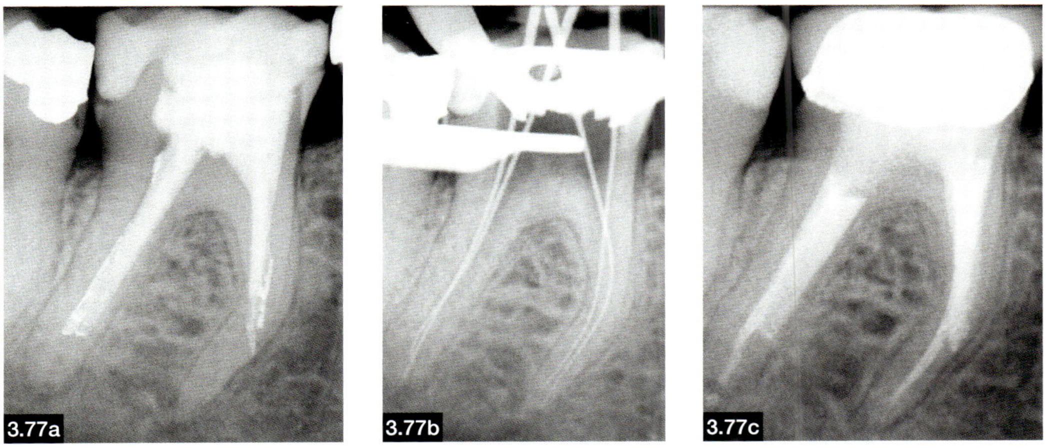

Fig. 3.77a: A retreatment process that is complicated by the development of a perforation in the mesial root and a corresponding mesial step.

Fig. 3.77b: The use of thin, pre-curved hand-tools made of steel makes it possible to by-pass the step and measure the working length.

Fig. 3.77c: The retreatment process is performed.

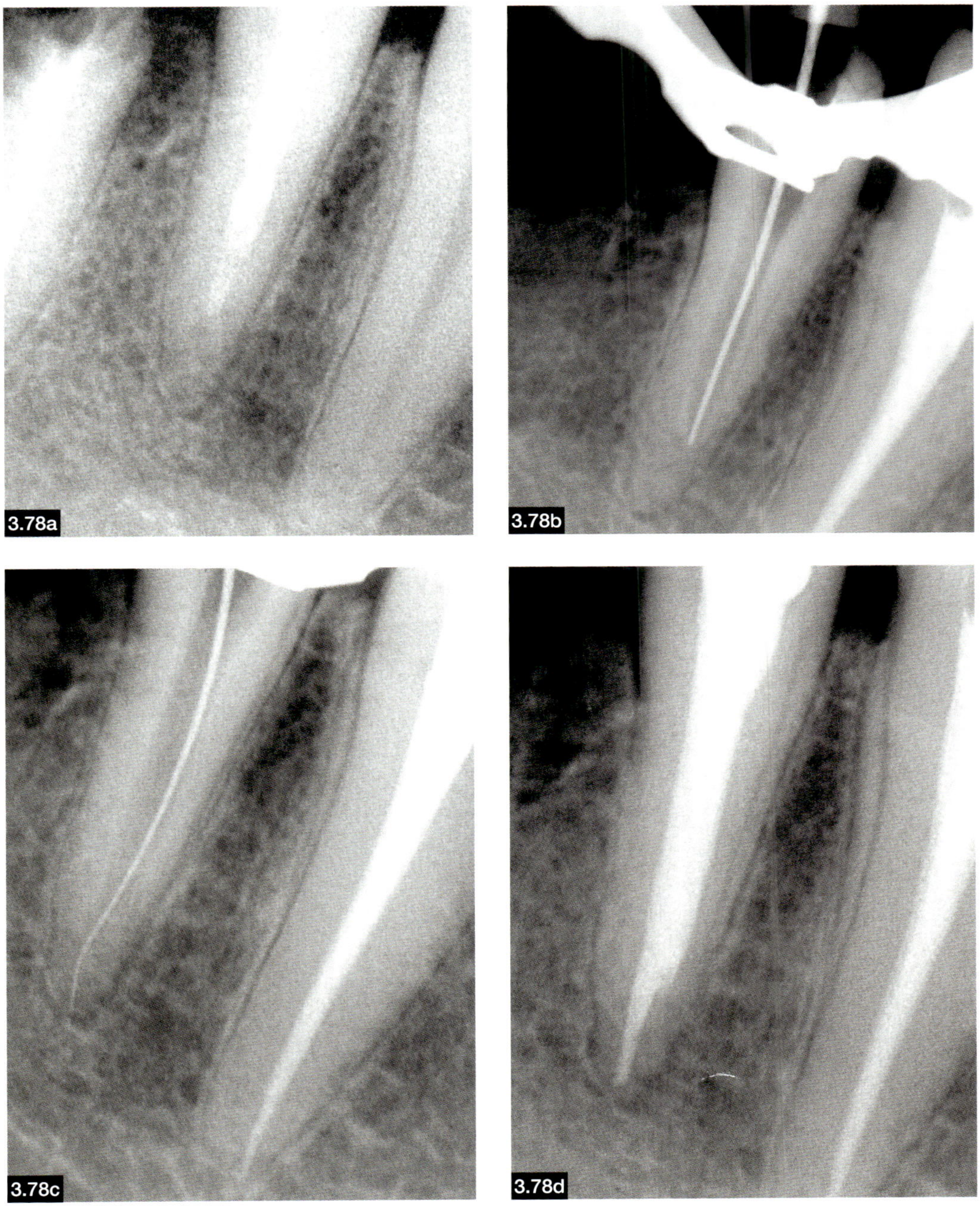

Fig. 3.78a: A clearly short paste filling indicates retreatment. The distal tooth was extracted before this procedure.

Fig. 3.78b: The file path does not seem to be easy within the canal.

Fig. 3.78c: Pre-curving the steel instrument allows the clinician to by-pass the obstacle and reach the apical limit.

Fig. 3.78d: The canal is now perfectly sealed.

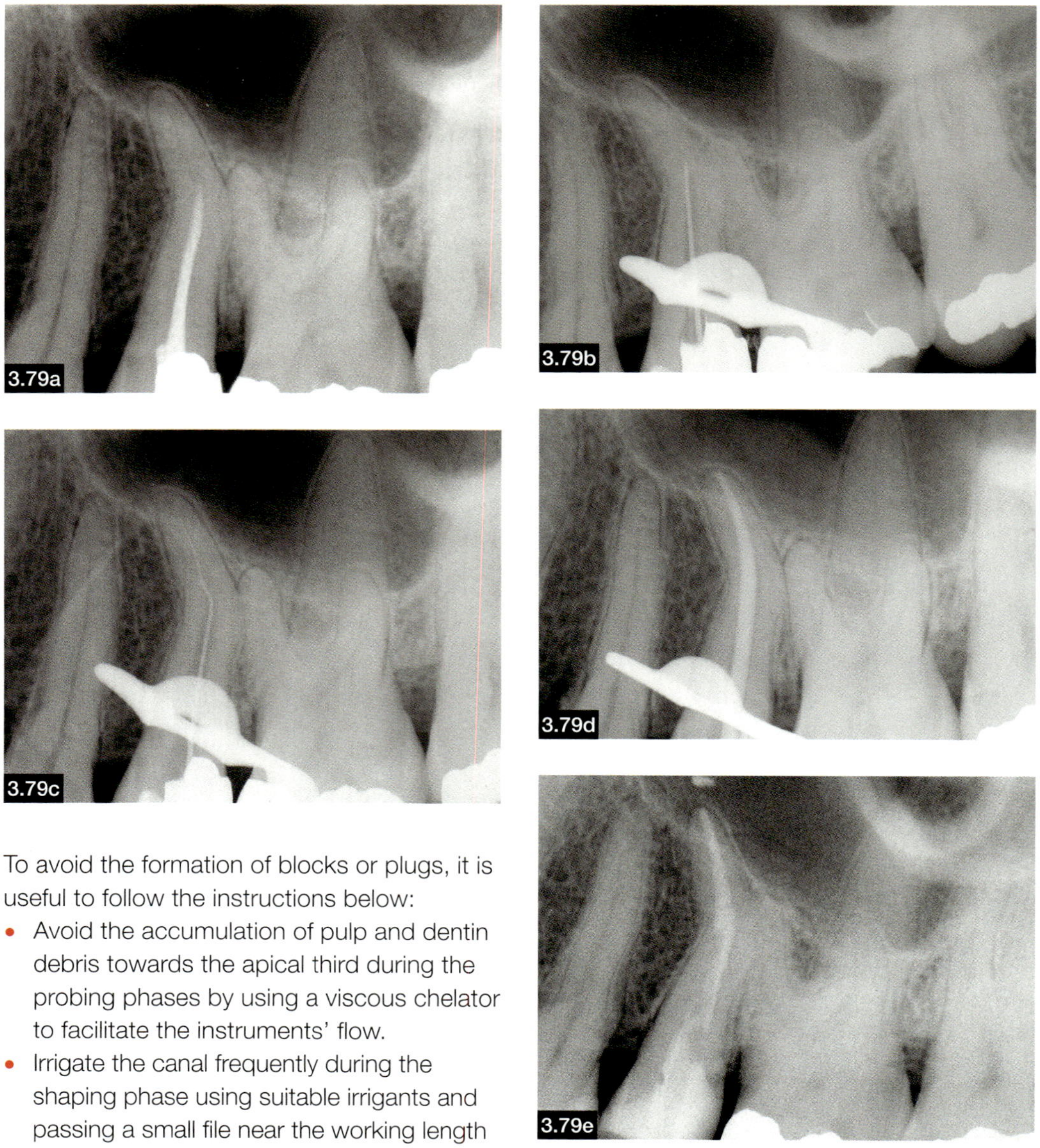

Fig. 3.79a: A previous endodontic treatment had not been performed owing to an inadequate interpretation of the canal morphology.

Fig. 3.79b: The distance of the remaining part of the canal seems to be difficult.

Fig. 3.79c: Bending the small diameter steel instrument makes it possible to by-pass the step.

Fig. 3.79d: The ideal shape confirms the good adaptation of the gutta-percha cone.

Fig. 3.79e: The filling is now completed and seems to be satisfactory.

To avoid the formation of blocks or plugs, it is useful to follow the instructions below:

- Avoid the accumulation of pulp and dentin debris towards the apical third during the probing phases by using a viscous chelator to facilitate the instruments' flow.
- Irrigate the canal frequently during the shaping phase using suitable irrigants and passing a small file near the working length to ensure effective apical and canal patency.
- In the case of a stop or block, first use larger instruments coronally with respect to the block, then rinse and work in the root canal with low taper instruments combined with viscous chelator.

Whether it is a block of collagen or dentin, the cap is generally made up of a harder surface layer in which the material is densely compacted. It is, therefore, this layer that makes it more difficult for instruments to pass and leads to a sense of retraction. On the other hand, the lower part, is made up of debris that is arranged loosely and it is easier to cross. Usually, once the instrument has passed the first layer, it can feel as if something has fallen into a void.

The maneuver that makes it possible to by-pass a collagen or dentin block, is called unblocking. Consequently, the best operational sequence is as follows:

1. Insert small files such as ISO 08 or ISO 10 with a watch-winding movement, in the presence of viscous chelating agent, thus exerting a slight pressure in the apical direction.
2. When the instrument feels as if it is inside the block, try to gain the presumed working length.
3. Once you have reached the presumed working length, use a "to and fro" movement with short excursions of about 0.5 mm.

4. Insert an instrument smaller than the one used to reach the working length.
5. Use an ISO10 k-file to reach the working length and, only when this falls freely to the desired length, commence the next shaping steps.

Dentinal cracks: can you prevent apical fractures?

In severely damaged teeth such as teeth that have undergone more than one root canal shaping operation, dentinal integrity appears to be severely impaired[118]. Therefore, the use ultrasound and of rotating instruments made of Ni-Ti alloy is not a risk-free process[119].
Many studies have reported a high incidence of cracks, of varying sizes, within the dentin compartment that can become accentuated and facilitate root fractures when the tooth is subjected to masticatory load, following treatment[120]. Needless to say, this phenomenon is difficult to predict.
However, it can be avoided with an appropriate use of mechanical and ultrasonic instruments. There are no certain elements in the literature providing clinical information for the prevention of dentinal fractures, whether they are complete or incomplete.

About perforations

Perforations are communications between the root canal system and periodontal tissues due to errors performed during canal treatment. Perforation can cause inflammation of periradicular tissues as a result of mechanical trauma and bacterial contamination. We will examine this subject in detail in chapter 7, however it seems appropriate to clarify a few key points here. The parameters to be considered when a perforation is identified are the following:

1. **Drilling position**. Perforations of the apical third or middle third of the root have a worse prognosis than others located at the floor multiradicular teeth of the pulp chamber of the multiradiculated elements. This is because these perforations are significantly more complex to treat.
2. **Size and shape**. The perforations must have a round shape and be retentive. Consequently, it is necessary that there is a minimum dentin thickness that favors the stabilization of the material.
3. **Time**. Timely repair of the perforation is recommended because an unrepaired perforation may result in periodontal damage over time.
4. **Periodontal probing**. If periodontal probing is found, the prognosis is generally worse.

It is always better, if clinicians decide to repair the perforation, to reduce the number of appointments needed to complete the endodontic therapy[121].
It is important to have the capacity to seal the perforation in a stable manner with a material that is biocompatible and, possibly, radiopaque, in order to facilitate radiographic control. Adequate magnification and illumination are essential: for this reason, the use of a surgical microscope is strongly recommended. The perforation must be cleaned and prepared as if it were an additional root canal; an ultrasonic drill or a small multi-blade bur can help. Before proceeding with the filling, it is important to ensure good hemostasis. In some cases, to prevent the filling from being pushed into the periodontium, it is possible to place

Fig. 3.80: Cracks are probably caused by over-energetic use of the Ni-Ti alloy instruments in the apical area.

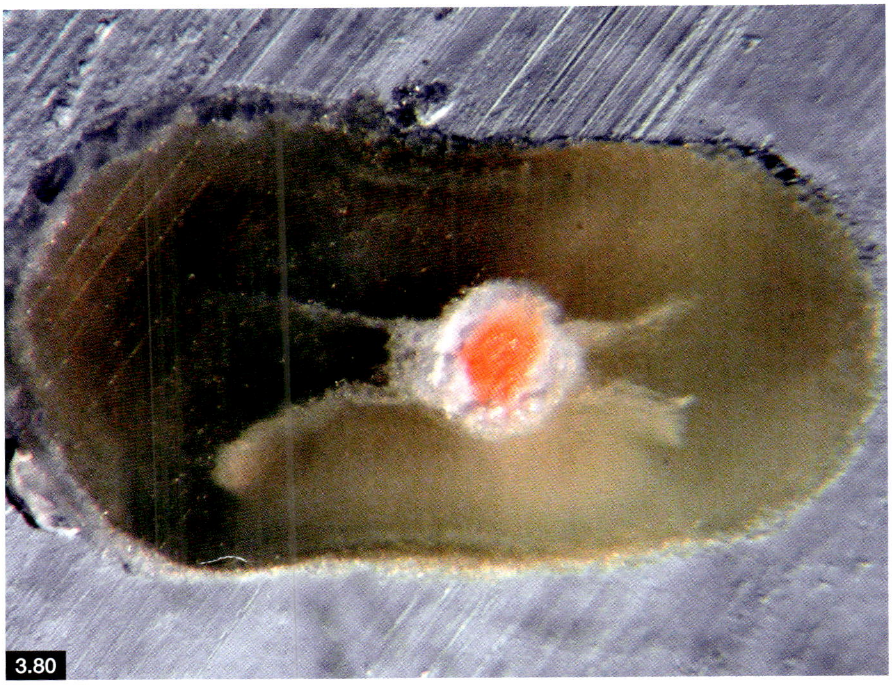

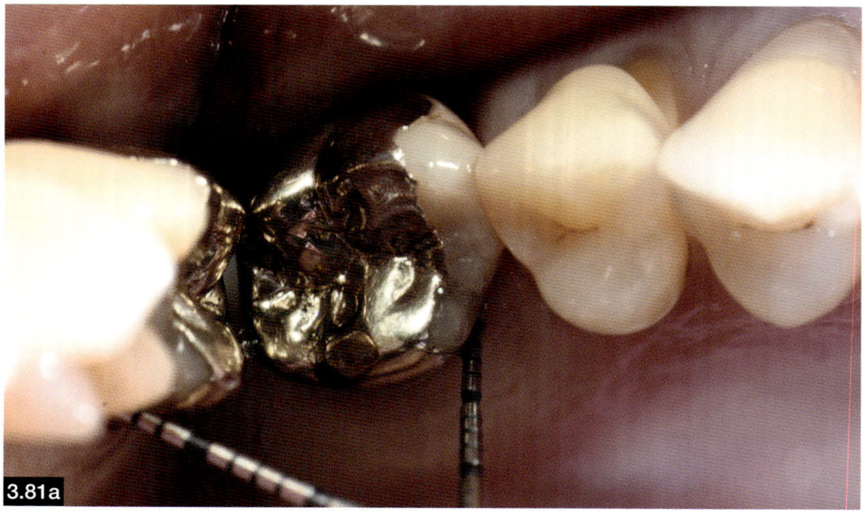

Fig. 3.81a: A case of an endodontically treated tooth that does not seem to present any problems except for a small mesial periodontal lesion.

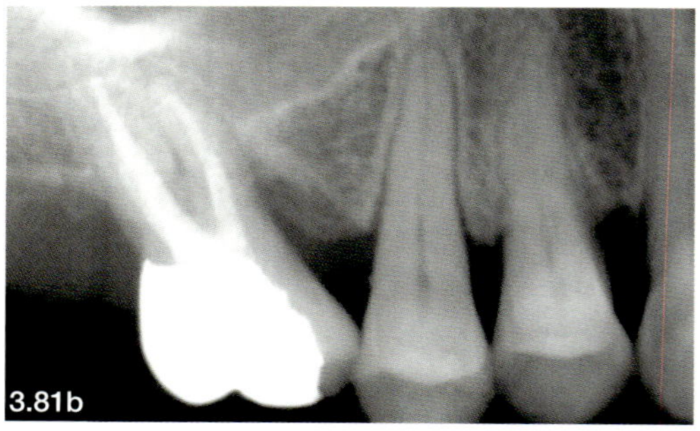

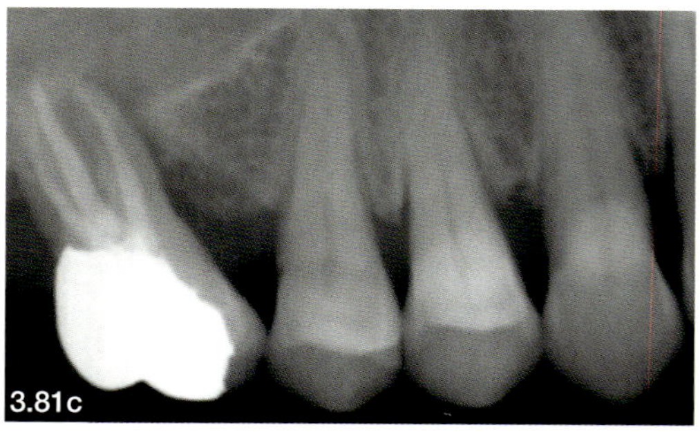

Fig. 3.81b-c: b) The radiological picture at the time of probing; c) The radiological picture approximately one year after the previous check.

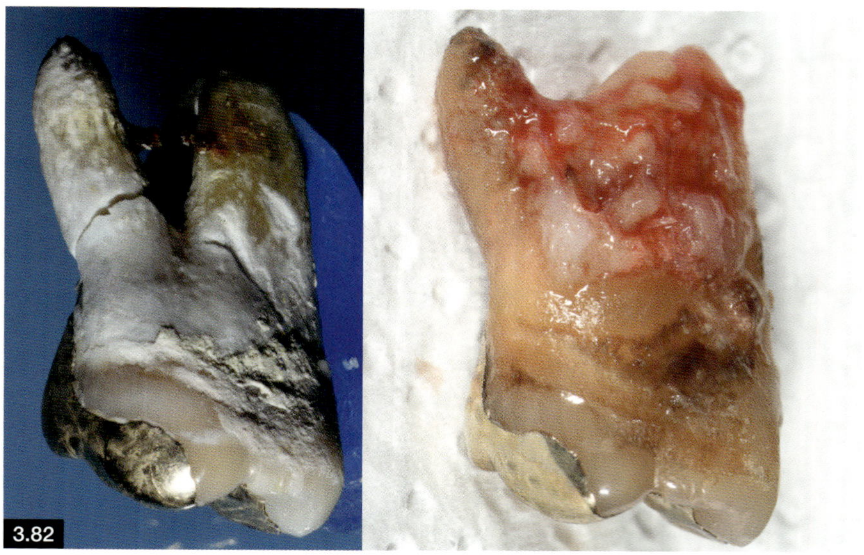

Fig. 3.82: The extracted tooth. The periodontal involvement is evident and is attributed to a root fracture.

resorbable and biocompatible extraradicular matrices (e.g. fibrin sponges) in the bone defect, after which the biocompatible sealer can be compacted[122].
Literature findings reveals that the materials of choice for filling perforations are[123-125]:

- Reinforced zinc oxide eugenol (SuperEba, Bosworth Co., Skokie, Illinois, USA)
- Mineral Trioxide Aggregate (MTA; ProRoot, Maillefer, Switzerland)
- Calcium silicate sealers (Biodentine, Septodont, France)
- Composites with adhesives.

The choice of the most suitable material is dictated, as highlighted above, by:

- The position of the perforation
- The size of perforation
- The possibility of moisture control
- The possibility of homeostasis.

If the perforation is adjacent to the gum, and hence outside the bone component of the periodontal tissue, it can be repaired with adhesive composites without changing the protocol that is normally followed in retreatment processes. Once the perforation is closed, endodontic therapy is then resumed.
In cases where perforations of the pulp chamber floor or along the canal walls have to be sealed, the use of Mineral Trioxide Aggregate (MTA) seems to be a very suitable option[126-129]. Currently, other materials have also shown promising potential for this process, and have active ingredients that are similar to those mentioned previously[123, 129].
In some circumstances, especially in the case of small drillings in areas where moisture can be controlled, the use of sealers such as SuperEBA seems to be a viable alternative solution.
We recommend referring to Chapter 7 for a more detailed analysis of the related clinical procedures.

References

1. Derhalli M and Mounce RE. *Clinical decision making regarding endodontics versus implants*. Compend Contin Educ Dent. 2011; 32(4):24-26, 28-30, 32-35.
2. Azarpazhooh A, Dao T, Ungar WJ et al. *Clinical decision making for a tooth with apical periodontitis: the patients' preferred level of participation*. J Endodont. 2014; 40(6):784-789.
3. Chercoles-Ruiz A, Sanchez-Torres A and Gay-Escoda C. *Endodontics, Endodontic Retreatment, and Apical Surgery Versus Tooth Extraction and Implant Placement: A Systematic Review*. J Endodont. 2017; 43(5):679-686.
4. Burns LE, Visbal LD, Kohli MR et al. *Long-term Evaluation of Treatment Planning Decisions for Nonhealing Endodontic Cases by Different Groups of Practitioners*. J Endodont. 2018; 44(2):226-232.
5. Torabinejad M, Salha W, Lozada JL et al. *Degree of patient pain, complications, and satisfaction after root canal treatment or a single implant: a preliminary prospective investigation*. J Endodont. 2014; 40(12): 1940-1945.
6. Peikoff MD. *Treatment planning dilemmas resulting from failed root canal cases*. Aust Endod J. 2005; 31(1):15-20.
7. Gillen BM, Looney SW, Gu LS et al. *Impact of the quality of corcnal restoration versus the quality of root canal fillings on success of root canal treatment: a systematic review and meta-analysis*. J Endodont. 2011; 37(7):895-902.
8. Chandra A. *Discuss the factors that affect the outcome of endodontic treatment*. Aust Endod J. 2009; 35(2):98-107.
9. Del Fabbro M, Corbella S, Sequeira-Byron P et al. *Endodontic procedures for retreatment of periapical lesions*. Cochrane Db Syst Rev. 2016; (10):Art no. CD005511.
10. Castellucci A. *Compendio di Endodonzia*. 1 ed. Bologna: Martina; 2018.
11. Oliveira MT, Constantino HV, Molina GO et al. *Evaluation of mercury contamination in patients and water during amalgam removal*. J Contemp Dent Pract. 2014; 15(2):165-168.
12. Vermelho PM, Reis AF, Ambrosano GMB et al. *Adhesion of multimode adhesives to enamel and dentin after one year of water storage*. Clin Oral Invest. 2017; 21(5):1707-1715.
13. Tartari T, Wichnieski C, Bachmann L et al. *Effect of the combination of several irrigants on dentine surface properties, adsorption of chlorhexidine and adhesion of microorganisms to dentine*. Int Endod J. 2018.
14. Pisacane C e Gerosa R. *Le fasi iniziali del ritrattamento endodontico*. In: Berutti E, Gagliani M, editors. *Manuale di Endodonzia*. Milano: EDRA; 2013; 144-149.
15. Addy LD, Bartley A and Hayes SJ. *Crown and bridge disassembly – when, why and how*. SADJ. 2008; 63(8):432, 434-438.
16. Rhodes JS. *Disassembly techniques to gain access to pulp chambers and root canals during non-surgical root canal re-treatment*. Endodontic Topics. 2011; 19(1):22-32.
17. Gorni F. *La chirurgia endodontica*. In: Berutti E, Gagliani M, editors. *Manuale di Endodonzia*. Milano, EDRA; 2013; 144-149.
18. Martin H. *Ultrasonic disinfection of the root canal*. Oral Surg Oral Med Oral Pathol. 1976; 42(1):92-99.
19. Martin H and Cunningham W. *Endosonics – the ultrasonic synergistic system of endodontics*. Endod Dent Traumatol. 1985; 1(6):201-206.
20. Laird WR and Walmsley AD. *Ultrasound in dentistry. Part 1 – Biophysical interactions*. J Dent. 1991; 19(1):14-17.
21. Walmsley AD, Laird WR and Lumley PJ. *Ultrasound in dentistry. Part 2 – Periodontology and endodontics*. J Dent. 1992; 20(1):11-17.
22. Lea SC, Walmsley AD and Lumley PJ. *Analyzing endosonic root canal file oscillations: an in vitro evaluation*. J Endodont. 2010; 36(5):880-883.
23. Plotino G, Pameijer CH, Grande NM et al. *Ultrasonics in endodontics: a review of the literature*. J Endodont. 2007; 33(2):81-95.
24. Johnson WB and Beatty RG. *Clinical technique for the removal of root canal obstructions*. J Am Dent Assoc. 1988; 117(3):473-476.
25. Hulsmann M. *Methods for removing metal obstructions from the root canal*. Endod Dent Traumatol. 1993; 9(6):223-237.
26. Fors UG and Berg JO. *Endodontic treatment of root canals obstructed by foreign objects*. Int Endod J. 1986; 19(1):2-10.
27. Weisman MI. *The removal of difficult silver cones*. J Endodont. 1983; 9(5):210-211.
28. Chenail BL and Teplitsky PE. *Orthograde ultrasonic retrieval of root canal obstructions*. J Endodont. 1987; 13(4):186-190.
29. Meidinger DL and Kabes BJ. *Foreign object removal utilizing the Cavi-Endo ultrasonic instrument*. J Endodont. 1985; 11(7):301-304.
30. Hulsmann M. *Retrieval of silver cones using different techniques*. Int Endod J.1990; 23(6):298-303.

31. Spriggs K, Gettleman B and Messer HH. *Evaluation of a new method for silver point removal*. J Endodont. 1990; 16(7):335-338.
32. Masseran J. *The extraction of posts broken deeply in the roots*. Actual Odontostomatol (Paris). 1986; 75:392-402.
33. Roig-Greene JL. *The retrieval of foreign objects from root canals: a simple aid*. J Endodont. 1983; 9(9):394-397.
34. Gettleman BH and Deemer JP. *Removal of solid intracanal fragments and silver points: technique survey and evaluation*. Endod Rep. 1991; 6(2):15-18.
35. Gettleman BH, Spriggs KA, ElDeeb ME et al. *Removal of canal obstructions with the Endo Extractor*. J Endodont. 1991; 17(12):608-611.
36. Suter B. *A new method for retrieving silver points and separated instruments from root canals*. J Endodont. 1998; 24(6):446-448.
37. Shahabinejad H, Ghassemi A, Pishbin L et al. *Success of ultrasonic technique in removing fractured rotary nickel-titanium endodontic instruments from root canals and its effect on the required force for root fracture*. J Endodont. 2013; 39(6):824-828.
38. Ling JQ, Wei X and Gao Y. [*Evaluation of the use of dental operating microscope and ultrasonic instruments in the management of blocked canals*]. Zhonghua kou qiang yi xue za zhi = Zhonghua kouqiang yixue zazhi = *Chinese journal of stomatology*. 2003; 38(5):324-326.
39. Castrisos T and Abbott PV. *A survey of methods used for post removal in specialist endodontic practice*. Int Endod J. 2002; 35(2):172-180.
40. McLaren JD, McLaren CI, Yaman P et al. *The effect of post type and length on the fracture resistance of endodontically treated teeth*. J Prosthet Dent. 2009; 101(3):174-182.
41. Soares JA, Brito-Junior M, Fonseca DR et al. *Influence of luting agents on time required for cast post removal by ultrasound: an in vitro study*. J Appl Oral Sci. 2009; 17(3):145-149.
42. Brady E, Mannocci F, Brown J et al. *A comparison of cone beam computed tomography and periapical radiography for the detection of vertical root fractures in nonendodontically treated teeth*. Int Endod J. 2014; 47(8):735-746.
43. Mota de Almeida FJ, Knutsson K and Flygare L. *The impact of cone beam computed tomography on the choice of endodontic diagnosis*. Int Endod J. 2015; 48(6):564-572.
44. Caputo BV, Noro Filho GA, de Andrade Salgado DM et al. *Evaluation of the Root Canal Morphology of Molars by Using Cone-beam Computed Tomography in a Brazilian Population: Part I*. J Endodont. 2016; 42(11):1604-1607.
45. Dixon EB, Kaczkowski PJ, Nicholls JI et al. *Comparison of two ultrasonic instruments for post removal*. J Endodont. 2002; 28(2):111-115.
46. Smith BJ. *Removal of fractured posts using ultrasonic vibration: an in vivo study*. J Endodont. 2001; 27(10):632-634.
47. Scotti N, Bergantin E, Alovisi M et al. *Evaluation of a simplified fiber post removal system*. J Endodont. 2013; 39(11):1431-1434.
48. Romeiro K, de Almeida A, Cassimiro M, Gominho L, Dantas E, Chagas N, et al. *Reciproc and Reciproc Blue in the removal of bioceramic and resin-based sealers in retreatment procedures*. Clin Oral Invest. 2019:1-12
49. Gound TG, Marx D and Schwandt NA. *Incidence of flare-ups and evaluation of quality after retreatment of resorcinol-formaldehyde resin ("Russian Red Cement") endodontic therapy*. J Endodont. 2003; 29(10):624-626.
50. Lenherr P, Allgayer N, Weiger R et al. *Tooth discoloration induced by endodontic materials: a laboratory study*. Int Endod J. 2012; 45(10):942-949.
51. Krastl G, Allgayer N, Lenherr P et al. *Tooth discoloration induced by endodontic materials: a literature review*. Dent Traumatol. 2013; 29(1):2-7.
52. Cavenago BC, Ordinola-Zapata R, Duarte MA et al. *Efficacy of xylene and passive ultrasonic irrigation on remaining root filling material during retreatment of anatomically complex teeth*. Int Endod J. 2014; 47(11):1078-1083.
53. Arslan H, Akcay M, Capar ID et al. *Efficacy of needle irrigation, EndoActivator, and photon-initiated photoacoustic streaming technique on removal of double and triple antibiotic pastes*. J Endodont. 2014; 40(9):1439-1442.
54. Schwandt NW and Gound TG. *Resorcinol-formaldehyde resin "Russian Red" endodontic therapy*. J Endodont. 2003; 29(7):435-437.
55. Hoen MM and Pink FE. *Contemporary endodontic retreatments: an analysis based on clinical treatment findings*. J Endodont. 2002; 28(12):834-836.
56. Duncan HF and Chong B.S. *Removal of root filling materials*. Endodontic Topics. 2008; 19(1):33–57.
57. Iqbal A. *The Factors Responsible for Endodontic Treatment Failure in the Permanent Dentitions of the Patients Reported to the College of Dentistry, the University of Aljouf, Kingdom of Saudi Arabia*. J Clin Diagn Res. 2016; 10(5):ZC146-148.
58. Hülsmann MT and Tulus G. *Non-surgical retreatment of teeth with persisting apical periodontitis following*

apicoectomy: decision making, treatment strategies and problems, and case reports. Endodontic Topics. 2016; 34(1):64-89.

59. Dincer AN, Er O and Canakci BC. *Evaluation of apically extruded debris during root canal retreatment with several NiTi systems*. Int Endod J. 2015; 48(12):1194-1198.
60. Kasikci Bilgi I, Koseler I, Guneri P et al. *Efficiency and apical extrusion of debris: a comparative ex vivo study of four retreatment techniques in severely curved root canals*. Int Endod J. 2016.
61. Topcuoglu HS, Akti A, Tuncay O et al. *Evaluation of debris extruded apically during the removal of root canal filling material using ProTaper, D-RaCe, and R-Endo rotary nickel-titanium retreatment instruments and hand files*. J Endodont. 2014; 40(12):2066-2069.
62. Yilmaz K and Ozyurek T. *Apically Extruded Debris after Retreatment Procedure with Reciproc, ProTaper Next, and Twisted File Adaptive Instruments*. J Endodont. 2017; 43(4):648-651.
63. Yuruker S, Gorduysus M, Kucukkaya S et al. *Efficacy of Combined Use of Different Nickel-Titanium Files on Removing Root Canal Filling Materials*. J Endodont. 2016; 42(3):487-492.
64. Zanettini PR, Barletta FB and de Mello Rahde N. *In vitro comparison of different reciprocating systems used during endodontic retreatment*. Aust Endod J. 2008; 34(3):80-85.
65. Pirovano AM, Grassi M, Colombo M et al. *Strumenti rotanti in lega nichel-titanio per il ritrattamento: un'analisi pre-clinica*. Giornale Italiano di Endodonzia. 2011; 25(3):145-151.
66. de Siqueira Zuolo A, Zuolo ML, da Silveira Bueno et al. *Evaluation of the Efficacy of TRUShape and Reciproc File Systems in the Removal of Root Filling Material: An Ex Vivo Micro-Computed Tomographic Study*. J Endodont. 2016; 42(2):315-319.
67. Fruchi Lde C, Ordinola-Zapata R, Cavenago BC et al. *Efficacy of reciprocating instruments for removing filling material in curved canals obturated with a single-cone technique: a micro-computed tomographic analysis*. J Endodont. 2014; 40(7):1000-1004.
68. Kfir A, Tsesis I, Yakirevich E et al. *The efficacy of five techniques for removing root filling material: microscopic versus radiographic evaluation*. Int Endod J. 2012; 45(1):35-41.
69. Ma J, Al-Ashaw AJ, Shen Y et al. *Efficacy of ProTaper Universal Rotary Retreatment system for gutta-percha removal from oval root canals: a micro-computed tomography study*. J Endodont. 2012; 38(11):1516-1520.
70. Silva E, Belladonna FG, Zuolo AS et al. *Effectiveness of XP-endo Finisher and XP-endo Finisher R in removing root filling remnants: a micro-CT study*. Int Endod J. 2018; 51(1):86-91.
71. Nevares G, de Albuquerque DS, Freire LG et al. *Efficacy of ProTaper NEXT Compared with Reciproc in Removing Obturation Material from Severely Curved Root Canals: A Micro-Computed Tomography Study*. J Endodont. 2016; 42(5):803-808.
72. Ozyurek T and Demiryurek EO. *Efficacy of Different Nickel-Titanium Instruments in Removing Gutta-percha during Root Canal Retreatment*. J Endodont. 2016; 42(4):646-649.
73. Gergi R and Sabbagh C. *Effectiveness of two nickel-titanium rotary instruments and a hand file for removing gutta-percha in severely curved root canals during retreatment: an ex vivo study*. Int Endod J. 2007; 40(7):532-537.
74. Yadav P, Bharath MJ, Sahadev CK et al. *An in vitro CT Comparison of Gutta-Percha Removal with Two Rotary Systems and Hedstrom Files*. Iran Endod J. 2013; 8(2):59-64.
75. Guess GM. *Predictable Therma-fil removal technique using the system-B heat source*. J Endodont. 2004; 30(1):61.
76. Hwang JI, Chuang AH, Sidow SJ et al. *The effectiveness of endodontic solvents to remove endodontic sealers*. Mil Med. 2015; 180(3 Suppl):92-95.
77. Rehman K, Khan FR and Aman N. *Comparison of orange oil and chloroform as gutta- percha solvents in endodontic retreatment*. J Contemp Dent Pract. 2013; 14(3):478-482.
78. De Deus G, Belladona FG, Zuolo AS, Simoes-Carvalho M, Santos CB, Oliveira DS, et al. *Effectiveness of Reciproc Blue in removing canal filling material and regaining apical patency*. Int Endod J. 2019;52:250–7.
79. Delai D, Pompermayer Jardine A, Boldrin Mestieri L, Boijink D, Camargo Fontanella VR, Soares Grecca F, et al. *Efficacy of a thermally treated single file compared with rotary systems in endodontic retreatment of curved canals: a micro-CT study*. Clin Oral Invest. 2019; 23:1837-1844.
80. Machado AG, Guilherme BP, Provenzano JC, Marceliano-Alves M, Goncalves LS, Siqueira JFJ, et al. *Effects of preparation with the Self-Adjusting File, TRUShape and XP-endo Shaper systems, and a supplementary step with XP-endo Finisher R on filling material removal during retreatment of mandibular molar canals*. Int Endod J. 2019; 52,:709-715.
81. Neelakantan P, Ahmed HMA, Chang JWW, Nabhan MS, Wei X, Cheung GSP, et al. *Effect of instrumentation systems on endotoxin reduction from root canal systems: A systematic review of clinical studies and meta-analysis. Australian endodontic journal*: the journal of the Australian Society of Endodontology Inc. 2018.
82. Hayakawa T, Tomita F and Okiji T. *Influence of the diameter and taper of root canals on the removal efficiency of Thermafil Plus plastic carriers using ProTaper Retreatment Files*. J Endodont. 2010; 36(10):1676-1678.
83. Pirani C, Pelliccioni GA, Marchionni S et al. *Effectiveness of three different retreatment techniques in canals filled with compacted gutta-percha or Thermafil: a scanning electron microscope study*. J Endodont. 2009; 35(10):1433-1440.

84. Beasley RT, Williamson AE, Justman BC et al. *Time required to remove guttacore, thermafil plus, and thermoplasticized gutta-percha from moderately curved root canals with protaper files*. J Endodont. 2013; 39(1):125-128.
85. Cantatore GB, Berutti E and Castellucci A. *Missed anatomy: frequency and clinical impact*. Endodontic Topics. 2006; 15(1):3-31.
86. Gorni F e Cerutti F. *Il ruolo degli ultrasuoni nel ritrattamento ortogrado*. Dentista Moderno. 2013; 17(1):86-93.
87. Mirmohammadi H, Mahdi L, Partovi P et al. *Accuracy of Cone-beam Computed Tomography in the Detection of a Second Mesiobuccal Root Canal in Endodontically Treated Teeth: An Ex Vivo Study*. J Endodont. 2015; 41(10):1678-1681.
88. Reis AG, Grazziotin-Soares R, Barletta FB et al. *Second canal in mesiobuccal root of maxillary molars is correlated with root third and patient age: a cone-beam computed tomographic study*. J Endodont. 2013; 39(5):588-592.
89. Hasan M and Raza Khan F. *Determination of frequency of the second mesiobuccal canal in the permanent maxillary first molar teeth with magnification loupes (x 3.5)*. Int J Biomed Sci. 2014; 10(3):201-207.
90. Karabucak B, Bunes A, Chehoud C et al. *Prevalence of Apical Periodontitis in Endodontically Treated Premolars and Molars with Untreated Canal: A Cone-beam Computed Tomography Study*. J Endodont. 2016; 42(4):538-541.
91. Ramos Brito AC, Verner FS, Junqueira RB et al. *Detection of Fractured Endodontic Instruments in Root Canals: Comparison between Different Digital Radiography Systems and Cone-beam Computed Tomography*. J Endodont. 2017; 43(4):544-549.
92. Rosen E, Azizi H, Friedlander C et al. *Radiographic identification of separated instruments retained in the apical third of root canal-filled teeth*. J Endodont. 2014; 40(10):1549-1552.
93. Madarati AA, Hunter MJ and Dummer PM. *Management of intracanal separated instruments*. J Endodont. 2013; 39(5):569-581.
94. Ungerechts C, Bardsen A and Fristad I. *Instrument fracture in root canals - where, why, when and what? A study from a student clinic*. Int Endod J. 2014; 47(2):183-190.
95. Nevares G, Cunha RS, Zuolo ML et al. *Success rates for removing or bypassing fractured instruments: a prospective clinical study*. J Endodont. 2012; 38(4):442-444.
96. Suter B. *Separated Root Canal Instruments - An overview of incidence, localisation, treatment strategies and outcome*. Swiss Dent J. 2017; 127(3):233-237.
97. Suter B, Lussi A and Sequeira P. *Probability of removing fractured instruments from root canals*. Int Endod J. 2005; 38(2):112-123.
98. Panitvisai P, Parunnit P, Sathorn C et al. *Impact of a retained instrument on treatment outcome: a systematic review and meta-analysis*. J Endodont. 2010; 36(5):775-780.
99. Agrawal V, Kapoor S and Patel M. *Ultrasonic Technique to Retrieve a Rotary Nickel-Titanium File Broken Beyond the Apex and a Stainless Steel File from the Root Canal of a Mandibular Molar: A Case Report*. J Dent (Tehran). 2015; 12(7):532-536.
100. Heydari A, Rahmani M and Heydari M. *Removal of a Broken Instrument from a Tooth with Apical Periodontitis Using a Novel Approach*. Iran Endod J. 2016; 11(3):237-240.
101. Madarati AA, Qualtrough AJ and Watts DC. *Endodontists experience using ultrasonics for removal of intra-canal fractured instruments*. Int Endod J. 2010; 43(4):301-305.
102. Ormiga F, da Cunha Ponciano Gomes JA and de Araujo MC. *Dissolution of nickel-titanium endodontic files via an electrochemical process: a new concept for future retrieval of fractured files in root canals*. J Endodont. 2010; 36(4):717-720.
103. Ormiga F, da Cunha Ponciano Gomes JA, de Araujo MC et al. *An initial investigation of the electrochemical dissolution of fragments of nickel-titanium endodontic files*. J Endodont. 2011; 37(4):526-530.
104. Aboud LR, Ormiga F and Gomes JA. *Electrochemical induced dissolution of fragments of nickel-titanium endodontic files and their removal from simulated root canals*. Int Endod J. 2014; 47(2):155-162.
105. Al-Sudani D, Grande NM, Plotino G et al. *Cyclic fatigue of nickel-titanium rotary instruments in a double (S-shaped) simulated curvature*. J Endodont. 2012; 38(7):987-989.
106. Adiguzel M and Capar ID. *Comparison of Cyclic Fatigue Resistance of WaveOne and WaveOne Gold Small, Primary, and Large Instruments*. J Endodont. 2017; 43(4):623-627.
107. Testarelli L, Plotino G, Al-Sudani D et al. *Bending properties of a new nickel-titanium alloy with a lower percent by weight of nickel*. J Endodont. 2011; 37(9):1293-1295.
108. Yang Q, Shen Y, Huang D et al. *Evaluation of Two Trephine Techniques for Removal of Fractured Rotary Nickel-titanium Instruments from Root Canals*. J Endodont. 2017; 43(1):116-120.
109. Cheung GS. *Instrument fracture: mechanisms, removal of fragments, and clinical outcomes*. Endodontic Topics. 2007; 16(1):1-26.
110. Cuje J, Bargholz C and Hulsmann M. *The outcome of retained instrument removal in a specialist practice*. Int Endod J. 2010; 43(7):545-554.

111. Lambrianidis T. *Ledging and blockage of root canals during canal preparation: causes, recognition, prevention, management, and outcomes*. Endodontic Topics. 2009; 15(1):56-74.
112. Burklein SS and Schäfer E. *Critical evaluation of root canal transportation by instrumentation*. Endodontic Topics. 2014; 29(1):110-124.
113. Gonzalez Sanchez JA, Duran-Sindreu F, de Noe S et al. *Centring ability and apical transportation after overinstrumentation with ProTaper Universal and ProFile Vortex instruments*. Int Endod J. 2012; 45(6):542-551.
114. Schäfer ED and Dammaschke T. *Development and sequelae of canal transportation*. Endodontic Topics. 2009; 15(1):75-90.
115. Peters OA. *Complications and procedural mishaps during root canal treatment: Part I*. Endodontic Topics. 2006; 15(1):1-2.
116. Hulsmann MD, Drebenstedt S and Holscher C. *Shaping and filling root canals during root canal re-treatment*. Endodontic Topics. 2008; 19(1):74-124.
117. Jafarzadeh H and Abbott PV. *Ledge formation: review of a great challenge in endodontics*. J Endodont. 2007; 33(10):1155-1162.
118. Perez AR, Alves FRF, Marceliano-Alves MF et al. *Effects of increased apical enlargement on the amount of unprepared areas and coronal dentine removal: a micro-computed tomography study*. Int Endod J. 2017.
119. Versiani MS, Souza E and De-Deus G. *Critical appraisal of studies on dentinal radicular microcracks in endodontics: methodological issues, contemporary concepts, and future perspectives*. Endodontic Topics. 2015; 33(1):87-156.
120. Madarati AA, Qualtrough AJ and Watts DC. *Vertical fracture resistance of roots after ultrasonic removal of fractured instruments*. Int Endod J. 2010; 43(5):424-429.
121. Pontius V, Pontius O, Braun A et al. *Retrospective evaluation of perforation repairs in 6 private practices*. J Endodont. 2013; 39(11):1346-1358.
122. Roda RS. *Root perforation repair: surgical and nonsurgical management*. Pract Proced Aesthet Dent. 2001; 13(6):467-472; quiz 474.
123. Dawood AE, Parashos P, Wong RHK et al. *Calcium silicate-based cements: composition, properties, and clinical applications*. J Invest Clin Dent. 2017; 8(2).
124. Balachandran J and Gurucharan. *Comparison of sealing ability of bioactive bone cement, mineral trioxide aggregate and Super EBA as furcation repair materials: A dye extraction study*. J Conserv Dent. 2013; 16(3):247-251.
125. Kakani AK, Veeramachaneni C, Majeti C et al. *A Review on Perforation Repair Materials*. J Clin Diagn Res. 2015; 9(9):ZE09-13.
126. Tawil PZ, Duggan DJ and Galicia JC. *Mineral trioxide aggregate (MTA): its history, composition, and clinical applications*. Compend Contin Educ Dent. 2015; 36(4):247-252; quiz 254, 264.
127. Parirokh M and Torabinejad M. *Mineral trioxide aggregate: a comprehensive literature review – Part III: Clinical applications, drawbacks, and mechanism of action*. J Endodont. 2010; 36(3):400-413.
128. Parirokh M, Torabinejad M. *Mineral trioxide aggregate: a comprehensive literature review- Part I: chemical, physical, and antibacterial properties.* Journal of endodontics. 2010; 36(1):16-27.
129. Torabinejad M, Parirokh M and Dummer PMH. *Mineral trioxide aggregate and other bioactive endodontic cements: an updated overview - part II: other clinical applications and complications*. Int Endod J. 2018; 51(3):284-317.

- Describe the **irrigants** and their properties.
- Illustrate the **activation methodologies** of the chemical agents used in the retreatments.
- Identify the set of **clinical protocols** that can be adopted in different pathological situations.

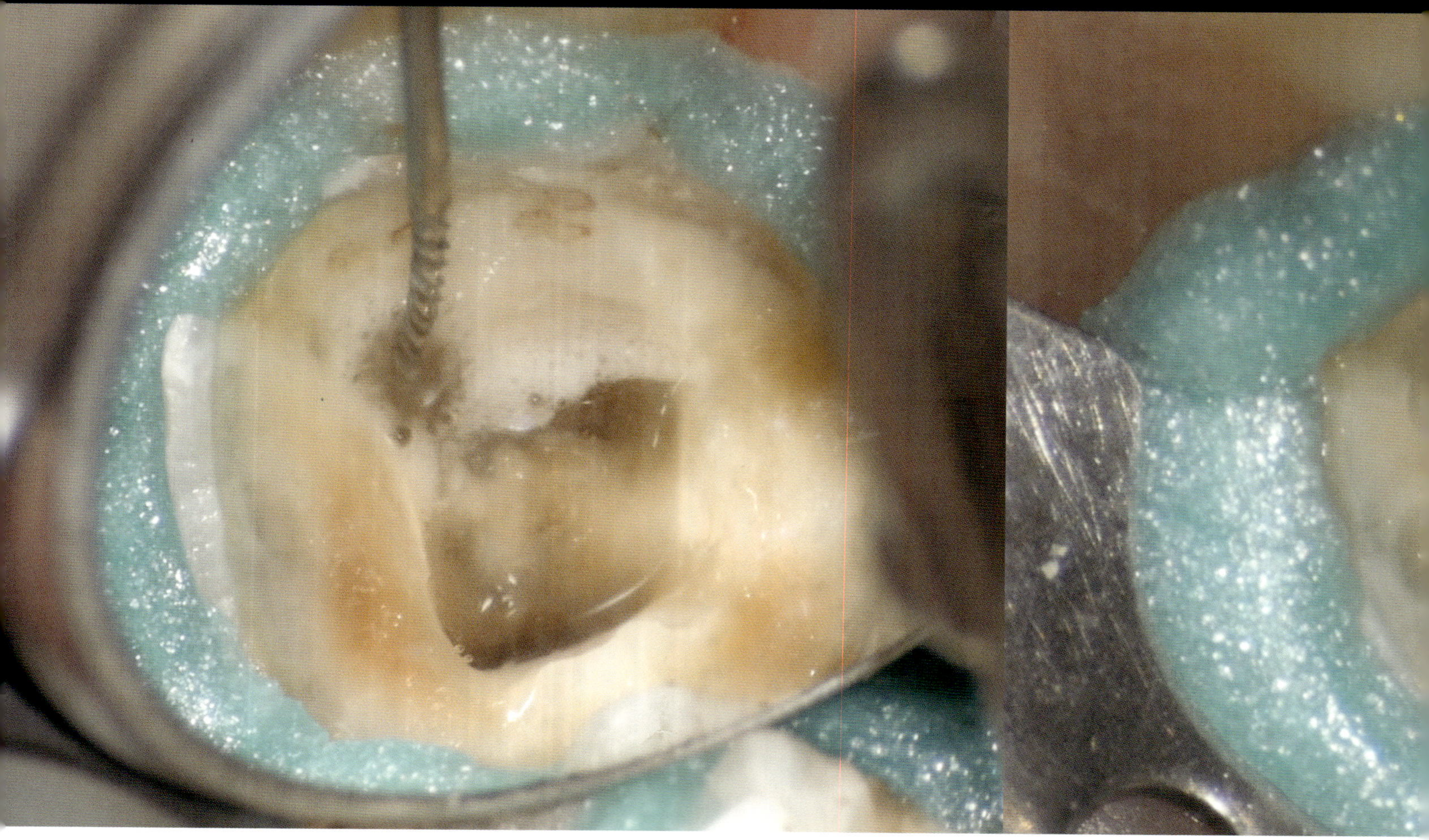

Riccardo Tonini, Francesca Cerutti

04

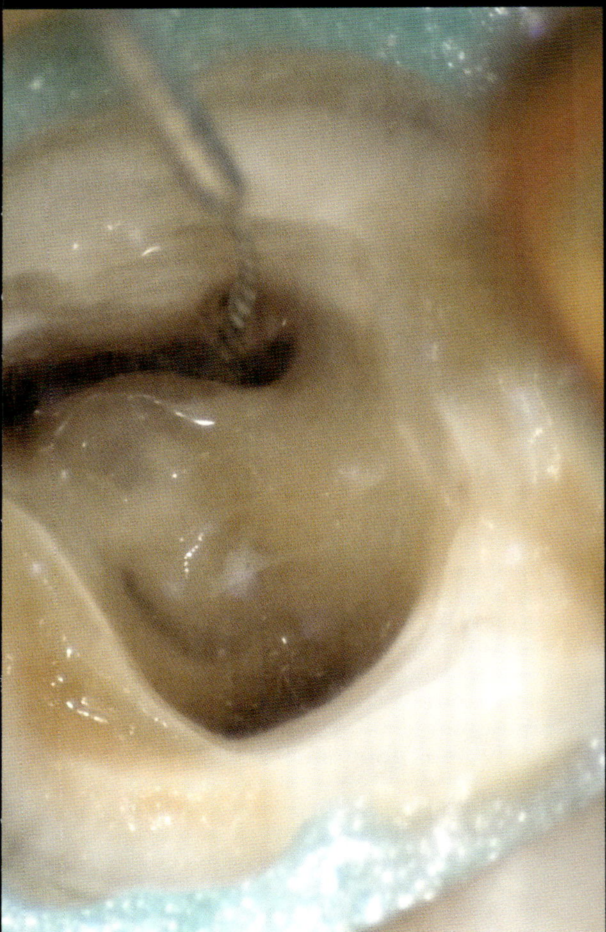

Disinfection and clinical protocols in retreatments

Instruments and clinical protocols for endodontic space disinfection

Introduction

The main cause of endodontic failure is the persistence of microorganisms in the canal system; this can happen even though the primary treatment has been characterized by the correct execution of all disinfection procedures with irrigants, because some microorganisms can survive even in 3D filled canals[1].
Another possible cause of endodontic failure is secondary infection caused by bacterial recolonization of the root canal system due to an inadequate coronal seal. Scientific studies have also shown that the result of endodontic treatment is significantly influenced by the presence of bacteria at the time of canal filling[2, 3]. Therefore, eradication of bacteria is a key element in achieving endodontic success. The importance of canal disinfection in the success of endodontic therapy is supported by the literature, which shows that neither the shaping nor the canal filling can guarantee a sufficient and ideal reduction of the bacterial load for the long-term success of endodontic therapy[4]. The instrumentation phase is essential to remove the filling material placed in the primary treatment[5], but cleaning is particularly important to eradicate bacteria that have contributed to the failure of the therapy (Figs. 4.1–4.3).
Given that some areas of the root canal system are inaccessible to root canal instruments, efforts have been made to improve the effectiveness of irrigation by studying new methods for bringing them into the canal system and activating them. In vitro studies have shown that cleaning of canal walls is better when using methods to improve irrigation action compared with using a conventional syringe and needle[6].
Another element that can improve

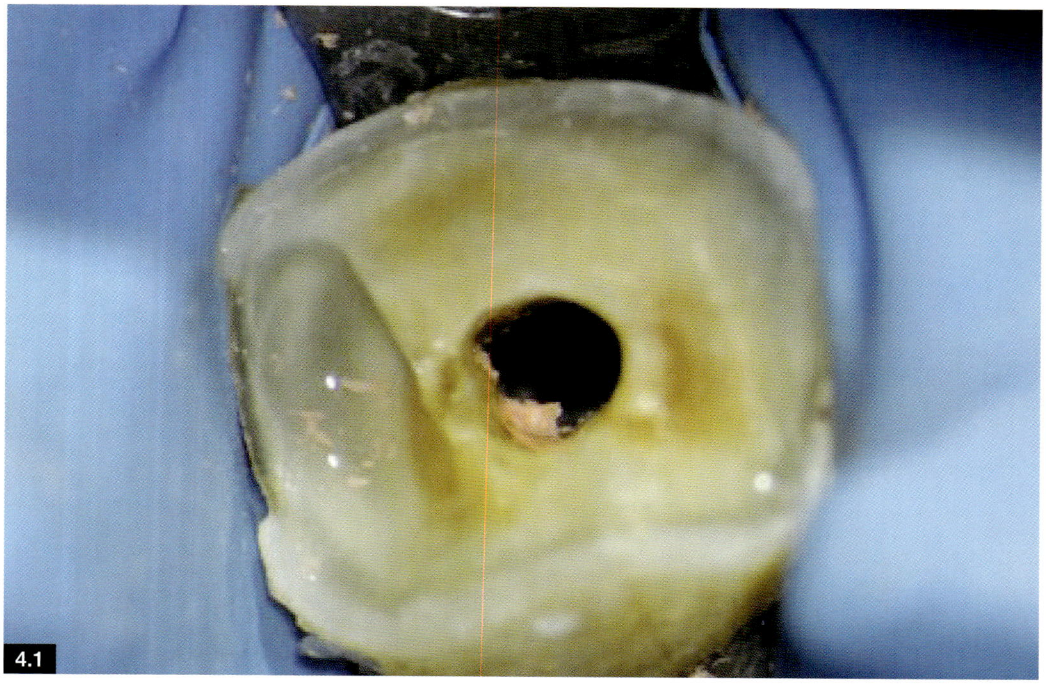

4.1

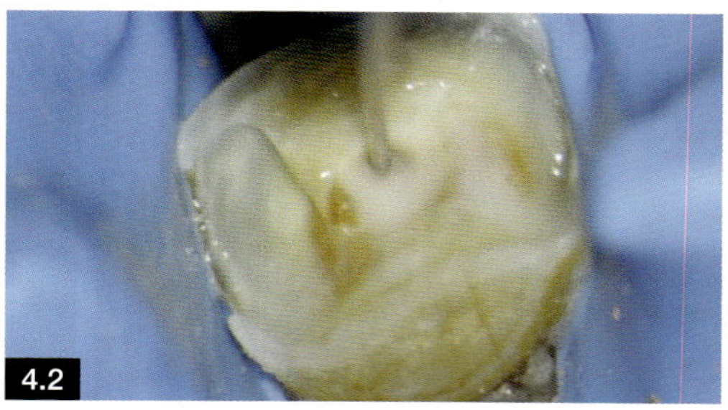

4.2

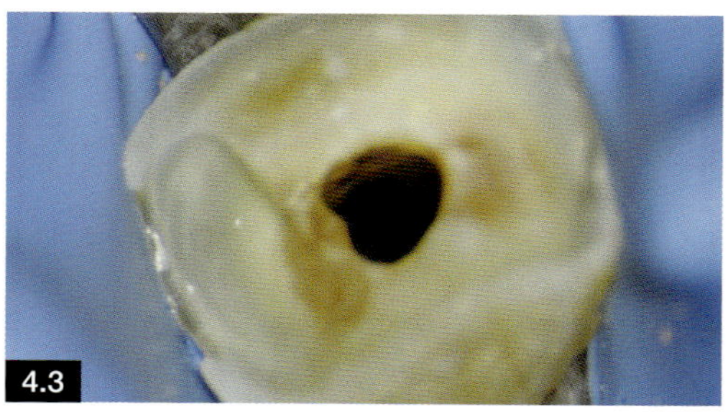

4.3

Figs. 4.1-4.3: This sequence shows the removal of residues of the gutta-percha from a canal during retreatment.
Part of the gutta-percha has remained attached to the walls, despite the action of mechanical instruments (Fig. 4.1). By ultrasonic activation, the gutta-percha detaches from the canal walls, and the irrigants are able to penetrate into the areas untouched by the rotating instruments and previously filled with the filling (Fig. 4.2). At the end of the operation, the canal is free of residues from the previous treatment (Fig. 4.3).

the effectiveness of irrigants and allow them to penetrate areas that are difficult to reach is the modulation of surface tension[7] (the ability of a liquid to distribute itself on a surface and penetrate into capillaries)[8]. The addition of surfactants promotes the reduction in surface tension of the irrigant and increase in the ability to remove debris from the canal dentin, as the solution adheres better to the dentinal walls and penetrates deeper into the tubules[7].
To be effective, cleaning must be carried out following strict protocols and cannot simply be considered a way to remove debris between one passage and the next of rotary instruments. Disinfection requires rules that must be followed and repeated step-by-step in every clinical situation; these protocols must be independent from the operator's capabilities.
Success is not mathematical but follows the following formula:

SUCCESS
=
SHAPING + CLEANING
+ FILLING - X

where × is the most unpredictable and important external factor, namely, the operator.

The disinfection protocol used for retreatment is similar to that used during conventional endodontic treatment, but the time factor plays a key role because complete complex retreatment requires numerous sessions and consequent intermediate medication.

Sterility or canal disinfection?

One of the few certainties we have in endodontics is the impossibility of achieving sterility of the canal system, despite the adoption of the most modern procedures and protocols of disinfection. This scenario applies to both the treatment and the retreatment of root canals, so we focus on the disinfection of the endodontic system, which means reducing the bacterial load below the critical threshold[9].

Bacterial load in retreatment

Recent publications have reported that the failure rate of initial treatment is between 14% and 16%[10-12].
Part of these failures stems from the fact that some bacterial colonies can nest in areas unaffected by endodontic instruments and irrigators, such as isthmuses, lateral canals, and apical ramifications. Bacteria that cause persistent infections can be identified as those present in the canal at the time of filling and can trigger a persistent infection.
The taxonomy of bacteria is a discriminating factor for the development or persistence of apical infections[13].
These infections only occur when the bacterial count exceeds the host's defense threshold. Effective treatment reduces bacterial populations and promotes healing (Figs. 4.4a and 4.4b)[9].

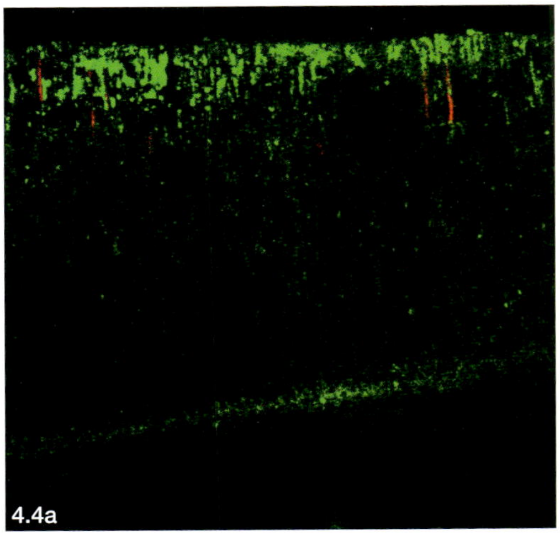

4.4a

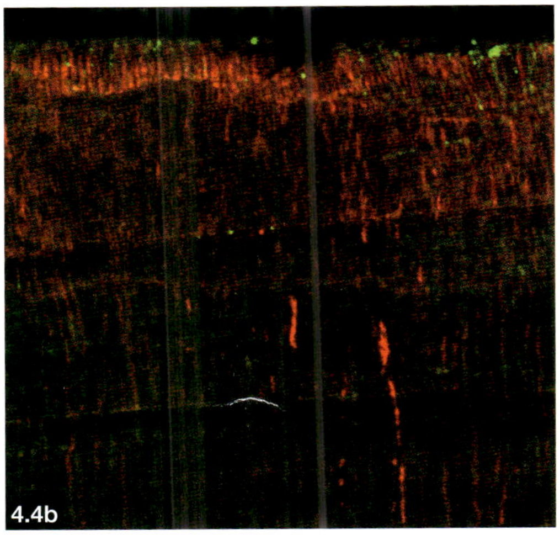

4.4b

Figs. 4.4a-b: The images show an example of bacterial persistence. Under the confocal laser microscope, live (green) and dead (red) bacteria can be seen. In the first image, the sample has been cleaned with physiological solution. In the second image, we can see how hypochlorite has decreased the bacterial load, but is unable to penetrate deep into the dentinal tubules, leaving the possibility of subsequent bacterial recolonization (our thanks to Dr. Francesca Carrara for providing the image).

Table 4.1 **IDEAL FEATURES OF A CANAL IRRIGANT**	
Antibacterial	Able to disinfect dentin and dentinal tubules
Non-cytotoxic	Must not interfere with the healing of periapical tissues
Stable solution	Must leave no residue
Prolonged antibacterial effect	Must not modify the dentin
Active in the presence of blood/serum	Economical
Able to remove the smear layer	Easy to use
Low surface tension	

Canal irrigants

Canal irrigants used during retreatment must be able to perform multiple functions (Table 4.1):

- help in the removal of previously used filling material;
- perform a biological action against residual bacteria and biofilms (Figs. 4.5 and 4.6);
- chemically remove the dentin debris produced during the reshaping of the canal system;
- have low tissue toxicity[14].

Irrigation solutions most commonly used during retreatment can be classified as antibacterial, chelating, and solvent.

Figs. 4.5 and 4.6: Having been cleaned with sodium hypochlorite, the tooth presents residues of the smear layer. Only the combined use of irrigants allows the complete removal of all residues from the canal.

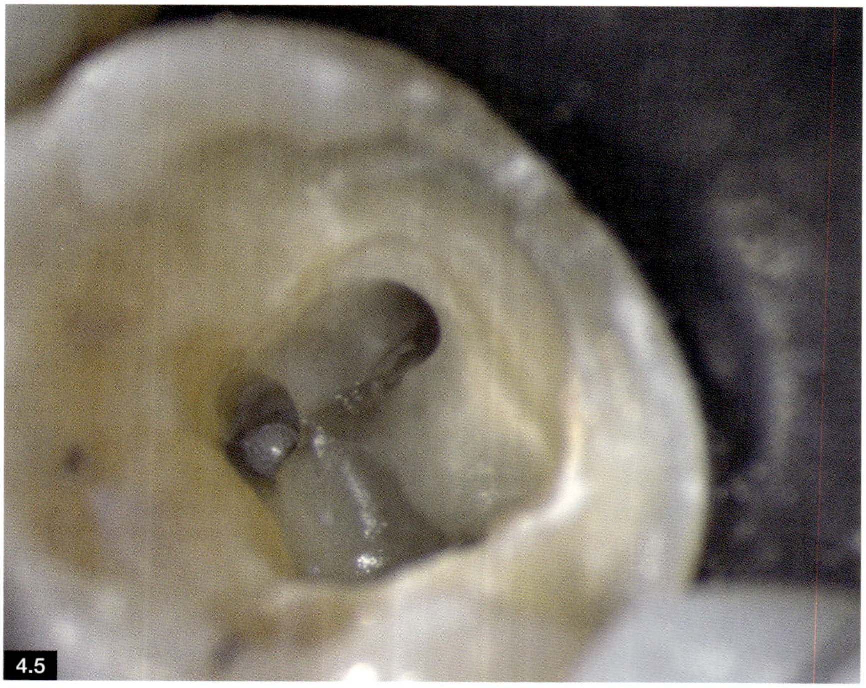

4.5

Below is a selection of the different types of irrigants, with the intention of providing an easily repeatable and applicable clinical guide.

Sodium hypochlorite

Sodium hypochlorite (NaOCl) is the most commonly used irrigation agent in endodontics as a primary disinfectant due to its broad antimicrobial proteolytic efficacy and ability to dissolve organic tissue residues present in the endodontium[15, 16], which can be amplified by reducing its surface tension[17]. Sodium hypochlorite is an aqueous solution with a concentration ranging from 0.5% to 15%[7], and its active part is chlorine, an unstable ion that degrades rapidly when it reacts with collagen and bacteria. In clinical settings, hypochlorite loses its solvent and antibacterial capabilities in a few seconds. Biofilm bacteria can nest in inaccessible areas of the endodontium, on the root surface, or in cement gaps.
Given that they grow in an unfavorable environment, these bacteria have a very low metabolism and are resistant to antimicrobial products; the only agent capable of physically removing the biofilm and killing the bacteria is sodium hypochlorite (Figs. 4.7 and 4.8).
The dissolution capacity of sodium hypochlorite depends on its concentration, its volume, the contact time between the solution and the dentin walls, and the surface of the exposed tissue area[18].

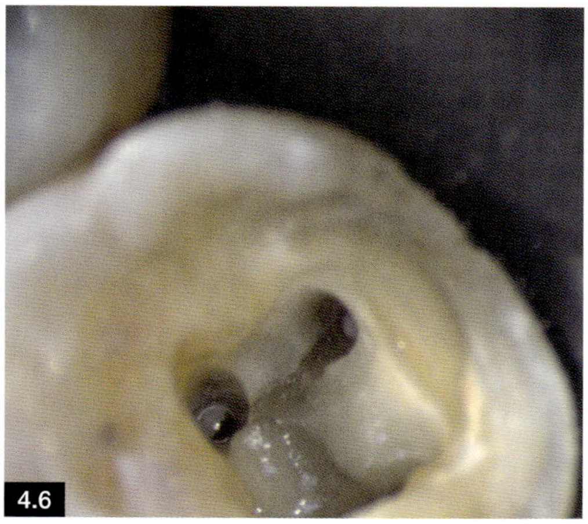

4.6

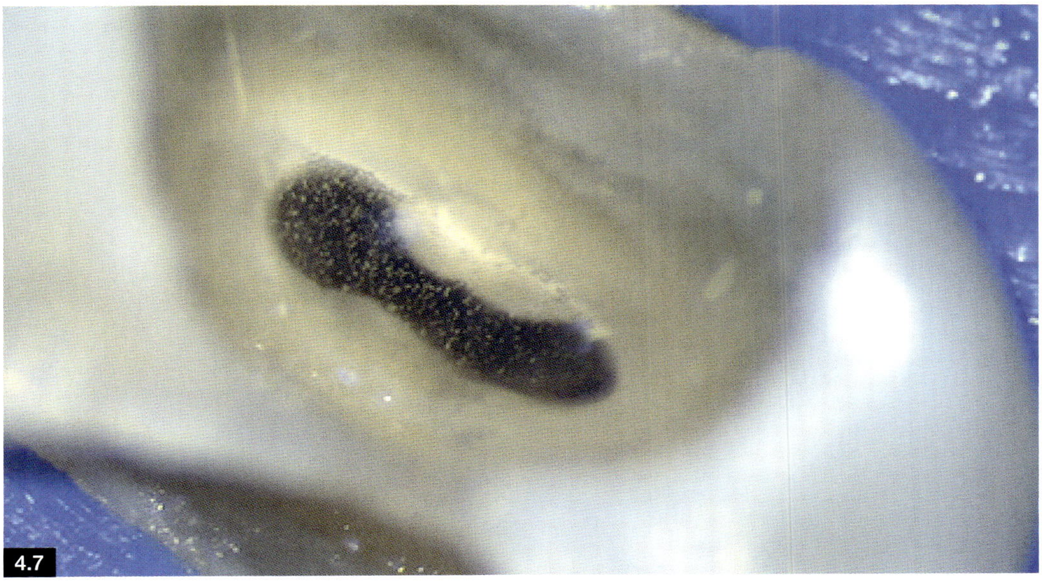

4.7

Figs. 4.7 and 4.8: Hypochlorite is a strong oxidant and continues its digestive action against collagen, pulp residue, and bacteria over time. Its action is macroscopically appreciable due to the formation of microbubbles coming to the surface.

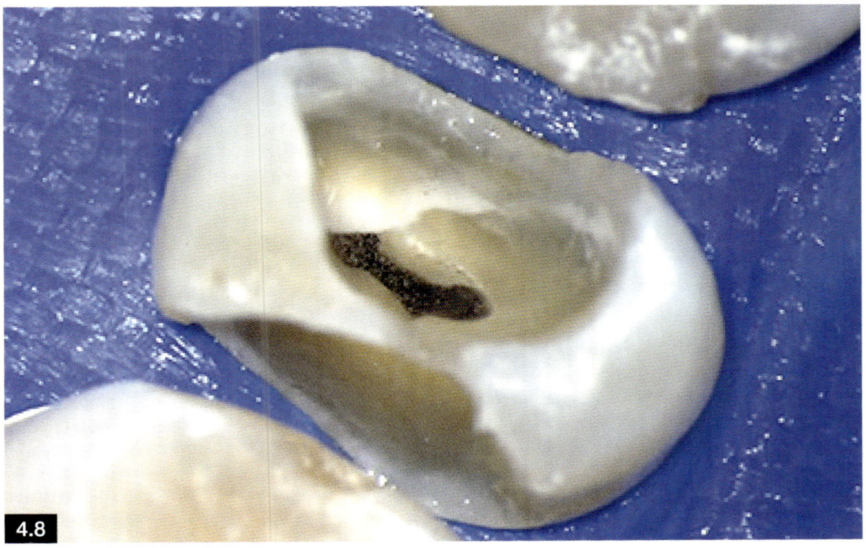

4.8

In vitro studies have shown that high concentrations of NaOCl are more effective on Candida albicans and *Enterococcus faecalis*[19] and may lead to higher tissue dissolution capabilities than low concentrations of NaOCl; the same effectiveness can be achieved with low concentration solutions used in large volumes[18, 20].
NaOCl penetrates the dentin tubules by 77–300 microns.
Parameters that influence this factor are concentration, solution temperature, and contact time.
However, excessive concentrations are potentially toxic for periapical tissues[21–23], and exposure to 2.5% and 5.25% sodium hypochlorite can change the mechanical properties of root dentin (e.g., high surface roughness and low microhardness)[24] through alterations in its organic components, due to the fragmentation of the long peptide chains and the chlorination of the protein end groups[25, 26].
The 5%–6% solutions are clinically recommended, as they combine good efficacy with relatively low toxicity, although extrusion of the irrigation agent in the periapical tissues should be avoided.
A study by Grossman[27] observed the dissolution of bovine dental pulp by different solutions of sodium hypochlorite (0.5%, 1%, 2.5%, and 5%) under different conditions and concluded that

- 5% hypochlorite dissolves the pulp in a time period between 20 min and 2 h;
- the rate of dissolution of the pulp is directly proportional to the concentration of sodium hypochlorite and is greater without the addition of surfactants;
- the variation in surface tension during pulp dissolution is directly proportional to the concentration of hypochlorite in the solution and is greater in surfactant-free solutions;
- the increase in temperature of the solution increases the rate of dissolution of the pulp;
- the most concentrated solutions have a low pH reduction after dissolution.

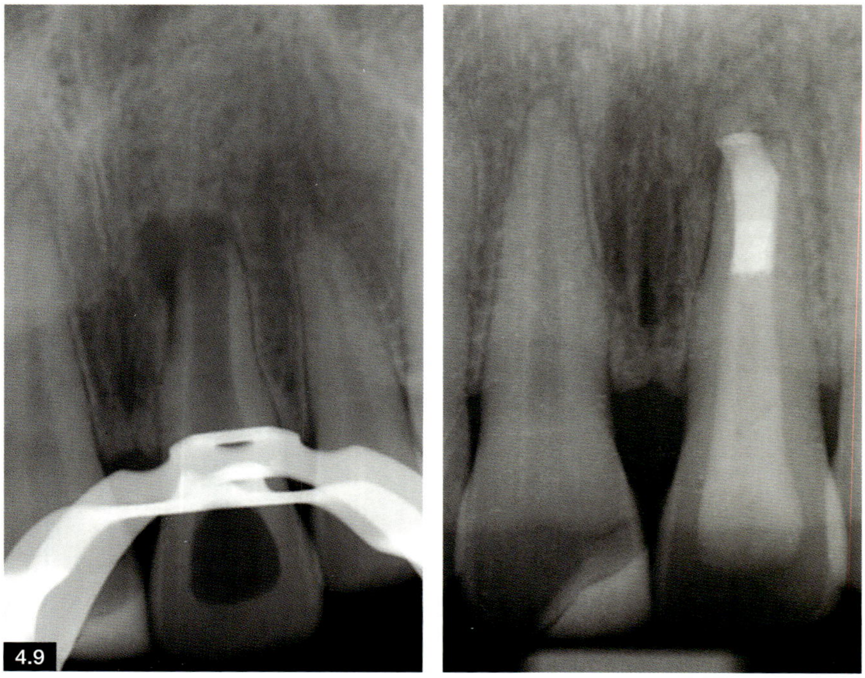

4.9

Table 4.2 **ACCIDENTAL INJECTION OF SODIUM HYPOCHLORITE IN PERIAPICAL/PERIRADICULAR TISSUES**

Symptoms	Immediate and intense pain
	Surrounding soft tissue edema
	Bleeding from the root canal
	Interstitial bleeding with skin and mucous membrane bleeding
	Chlorine taste in the mouth and irritation of the throat (after injection of hypochlorite into the maxillary sinus)
	Infection
	Reversible anesthesia
	Paresthesia
Therapy	Immediate irrigation of the canal with physiological adaptation and encourage bleeding
	Therapy with local anesthetics and analgesics
	Frequent rinsing and hot compresses to stimulate local circulation
	Reassure the patient and monitor improvements
Consequences	Hypochlorite damages the spongy bone, dissolving its architecture and causing cellular necrosis and apoptosis, while it has no effect on cortical excitability
Precautions	Insert a stop on the irrigation needle in order to determine the insertion depth
	Use needles designed specifically for irrigation
	Use a low pressure on the syringe plunger to reduce the risk of accidents

The effectiveness of tissue dissolution of hypochlorite can be increased by increasing the pH[28] and the temperature of the solution, activating the irrigation with ultrasonic sources, and increasing the contact time between hypochlorite and dentin wall[15]. However, the mechanism by which this enhancement occurs is not yet completely clear, and the relative importance of temperature, concentration, and stirring remains unknown.

Although there is consensus that raising the temperature enhances the effect of hypochlorite, only a few articles mention it[29-31]. Heating solutions with a low concentration of hypochlorite should increase their dissolution capacity and lower their systemic toxicity (when compared with that of solutions with a high concentration and low temperature) while maintaining the same efficacy[30], without affecting their short-term stability.

The literature has shown that raising the temperature of hypochlorite to 37 °C does not increase the effectiveness of tissue dissolution. Ideally, the working temperature should be a few degrees higher than the body temperature to improve the antibacterial action without having adverse effects on the cells of the periodontal ligament.

Moorer and Wesselink[18] were the first to emphasize the action of mechanical stirring of hypochlorite which, thanks to activation by ultrasonic sources that caused violent flow and strong oscillations, greatly increased its ability to dissolve tissues. Fabiani[32] demonstrated the greatest effectiveness of 5% hypochlorite in the apical third when it was stirred using ultrasonic sources.

Lowering the surface tension improves the action of hypochlorite solutions; for this reason, they may contain surfactants[33].

The surface tension values of hypochlorite preparations reported in the literature vary, due to differences in the concentration of the solutions tested, the temperature utilized, and the measurement method adopted[29,34].

Recently, surfactants have been added to conventional hypochlorite (Chlor-XTRATM, Vista Dental), with the intention of reducing

surface tension and facilitating the penetration of irrigants into the dentinal tubules.
The pH and the available chlorine remain unchanged, but the effectiveness is enhanced[35, 36].
However, hypochlorite is known to have poor ability in removing the smear layer from the canal walls, which is why several irrigators should be combined to achieve optimal cleaning of the endodontic space[37].
These measures will be extensively documented in the following pages; the interaction of sodium hypochlorite with other canal irrigants should be taken into account as adverse events, such as the orange coloring generated by the reaction between sodium hypochlorite and chlorhexidine, have effects that cannot be easily remedied.
Contact inactivation is present with the acids used for the removal of the smear layer, which we will discuss later[38].
The possibility of obtaining the required effects is governed by a precise irrigation sequence, which is to be carried out with suitable volumes.
Incorrect use of hypochlorite can lead to some unpleasant accidents; hypochlorite is a non-specific oxidizing agent, and oxidation products are corrosive[39].
Several adverse effects are known: the simplest and most harmless effects are related to the loss of drops of this liquid while carrying it to the mouth of the patient.
If adequate protection is not provided, the most common adverse effect is damage to the patient's clothing.
In the event that hypochlorite comes into contact with the skin, the subject will experience a sensation of burning that will go away with the application of water.
More serious damage could be caused to the eye if drops fall on the cornea of the patient. This may also occur due to the loss of contact with the injection needle; for this reason, the use of Luer-lock syringes is always advisable.
Finally, apical extrusion in teeth whose apex is shown is presented in Fig. 4.9.
Even in these cases, a careful injection with dedicated needles for lateral leakage can avoid unpleasant inconveniences.
The cases that are often presented in journals, which show the massive involvement of tegumentary tissues, are instead attributable to the particular anatomical conformations of the vascular venous bed. Fortunately, these cases are not found in the great majority of patients.
We have decided to dedicate a particular section of this chapter (see Box 4.1) to this aspect, in which detailed information is provided.
Refer to Table 4.2 for hypochlorite injection into periapical tissues.

Box 4.1 **SERIOUS SODIUM HYPOCHLORITE ACCIDENTS**

Although sodium hypochlorite (NaOCl) accidents, created by extruding the irrigant through the radical apexes, are relatively rare and not life-threatening, they create considerable morbidity when they occur.
They have only been published as isolated clinical cases. Although several previous studies have attempted to synthesize the symptoms involved in these clinical examples, no group has attempted to analyze the causes in depth.
In a review, we examined the paradigmatic signs of a classic NaOCl incident, which presents itself with facial swelling and bruising.
A new hypothesis has emerged, which foresees the anatomical involvement of a part of the vascular bed. The intravenous infusion of NaOCl in the facial vein occurs through non-collapsible venous sinusoids inside the spongy bone; this gives rise to a massive reaction of the entire maxilla-facial district. Therefore, the reactions from NaOCl of massive size are a result of anatomical complexity and present only in a small circle of individuals. These reactions would not be generally attributable to all subjects who have undergone an accidental injection of NaOCl beyond the apical limit.

Zhu WC, Gyamfi J, Niu LN, Schoeffel GJ, Liu SY, Santarcangelo F, Khan S, Tay KC, Pashley DH, Tay FR. *Anatomy of sodium hypochlorite accidents involving facial ecchymosis - a review*. J Dent. 2013 Nov;41(11):935-48.

EDTA

Ethylene diamine-tetraacetic acid, commonly called EDTA, is a chelating agent that can help remove the smear layer produced during mechanical shaping.
EDTA was introduced to address the paradox that mechanical shaping is more of a problem than a benefit, as debris is produced and pushed into all those areas of the endodontium that are not or cannot be touched by the instruments.
EDTA is an acid that removes the mineralized part of the dentin and the smear layer as it is able to bind the Ca^{2+} and Fe^{3+}[16] ions.
EDTA decalcifies dentin to a depth of 20–30 microns in 5 min[38], although Fraser has stated that the chelating effect is almost negligible in the apical third of the canal[40].
Paste chelators have been proved to be less effective than liquid EDTA in removing the smear layer, and the addition of surfactant does not improve the cleaning action of the solution[41].
Various formulations containing EDTA have been proposed. One of the most common, containing urea acid and EDTA, has been introduced to facilitate the leak of debris from the canal, but it contains a wax that deposits on the dentinal surfaces and cannot be removed either mechanically or with other irrigants, thereby compromising the hermetic seal of the root canal system.
Other formulations add antibacterial solutions (e.g., bis-dequalino-acetate [BDA]) or ethylene-glycol-bis (β-aminoethyl ether)-N,N,N′,N′-tetracetic acid (EGTA) to EDTA. These formulations may increase the effectiveness in removing the smear layer, but they are not always effective in the apical third.
EDTA should be allowed to work in the canal for 15 min; after this time, an increase in chelating action should not be expected[38].
For the removal of the smear layer to also be effective in the apical third, mechanical activation of EDTA inside the canal (by means of ultrasonic or sonic inserts) is advisable.
The recommended concentration for optimal use of EDTA is 17%: the solution removes the smear layer in less than 1 minute if it reaches the root canal wall.
The dentin decalcification process is self-limiting because the chelating agent is consumed[16].
During retreatment, removal of dentine blockages previously created within the canals is useful, but it must be used with caution because softening the dentine can cause the operator to create ledges and false paths[42].

Fig. 4.10: Phytic acid can release the dentin tubules. Unlike EDTA, the surface of the tubules is preserved and not corroded (our thanks to Dr. Diletta Forgione for providing the image).

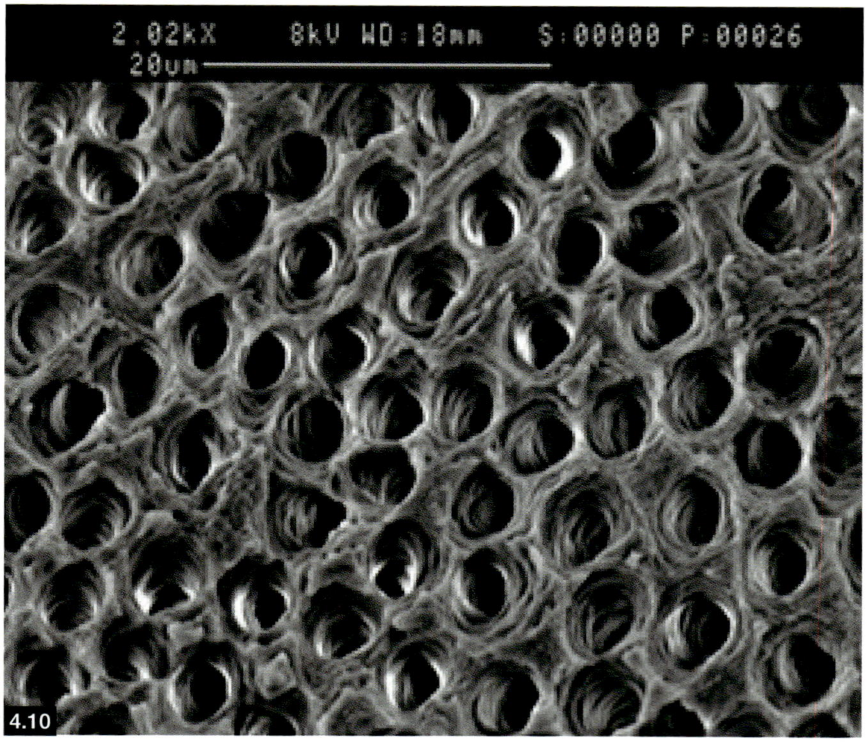

Phytic acid (IP6)

Considering that EDTA is not biodegradable, of synthetic origin, and not biocompatible, phytic acid (IP6) has recently been introduced as an alternative.
IP6 is a chelator of natural origin, easily extractable from rice, and able to bind calcium ions, magnesium, and iron because it is characterized by strong negative charges[43]. IP6, specifically, binds Ca^{2+} more than EDTA, so it is more effective at low concentrations.
Ca^{2+} ions are available in large quantities

at a low pH, but EDTA works at a pH between 6 and 10, while IP6 works at a pH of 1.2. Moreover, EDTA, when it binds to Ca^{2+} ions, generates a decrease in the pH of the solution and is rapidly inactivated (Fig. 4.10). 1% IP6 has an action equal to or greater than that of EDTA and is characterized by low cytotoxicity and low aggressiveness toward dentin (preserving the dentin tubules)[44].

Citric acid

Citric acid, at concentrations of between 5% and 50%, has also been tested as an alternative to EDTA to remove the smear layer[45]. Although citric acid performs slightly better than EDTA when the two products are used at similar concentrations, both agents are effective in removing the smear layer (in the middle and coronal third) and in improving penetration sealer in the dentinal tubules[46, 47].

Other irrigants

Other types of canal irrigants have been developed over time, and they can be used in substitution of those described above. Although allergic reactions to sodium hypochlorite (because both sodium and chlorine are essential elements in the physiology of the human body) are highly unlikely, there are documents in the literature of some allergic reactions to hypochlorite[48, 49], along with rare cases of hypersensitivity or contact dermatitis[50].
In case of hypersensitivity to sodium hypochlorite, not even chlorhexidine can act as a canal irrigation agent because of its chlorine content; instead, iodine potassium iodide is indicated after verifying the absence of allergies to iodides, because it has good antimicrobial properties.
Other irrigants mentioned in the literature are alcohol or water, even if they do not dissolve the vital or necrotic pulp tissue and are not very effective as an antibacterial agent.
In these cases, one can medicate the tooth with calcium hydroxide, a material that can dissolve vital and non-vital tissues[51, 52]. More recently, irrigants containing antibiotics have been introduced. Tetracyclines are broad-spectrum antibiotics that have excellent antimicrobial capabilities. When placed in concentrated solutions, tetracyclines have a low pH that allows them to chelate calcium and demineralize the surface of enamel and radicular dentin in a similar measure to that of *citric acid* (but with a lower demineralization).
According to some authors, doxycycline hydrochloride (100 mg/ml) is effective in removing the smear layer from the surface of the instrumented root canals, leaving a trail of antibacterial agents that can prevent a reinfection of the root canal system, because doxycycline can adhere to the root dentin and be released later.
In 2003, Torabinejad and colleagues developed an irrigation solution that could both remove the smear layer and disinfect the canal system: this solution, called MTAD, contains a mixture of isomers of tetracycline, citric acid, and a detergent.
The indication was to use it as a final irrigant after the chemomechanical preparation[53, 54].
A similar product on the market, namely, Tetraclean (Ogna Laboratori Farmaceutici, Muggiò, Italy), has an antibiotic concentration lower than MTAD (50 mg/5 ml *doxycycline* instead of 150 mg/5 ml) and uses a different detergent (polypropylene glycol instead of Tween 80)[16].
Given that bacteria isolated from the root canal system usually become resistant to tetracyclines, the use of antibiotics instead of biocides such as NaOCl or chlorhexidine is not recommended.
Hydrogen peroxide has long been used as an irrigant in concentrations usually between 3% and 5%. It is active against bacteria, viruses, and yeasts.
Hydroxyl-free radicals destroy protein and DNA. Its ability to dissolve tissues is certainly lower than that of sodium hypochlorite and has slight antibacterial activity, so it is no longer recommended as an endodontic irrigant, although it is still used in some countries[16].

CITRIC ACID

Like all acid compounds, citric acid can **demineralize** intracanal dentin.

DOXYCYCLINE

The use of specific antibiotics within **low surface tension** irrigants is a valid alternative to traditional irrigants.

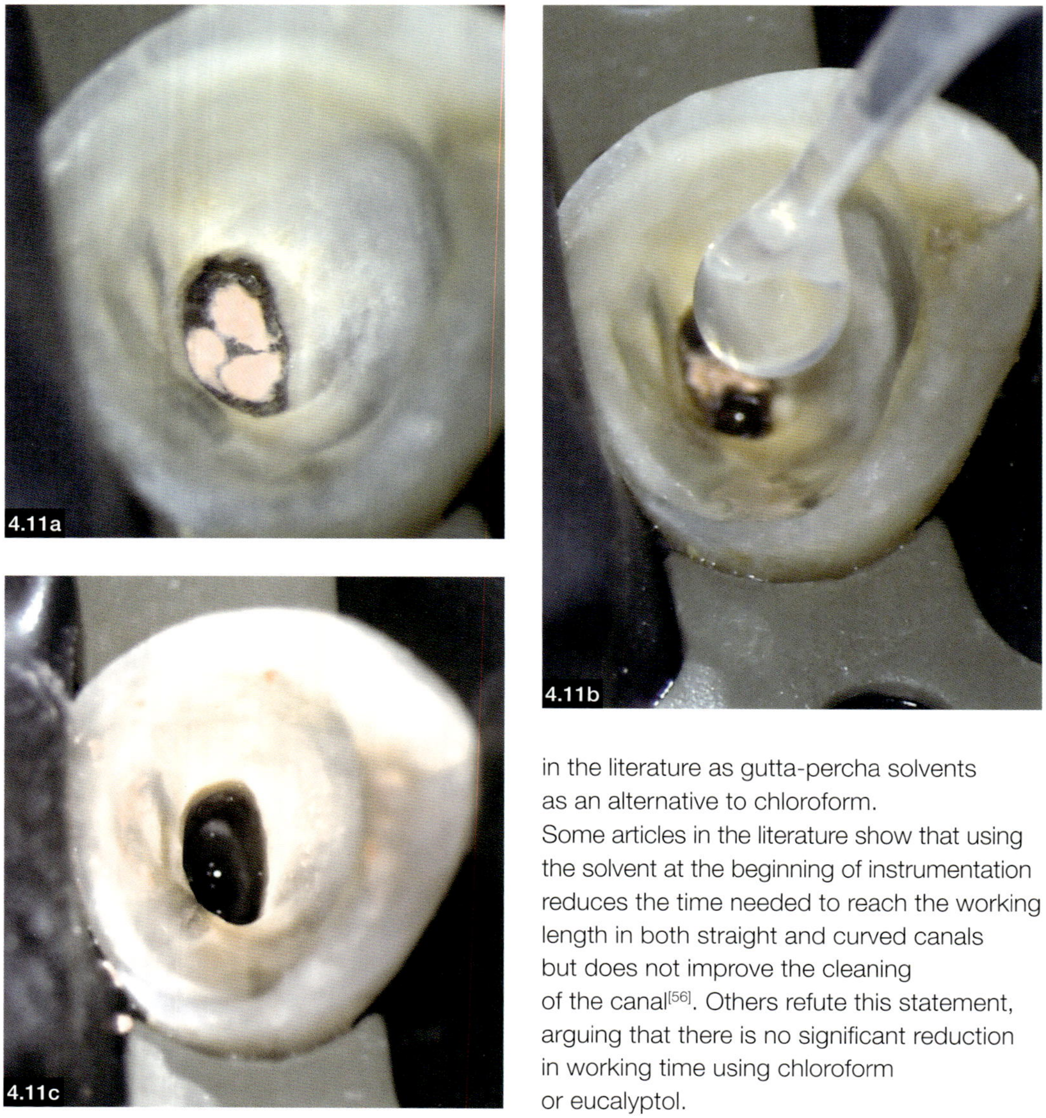

Fig. 4.11a-c: In the event that removal of root canal fillings with mechanical tools (a) is risky or difficult, a solvent may be used. This solvent is applied by means of a micropipette inside the pulp chamber (b).
In a few seconds, the gutta-percha is softened and its removal is simplified (c).

Solvents

To easily remove the gutta-percha inside the canals, the operator can use solvents that can soften the gutta-percha and dissolve the sealers.
In the past, chloroform, a very effective chemical agent, was used, but it was extremely toxic for periapical tissues and the operator. For this reason, the FDA has banned its use in drugs and cosmetics[55]. Alternatively, safer but less fast-acting solvents can now be used, such as xylol or essential oils of orange (e.g.. *orange solvent*) or eucalyptol.
Other solvents of natural origin that have good biocompatibility characteristics (e.g., limonene) have been proposed in the literature as gutta-percha solvents as an alternative to chloroform.
Some articles in the literature show that using the solvent at the beginning of instrumentation reduces the time needed to reach the working length in both straight and curved canals but does not improve the cleaning of the canal[56]. Others refute this statement, arguing that there is no significant reduction in working time using chloroform or eucalyptol.
However, the studies agree that the use of solvents increases the residues of the gutta-percha and sealer that are deposited on the canal walls and in the dentinal tubules, worsening the degree of cleansing achievable during the therapy[57, 58].
Thus, solvents should not be used as a standard procedure during retreatment, but they can be applied only when the working length cannot be objectively reached without their use[59].
The recommended application is drop by drop by means of a micropipette, which brings the solution directly into contact with the gutta-percha.
After a few moments, the surface of the filling will soften. It will be easy to remove with manual or mechanical endodontic instruments (Figs. 4.11a–4.11c).

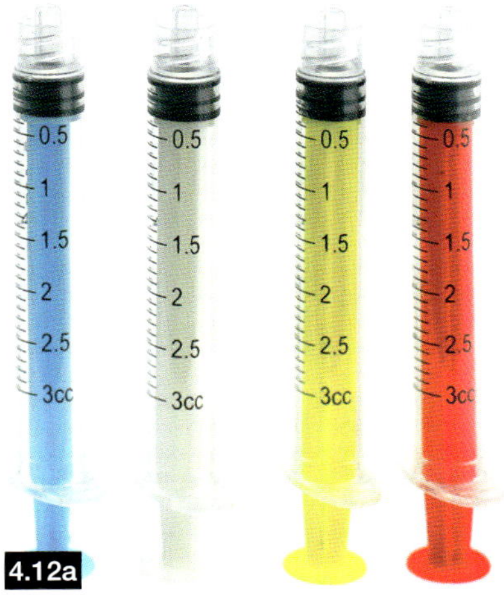

4.12a

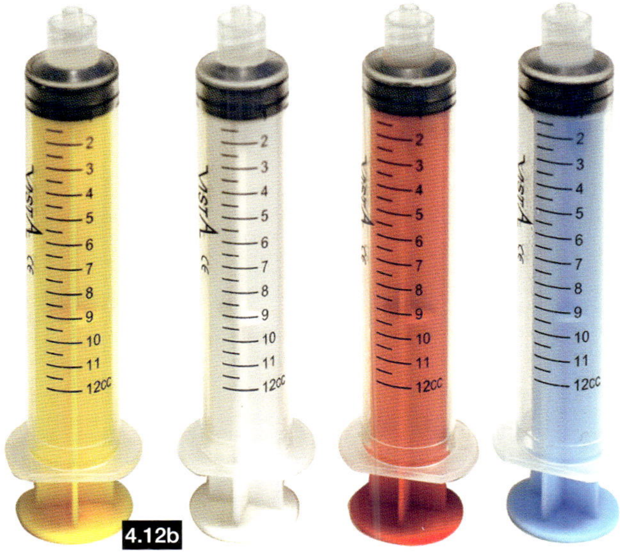

4.12b

Fig. 4.12a-b: Use of 3 cc and 5 cc colored syringes allows immediate distinction and facilitates the clinical procedure.

Irrigation methods

Factors that pose a challenge in root canal irrigation and disinfection include biofilm resistance, poor irrigation penetration, and irrigation exchange in the highly complex root canal anatomy.

The irrigants must come into direct contact with the surface to be treated to obtain the desired result.

To achieve this goal, over the years, several systems have been developed of which a small part has been selected to help carry out an effective, simple, and repeatable clinical practice.

Syringes and needles

Conventional syringes are the most common tool for positive endodontic irrigation.

Different types of syringes exist.

In endodontics, a 5 ml syringe with luer lock security attachment is advised.

Larger diameter syringes are more difficult to control than small diameter syringes, and the laminar flow produced is not continuous. If different irrigants are used, then syringes of different colors should be selected to distinguish them during the irrigation phases or single-patient kits with syringes coded for the different types of irrigants may be used (Figs. 4.12a and 4.12b).The effectiveness of irrigation is largely determined by the relative diameter of the needle and root canal[60]. The needle must be selected based on the principle of safety and be of such a size that it does not rub against the canal walls during irrigation, as this would increase the risk of extrusion of the irrigant into the periapical tissue[61, 62].

Needles must have dedicated openings and can be either open non-flat tip (notched) or closed tip with a side exit (side vented).

These particular shapes guarantee controlled laminar flow and allow the tip to be safely positioned in the apical areas, because the extruded liquid can always flow out coronally (Figs. 4.13a and 4.13b).

The dimensions of the needle diameter used in medicine are defined by the ISO 9626:199

Fig. 4.13a-b: Side-vented needles allow lateral extrusion of the liquid for coronal laminar flow and control of the liquid extrusion. Figure 4.13b shows two needles with side vents: 27G (yellow) and 30G (purple).

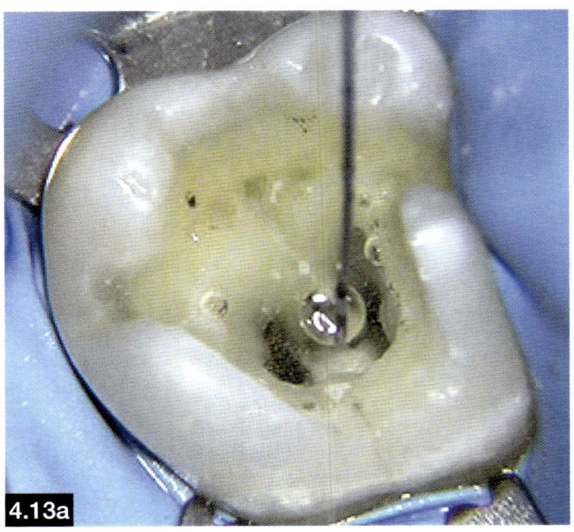

4.13a

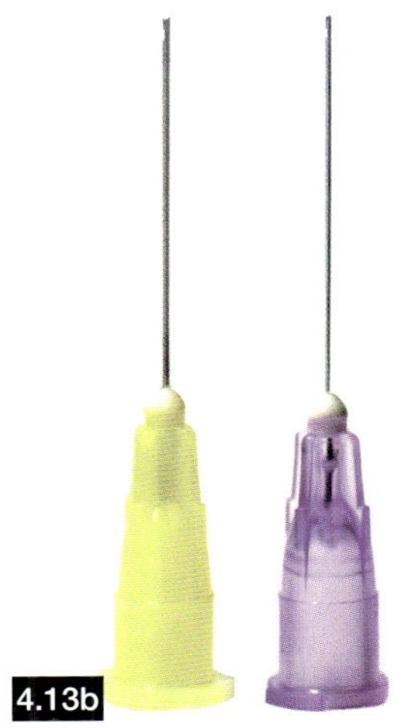

4.13b

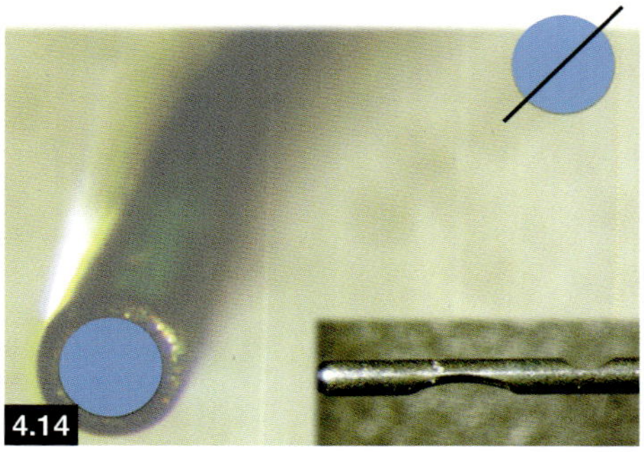

GAUGE	ISO
30	30
27	40
23	60-70
20	70-80

Fig. 4.14: Sample image showing the association between ISO diameters and Gauge, the universal system used to measure tubular diameters.

and the Amd 1:2001 specification (ISO 9626 2001)[63]. The needles selected for irrigation in endodontics have a small diameter, between 25 and 30 Gauge (G), although those used by specialists are those of 27 (ISO40) and 30G (ISO35; Fig. 4.14).
The anatomy of the periodontium provides a resistance of 25 mm/hg and is a permeable system. If this resistance is exceeded and there is no possibility of coronal flow, liquids extrude from the system.
A recent study[64] calculated the mean flow of irrigation through 26G, 27G, or 30G needles: the flow was 0.27 ml/s for 26G needles, 0.19 ml/s for 27G needles, and 0.09 ml/s for 30G needles.
The study found a statistically significant difference among the flow of needles ($P < 0.001$).
The 26G needle had a higher flow than the other two needles, followed by the groups of 27G and 30G.
However, the more violent the flow, the greater the risk that the debris present within the root canal system exudes in the periapical tissues, and the open needles exudes more product than *side-vented* needles[65].

Push–pull technique

Irrigation is meant by most clinicians as the extrusion of an irrigant from a syringe gripped by holding the index and middle fingers under the wings of the syringe and the thumb over the plunger.
Without requiring special devices, there is a technique that allows alternating positive and negative irrigation and obtains a better cleaning of the root canal system.
If, after injecting an amount of irrigant, the clinician places the thumb under the plunger and pushes upwards, a negative pressure develops that opposes the pressure used to inject the irrigant into the canal; this motion causes a suction of fluids into the canals, improving the fluid dynamics within the root canal system.
In this way, keeping the needle stationary and moving the plunger, the liquids have better penetration into the canals emptied and act more effectively (as the buffer effect is decreased by a constant exchange of solutions)[63, 65].
During the negative pressure phase, the fluids in the canal (now depotentiated) return to the syringe by capillarity and are reactivated, while any pathogens are eliminated thanks to the action of the irrigant.
An ideal condition for the next active irrigation phase is then created, because the new irrigant can come into contact with the entire dentine surface (Figs. 4.15a and 4.15b).
This technique is simple, effective, and able to show the operator any confluence

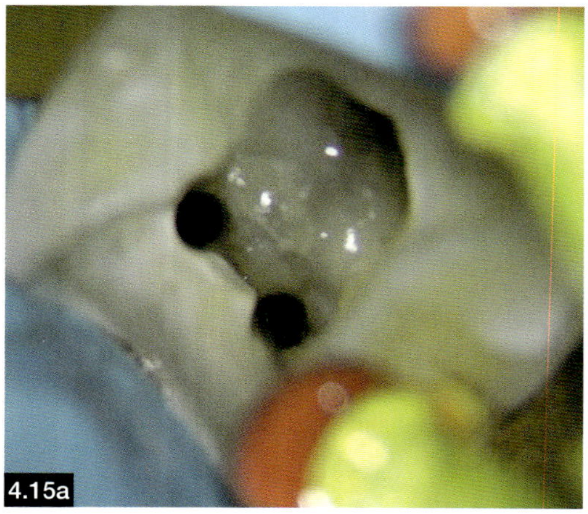

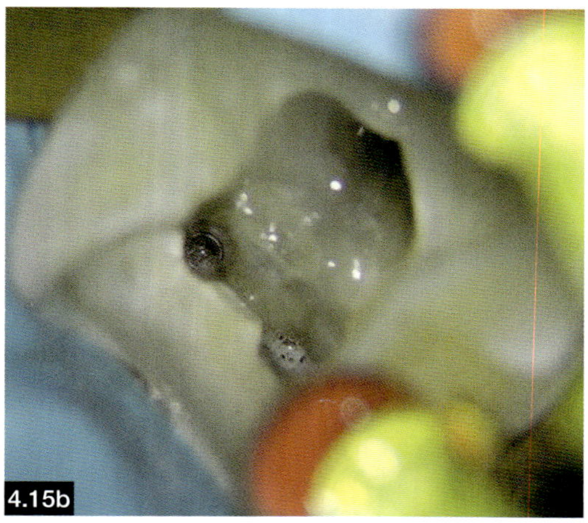

Fig. 4.15a-b: The push-pull technique is easy to apply and makes it possible to identify canal confluences. Its use also ensures better interchange between irrigants.

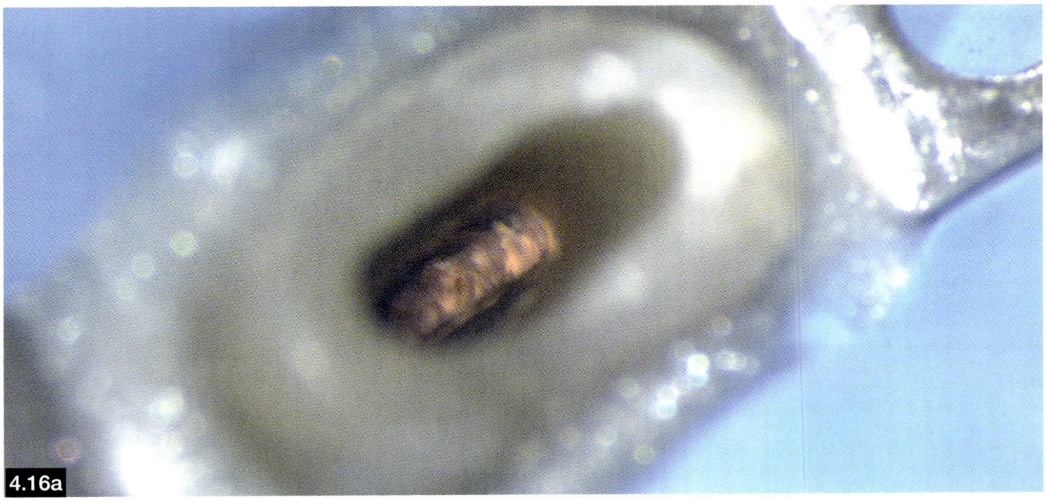

4.16a

of apparently independent canals. In this case, it is sufficient to observe whether during the suction phase carried out in one canal, the irrigant disappears from the adjacent canal. In retreatment, the push–pull technique allows for a greater removal of dentine debris and previous filling materials than active irrigation only.
The clinician, during the execution of the technique, should try not to introduce air into the root canal.

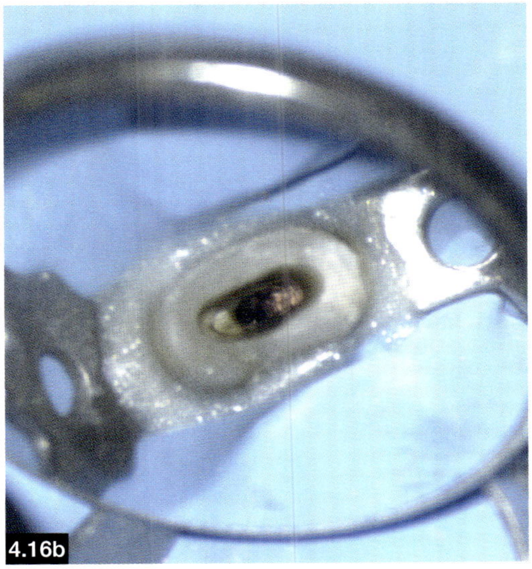

4.16b

Fig. 4.16a-c: During retreatment, all the material from the previous filling must be removed, as it can promote the persistence of bacteria within the body of the root canal system and create a barrier between the bacteria and the irrigants (preventing the optimal action of the latter). Complete removal of the previous filling material from the canal walls is the first step to achieving a good degree of cleanliness.

Activation of irrigants

The complexity of the canal anatomy makes the complete debridement of all the areas of the root canal complex. Numerous studies published in the literature have shown that an optimal level of cleansing is impossible to reach simply by letting the irrigation agent work within the root canal system. Isthmuses, lateral canals, and dentinal tubules often become areas in which microorganisms and residues of vital or necrotic pulp tissue can nest and remain undisturbed, supporting inflammatory and infectious processes[66].
A further obstacle to the correct cleansing of the canal system is represented by the previous filling material, especially when treating curved canals: this material can act as a protection for bacteria involved in secondary infections and prevent the eradication of the infection (Figs. 4.16a–4.16c)[67].

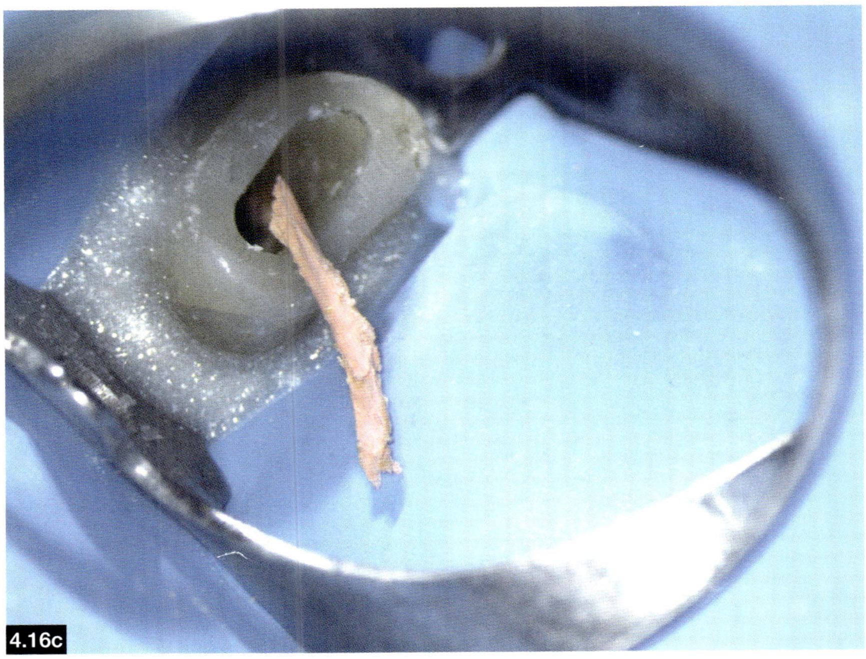

4.16c

Unfortunately, numerous studies have shown that complete removal of the gutta-percha, sealer, and other fillings is almost impossible with instrumentation (manual or mechanical) and conventional irrigation[68-70].
For this reason, the activation of the irrigants is the optimal solution for removing and detaching the residues of the previous filling from the canal walls and increasing the effectiveness of the cleaning[70, 71].
According to Cunningham[73], increasing the temperature of hypochlorite to 37 °C improves its ability to kill bacteria.
Basrani et al.[16] stated that raising the temperature of sodium hypochlorite has benefits, allowing bacteria to be killed faster, although it does not improve the effectiveness of tissue dissolution.
The ideal temperature is a few degrees above body temperature, because excessive temperatures can damage the cells of the periodontal ligament.
Various devices can increase the temperature of sodium hypochlorite. Given that syringe heaters do not keep the temperature constant, the best way to increase the temperature is to use ultrasound to activate hypochlorite.
A recent study compared the effects of concentration, temperature, and stirring on the tissue dissolution capacity of sodium hypochlorite; they concluded a linear relationship between the hypochlorite concentration and tissue dissolution, and the effects of stirring on tissue dissolution are greater than those of temperature[18].
Many techniques can be employed to activate sodium hypochlorite, but ultrasonic activation of irrigants is probably the most studied method in the literature and is now commonly used in dental practices[74]. It can increase the effectiveness of hypochlorite in the apical third by 5%[32].
From a clinical point of view, dedicated instruments that are easy to find but not necessarily expensive should be used[72, 76].
Stojicic et al.[77] showed that a continuous exchange of solution also increases the effectiveness of hypochlorite.

Fig. 4.17a-b: Ultrasonic tip: not activated (a) and activated (b). Note the energy that is transferred to the liquid without any movement of the tip.

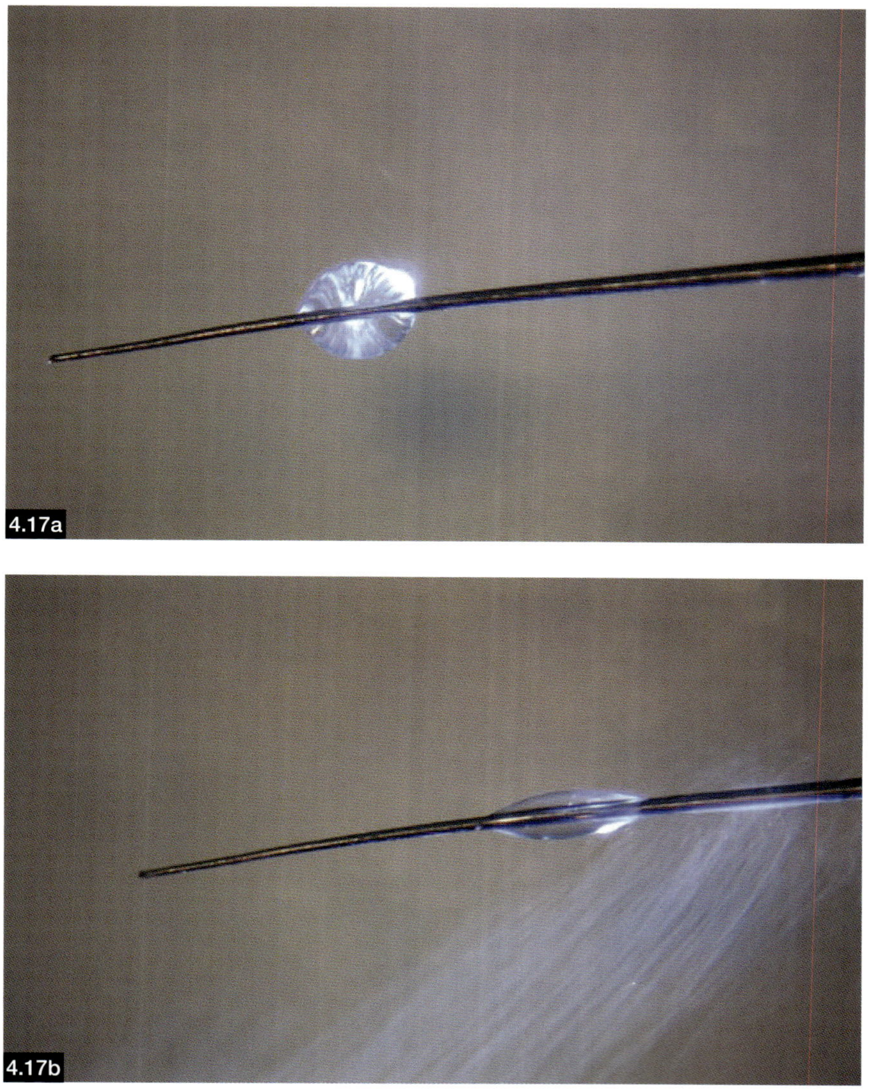

4.17a

4.17b

Ultrasonic activation of irrigants and passive ultrasonic irrigation

The activation of irrigants through dedicated ultrasonic tips occurs when the operator inserts these tips into the canals filled with irrigant.
Boutsioukis recently redefined the way to identify ultrasonic irrigation activation, generally labeled in the literature with the term passive ultrasonic irrigation (PUI). PUI identifies a smooth ultrasonic tip inserted "passively" into the canal, ideally floating in the middle, generating cavitation. Unfortunately, in clinical practice, the passivity of the tip does not occur, because it comes into contact with the walls of the canal, especially in curved canals, thereby changing the surface

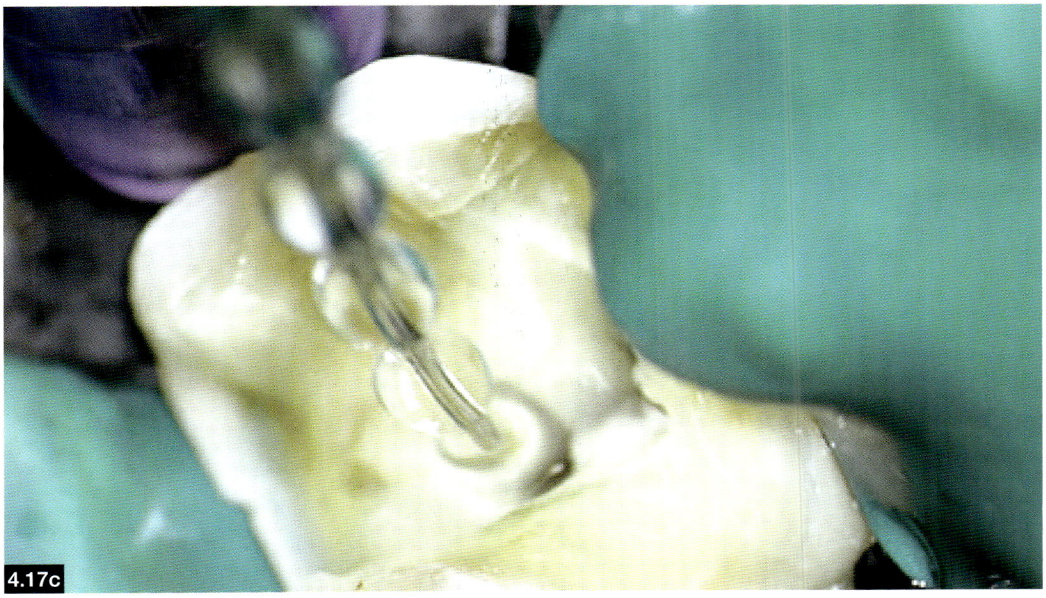
4.17c

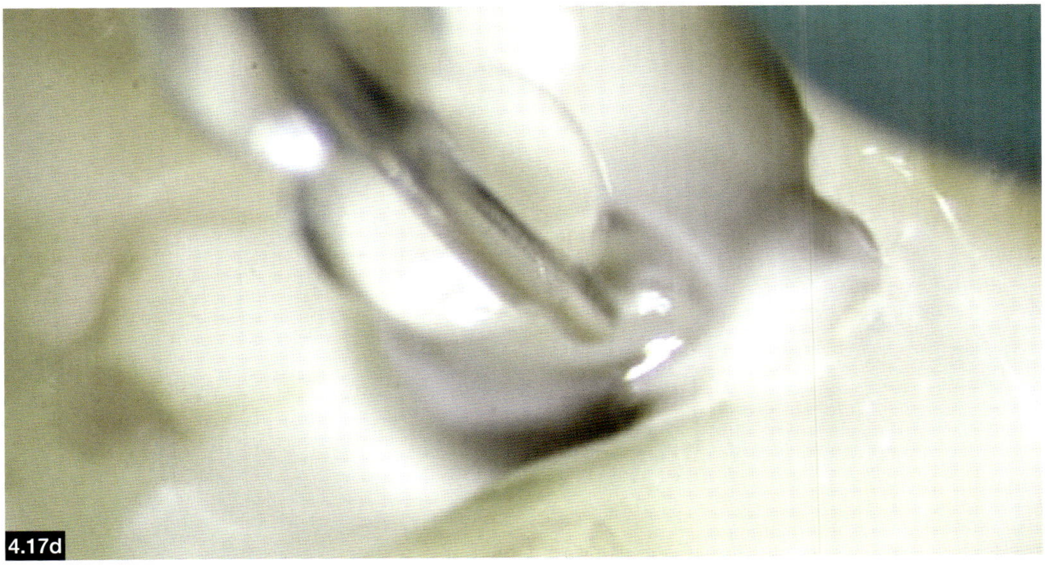
4.17d

Fig. 4.17c-d: Acoustic streaming in action around the ultrasonic tip.

with which it comes into contact.
For this reason, this technique should be defined in a general manner as passive ultrasonic irrigation (UAI), or ultrasonic activation of irrigants[78].
We talk about UAI when a blunt point with smooth walls is inserted into a canal filled with irrigants.
Once activated, the tip oscillates by transmitting at least 30 kHz of energy to the irrigant in the root canal via ultrasonic waves, chemically modifying the irrigants (*sonochemistry*) and causing acoustic streaming and cavitation (Figs. 4.17a and 4.17b).
Cavitation is defined as follows: when an ultrasonic wave is transmitted in a liquid, negative pressure is generated in the liquid itself. Cavitation creates unstable bubbles that follow the created acoustic waves. Their implosion generates energy waves through a current called acoustic streaming.
Cavitation and acoustic streaming allow the irrigant to perform better removal of the filling material and all debris present in the canal (Figs. 4.17c and 4.17d).
When the ultrasonic tip touches the canal walls, a low-frequency secondary wave (6 kHz) is generated, which is added to the tip frequency (30 kHz).
Therefore, contact with the walls does not cause a decrease in power but rather,

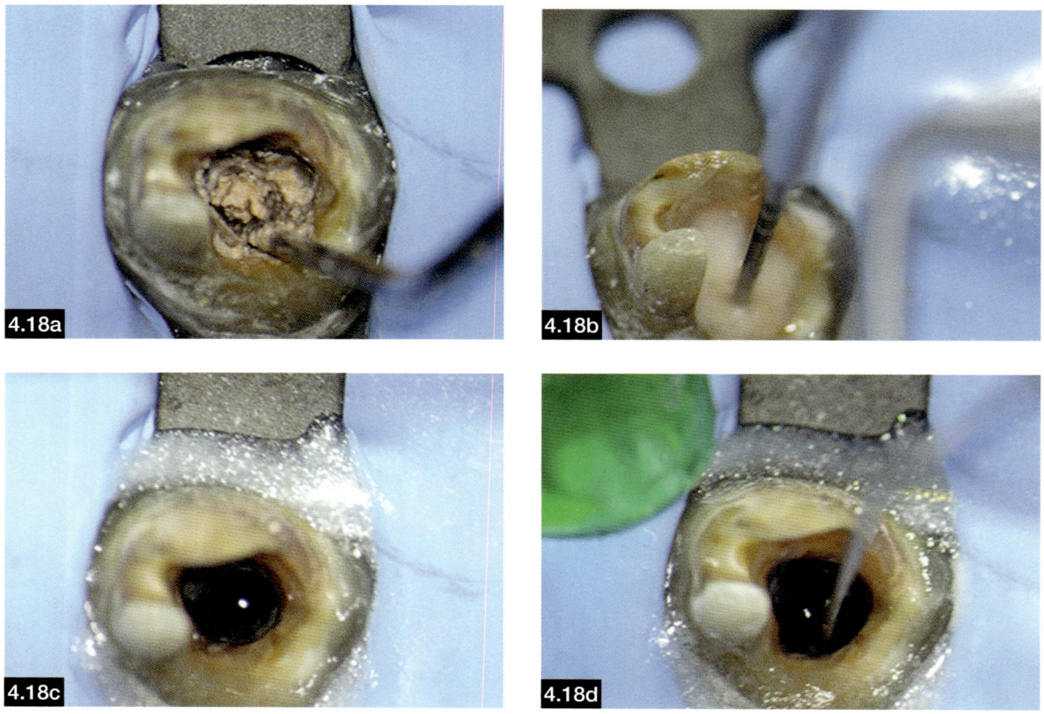

Fig. 4.18a-d: Root canal of large dimensions that presents an incongruous primary treatment. Shaping alone is unable to completely remove the filling material from the canal: for this reason, after extracting the main cone, ultrasonic cleaning with sodium hypochlorite is performed. After several 30-second activation cycles the walls are thoroughly cleaned and the ultrasonic tip is not weakened when it comes into contact with the canal walls.

in case of retreatment, encourages the mechanical removal of residues (Figs. 4.18a–4.18d). The chemistry of the irrigants is also changed during activation by ultrasound: NaOCl reacts by increasing the number of Cl- ions (chlorine): hypochlorite is enhanced but also must be renewed often as its action diminishes rapidly. As mentioned above, the UAI can heat the irrigants directly inside the canal and increase their effectiveness, because the preheated irrigants, after a few seconds from the introduction into the canal, decrease to body temperature (Figs. 4.19a–4.19c)[79].

From a clinical perspective, activation can be performed with any ultrasonic motor connected to thin tips (20/04). The power of the source should be adjusted appropriately to avoid excessive vibrations causing the fracture of the tip (particularly its terminal portion).

Excessive power also creates the risk of removing healthy dentin and causing step formation or iatrogenic damage.

To overcome these problems, the first cordless ultrasound handpiece (EndoUltra™, Vista Dental) was recently introduced (Fig. 4.20). The power generated is only one (40 kHz) and is delicate to the associated titanium tip (20/04), making the workflow particularly safe.

The cordless design also determines its ease of use[78].

Fig. 4.19a-c: UAI within the canals. The metal tip absorbs energy and is able to produce cavitation and acoustic streaming. The tip absorbs and transmits energy, so it is able to heat the irrigants directly on site, allowing the effective removal of debris (c).

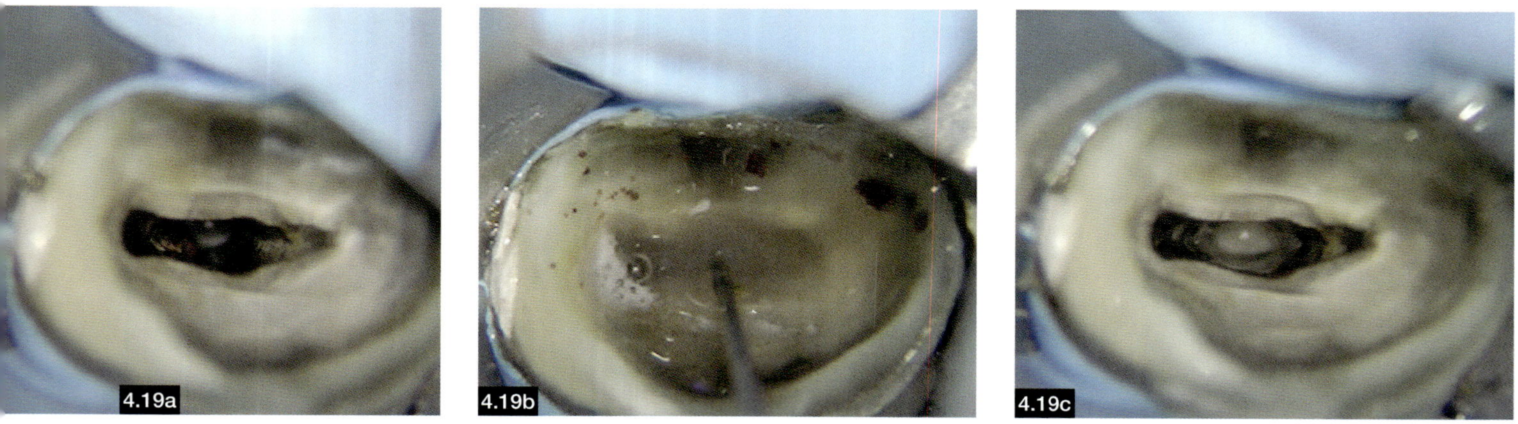

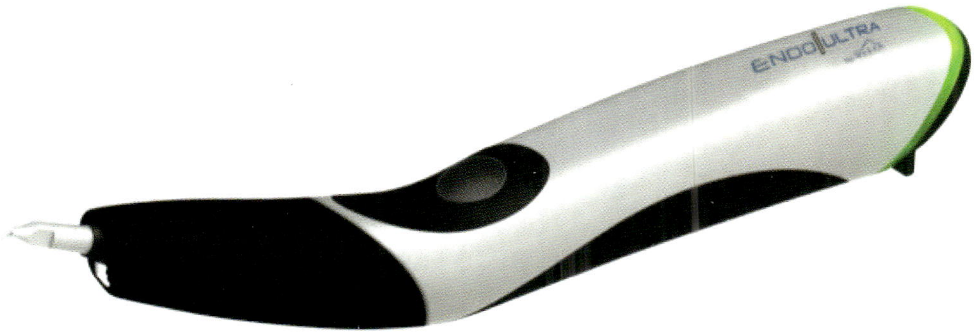

Fig. 4.20: EndoUltra™, cordless ultrasound handpiece with a delicate 20/02 titanium tip.

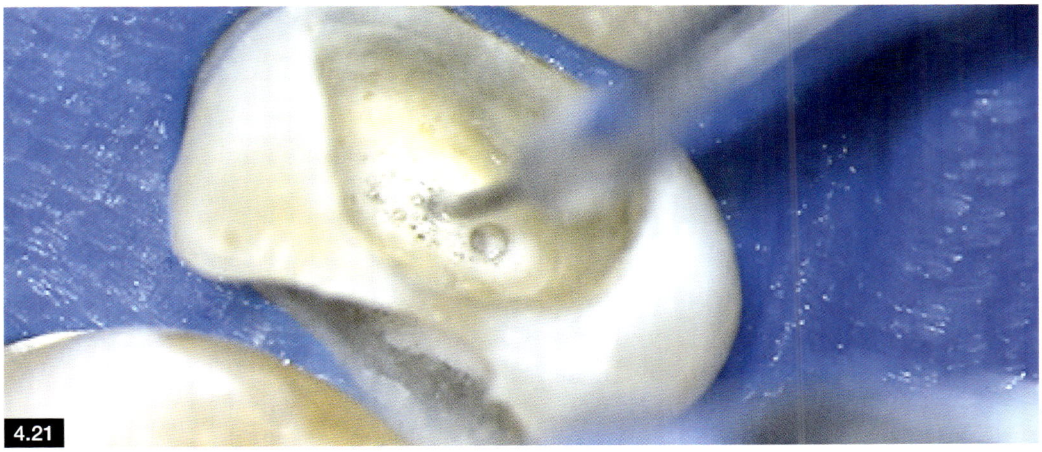

4.21

Fig. 4.21: Typical ultrasonic activation of sodium hypochlorite. After activating the ultrasonic source, microbubbles are produced and the liquid immediately becomes cloudy (indicating the need to change liquids frequently).

Accessories for canal irrigation

During the root canal cleaning phases, accessories help by simplifying the clinical procedures. During retreatment, the operating field must be as clean as possible; we often need instruments that are able to remove debris and moisture from the canals.
The best available instruments in the field are the Stropko syringe and the Elasti-Vac™ plastic cannulae (Vista Dental; Fig. 4.22).
The Stropko syringe allows air or water to be extruded from small needles.
It is a simple accessory but indispensable for cleaning the access cavity of the macro-detriti produced during the first stages of retreatment. It is also extremely useful for removing the debris that accumulates in the canal during the use of ultrasonic tips.
By contrast, plastic cannulae (Elasti-Vac™) are used to microevacuate moisture from endodontic canal systems, minimizing the need for paper tips.
They are made of a translucent material and can be bent at will. Another useful instrument is the rotating brush, which removes the gutta-percha and sealer macrodetritis from the coronal walls of the canal when used at low speed (Fig. 4.23).

Next-generation polymer needles

Thanks to the new industrial technologies of microinjection, new polymer needles with a design that can guarantee both effectiveness and safety during the phases of canal cleaning have recently been introduced. The plastic material allows optimal flexibility and greater penetration into the curved canals. Conventional steel needles are often too rigid and tend to engage with and lock onto the outer walls of the canal curves. One of these new generation needles (IrriFlex™, Produits Dentaires SA) has the ability to bend and flex easily due to its soft polypropylene body. These needles follow the anatomy of the canal to the apex and allow the operator to control the depth of irrigation due to the millimetric notches printed on the shaft of the needle.
The needle design is unique: the 30G diameter tapered tip has two apical outlets on both sides, which improve stress along the canal walls and provide superior cleanliness compared with needles with only one side outlet.
IrriFlex improves fluid dynamics throughout the root canal system, retaining the safety features of closed tip needles. The irrigant can

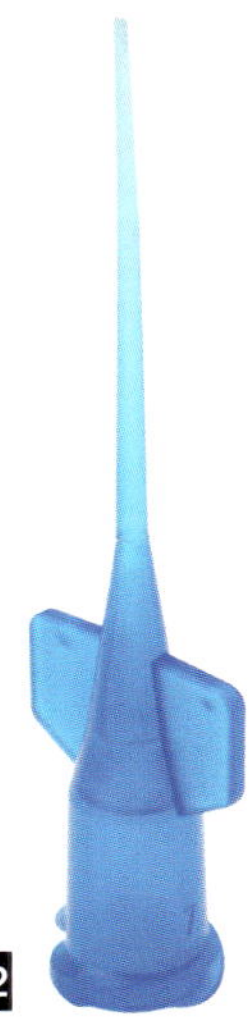

4.22

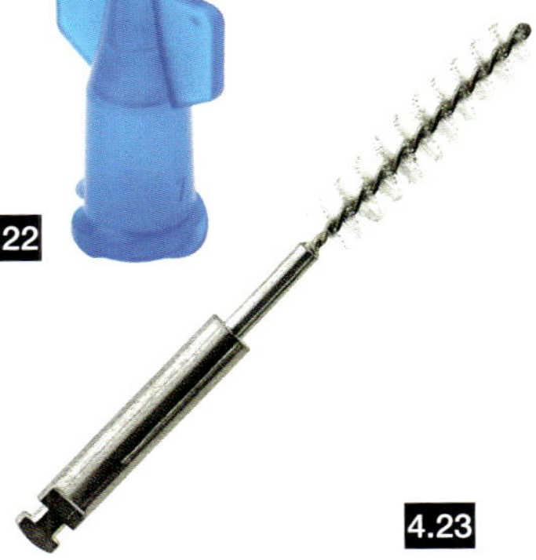

4.23

Fig. 4.22: Elasti-Vac™, polymer tip useful for microsuction of liquid and debris inside the canal.

Fig. 4.23: Versa-Brush™, micromotor toothbrush capable of removing macrodetrites from canal walls at 250 rpm.

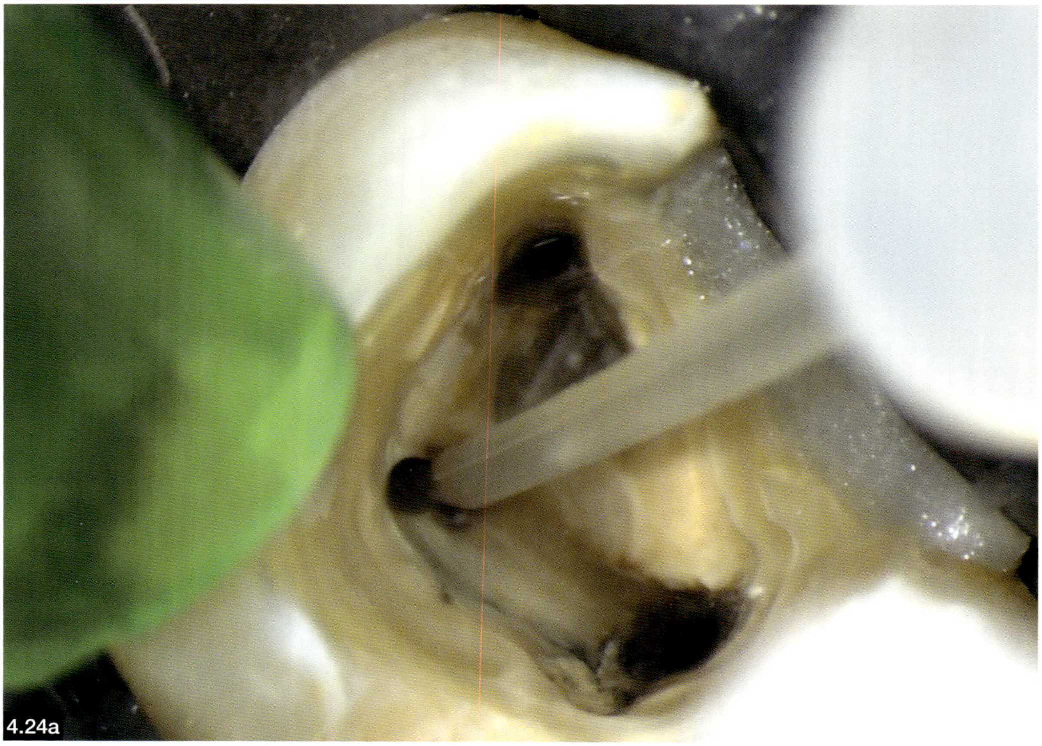

4.24a

Fig. 4.24a-b: IrriFlex® in action. The polymeric material allows better penetration of the needle in the root canal, ensuring the safe extrusion of liquid due to the two side vents.

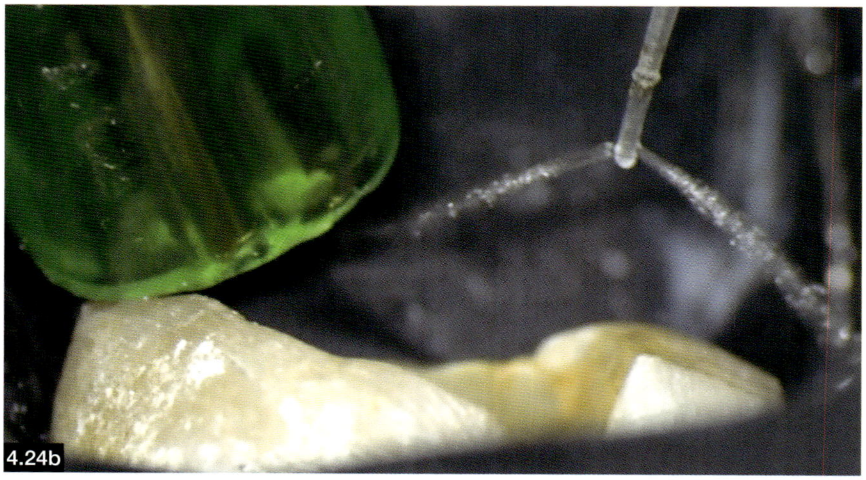

4.24b

only flow coronally; the two microscopic outlets induce atomization of the liquid, produce effective fluid dynamics turbulence for fluid replacement, and improve the removal of dentin debris (Figs. 4.24a and 4.24b).

Clinical protocols

Clinical procedures that are performed during retreatment can be divided into two phases:

1. removal of the filling. This happens thanks to the synergistic action of rotating instrumentation and solvents. The repeated application of drops of solvent removes most of the gutta-percha and canal cements within a short time period;
2. disinfection and removal of residual debris from the canal walls. This phase is essential for achieving deep disinfection of the endodontium and requires a well-defined clinical protocol. If there is any doubt about the actual removal of the gutta-percha, an x-ray may be performed for a macroscopic analysis.

The literature does not provide unambiguous indications on which protocol to follow for irrigation in retreatment, because clinical scenarios can vary considerably from case to case, given the large number of variables to be considered (particularly the operator's experience, the difficulty and variability of the canal anatomy, and any errors of the previous treatment to be remedied).

Therefore, until the shaping of the canals is completed, an effective protocol for proper cleaning cannot be proposed.

The irrigants used during the scouting, debris removal, and shaping phases cannot be considered efficient, as their action is weakened and buffered by the debris

4.25 **PROTOCOL FOR RETREATMENTS**

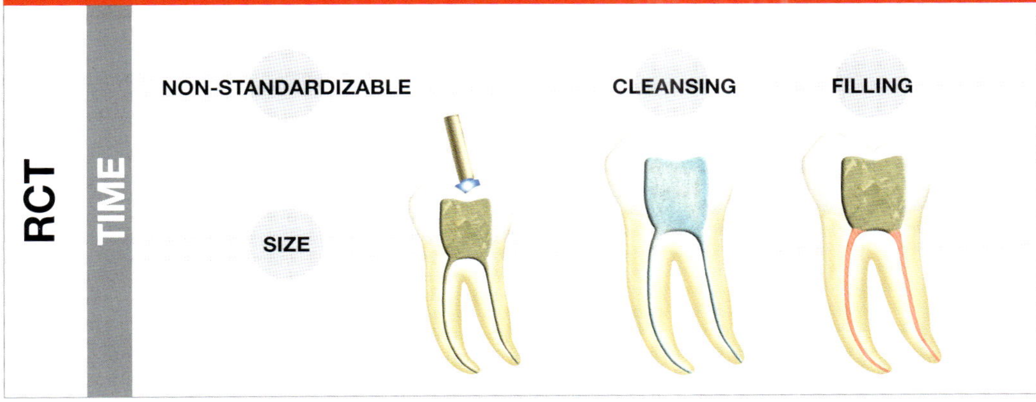

Fig. 4.25: Schematic division of the clinical phases of endodontic therapy. During the shaping process, irrigants are used. This phase is called chemomechanical shaping. Unfortunately, to standardize the protocol, the volume and time of application of the irrigants during this phase should not be counted, as they are not quantifiable.

produced; moreover, any type of ultrasonic activation of the irrigants is useless in this phase, because it must be performed once the shaping is completed.[80]
In the same way, the time of application of the irrigants and the volume used in this phase need not be considered, because the variables listed above (e.g., operator ability and anatomy) can significantly modify these values (Fig. 4.25).
Grawehr[81] studied the interactions between EDTA and NaOCl, concluding that when the two irrigators are mixed, EDTA retains its ability to chelate calcium, while NaOCl loses its ability to dissolve tissues.
Clinically, therefore, these irrigants should be used separately.
The optimal situations to obtain after irrigation are as follows: the canal is free from organic residues, microorganisms, and smear layers; the bacteria penetrated into the dentin tubules have been neutralized; and the physical and mechanical characteristics of the dentin have remained unchanged[16]. Correctly for achieving NaOCl and EDTA is crucial for achieving the ideal situation and controlling the demineralization of root dentin (considering that dentin erosion already occurs after 1 min of exposure to NaOCl in the final irrigation phase).
When attempting to devise a clinical protocol to be used during retreatment, the first step consists in not considering the liquids used during the first phases of therapy (thus eliminating the variables due to the anatomy, operator, and initial situation of the tooth).
The end of the shaping of the root canal system will be considered as time 0[82].

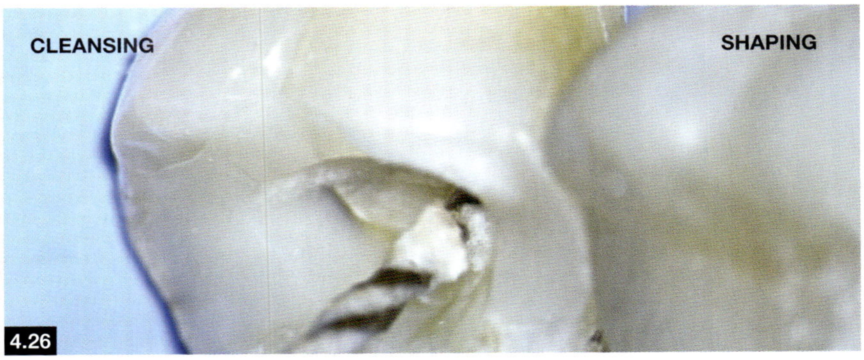

Fig. 4.26: Typical chemomechanical shaping performed with mechanical instruments in Ni-Ti in canals filled with irrigants.

On the basis of the data in the literature, to define a clinical irrigation protocol, three variables must be considered: irrigation volume, extrusion time, and activation time. Table 4.3 summarizes the indications to be followed.
The extrusion rate of the irrigant can be quantified in 2 ml/min, considering the use of a 5 ml syringe and a 27/30G needle, with drop by drop extrusion to ensure optimal safety (Fig. 4.27).
The literature indicates that the ideal volumes per canal of NaOcl and EDTA are 10 and 2 ml, respectively, and ultrasound can be used for up to 20–30 s, after which the liquids inside the canal should be renewed (Fig. 4.28).

Table 4.3 **INFORMATION FOR IRRIGATION EXECUTION**

Variable	Quantity
Irrigation volume per canal	10 ml NaOCl 2 ml EDTA
Extrusion speed	2 ml/min
Activation time	20-30 s

4.27 **CANAL CLEANING PROTOCOL**

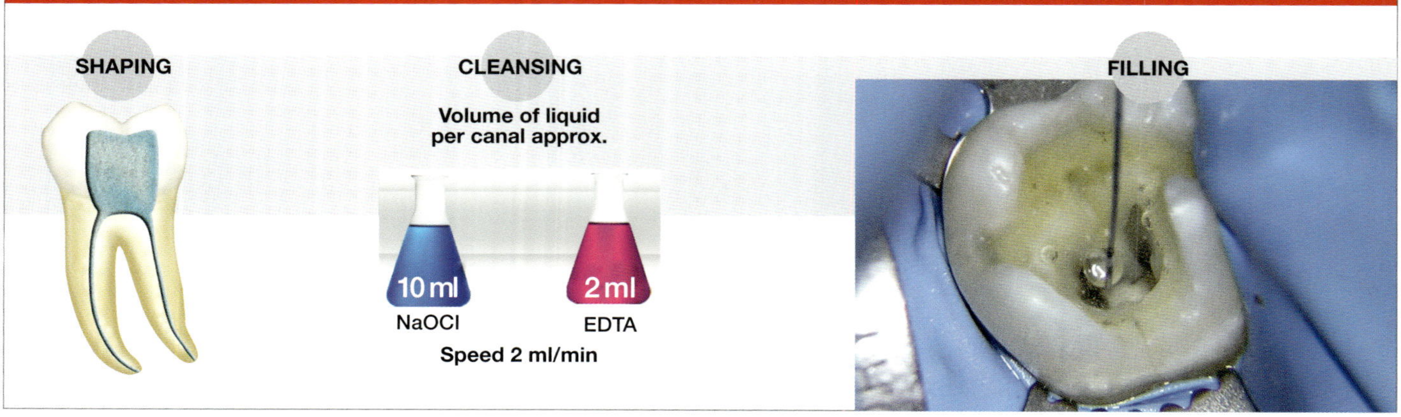

4.28 **FINAL CLEANING**

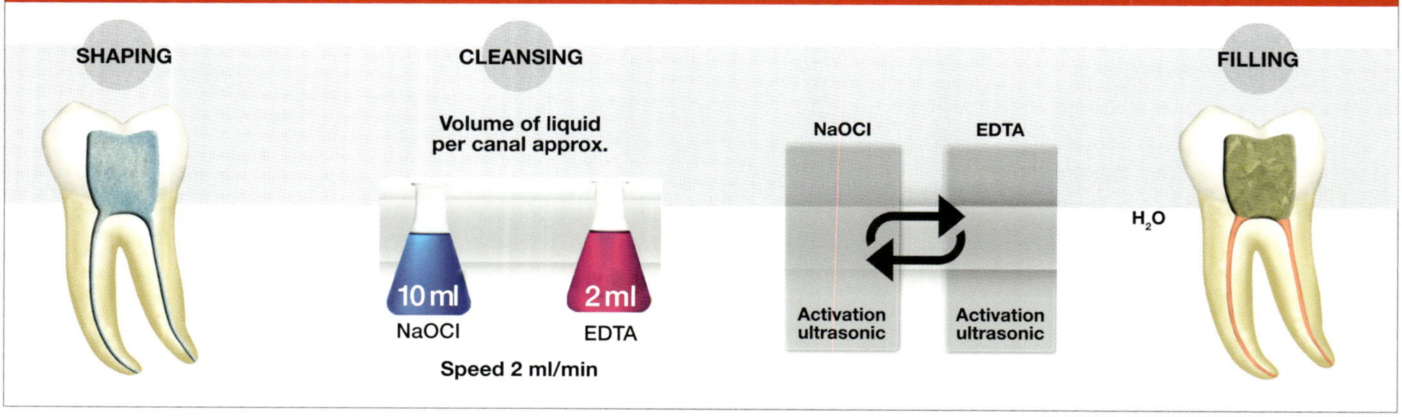

Fig. 4.27: Volume of irrigants needed for this phase of the clinical protocol: the speed of extrusion should always be 2 ml/min (i.e., drop by drop).

Fig. 4.28: The protocol begins at the end of the shaping, thereby providing for the indicated volume of the liquids to be used, the time required for the extrusion of these liquids, and ultrasonic activation of 20 s maximum per canal per cycle.

From this analysis, we may obtain the data needed to define an irrigation protocol, which must be carried out continuously, without leaving the static liquids inside the canal.
Six cycles of alternating extrusion and ultrasonic activation are planned (Table 4.4). The times vary when the number of canals to be treated increases.
If a volume of 30 ml is difficult to reach in multiradicular teeth then a volume of about 20 ml may be used instead (Figs. 4.29–4.31). As illustrated in the diagrams, EDTA must also be activated to guarantee a better result, because the chemical solution is unable to remove the smear layer on its own.
At the end of the suggested clinical protocol, the canal should be washed with sterile distilled water or alcohol to ensure the removal of irrigation residues.

Effect of tapering and apical diameter on irrigation efficiency

The penetration of the irrigant into the apical portion of the root canal system largely depends on the reaming achieved with the instrumentation.

Table 4.4 **TYPE OF TOOTH AND IRRIGATION METHOD**

Type of tooth	Total time	Extrusion	Ultrasonic activation
Single canal	10 min	1 min	30 s
Bicanalar	12 min	1.2 min	40 s
Multi-canalar	15 min	1.3–1.5 min	60 s

FINAL IRRIGATION PROTOCOL

Monoradicular

NaOCl 1 min	UAI 30 s
NaOCl 1 min	UAI 30 s
NaOCl 1 min	UAI 30 s
NaOCl 1 min	UAI 30 s
NaOCl 1 min	UAI 30 s
EDTA 1 min	UAI 30 s

10 min

Fig. 4.29: Clinical protocol recommended for monoradicular elements.

Biradicular

NaOCl 1.20 min	UAI 40 s
NaOCl 1.20 min	UAI 40 s
NaOCl 1.20 min	UAI 40 s
NaOCl 1.20 min	UAI 40 s
NaOCl 1.20 min	UAI 40 s
EDTA 1.20 min	UAI 40 s

12 min

Fig. 4.30: Clinical protocol recommended for biradicular elements.

Multiradicular

NaOCl 1.30 min	UAI 60 s
NaOCl 1.30 min	UAI 60 s
NaOCl 1.30 min	UAI 60 s
NaOCl 1.30 min	UAI 60 s
NaOCl 1.30 min	UAI 60 s
EDTA 1.30 min	UAI 60 s

15 min

Fig. 4.31: Clinical protocol recommended for multiradicular elements.

Many studies on the effectiveness of irrigation have concluded that an adequate apical preparation size and needle placement close to the working length have a direct effect on the flow of irrigation in the apical third of the canal[63]. In general, by increasing the preparation, the efficiency of the renewal of the irrigation system and the cleaning of the canal walls is improved and the distribution of stress within the structure is enhanced[83, 84]. However, given that the stress developed on the canal walls is primarily responsible for the removal of debris, dental tissue residues, microorganisms, and biofilm, an excessive enlargement of the canal does not lead to a significant improvement in cleaning, as demonstrated by previous studies[85, 86].

The *diameter of the apical preparation* affects the renewal of the irrigant, the stress developed on the canal walls, and the pressure recorded at the apical frame. The data suggest that an apical diameter greater than .25 improves irrigation performance, provided there is sufficient space between the tip of the needle and the canal walls (to ensure reverse flow of the irrigant through the canal orifice)[83, 85].

DIAMETER APICAL PREPARATION

The apical diameter of the shaping plays an important role in increasing the **volume of canal irrigants** and in improving their effectiveness.

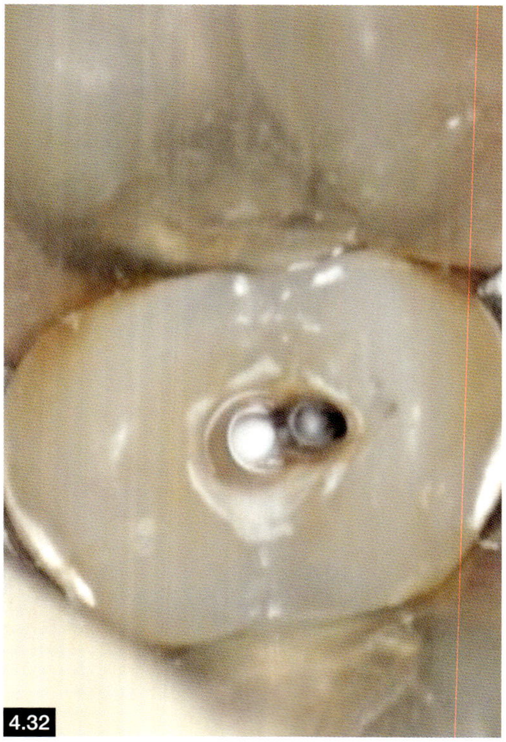

4.32

Fig. 4.32: Introduction of calcium hydroxide into the canal can be performed with many systems. One of the most commonly employed involves the use of a lentula which ensures an adequate distribution of the same in the endodontium.

Intermediate dressings

Intermediate dressings contribute to canal disinfection, promoting a significant decrease in bacterial counts after chemomechanical procedures and potentially reaching areas not affected by mechanical instrumentation and irrigation[87]. Intermediate dressings are used to counteract bacterial growth when endodontic treatment cannot be completed in a single session, as often is the case with retreatment.

In the 1930s, substances were used to "mummify" the pulp, such as paraformaldehyde, phenols, chlorophenols, and iodoformic paste. Given the toxicity of these compounds, calcium hydroxide, antibiotics, or phenolic antiseptics are currently used.

Calcium hydroxide

Calcium hydroxide, $Ca(OH)_2$, is used in endodontics as an intermediate dressing due to its good antimicrobial properties[16] resulting from the dissociation of OH- ions in an aqueous environment, which gives it a very high pH. Calcium hydroxide performs its action slowly; the literature suggests that it should remain in the canal for at least one week to achieve adequate antimicrobial activity[88].

Calcium hydroxide, when left to act for a sufficient time, can disinfect the canal; by contrast, in retreatment, where the microflora are different, two-thirds of the cases treated still present bacteria inside the canal[89, 90]. However, calcium hydroxide residues on the dentin walls may decrease the penetration sealers into the dentin tubules and increase apical leakage.

For these reasons, calcium hydroxide present inside the root canal system should first be removed before proceeding with the filling (this generally happens with the canal instrumentation and a copious irrigation with NaOCl and EDTA activated with ultrasound)[91].

Triple antibiotic paste (TAP)

TAP is a combination of three antibiotics (ciprofloxacin, metronidazole, and minocycline) used in vital tooth therapy, regeneration, and revascularization; it also has antimicrobial properties[90].
This combination of substances, when used at a concentration of 1 mg/ml, is active against Gram-positive and Gram-negative bacteria, making it an intermediate dressing to be used as an alternative to calcium hydroxide.

Effectiveness

None of the available root canal dressings are effective in completely eliminating optional aerobic and anaerobic microorganisms from the root canal system in the presence of necrotic pulp.
Thus, irrigation procedures are also essential in treatments that require more than one session. Research is moving toward active dressings against individual bacterial species and multi-species biofilms[92].

Treatment in single or multiple sessions

The use of calcium hydroxide[93-95] is a characteristic measure, which is adopted when treatment is spread out to several sessions of instrumentation, shaping, and disinfection of the endodontium[96-98].
It is especially useful in retreatment, where endodontic space disinfection in a relatively short time is challenging to achieve[99, 100].
Therefore, the so-called intermediate dressing, i.e., the use of calcium hydroxide inside the root canals, between one session and the next, is necessary by the time that retreatment is required.
The literature on treatment, or rather on retreatment, with several sessions or with a single session (appointment) is varied and full of contradictions[101-103].
Only a few objective evaluations remain, mainly of a practical clinical nature.
First, the time of day is a matter of concern. In a case of complex retreatment, which requires a procedure for the removal of coronal restorations, a root canal post, and residual endodontic content, the operating time often exceeds 1.5 h. Keeping the practitioner's concentration focused and allowing the patient to maintain an adequate buccal opening for this time is a very difficult task. Resorting to several sessions is not always, but often, a clinical necessity rather than a procedural obligation.
Numerous studies have been carried out on this subject, and none of them has come to considerations that can be considered conclusive[104]. Some authors favor single sessions on the basis of evidence obtained from the literature; others have obtained different and encouraging results in the treatments carried out in more than one session[105-108]. The use of calcium hydroxide *between one session and the next* does not seem to be harmful, although its use involves longer operating times, both for the introduction into the root canals and for its subsequent removal, which are not negligible. In a systematic review of the literature conducted by the authors, the use of a multi-session scheme in dental elements with periapical lesions would result in a non-negligible decrease in transient postoperative sequelae[105-107].

MULTIPLE SESSIONS

The use of **hydroxide calcium** is still a useful alternative for maintaining the decontaminated root canal.

As an immediate consequence, patients have been shown to take fewer drugs to alleviate pain and to counteract septic processes. The exacerbation of periapical inflammatory processes after treatment is in the order of 5–12% depending on the case history, and this acute phase must be controlled by systematic administration of antibiotic drugs. Several authors have shown that the use of calcium hydroxide can reduce or eradicate the bacterial load.
More than one study has confirmed the hypothesis that the use of calcium hydroxide may decrease the bacterial load in dental elements with infections inside the root canal[109-113].
In conclusion, the use of calcium hydroxide is unable to change the final fate of endodontic treatment but is a useful clinical aid.

CASE REPORT 1

Large periapical lesion in the upper cuspid, bridge abutment

The case involves a patient who, having come to the consult with the suspicion of a root fracture, has undergone a new diagnostic procedure on a severe periapical lesion, since the canal has not benn filled properly. In these cases, the periapical reaction appears proportional to the insufficient canal filling.

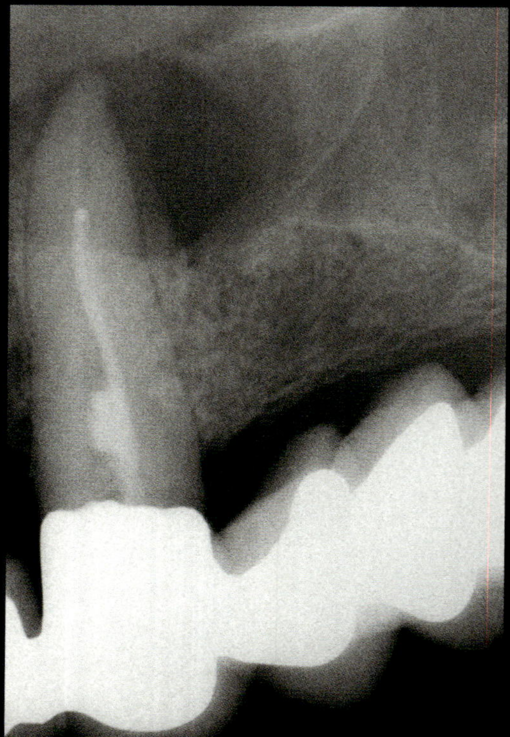

1

Figure 1: The cuspid, a bridge abutment, has a large periapical lesion and incomplete canal treatment.

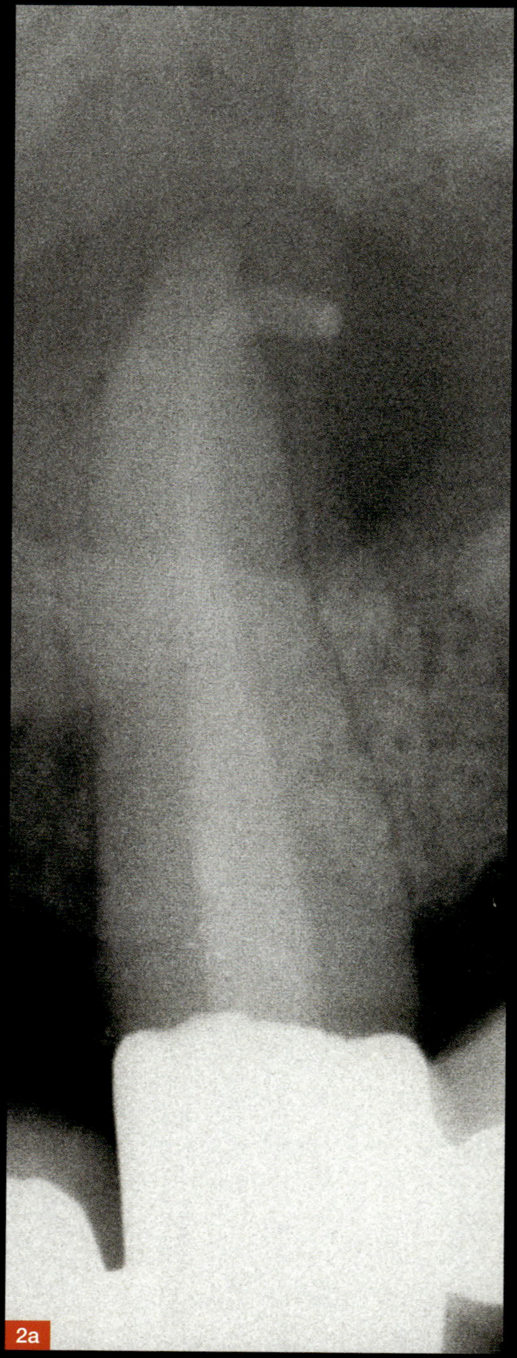

2a

Figure 2a-b: Removal of the material inside the canal led to a shaping with an apical size of 120 ISO; the canal was filled with calcium hydroxide; a slight apical excess was rapidly reabsorbed.

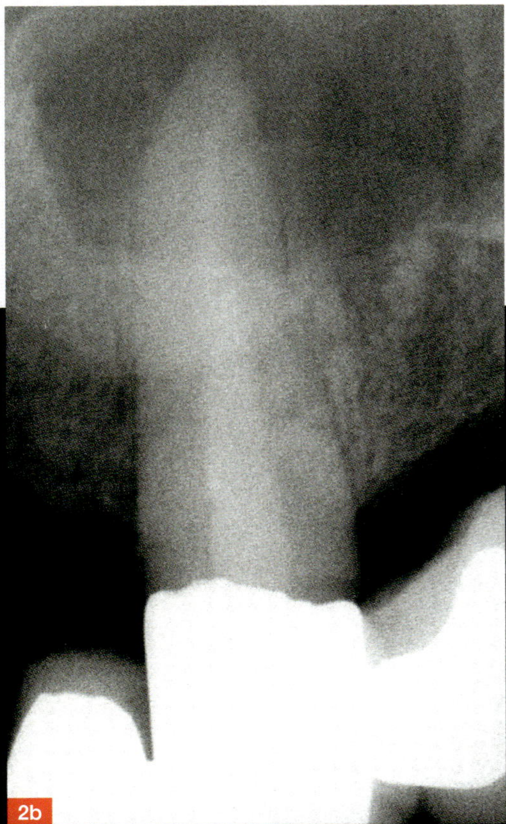

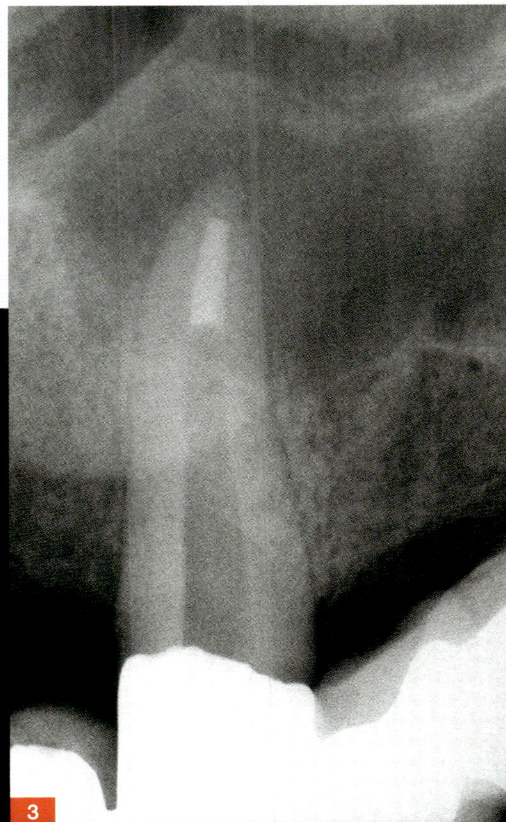

Figure 3: The apical closure with an MTA cap has become crucial for the canal size at this level.

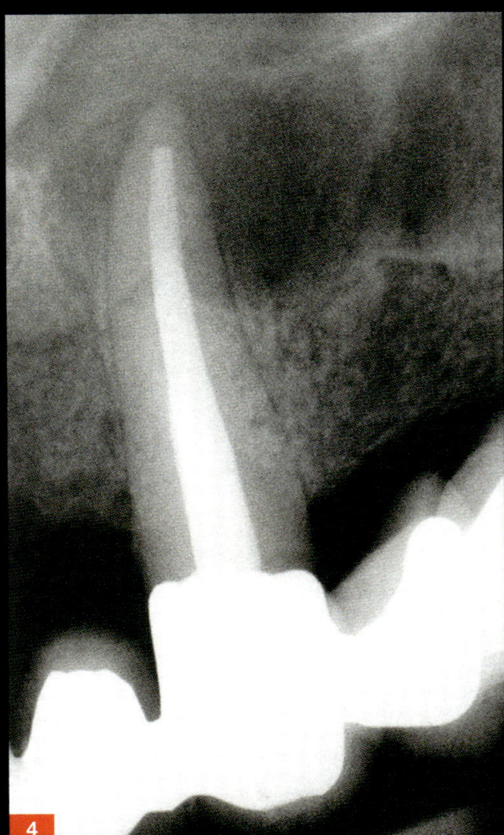

Figure 4: Complete sealing of the remaining part of the canal with zinc-oxyphosphate cement and gutta-percha.

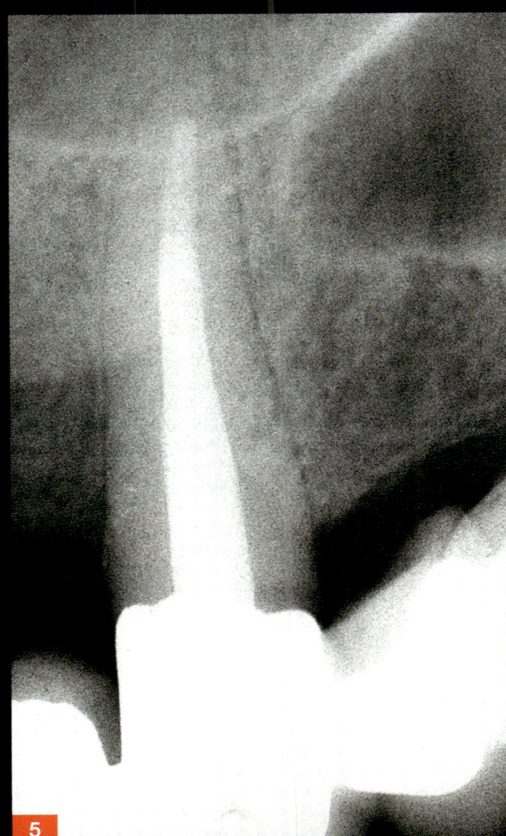

Figure 5: The 3-year follow-up demonstrates the excellent resolution of the periapical disease, with good representation of the periradicular cortical bone, a characteristic sign of bone reintegration.

References

1. Antunes HS, Rocas IN, Alves FR, Siqueira JF, Jr. *Total and Specific Bacterial Levels in the Apical Root Canal System of Teeth with Post-treatment Apical Periodontitis*. J Endod. 2015;41(7):1037-42.
2. Rocas IN, Jung IY, Lee CY, Siqueira JF, Jr. *Polymerase chain reaction identification of microorganisms in previously root-filled teeth in a South Korean population*. J Endod. 2004;30:504-8.
3. Fabricius L, Dahlen G, Sundqvist G, Happonen RP, Möller AJR. *Influence of residual bacteria on periapical tissue healing after chemomechanical treatment and root filling of experimentally infected monkey teeth*. European journal of oral sciences. 2006;114:278-85.
4. Lacerda M, Marceliano-Alves MF, Perez AR, Provenzano JC, Neves MAS, Pires FR, et al. *Cleaning and Shaping Oval Canals with 3 Instrumentation Systems: A Correlative Micro-computed Tomographic and Histologic Study*. J Endod. 2017;43(11):1878-84.
5. Abramovitz I, Relles-Bonar S, Baransi B, Kfir A. *The effectiveness of a self-adjusting file to remove residual gutta-percha after retreatment with rotary files*. Int Endod J. 2012;45(4):386-92.
6. Gu LS, Kim JR, Ling J, Choi KK, Pashley DH, Tay FR. *Review of contemporary irrigant agitation techniques and devices*. J Endod. 2009;35:791-804.
7. Rossi-Fedele G, Prichard JW, Steier L, de Figueiredo JA. *The effect of surface tension reduction on the clinical performance of sodium hypochlorite in endodontics*. Int Endod J. 2013;46(6):492-8.
8. Cameron JA. *The effect of a fluorocarbon surfactant on the surface tension of the endodontic irrigant, sodium hypochlorite*. Aust Dent J 1986;31:364-8.
9. Siqueira JF, Jr., Rocas IN. *Clinical Implications and Microbiology of Bacterial Persistence after Treatment Procedures*. J Endod. 2008;34:1291–301.
10. Ng Y, Mann V, Rahbaran S, Lewsey J, Gulabivala K. *Outcome of primary root canal treatment: systematic review of the literature - Part 1. Effects of study characteristics on probability of success*. Int Endod J. 2007;40(12):921-39.
11. Torabinejad M, Anderson P, Bader J, Brown LJ, Chen LH, Goodacre CJ, et al. *Outcomes of root canal treatment and restoration, implant-supported single crowns, fixed partial dentures, and extraction without replacement: a systematic review*. J Prosthet Dent. 2007;98(4):285-311.
12. Ng YL, Mann V, Rahbaran S, Lewsey J, Gulabivala K. *Outcome of primary root canal treatment: systematic review of the literature - Part 2. Influence of clinical factors*. Int Endod J. 2008;41(1):6-31.
13. Rocas IN, Siqueira JF, Jr. *Identification of bacteria enduring endodontic treatment procedures by a combined reverse transcriptase-polymerase chain reaction and reverse-capture checkerboard approach*. J Endod. 2010;36(1):45-52.
14. Al-Ali M, Sathorn C, Parashos P. *Root canal debridement efficacy of different final irrigation protocols*. Int Endod J. 2012;45(10):898-906.
15. Zehnder M. *Root canal irrigants*. J Endod. 2006;32:389-98.
16. Basrani B, Haapasalo M. *Update on endodontic irrigating solutions*. Endo Topics. 2012;27:74-102.
17. Palazzi F, Morra M, Mohammadi Z, Grandini S, Giardino L. *Comparison of the surface tension of 5.25% sodium hypochlorite solution with three new sodium hypochlorite-based endodontic irrigants*. Int Endod J. 2012;45(2):129-35.
18. Moorer WR, Wesselink PR. *Factors promoting the tissue dissolving capability of sodium hypochlorite*. Int Endod J. 1982;15:187-96.
19. Gomes B, Ferraz C, Vianna M, Berber V, Teixeira F, Souza-Filho F. *In vitro antimicrobial activity of several concentrations of sodium hypochlorite and chlorhexidine gluconate in the elimination of Enterococcus faecalis*. Int Endod J. 2001;34:424-8.
20. Siqueira JFJ, Rôças IN, Favieri A, Lima KC. *Chemomechanical reduction of the bacterial population in the root canal after instrumentation and irrigation with 1%, 2.5%, and 5.25% sodium hypochlorite*. J Endod. 2000;26:331-4.
21. Mehra P, Clancy C, Wu J. *Formation of a facial hematoma during endodontic therapy*. J Am Dent Assoc. 2000;131:67-71.
22. Gernhardt CR, Eppendorf K, Kozlowski A, Brandt M. *Toxicity of concentrated sodium hypochlorite used as an endodontic irrigant*. Int Endod J. 2004;37:272-80.
23. Barnhart BD, Chuang A, Lucca JJ, Roberts S, Liewehr F, Joyce AP. *An in vitro evaluation of the cytotoxicity of various endodontic irrigants on human gingival fibroblasts*. J Endod. 2005;31:613-5.
24. Ari H, Erdemir A, Belli S. *Evaluation of the effect of endodontic irrigation solutions on the microhardness and the roughness of root canal dentin*. J Endod.30:792-5.
25. Stoward PJ. *A histochemical study of the apparent deamination of proteins by sodium hypochlorite*. Histochemistry. 1975;45:213-26.
26. Oyarzun A, Cordero AM, Whittle M. *Immunohistochemical evaluation of the effects of sodium hypochlorite on dentin collagen and glycosaminoglycans*. J Endod. 2002;28:152-6.
27. Grossman L, Meiman B. *Solution of pulp tissue by chemical agent*. J Amer Dent Ass. 1941;28:223-32.
28. Christensen CE, McNeal SF, Eleazer P. *Effect of lowering the pH of sodium hypochlorite on dissolving tissue in vitro*. J Endod. 2008;34:449-52.

29. Abou-Rass M, Oglesby SW. *The effects of temperature, concentration, and tissue type on the solvent ability of sodium hypochlorite*. J Endod. 1981;7:376-7.
30. Sirtes G, Waltimo T, Schaetzle M, Zehnder M. *The effects of temperature on sodium hypochlorite short-term stability, pulp dissolution capacity, and antimicrobial efficacy*. J Endod. 2005;31:669-71.
31. Rossi-Fedele G, De Figueiredo JA. *Use of a bottle warmer to increase 4% sodium hypochlorite tissue dissolution ability on bovine pulp*. J Endod. 2008;34:39-42.
32. Fabiani C, Mazzoni A, Nato F, Tay FR, Breschi L, Grandini S, et al. *Final rinse optimization: influence of different agitation protocols*. J Endod. 2010;36:282-5.
33. Clarkson RM, Podlich HM, Moule AJ. *Influence of ethylenediaminetetraacetic acid on the active chlorine content of sodium hypochlorite solutions when mixed in various proportions*. J Endod. 2011;37(4):538-43.
34. Giardino L, Ambu E, Becce C, Rimondini L, Morra M. *Surface tension of four common root canal irrigants and two new irrigants containing antibiotics*. J Endod. 2006;32:1091-3.
35. Clarkson RM, Kidd B, Evans GE, Moule AJ. *The effect of surfactant on the dissolution of porcine pulpal tissue by sodium hypochlorite solutions*. J Endod. 2012;38(9):1257-60.
36. Baron A, Lindsey K, Sidow SJ, Dickinson D, Chuang A, McPherson JC, 3rd. *Effect of a Benzalkonium Chloride Surfactant-Sodium Hypochlorite Combination on Elimination of Enterococcus faecalis*. J Endod. 2016;42(1):145-9.
37. Violich DR, Chandler NP. *The smear layer in endodontics - a review*. Int Endod J. 2010;43(1):2-15.
38. Arias-Moliz MT, Morago A, Ordinola-Zapata R, Ferrer-Luque CM, Ruiz-Linares M, Baca P. *Effects of Dentin Debris on the Antimicrobial Properties of Sodium Hypochlorite and Etidronic Acid.* J Endod, 2016. 42(5):771-5.
39. Hülsmann M, Rödig T, Nordmeyer S. *Complications during root canal irrigation.* Endo Topics. 2007;16:27-63.
40. Fraser J. *Chelating agents: their softening effect on root canal dentin*. Oral Surg Oral Med Oral Pathol. 1974;37:803-11.
41. Lui J-N, Kuah H-G, Chen N-N. *Effects of EDTA with and without surfactants or ultrasonics on removal of smear layer*. J Endod. 2007;33:472-5.
42. Biesterfeld RC, Taintor JF. *A comparison of periapical seals of root canals with RC-Prep or Salvizol*. Oral Surg Oral Med Oral Pathol. 1980;49:532-7.
43. Jagzap JB, Patil SS, Gade VJ, Chandhok DJ, Upagade MA, Thakur DA. *Effectiveness of three different irrigants - 17% ethylenediaminetetraacetic acid, Q-MIX and phytic acid in smear layer removal: A comparative scanning electron microscope study*. Contemp Clin Dent. 2017;8(3):459-63.
44. Nassar M, Hiraishi N, Tamura Y, Otsuki M, Aoki K, Tagami J. *Phytic acid: an alternative root canal chelating agent*. J Endod. 2015;41(2):242-7.
45. Prado M, de Assis DF, Gomes BP, Simao RA. *Effect of disinfectant solutions on the surface free energy and wettability of filling material.* J Endod. 2011;37(7):980-2.
46. Di Lenarda R, Cadenaro M, Sbaizero O. *Effectiveness of 1 mol L-1 citric acid and 15% EDTA irrigation on smear layer removal*. Int Endod J. 2000;33(1):46-52.
47. Machado R, Garcia LDFR, da Silva Neto UX, Cruz Filho AMD, Silva RG, Vansan LP. *Evaluation of 17% EDTA and 10% citric acid in smear layer removal and tubular dentin sealer penetration. Microscopy research and technique*. 2018;81(3):275-82.
48. Eun H, Lee A, Lee Y. *Sodium hypochlorite dermatitis*. Contact Dermatitis. 1984;11:45-7.
49. Zou L, Shen Y, Li W, Haapasalo M. *Penetration of sodium hypochlorite into dentin*. J Endod. 2010;36(5):793-6.
50. Habets JM, Geursen-Reitsma AM, Stolz E, Van Joost T. *Sensitization to sodium hypochlorite causing hand dermatitis*. Contact Dermatitis. 1986;15:140-57.
51. Hasselgren G, Olsson B, Cvek M. *Effects of calcium hydroxide and sodium hypochlorite on the dissolution of necrotic porcine muscle tissue.* J Endod. 1988;14:125-8.
52. Andersen M, Lund A, Andreasen J, Andreasen F. *In vitro solubility of human pulp tissue in calcium hydroxide and sodium hypochlorite*. Endodontics & dental traumatology. 1992;8:104-8.
53. Torabinejad M, Shabahang S, Aprecio RM, Kettering JD. *The antimicrobial effect of MTAD: an in vitro investigation*. J Endod. 2003;29:400-3.
54. Baumgartner JC, Johal S, Marshall JG. *Comparison of the antimicrobial efficacy of 1.3% NaOCl/Biopure MTAD to 5.25% NaOCl/15% EDTA for root canal irrigation*. J Endod. 2007;33:48-51.
55. Keskin C, Sariyilmaz E, Sariyilmaz O. *Effect of solvents on apically extruded debris and irrigant during root canal retreatment using reciprocating instruments*. Int Endod J. 2017;50(11):1084-8.
56. Rossi-Fedele G, Ahmed HM. *Assessment of Root Canal Filling Removal Effectiveness Using Microcomputed Tomography: A Systematic Review*. J Endod. 2017;43(4):520-6.
57. Ferreira JJ, Rhodes JS, Ford TR. *The efficacy of guttapercha removal using ProFiles*. Int Endod J. 2001;34:267-74.
58. Hülsmann M, Bluhm V. *Efficacy, cleaning ability and safety of different rotary NiTi instruments in root canal retreatment*. Int Endod J. 2004;37:468-76.
59. Horvath SD, Altenburger M, Naumann M, Wolkevitz M, Schirrmeister JF. *Cleanliness of dentinal tubules following gutta-percha removal with and without solvents: a scanning electron microscopic study*. Int Endod J. 2009;42:1032-8.
60. Ram Z. *Effectiveness of root canal irrigation*. Oral Surg Oral Med Oral Pathol. 1977;44:306–12.

61. Lambrianidis TP. *Risk Management in Root Canal Treatment*, 1st edn. Thessaloniki, Greece: University Studio Press; 2001.
62. Ingle JI, Himel VT, Hawrish CEea. *Endodontic cavity preparation*. Endodontics. Ontario, Canada: BC Decker; 2002. p. 502.
63. Boutsioukis C, Lambrianidis T, Verhaagen B, Versluis M, Kastrinakis E, Wesselink PR, et al. *The effect of needle-insertion depth on the irrigant flow in the root canal: evaluation using an unsteady computational fluid dynamics model.* J Endod. 2010;36(10):1664-8.
64. Gopikrishna V, Sibi S, Archana D, Pradeep Kumar AR, Narayanan L. *An in vivo assessment of the influence of needle gauges on irrigation flow rate.* J Conserv Dent JCD. 2016;19(2):189-93.
65. Boutsioukis C, Psimma Z, Kastrinakis E. *The effect of flow rate and agitation technique on irrigant extrusion ex vivo.* Int Endod J. 2014;47(5):487-96.
66. Burleson A, Nusstein J, Reader A, Beck M. *The in vivo evaluation of hand/rotary/ultrasound instrumentation in necrotic, human mandibular molars.* J Endod. 2007;33(7):782-7.
67. Yilmaz F, Koc C, Kamburoglu K, Ocak M, Geneci F, Uzuner MB, et al. Evaluation of 3 Different Retreatment Techniques in Maxillary Molar Teeth by Using Micro-computed Tomography. J Endod. 2018;44(3):480-4.
68. Alves FR, Ribeiro TO, Moreno JO, Lopes HP. *Comparison of the efficacy of nickel-titanium rotary systems with or without the retreatment instruments in the removal of gutta-percha in the apical third.* BMC Oral Health. 2014;14:102.
69. Capar ID, Ozcan E, Arslan H, Ertas H, Aydinbelge HA. *Effect of different final irrigation methods on the removal of calcium hydroxide from an artificial standardized groove in the apical third of root canals.* J Endod. 2014;40(3):451-4.
70. Alves FR, Marceliano-Alves MF, Sousa JC, Silveira SB, Provenzano JC, Siqueira JF, Jr. *Removal of Root Canal Fillings in Curved Canals Using Either Reciprocating Single- or Rotary Multi-instrument Systems and a Supplementary Step with the XP-Endo Finisher.* J Endod. 2016;42(7):1114-9.
71. Akcay M, Arslan H, Mese M, Durmus N, Capar ID. *Effect of photon-initiated photoacoustic streaming, passive ultrasonic, and sonic irrigation techniques on dentinal tubule penetration of irrigation solution: a confocal microscopic study.* Clin Oral Investig. 2017;21(7):2205-12.
72. Barreto MS, Rosa RA, Santini MF, Cavenago BC, Duarte MA, Bier CA, et al. *Efficacy of ultrasonic activation of NaOCl and orange oil in removing filling material from mesial canals of mandibular molars with and without isthmus. Journal of applied oral science: revista FOB*. 2016;24(1):37-44.
73. Cunningham W, Joseph SW. *Effect of temperature on the bactericidal action of sodium hypochlorite endodontic irrigant.* Oral Surg Oral Med Oral Pathol. 1980;50:569-71.
74. Conde AJ, Estevez R, Lorono G, Valencia de Pablo O, Rossi-Fedele G, Cisneros R. *Effect of sonic and ultrasonic activation on organic tissue dissolution from simulated grooves in root canals using sodium hypochlorite and EDTA*. Int Endod J. 2017;50(10):976-82.
75. Bernardes RA, Duarte MA, Vivan RR, Alcalde MP, Vasconcelos BC, Bramante CM. *Comparison of three retreatment techniques with ultrasonic activation in flattened canals using micro-computed tomography and scanning electron microscopy*. Int Endod J. 2015.
76. Jiang S, Zou T, Li D, Chang JW, Huang X, Zhang C. *Effectiveness of Sonic, Ultrasonic, and Photon-Induced Photoacoustic Streaming Activation of NaOCl on Filling Material Removal Following Retreatment in Oval Canal Anatomy. Photomedicine and laser surgery*. 2016;34(1):3-10.
77. Stojicic S, Zivkovic S, Qian W, Zhang H, Haapasalo M. *Tissue dissolution by sodium hypochlorite: effect of concentration, temperature, agitation, and surfactant*. J Endod. 2010;36(9):1558-62.
78. Boutsioukis C, Verhaagen B, Walmsley AD, Versluis M, van der Sluis LW. *Measurement and visualization of file-to-wall contact during ultrasonically activated irrigation in simulated canals*. Int Endod J. 2013;46(11):1046-55.
79. de Hemptinne F, Slaus G, Vandendael M, Jacquet W, De Moor RJ, Bottenberg P. *In Vivo Intracanal Temperature Evolution during Endodontic Treatment after the Injection of Room Temperature or Preheated Sodium Hypochlorite*. J Endod. 2015;41(7):1112-5.
80. Neelakantan P, Herrera DR, Pecorari VGA, Gomes B. *Endotoxin levels after chemomechanical preparation of root canals with sodium hypochlorite or chlorhexidine: a systematic review of clinical trials and meta-analysis.* Int Endod J. 2019;52(1):19-27.
81. Grawehr M, Sener B, Waltimo T, Zehnder M. *Interactions of ethylenediamine tetraacetic acid with sodium hypochlorite in aqueous solutions*. Int Endod J. 2003;36:411-7.
82. Paragliola R, Franco V, Fabiani C, Mazzoni A, Nato F, Tay FR, et al. *Final rinse optimization: influence of different agitation protocols*. J Endod. 2010;36(2):282-5.
83. Boutsioukis C, Gogos C, Verhaagen B, Versluis M, Kastrinakis E, Van der Sluis LW. *The effect of apical preparation size on irrigant flow in root canals evaluated using an unsteady Computational Fluid Dynamics model.* Int Endod J. 2010;43(10):874-81.
84. Boutsioukis C, Verhaagen B, Versluis M, Kastrinakis E, Wesselink PR, van der Sluis LW. *Evaluation of irrigant flow in the root canal using different needle types by an unsteady computational fluid dynamics model*. J Endod. 2010;36(5):875-9.
85. Boutsioukis C, Gogos C, Verhaagen B, Versluis M, Kastrinakis E, Van der Sluis LW. *The effect of root canal taper on the irrigant flow: evaluation using an unsteady Computational Fluid Dynamics model*. Int Endod J. 2010;43(10):909-16.

86. Arvaniti IS, Khabbaz MG. *Influence of root canal taper on its cleanliness: a scanning electron microscopic study*. J Endod. 2011;37(6):871-4.
87. Akcay M, Arslan H, Topcuoglu HS, Tuncay O. *Effect of calcium hydroxide and double and triple antibiotic pastes on the bond strength of epoxy resin-based sealer to root canal dentin*. J Endod. 2014;40(10):1663-7.
88. Martinho FC, Gomes CC, Nascimento GN, Gomes APM, Leite FRM. *Clinical comparison of the effectiveness of 7- and 14-day intracanal medications in root canal disinfection and inflammatory cytokines. Clin Oral Investig*. 2018;22(1):523-30.
89. Spångberg LSW, Haapasalo M. *Rationale and efficacy of root canal medicaments and root filling materials with emphasis on treatment outcome*. Endo Topics. 2002;2:35-58.
90. Parhizkar A, Nojehdehian H, Asgary S. *Triple antibiotic paste: momentous roles and applications in endodontics: a review*. Restor Dent Endod. 2018;43(3):e28.
91. Capar ID, Ozcan E, Arslan H, Ertas H, Aydinbelge HA. *Effect of Different Final Irrigation Methods on the Removal of Calcium Hydroxide from an Artificial Standardized Groove in the Apical Third of Root Canals*. J Endod. 2014;40:451-4.
92. Paikkatt JV, Aslam S, Sreedharan S, Philomina B, Kannan VP, Madhu S. *Efficacy of various intracanal medicaments against aerobic and facultative anaerobic microorganism*. J Indian Soc Pedod Prev Dent. 2018;36(3):268-72.
93. Farhad A, Mohammadi Z. *Calcium hydroxide: a review*. International Dental Journal. 2005;55(5):293-301.
94. Zehnder MP, Paquè F. *Disinfection of the root canal system during root canal re-treatment*. Endodontic Topics. 2008;19(1):58–73.
95. Sjogren U, Figdor D, Spangberg L, Sundqvist G. *The antimicrobial effect of calcium hydroxide as a short-term intracanal dressing*. International Endodontic Journal. 1991;24(3):119-125.
96. Sathorn C, Parashos P, Messer H. Antibacterial efficacy of calcium hydroxide intracanal dressing: a systematic review and meta-analysis. International Endodontic Journal. 2007;40(1):2-10.
97. Sathorn C, Parashos P, Messer HH. *Effectiveness of single- versus multiple-visit endodontic treatment of teeth with apical periodontitis: a systematic review and meta-analysis. International Endodontic Journal*. 2005;38(6):347-355.
98. Orstavik D. *Root canal disinfection: a review of concepts and recent developments*. Australian Endodontic Journal. 2003;29(2):70-74.
99. Haapasalo MS, Shen Y. *Current therapeutic options for endodontic biofilms*. Endodontic Topics. 2010;22(1):79–98.
100. Kishen A. *Advanced therapeutic options for endodontic biofilms*. Endodontic Topics 2010;22(1):99–123.
101. Vera J, Siqueira JF, Jr., Ricucci D, Loghin S, Fernandez N, Flores B, et al. *One- versus two-visit endodontic treatment of teeth with apical periodontitis: a histobacteriologic study*. Journal of Endodontics. 2012;38(8): 1040-1052.
102. Kawashima N, Wadachi R, Suda H, Yeng T, Parashos P. *Root canal medicaments. International Dental Journal*. 2009;59(1):5-11.
103. Huffaker SK, Safavi K, Spangberg LS, Kaufman B. *Influence of a passive sonic irrigation system on the elimination of bacteria from root canal systems: a clinical study*. Journal of Endodontics. 2010;36(8):1315-1318.
104. Kvist T, Molander A, Dahlen G, Reit C. *Microbiological evaluation of one- and two-visit endodontic treatment of teeth with apical periodontitis: a randomized, clinical trial*. Journal of Endodontics. 2004;30(8):572-576.
105. Figini L, Lodi G, Gorni F, Gagliani M. *Single versus multiple visits for endodontic treatment of permanent teeth. The Cochrane database of systematic reviews*. 2007(4):CD005296.
106. Figini L, Lodi G, Gorni F, Gagliani M. *Single versus multiple visits for endodontic treatment of permanent teeth: a Cochrane systematic review. Journal of Endodontics*. 2008;34(9):1041-1047.
107. Manfredi M, Figini L, Gagliani M, Lodi G. *Single versus multiple visits for endodontic treatment of permanent teeth. The Cochrane database of systematic reviews*. 2016;12:CD005296.
108. Paredes-Vieyra J, Enriquez FJ. *Success rate of single- versus two-visit root canal treatment of teeth with apical periodontitis: a randomized controlled trial*. Journal of Endodontics. 2012;38(9):1164-1169.
109. Mohammadi Z, Abbott PV. *Antimicrobial substantivity of root canal irrigants and medicaments: a review. Australian Endodontic Journal*. 2009;35(3):131-139.
110. Mohammadi Z, Dummer PM. *Properties and applications of calcium hydroxide in endodontics and dental traumatology. International Endodontic Journal*. 2011;44(8):697-730.
111. Rocas IN, Siqueira JF, Jr. *Identification of bacteria enduring endodontic treatment procedures by a combined reverse transcriptase-polymerase chain reaction and reverse-capture checkerboard approach*. Journal of Endodontics. 2010;36(1):45-52.
112. Rocas IN, Siqueira JF, Jr. *In vivo antimicrobial effects of endodontic treatment procedures as assessed by molecular microbiologic techniques*. Journal of Endodontics. 2011;37(3):304-310.
113. Schirrmeister JF, Liebenow AL, Braun G, Wittmer A, Hellwig E, Al-Ahmad A. *Detection and eradication of microorganisms in root-filled teeth associated with periradicular lesions: an in vivo study*. Journal of Endodontics. 2007;33(5):536-540.

- Underline the importance of the **sealing phase** in the retreatment procedure.
- Examine the techniques available to identify the most effective way to **seal** the root canals after shaping and decontamination.
- Present alternative techniques that can guarantee an **airtight filling** of the endodontic compartment.

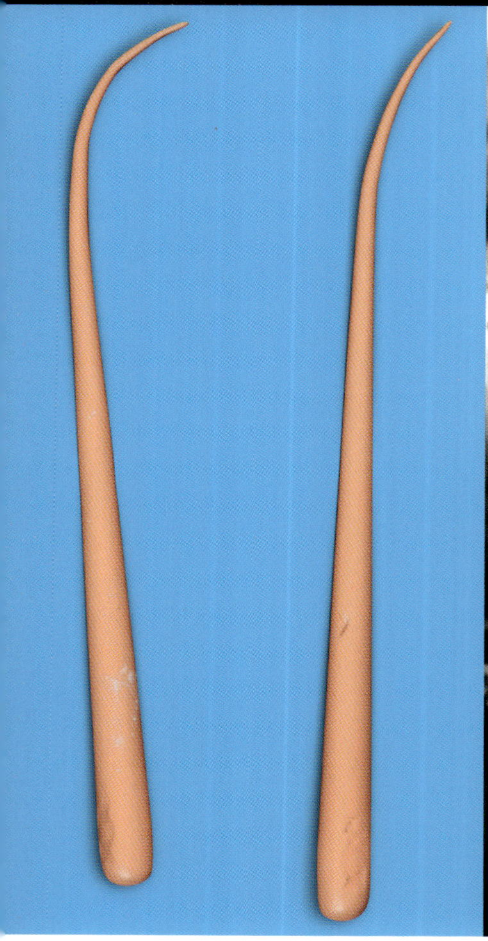

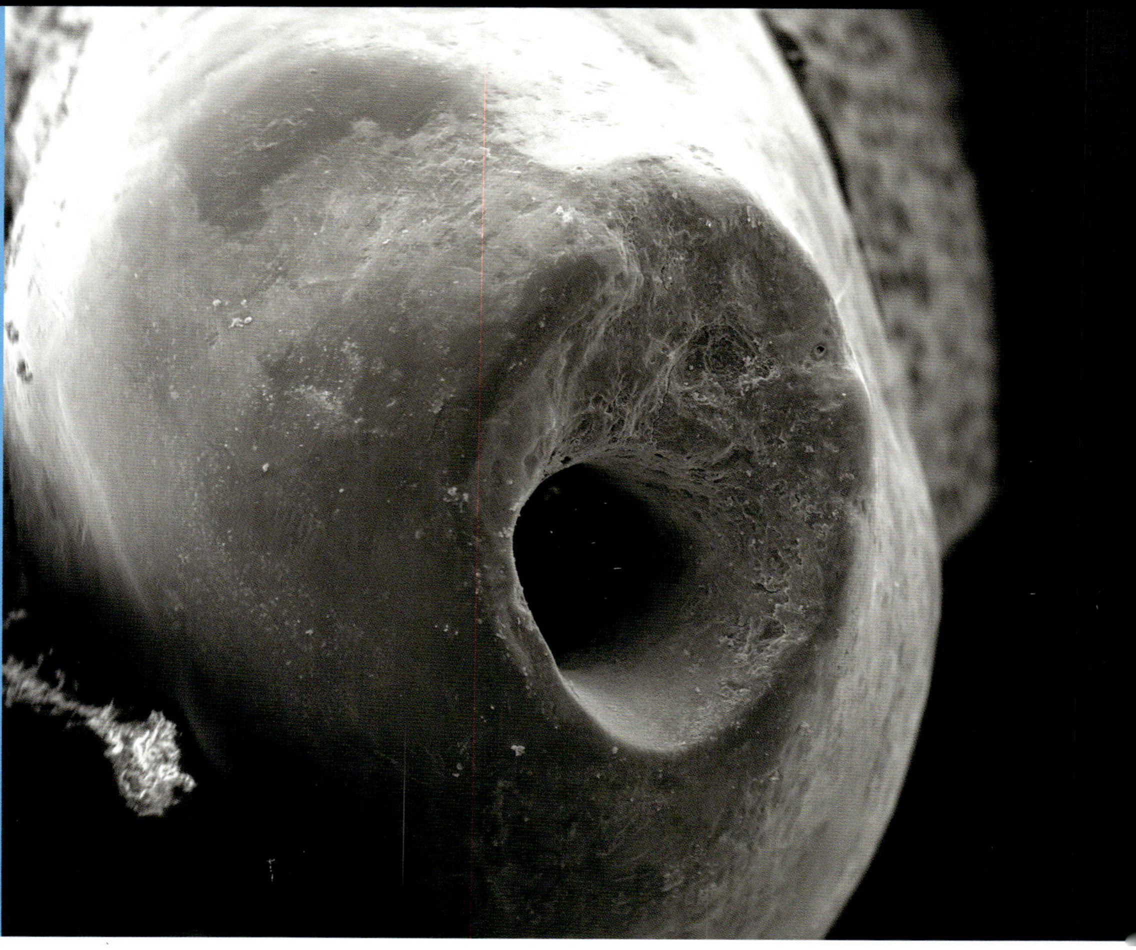

Calogero Bugea, Arnaldo Castellucci

05

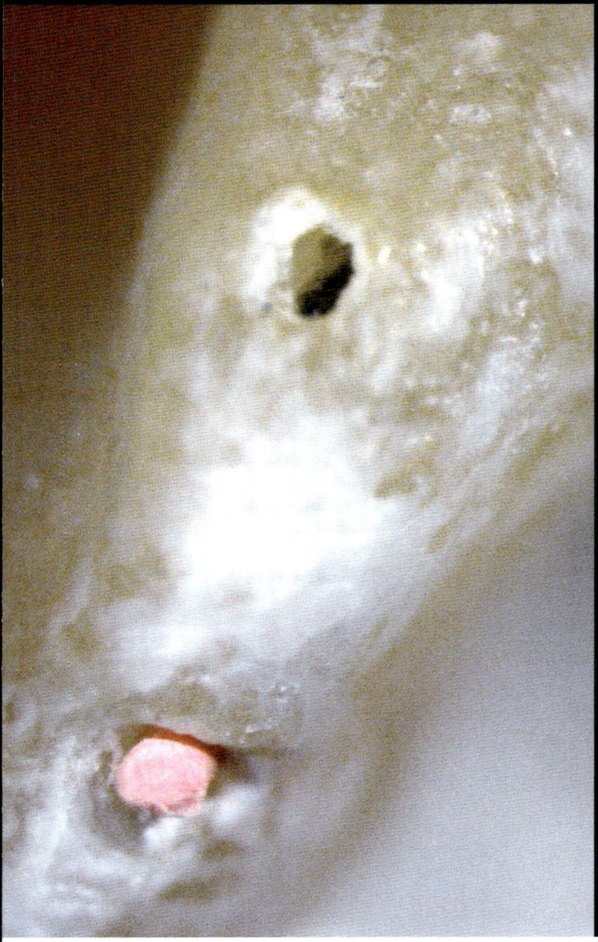

Filling methods in retreatment

Traditional and alternative techniques for sealing the endodontic space

Root canal filling and root canal morphology

The phase of root canal filling is crucial for the success of endodontic treatment; it becomes neuralgic in retreatment because of the septic and anatomical implications of these cases[1].

Shaping determines good filling; however, in retreatment cases, shaping may not have been carried out in accordance with the normal criteria because the canal morphology obtained will not always be an ideal one.

As described in many other parts of this text (Chapters 2 and 3), the previous treatments[2] and alterations of apical morphologies[3-5], which are consequent to inflammatory processes in such areas[6, 7], often present the clinician with particular solutions that differ from normal practice during the filling phase when dealing with teeth that have never been treated[8-10]. Therefore, the preoperative state of a tooth and the morphological evaluations on the obtained shape will help the clinician to choose the most suitable method for root canal filling[11, 12]. Consequently, a dentist must have the necessary knowledge to adopt two or more techniques for filling an endodontic space because outlining a universally valid technique is impossible. A series of clinical situations should be indicated in relation to the following distinctive elements to make more comprehensible choices:

- the apical diameter obtained at the end of the cleaning and shaping process;
- the taper determined at the end of this process (Box 5.1).

We try to outline the clinical opportunities through anarbitrary classification that is considered useful for clinical purposes (Table 5.1).

Although we should also consider the taper, which we will discuss later, the size of the apical diameter affects the selection of appropriate root canal filling methods because the control at the end of the filling is crucial to the success of the treatment. Gesi et al.[13] and other researchers[14]

Box 5.1 TAPER

The shape given to the root canal during treatments and retreatment can be defined as a truncated cone shape in which the bases of the truncated cone can be figuratively placed at the entrance of the root canal and at its apical limit. The progressive decrease in apical diameters from the coronal mouth to the apical end can be very small or very high. Therefore, low truncated conicity (lower values at 4 ISO), average taper (ISO values between 4 and 8), and high ISO values above 8, are discussed. ISO values are determined by the difference between the apical diameter (lower base of the cone) and the diameter 1 mm higher in the coronal direction.

For example, if the size of the apex is ISO 30, and the channel has ISO 35 size 1 mm from the apex and an ISO 40 dimension in the upper millimeter, the taper is equal to 5. The lower the taper, the straighter the canal walls will be. As the value increases, the lower the taper is, the straighter the canal walls will be. As the taper value increases, the walls increasingly converge toward the apical limit, starting from larger coronal diameters.

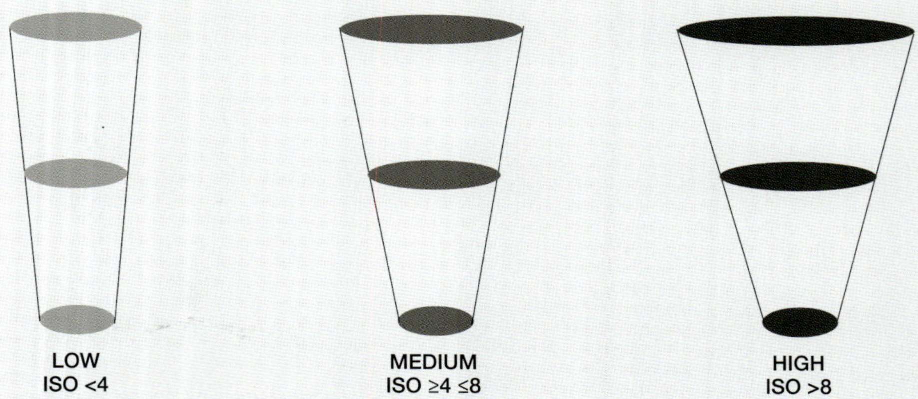

Table 5.1 **CANAL FILLING TECHNIQUE ACCORDING TO CANAL MORPHOLOGY**

Canal anatomy	Apex diameter (ISO)	Type	Recommended filling technique(*)
Preserved	More than 50	Straight[(a)]	Apical Plug in MTA
		Curvilinear[(b)]	Warm Gutta-Percha / Single Cone with Bioactive Sealer(*)
	Not exceeding 50	Straight	Warm Gutta-Percha / Single Cone with Bioactive Sealer(*)
		Curvilinear	Warm Gutta-Percha / Warm Gutta-Percha with Carrier
Altered	More than 50	Straight	Apical Plug in MTA
		Curvilinear	Apical Plug in MTA
	Not exceeding 50	Straight	Warm Gutta-Percha / Single Cone with Bioactive Sealer(*)
		Curvilinear	Warm Gutta-Percha / Single Cone with Bioactive Sealer(*)

(*) The use of bioactive sealer(*) is recommended as a future possibility because the studies available are still limited; however, promising results allow us to justify the use of these sealers, especially in retreatment.

(a) A straight canal is a root canal characterized by a parallel course between the longitudinal axis of the canal and the walls; it has a taper of less than 5 ISO.

(b) Curvilinear refers to a root canal that has a root canal entry axis that does not coincide with the axis that can be traced from the apex toward the most coronal limit. It is characterized by a taper greater than 5 ISO.

demonstrated that the apical size that deviates from the shaping procedures in retreatment is greater than that found in similar elements that have never been treated; in these teeth, apical diameters are often large because a greater shaping action is necessary to ensure bacterial decontamination[14]. At this stage, some indications regarding the taper should be given. NiTi alloy instruments can provide a predetermined taper to the root canal that is responsible for the final shaping. However,

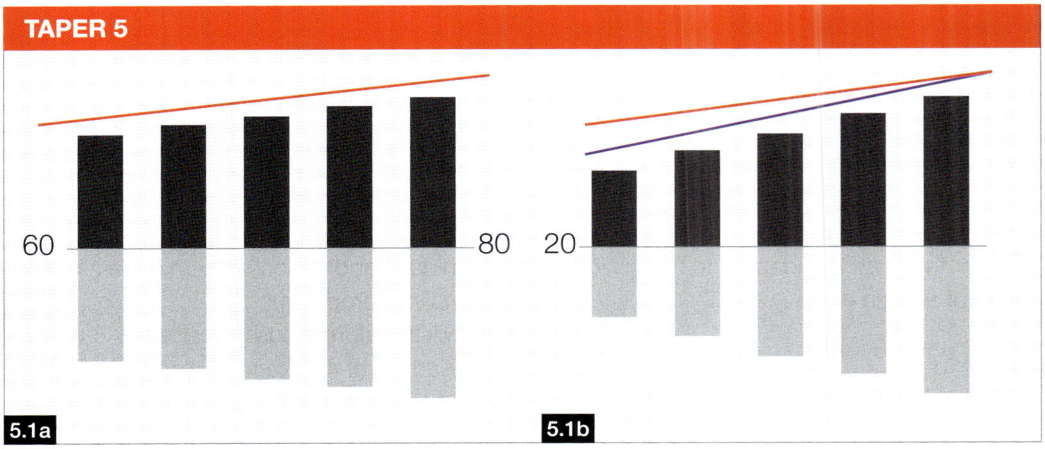

Fig. 5.1a-b:
a) A taper of ISO 5 with a starting diameter of ISO 60;

b) the taper of ISO 5 with a starting diameter of ISO 20.

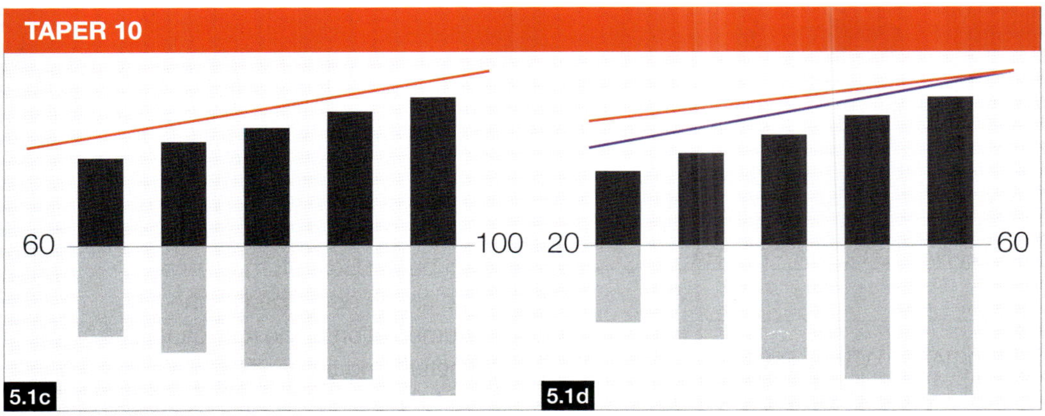

Fig. 5.1c-d:
c) A taper of ISO 10 with a starting diameter of ISO 60.

d) the taper of ISO 10 with a starting diameter of ISO 20.

apical diameters often exceed ISO 50, so techniques involving NiTi instruments do not always have elements with such a diameter at the tip. Therefore, the apical parts of the endodontic space when using steel instruments with diameters greater than ISO 60 should be carefully shaped. Not infrequently, conferring a taper greater than ISO 5 (Fig. 5.1a) and lower than ISO 10, to avoid weakening the root canal, will result in a cylindrical and non-truncated canal shape (Fig. 5.1b). Hence, materials and methods that are dependent on the condensation of sealer and gutta-percha should be developed to guarantee a safe apical seal. Therefore, the most cylindrical preparation is that with the largest apical diameter (compare red and purple lines in the figures on page 287). As such, it is much less suitable for condensation manuevers in an apical direction to compact sealer and gutta-percha. In short, canal morphologies resulting from shaping processes carried out in retreatments are often inconsistent with those found in teeth that have never been treated. Pathological transformations and iatrogenic damage further contribute to the complexity and difficulty in standardizing this morphology. It is therefore necessary, as shown in Table 5.1, to be familiar with a set of techniques for canal filling and their corresponding advantages and disadvantages should be examined to verify whether they can be adapted to the clinical needs of a given case.

Canal filling techniques

The canal filling techniques associated with retreatment are shown in Table 5.2.

Table 5.2. **SUITABLE ROOT CANAL FILLING TECHNIQUES IN RETREATMENT**
• LATERAL OR VERTICAL CONDENSATION OF THE GUTTA-PERCHA WITH SEALER
• FILLING WITH PREHEATED CARRIER-BASED GUTTA-PERCHA
• APICAL PLUG WITH MTA
• USE OF BIOACTIVE SEALERS ASSOCIATED WITH A SINGLE CALIBRATED GUTTA-PERCHA CONE

Box 5.2 **CLASSICAL FILLING MATERIALS**

The materials used in the root canal filling process do not differ from those available for untreated cases and are represented by gutta-percha and endodontic sealer.
Below is a brief description.

Gutta-percha

Gutta-percha is universally chosen as the material for the filling of the root canal system. That for dental use is not "pure," rather it is obtained by mixing isoprene (18.9%–21.8%) with zinc oxide (59.1%–78.3%), heavy metal sulfates (2.5%–17.3%), waxes and resins (1%–4.1%), dyes and antioxidants (3%), and fatty acids (traces). Each brand of gutta-percha differs from the others because cones with different levels of radiopacity, softness, and color can be obtained by changing the percentages of the materials listed above.
In general, the more consistent the gutta-percha cone is, the higher the zinc oxide content will be; the softer the cone is, the higher the concentration of isoprene will be. It is available in cones with different morphologies. The most frequently used cones are those with known taper and diameters at the tip classifiable in accordance with ISO

Lateral or vertical condensation of the gutta-percha with sealer

In this situation, making a digression to compare the two best known canal filling techniques and describe them in detail seems inappropriate.
We will therefore focus on certain peculiarities of the warm vertical condensation of gutta-percha, but will disregard the aspects related to the lateral condensation technique, even though they are still valid and widely used[2, 15, 16].
The original statement does not express a complete thought. Provide additional information to construct a sentence with a complete thought or rewrite to improve expression/structure[17, 18].
The cone, whose characteristics[19] are described in Box 5.1, must adapt to the shape developed by the instrumentation of the root canal; the diameters and the taper of the instruments used for shaping should be determined

standards, which correspond to the instruments used in the shaping process; however, there are equally valid "nonstandard" cones that differ in taper only and can be properly calibrated with appropriate instruments.

Endodontic sealer

Endodontic sealer is an essential element for successful filling because it improves the otherwise labile seal produced by gutta-percha. Many sealers have given a proven effectiveness, and the most commonly used sealers are based on zinc oxide and eugenol. Those containing epoxy resins are also popular, but the advantages compared with those mentioned previously do not appear particularly relevant. The sealer, which is marketed in a powder-liquid form, is mixed and inserted into root canals either with paper cones or the same gutta-percha cones used for filling.
In retreatment, clinical situations in which the apical control of the filling must be doubly scrupulous, the mixing and placement of the sealer in the root canal must be performed with great care.
Bioactive sealers, which will be discussed later in this chapter, have an interesting role to play.

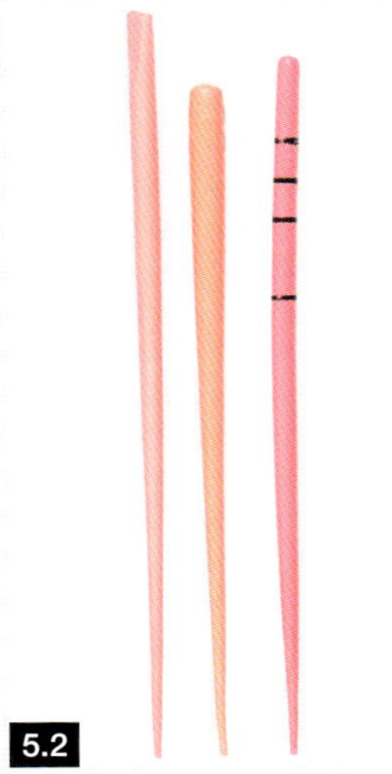

5.2

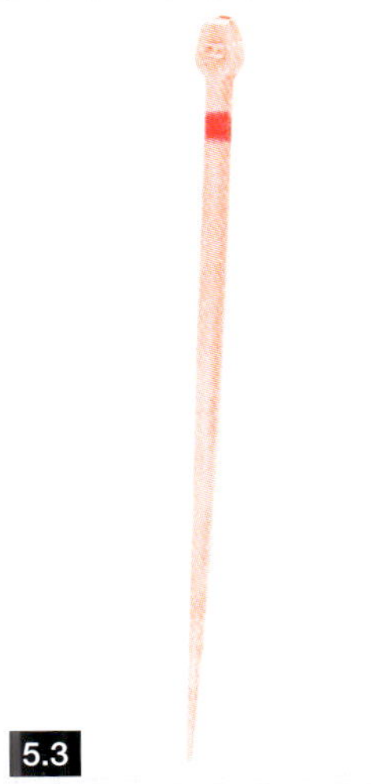

5.3

Fig. 5.2: Three examples of nonstandardized cones. Note the different tapers and the small tip diameters.

Fig. 5.3: Example of a cone with a known tip diameter (25 ISO) and predefined taper that is ideal for vertical condensation fillings in canals shaped with the corresponding NiTi instruments.

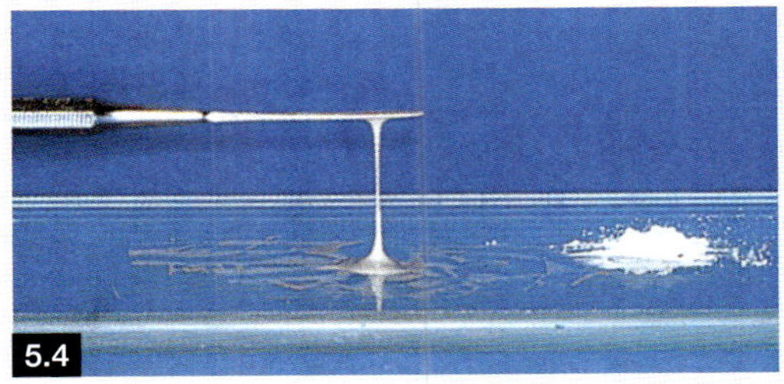

5.4

Fig. 5.4: Method for mixing the zinc oxide eugenol sealer that is ideal for insertion into in a shaped canal.

to easily select the cone with the correct size[20]. A preliminary step is the final verification of the working length used, which can be further tested by using a paper cone, in a roughly dried root canal.
Subsequently, the gutta-percha cone is tested in a canal that has been rehydrated with hypochlorite. The main points of a correct test of the cone are as follows:

- the decontamination of cones before the test process and before the filling phase
- the choice of the apical diameter corresponding to that of the canal to be filled
- intracanal adaptation
- length check
- apical resistance or "tug back"

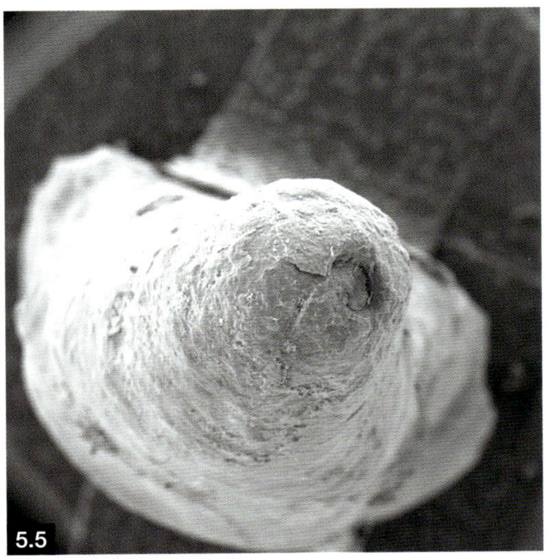

5.5

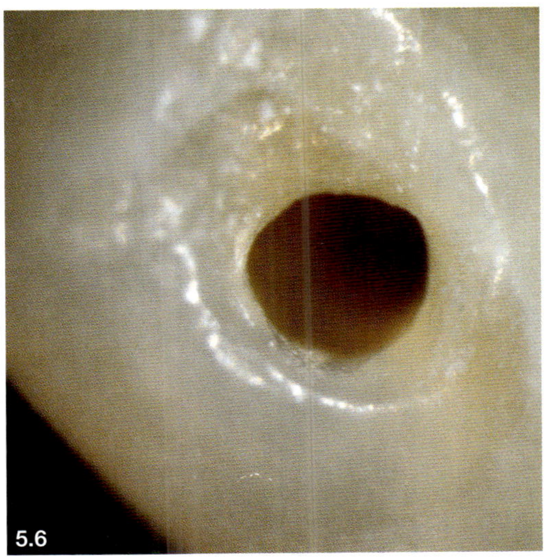

5.6

Fig. 5.5: Electron microscopic image of a mesial root of an extensively calcified upper molar, which does not show any foramen.

Fig. 5.6: The main apical foramen is well represented despite showing signs of resorption; both cases verify the clinical difficulties in reaching a certain dimensional concordance between the cone and the apical limit.

Verification of the working length and the apical limit of filling

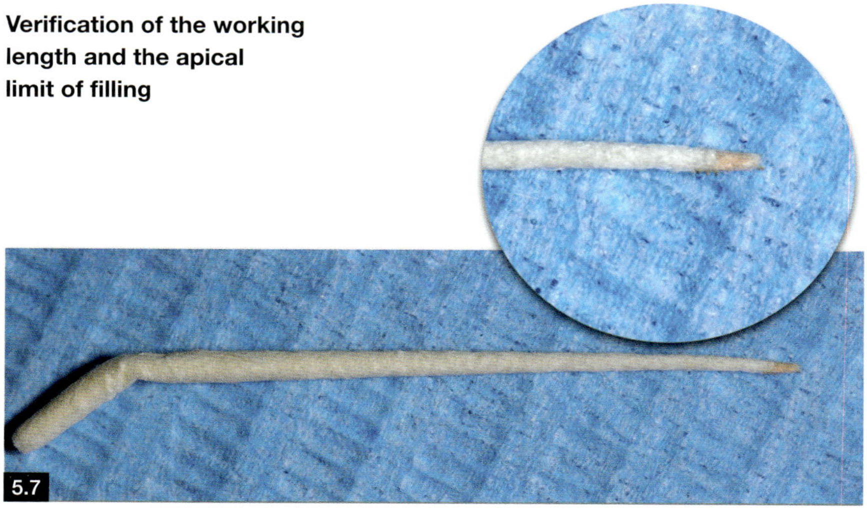

Fig. 5.7: Trying a paper cone in a roughly dried canal makes it possible to establish the boundary between the endodontium and periodontium (dark area).

Decontamination

Cones should be immersed in a 5% sodium hypochlorite bath in a Petri dish. For example, 60 seconds is sufficient to eradicate *Bacillus subtilis* spores[21]. During intracanal test steps, canals should be filled with sodium hypochlorite to prevent cone contamination[22].

Known apical diameter

A "nonstandardized" cone can be adapted, and the proximal part can be resected using a scalpel with a special caliber. The cut must be precise.
Cones with known apical diameter and taper may also be used. However, these cones should still be tested by an operator.

Intracanal adaptation

Intracanal adaptation is perhaps a crucial phase. This test must be carried out with an irrigation-filled root canal because a humid environment favors the flow of water in the cone and avoids the septic contamination of the endodontium.
A cone is considered adequate if it

- reaches the apical end of the canal determined during the shaping phase and does not exceed it;
- perceives a certain resistance in the apical area, in the insertion phase, and in the extraction phase (tug back);
- allows repeatable insertion;
- does not show creases or curls when extracted.

In retreatment, the presence of intracanal obstacles or inorganic material (e.g., gutta-percha residues, pastes and sealers, steps, or dentin blocks) can make the shaping of the endodontic space complex; at the end of this process, the acquired canal morphology does not always allow an easy adaptation of the gutta-percha cone. Understanding the errors of previous root canal shaping allows the re-evaluation of the phase of further re-instrumentation. This initiative leads to the modification of canal

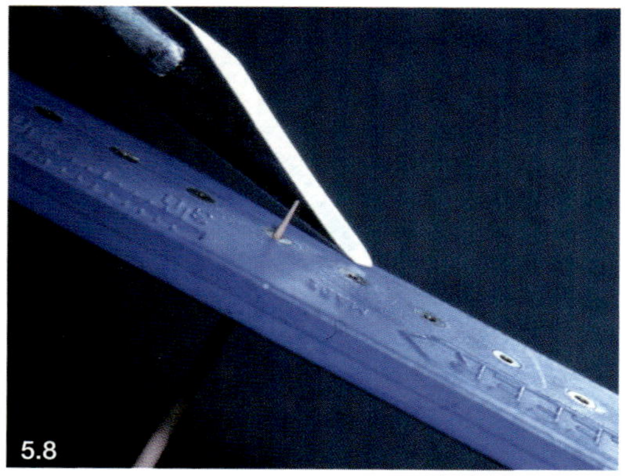

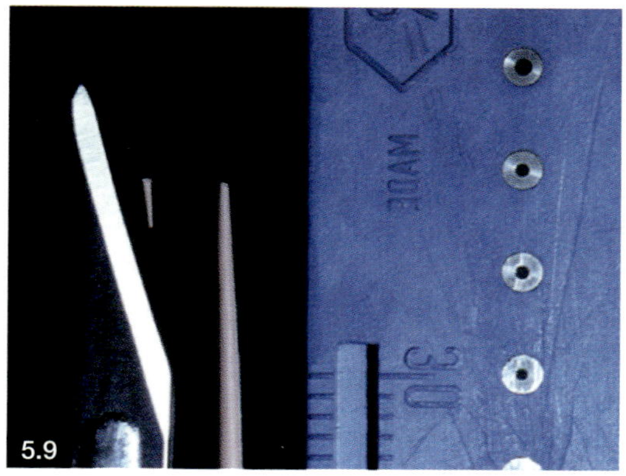

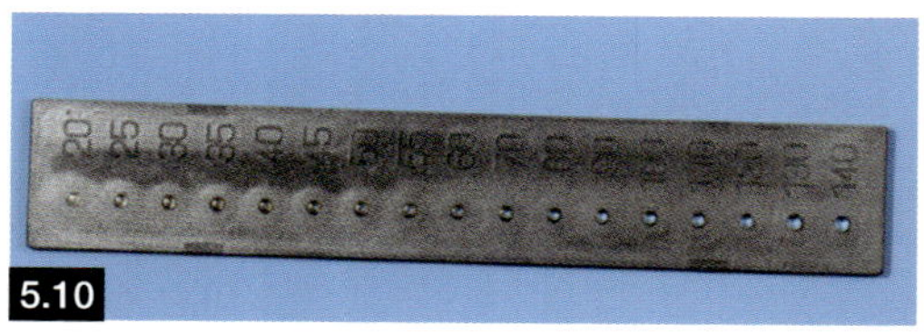

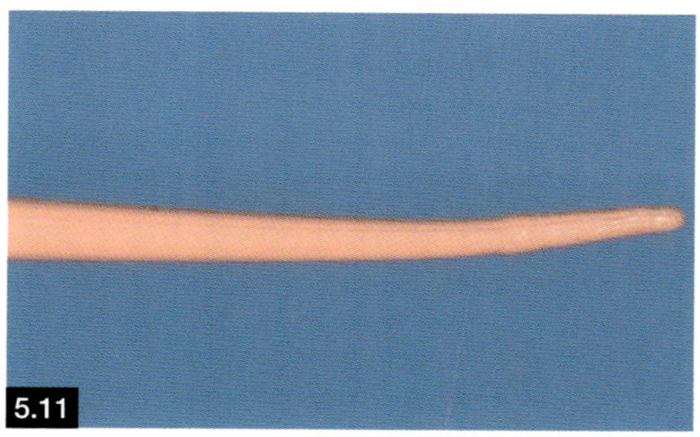

Fig. 5.8: Cone inserted in the hole of the corresponding ISO diameter ready to be cut.

Fig. 5.9: Cone cut for measurement.

Fig. 5.10: Tool required to perform the cut to the desired ISO diameter.

Fig. 5.11: Perfectly adapted cone with an apical incision, which is an indication of good adaptation to the end of the root canal.

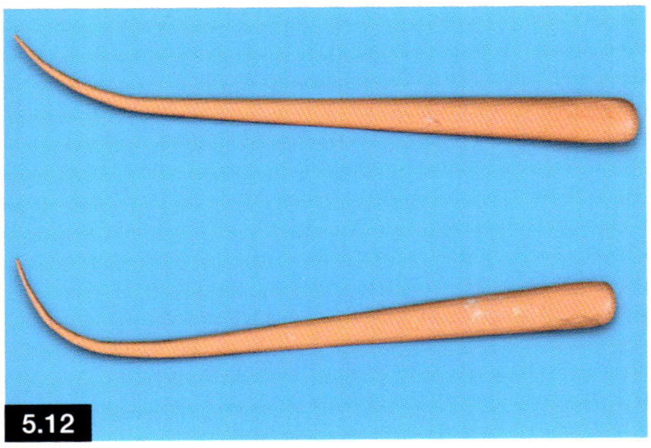
5.12

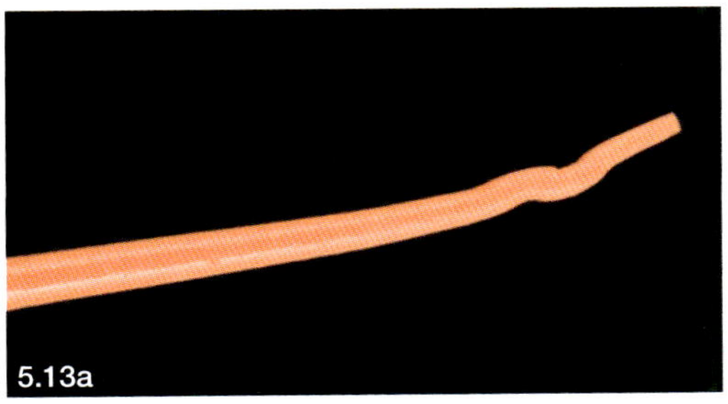
5.13a

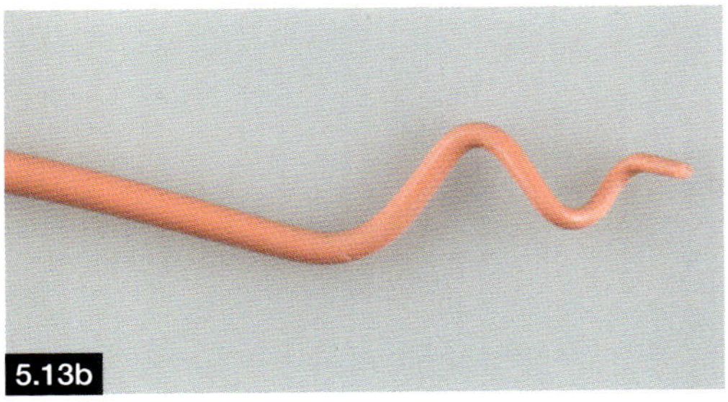
5.13b

diameters and apical diameters and consequently allows further decontamination of the endodontium and better adaptation of the filling material. In the latter case, ultrasound is a valuable aid, especially when an operation is carried out with the aid of a surgical microscope. Ultrasound is also particularly useful when a tooth has been extensively prepared because an additional shaping action would weaken an already fragile root. In all these cases, gutta-percha cones with different tapers or with different consistencies should be used. Immersion in pure alcohol for at least 1 min increases the hardness of the gutta-percha cone. Obtaining stiffer cones or cones with an already well-defined shape will make it possible to reach anatomically complex areas of the apical endodontium in the test phase.
The good containment of a filling within the endodontium is guaranteed by a snug fit of the gutta-percha against the canal walls; this process should occur in the apical part and not in the coronal part to develop a three-dimensional filling that avoids over- or underfilling[23, 24].
In the test phase, the unwanted contact of the cone along the canal walls causes the presence of small visible streaks on the surface; the streaks located in the third apical part confirm the good adaptation of the cone to the canal, and its resistance to extraction (tug back in Schilder's original conception[25]) definitively establishes a snug fit between gutta-percha and dentin in this region. Adaptation problems highlighted by curls or folds of the cone in the apical area must

Fig. 5.12: Immersion in pure alcohol makes it possible to shape the cones and provide greater stiffness and a higher degree of curvature suited to the canal to be filled.

Fig. 5.13a-b: Two examples of cones that are curled at the tip and do not meet the requirements of the test.

Fig. 5.14a-d: a-c) A correct cone test allows a good vertical comparison, as shown by the presence of a lateral canal in the apical third; (d) the 1-year radiographic examination shows recovery.

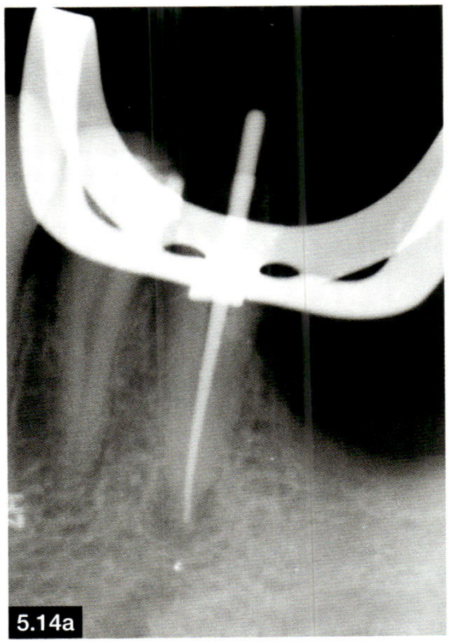
5.14a

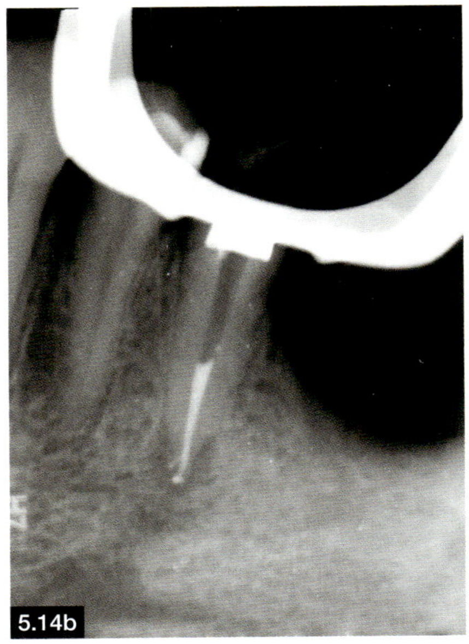
5.14b

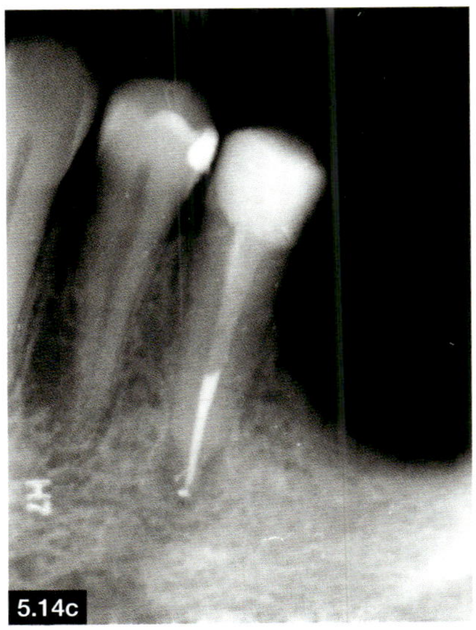
5.14c

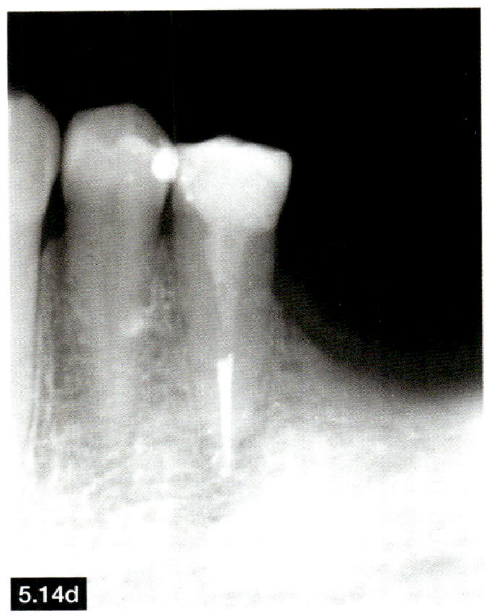
5.14d

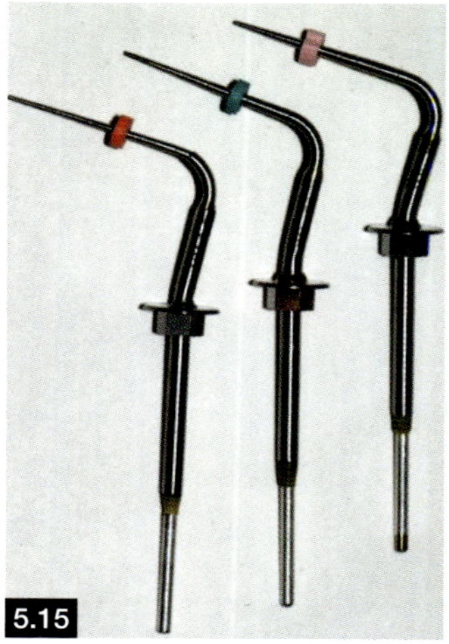

5.15

Fig. 5.15: Heat carriers and/or condensers. Today, electronically controlled instruments are available that deliver a precise amount of heat inside the canal, i.e., sufficient to soften the gutta-percha. Thin flexible drills with diameters of around ISO 30 are also available to reach the depths of the most complex channels.

be overcome by re-shaping the root canal, perhaps increasing the taper of the canal treated with appropriate instruments or with different sequences of it. A microscope or magnifiers with a coaxial light source can be used to visualize these areas and visually improve the morphological characteristics of the apical limit[12-13, 19].

Performing an X-ray test

An X-ray of an individual with inserted cones may be performed to evaluate some of the previous points, verify the working lengths, and preview the canal filling. If the X-ray confirms that the selected cone is suitable, the final canal filling can be performed.

Compaction techniques

Some instruments are necessary in warm gutta-percha vertical condensation techniques to adapt the gutta-percha to the canal morphology obtained:

- heat carriers to heat the gutta-percha at root canal depth (Fig. 5.15)
- compactors to reach the most apical parts of the root canal and condense the previously heated gutta-percha (Fig. 5.16)

Currently available systems with a single instrument of known size and morphology can combine the two roles, i.e., simultaneously heat and pack gutta-percha; they are not the only ones because various other methods have been reported in the literature for effectively heating gutta-percha in the most apical parts of the root canal[26-30].
The details of these operations are excluded from this text, but available tools and methods for obtaining a good sealing of the endodontic space are described using images. A final consideration should be made regarding cases of retreatment when the vertical condensation of gutta-percha is applied. The apical seal is a consequence of a scrupulous preparation of the apical limit. Consequently, sealing methods should be varied as appropriate in uncertain situations.

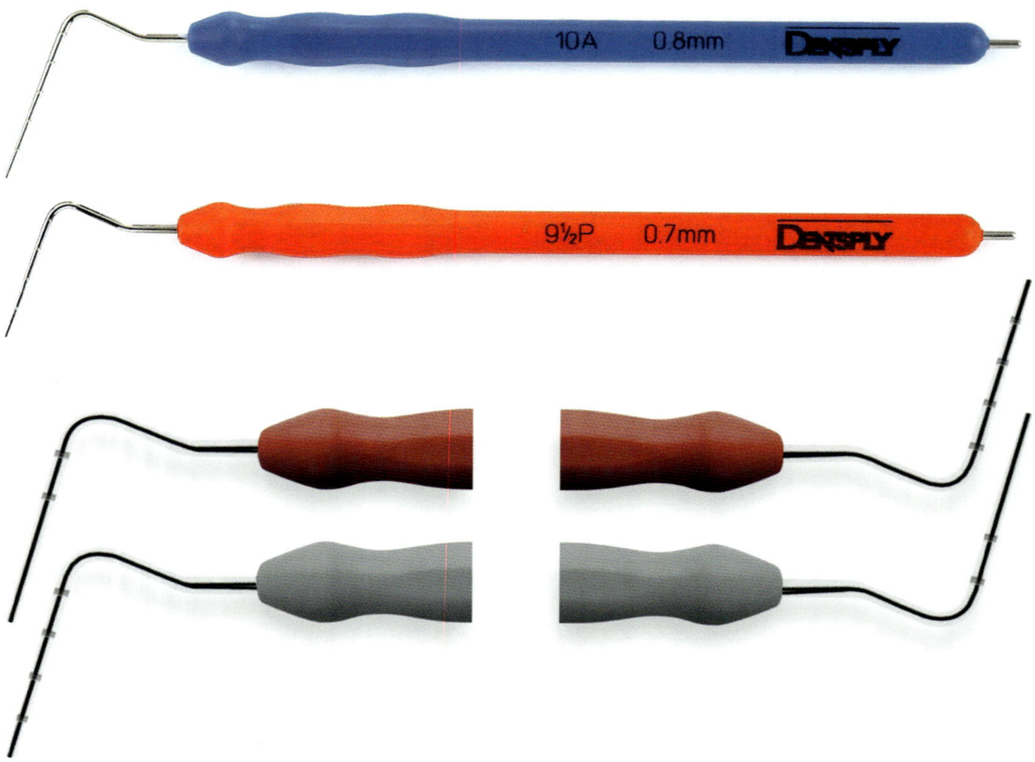

5.18

Fig. 5.16: Two examples of pluggers for heated gutta-percha (Maillefer, Switzerland). Pluggers are marked with notches placed at 5 mm intervals and provided with a stop so that an operator can have a guide as to the depth at which a plugger is working inside the root canal. Pluggers must be introduced passively into the canal to avoid root fractures caused by the wedge effect resulting from the application of a force.

▶ continue to page 298

Retreatment through vertical condensation of the gutta-percha

CASE REPORT 1

The canal morphology of the cases represented here is not very different from that which can be found in similar never previously treated cases, a sign that the previous treatment had not changed the anatomy much, particularly at apical level. The choice of shaping the channels and filling them using the vertical condensation technique was therefore possible for the reasons listed above.

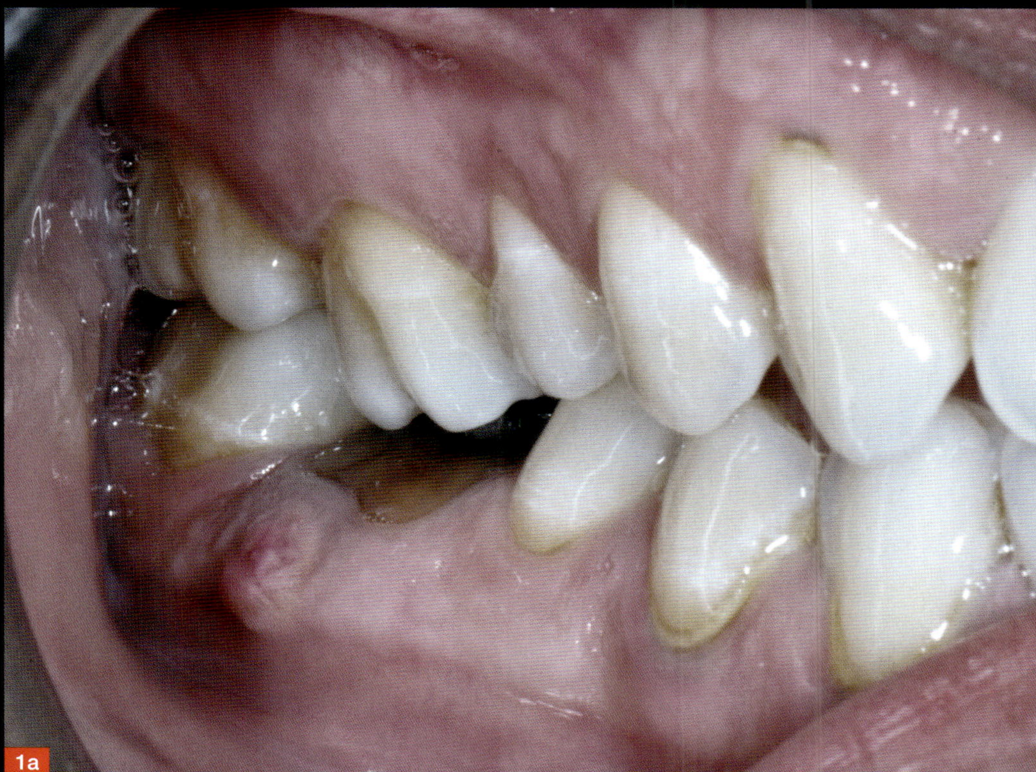

1a

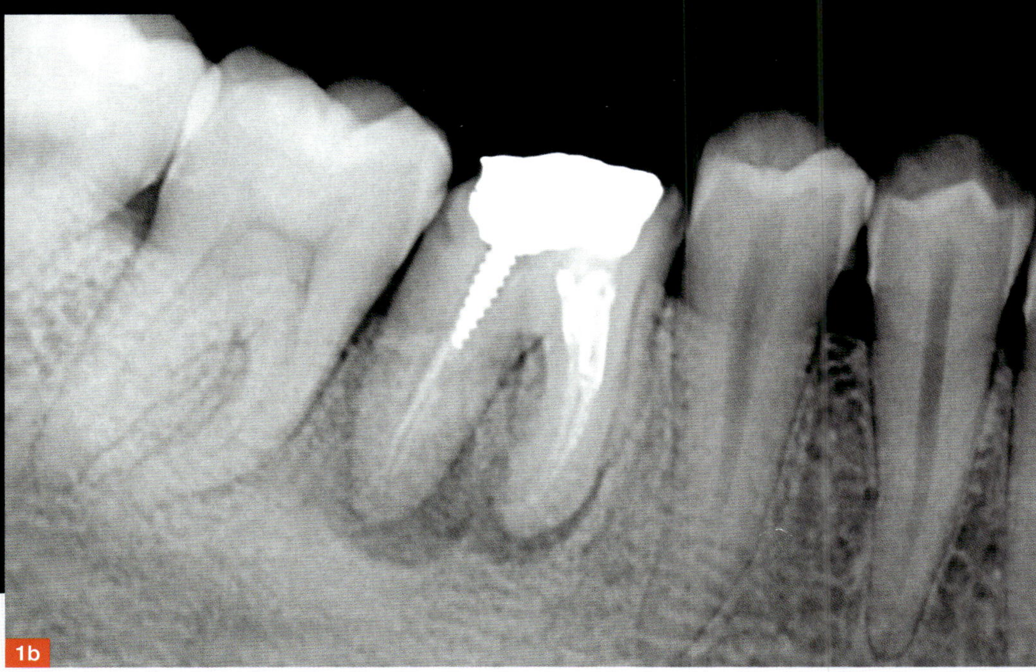

1b

Figure 1a-b: A high fistula (a) in the molar area testifies to a periodontal involvement in an unsuitable endodontic treatment; (b) it also shows a reconstruction anchored to a threaded pin.

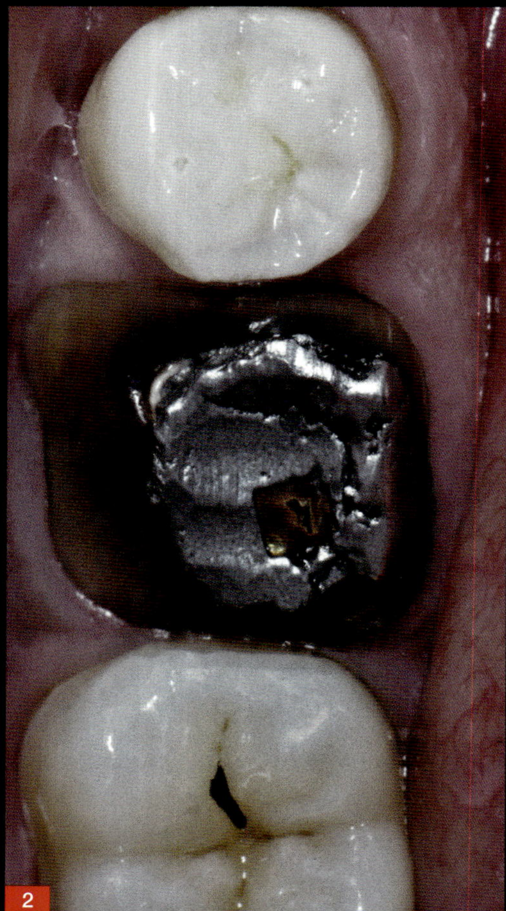

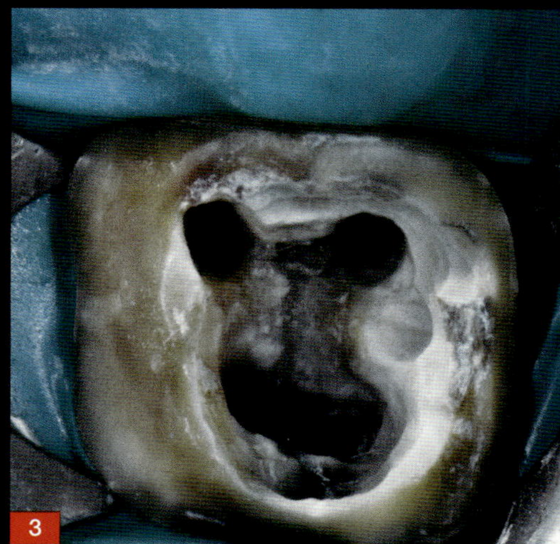

Figure 2: Occlusal view of the tooth.

Figure 3: The cavity shape once all the amalgam has been removed.

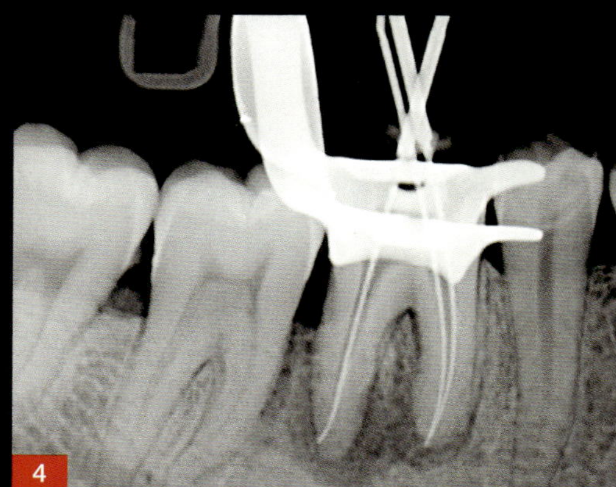

Figure 4: The empty root canals with the tools inserted to verify the length.

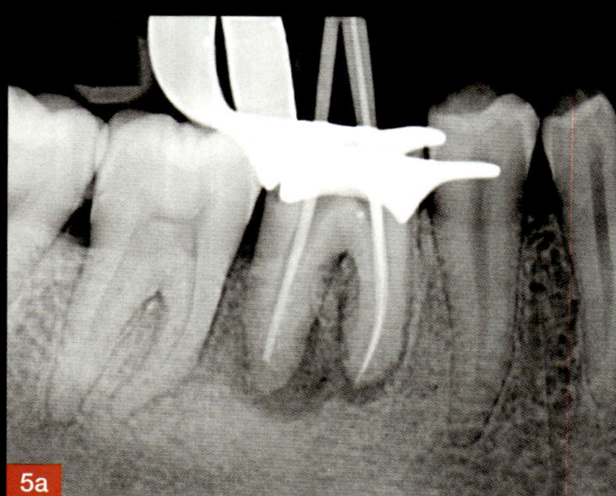

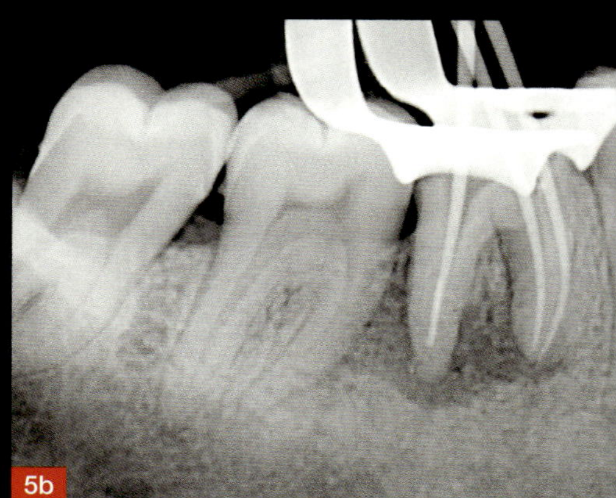

Figure 5a-b: Image showing the cones; note the different projections.

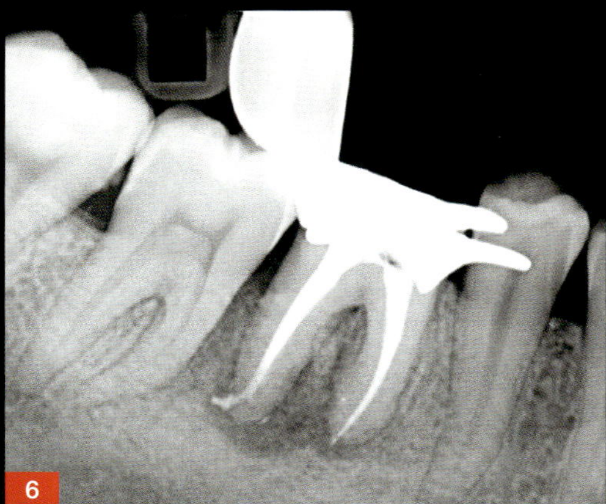

6

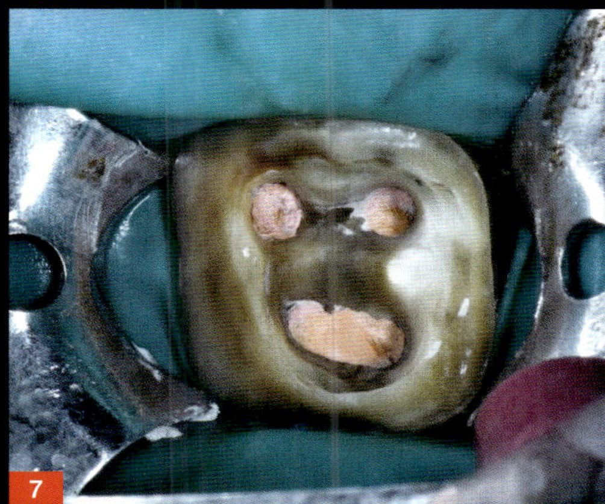

7

Figure 6: Final x-ray showing the good fit of the closure.

Figure 7: Occlusal view.

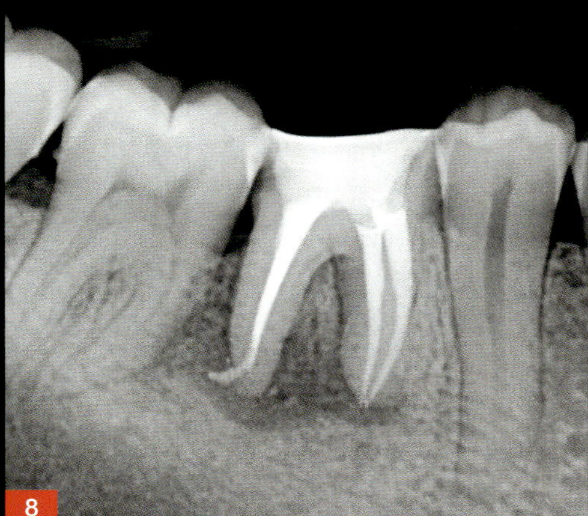

8

Figure 8: Radiographic images at the end of the treatment with the retreatment.

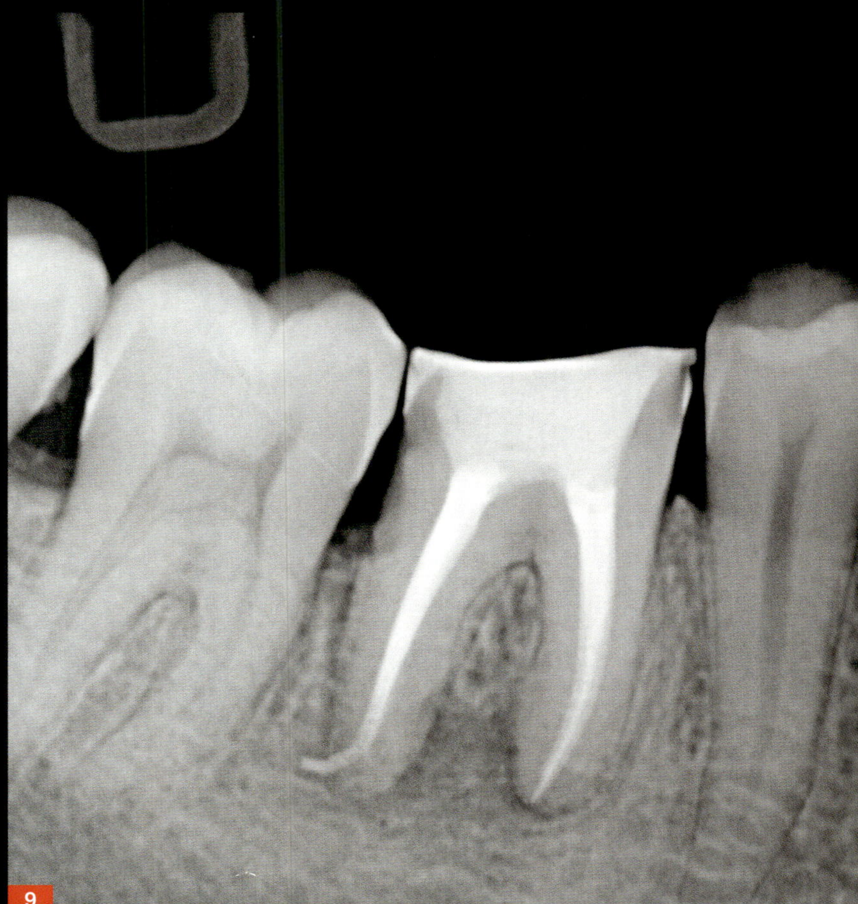

9

Figure 9: The follow-up x-ray after 3 years.

CASE REPORT 2

Retreatment of a lower molar with wide curvatures

When analyzing the anatomy of root canals, understanding the morphology from the beginning is very important: this will help us choose the exact filling technique to be used once the root canals have been shaped. The morphology, with continuous curvature, suggests a preheated gutta-percha filling techniques should be used.

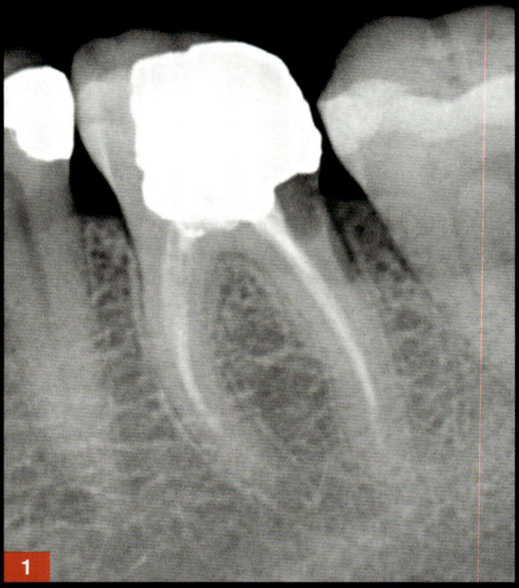

Figure 1: A distal cervical lesion requires the restoration of a very extensive restoration on a lower molar.

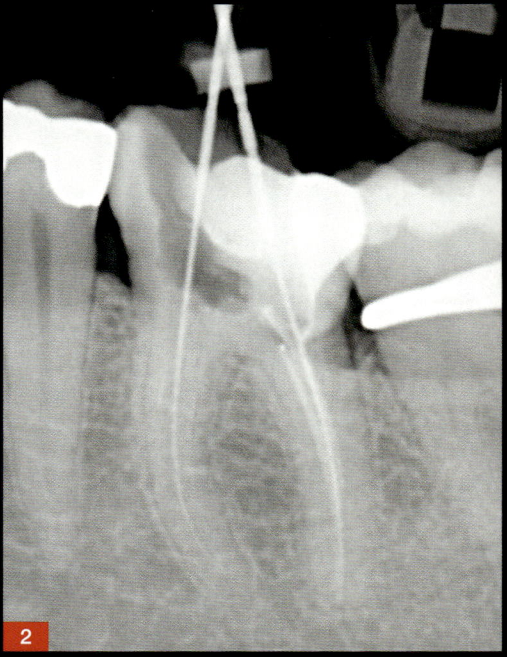

Figure 2: Once the old filling had been removed and the previous content had been removed, the root canals were re-scanned.

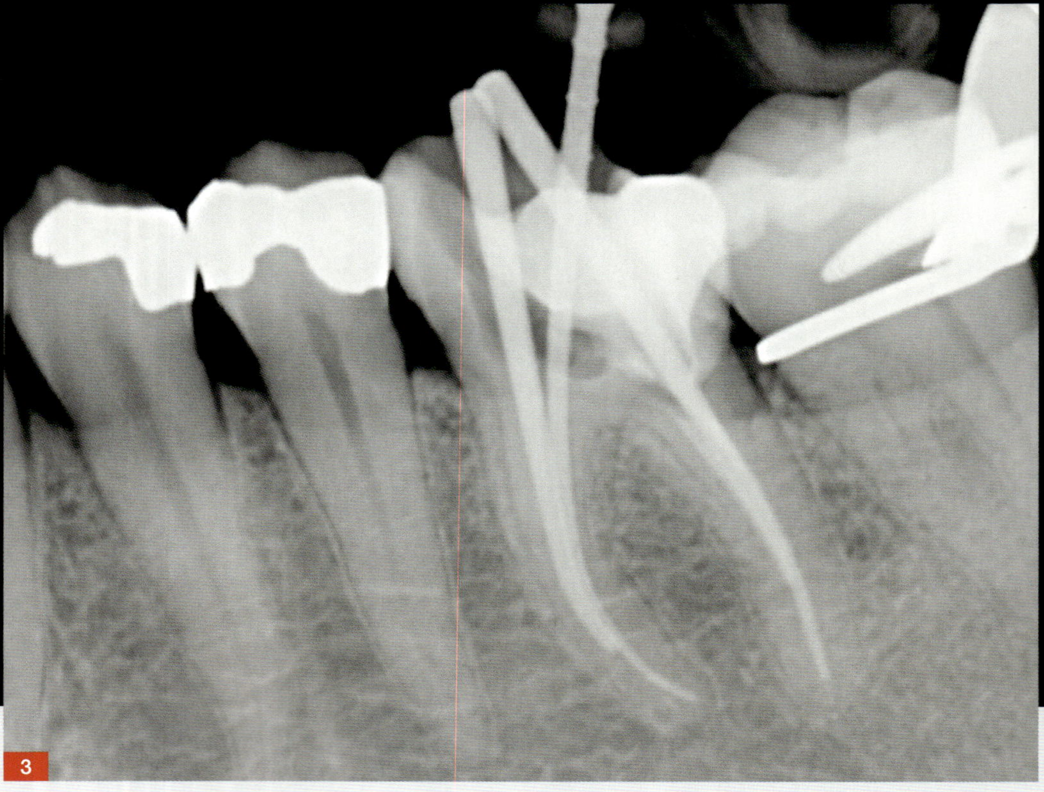

Figure 3: The cone test with the preheated gutta-percha checker demonstrates how well shaped the canals are, especially towards the apical area.

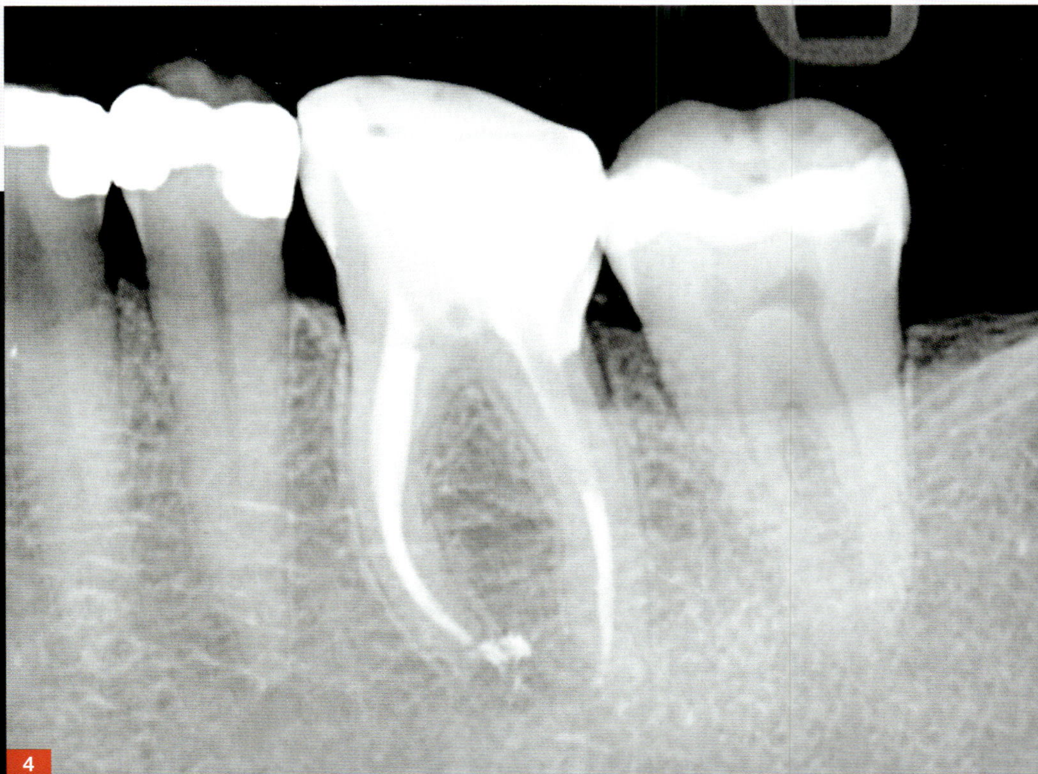

Figure 4: Radiograph at the end of the treatment.

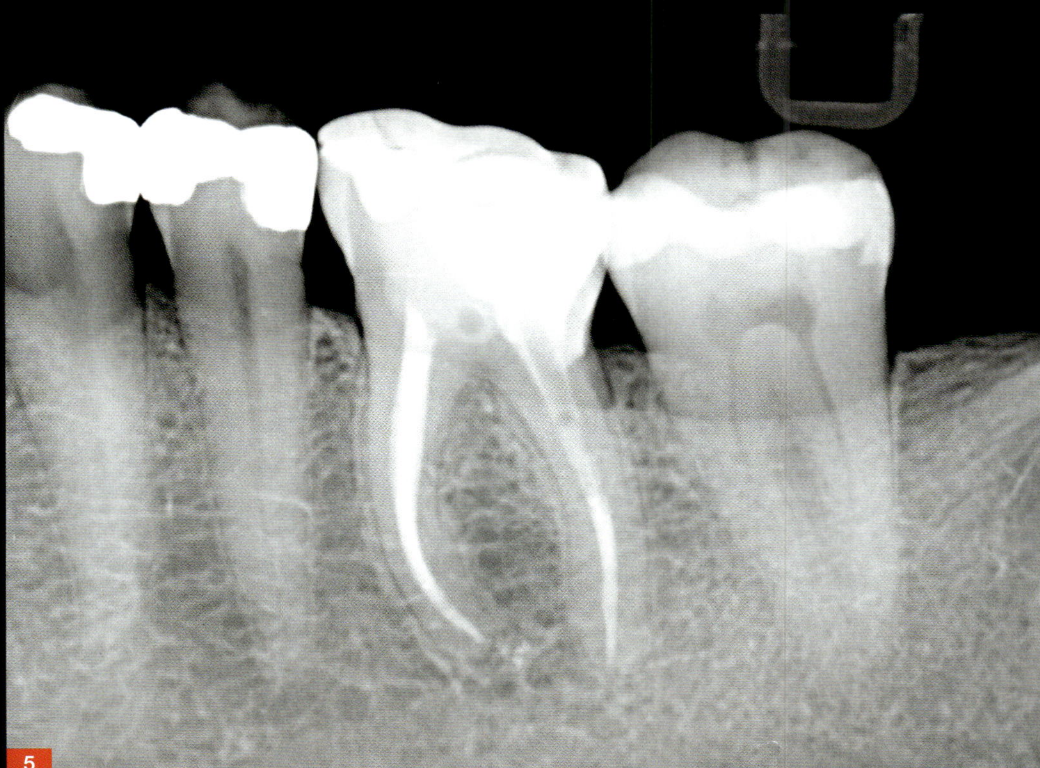

Figure 5: The 2-year follow-up testifies to the success of the retreatment.

Filling using preheated gutta-percha on a carrier

Since the development of systems using preheated gutta-percha on a central core of a radiopaque plastic (carrier) at the end of the 1970s[31], they have become increasingly popular[32-34] (Fig. 5.17a-c).

Carriers have a colored handle, which follows the sizes and colors of the ISO standardization.
They are ideal for filling curved root canals that do not have excessively large apical diameters[35]. A precise sequence should be followed to obtain a good adaptation of the filling; the corresponding apical diameter that is slightly larger than that used at the limit of instrumentation should be selected by using a carrier without gutta-percha[36]. However, the position and adaptation of a plastic carrier should be verified with a periapical X-ray. Filling involves the use of even small amounts of sealer, which is introduced into the canal with a sterile paper cone. Excess sealer is then eliminated with dry sterile paper cones.
Once it has been heated in a special oven, a carrier-based gutta-percha system should be slowly introduced into the canal until it reaches the length set during the test phase. In this process, slight pressure is exerted for 8-10 s. This system represents a simple and effective method for obtaining a correct three-dimensional filling of the complex root canal system.
In particular, this system seems to be effective in the filling of narrow, long, and curved canals, where it is difficult to insert a heat carrier or a plugger in the last 4 mm of the canal in order to properly thermoplasticize the gutta-percha cones. Unlike "cold"[37, 38] techniques, which do not involve heat for the adaptation of gutta-percha inside the endodontium, thermoplasticized gutta-percha can be used to seal the endodontium with all its complexities in a three-dimensional way[39].

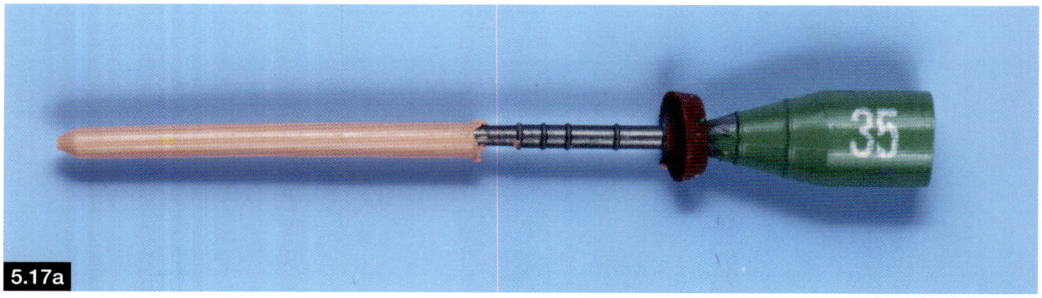

Fig. 5.17a: Instrument for canal fillings with thermoplasticized gutta-percha (Thermafil, Maillefer, Switzerland).

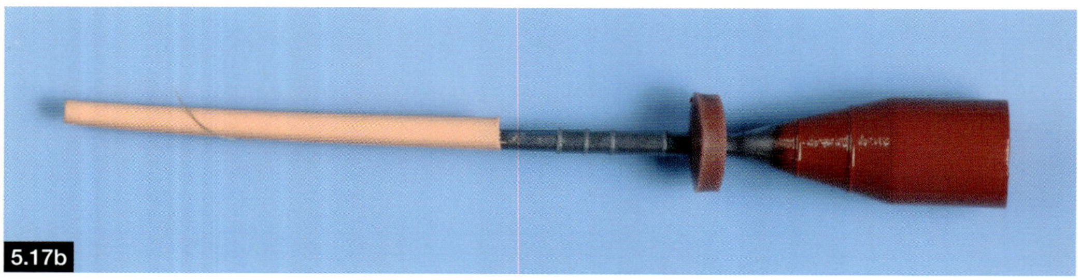

Fig. 5.17b: Same tool with different apex sizes (25 ISO).

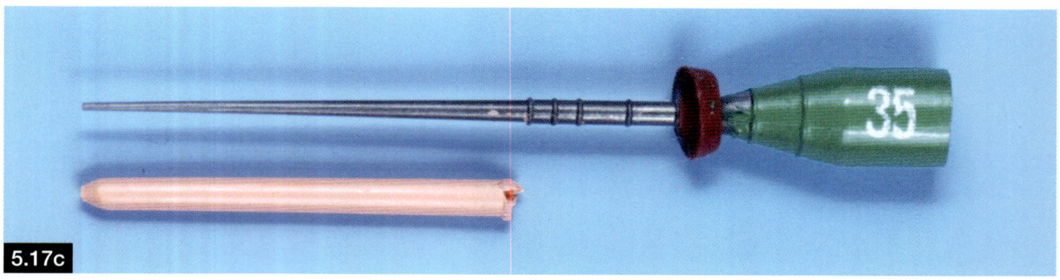

Fig. 5.17c: Using a carrier stripped of gutta-percha is a good way to verify the correctness of the working length.

▶ continue to page 302

Obturation of lower molar with preheated gutta-percha

CASE REPORT 3

The lower molar examined was ideal for re-shaping and filling with a method using preheated gutta-percha introduced inside the canal using a “carrier”. There were many reasons for this: the apical morphology, the length of the canals and their size would have been poorly suited to vertical gutta-percha condensation.

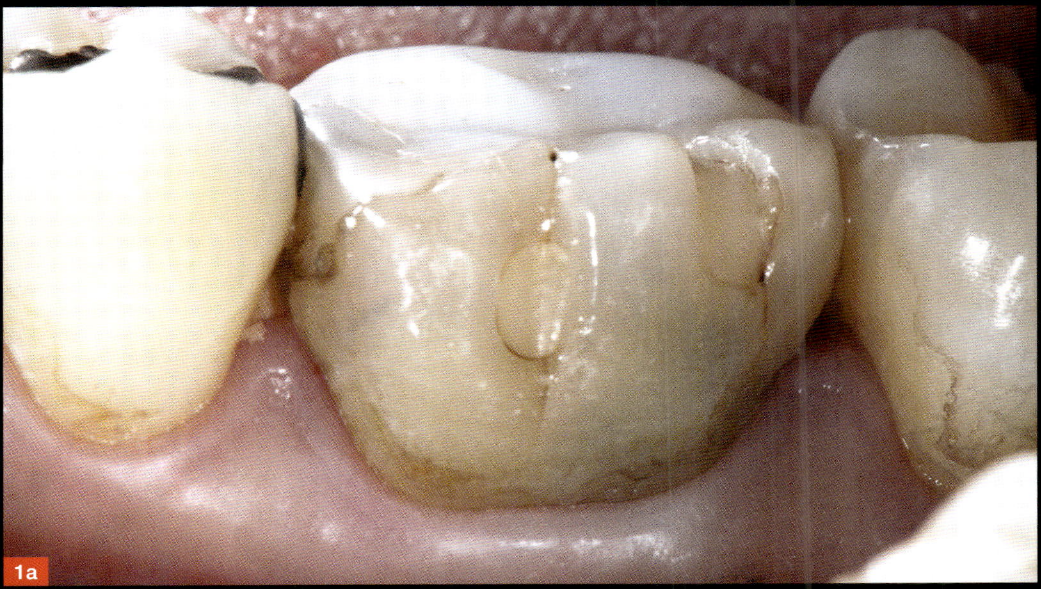

Figure 1a: Lower molar with a good amount of residual dental tissue.

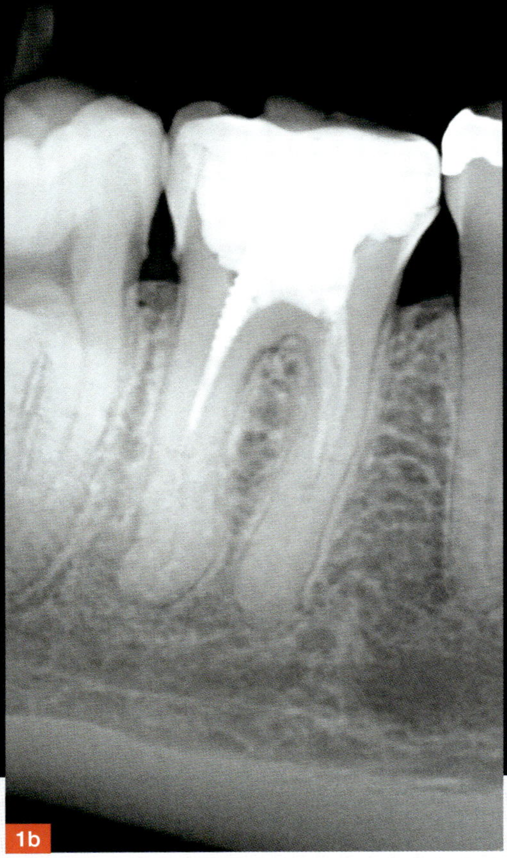

Figure 1b: Radiographic examination showing incorrect root canal instrumentation and incorrect closure; the profiles of the root canals can be seen beyond the limits of the current fillings. There is an indication for retreatment.

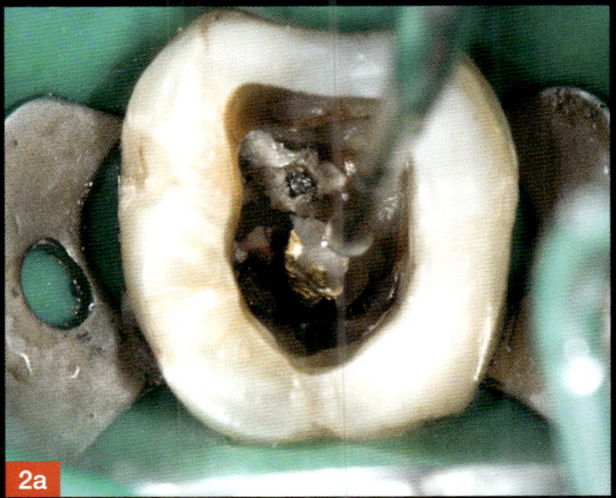

Figure 2a: Appearance of the pulp chamber.

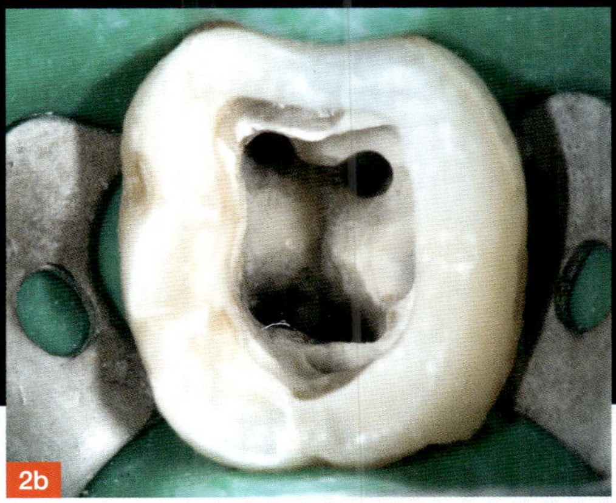

Figure 2b: The same after proper cleansing.

In these cases, the elective choice is precisely that of being conservative, when performing the shaping manoeuvres, as the canal itself is narrow. An extension seems critical but, however it is considered, the small size of the root does not allow the introduction of compactors and heat carriers without touching the walls up to the depth required to achieve a perfect fit of the filling material.

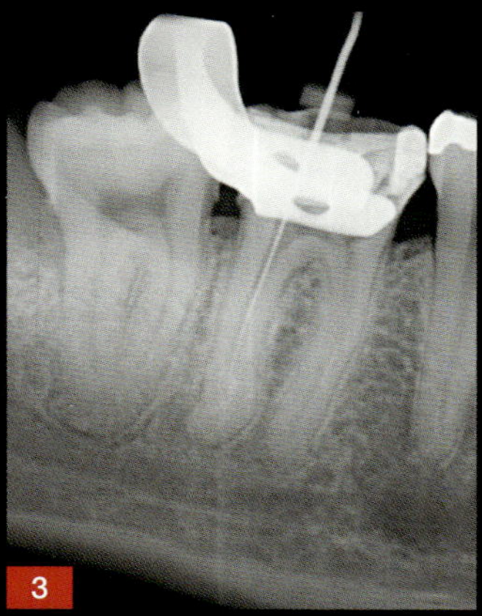

Figure 3: The probing of the distal canal.

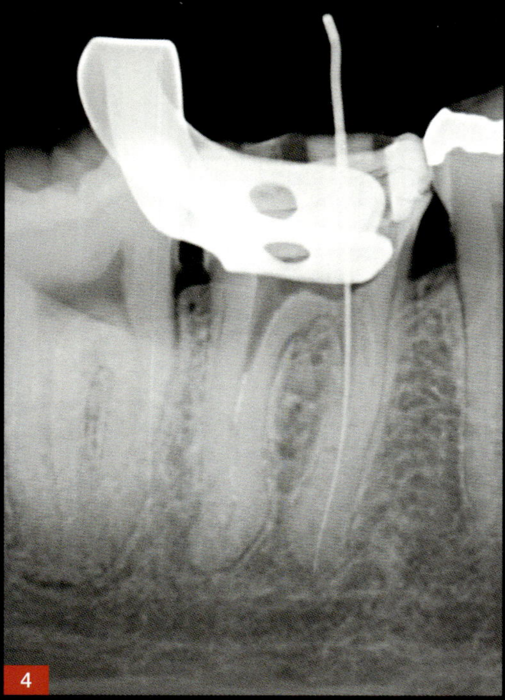

Figure 4: The probing of the mesial channel.

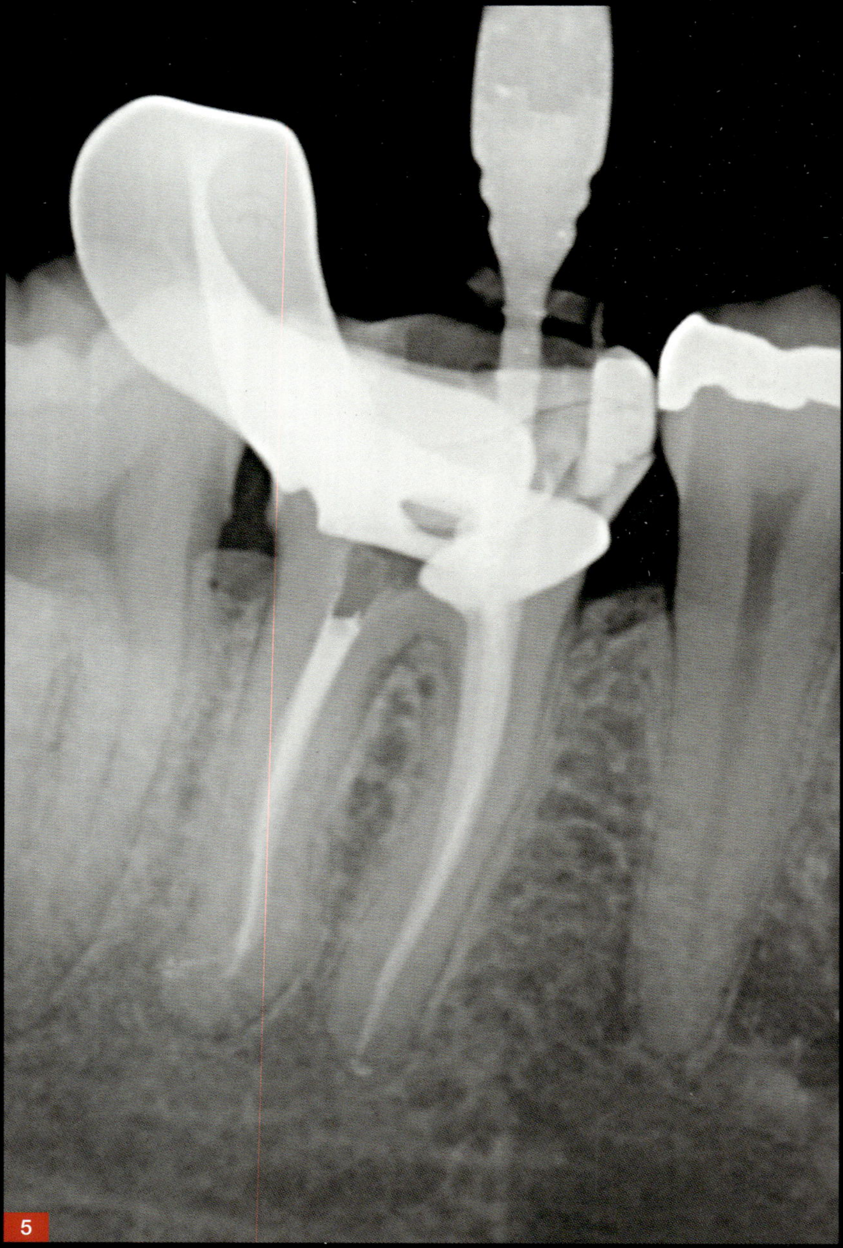

Figure 5: Proof of closure with a "carrier" still inserted.

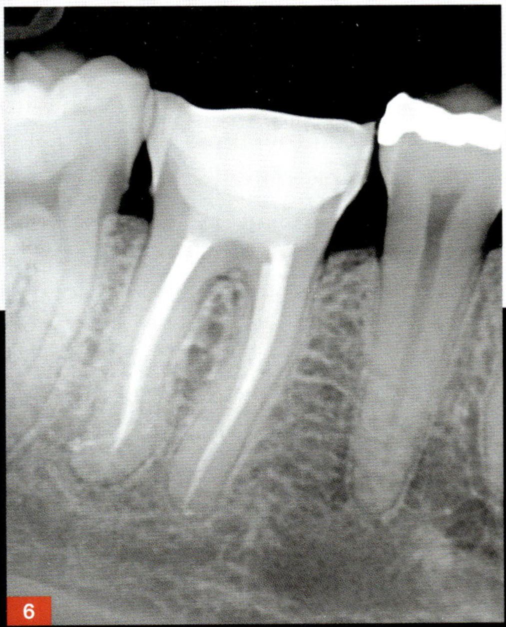

6

Figure 6: Check performed a short time after closure.

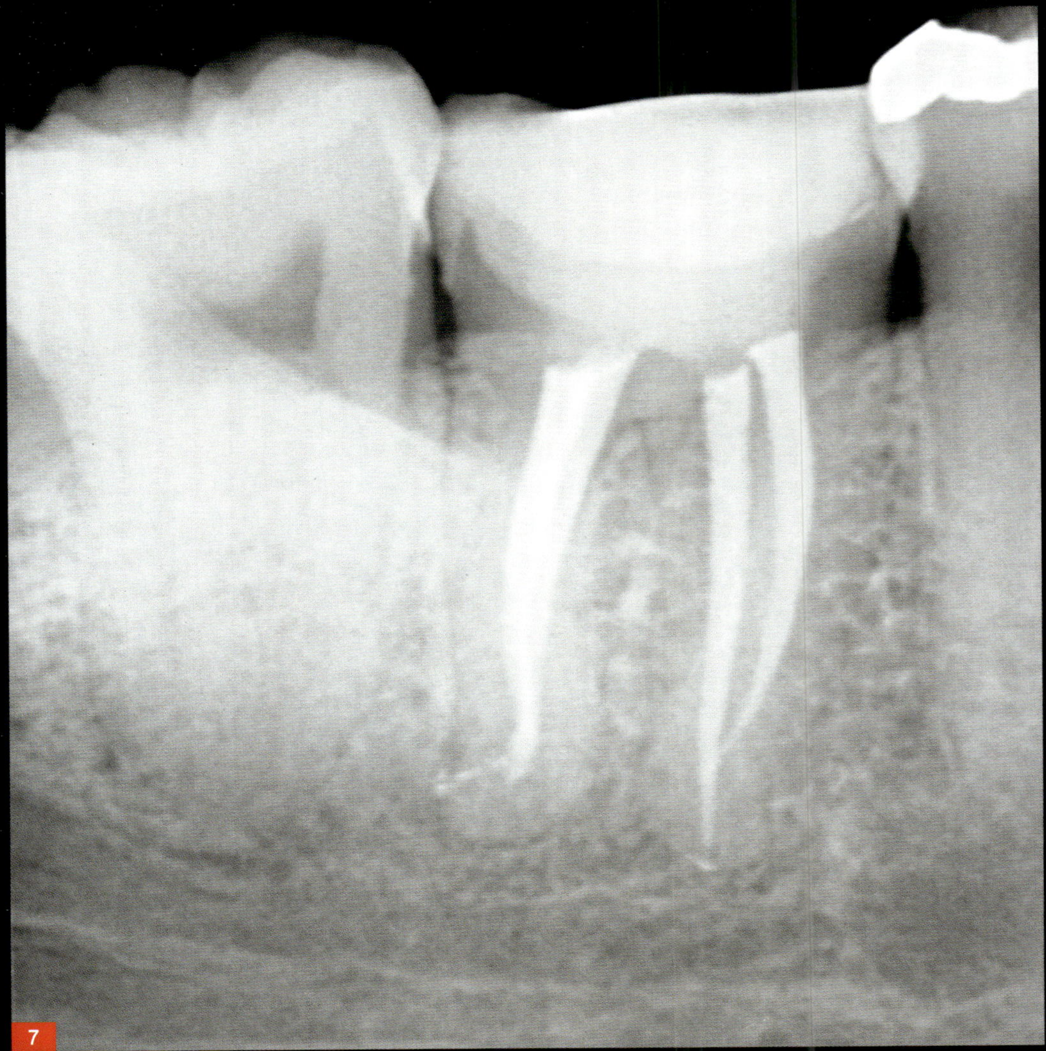

7

Figure 7: Follow-up 2 years after surgery.

Comparison of filling methods

Most studies on this topic compare the most recent methodologies, including warm vertical gutta-percha condensation and preheated gutta-percha, with cold lateral techniques[40] whose only advantage would be the ease of use and wide diffusion. Jarrett et al.[41] examined the palatal roots of the upper molars and demonstrated an excellent adaptation of the thermoplasticized gutta-percha using a carrier and applying vertical condensation. Gençoglu et al.[42] performed an in vitro study and showed good resistance to dye infiltration. Gulabivala et al.[43] and Leung et al.[44] reported a better result than that obtained with the lateral gutta-percha condensation technique. In the latter study, the best results are obtained in canals with an angle of curvature greater than 25°. Not all the results have been positive in fact, Lares et al.[45] demonstrated that the efficacy of the *lateral technique* is better than that of vertical condensation. Bhambhani et al. found no statistically significant differences between lateral and thermoplastic gutta-percha carrier-based canal filling[40].
They appear to be superimposable in bacterial infiltration studies[46-48]. In 2001, Pommel et al.[49] compared the apical infiltration of closed roots with the continuous wave condensation technique, lateral condensation and preheated gutta-percha with a carrier, and vertical condensation using a fluid filtration system. They showed that the preheated carrier gutta-percha method provides an immediate seal comparable with that obtained with other methods.
After 1 month, the same experiment revealed an increased infiltration level in the lateral technique.
The authors hypothesized that this result is due to the greater presence of sealers in the last millimeter than in other techniques. Another study evaluated the effectiveness of the method with or without a sealer and showed that the infiltration of the dye is greater than that of the use of the sealer technique[50, 51].
This result confirms the usefulness of the latter during the filling phases.

FILLING TECHNIQUES

New techniques do not seem to provide clear advantages in terms of endodontic therapeutic success.

However, adaptation to particular canal morphologies seems to be a pivotal element that can lead to the development of favorable methods of filling with warm gutta-percha compaction.
Some studies have demonstrated that the percentage of endodontic space filled with carrier-based gutta-percha is higher than that measured in cases sealed with lateral compaction[52, 53]. This result highlights how the use of a sealer in the preheated gutta-percha technique can be minimized compared with that of other techniques[54, 55].
In a similar study, De-Deus et al.[48] used oval canals and found a better fit of gutta-percha in cases filled using the preheated gutta-percha technique (98.16% ± 0.50%) than those filled using the lateral technique (82.60% ± 10.67); furthermore, it is difficult to fill the entire volume of oval canals using any method[48]. Many studies have emphasized the importance of the role played by sealer[56], suggesting that the synergy between the two components is fundamental[57, 58].
In conclusion, a universal shaping and filling method may be established a priori, especially in cases of retreatment where previous manuevers have caused more or less significant variations in the canal lumen. Owing to the frequent variations in apex morphology caused by inflammatory processes, it is easy to understand that having the knowledge to use the methods best-suited to the case – pre-heated or warm gutta-percha compaction – allows good sealer and gutta-percha, even in root canals that are not rounded. Both techniques are well suited to filling root canals with apices below ISO 50–60, although maintaining a precise root canal filling in the case of endodontic spaces with apices above ISO 50 or with a poor taper seems more complex. Pirani et al.[59] showed that teeth filled using a carrier-based technique in a specialist master's program presented survival and a periapical health comparable with those of cohorts whose root canals are filled with other obturation techniques after 10 years. In these cases, different techniques using bioactive sealers should be applied.

▶ *continue to page 310*

Is the extrusion of apical cement a real drawback?

CASE REPORTS 4-5

The extrusion of material beyond the root apex should not always be interpreted in a negative way; although the immunocompetent cells will be stimulated to remove the cement and the gutta-percha, this release of material beyond the apical limit of instrumentation must also be understood as the expression of a correct sealing of the entire endodontic space.

CASE REPORT 4

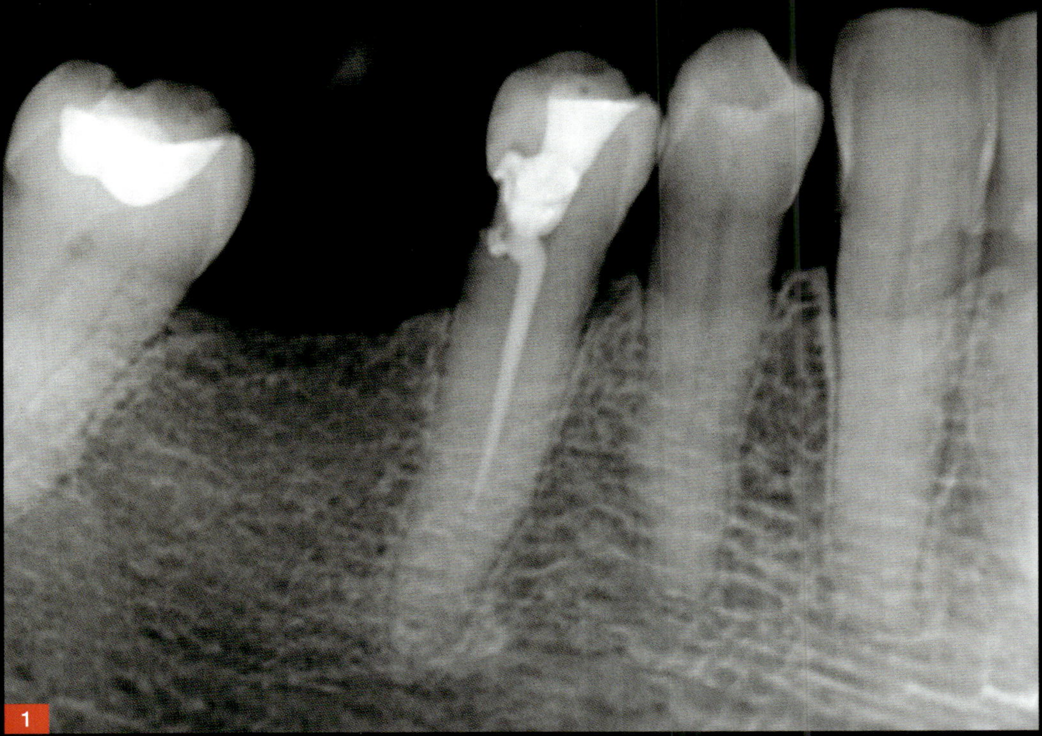

1

Figure 1: A lower premolar in which the previous endodontic treatment has left an obvious gap.

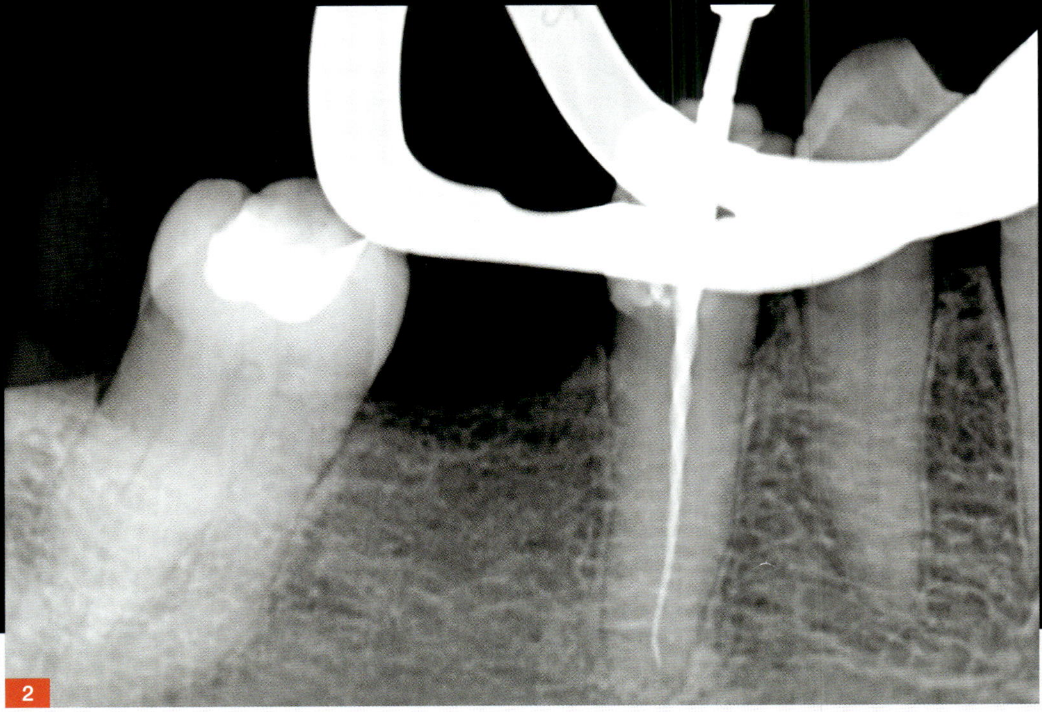

2

Figure 2: The instrumentation of the root canal, which was not previously traversed, leads to the achievement of the working length.

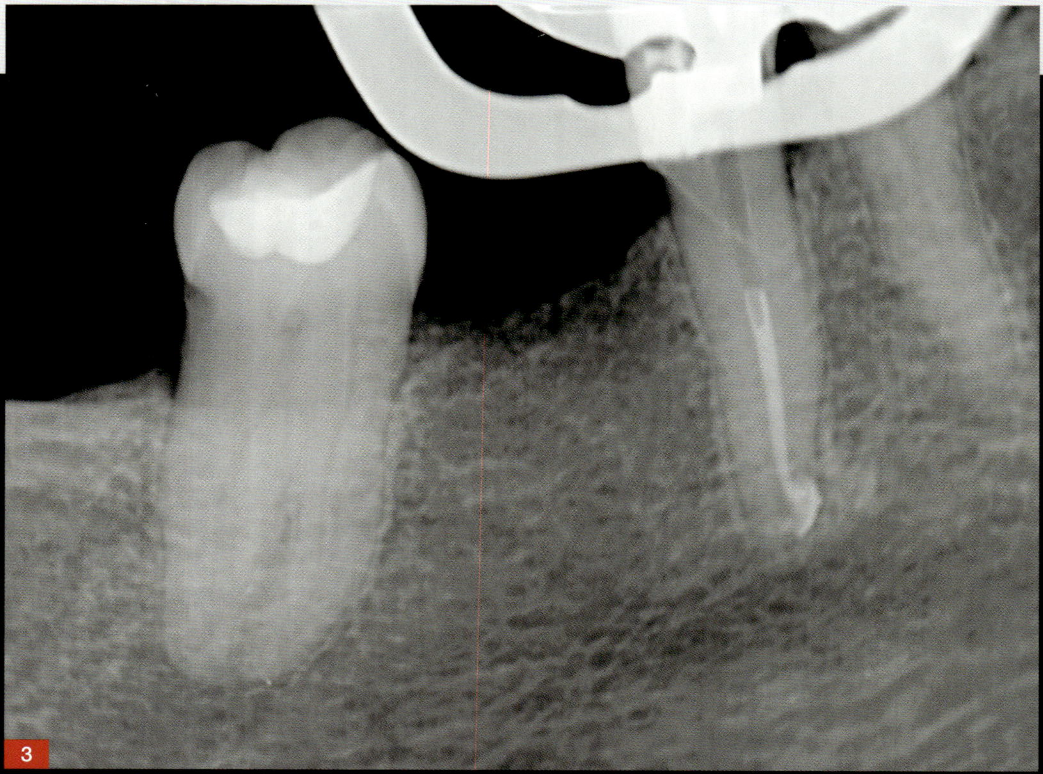

Figure 3: The apex closure gives a glimpse of an apical extrusion of filling material.

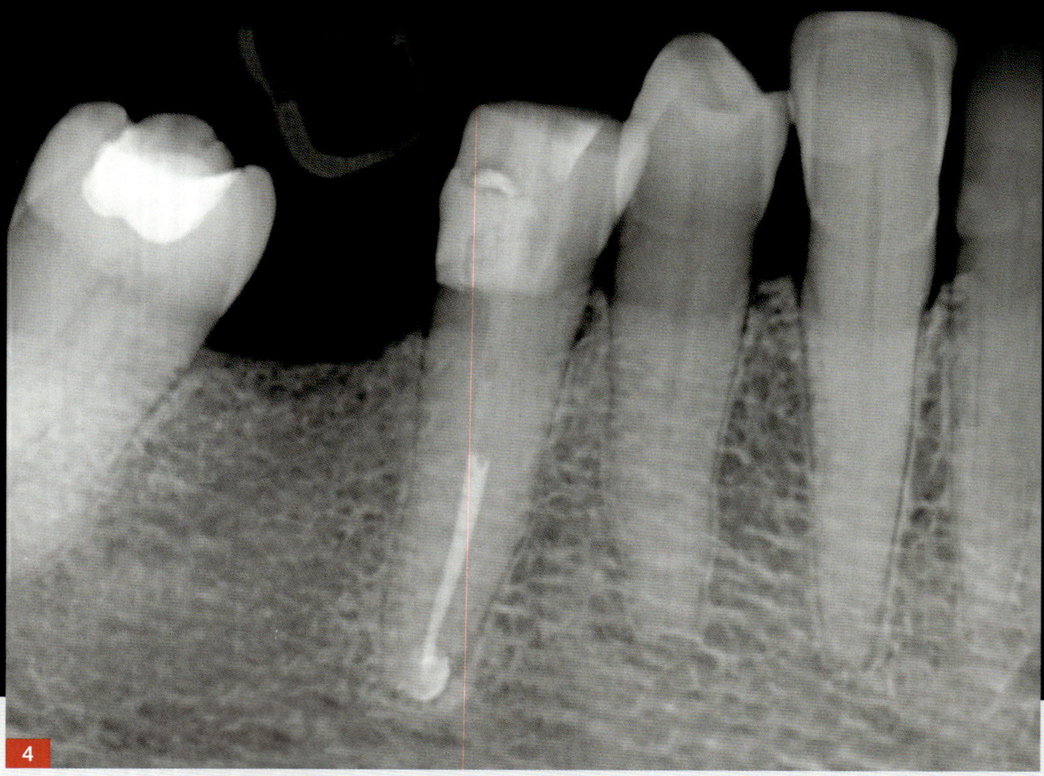

Figure 4: The 3-year follow-up certifies the success of the case.

CASE REPORT 5

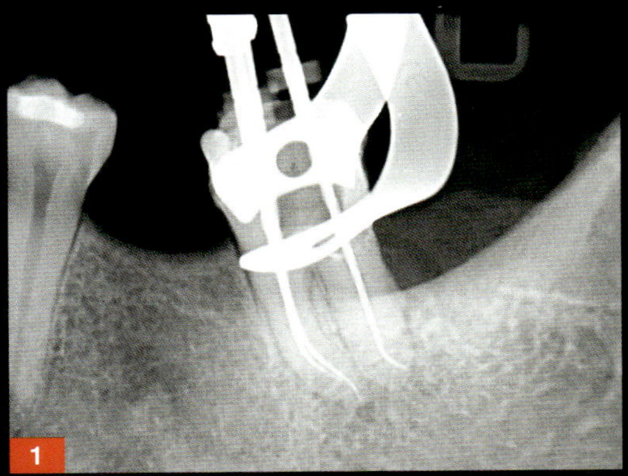

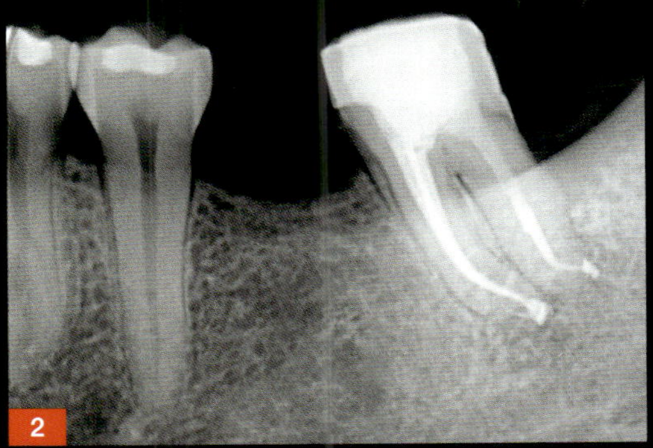

Figure 1: Lower molar with particularly curved apexes.

Figure 2: Closure of the case.

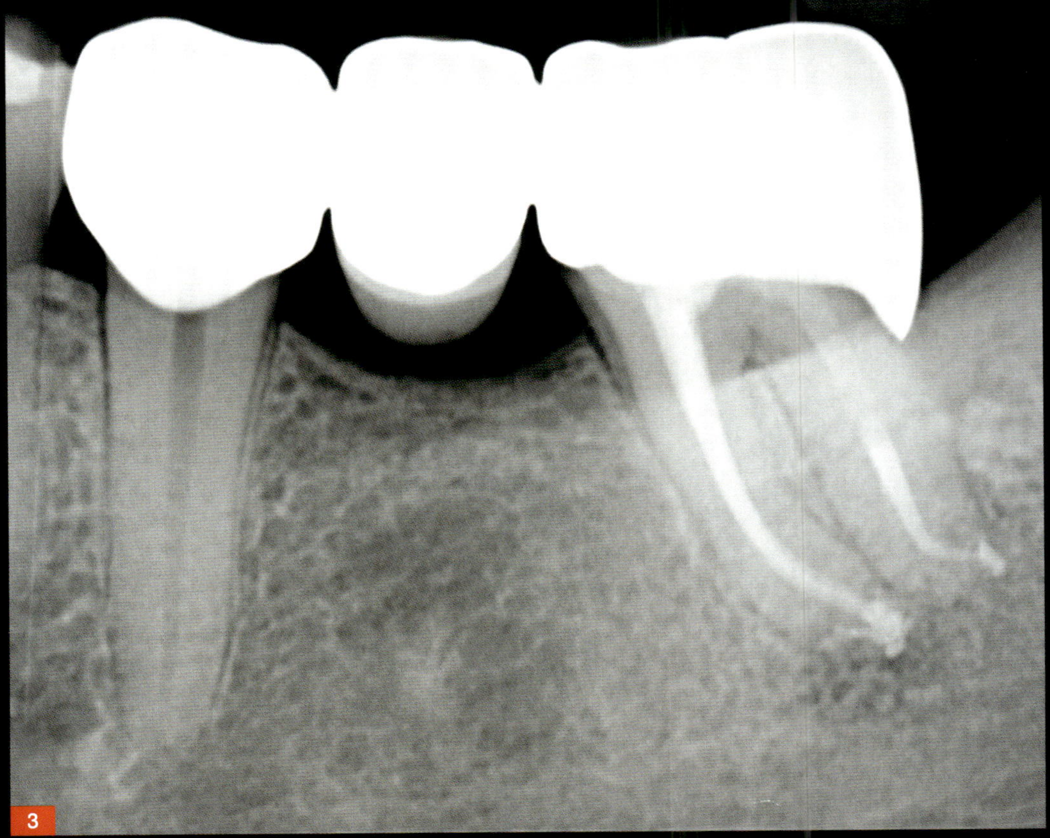

Figure 3: Follow-up after 3 years.

Box 5.3 CLINICAL SIGNIFICANCE OF OVERFILLING

Overfilling means an excess of filling material beyond a radiographically identifiable apical limit. It can be simply a canal sealer, a gutta-percha cone, a carrier bearing gutta-percha, or a combination of these components.

Studies have shown a decrease in endodontic success in the case of overfilling[1-3] without specifying the underlying reason. Other studies have divided the term overfilling into two subsections: overfilling and overextension. Some scholars argued that overfilling should be considered when root canal filling is complete, but results in material expulsion beyond the apical foramen, whereas overextension is defined as the extrusion of a filling material but with a deficient filling of the root canal[4]. In any case, clinical results are often inevitable[5, 6]; the fate of an extruded material depends on its solubility and susceptibility to phagocytosis, which depends on the biocompatibility of the components. A decrease in the success rate due to the cytotoxicity of a material or a foreign body reaction is also evaluated[7-9]. Overfilling is linked to the incorrect shaping of the apical tract, so the filling does not seal the apex, rather it escapes into the periapical tissues[10], slowing down the healing process[11]. Material extrusion is not the only cause of failure[12, 13] unless it affects the neurovascular structures[14]. However, incorrect filling control associated with incorrect instrumentation can be a source of extraradicular bacterial contamination[15] and detrimental to the final prognosis.

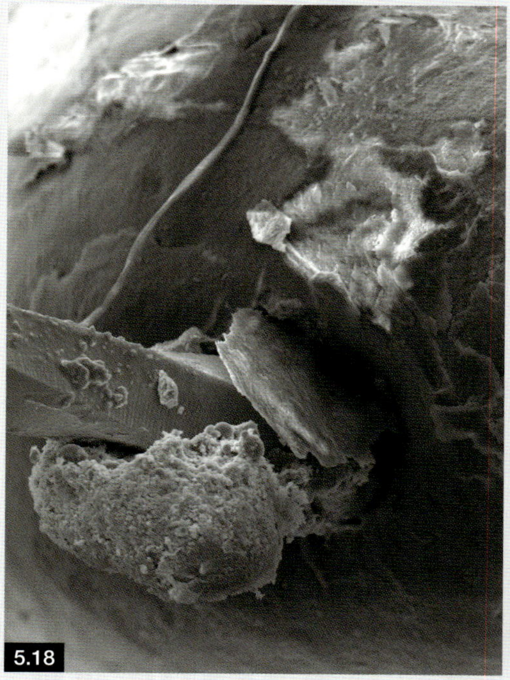

5.18

Fig. 5.18: This electron microscopy image shows the damage that overinstrumentation and overfilling can produce. Dentin fragments are probably infected and expelled, and the lacerations of the entire contour of the foramen are visible. Overinstrumentation almost always corresponds with overfilling.

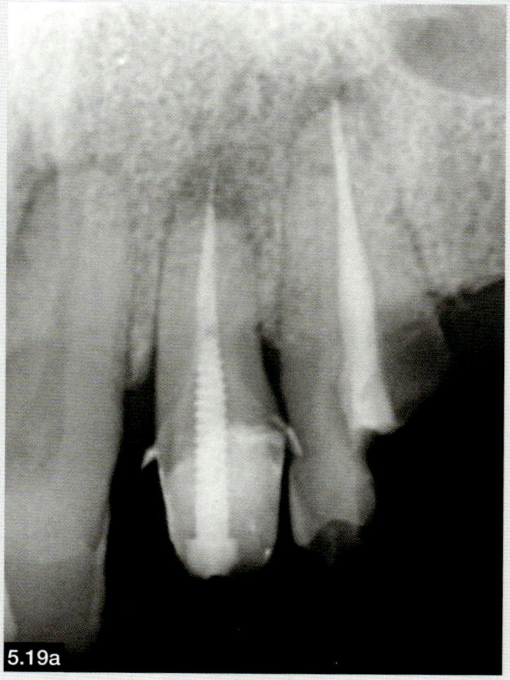

5.19a

1. Schaeffer MA, White RR, Walton RE. *Determining the optimal obturation length: a meta-analysis of literature*. J Endod. 2005;31:271–4.
2. Sjögren U, Hagglund B, Sundqvist G, Wing K. *Factors affecting the long-term results of endodontic treatment*. J Endod. 1990;16:498–504.
3. Ricucci D, Russo J, Rutberg M, et al. *A prospective cohort study of endodontic treatments of 1,369 root canals: results after 5 years*. Oral Surg Oral Med Oral Pathol Oral Radiol Endod. 2011;112:825–42.
4. American Association of Endodontists. *Glossary of terms used in endodontics*. 4th ed. Chicago (IL): American Association Endodontists. 1984. p 10.
5. Schilder H. *Filling root canals in three dimensions*. Dent Clin North Am. 1967;11: 723–44.
6. Farzaneh M, Abitbol S, Lawrence HP, Friedman S; Toronto Study.*Treatment outcome in endodontics-the Toronto Study*. Phase II: initial treatment. J Endod. 2004 May;30(5):302-9.
7. Muruz Abal M, Erasquin J, DeVoto FCH. *A study of periapical overfilling in root canal treatment in the molar of rat*. Arch Oral Biol 1966;11:373–83.
8. Nair PN, Sjögren U, Krey G, Sundqvist G. *Therapy-resistant foreign body giant cell granuloma at the periapex of a root-filled human tooth*. J Endod 1990; 16:589–95.
9. Ricucci D, Siqueira JF Jr, Bate AL, Pitt Ford TR. *Histologic investigation of root canal treated teeth*

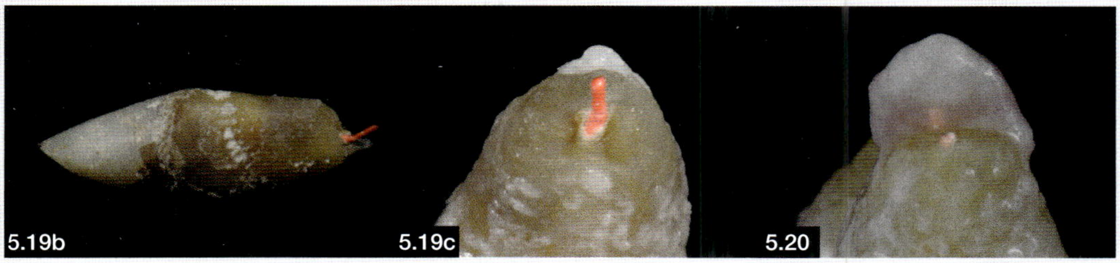

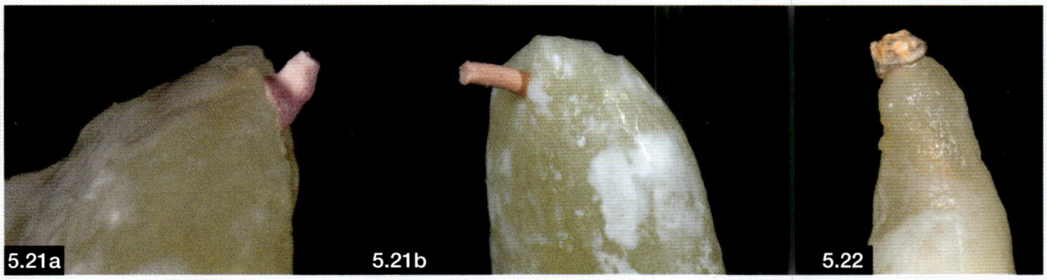

Fig. 5.19a: Image of overfilling with periapical lesions.

Fig. 5.19b-c: The extracted tooth shows root resorption and a gutta-percha cone beyond the apex.

Fig. 5.20: Long cone with connected inflammatory tissue.

Fig. 5.21a-b: Typical overfill that is not radiographically visible because it is masked by the shape of the dental apex (early foramen).

Fig. 5.22: Extensive overfilling due to the improper use of the Thermafil technique or the hot gutta-percha without cone injection technique.

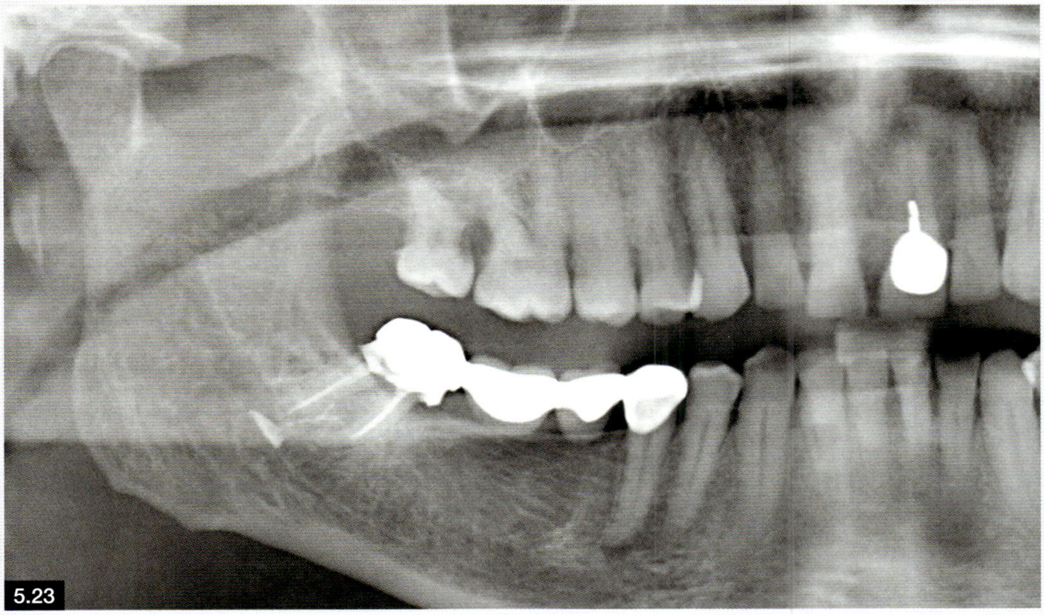

Fig. 5.23: Massive overfilling: the careless use of root canal sealers has led to the penetration of the material beyond the apical limit up to the lower alveolar nerve channel. Such cases can progress silently or generate worrying nerve lesions that often result in medicolegal disputes.

with apical periodontitis: a retrospective study from twenty-four patients. J Endod. 2009;35:493–502.

10. Siqueira JF Jr, Rocas IN, Ricucci D, Hulsmann M. *Causes and management of post-treatment apical periodontitis*. Br Dent J. 2014;216:305–12.
11. Fristad I, Molven O, Halse A. *Nonsurgically retreated root filled teeth–radiographic findings after 20-27 years*. Int Endod J. 2004;37:12–8.
12. Augsburger RA, Peters DD. *Radiographic evaluation of extruded obturation mate- rials*. J Endod. 1990;16:492–7.
13. Deemer JP, Tsaknis PJ. *The effects of overfilled polyethylene tube intraosseous implants in rats*. Oral Surg Oral Med Oral Pathol. 1979 Oct;48(4):358-73.
14. Kim JE, Cho JB, Yi WJ, Heo MS, Lee SS, Choi SC, Huh KH. *Accidental overextension of endodontic filling material in patients with neurologic complications: a retrospective case series*. Dentomaxillofac Radiol. 2016;45(5):20150394
15. Ricucci D, Candeiro GT, Bugea C, Siqueira JF Jr. *Complex Apical Intraradicular Infection and Extraradicular Mineralized Biofilms as the Cause of Wet Canals and Treatment Failure: Report of 2 Cases*. J Endod. 2016 Mar;42(3):509-15

▸ *continue to page 310*

CASE REPORT 6

Retreatment on overfilling

Retreatment procedures often have to be carried out on teeth with overfills; as such, these cannot always be eliminated. However, good shaping and re-disinfection of the endodontium should be sufficient to improve the overall microbiological situation and promote the healing of periapical lesions of endodontic origin.

The case shown here, concerning a complex tooth such as the second lower molar, gives tangible proof of this.

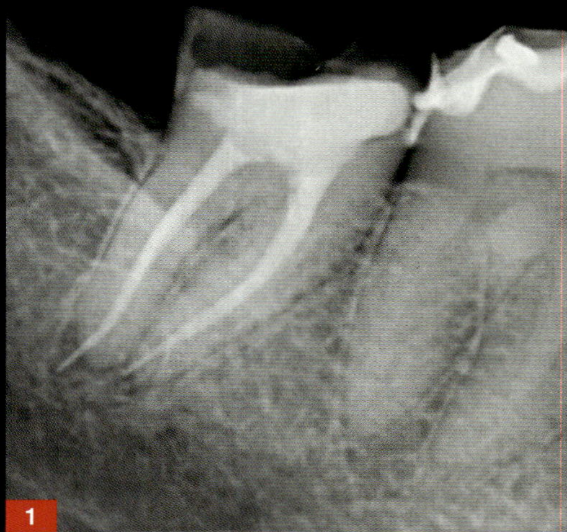

1

Figure 1: The initial case which reveals a franc overfill in the distal channel; in these cases it is not easy to remove. On the other hand, it is an expression of a lack of control of the apical shaping and of an inconsistency between apex diameter and the material chosen filling.

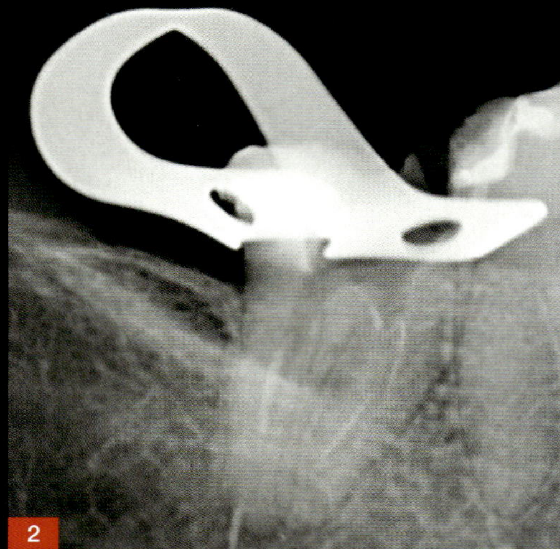

2

Figure 2: Removal of the filling material: the final part remains in the periodontium.

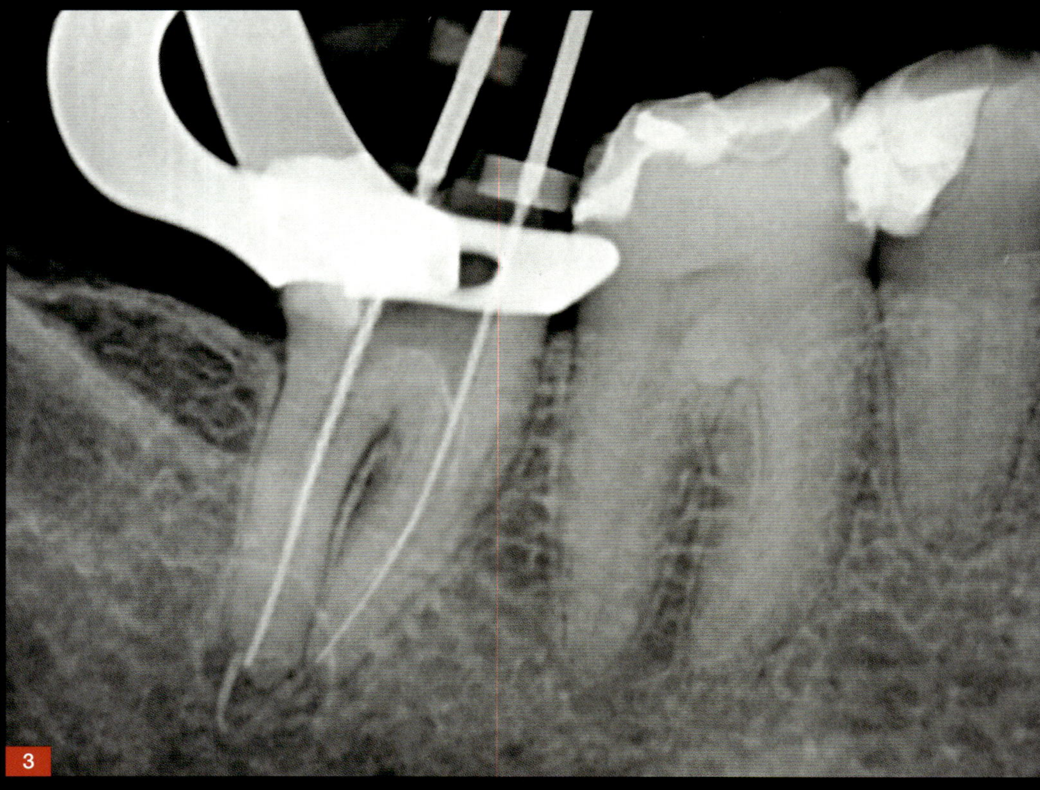

3

Figure 3: The new working length.

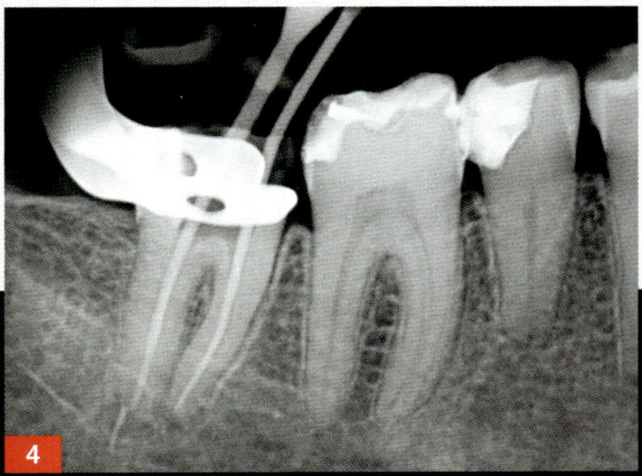

4

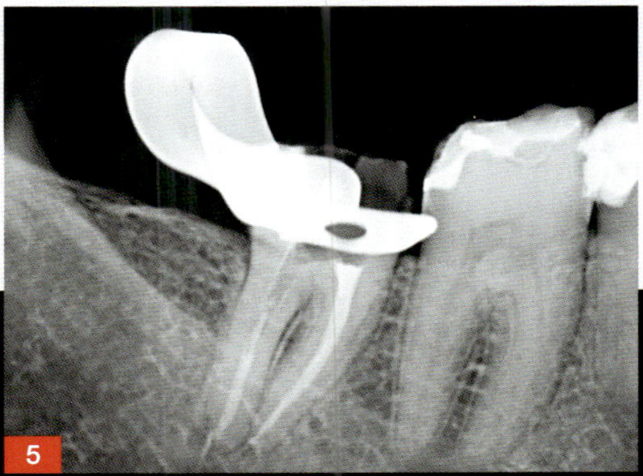

5

Figure 4: Carrier testing in the distal canal and gutta-percha cone in the mesial root.

Figure 5: Closure with MTA in the distal root and with the vertical condensation technique in the mesial root.

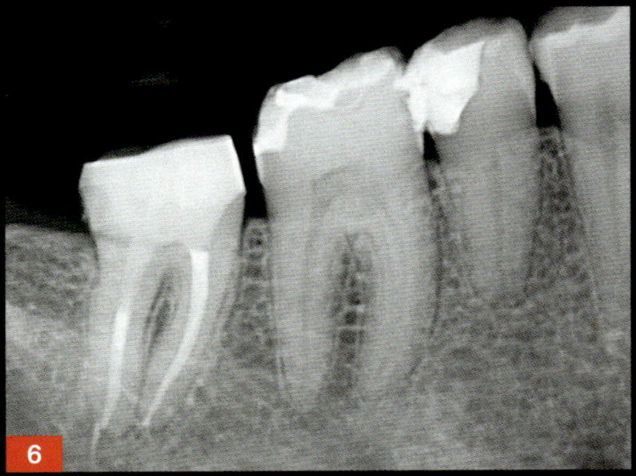

6

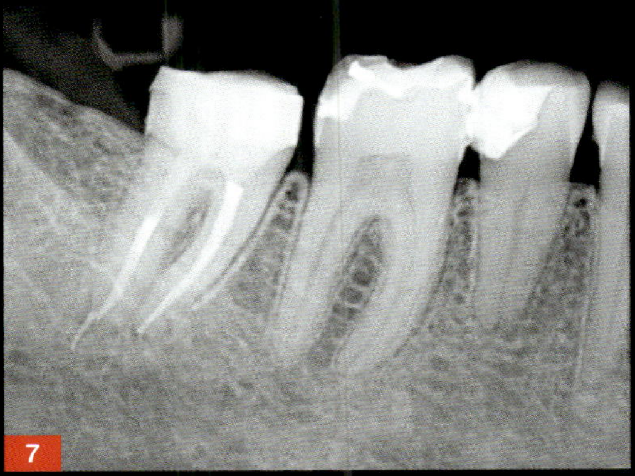

7

Figure 6: Completion of the endodontic treatment with composite reconstruction and fiber post.

Figure 7: Follow-up x-ray at 6 months: a decrease in the radio transparent area is noted and no clinical symptoms are noted.

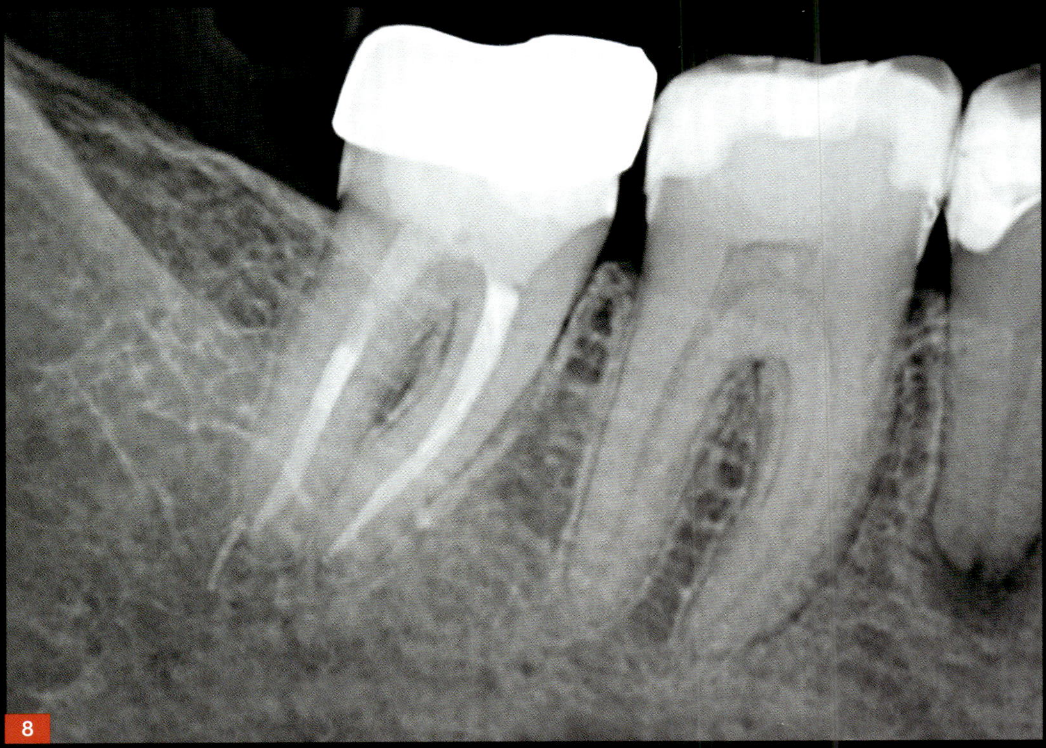

8

Figure 8: The follow-up x-ray after 2 years, in this asymptomatic patient, certifies the good result achieved – note the contour of the lamina dura around the distal root – although it was necessary to compromise by keeping the filling beyond the apex.

Apical plug, i.e. the use of bioactive sealers for the apical seal

Directions

In root canals with an apical diameter of more than ISO 50-60, including those that are larger than ISO 80, controlling the apical area of the filling is difficult. The taper obtained at the end of the shaping procedure is often not ideal, and root resorption processes give the apical portion of the canal an irregular shape and size. With these situations, all the filling methods that have been examined present clinicians with various problems in performing a three-dimensional filling that is airtight and well confined within the endodontic space. Various materials, such as mineral trioxide aggregate (MTA, Box 5.4) or those of a similar nature, whose active ingredient is calcium silicate, have been used to seal root canals with the morphological characteristics described above using an orthograde approach. These materials have high biocompatibility and are designed to harden in a moist environment, and they are an ideal choice for occluding the apical endodontic space in these cases.
The procedure to be used in these clinical circumstances is known as "apical plugging."

Fig. 5.24a-b: a) Size of the inserted instruments showing how large the apical limits of these teeth are; (b) microscopic vision.

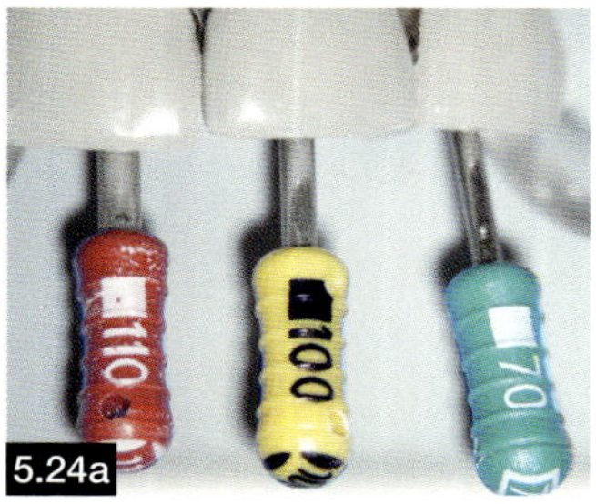

5.24a

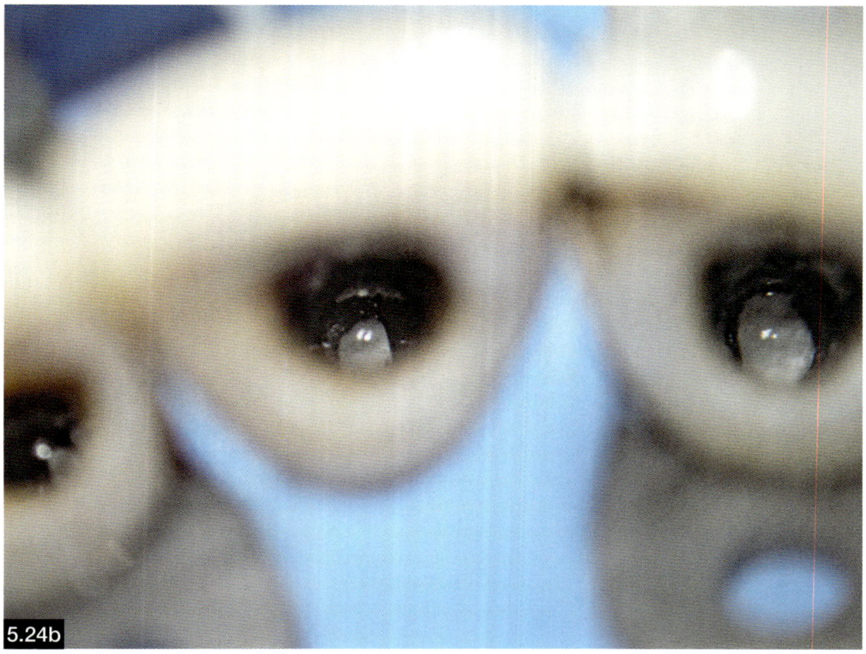

5.24b

MTA, which was developed by Torabinejad and White at Loma Linda University[1-3], is an endodontic sealer composed mainly of three oxides: calcium oxide (CaO), silica oxide (SiO_2), and aluminum oxide (Al_2O_3). They form calcium trisilicate, calcium disilicate, and tricalcium aluminium when mixed together. Bismuth oxide, which guarantees radiopacity, gypsum, which interacts with aluminium oxide, and some heavy metals, such as arsenic, barium, cadmium, chlorine, chrome, copper, gallium, indium, potassium, lithium, magnesium, molybdenum, nickel, lead, strontium, titanium oxide, thallium, and zinc, have also been used[4-9].

Chemical reaction

The chemical reaction that distinguishes MTA is a hydration reaction in which calcium disilicate and trisilicate, when mixed with water produces calcium disilicate and calcium hydroxide.
Tricalcium aluminum, together with plaster and water, forms concrete and monosulfate.
At the end of the hardening process, a homogeneous honeycomb structure constituted is formed and by calcium silicate islands of calcium hydroxide are also produced. The presence of other metal oxides can affect the workability, setting time, and kinetics of a material[10-11].

Properties

MTA is a compound with a strong basic component; the initial pH immediately after mixing is equal to 10.2 and reaches 12.5 a few hours after positioning[12].
MTA manufacturers generally recommend mixing at a ratio of 1:3[13].
The setting time depends on the other ingredients and has been modified to achieve faster curing times, that are compatible with the clinical activities to be performed.

Mechanical characteristics

24 hours after mixing, the compressive strength (40 MPa) of MTA is lower than that of SuperEBA (Bosworth, US) and IRM® (Dentsplay DeTrey, Germany); after 21 days, the difference between these materials becomes similar.
MTA increases the fracture resistance of endodontically treated immature teeth and inhibits metalloproteinase-2 (TIMP-2)[14].
The adhesive ability of the MTA ProRoot varies from 4.7 MPa to 7 MPa when immersed in a solution for 2 months; if the solution is covered with a cotton pellet, the initial resistance is lower (3 MPa), and it reaches 10 MPa 2 months later.

Box 5.4 **MINERAL TRIOXIDE AGGREGATE (MTA): SEALER FOR ENDODONTICS**

This shows that MTA needs to be hydrated to implement its mechanical characteristics[15-17].
pH is another factor that can interfere with MTA hardening. Several studies have shown that the higher the pH, the greater the adhesion capacity.
Studies have been carried out on dental samples with MTA immersed in a solution with different pH levels; they have shown that pH plays an important role in terms of greater adhesion to a substrate[18,19].

Microhardness

Microhardness ranges from 37.43 to 53.56[20-22]. These values can be influenced by a number of factors: pH, material thickness, mixing technique, condensation force, particle morphology, contact with blood, fluids, and temperature, are factors that can be considered. pH, blood, and low temperature tend to decrease this parameter. Particle size plays a fundamental role: the smaller the particle size the more compact the material will be[23-27]. For this reason, many authors recommend restoring teeth after at least 96 h[27].

Dimensional stability

MTA is stable, but pH, mixing mode and MTA type also influence dimensional stability and solubility. During the curing process, MTA undergoes hygroscopic expansion in the presence of humidity[28, 29] and contraction in a dry environment[28]. This expansion during setting increases the sealing power[30, 31].

Solubility

Studies have reported a very low or absent solubility[32, 33] influenced by the powder/liquid ratio. White MTA is more soluble than the gray MTA[34].

Sealing capacity

Since the development of this material, MTA has been demonstrated to have less infiltration in laboratory tests regardless of contact with blood than amalgam, sealers, and oxide zinc eugenol reinforced with the introduction of ethoxybenzoic acid (IRM® or Super EBA)[35, 36], making it the material of election for surgical endodontics and puncture repair.

Antibacterial properties

MTA has an antibacterial capacity[37]. EndoSequence BC Sealer more significantly kills *E. faecalis* in biofilm attached to canal surfaces than AH plus sealer. During the curing reaction, it exerts activity against *C. albicans*.

Biocompatibility

The excellent biocompatibility[39] of MTA promotes cell growth and increases cytokine levels[40]. Histological evaluations have shown that the tissue behavior of MTA is better than that of SuperEBA or amalgam. An in vivo study has revealed that a layer of the sealer grows over retrograde fillings performed with MTA, but it does not form in retrograde fillings performed with amalgam[41,42]. Bioceramics positively affects the adhesion, proliferation, and biomineralization of human periodontal ligament cells[43].

Interactions

The irrigation protocol can negatively affect the behavior of MTA, and the use of EDTA reduces the performance described above[44, 45].

5.25a: The mixed material has a nonliquid consistency that must be achieved with a powder to liquid mixing ratio of 3:1.

5.25b: MTA carriers have a known diameter at the tip as shown on the color-coded handle.

5.25c: MTA cylinders released by carriers of various sizes (from the left): 1.1, 0.9, and 0.7 mm.

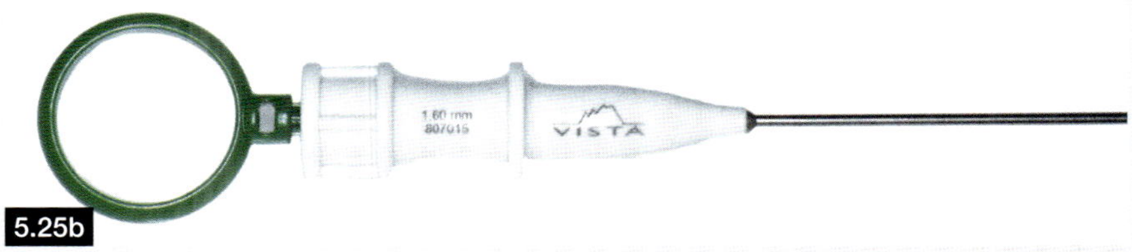

5.25b

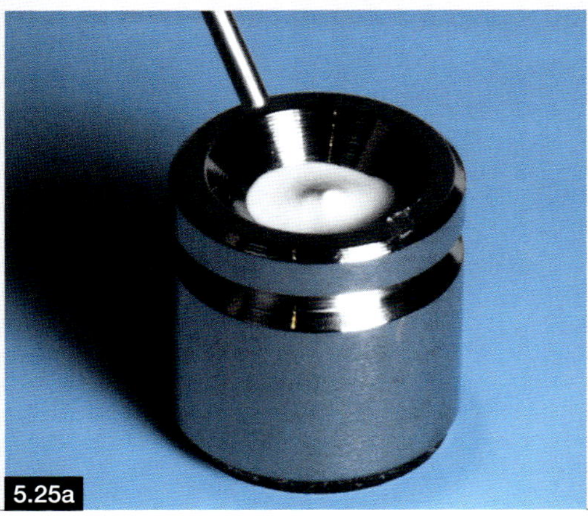

5.25a

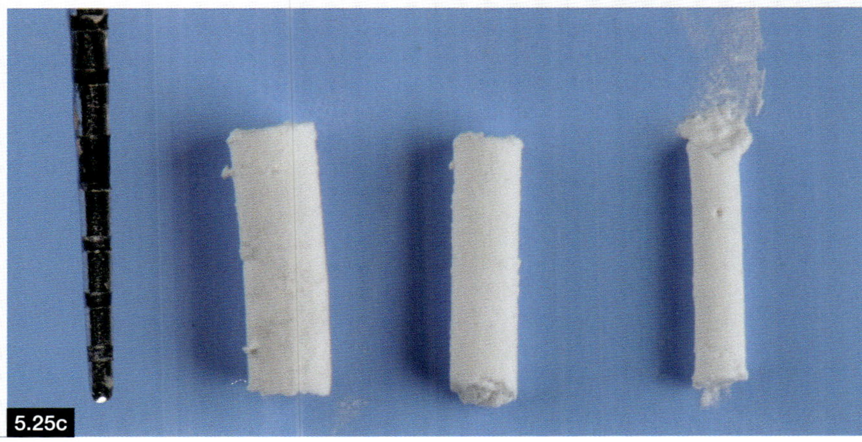

5.25c

Table 5.3 **INDICATIONS FOR THE USE OF BIOLOGICALLY ACTIVE SEALERS FOR APICAL FILLING (APICAL PLUG)**

• APICAL DIAMETER OF MORE THAN ISO 50-60	• PARALLEL-WALLED CANAL MORPHOLOGY
• IMMATURE APICES	• INTERNAL RESORPTION
• IRREGULAR APICAL MORPHOLOGIES	

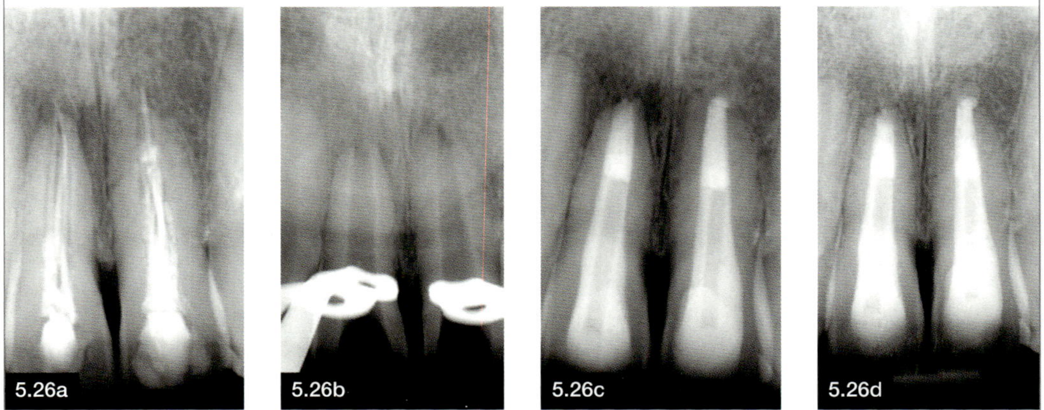

Fig. 5.26a-d: a) Emblematic case of periapical lesion caused by poor canal therapy; (b) the emptied channels show that it is impossible to obtain a taper suitable for containing any traditional filling; c) the apical caps in MTA with the subsequent positioning of fiber posts; (d) the 2-year follow-up confirming the success of the case.

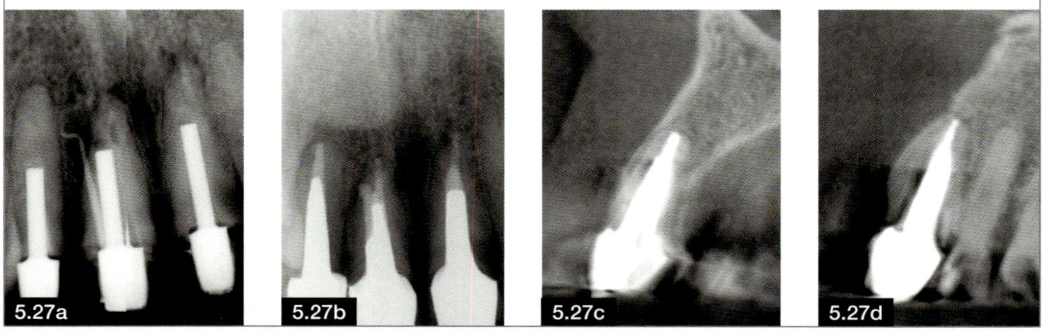

Fig. 5.27a-d:
a) Multiple periapical lesions complicated by the presence of pins and false paths;
b) channels filled with MTA apical plugs and metal posts;
c-d) CBCT evaluation confirming the effectiveness of the treatment performed.

Filling technique with an apical plug

The clinical conditions for this filling type are peculiar but frequent in retreatment cases. If the chosen material is MTA or a homologous calcium silicate sealer, it is important to consider a disadvantage represented by difficulties handling the material because it has a "wet sand" consistency, and conveying it into canals is not easy.
Some instruments have been designed, but their use has been limited to surgery only since they were conceived.
Subsequently, Giovarruscio et al.[60] developed an MTA transport system that applies instruments usually used for surgical endodontics, associated with the use of the plastic Thermafil carrier (Maillefer, Switzerland) as a plugger. Another similar and more versatile system is a micro apical placement system (MAP, Produits Dentaires SA, Switzerland).
The system is equipped with tips dedicated to different clinical situations in orthograde and surgical endodontics. The MAP system consists of a steel applicator with a piston composed of a terminal bayonet through which a plastic plunger that pushes the material is inserted and a screw connection through which a tip specific to each clinical situation is inserted. Straight or slightly curved inserts are used for orthograde endodontics. An elastic NiTi tip, which can be easily shaped manually, returns to its original shape when it is heated.
The outer diameters of the inserts are 0.9 (yellow), 1.10 (red), and 1.30 mm (blue).
The internal plunger made of a flexible polymer that is longer than the tip itself allows the sealer to be inserted and compacted inside the root canal.
When the MAP tool is correctly loaded,

a cylindrical amount of material, approximately 6 mm long and slightly smaller in diameter than the outer diameter of the insert used, is released by the MAP tool. Technically, this method can also be used with all sealers other than MTA.

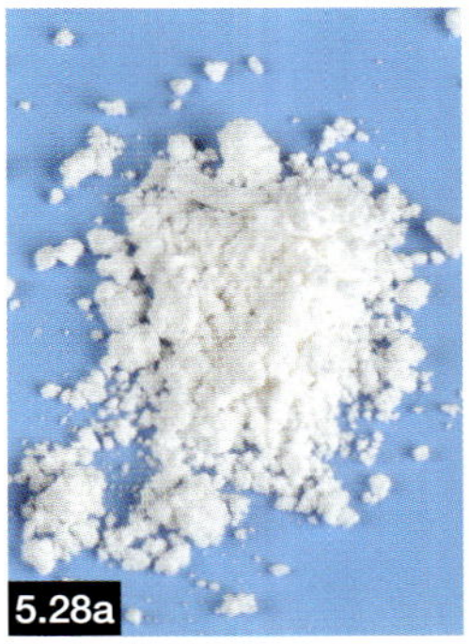
5.28a

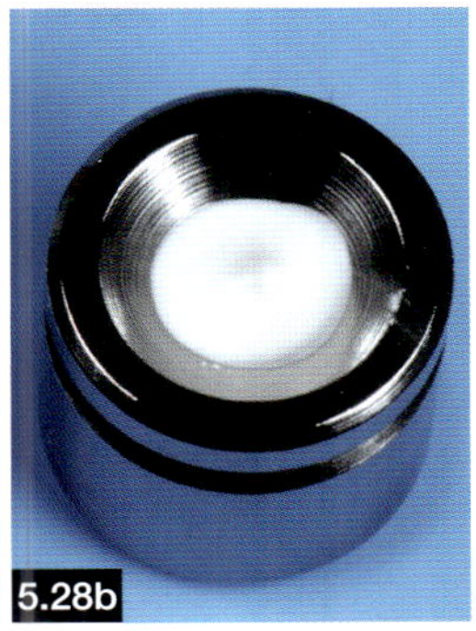
5.28b

Fig. 5.28a: MTA powder before it is mixed.

Fig. 5.28b: Small metal mortar used for mixing.

Fig. 5.28c: Graphic example of the positioning of "apical plug" with a bare Thermafil system carrier.

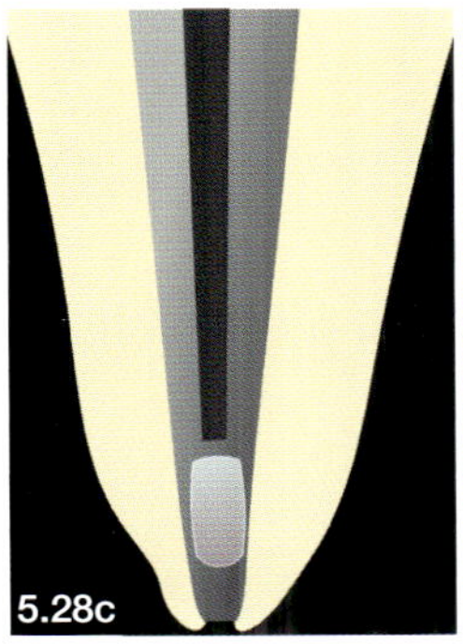
5.28c

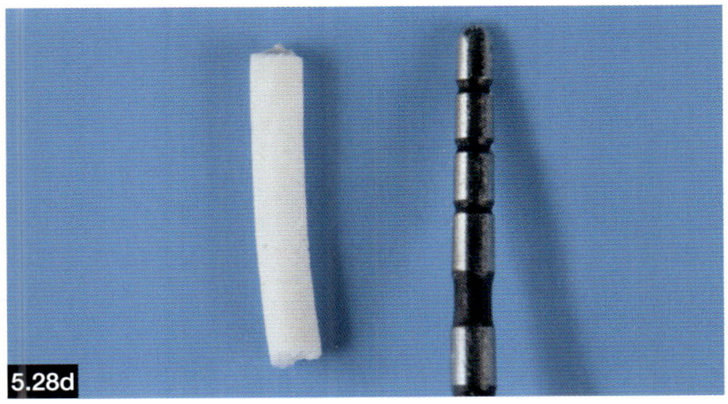
5.28d

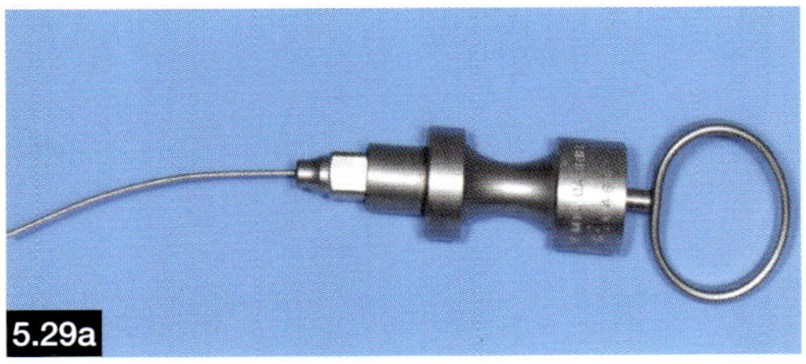
5.29a

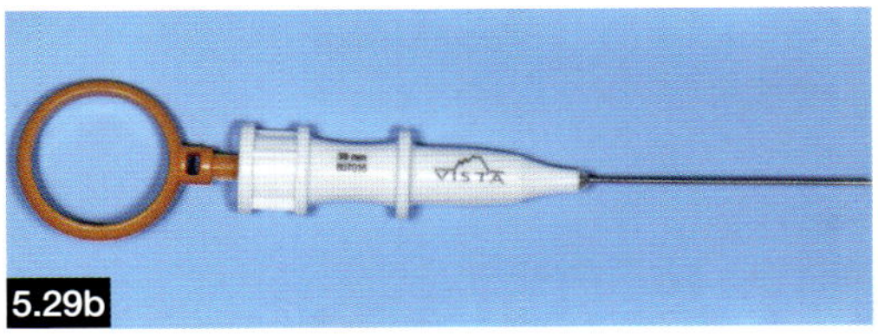
5.29b

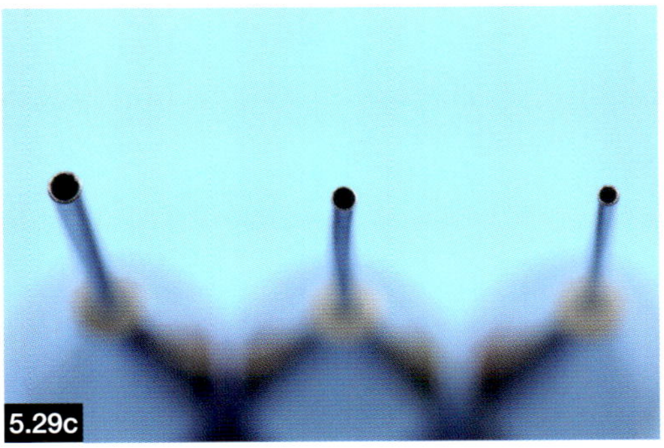
5.29c

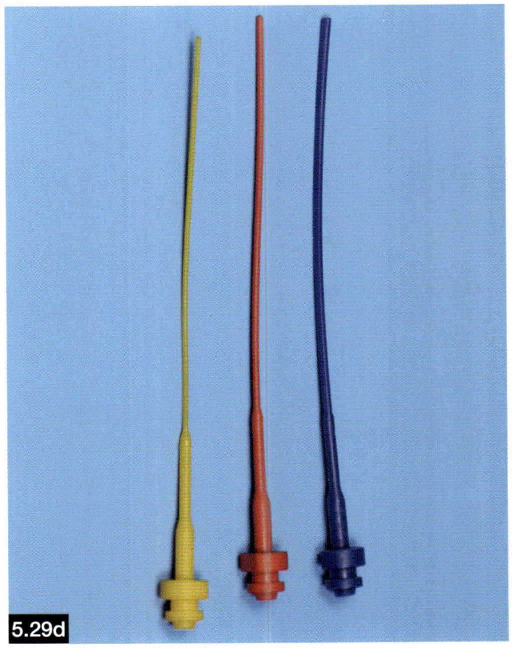
5.29d

Fig. 5.28d: MTA cylinder produced by the MAP system with a red tip.

Fig. 5.29a-b: Two examples of MTA carriers.

Fig. 5.29c: Diameters of the tips used in the MAP system.

Fig. 5.29d: Plungers of Fig. 5.29c.

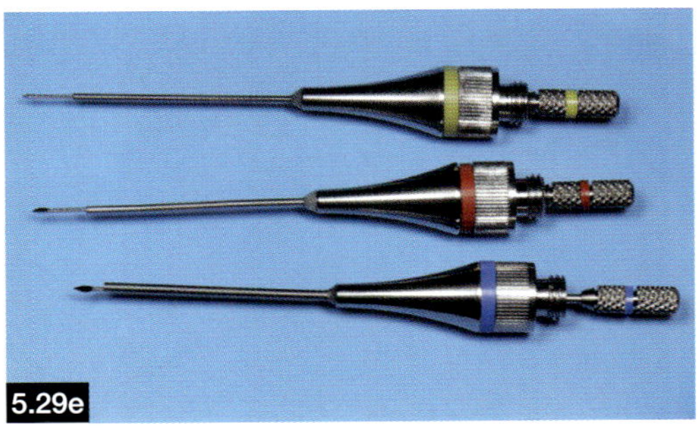
5.29e

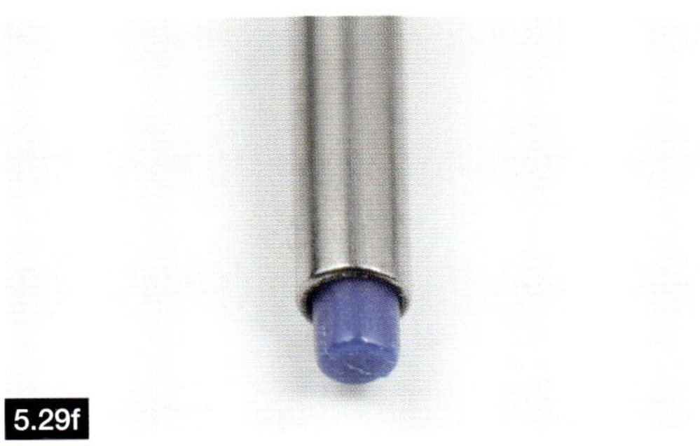
5.29f

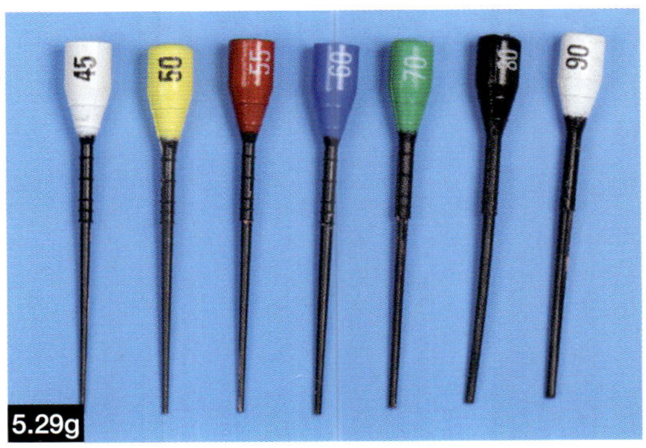

5.29g

Fig. 5.29e: MAP system tips with cleaning curettes.

Fig. 5.29f: Plunger that protrudes from the syringe by about 1 mm and acts as a plugger.

Fig. 5.29g: Thermafil system carriers (Maillefer, Baillegues, Switzerland) for apical diameters over ISO 50; they can also be very effective compactors of MTA inserted in the root canal.

▶ *continue to page 320*

CASE REPORT 7

Complex rehabilitation on central incisors

Functional recovery of anterior teeth presents many difficulties, especially if the degree of endodontic impairment is high. These central incisors have a compromised prosthetic and endodontic situation; synergistic intervention leads to healing, thus improving the patient's personal life.

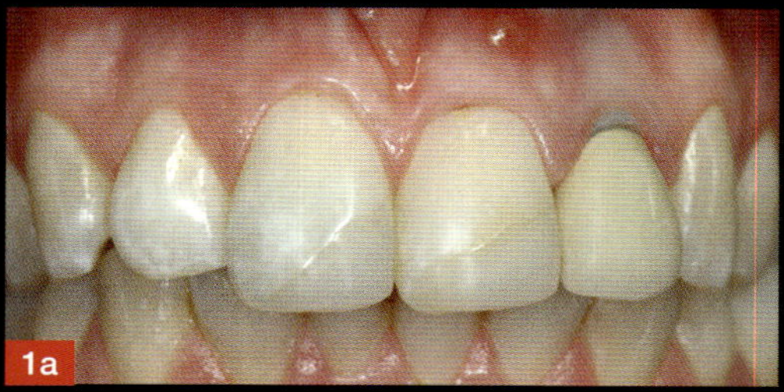

1a

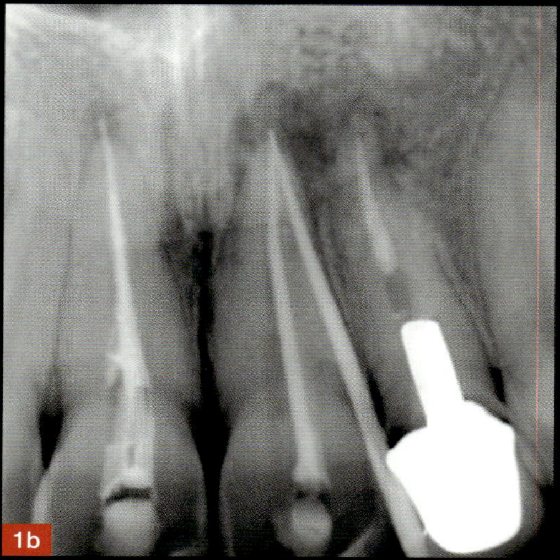

1b

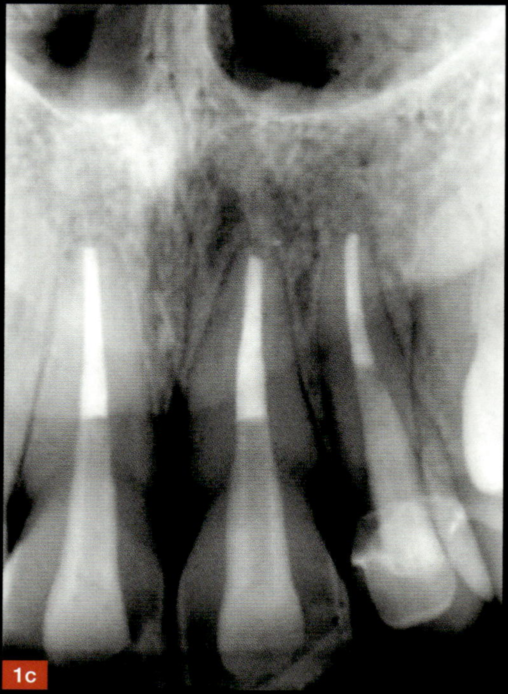

1c

Figure 1a-c: a) The case at the beginning;
b) the radiographic analysis reveals multiple periapical involvement;
c) the case completed with the controlled vertical condensation technique.

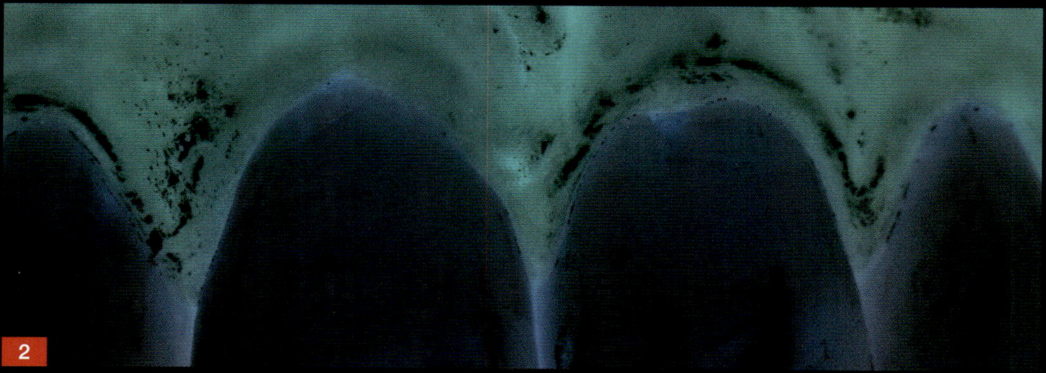

2

Figure 2: The gumline.

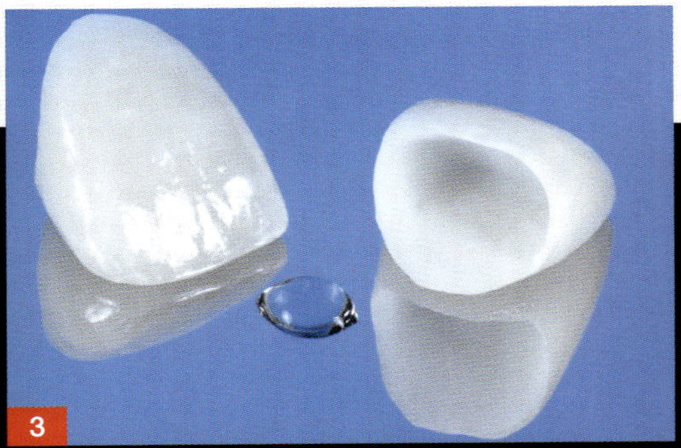

3

Figure 3: Lithium disilicate crowns.

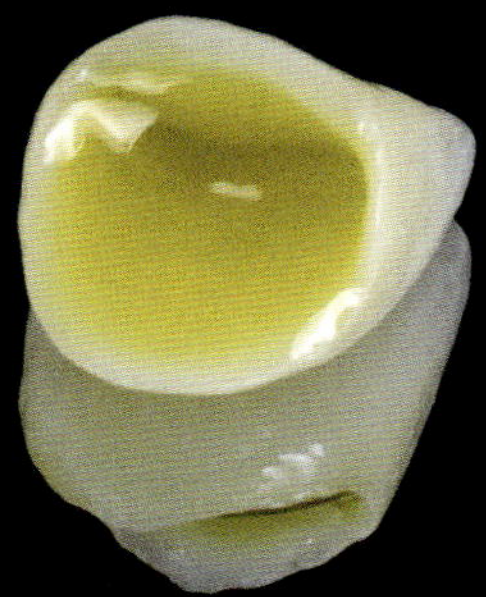

4

Figure 4: Conditioning with 5% hydrofluoric acid.

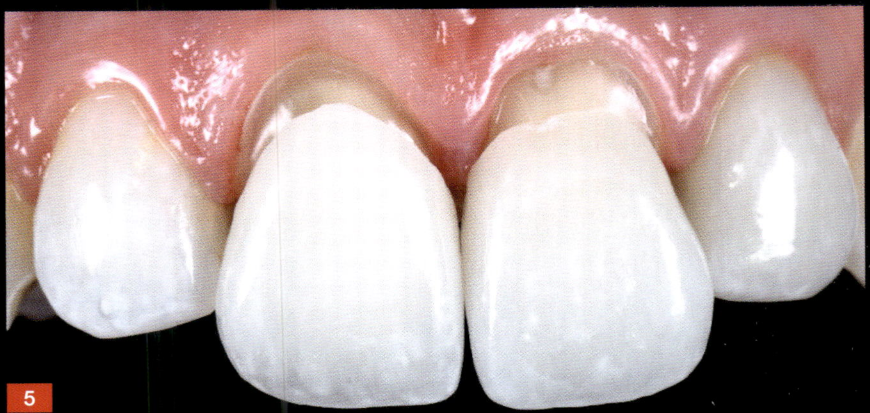

5

Figure 5: The testing of the crowns.

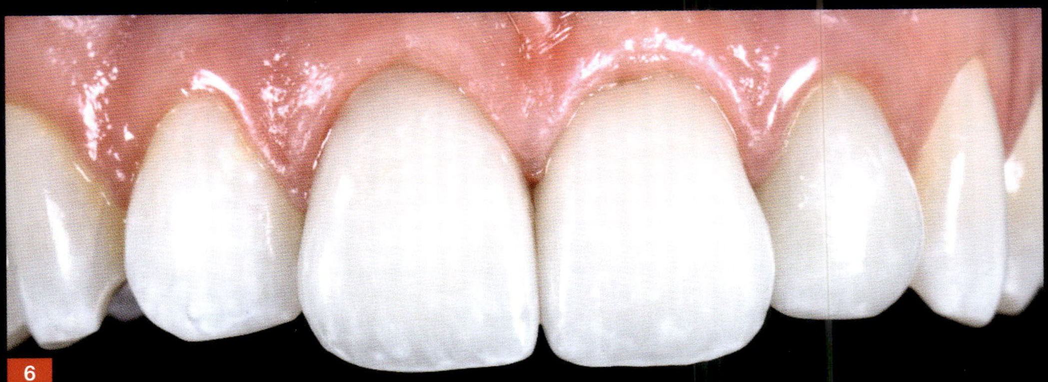

6

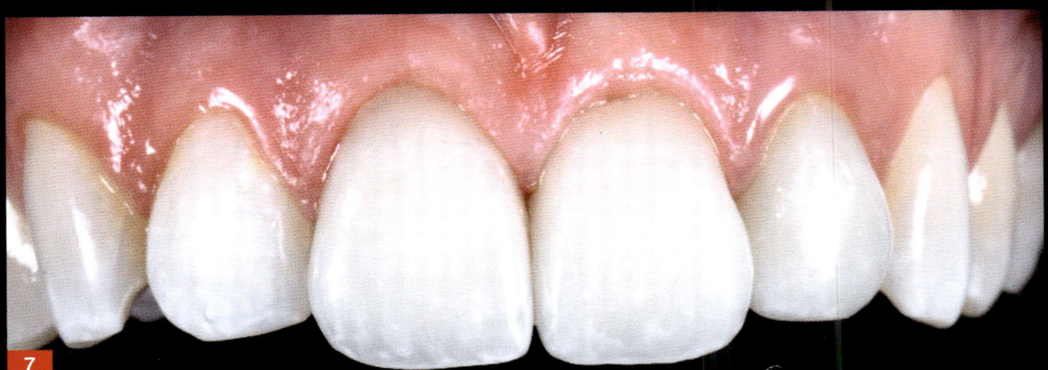

7

Figure 6: Crowns in place.

Figure 7: Follow-up after 2 years.

CASE REPORT 8

Complex retreatment of canal erosion on lower molar

Erosion, also known as stripping, of the inner surface of the mesial roots of the lower molars is a major complication. These lesions should always be suspected when there is a lesion of the intraradicular furcation. In this case, the deep endodontic space is closed before the erosion is sealed.

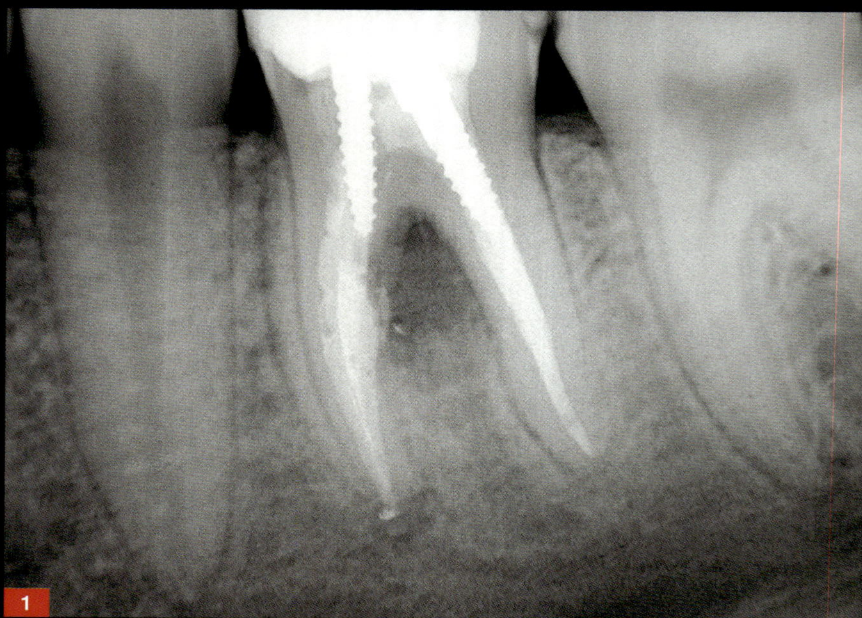

1

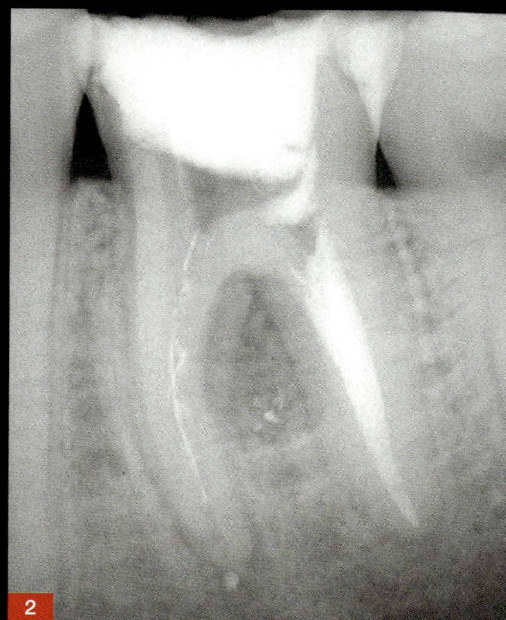

2

Figure 1: Preoperative X-ray of the first lower left molar. The introduction of the screw caused a perforation in a canal of the mesial root. There is a bifurcation lesion and a fistulous vestibular path.

Figure 2: The screws were removed and the channels of the mesial root were medicated with calcium iodide for a week, in order to restore the pH to a basic value.

Figure 3: Cone test. The gutta-percha cone has been partially pre-sectioned at an apical height above the drilling site.

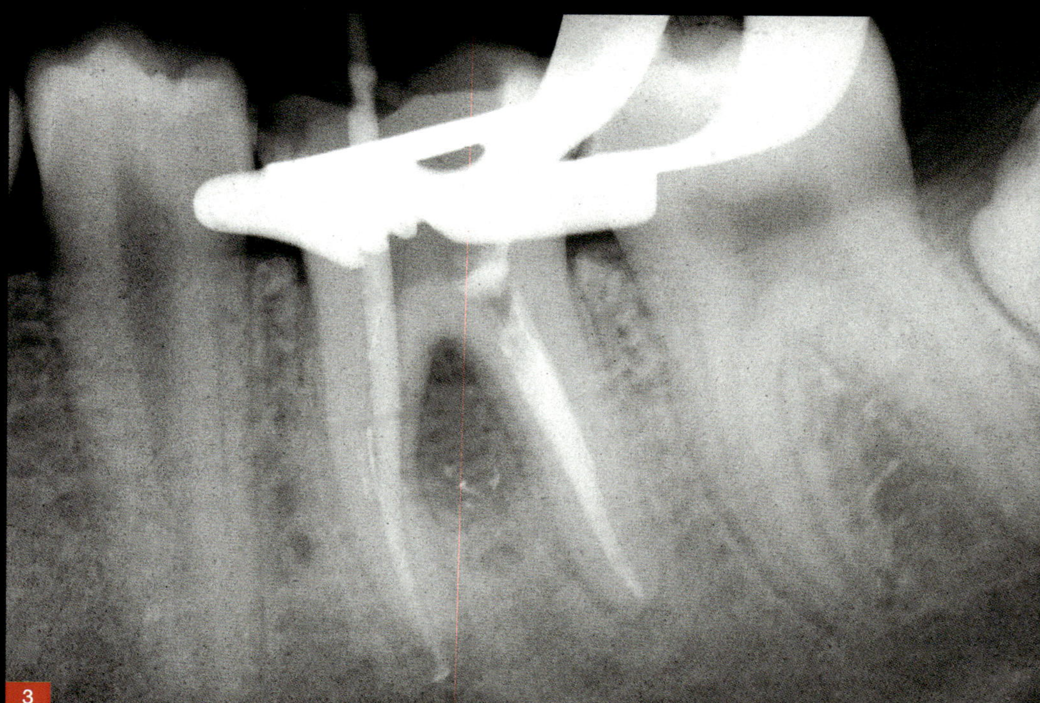

3

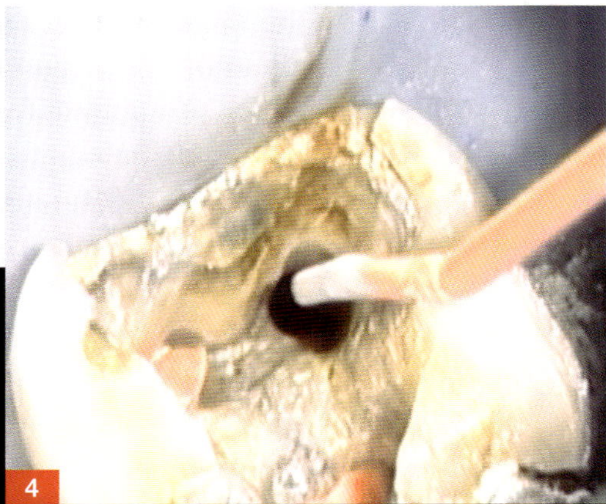

Figure 4: The clinical photo shows the pre-cut gutta-percha cone, covered with pulp canal sealer canal cement only in the apical area and folded mesially so as not to soil the perforation area.

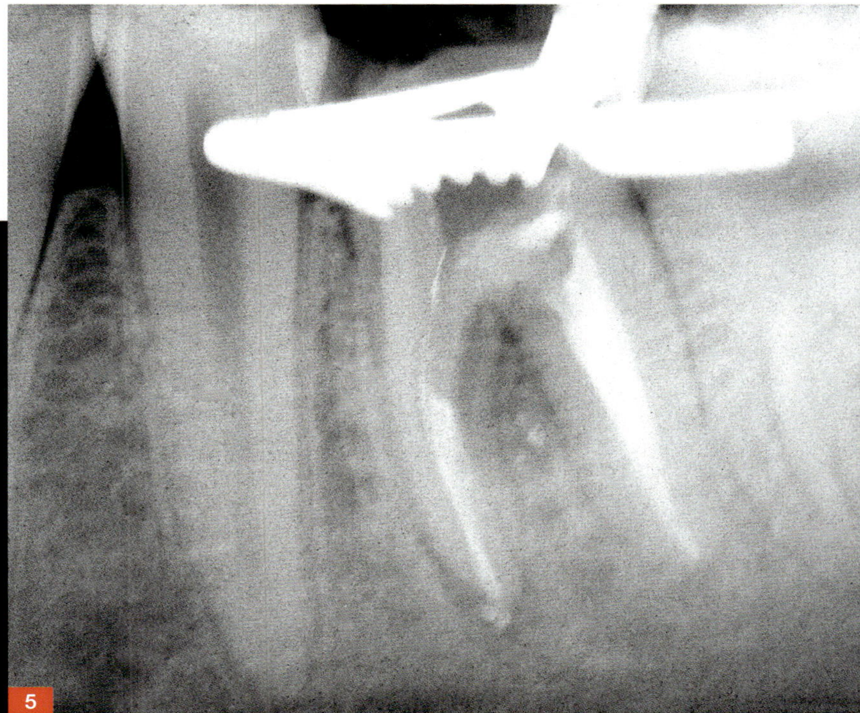

Figure 5: Down-packing was performed in the mesial channels with vertical compaction of the hot gutta-percha (Warm Vertical Compaction, WVC), so as not to disturb the drilling site with cement or gutta-percha.

Figure 6: The back-packing of the perforated canal was entirely performed with MTA gray. The image on the right shows the post-operative X-ray.

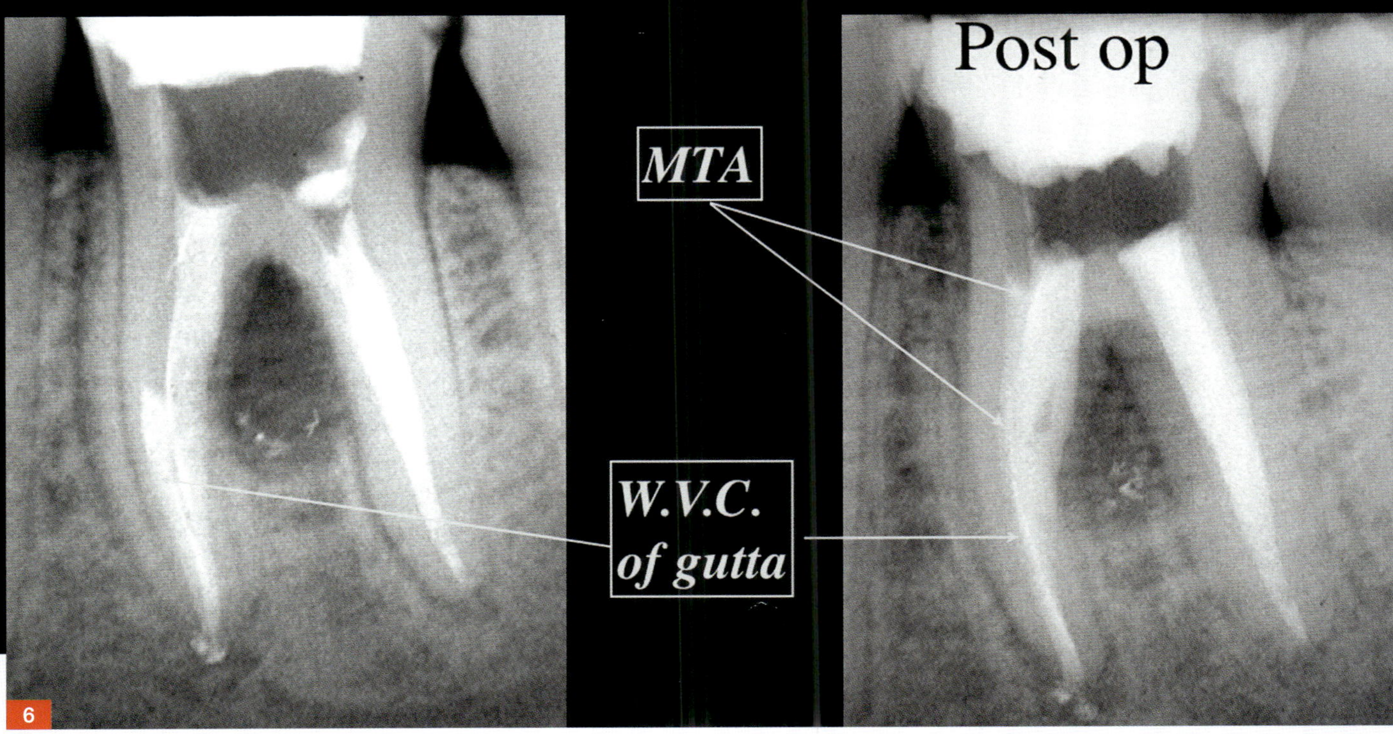

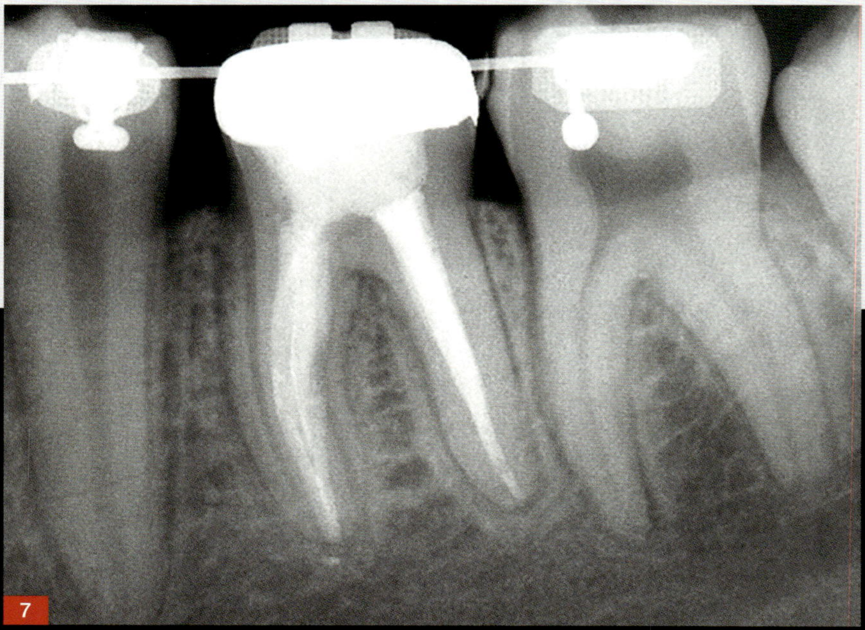

7

Figure 7: The follow-up after 24 months shows complete recovery. Meanwhile the young patient commenced orthodontic care.

Figure 8: Orthodontic traction certainly compromised the seal of the MTA and caused recurrence of the lesion.

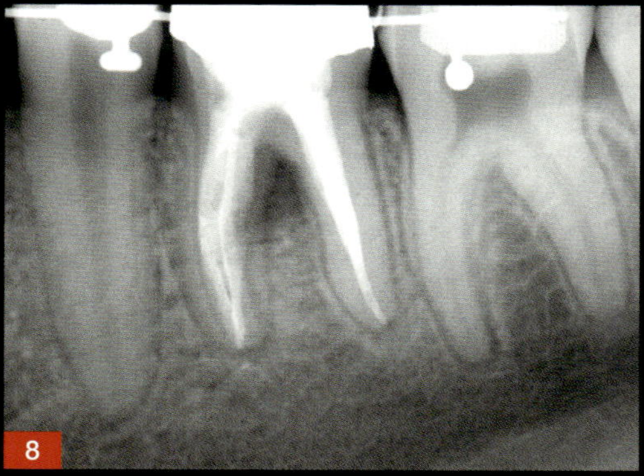

8

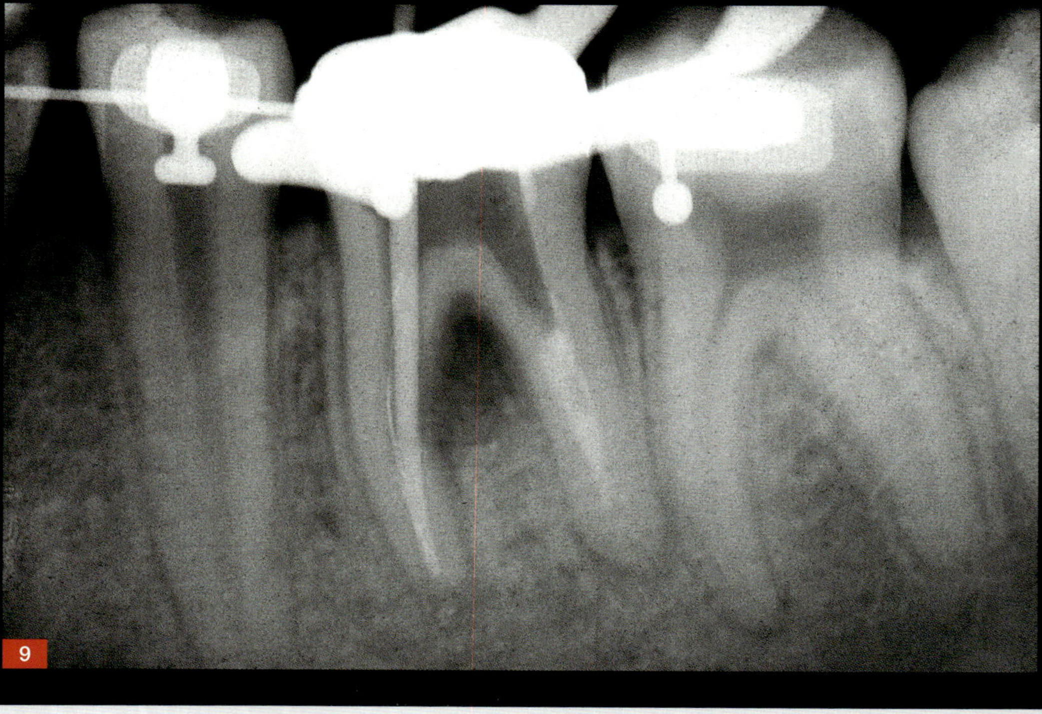

9

Figure 9: The tooth was retreated and re-medicated with calcium hydroxide for a week. The previous protocol was then repeated. The X-ray shows the cone test in the course of retreatment.

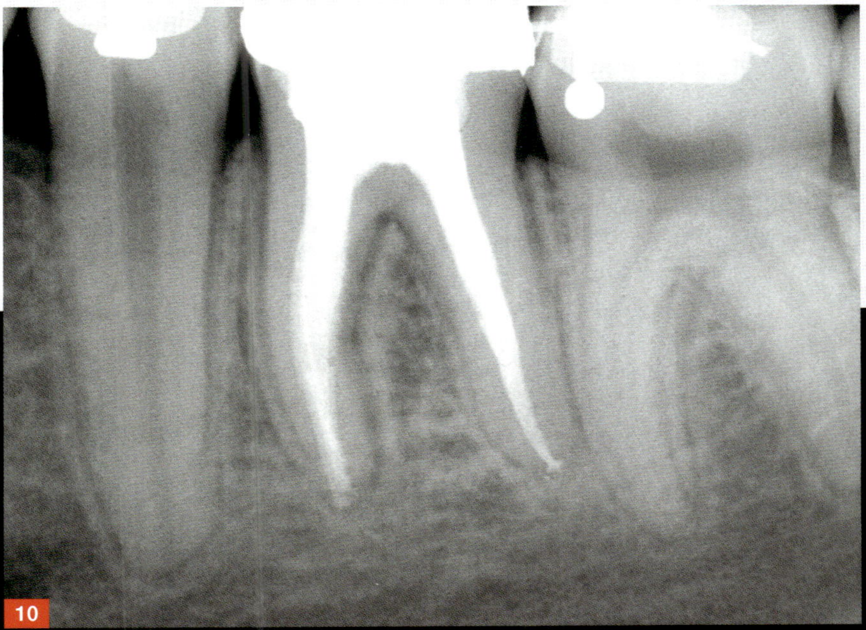

10

Figure 10: Postoperative X-ray. In the meantime, the orthodontist was asked to stabilize the tooth and remove any traction.

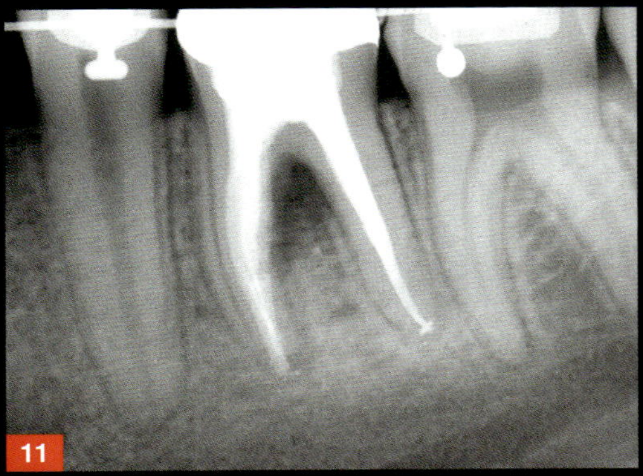

11

Figure 11: The X-ray 2 years after retreatment again shows complete recovery.

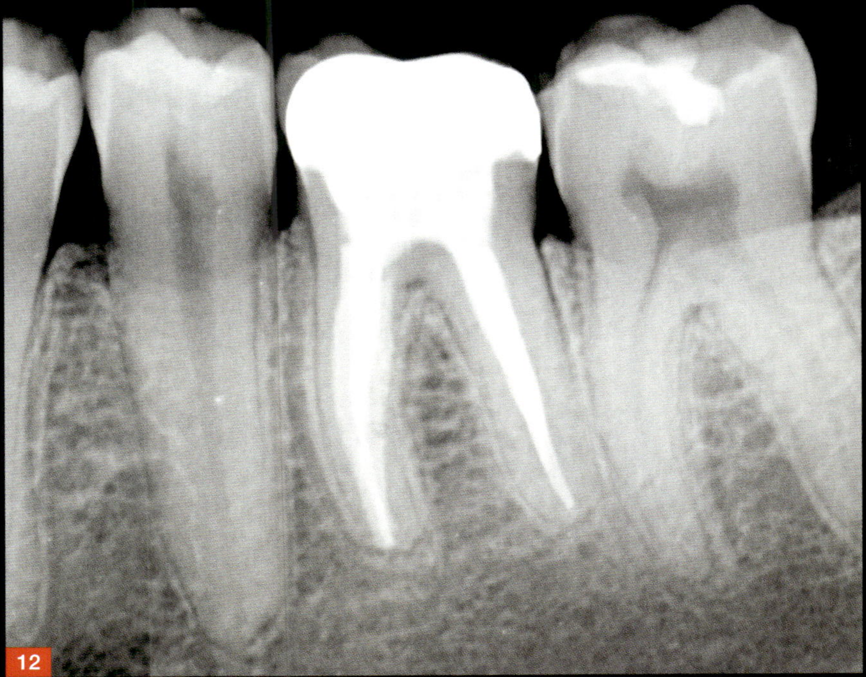

12

Figure 12: Follow-up x-ray 18 years after the start of therapy.

APPLYING AN APICAL PLUG

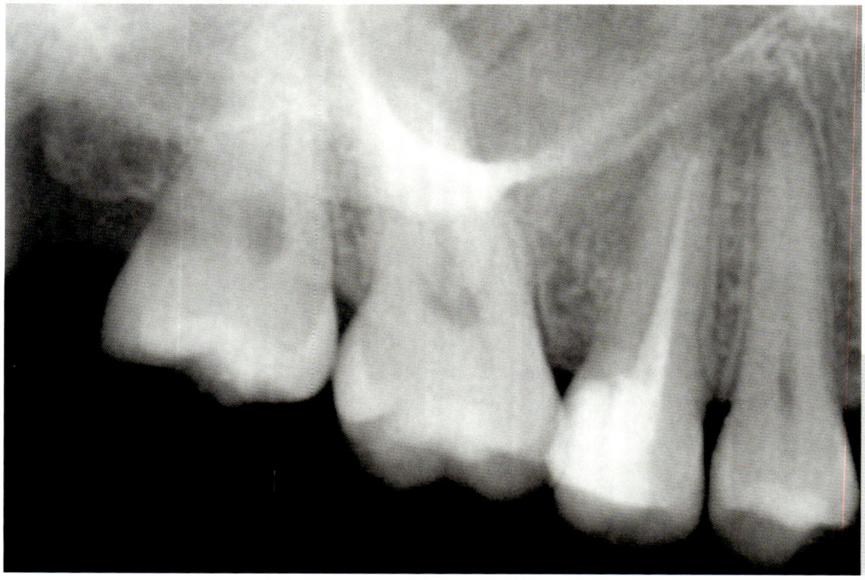

1

A case of retreatment on an upper premolar with a poor endodontic treatment leading to periapical lesions is shown; given the disease, the apical size can be expected to be larger than ISO 50-60, and therefore very difficult to seal.

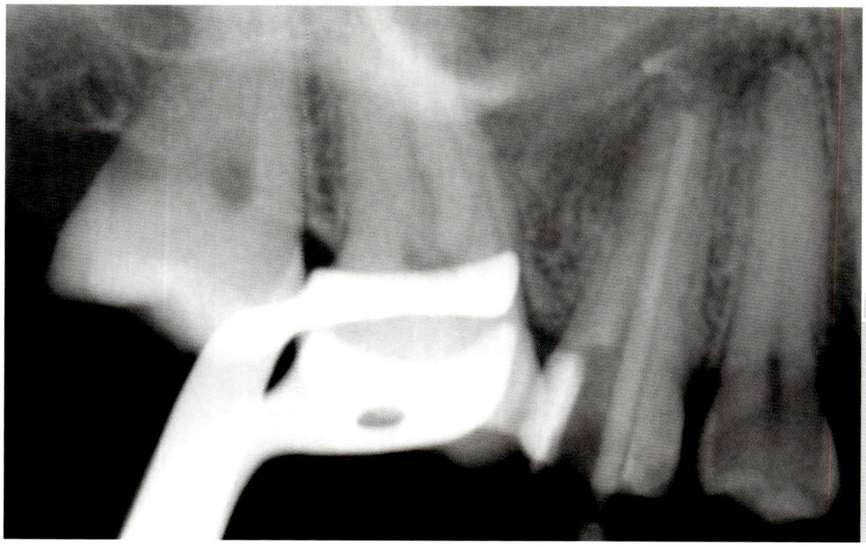

2

Once all the materials in the endodontic space have been removed and all the walls have been reamed congruously, one realizes that the size of the apical limit may allow the use of the an "apical plug".

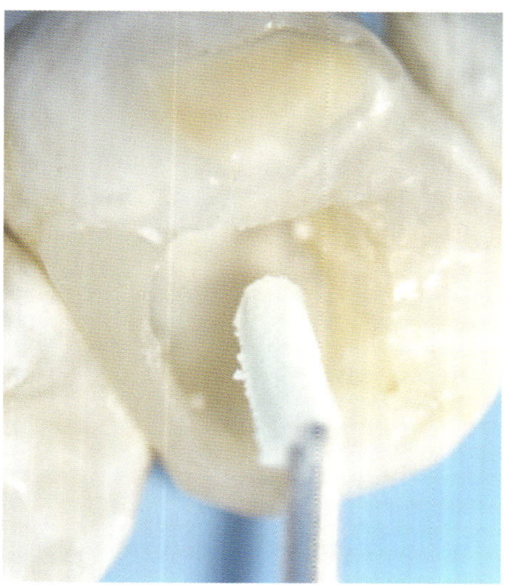

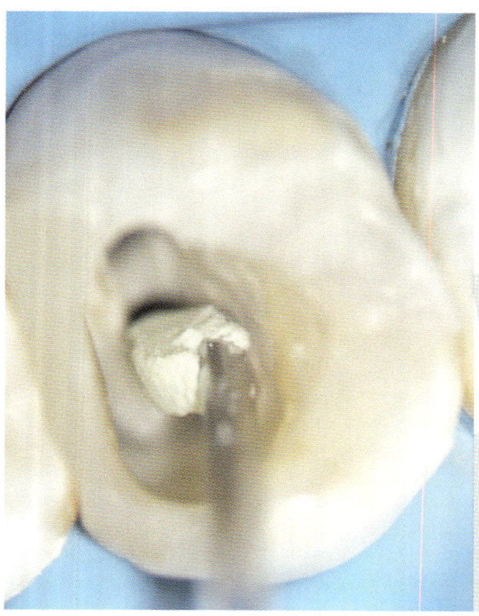

3

The method of inserting MTA into the root canal is quite simple. It depends on the mixing of the material, which must have a such as that shown in the image.

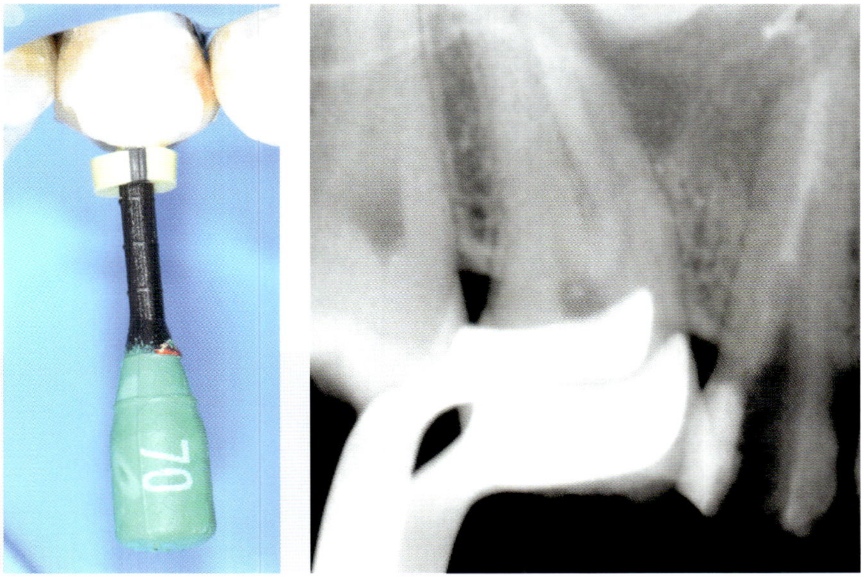

An example of apical compaction with the Thermafil system carrier (Maillefer, Baillegues, Switzerland) shows that the known size allows a gradual and measured compression without breaching the apical limit.

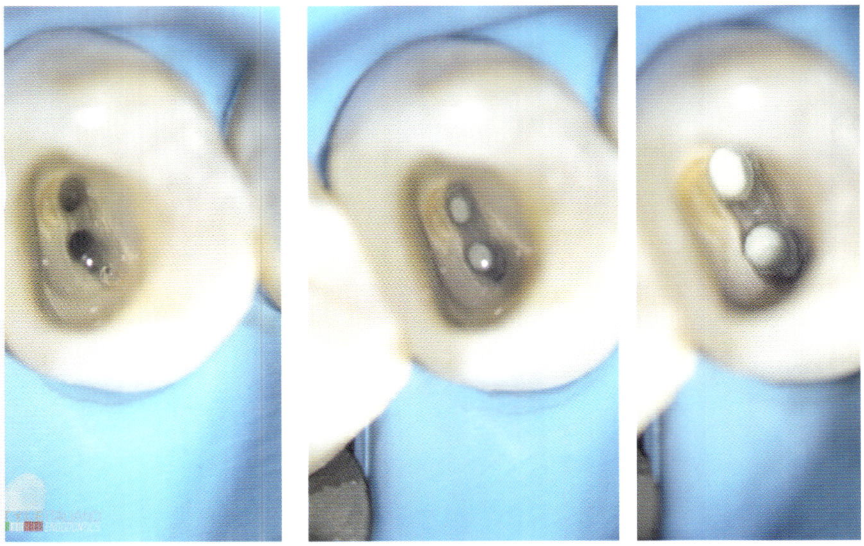

View through the optical microscopy of the apical limit filled to about 4-5 mm with MTA.

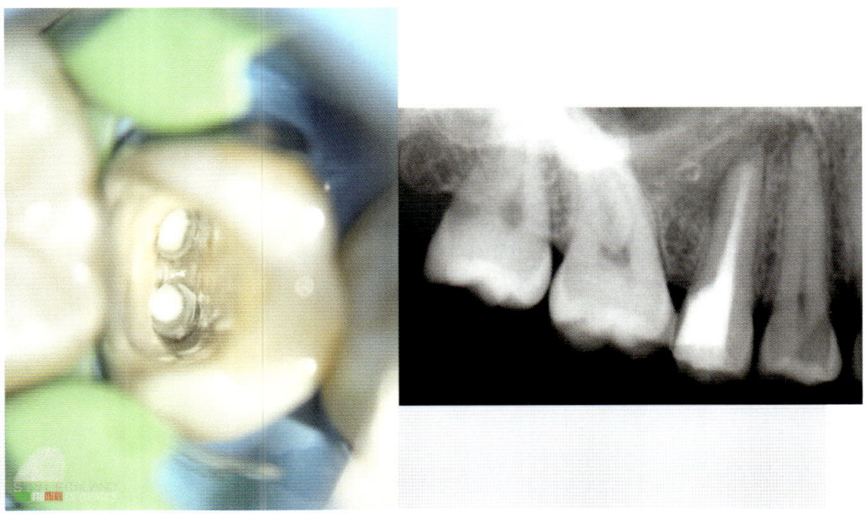

Closing the case with a perfect fit of the apical part and subsequent filling of the rest of the root canal.

▶ *continue to page 324*

CASE REPORT 9

Closure with single "apical plug"

Placing a single apical cap of MTA can be a valid alternative in cases where the root size is short and the apical diameter is wide; the material alone is able to provide a valid seal, as shown by this case.
A bridge that had to be preserved had a clear periradicular lesion, at the level of the anterior abutment; this was associated with incomplete treatment and the apical lesion had already caused overt symptoms.

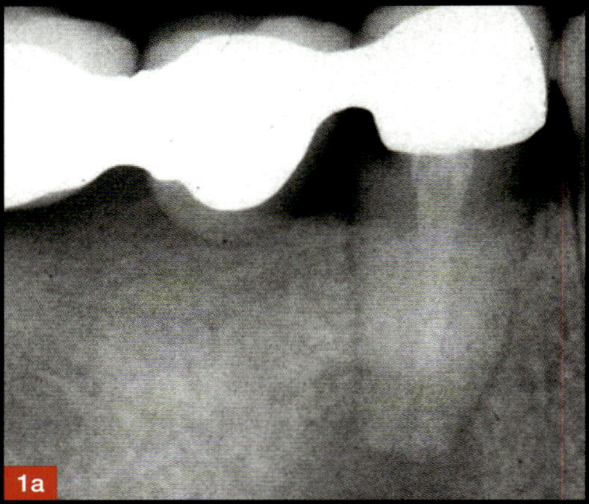

1a

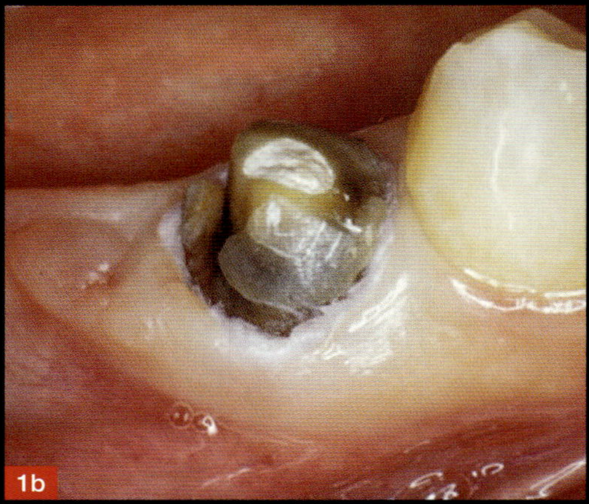

1b

Figure 1a-b: The initial case with the X-ray and the clinical appearance of the abutment.

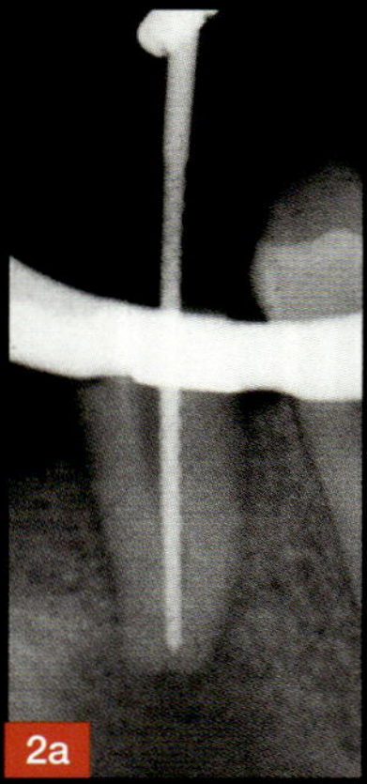

2a

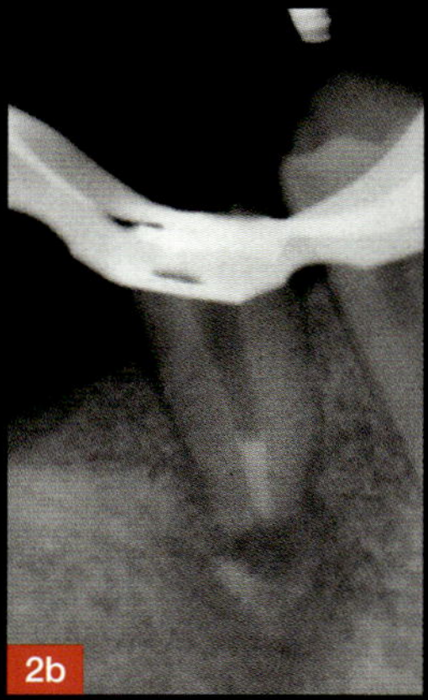

2b

Figure 2a-b: Access to the root apex and closure with the "apical plug".

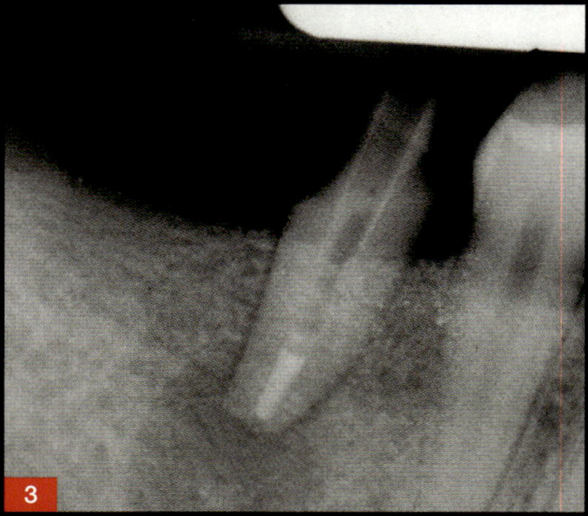

3

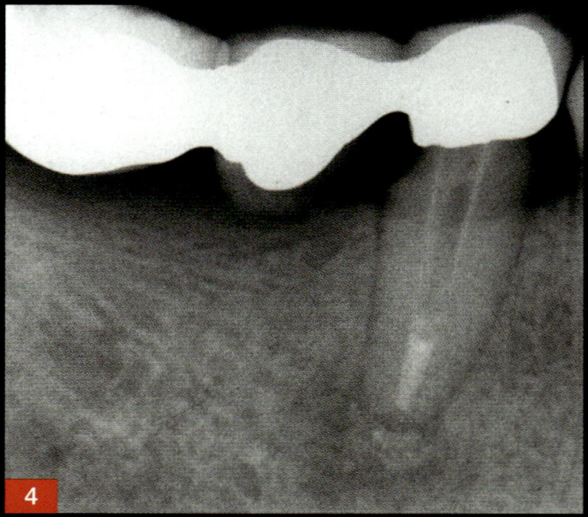

4

Figure 3: The tooth reconstructed with a composite post.

Figure 4: The resolution of the disease at a distance of almost 1 year.

Filling of an upper cuspid with an “apical plug”

CASE REPORT 10

Cuspids are complex teeth to treat due to the size of the root canal, particularly when accompanied by periradicular lesions. In this example, the rarefaction induced the clinician to also carry out a three-dimensional radiographic examination to verify whether there were other concomitant situations, such as occult root fractures.

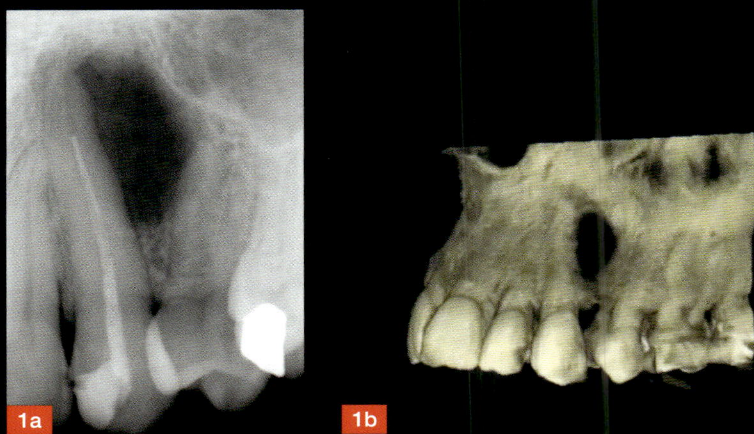

Figure 1a-b: Radiographic examination of an upper canine with evident periradicular lesion in a distal direction; the three-dimensional X-ray confirms the extent of the lesion.

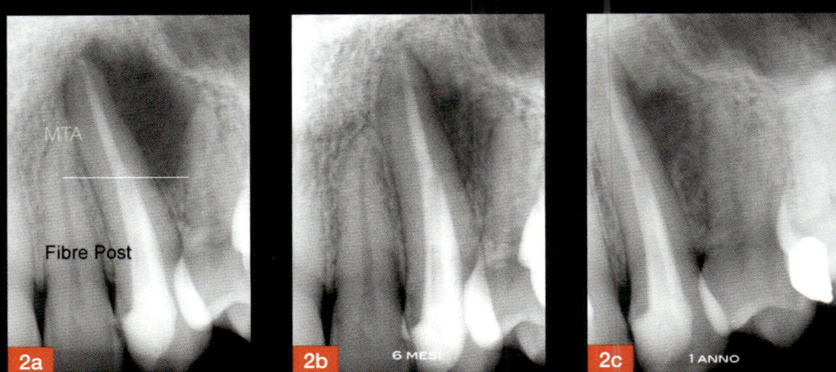

Figure 2a-c: The endodontic treatment is performed with an “apical plug” to which thermoplastic gutta-percha was subsequently added.

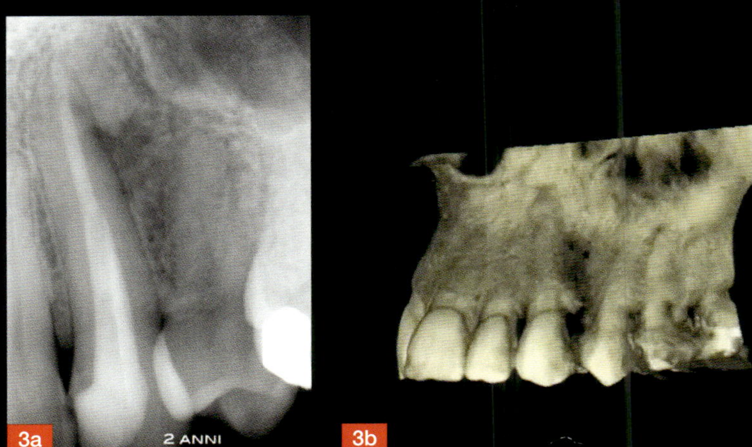

Figure 3a-b: The pathway to complete recovery and integrity ends after almost 2 years with a reconstitution of the periradicular lamina dura verified by the two-dimensional and three-dimensional radiographic examination.

Use of bioactive sealers associated with a single gutta-percha cone

Bioactive sealers are derived, as regards their composition, from calcium silicate which constitutes the basis of one of the most famous materials of the last 20 years, i.e., MTA (Box 5.4) [60-63].
Sealers suitable for root canal filling have been designed on the basis of chemical formulation, with a consistency that can be used in combination with gutta-percha cones[65].

One of the main characteristics is an excellent biocompatibility[66, 67]; a sealer releases different compounds, including hydroxyapatite, during the setting phase. When sealers are placed in contact with the bone, they have an osteoconductive power[68, 69], which guarantees bone neoformation along the surface of the sealer[70, 71]; this intrinsic ability is determined in accordance with the active ingredient, i.e., calcium silicate, and it likely favors the healing of bone tissues in the immediate vicinity of inflammatory lesions because of numerous factors[72-74].
In addition to their excellent biocompatibility,

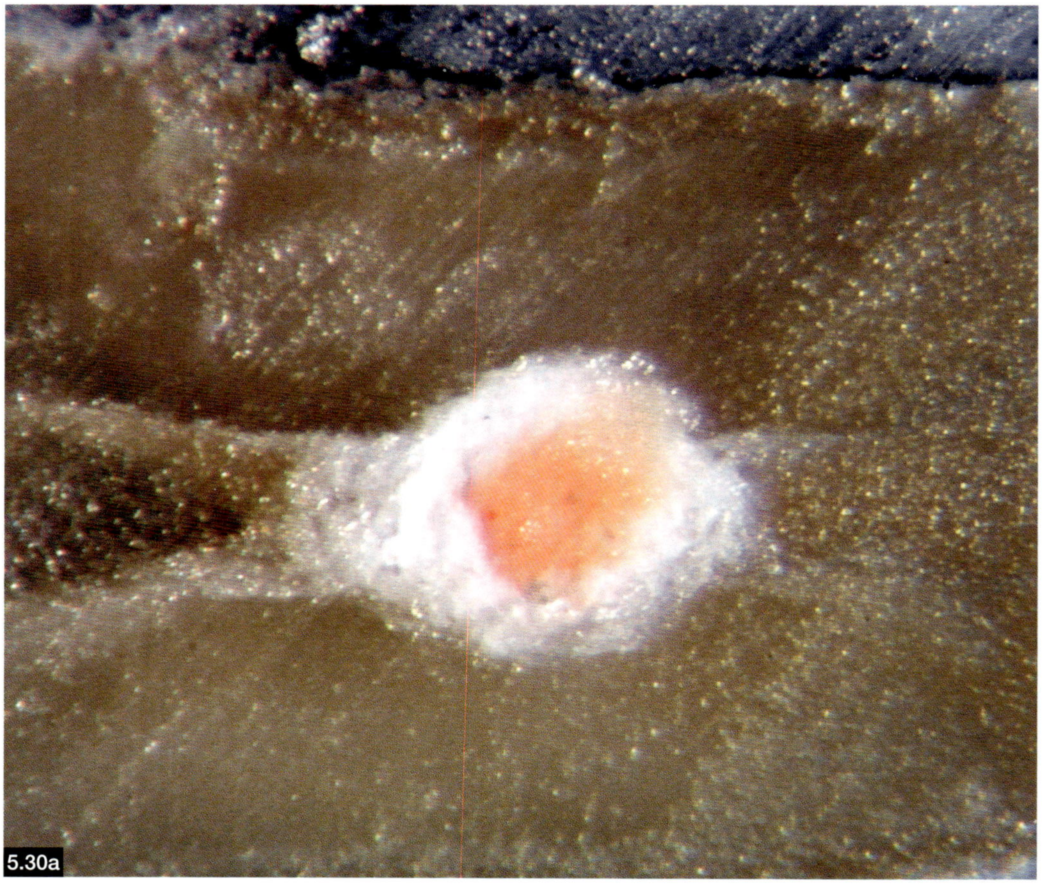

Fig. 5.30a: Distribution of a bioactive sealer in a particularly narrow root canal.

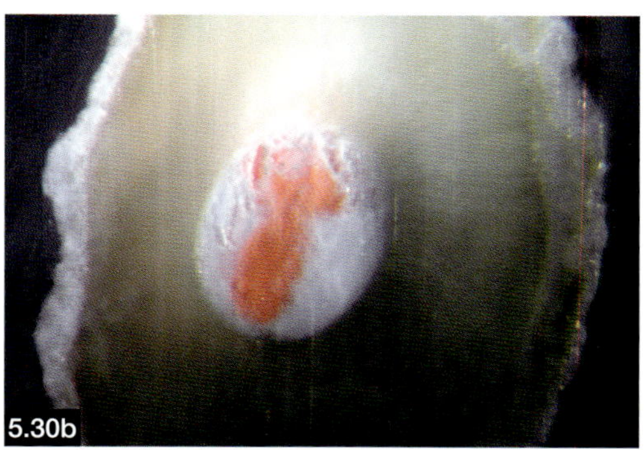

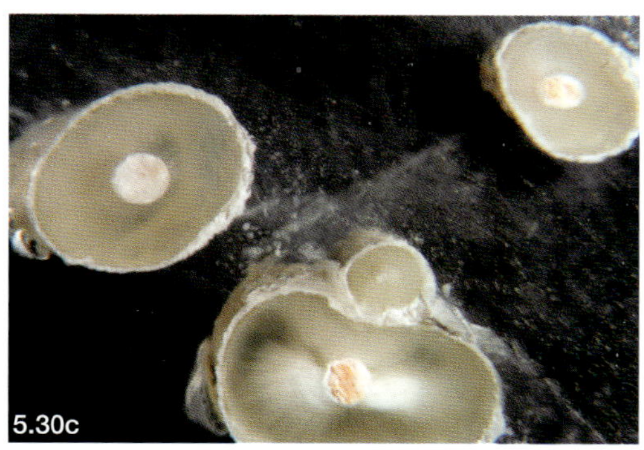

Fig. 5.5.30b-c: b) Distribution of the sealer in an ogival canal. (c) very good distribution in the mesial canals; (d) very good distribution in the mesial and disto-vestibular canals.

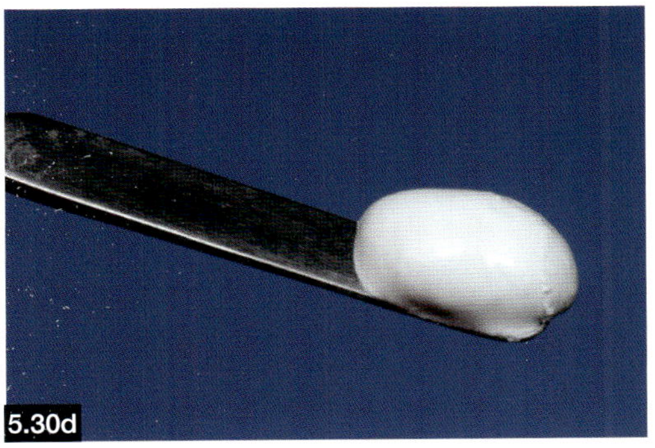

5.30d

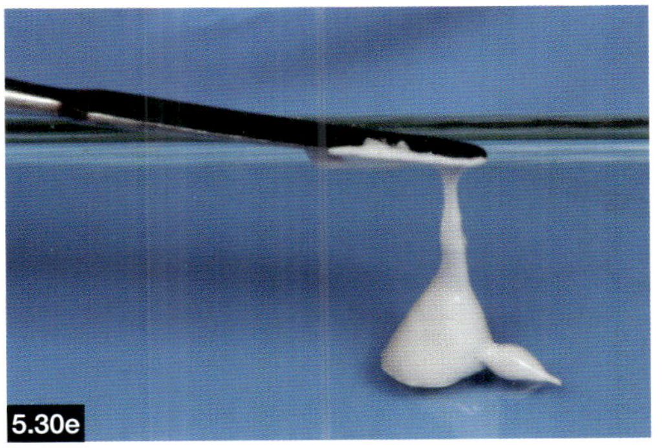

5.30e

Fig. 5.30d-e: Sealers must be mixed carefully, possibly with the aid of mixers for a glass ionomer or amalgam. At the end of the process, the sealer must have a cohesion that does not detach the sealer during traction.

sealers have antibacterial properties[75, 76], due to: the high pH – about 12 – during the hardening phase; the presence of nanocrystals with a diameter of between 1 and 3 nm, which hinders bacterial adhesion, and the presence of some fluoride ions, making up the crystals of hydroxyapatite, which have potent antibacterial properties[77-80].

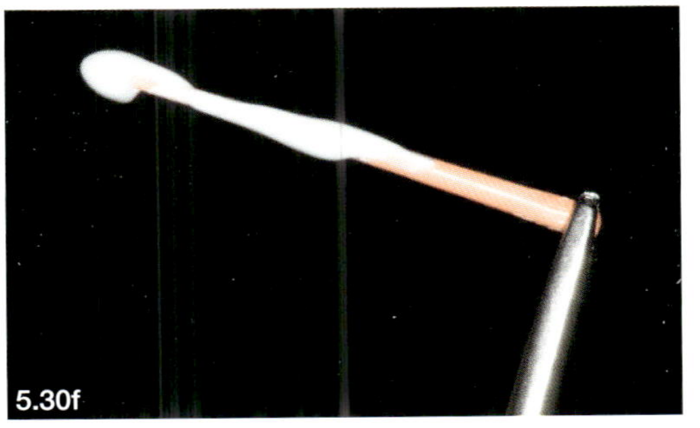

5.30f

Fig. 5.30f: The sealer can be inserted in the endodontic space using a cement-stained cone that must not rub against the walls.

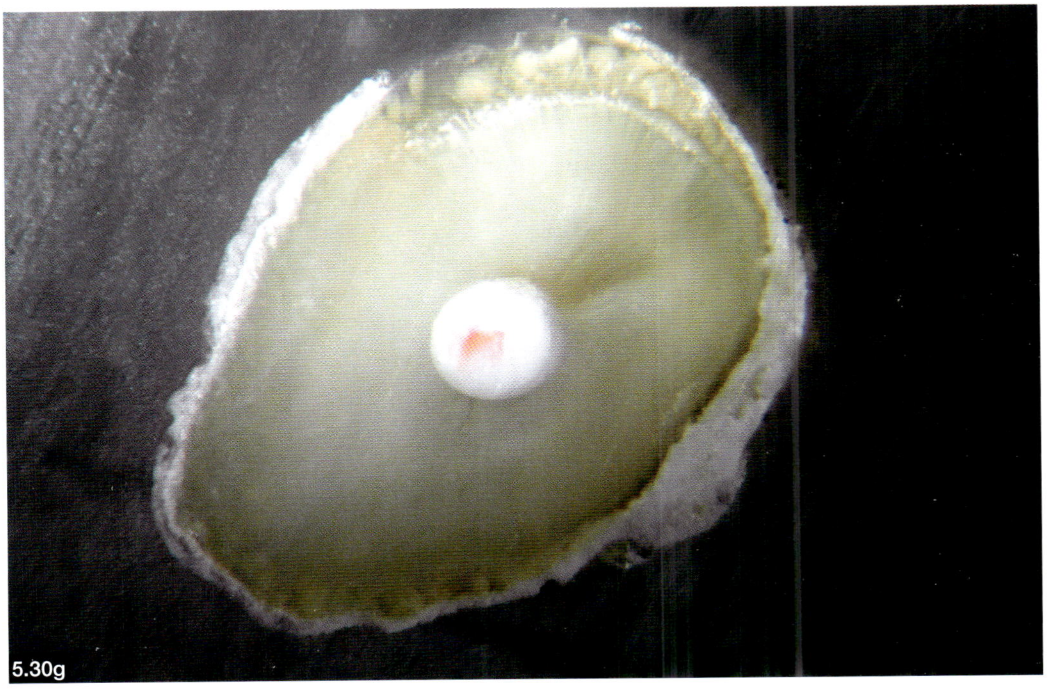

5.30g

5.30g: In this image the sealer is well adapted to the endodontium; it is imperative that the cone has no canal engagement.

Some studies investigating its effectiveness observed it to be effective against *Enterococcus faecalis*[81]. Various studies[82-84] have shown that these sealers are able to maintain a valid long-term seal[85-88], are chemically stable and have no corrosive action. They are hydrophilic materials, and therefore insensitive to moisture and blood contamination, and they do not undergo significant dimensional changes over time; on the contrary, they expand slightly during the setting phase[89-93]. In numerous studies, the structural characteristics of these sealers seem to be interesting; however, high-level clinical studies that demonstrate the superiority of these materials compared with those used in conventional techniques remain limited. De-Deus et al.[48] showed that oval channels filled with a single cone technique associated with bioceramic sealers can be filled effectively in the middle and coronal third, but voids may be visible in the apical third.

Studies have shown that the use of bioceramic sealers can positively influence the fracture resistance of teeth[94, 95]. Ghoneim et al.[96] reported that teeth sealed with this type of sealer associated with gutta-percha cones coated with a glass ionomer layer can potentially have a fracture resistance comparable with that of untreated teeth.

A slight difference in fracture resistance in teeth under vertical loading was observed between teeth filled with the same technique (cold lateral), varying the type of endodontic sealers[97].

Celikten et al.[98] revealed an insignificant difference by measuring fracture resistance in teeth filled with different sealers.

Opinions regarding solubility are controversial. Some studies have shown controlled stability over time, and other studies have reported conflicting data, i.e., complete material hardening is not achieved[83]. The discrepancies that emerged can be explained by various factors, such as different moisture analysis methods; they can also be described by different authors, and these contradictory findings are considered of minimal clinical relevance[86, 87]. The properties of bioceramic-based sealers can be considered to be similar to those of MTA.

However, the main difference between the two is composition, because the former does not contain heavy metals, such as aluminum, lead, chromium, and arsenic. The absence of bismuth oxide, used as a radiopacity mean in the composition of MTA, can limit dyschromia, which is difficult to eliminate if it is caused by sealers, such as MTA[85].

Bioceramic-based sealers, such as MTA, can be used either as the only component for root canal filling or in combination with gutta-percha cones[81].

Compared to MTA, curing times are short, and some of them have average hardening times of about 4 hours. This characteristic is a huge clinical advantage.

The elective use of the filling of the teeth subjected to retreatment has been suggested by several authors[99]; as often reported in this text, the shaping of previously treated root canals involves the formation of endodontic spaces with apices larger than ISO 50.

Many may also be irregular, particularly in large periapical inflammatory lesions, because root resorptions can often be observed. Sealers are placed "cold," with a single gutta-percha cone or with the lateral gutta-percha condensation technique. In these filling techniques, the sealer/gutta-percha ratio is in favor of the former, making gutta-percha a carrier for bioceramic sealers.

From a clinical point of view, a partial contraindication may be that carrying out an immediate restoration, especially if endocanal retention is required to complete restoration, is not advisable. Studies have shown a negative interaction between bioceramic sealers and adhesion processes[100].

Ultimately, it constitutes a promising alternative to traditional filling methods that at the current time has limited but authoritative supporting literature[101].

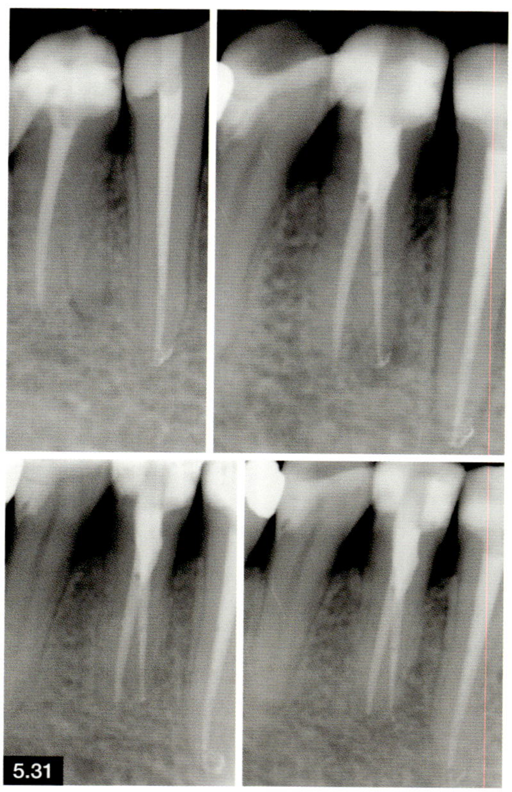
5.31

Fig. 5.31: A case of a forgotten canal in a lower premolar with an abnormal anatomy. Identification, shaping, and the filling with a bioactive sealer allowed the resolution of the condition in just 12 months.

Endodontic retreatment for an upper left central incisor

CASE REPORT 11

A 39-year-old male presented complaining of a discolored UL1. His history included a trauma when he was 8 years old; however, since that time, he had not experienced any pain or tenderness on percussion. Patient reported an intermittent labial sinus tract. The diagnosis was a previously treated UL1. The treatment was carried out over three appointments.

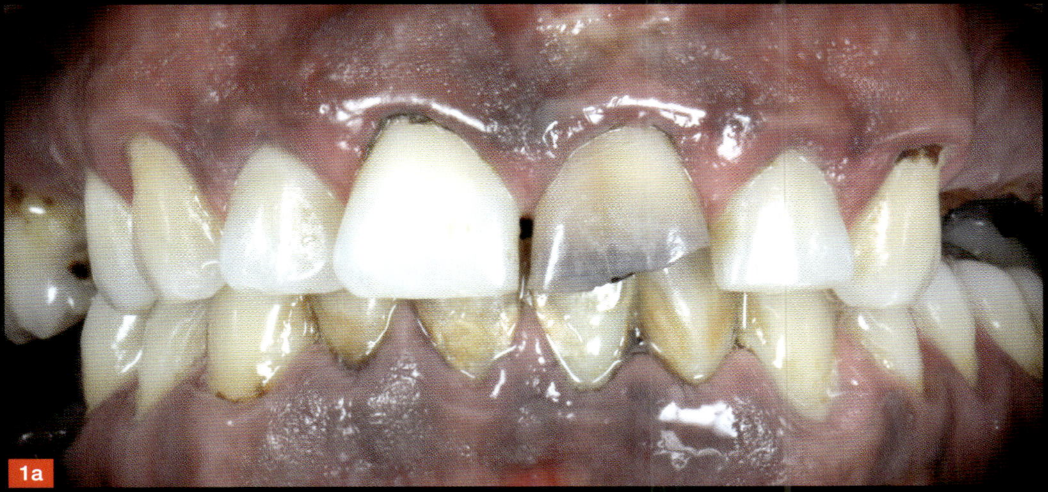

1a

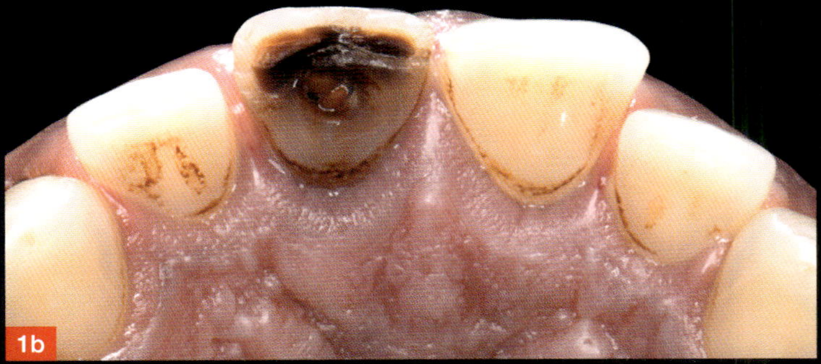

1b

Figs. 1a-b: The clinical examination shows dark discolouration of UL1 with CL IV decay. Lingually, there was an absence of coronal restoration. The tooth was negative for tenderness and gingival probing around the tooth was normal.

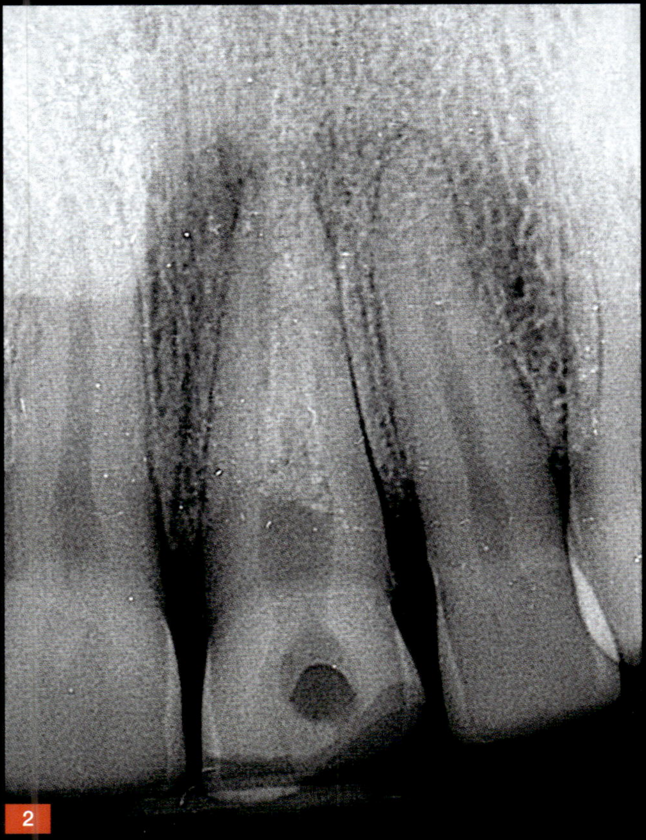

2

Fig. 2: The intraoral periapical X-ray revealed poor quality root canal treatment with absence of coronal restoration.

First appointment

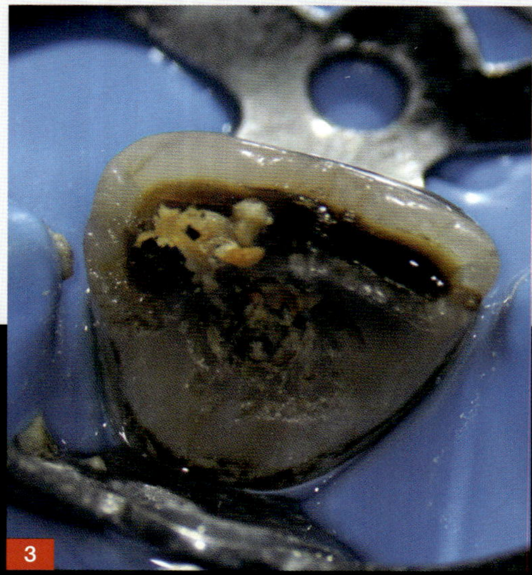

Fig. 3: The teeth were isolated with a rubber dam using a butterfly clamp.

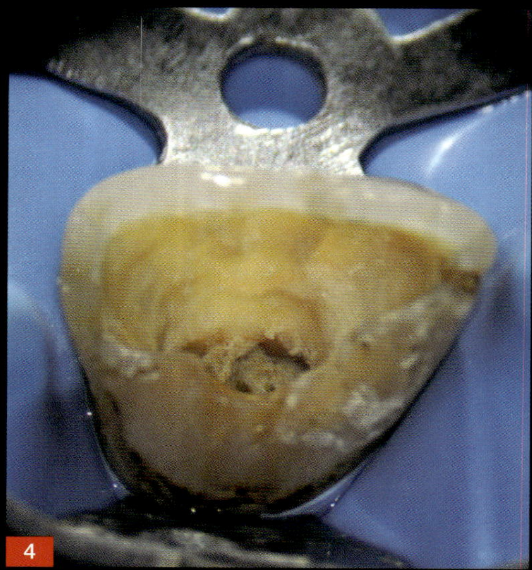

Fig. 4: The coronal decay was removed using a round bur with a slow hand piece. The pulp chamber was disinfected using 5.25% NaOCl.

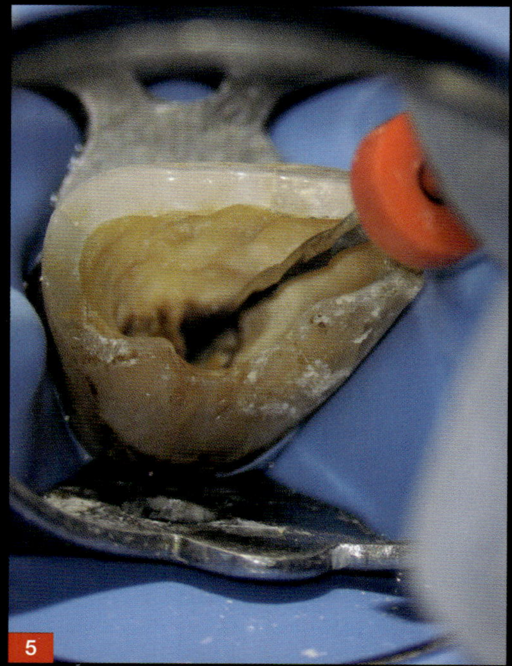

Fig. 5: The old root canal filling was removed using a Fanta F One file #25/0.06 (speed 500 rpm).

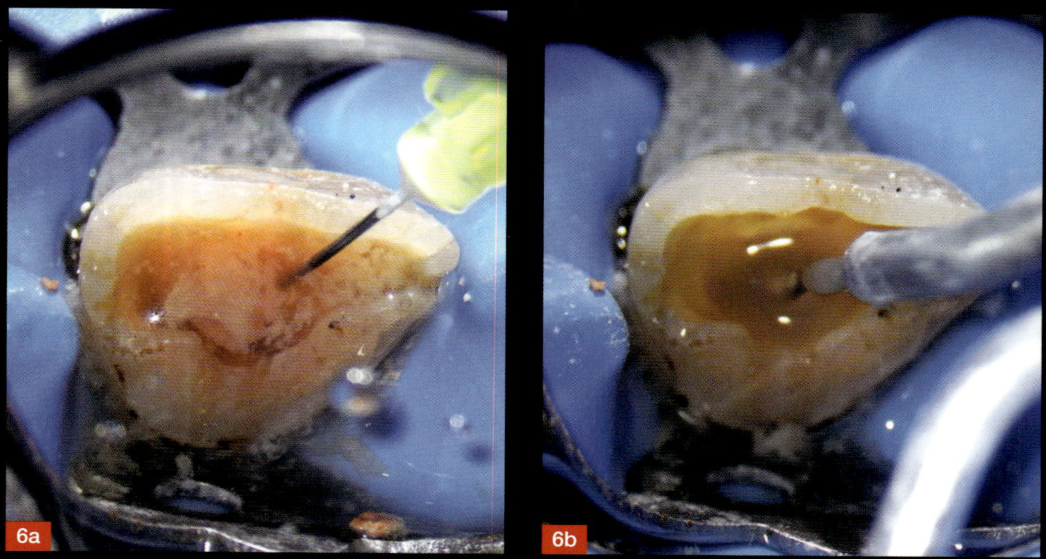

Fig. 6a-b: Copious amount of saline (as the tooth had an open apex and the working length was not confirmed at the time of treatment) aided by ultrasonic activation using Eighteeth Ultra was used to remove as much as debris, necrotic tissues and root canal filling remnants as possible.

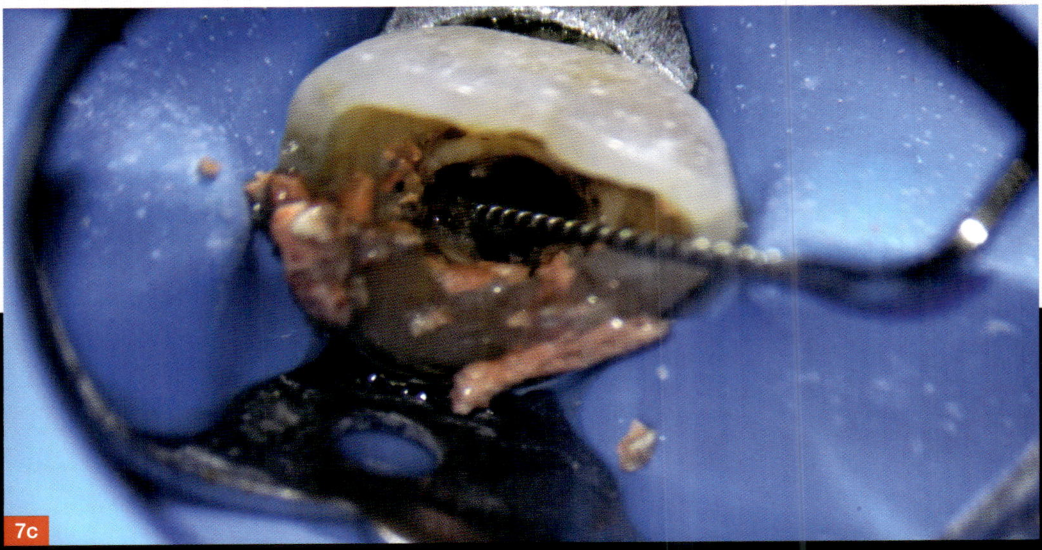

7c

Fig. 7a-c: The rest of the old gutta-percha was removed and pulled out using a Fanta MC-Shaper #30/0.02.

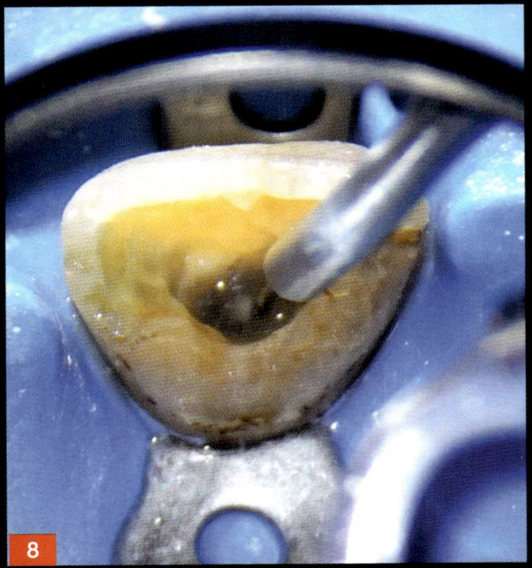

8

Fig. 8: The working length was measured using an E-Connect S built-in apex locator manufactured by Eighteeth. Copious irrigation with 5.25% NaOCl and 17% EDTA activated Ultra X.

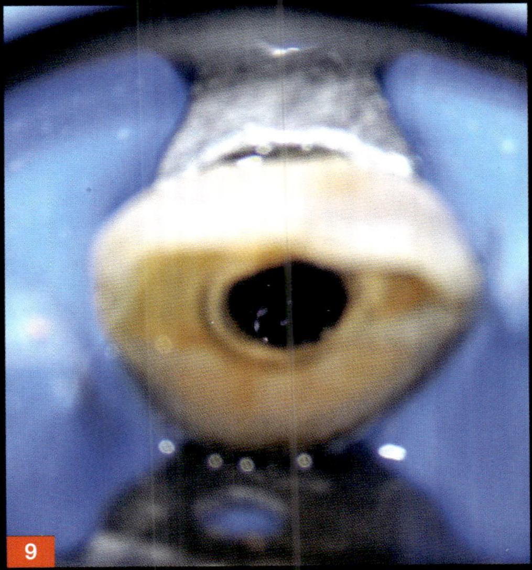

9

Fig. 9: The root canal system was dried with paper tips.

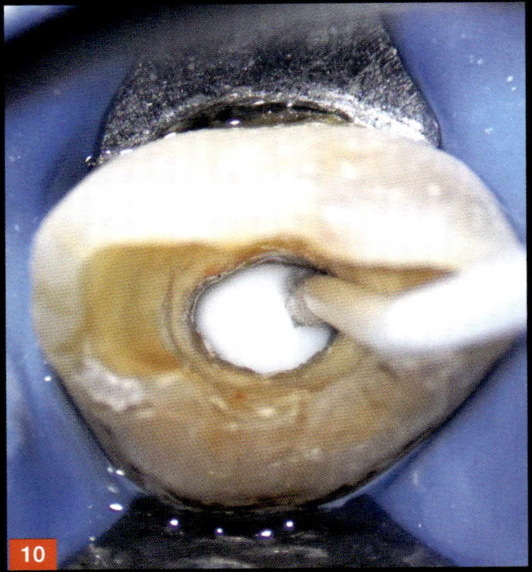

10

Fig. 10: The root canal system was filled with a non-setting intracanal sodium hypochlorite dressing (Metapaste by Meta Biomed).

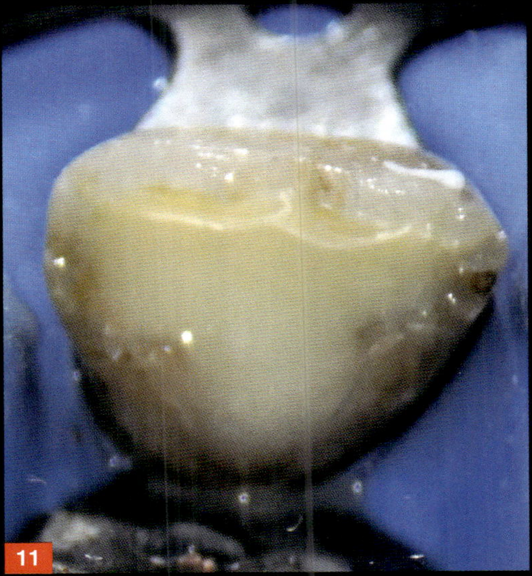

11

Fig. 11: The tooth was restored with a temporary GIC.

Second appointment
(one week later)

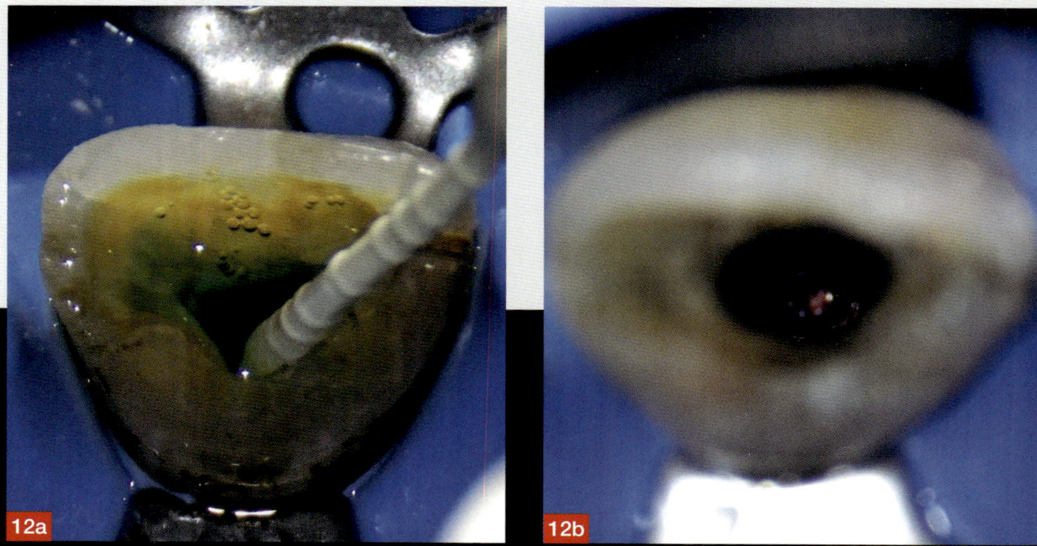

Fig. 12a-b: Copious irrigation with saline solution, activated by ultrasonic device, was utilized to flush out the dressing material and a chlorhexidine solution was utilized for final disinfection.

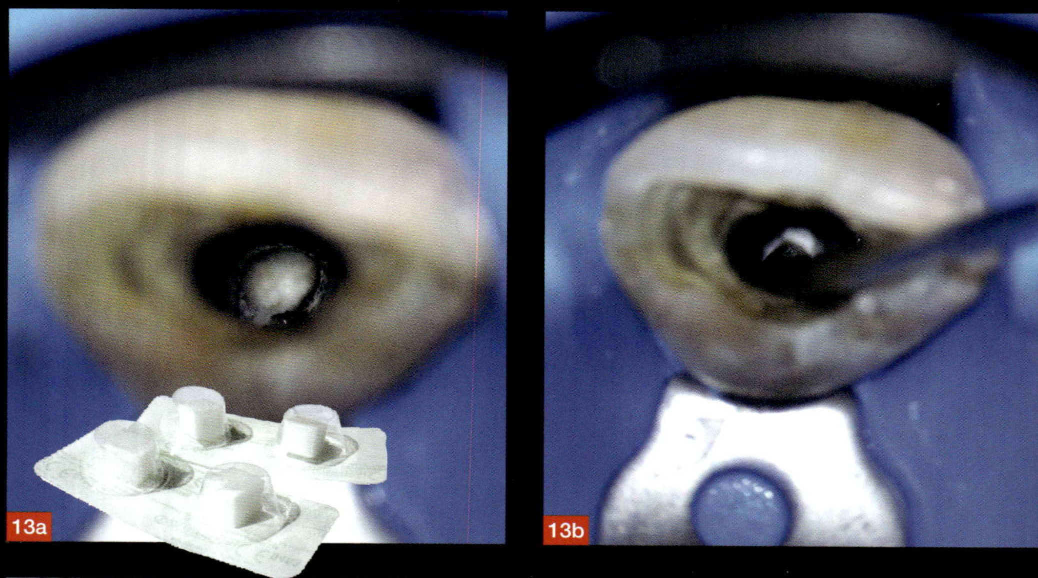

Fig. 13 a-b: An absorbable gelatin hemostatic sponge was introduced into the periradicular area, through the canal by a plugger, to act as a platform for MTA condensation.

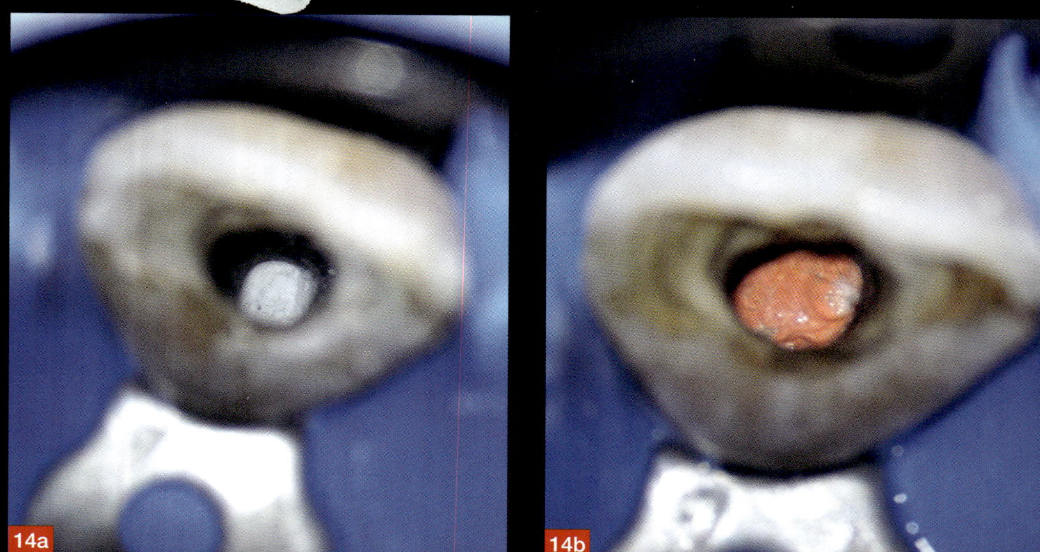

Fig. 14 a-b: The root canal was filled with gutta-percha. The pulp chamber was cleaned using a 75% alcohol solution applied utilizing microbrushes, the rest of the canal was restored and sealed using dual cure resin cement. An internal bleaching agent (OpalescenceTM Endo, Ultradent) was introduced into the cavity and the tooth was restored with temporary glass ionomer cement.

Third appointment
(5 days later)

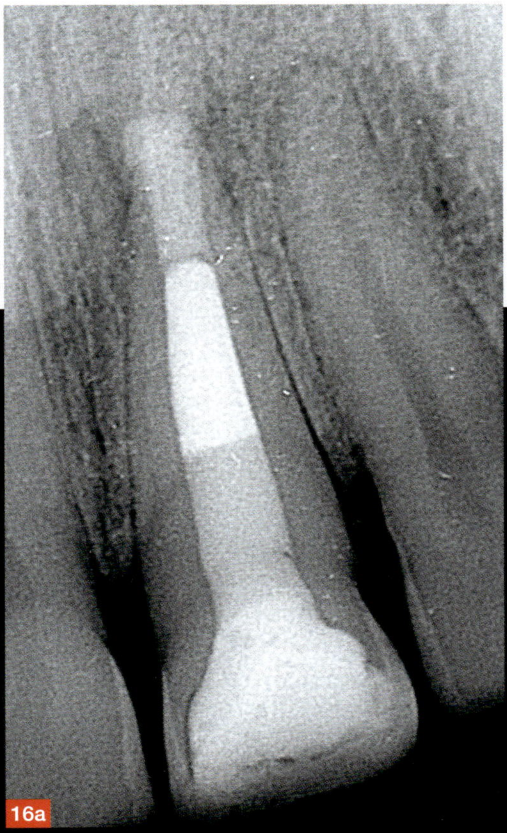
16a

Fig. 16a-b:
The tooth was isolated using a rubber dam.
The temporary GIC was removed and the cavity was cleaned of the bleaching agent.
The tooth was restored with a composite restoration using layering technique and IPS Empress direct (Ivoclar) to mimic the adjacent central incisor.

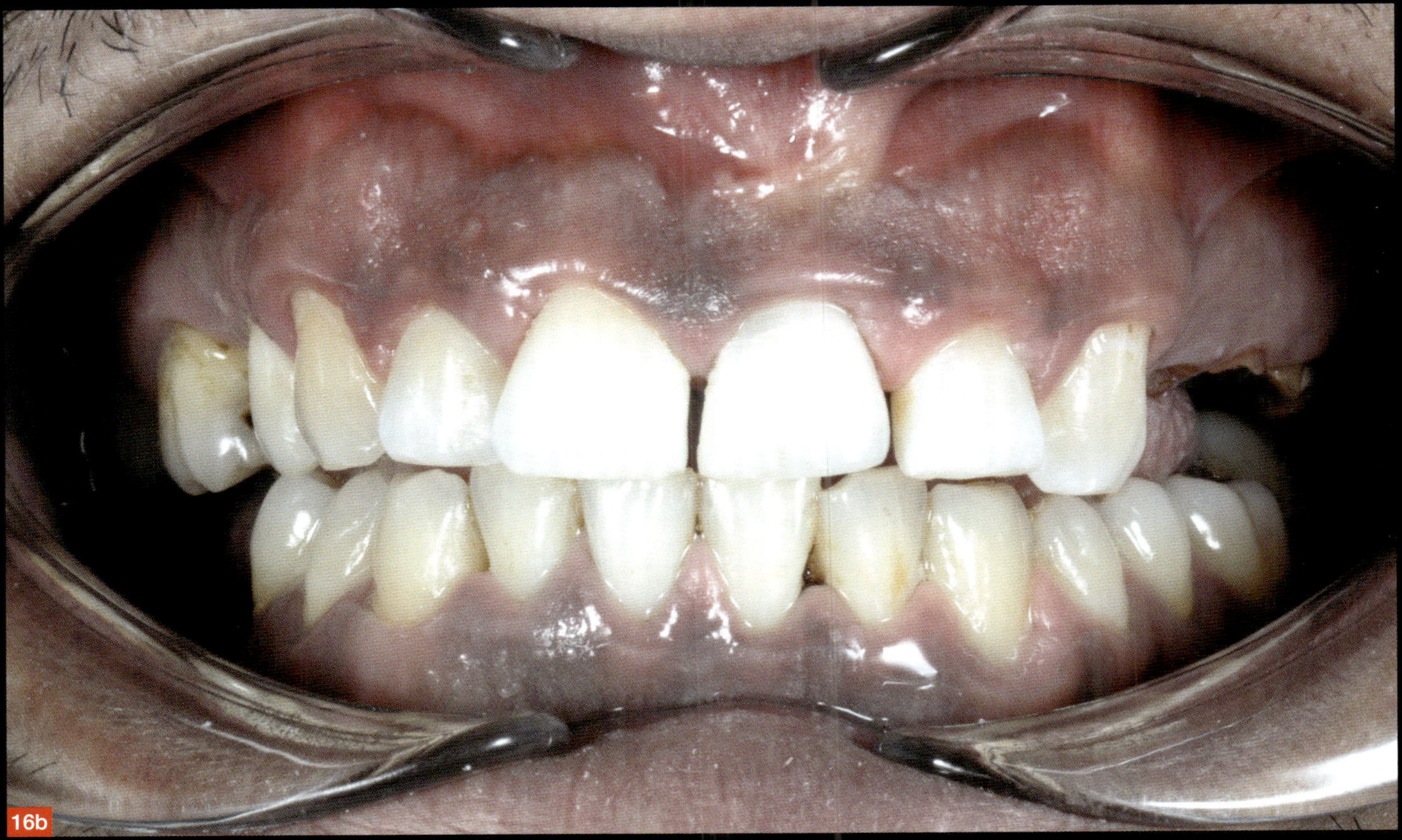
16b

CASE REPORT 12

Apical plug in a large periapical lesion

This case describes an emergency treatment on a 48-year-old female patient presenting an acute swelling and a vestibular fistula between the elements 1.2-1.3 (Figs. 1 and 2). The radiographic examination revealed a large periapical lesion of endodontic origin associated with the previously treated tooth 1.2 (Figs. 3-7). No periodontal probing was assessed. The patient reported an endodontic treatment two years earlier and severe sensitivity in this area immediately after the treatment.

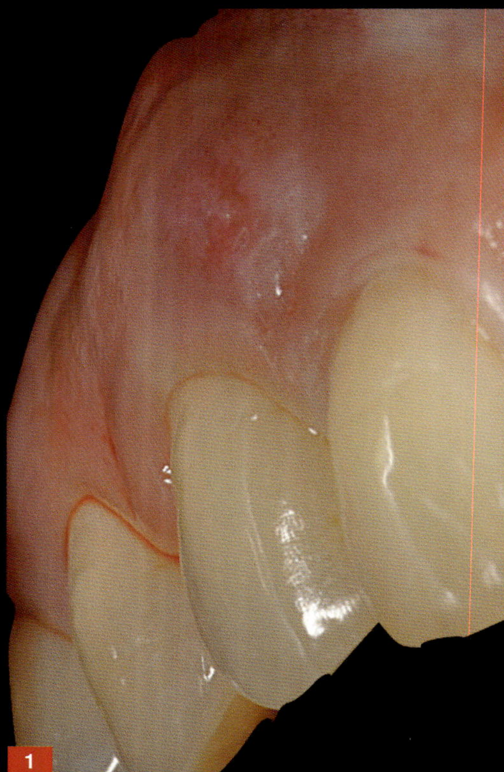

1

Figure 1: Clinical view of the buccal area between the lateral incisor and cuspid; a fistula is clearly visible, although it is still unclear which tooth it originates from.

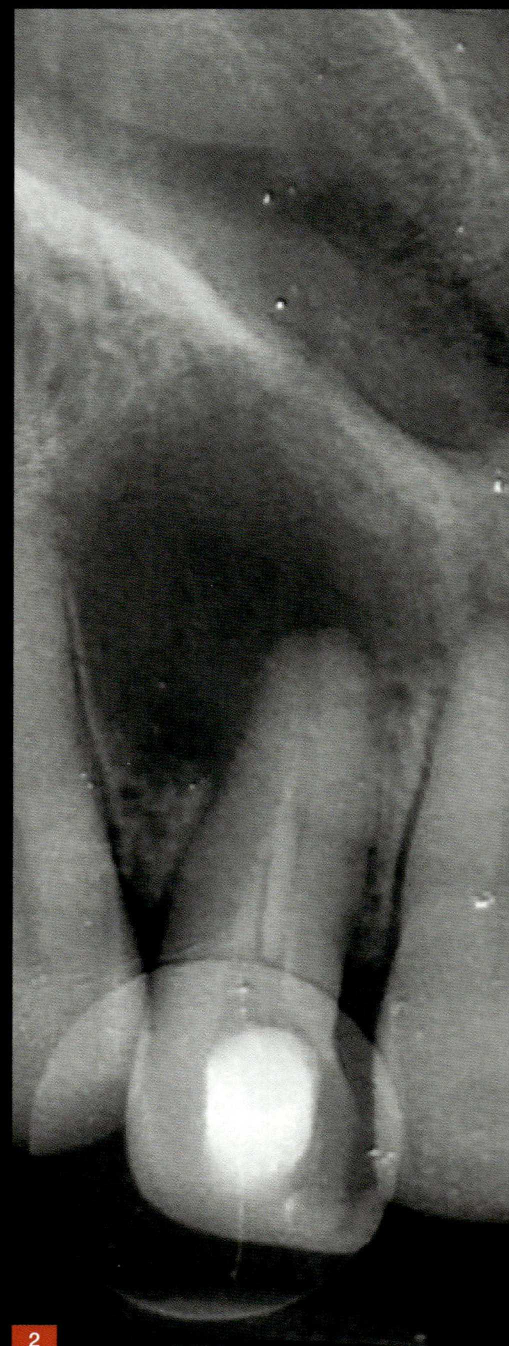

2

Figure 2: The intraoral two-dimensional X-ray reveals a clear periapical lesion of endodontic origin associated with the previously poorly treated upper right incisor.

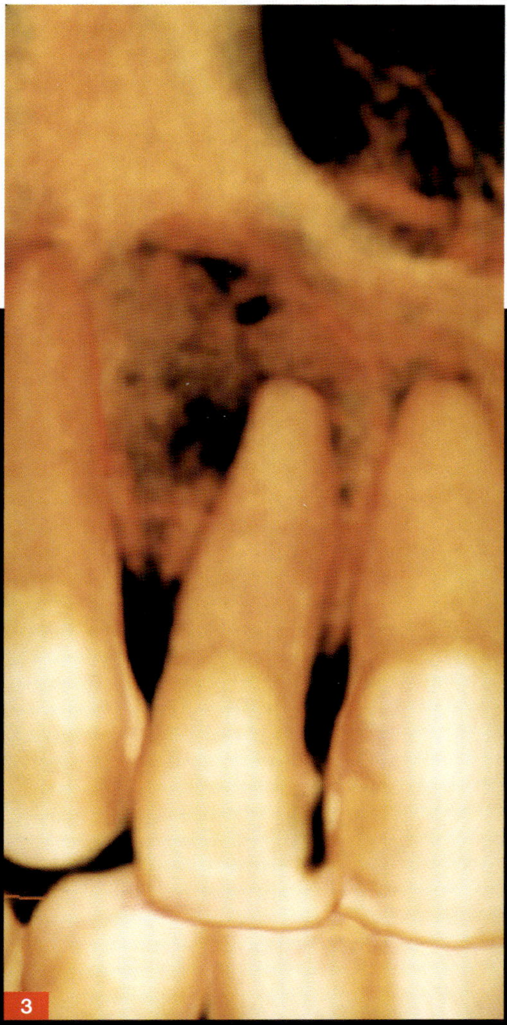

3

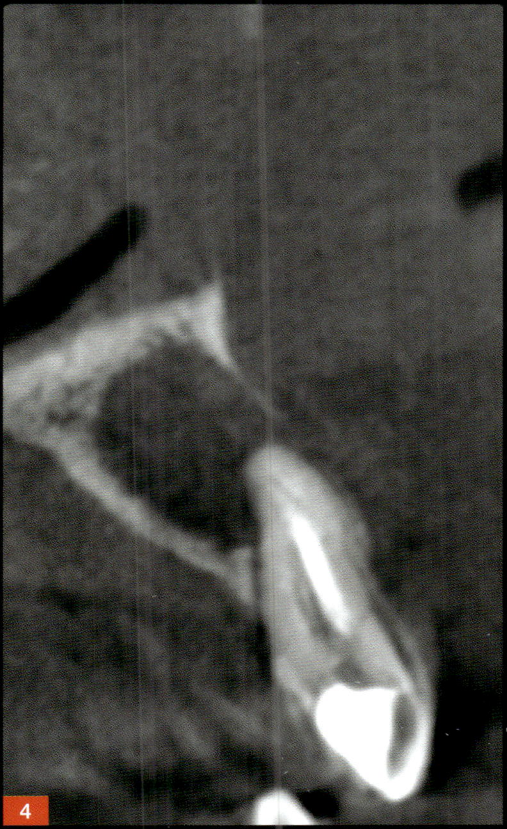

4

Figures 3-5: A CBCT analysis was performed to exclude root fractures or pathological resorption; the root canal treatment was inadequate in terms of both apical length and filling volume.

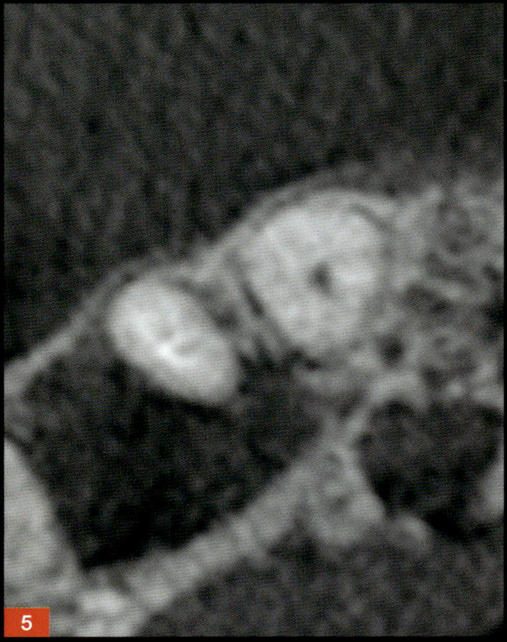

5

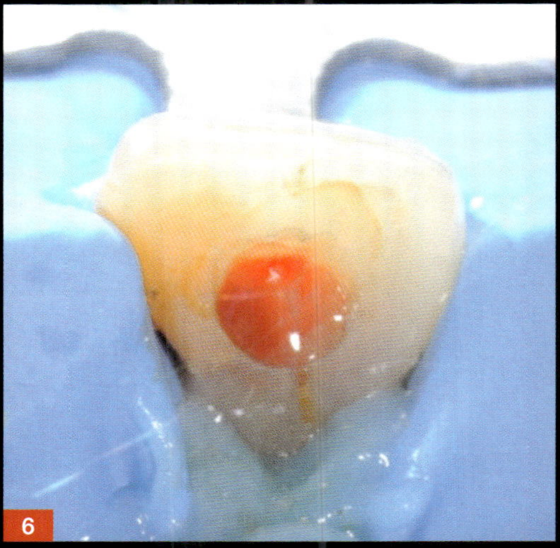

6

Figure 6: During the first phase of the endodontic orthograde retreatment copious drainage was present, suggesting a two-step root canal pretreatment.

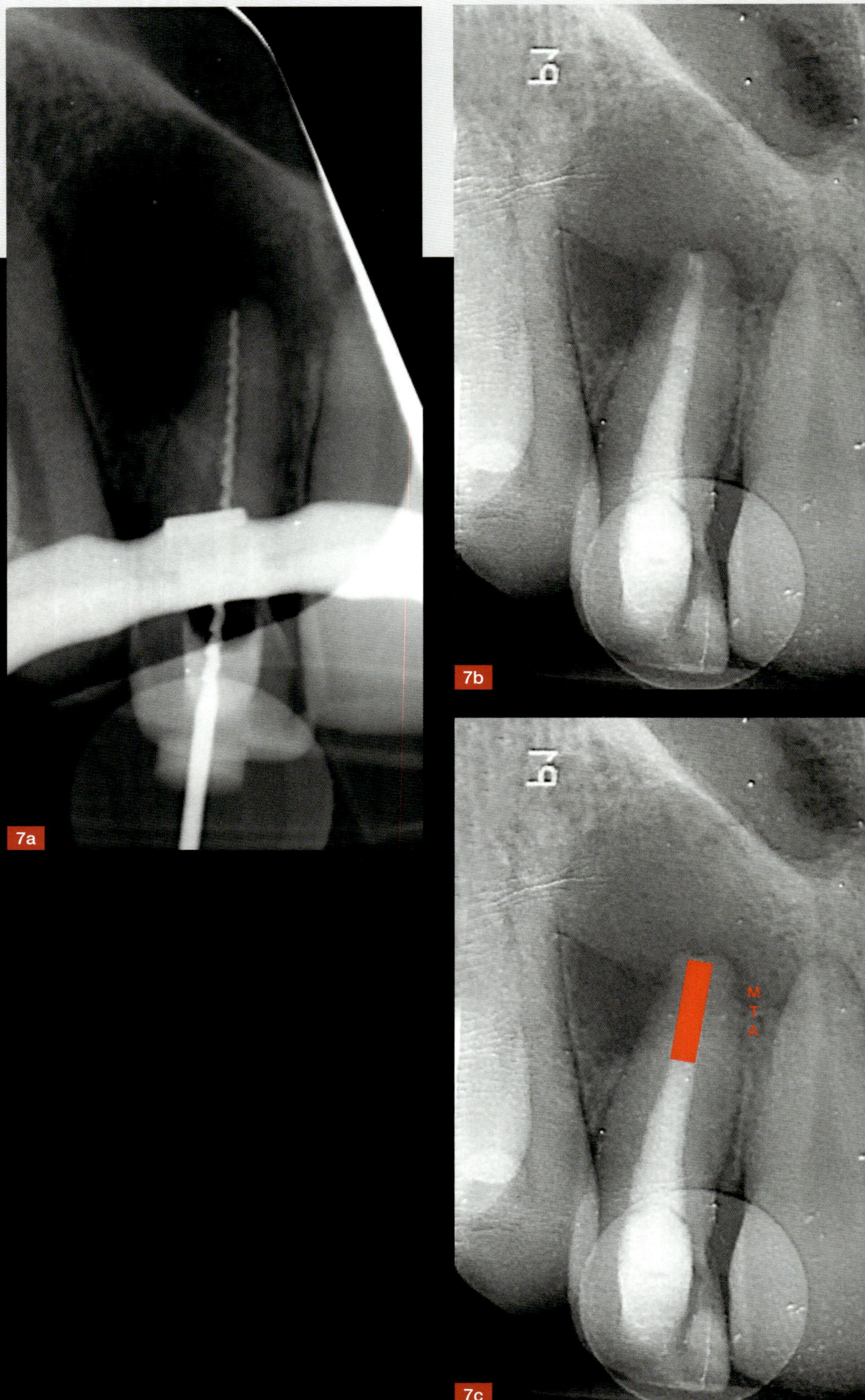

Figure 7a-c: The root canal retreatment was accomplished in two stages and a huge ISO diameter was verified utilizing a stainless steel instrument; in accordance with previously reported data, an apical plug with bio-active material was planned, a further warm gutta-percha vertical compaction was utilized to finish the sealing procedures.

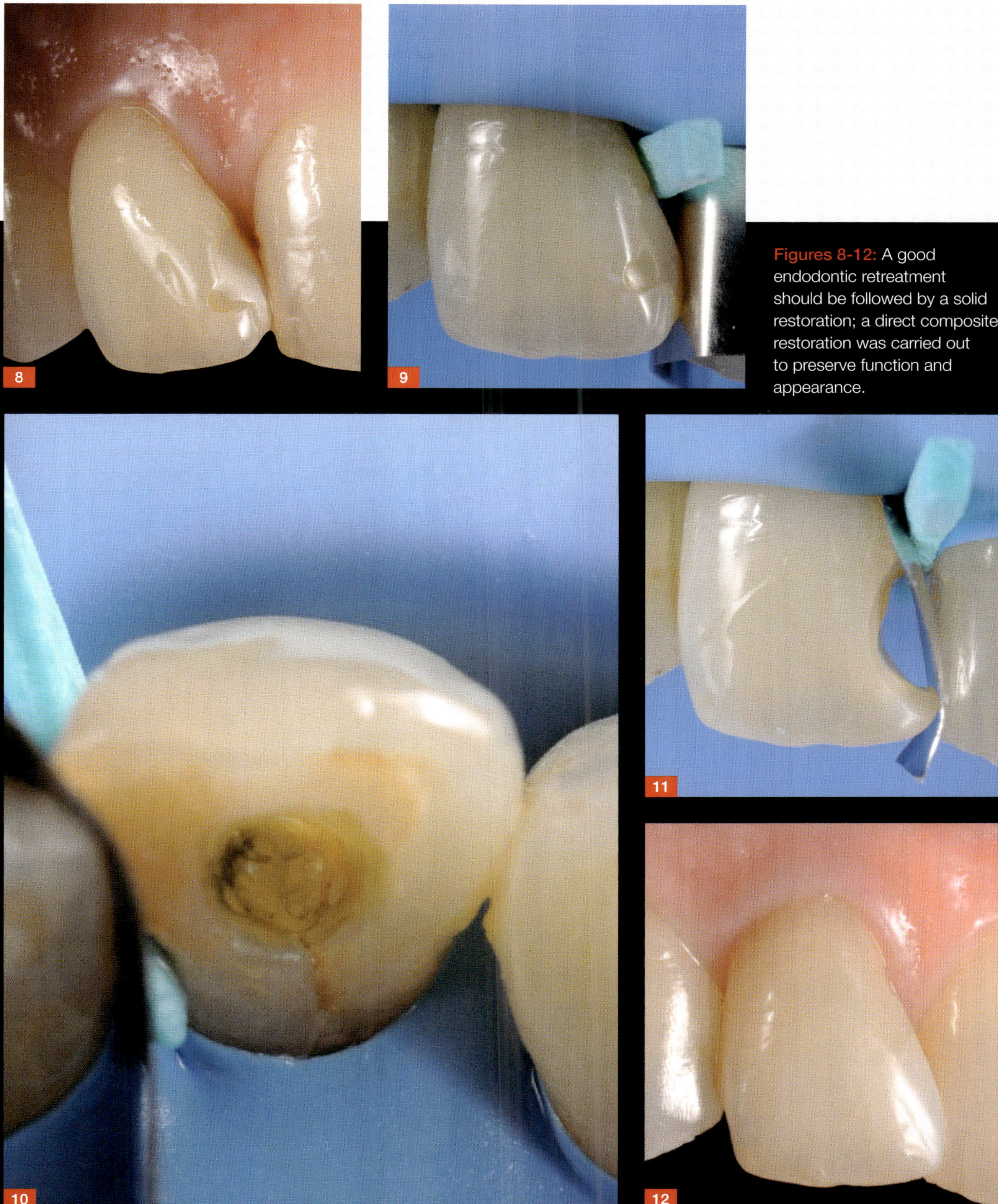

Figures 8-12: A good endodontic retreatment should be followed by a solid restoration; a direct composite restoration was carried out to preserve function and appearance.

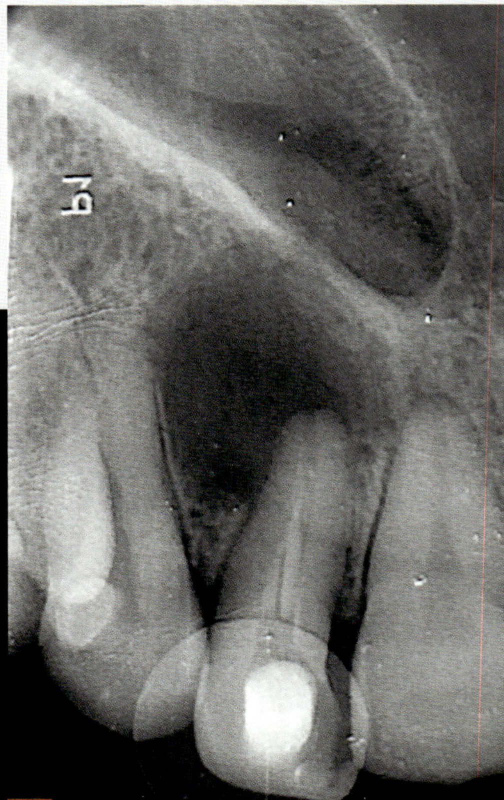

13a

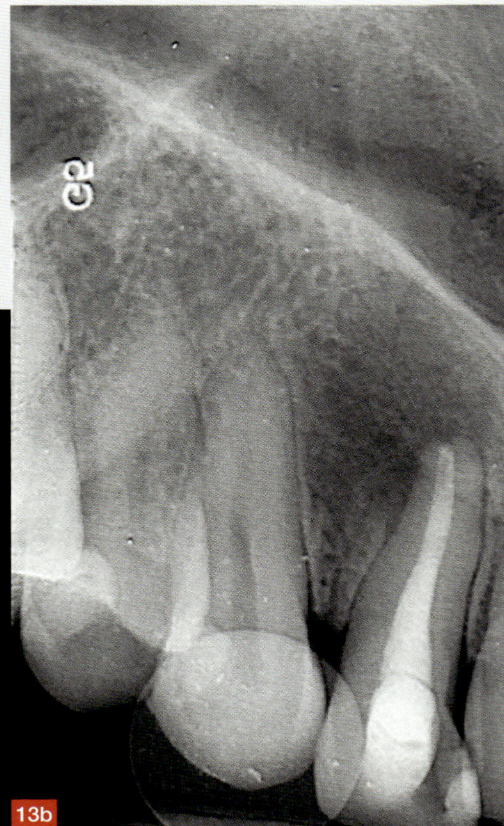

13b

Figure 13a-c: Three images taken at different times from the beginning of the retreatment; a clear improvement was assessed as soon as the endodontic procedure was finished. A one-year follow-up radiographic examination confirmed the perfect healing of the surrounding bone.

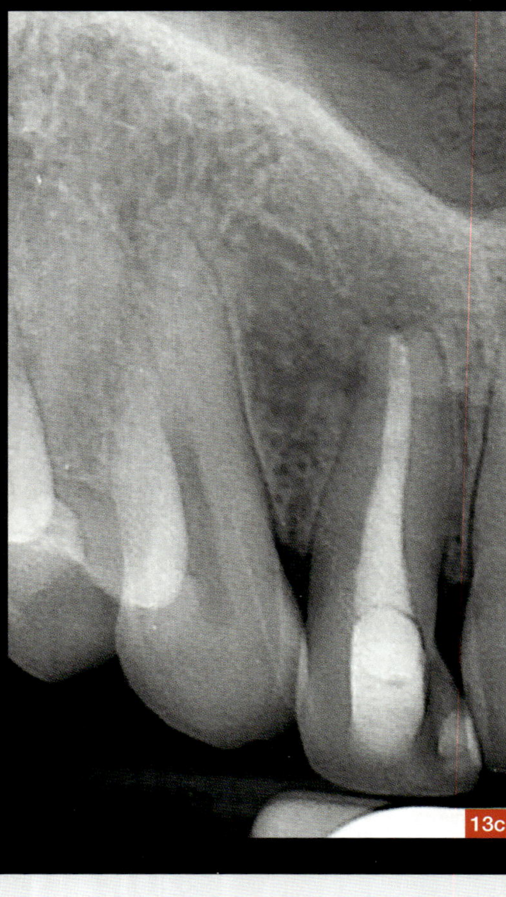

13c

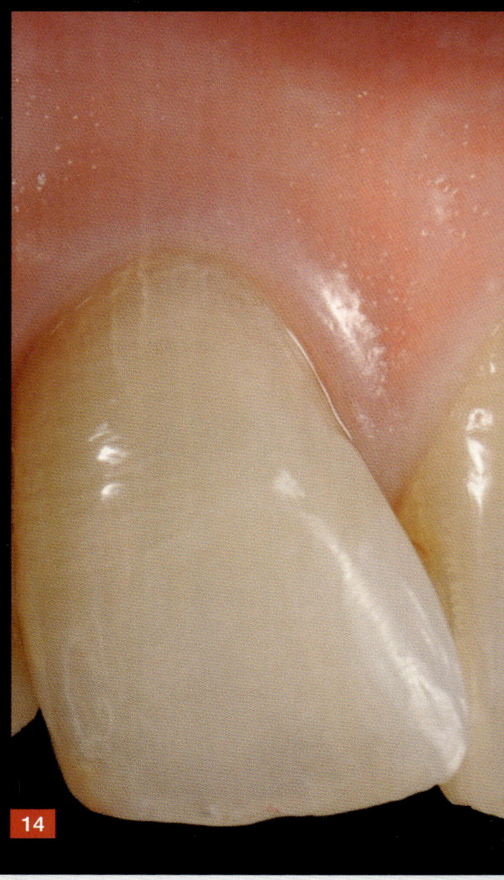

14

Figure 14: A clinical view of the dental-periodontal integration of the endodontically retreated upper lateral incisor, demonstrating the importance of a correct postendodontic restoration.

Some cases of canal closure with bioactive sealers

CASE REPORTS 13-18

The following sequence of cases belongs to one of the leading experts in this canal closure technique: Prof. Gilberto Debelian. The review consists of some very common clinical situations, where the choice of the canal filling method was guided by the evaluations that the Author carried out before starting the treatment.

CASE REPORT 13

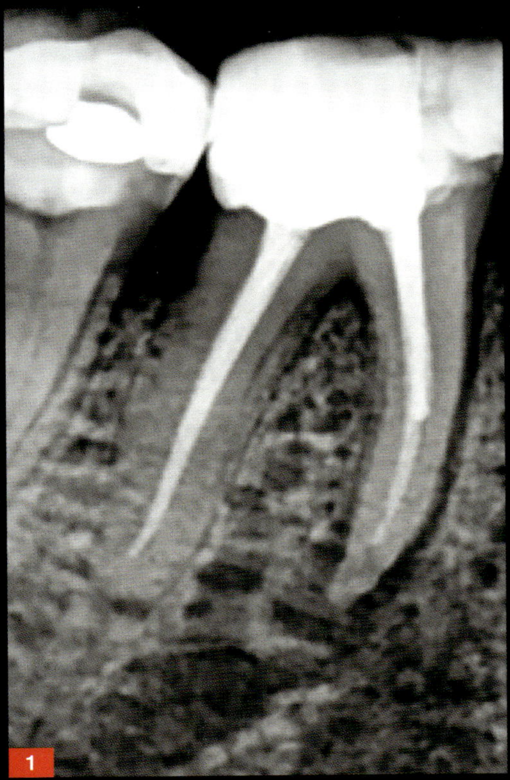

1

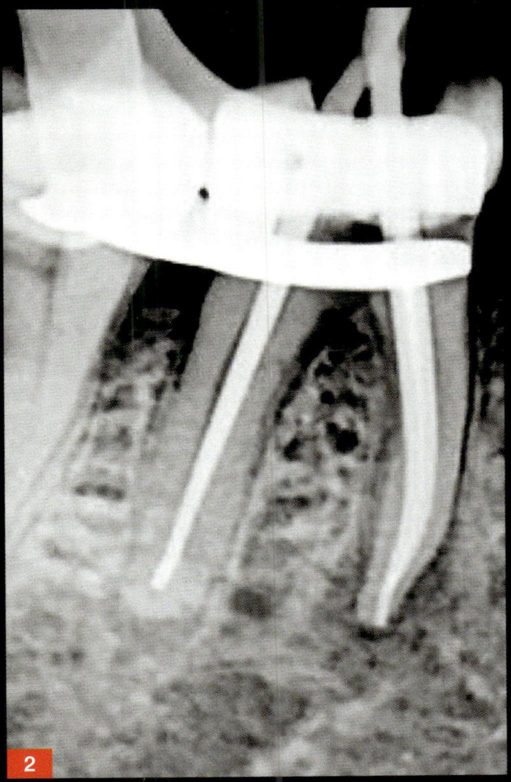

2

Figure 1: An inferior molar with a clear periapical lesion requiring retreatment.

Figure 2: Once the old filling material has been removed and the canal has been reshaped, the gutta-percha cone test is performed.

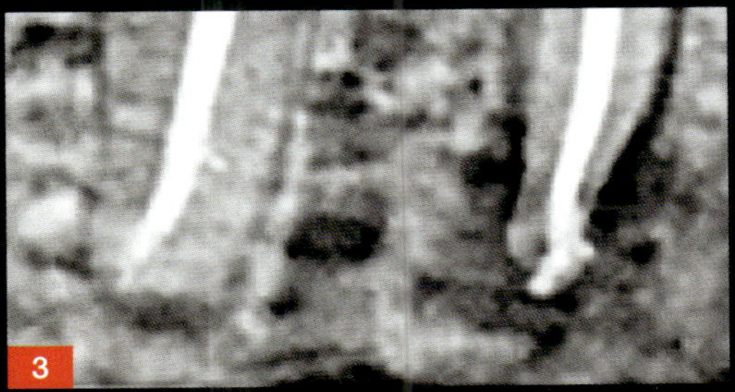

3

Figure 3: Adaptation of bioactive sealer and cones at apical level; note the various apical branches.

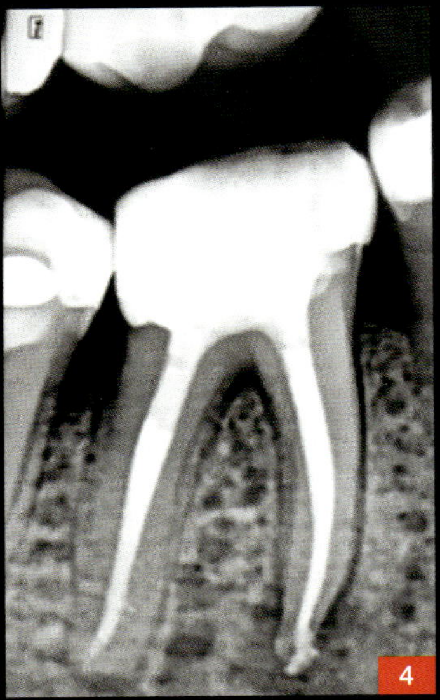

4

Figure 4: The final closure with slight overfilling.

CASE REPORT 14

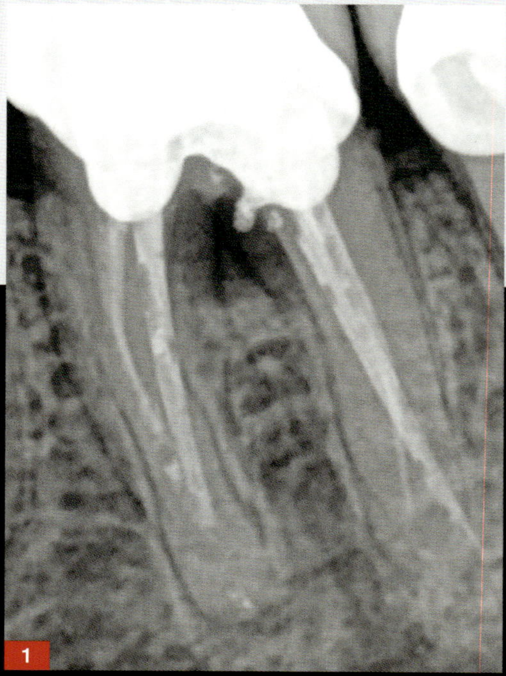

1

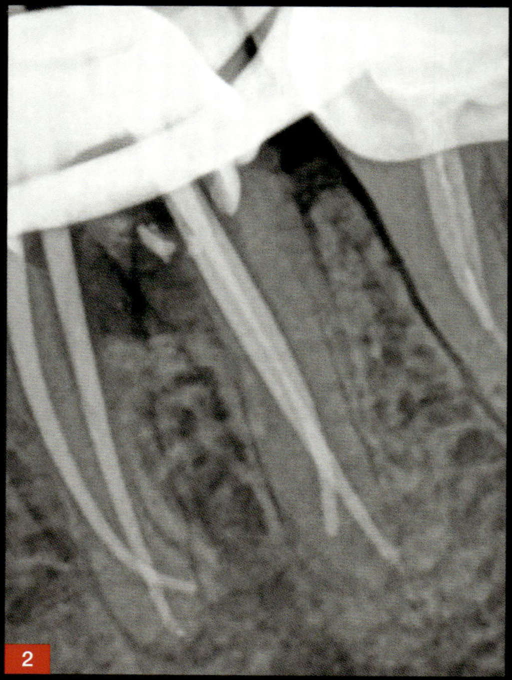

2

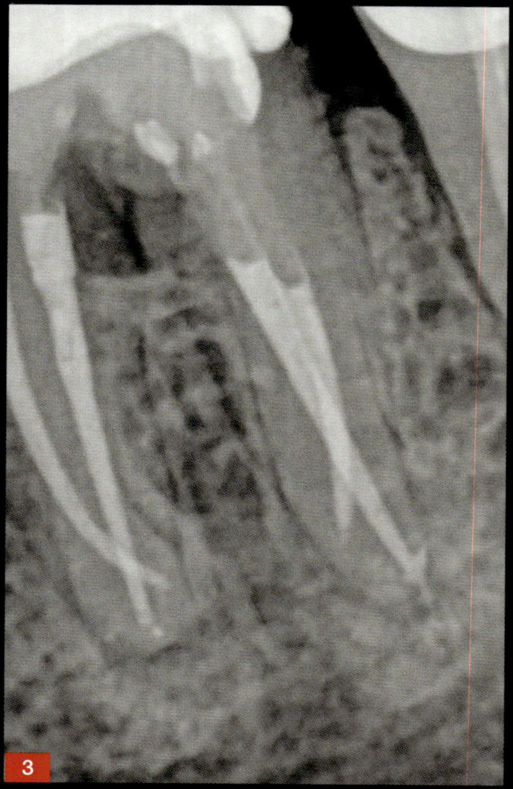

3

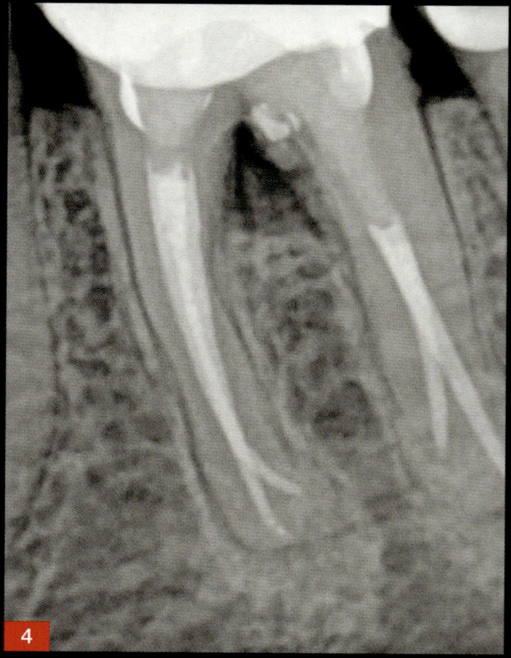

4

Figure 1: An incorrect endodontic treatment requiring re-intervention.

Figure 2: Once the endodontium has been emptied and expertly shaped, the cones can be adapted in the best possible way.

Figure 3: The final canal closure.

Figure 4: The result after time confirming the success of the treatment.

CASE REPORT 15

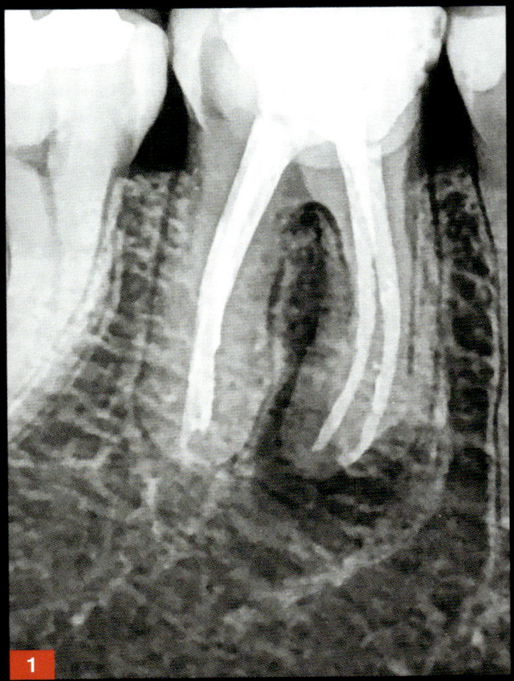

1

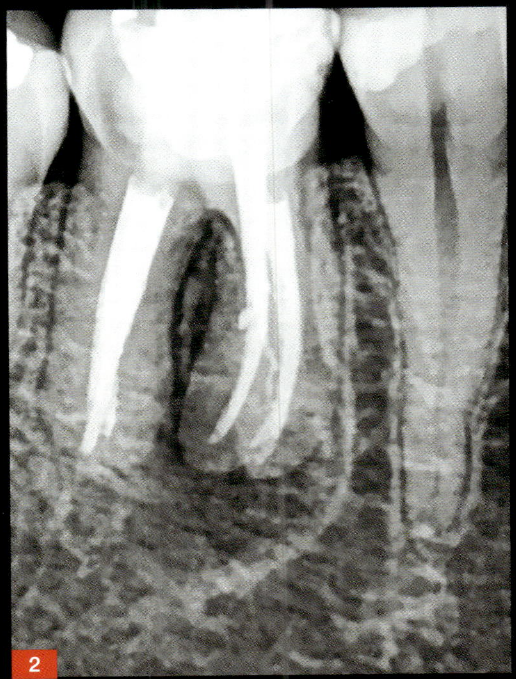

2

Figure 1: Endodontic treatment with bioactive sealer; note the perfect interpenetration of the material in the root canalspace.

Figure 2: Same image from a different angle.

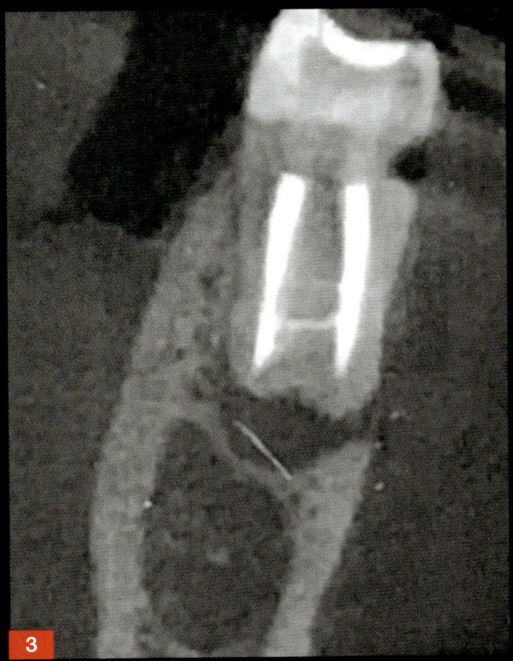

3

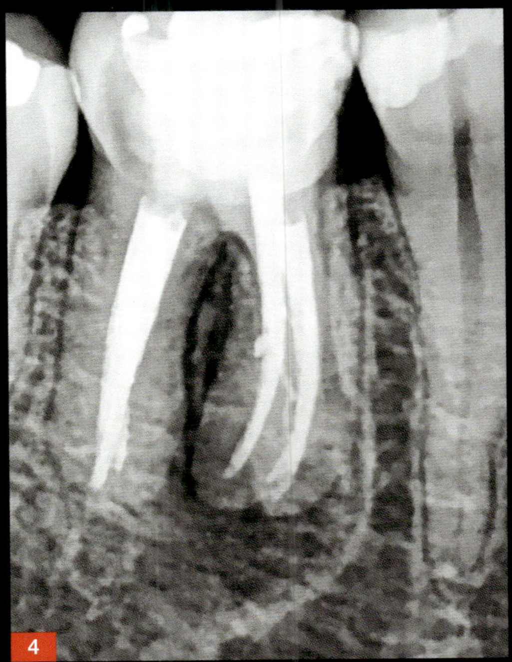

4

Figure 3: The mesio-distal view highlighting intra-canal communications (CBCT).

Figure 4: The resolution about 8 months after treatment.

Complex orthograde sealing with or without retrograde filling

In some cases, the desired result cannot be achieved with filling alone.
In some clinical situations[102-105], operating sequences typical of perforation repair may be utilized (Chapter 7), but endodontic space filling performed in accordance with criteria[106-108] can be combined with surgical endodontics to obtain the best final solution (Chapter 8)[109-111]. Therefore, a clinician can provide orthograde treatment followed by a surgical treatment that accelerates healing times[112].

CASE REPORT 16

The wide channels of the central incisors frequently require apical revision.

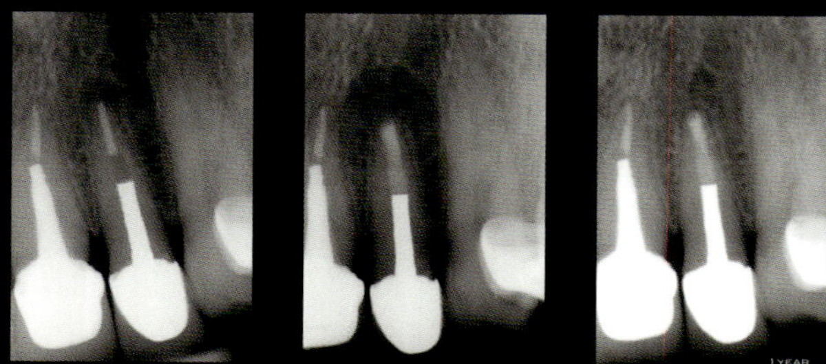

CASE REPORT 17

The decision to preserve the premolars, mainly for aesthetic reasons, passes through this synergy between orthograde and retrograde.

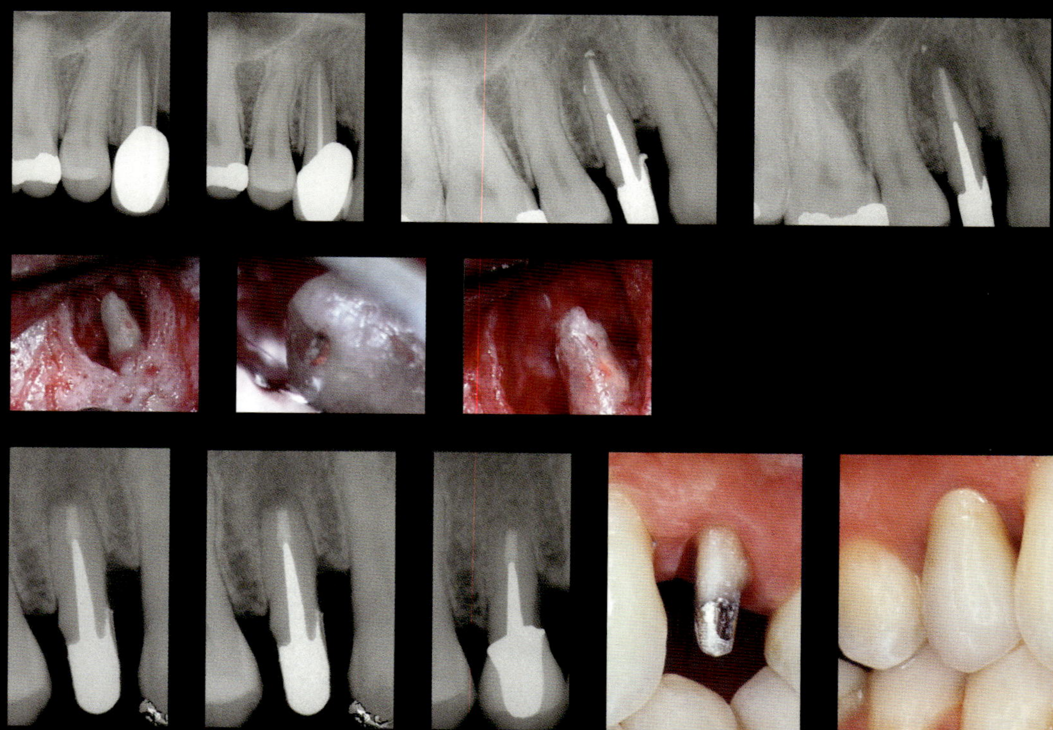

CASE REPORT 18

An evident apical lateral perforation forces the clinician to take the surgical option.

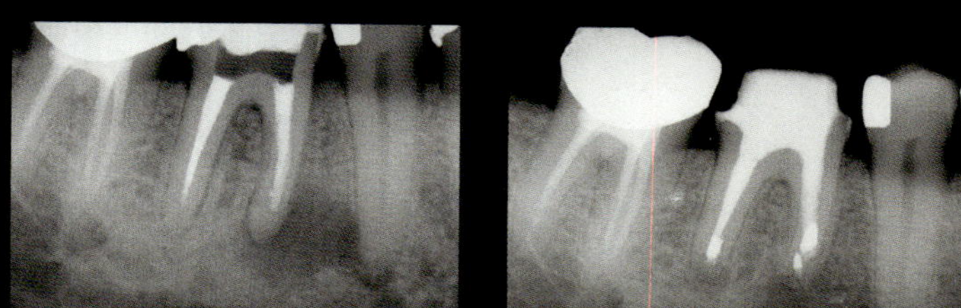

Orthograde and retrograde therapies

These cases present solutions that have given excellent results even years later and have more than one thing to teach us, i.e. that the endodontic orthodontic solution has objective difficulties of success because the determinants cannot be restricted to the endodontium alone and, in addition, the natural or induced anatomical deformities are difficult to overcome with treatment alone. A combination of orthograde and retrograde therapy will make it possible to achieve the desired final result.

CASE REPORT 19

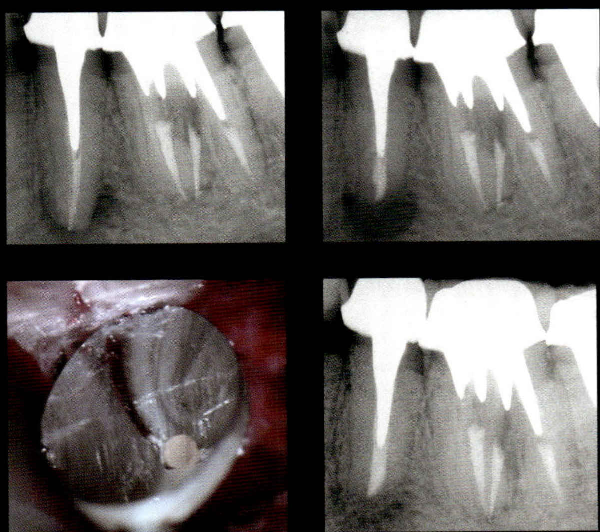

Failure determined by an unpredictable anatomy: only surgery can solve this kind of condition.

CASE REPORT 20

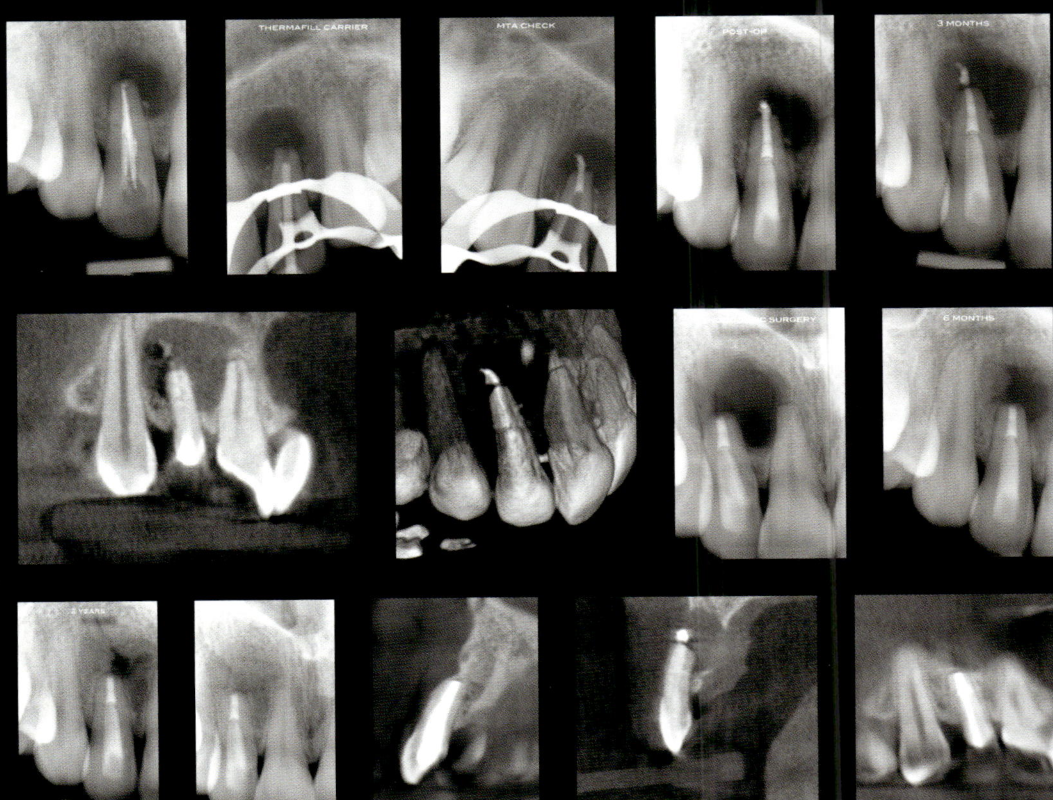

Such complex situations, with large lesions that probably date back years, must be considered solvable only with a combination of orthograde and retrograde retreatment.

References

1. Seltzer S. *Long-term radiographic and histological observations of endodontically treated teeth.* J Endod. 1999; 25(12):818-822.
2. Friedman S, Abitbol S and Lawrence HP. *Treatment outcome in endodontics: the Toronto Study. Phase 1: initial treatment*. J Endod. 2003; 29(12):787-793.
3. Gorni FG and Gagliani MM. *The outcome of endodontic retreatment: a 2-yr follow-up*. J Endod. 2004; 30(1):1-4.
4. Farzaneh M, Abitbol S and Friedman S. *Treatment outcome in endodontics: the Toronto study. Phases I and II: Orthograde retreatment.* J Endod. 2004; 30(9):627-633.
5. Farzaneh M, Abitbol S, Lawrence HP et al. *Treatment outcome in endodontics-the Toronto Study. Phase II: initial treatment.* J Endod. 2004; 30(5):302-309.
6. Nair PN. *Pathogenesis of apical periodontitis and the causes of endodontic failures*. Crit Rev Oral Biol Med. 2004; 15(6):348-381.
7. Nair PN. *On the causes of persistent apical periodontitis: a review*. Int Endod J. 2006; 39(4):249-281.
8. Friedman S. *Expected Outcomes in the Prevention and Treatment of Apical Periodontitis*. In: Orstavik D, Pitt Ford TR, editors. *Essential Endodontology*. 2nd ed. Oxford, UK: Blackwell Munksgaard Ltd; 2008. 408-471.
9. Garcia CC, Sempere FV, Diago MP et al. *The post-endodontic periapical lesion: histologic and etiopathogenic aspects*. Med Oral Patol Oral Cir Bucal. 2007; 12(8):E585-590.
10. Philpott R, Gulabivala K, Leeson R et al. *Prevalence, predictive factors, and clinical course of persistent pain associated with teeth displaying periapical healing following non-surgical root canal treatment: a prospective study*. Int Endod J. 2018.
11. Ng YL, Mann V and Gulabivala K. *Tooth survival following non-surgical root canal treatment: a systematic review of the literature.* Int Endod J. 2010; 43(3):171-189.
12. Ng YL, Mann V, Rahbaran S et al. *Outcome of primary root canal treatment: systematic review of the literature - Part 2. Influence of clinical factors*. Int Endod J. 2008; 41(1):6-31.
13. Gesi A, Mareschi P, Doldo T et al. *Apical Dimension of Root Canal Clinically Assessed with and without Periapical Lesions.* Int J Dent. 2014; 2014:374971.
14. Rodrigues RCV, Zandi H, Kristoffersen AK et al. *Influence of the Apical Preparation Size and the Irrigant Type on Bacterial Reduction in Root Canal-treated Teeth with Apical Periodontitis*. J Endod. 2017; 43(7):1058-1063.
15. Blum JY, Esber S and Micallef JP. *Analysis of forces developed during obturations. Comparison of three gutta-percha techniques*. J Endod. 1997; 23(5):340-345.
16. Peak JD, Hayes SJ, Bryant ST et al. *The outcome of root canal treatment. A retrospective study within the armed forces (Royal Air Force).* Br Dent J. 2001; 190(3):140-144.
17. Blum JY, Parahy E and Machtou P. *Warm vertical compaction sequences in relation to gutta-percha temperature*. J Endod. 1997; 23(5):307-311.
18. Blum JY, Parahy E and Micallef JP. *Analysis of the forces developed during obturation: warm vertical compaction.* J Endod. 1997; 23(2):91-95.
19. Friedman CM, Sandrik JL, Heuer MA et al. *Composition and mechanical properties of gutta-percha endodontic points.* J Dent Res. 1975; 54(5):921-925.
20. Buchanan LS. *Continuous wave of condensation technique*. Endod Prac. 1998; 1(4):7-10, 13-16, 18 passim.
21. Siqueira JF Jr., da Silva CH, Cerqueira MdD et al. *Effectiveness of four chemical solutions in eliminating Bacillus subtilis spores on gutta-percha cones*. Endod Dent Traumatol. 1998; 14(3):124-126.
22. Seabra Pereira OL, Siqueira JF Jr. *Contamination of gutta-percha and Resilon cones taken directly from the manufacturer*. Clin Oral Investig. 2010; 14(3):327-330.
23. Zhang C, Huang W, Sun Z et al. *A comparison of two gutta-percha master points consisting of different phases in filling of artificial lateral canals and depressions in the apical region of root canals when using a warm vertical compaction technique*. Int Endod J. 2011; 44(11):1041-1046.
24. Zhang W, Suguro H, Kobayashi Y et al. *Effect of canal taper and plugger size on warm gutta-percha obturation of lateral depressions*. J Oral Sci. 2011; 53(2):219-224.
25. Schilder H. *Cleaning and shaping the root canal*. Dent Clin North Am. 1974; 18(2):269-296.
26. Venturi M, Pasquantonio G, Falconi M et al. *Temperature change within gutta-percha induced by the System-B Heat Source*. Int Endod J. 2002; 35(9):740-746.
27. Venturi M, Prati C, Capelli G et al. *A preliminary analysis of the morphology of lateral canals after root canal filling using a tooth-clearing technique*. Int Endod J. 2003; 36(1):54-63.
28. Venturi M and Breschi L. *Evaluation of apical filling after warm vertical gutta-percha compaction using different procedures.* J Endod. 2004; 30(6):436-440.
29. Collins J, Walker MP, Kulild J et al. *A comparison of three gutta-percha obturation techniques to replicate canal irregularities.* J Endod. 2006; 32(8):762-765.
30. Venturi M. *Evaluation of canal filling after using two warm vertical gutta-percha compaction techniques in vivo: a preliminary study*. Int Endod J. 2006; 39(7):538-546.

31. Johnson WB. *A new gutta-percha technique*. J Endod. 1978; 4(6):184-188.
32. Gutmann JL, Saunders WP, Saunders EM et al. *An assessment of the plastic Thermafil obturation technique. Part 2. Material adaptation and sealability*. Int Endod J. 1993; 26(3):179-183.
33. Weller RN, Kimbrough WF and Anderson RW. *A comparison of thermoplastic obturation techniques: adaptation to the canal walls.* J Endod. 1997; 23(11):703-706.
34. Cantatore G. *Thermafil vs System B*. Endod Prac. 2001; 4(5):30-39.
35. Kytridou V, Gutmann JL and Nunn MH. *Adaptation and sealability of two contemporary obturation techniques in the absence of the dentinal smear layer*. Int Endod J. 1999; 32(6):464-474.
36. Pirani C, Iacono F, Gatto MR et al. *Outcome of secondary root canal treatment filled with Thermafil: a 5-year follow-up of retrospective cohort study.* Clin Oral Investig. 2018; 22(3):1363-1373.
37. Da Silva D, Endal U, Reynaud A et al. *A comparative study of lateral condensation, heat-softened gutta-percha, and a modified master cone heat-softened backfilling technique.* Int Endod J. 2002; 35(12):1005-1011.
38. Clinton K and Van Himel T. *Comparison of a warm gutta-percha obturation technique and lateral condensation.* J Endod. 2001; 27(11):692-695.
39. Neuhaus KW, Schick A and Lussi A. *Apical filling characteristics of carrier-based techniques vs. single cone technique in curved root canals*. Clin Oral Investig. 2016; 20(7):1631-1637.
40. Bhambhani SM and Sprechman K. *Microleakage comparison of thermafil versus vertical condensation using two different sealers*. Oral Surg Oral Med Oral Pathol. 1994; 78(1):105-108.
41. Jarrett IS, Marx D, Covey D et al. *Percentage of canals filled in apical cross sections - an in vitro study of seven obturation techniques*. Int Endod J. 2004; 37(6):392-398.
42. Gençoglu N, Garip Y, Bas M et al. *Comparison of different gutta-percha root filling techniques: Thermafil, Quick-fill, System B, and lateral condensation*. Oral Surg Oral Med Oral Pathol Oral Radiol Endod. 2002; 93(3):333-336.
43. Gulabivala K, Holt R and Long B. *An in vitro comparison of thermoplasticised gutta-percha obturation techniques with cold lateral condensation*. Endod Dent Traumatol. 1998; 14(6):262-269.
44. Leung SF and Gulabivala K. *An in-vitro evaluation of the influence of canal curvature on the sealing ability of Thermafil.* Int Endod J. 1994; 27(4):190-196.
45. Lares C and elDeeb ME. *The sealing ability of the Thermafil obturation technique*. J Endod. 1990; 16(10):474-479.
46. Siqueira JF Jr., Rocas IN, Favieri A et al. *Bacterial leakage in coronally unsealed root canals obturated with 3 different techniques.* Oral Surg Oral Med Oral Pathol Oral Radiol Endod. 2000; 90(5):647-650.
47. De-Deus G, Murad CF, Reis CM et al. *Analysis of the sealing ability of different obturation techniques in oval-shaped canals: a study using a bacterial leakage model.* Braz Oral Res. 2006; 20(1):64-69.
48. De-Deus G, Murad C, Paciornik S et al. *The effect of the canal-filled area on the bacterial leakage of oval-shaped canals.* Int Endod J. 2008; 41(3):183-190.
49. Pommel L and Camps J. *In vitro apical leakage of system B compared with other filling techniques.* J Endod. 2001; 27(7):449-451.
50. De-Deus G, Gurgel-Filho ED, Magalhaes KM et al. *A laboratory analysis of gutta-percha-filled area obtained using Thermafil, System B and lateral condensation*. Int Endod J. 2006; 39(5):378-383.
51. Bertacci A, Baroni C, Breschi L et al. *The influence of smear layer in lateral channels filling*. Clin Oral Investig. 2007; 11(4):353-359.
52. Xu Q, Ling J, Cheung GS et al. *A quantitative evaluation of sealing ability of 4 obturation techniques by using a glucose leakage test.* Oral Surg Oral Med Oral Pathol Oral Radiol Endod. 2007; 104(4):e109-113.
53. Stratul SI, Didilescu A, Grigorie M et al. *How accurate replicates the Thermafil System the morphology of the apical endodontic space? An ex vivo study*. Rom J Morphol Embryol. 2011; 52(1):145-151.
54. Gambarini G, Piasecki L, Schianchi G et al. *In vitro evaluation of carrier based obturation technique: a CBCT study*. Ann Stomatol (Roma). 2016; 7(1-2):11-15.
55. Yilmaz A and Karagoz-Kucukay I. *In vitro comparison of gutta-percha-filled area percentages in root canals instrumented and obturated with different techniques*. J Istanb Univ Fac Dent. 2017; 51(2):37-42.
56. Poggio C, Arciola CR, Dagna A et al. *Solubility of root canal sealers: a comparative study*. Int J Artif Organs. 2010; 33(9):676-681.
57. Siqueira JF Jr., Rocas IN and Valois CR. *Apical sealing ability of five endodontic sealers*. Aust Endod J. 2001; 27(1):33-35.
58. Schafer E and Olthoff G. *Effect of three different sealers on the sealing ability of both thermafil obturators and cold laterally compacted Gutta-Percha*. J Endod. 2002; 28(9):638-642.
59. Pirani C, Zamparini F, Peters OA, et al *The fate of root canals obturated with Thermafil: 10-year data for patients treated in a master's program*. Clin Oral Investig. 2019 Aug. 23(8): p. 3367-77
60. Giovarruscio M, Uccioli U, Malentacca A et al. *A technique for placement of apical MTA plugs using modified Thermafil carriers for the filling of canals with wide apices*. Int Endod J. 2013; 46(1):88-97.

61. Prati C and Gandolfi MG. *Calcium silicate bioactive cements: Biological perspectives and clinical applications.* Dent Mater. 2015; 31(4):351-370.
62. Mohammadi Z, Shalavi S and Soltani MK. *Mineral trioxide aggregate (MTA)-like materials: an update review.* Compend Contin Educ Dent. 2014; 35(8):557-561: quiz 562.
63. Jefferies S. *Bioactive and biomimetic restorative materials: a comprehensive review. Part II.* J Esthet Restor Dent. 2014; 26(1):27-39.
64. Jefferies SR. *Bioactive and biomimetic restorative materials: a comprehensive review. Part I.* J Esthet Restor Dent. 2014; 26(1):14-26.
65. Ree M and Schwartz R. *Clinical application of bioceramics materials in endodontics*. Endod Prac. 2014; 7:32-40.
66. Parirokh M, Torabinejad M and Dummer PMH. *Mineral trioxide aggregate and other bioactive endodontic cements: an updated overview - part I: vital pulp therapy*. Int Endod J. 2018; 51(2):177-205.
67. Torabinejad M, Parirokh M and Dummer PMH. *Mineral trioxide aggregate and other bioactive endodontic cements: an updated overview - part II: other clinical applications and complications*. Int Endod J. 2018; 51(3):284-317.
68. Castro-Raucci LMS, Teixeira LN, Oliveira IR et al. *Osteogenic cell response to calcium aluminate-based cement*. Int Endod J. 2017; 50(8):771-779.
69. Gandolfi MG, Iezzi G, Piattelli A et al. *Osteoinductive potential and bone-bonding ability of ProRoot MTA, MTA Plus and Biodentine in rabbit intramedullary model: Microchemical characterization and histological analysis.* Dent Mater. 2017; 33(5):e221-238.
70. Maeda H, Nakano T, Tomokiyo A et al. *Mineral trioxide aggregate induces bone morphogenetic protein-2 expression and calcification in human periodontal ligament cells*. J Endod. 2010; 36(4):647-652.
71. Oliveira IR, Pandolfelli VC and Jacobovitz M. *Chemical, physical and mechanical properties of a novel calcium aluminate endodontic cement*. Int Endod J. 2010; 43 12):1069-1076.
72. Mohapatra S, Patro S and Mishra S. *Bioactive Materials in Endodontics: An Evolving Component of Clinical Dentistry*. Journal of esthetic and restorative dentistry. 2016; 28(6):376-381; quiz 382.
73. Bartols A, Roussa E, Walther W et al. *First Evidence for Regeneration of the Periodontium to Mineral Trioxide Aggregate in Human Teeth*. J Endod. 2017; 43(5):715-722.
74. Huang XQ, Camba J, Gu LS et al. *Mechanism of bioactive molecular extraction from mineralized dentin by calcium hydroxide and tricalcium silicate cement*. Dent Mater. 2018; 34(2):317-330.
75. Singh G, Elshamy FM, Homeida HE et al. *An in vitro Comparison of Antimicrobial Activity of Three Endodontic Sealers with Different Composition*. J Contemp Dent Pract. 2016; 17(7):553-556.
76. Singh G, Gupta I, Elshamy FM et al. *In vitro comparison of antibacterial properties of bioceramic-based sealer, resin-based sealer and zinc oxide eugenol based sealer and two mineral trioxide aggregates*. Eur J Dent. 2016; 10(3):366-369.
77. Zhang H, Pappen FG and Haapasalo M. *Dentin enhances the antibacterial effect of mineral trioxide aggregate and bioaggregate*. J Endod. 2009; 35(2):221-224.
78. Zhang H, Shen Y, Ruse ND et al. *Antibacterial activity of endodontic sealers by modified direct contact test against Enterococcus faecalis*. J Endod. 2009; 35(7):1051-1055.
79. Candeiro GT, Correia FC, Duarte MA et al. *Evaluation of radiopacity, pH, release of calcium ions, and flow of a bioceramic root canal sealer*. J Endod. 2012; 38(6):842-845.
80. Prestegaard H, Portenier I, Orstavik D et al. *Antibacterial activity of various root canal sealers and root-end filling materials in dentin blocks infected ex vivo with Enterococcus faecalis*. Acta Odontol Scand. 2014; 72(8):970-976.
81. Wang Z, Shen Y and Haapasalo M. *Dentin extends the antibacterial effect of endodontic sealers against Enterococcus faecalis biofilms*. J Endod. 2014; 40(4):505-508.
82. Dawood AE, Parashos P, Wong RHK et al. *Calcium silicate-based cements: composition, properties, and clinical applications*. J Investig Clin Dent. 2017; 8(2).
83. Poggio C, Dagna A, Ceci M et al. *Solubility and pH of bioceramic root canal sealers: A comparative study.* J Clin Exp Dent. 2017; 9(10):e1189-1194.
84. Siboni F, Taddei P, Prati C et al. *Properties of NeoMTA Plus and MTA Plus cements for endodontics*. Int Endod J. 2017; 50 Suppl 2:e83-94.
85. Vasconcelos BC, Bernardes RA, Duarte MA et al. *Apical sealing of root canal fillings performed with five different endodontic sealers: analysis by fluid filtration*. J Appl Oral Sci. 2011; 19(4):324-328.
86. Borges RP, Sousa-Neto MD, Versiani MA et al. *Changes in the surface of four calcium silicate-containing endodontic materials and an epoxy resin-based sealer after a solubility test*. Int Endod J. 2012; 45(5):419-428.
87. Zhou HM, Shen Y, Zheng W et al. *Physical properties of 5 root canal sealers*. J Endod. 2013; 39(10):1281-1286.
88. Antunes HS, Gominho LF, Andrade-Junior CV et al. *Sealing ability of two root-end filling materials in a bacterial nutrient leakage model*. Int Endod J. 2016; 49(10):960-965.
89. Castro-Raucci LM, Oliveira IR, Teixeira LN et al. *Effects of a novel calcium aluminate cement on the early events of the progression of osteogenic cell cultures.* Braz Dent J. 2011; 22(2):99-104.

90. Darvell BW and Wu RC. *"MTA" - an Hydraulic Silicate Cement: review update and setting reaction*. Dent Mater. 2011; 27(5):407-422.
91. Gandolfi MG, Taddei P, Siboni F et al. *Fluoride-containing nanoporous calcium-silicate MTA cements for endodontics and oral surgery: early fluorapatite formation in a phosphate-containing solution.* Int Endod J. 2011; 44(10):938-949.
92. Wang CW, Chiang TY, Chang HC et al. *Physicochemical properties and osteogenic activity of radiopaque calcium silicate-gelatin cements*. J Mater Sci Mater Med. 2014; 25(9):2193-2203.
93. Han L, Kodama S and Okiji T. *Evaluation of calcium-releasing and apatite-forming abilities of fast-setting calcium silicate-based endodontic materials*. Int Endod J. 2015; 48(2):124-130.
94. Butt N, Talwar S, Chaudhry S et al. *Comparison of physical and mechanical properties of mineral trioxide aggregate and Biodentine.* Indian J Dent Res. 2014; 25(6):692-697.
95. Viapiana R, Flumignan DL, Guerreiro-Tanomaru JM et al. *Physicochemical and mechanical properties of zirconium oxide and niobium oxide modified Portland cement-based experimental endodontic sealers*. Int Endod J. 2014; 47(5):437-448.
96. Ghoneim AG, Lutfy RA, Sabet NE et al. *Resistance to fracture of roots obturated with novel canal-filling systems*. J Endod. 2011; 37(11):1590-1592.
97. Cauwels RG, Pieters IY, Martens LC et al. *Fracture resistance and reinforcement of immature roots with gutta percha, mineral trioxide aggregate and calcium phosphate bone cement: a standardized in vitro model.* Dent Traumatol. 2010; 26(2):137-142.
98. Celikten B, Uzuntas CF, Orhan AI et al. *Evaluation of root canal sealer filling quality using a single-cone technique in oval shaped canals: An In vitro Micro-CT study*. Scanning. 2016; 38(2):133-140.
99. Debelian G and Trope M. *The use of premixed bioceramic materials in endodontics*. G Ital Endod. 2016; 30(2):70-80.
100. Scotti N, Rota R, Berutti E. *Otturazione endodontica e restauri adesivi: esiste un legame?* G Ital Endod. 2013; 27(1):59-62.
101. Watson TF, Atmeh AR, Sajini S et al. *Present and future of glass-ionomers and calcium-silicate cements as bioactive materials in dentistry: biophotonics-based interfacial analyses in health and disease*. Dent Mater. 2014; 30(1):50-61.
102. Del Fabbro M, Corbella S, Sequeira-Byron P et al. *Endodontic procedures for retreatment of periapical lesions.* Cochrane Database Syst Rev. 2016; 10:CD005511.
103. Friedman S. *Retrograde approaches in endodontic therapy*. Endod Dent Traumatol. 1991; 7(3):97-107.
104. Molven O, Halse A and Grung B. *Surgical management of endodontic failures: indications and treatment results.* Int Dent J. 1991; 41(1):33-42.
105. Riccitiello F, Stabile P, Amato M et al. *The treatment of the large periradicular endodontic injury*. Minerva Stomatol. 2011; 60(9):417-426.
106. Brito-Junior M, Faria-e-Silva AL, Quintino AC et al. *Orthograde retreatment failure with extruded MTA apical plug in a large periradicular lesion followed by surgical intervention: case report*. Gen Dent. 2012; 60(2):e96-100.
107. Carrotte PV. *Current practice in endodontics: 6. Retreatments and periradicular surgery*. Dent Update. 2001; 28(2):92-96.
108. Hepworth MJ and Friedman S. *Treatment outcome of surgical and non-surgical management of endodontic failures*. J Can Dent Assoc. 1997; 63(5):364-371.
109. Christiansen R, Kirkevang LL, Horsted-Bindslev P et al. *Randomized clinical trial of root-end resection followed by root-end filling with mineral trioxide aggregate or smoothing of the orthograde gutta-percha root filling - 1 year follow-up.* Int Endod J. 2009; 42(2):105-114.
110. Kahler B. *Microsurgical endodontic retreatment of post restored posterior teeth: a case series.* Aust Endod J. 2010; 36(3):114-121.
111. von Arx T. *Frequency and type of canal isthmuses in first molars detected by endoscopic inspection during periradicular surgery*. Int Endod J. 2005; 38(3):160-168.
112. Beck-Broichsitter BE, Schmid H, Busch HP et al. *Long-term survival of teeth in the posterior region after apical surgery.* J Craniomaxillofac Surg. 2018 (e-pub before publication).

References Box 5.4

1. Torabinejad M. Historical and contemporary perspectives on root-end filling materials. J Endod. 1993;19(8):432–3.
2. Torabinejad M, White DJ. Tooth filling material and method of use. US Patent 5415547. 1993.
3. Torabinejad M, White DJ, inventors; Loma Linda University, assignee. Tooth filling material and method of use. United States Patent 5769638; 23rd June 1998.
4. Funteas UR, Wallace JA, Fochtman EW. A comparative analysis of mineral trioxide aggregate and Portland cement. Australian Endodontics Journal. 2003;29:43–4.
5. Monteiro Bramante C, Demarchi AC, De Moraes IG, et al. Presence of arsenic in different types of MTA

and white and gray Portland cement. Oral Surgery, Oral Medicine, Oral Pathology, Oral Radiology, and Endodontics. 2008;106:909–13.
6. Comin-Chiaramonti L, Cavalleri G, Sbaizero O et al. Crystallochemical comparison between Portland cements and mineral trioxide aggregate (MTA). Journal of Applied Biomaterials and Biomechanics. 2009;7:171–8.
7. Dammaschke T, Gerth HU, Züchner H., et al. Chemical and physical surface and bulk material characterization of white ProRoot MTA and two Portland cements. Dental Materials. 2005;21:731-8.
8. Schembri M, Peplow G, Camilleri J. Analyses of heavy metals in mineral trioxide aggregate and Portland cement. Journal of Endodontics. 2010;36:1210–5.
9. Chang SW, Shon WJ, Lee W, et al. Analysis of heavy metal contents in gray and white MTA and 2 kinds of Portland cement: a preliminary study. Oral Surgery, Oral Medicine, Oral Pathology, Oral Radiology, and Endodontics. 2010;109:642–6.
10. Camilleri J. Hydration mechanisms of mineral trioxide aggregate. Int Endod J. 2007;40(6):462-70.
11. Camilleri J, Kralj P, Veber M, Sinagra E. Characterization and analyses of acid-extractable and leached trace elements in dental cements. Int Endod J. 2012;45(8):737–43.
12. Torabinejad M, Hong CU, McDonald F, Pitt Ford TR. Physical and chemical properties of a new root- end filling material. J Endod. 1995;21:349–53.
13. Torabinejad M, Watson TF, Pitt Ford TR. Sealing ability of a mineral trioxide aggregate when used as a root end filling material. J Endod. 1993;19:591–5.
14. Hatibovic ⊠-Kofman S, Raimundo L, Zheng L, Chong L, Friedman M, Andreasen JO. Fracture resistance and histological findings of immature teeth treated with mineral trioxide aggregate. Dent Traumatol. 2008;24:272–6.
15. Dammaschke T, Gerth HU, Züchner H, Schäfer E E. Chemical and physical surface and bulk material characterization of white ProRoot MTA and two Portland cements. Dent Mater. 2005;21:731–8.
16. Gancedo-Caravia L, Garcia-Barbero E. Influence of humidity and setting time on the push-out strength of mineral trioxide aggregate obturations. J Endod. 2006;32(9):894–6.
17. Reyes-Carmona JF, Felippe MS, Felippe WT. The biomineralization ability of mineral trioxide aggre- gate and Portland cement on dentin enhances the push-out strength. J Endod. 2010;36(2):286–91.
18. Saghiri MA, Shokouhinejad N, Lotfi M, Aminsobhani M, Saghiri AM. Push-out bond strength of mineral trioxide aggregate in the presence of alkaline pH. J Endod. 2010;36(11):1856–9.
19. Shokouhinejad N, Nekoofar MH, Iravani A, Kharrazifard MJ, Dummer PM. Effect of acidic environment on the push-out bond strength of min- eral trioxide aggregate. J Endod. 2010;36(5):871–4.
20. Saghiri MA, Lotfi M, Joupari MD, Aeinehchi M, Saghiri AM. Effects of storage temperature on sur- face hardness, microstructure, and phase formation of white mineral trioxide aggregate. J Endod. 2010;36(8):1414–8.
21. Namazikhah MS, Nekoofar MH, Sheykhrezae MS, Salariyeh S, Hayes SJ, Bryant ST, Mohammadi MM, Dummer PM. The effect of pH on surface hardness and microstructure of mineral trioxide aggregate. Int Endod J. 2008;41(2):108–16.
22. Giuliani V, Nieri M, Pace R, Pagavino G. Effects of pH on surface hardness and microstructure of mineral trioxide aggregate and Aureoseal: an in vitro study. J Endod 2010;36(11):1883–6.
23. Namazikhah MS, Nekoofar MH, Sheykhrezae MS, Salariyeh S, Hayes SJ, Bryant ST, Mohammadi MM, Dummer PM. The effect of pH on surface hardness and microstructure of mineral trioxide aggregate. Int Endod J. 2008;41(2):108–16.
24. Nekoofar MH, Oloomi K, Sheykhrezae MS, Tabor R, Stone DF, Dummer PM. An evaluation of the effect of blood and human serum on the surface microhardness and surface microstructure of mineral trioxide aggregate. Int Endod J. 2010;43(10): 849–58.
25. Saghiri MA, Asgar K, Lotfi M, Garcia-Godoy F. Nanomodification of mineral trioxide aggregate for enhanced physiochemical properties. Int Endod J. 2012;45(11):979–88.
26. Matt GD, Thorpe JR, Strother JM, McClanahan SB. Comparative study of white and gray mineral triox- ide aggregate (MTA) simulating a one- or two-step apical barrier technique. J Endod. 2004;30:876–9.
27. Kayahan MB, Nekoofar MH, Kazandağ M, Canpolat C, Malkondu O, Kaptan F, Dummer PM. Effect of acid-etching procedure on selected physical proper- ties of mineral trioxide aggregate. Int Endod J. 2009;42(11):1004–14.
28. Camilleri J. Evaluation of the effect of intrinsic mate- rial properties and ambient conditions on the dimen- sional stability of white mineral trioxide aggregate and Portland cement. J Endod. 2011;37(2):239–45.
29. Storm B, Eichmiller FC, Tordik PA, Goodell GG. Setting expansion of gray and white mineral trioxide aggregate and Portland cement. J Endod. 2008;34:80–2.
30. Islam I, Chng HK, Yap AU. Comparison of the physical and mechanical properties of MTA and Portland cement. J Endod. 2006;32:193–7.
31. Chng HK, Islam I, Yap AU, Tong YW, Koh ET. Properties of a new root-end filling material. J Endod. 2005;31:665–8.
32. Danesh G, Dammaschke T, Gerth HU, Zandbiglari T, Schäfer E. A comparative study of selected properties of ProRoot mineral trioxide aggregate and two Portland cements. Int Endod J. 2006;39:213–9.

33. Torabinejad M, Hong CU, McDonald F, Pitt Ford TR. Physical and chemical properties of a new root- end filling material. J Endod. 1995;21:349–53.
34. Fridland M, Rosado R. Mineral trioxide aggregate (MTA) solubility and porosity with different water-to-powder ratios. J Endod. 2003;29(12):814–7.
35. Torabinejad M, Watson TF, Pitt Ford TR. Sealing ability of a mineral trioxide aggregate when used as a root end filling material. J Endod. 1993;19:591–5.
36. Torabinejad M, Higa RK, McKendry DJ, Pitt Ford TR. Dye leakage of four root end filling materials: effects of blood contamination. J Endod. 1994; 20(4):159–63.
37. Torabinejad M, Parirokh M. Mineral trioxide aggre- gate: a comprehensive literature review part II: leakage and biocompatibility investigations. J Endod. 2010;36(2):190–202.
38. Bukhari S, Karabucak B. Antimicrobial Effect of Bioceramic Sealer on an 8-Week Matured Enterococcus faecalis Biofilm Attached to a Root Canal Dentinal Surface J Endod. 2019 Aug;45(8):1047-1052.
39. Camilleri J, Pitt Ford TR. Mineral trioxide aggregate: a review of the constituents and biological properties of the material. Int Endod J. 2006;39(10):747–54.
40. Haglund R, He J, Jarvis J, Safavi KE, Spångberg LS, Zhu Q. Effects of root-end filling materials on fibroblasts and macrophages in vitro. Oral Surg Oral Med Oral Pathol Oral Radiol Endod. 2003;95(6): 739–45.
41. Holland R, Filho JA, de Souza V, Nery MJ, Bernabé PF, Junior ED. Mineral trioxide aggregate repair of lateral root perforations. J Endod. 2001;27(4):281–4.
42. Torabinejad M, Pitt Ford TR, McKendry DJ, Abedi HR, Miller DA, Kariyawasam SP. Histologic assessment of mineral trioxide aggregate as a root-end filling in monkeys. J Endod. 1997;23(4):225–8.
43. Luo T, Liu J, Sun Y, Shen Y, Zou L, Cytocompatibility of Biodentine and iRoot FS with human periodontal ligament cells: an in vitro study. Int Endod J, 2018. 51: p. 779–88
44. UyanikMO,NagasE,SahinC,DagliF,CehreliZC. Effects of different irrigation regimens on the sealing properties of repaired furcal perforations. Oral Surg Oral Med Oral Pathol Oral Radiol Endod. 2009;107(3):e91–5.
45. Yildirim T, Oruçoğlu H, Cobankara FK. Long-term evaluation of the influence of smear layer on the api- cal sealing ability of MTA. J Endod. 2008;34(12):1537–40.

- Review the **pre- or intraoperative causes** that can generate postoperative problems.
- Describe the **clinical situations** associated with the minor or serious complications that occur at the end of retreatments.
- Identify the most suitable **therapeutic measures** for dealing with the complications.
- Define a correct **time path** to assess complications and determine the general success of a retreatment.

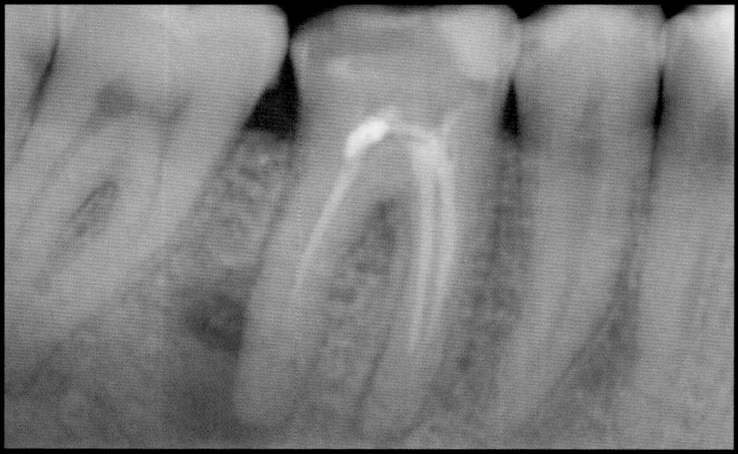

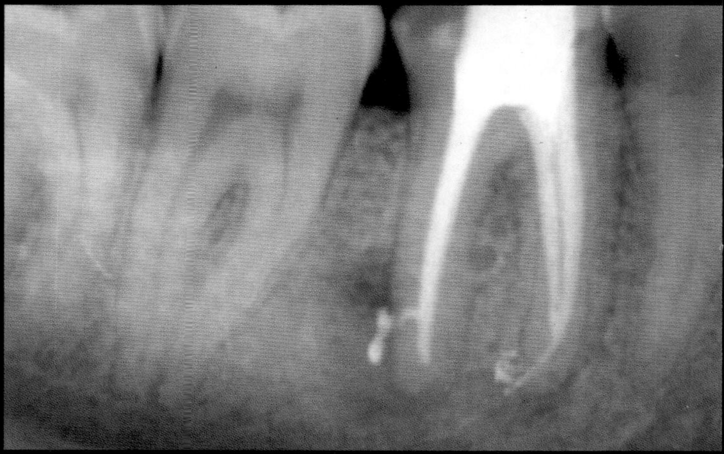

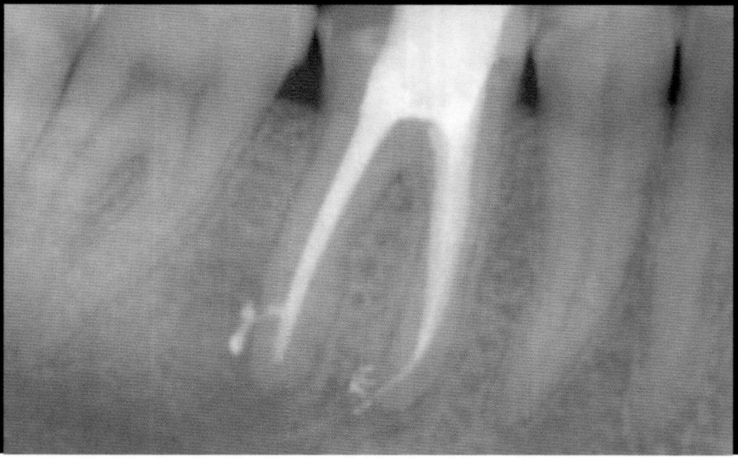

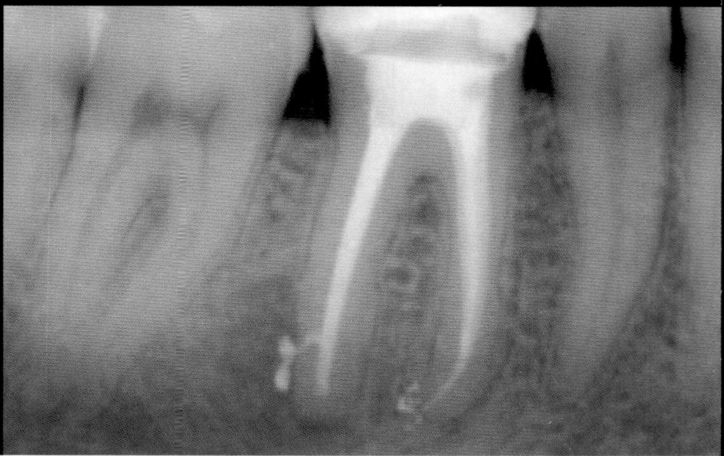

Massimo Gagliani, Fabio Gorni,
Marco Martignoni

06

Post-retreatment phase: a guided plan

Temporal evolution of therapies: evaluation tools and methods

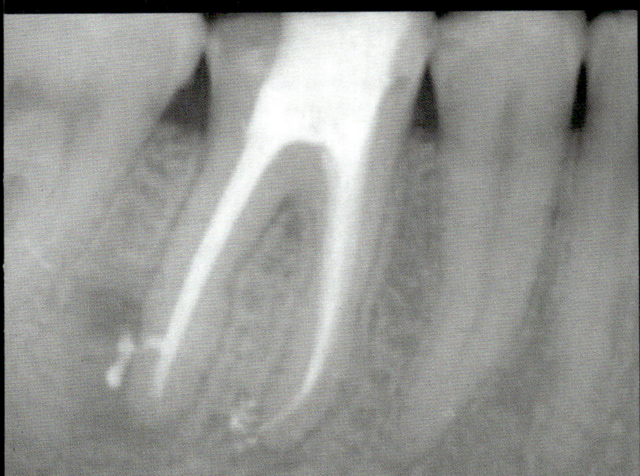

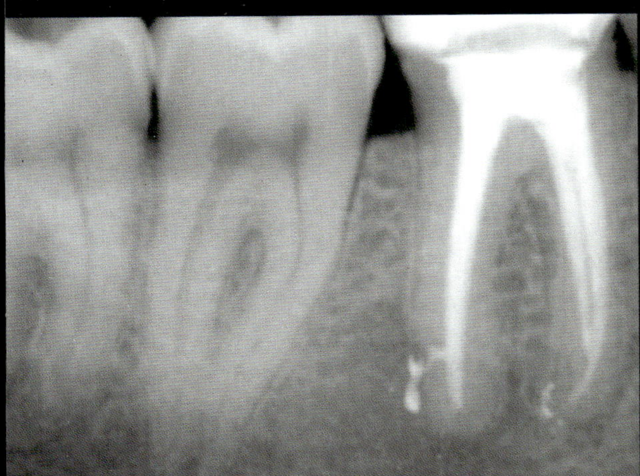

Preliminary remarks

Endodontic treatment is an unpleasant experience in some patients[1]; retreatment procedures entail certain risks[2], and the scenario is complex. As specified by the authors, some elements can be considered predictive. The presence of an established radiolucent lesion at an apical level, treatment complexity, and clinical symptoms should also be addressed.
In any case, dealing with a canal content rich in bacteria containing filling and reconstruction materials can generate many problems, albeit in a small number of cases[3].
In this chapter, various situations are examined: (1) events that lead to the incorrect completion of a retreatment and (2) general clinical scenarios that may arise after a correct or incorrect retreatment procedure.
Among the latter, the most common scenarios are represented by spontaneous or provoked pain[4] [5] and by more or less marked swelling, which oblige a dentist to prescribe supportive pharmacological therapy.
All the problems resulting from these clinical cases are considered, i.e., reconstruction types and strategies to be adopted to observe the evolution of postendodontic treatment disease (Figs. 6.1a–c).

Fig. 6.1a: Painful palatine swelling is highlighted by clinical examination.

Fig. 6.1b: The signs of the fracture of the restoration are visible at higher magnification.

Fig. 6.1c: The radiographic image does not show signs of apical rarefaction, so the case is diagnosed as deep corono-radical fracture possibly requiring the extraction of the molar.

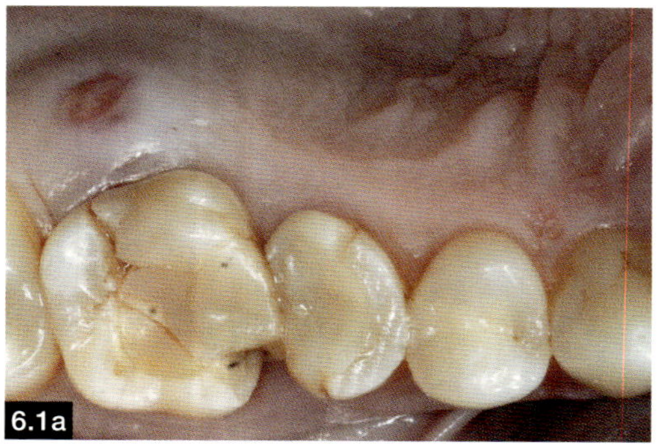
6.1a

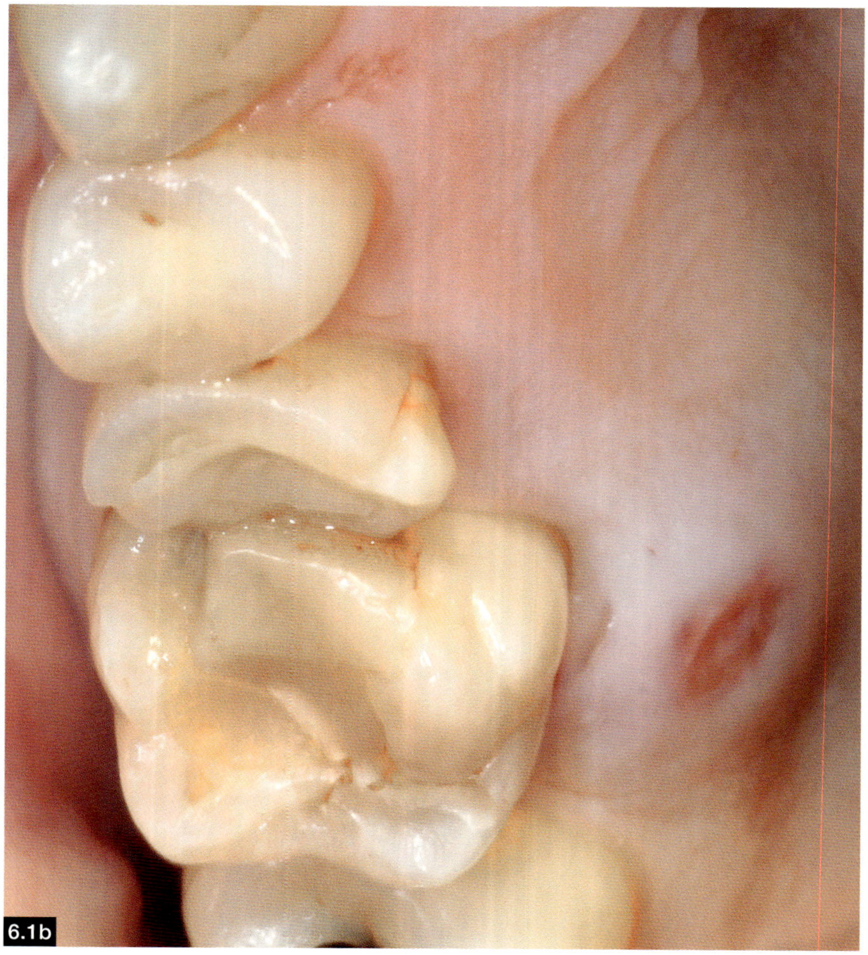
6.1b

Completion of incorrect therapy

In some instances, the endodontic space is practicable, but the desired technical quality of retreatment is not achieved. These situations are predictable in the diagnostic phase but are not precisely quantified in some cases.
The clinical case presented below is emblematic in this respect.

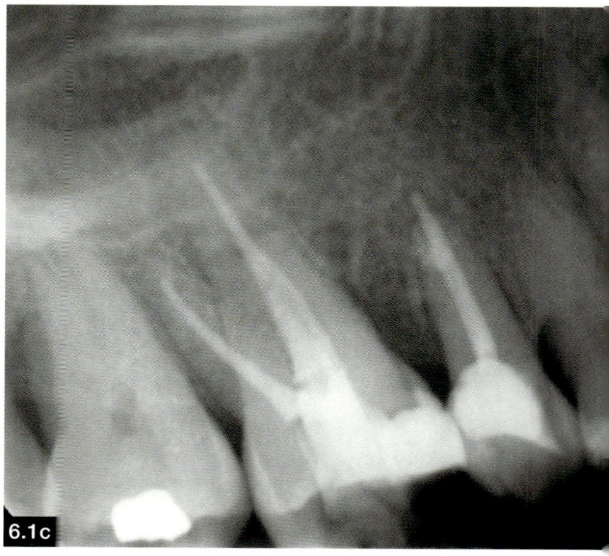
6.1c

Fracture starting from the apex

CASE REPORT 1

Follow-up on a tooth treated previously for pulp disease presents a double lingual and vestibular fistula; the patient complains of a severe pain while chewing.
The x-ray reveals an endodontic treatment with two small voids but that is otherwise acceptable; the periapical radiotransparency appears very large in relation to the quality of the previous treatment. The periradicular probing appears abnormal and punctiform, a clear sign of a suspected longitudinal root fracture.

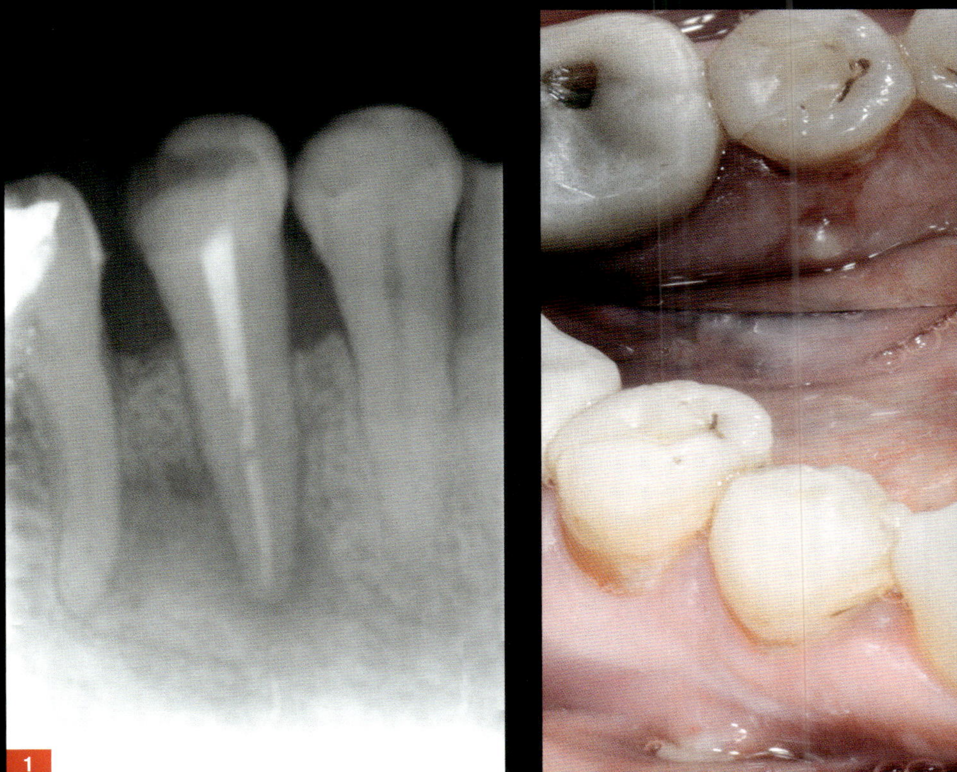

Figure 1: The clinical scenario of a double lingual and vestibular fistula arouses suspicion in the endodontically treated premolar; the radiological picture reveals a radiolucent area that follows the entire root contour and is disproportionately wide in relation to the quality of the endodontic therapy which, although with two small voids, appears to be well performed.

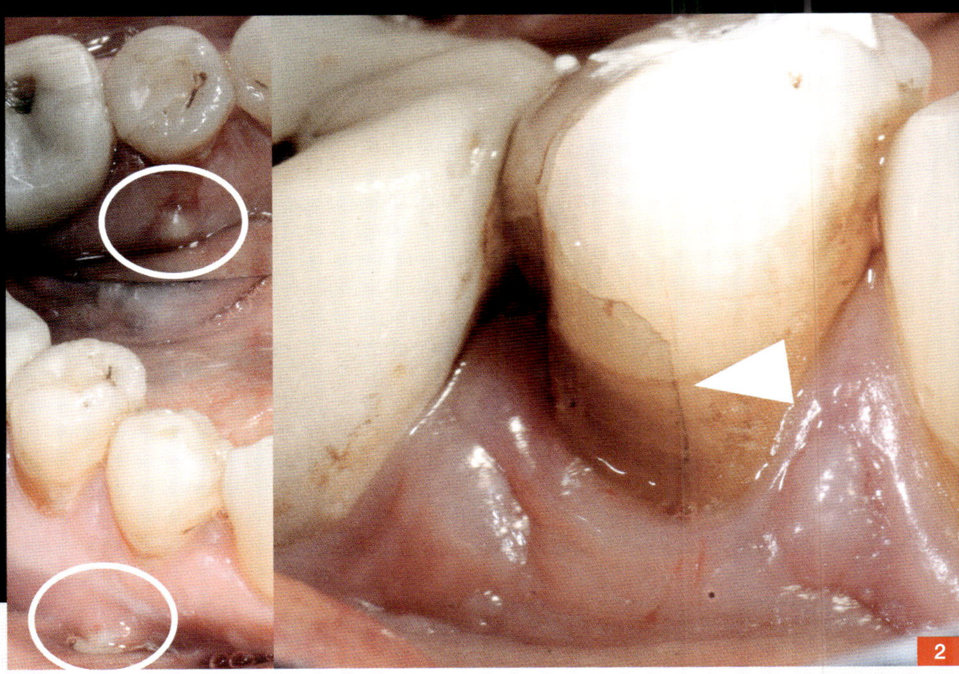

Figure 2: A more careful analysis reveals a longitudinal crack involving the vestibular and distal area of the tooth.

This is confirmed by the extraction; it could be due to an apical-crack that started from the apical zone and spread along the root in a coronal sense.

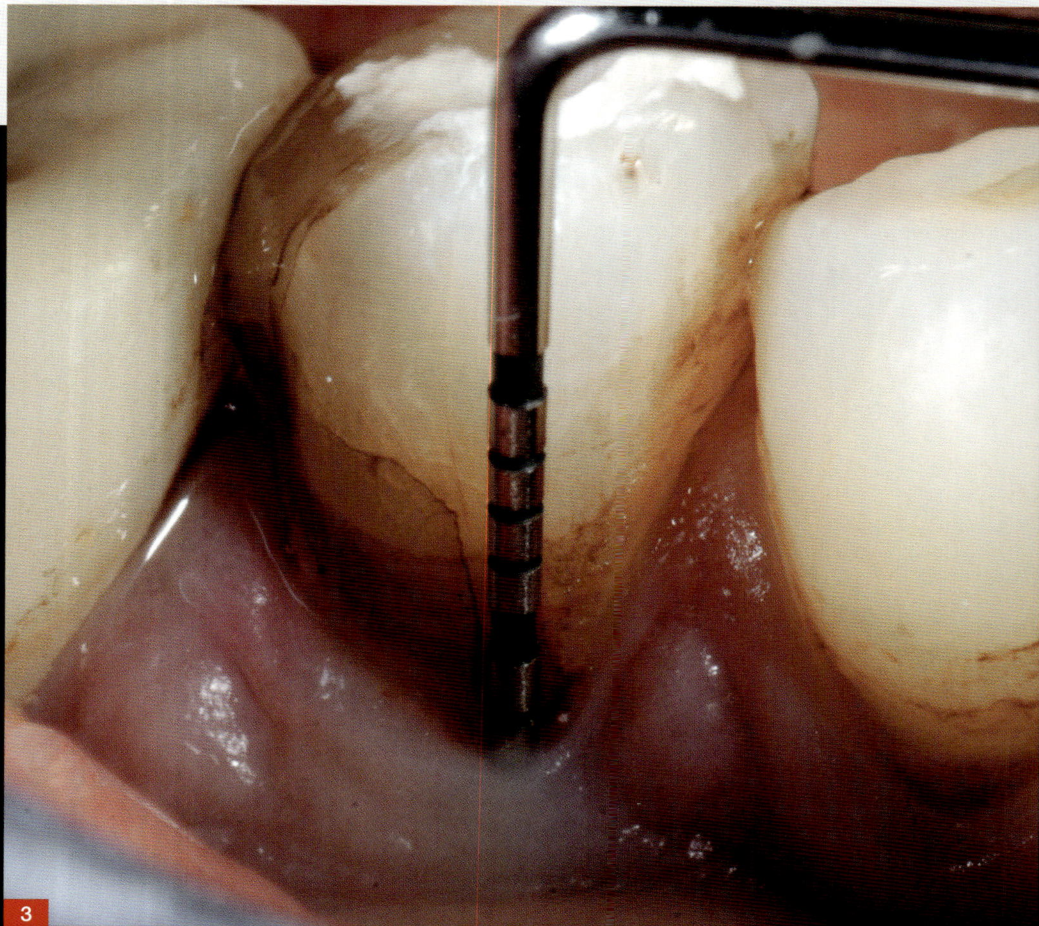

3

Figure 3: In these cases, periodontal probing is often not conclusive, since it is only present near the line of supposed fracture.

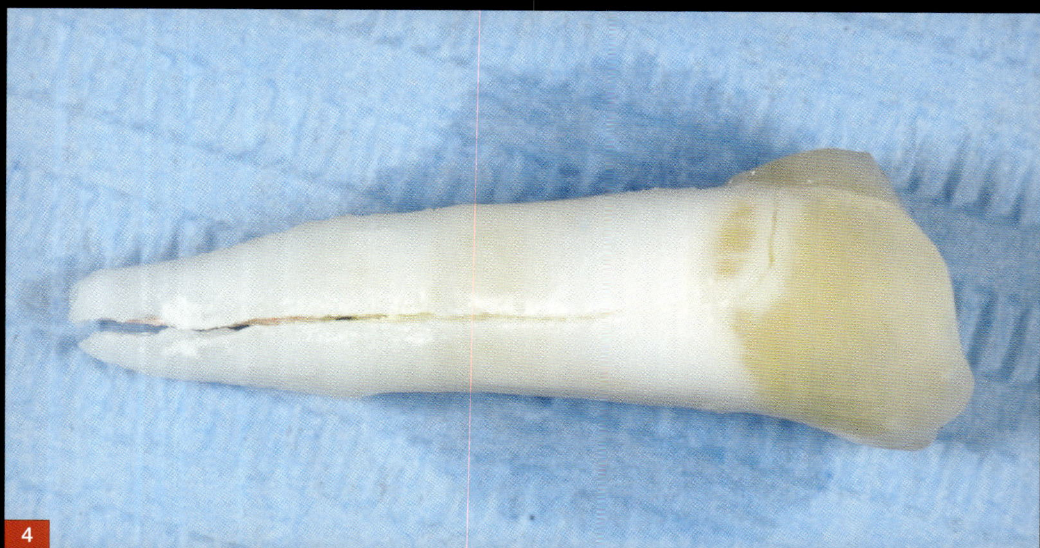

4

Figure 4: The extracted tooth shows a frank longitudinal fracture, beginning at the apex, the origin now is clear.

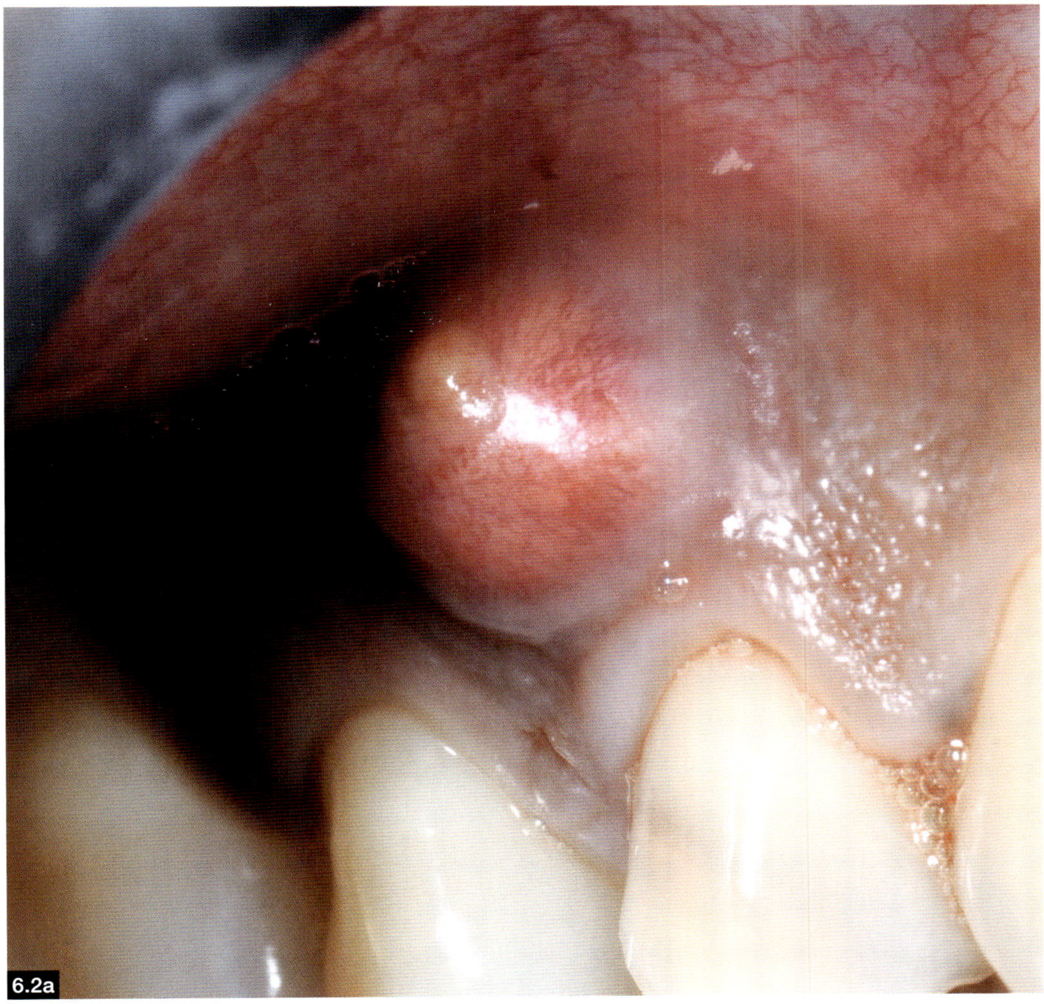

6.2a

Fig. 6.2a: One of the most characteristic signs of negative developments in endodontic treatments is represented by septic recrudescence that results in clinically visible swellings.

Fig. 6.2b: Uncomplicated coronal fracture is a visible sign of endodontium contamination by oral fluids rich in bacteria.

Septic situations after treatment

At the end of a retreatment, a patient may have more or less intense pain symptoms that may last several days[6].
In percentage terms, this eventuality varies according to the case considered but almost never exceeds 10% of the cases treated. Certain conditions may favor a negative and completely reversible post-treatment phase. Some authors[7] suggest focussing on canal overfilling, which may lead to postoperative pain but has no influence on the final outcome. Postoperative pain is sometimes associated with swelling. Alves[7] argued that the preoperative situation should guide the clinician and allow him or her to consider patterns of therapeutic behavior that provide the correct number of sessions to avoid these eventualities[8, 9] (Fig. 6.2a–b).

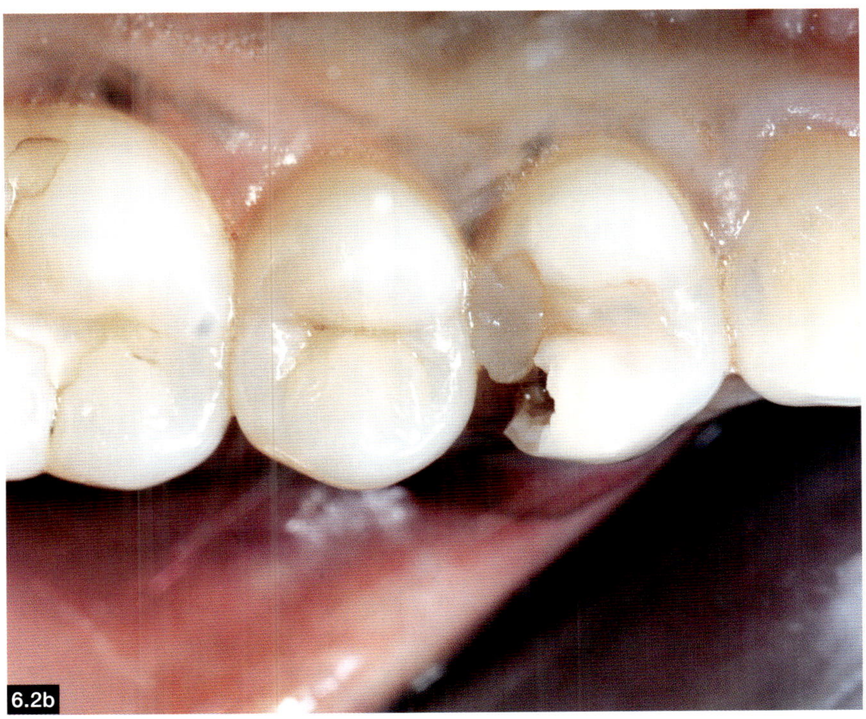

6.2b

Causes

OVERINSTRUMENTATION

Postoperative pain is frequently attributable to the use of instruments **beyond the apical limit**

Postoperative sequelae can be linked to *overinstrumentation* or to the extrusion of infected dentin debris or canal fillers, which are also contaminated by bacteria invading the periodontal space. Although many precautions are taken in this regard, this shaping effect is almost inevitable[10].

Symptoms

Inflammatory reactions are an inevitable element at the end of a retreatment; they may be limited to the periradicular region only, where they cause mild pain when chewing or assume the connotations of fully-blown periodontitis, which requires a specific causal therapy.
In the first postoperative phase, releasing a tooth from its occlusal contacts seems to be only weakly indicated to prevent this effect[11].

Prevention

PREVENTING PAIN

A **lower incidence of postoperative pain** will be determined by an adequate opening of more coronal areas

Many studies have been conducted to *prevent postoperative pain*, and all the causes of this pain have been investigated. The instrumentation of infected canals can generate an extrusion of infected dentinal debris beyond the apical limit and consequently induce an inflammatory process in the periapical area near the highly innervated periodontal ligament[6].
As such, many authors have evaluated the factors that can reduce this phenomenon.

Arora et al.[12] demonstrated that the maintenance of apical patency seems irrelevant. Pasqualini et al.[13] reiterated this assumption. They compared the operation of maintaining apical patency with rotary instruments in NiTi alloy and with steel instruments and concluded that the former are less traumatic than the latter. Kherlakian et al.[14] observed similar results. Conversely, Pasqualini et al.[15] reported that patients treated with NiTi instruments activated by reciprocal movement experience a greater degree of discomfort than patients treated with steel instruments. Comparin et al.[16] compared to NiTi rotary instruments with reciprocating motion analogs and found no significant differences. Saumya-Rajesh et al.[17] obtained similar data with different instruments.
Postoperative pain can be affected by another element related to the precision of a treatment performed at apical foramen level; for this reason, performing a treatment with the electronic control of the length of work activated can result in a low incidence of postoperative pain[18].
The enlargement of the apical foramen, often dictated by the disease dealt with during retreatment, may also play a role, although an enlargement of untreated teeth of up to ISO 40 with new-generation reciprocating NiTi instruments may not generate marked pain compared with that of the controls[19].
Silva et al.[20] had similar opinions, whereas Saini et al.[21] were of the opposite opinion.
The precautions used when enlarging the apical foramen may differ for various reasons, and this variability can be associated with instrumentation types and operators.
Cryotherapy with an EndoVac system (Kerr Endo, CA, USA) has also been suggested; this procedure involves washing with a physiological solution at 2.5 °C and the preliminary clinical findings would appear very promising[22].
Similarly, exposure to low-intensity laser irradiation at the end of retreatment procedures leads to a significant reduction in postoperative pain symptoms in teeth that need retreatment [23].

Injury exacerbated by the load on an upper lateral

CASE REPORT 2

As has often been mentioned, swelling, indicating the presence of an abscess, is undoubtedly a sequela incorrectly performed of endodontic treatment. In this case, a lateral incisor, treated with root canal paste, shows a very extensive apical rarefaction that seems to compromise its permanence in the patient's mouth. It is clear that these teeth, before being extracted,

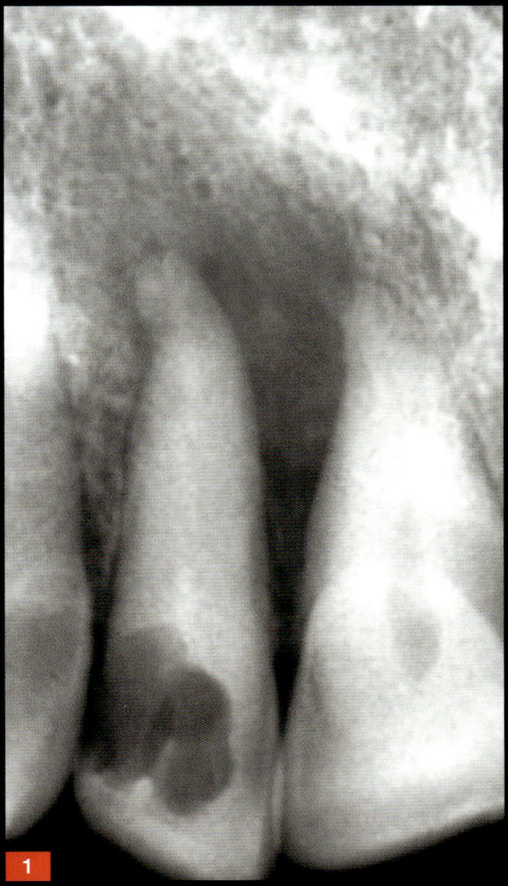

1

Figure 1: An upper lateral with an extensive previously treated palatine caries and an inappropriate canal filling results, after several years from the first treatment, in a very large abscess.

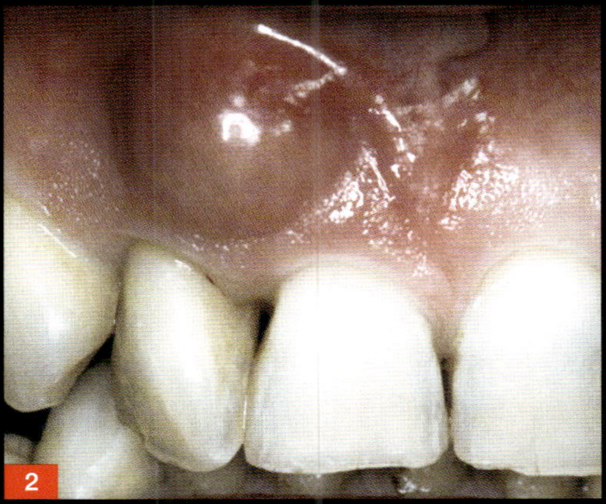

2

Figure 2: The abscess easily attributable to tooth no. 12.

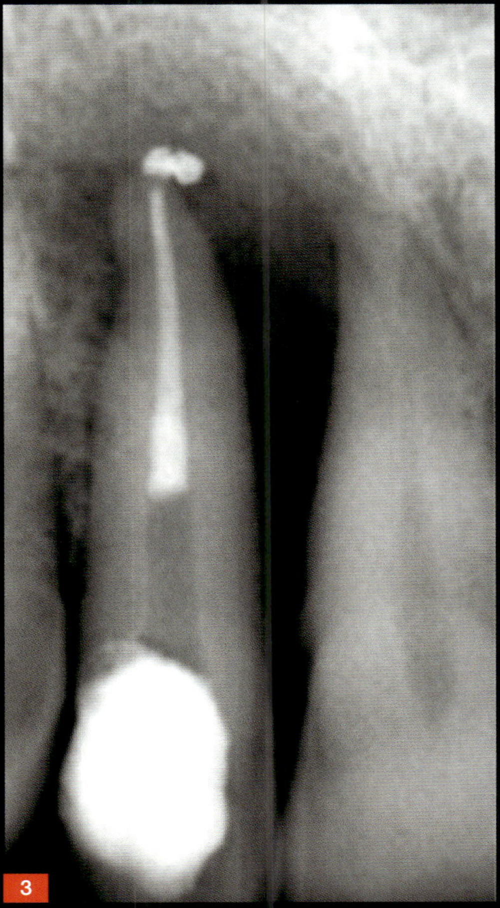

3

Figure 3: The endodontic treatment ended with a slight overfill.

must be evaluated with special attention regarding all the implications – functional and aesthetic – that they involve. The treatment plan involves technically modifying the canal access and shaping that respects the apical anatomical peculiarities that this tooth often presents. We can note the slight, but well defined, curvature that has allowed the sealing with a slight overfill, of the apical area of tooth no. 12. The 14-year x-ray shows consistent recovery of alveolar bone around the lateral.

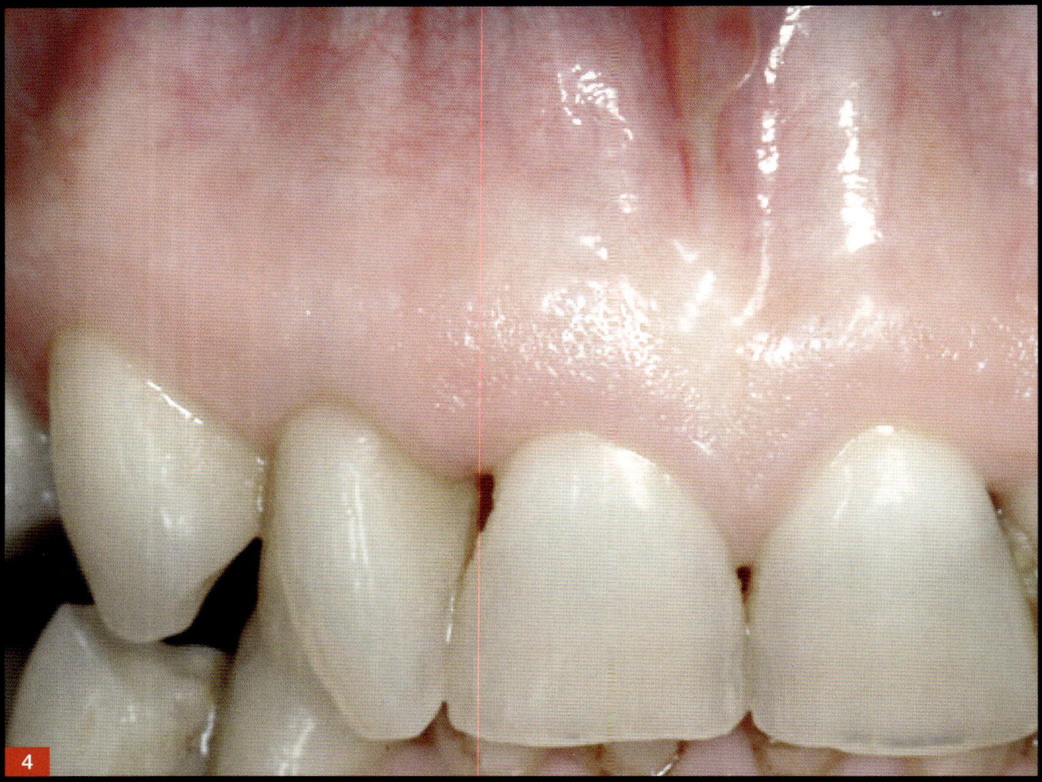

Figure 4: The resolution of the abscess with perfect reintegration of the soft tissue.

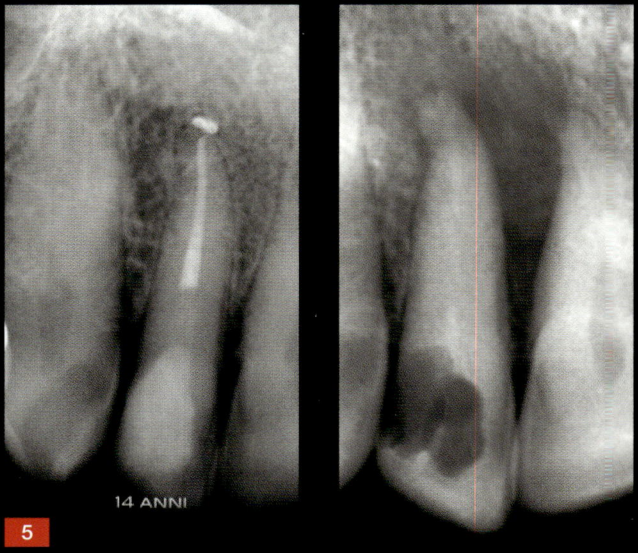

Figure 5: The X-ray performed 14 years later shows a perfect resolution of periapical inflammation with a remodelling of extruded periradicular cement.

Multisession treatments

As discussed in Chapter 4, treatment should be carried out in several sessions to separate the instrumentation phase from the filling phase and consequently prevent this kind of postoperative complication. The use of disinfectants inside the root canal can limit the onset of such reactions due to their direct effect on bacteria and the effect generated by emptying a canal. The latter possibly acts as an outlet chamber for extraradicular edema which does not, therefore, compress the richly innervated structures of the periodontal ligament because it can flow into the canal. This effect cannot therefore be attributed to the antibacterial action of the medicinal product introduced into the root canal alone, but this is of little importance to the final result. A systematic review has shown that an analgesic effect is attributable to this reason regardless of the use of drugs[24]. Although multisession treatments are discussed in Chapter 4, it would seem interesting to discuss the results of studies evaluating the influence of temporary treatment on postoperative pain. Figini et al.[25] and Manfredi et al.[26] conducted a systematic review and found that postoperative use of painkillers and antibiotics is lower in patients who receive treatment in several sessions than in patients who take other drugs for nondental reasons. Therefore, this treatment seems advisable in terms of final effectiveness compared with that of a single session. El Mubarak et al.[27] studied more than 200 patients and found postoperative pain in about 9% of the patients treated. The relative percentage is higher in patients who are already suffering from pain before treatment than in patients who experience pain after treatment. The authors did not find significant differences between the two types of treatment, i.e., whether they are performed in a single session or multiple sessions. Su et al.[28] systematically analyzed related studies and reported substantial equality between the two treatments. However, there was slightly higher incidence of pain immediately after treatment in several sessions.

Pharmaceutical remedies

Pretreatment drugs

To improve postoperative conditions, several clinicians have used pharmacological therapies before endodontic treatment. In this regard, Jalalzadeh et al.[29] proposed using 30 mg of prednisolone 30 min before the treatment. Use of cortisone led to a significant decrease in postoperative pain. These results have been confirmed by other authors[30], although they were based on studies carried out on previously untreated teeth with periapical lesions. One interesting solution could be treatment, which has been seen to be prior to endodontic treatment; this procedure has been proven effective in reducing postoperative pain[31].

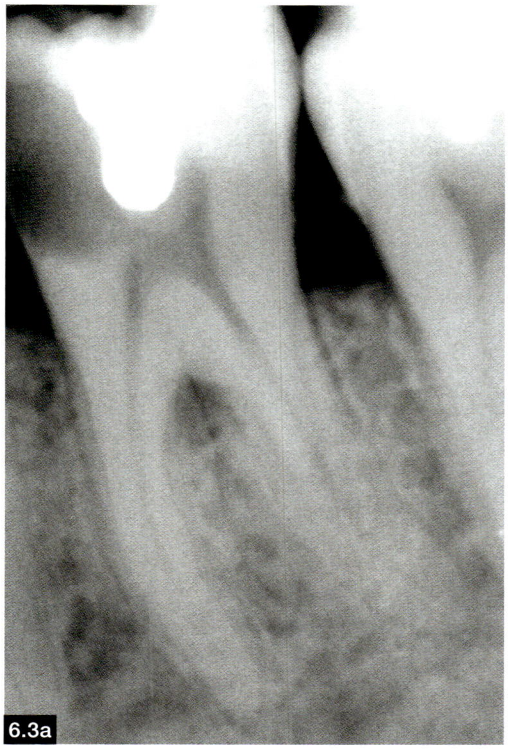

6.3a

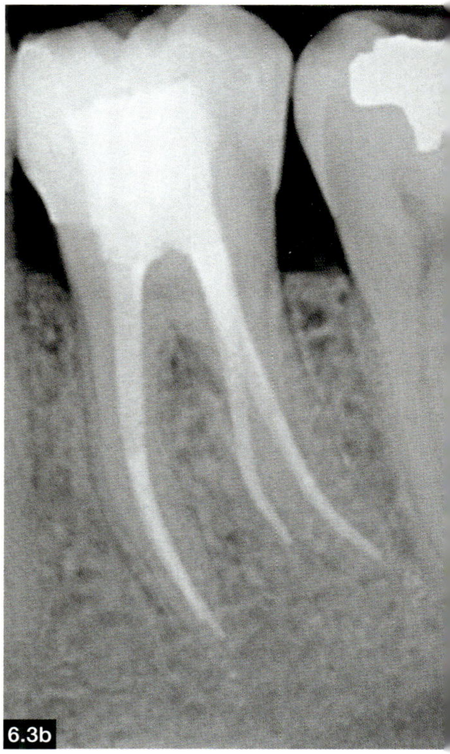

6.3b

Fig. 6.3a-b: Complex retreatment requires several sessions. The previous therapy did not consider the typical canal morphology of *radix entomolaris*.

CASE REPORT 3

Molar with severe destruction of periodontal and endodontic origin

A case intended for extraction with a double periapical lesion and a previous treatment attempt is reconsidered because of the young age of the patient and the good health of the surrounding teeth. The isolation of the operating field is extremely complicated, but a simple apical repositioning of the gingival flap, together with the use of light-curing

Figure 1-2: The radiographic (Figure 1) and clinical (Figure 2) pictures show a previously incorrectly treated molar tooth, without a coronal reconstruction and with a few clear periapical lesions of endodontic origin.

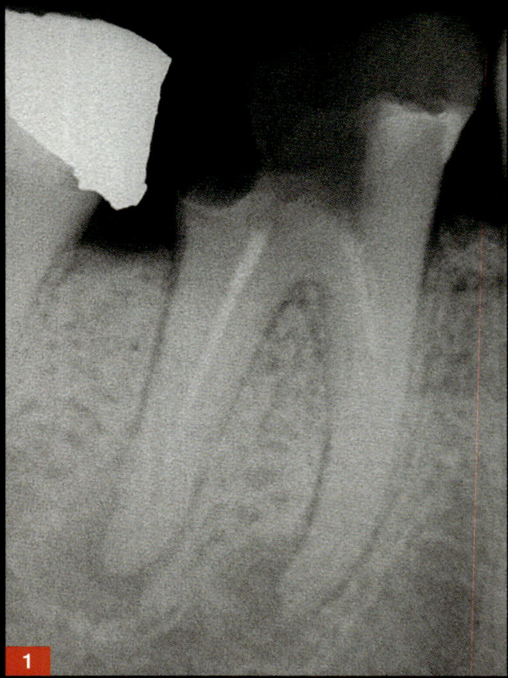

1

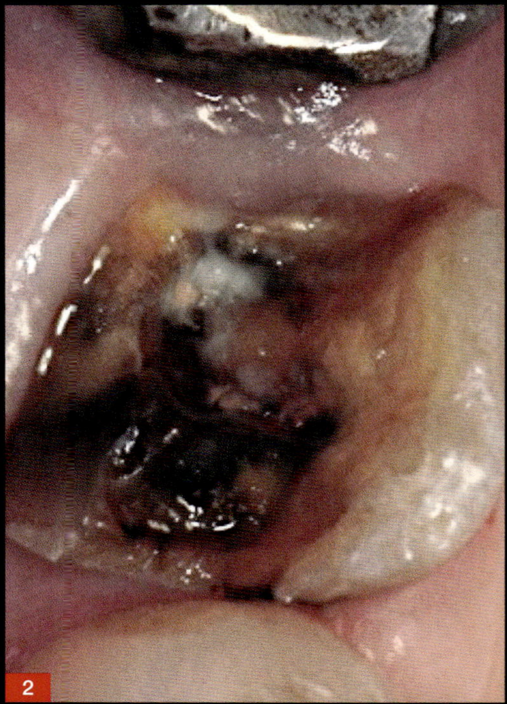

2

Figure 3: A purulent exudate is visible as soon as vestibular palpation is performed.

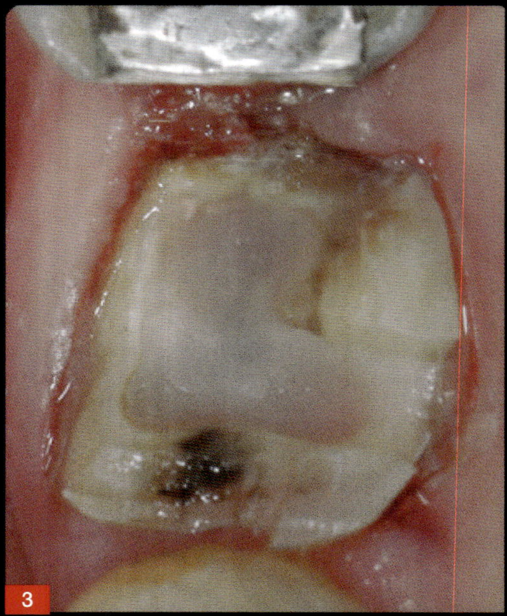

3

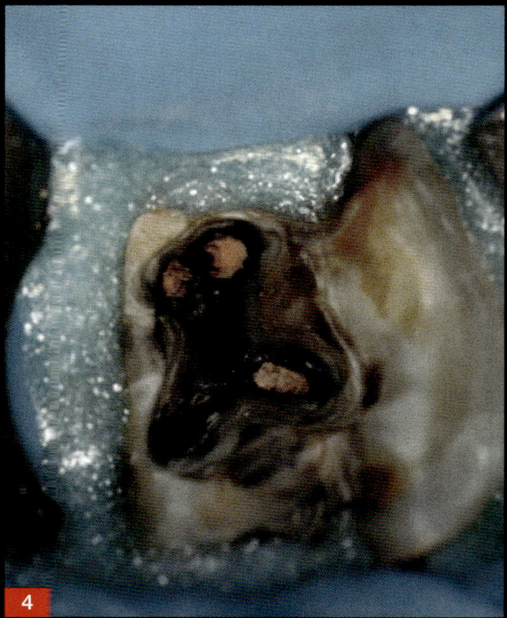

4

Figure 4: The tooth is isolated using resinous material to perfectly seal the access.

polymers to improve the seal of the dam, made it possible to perform an effective retreatment and closure of the endodontic space that, 7 years later, shows excellent health, radiologically highlighted by the periradicular contour, which is well trabeculated and without radiotransparency.

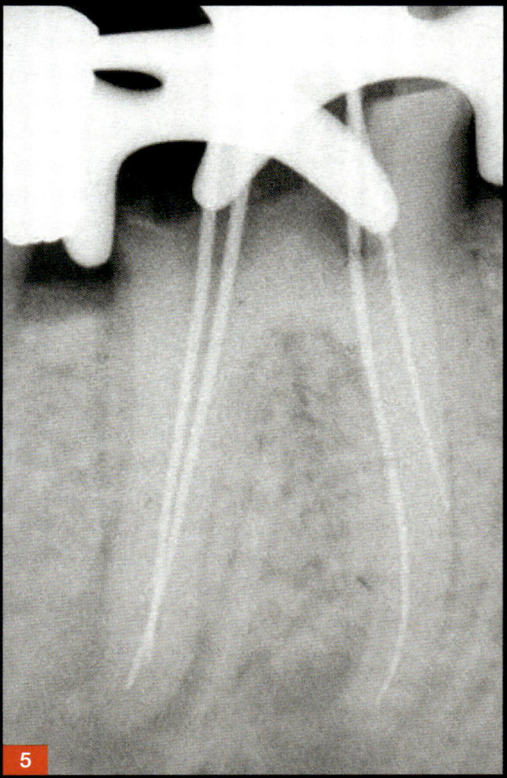

5

Figure 5: Radiographic verification of canal patency and the working length.

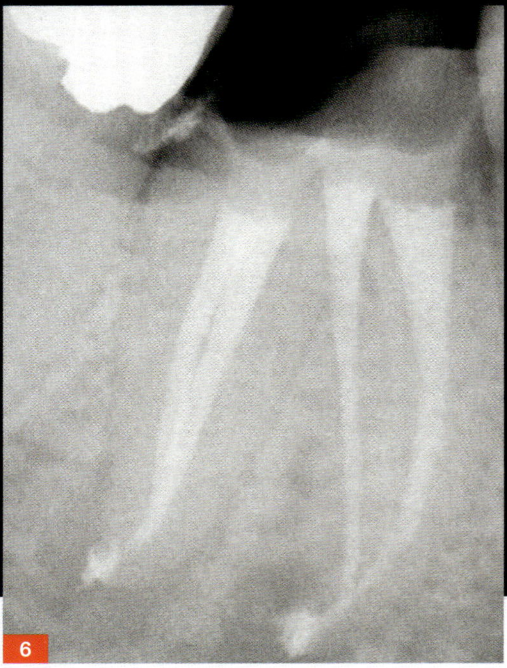

6

Figure 6: Closure of the root canal: note the apical confluence of the four root canals.

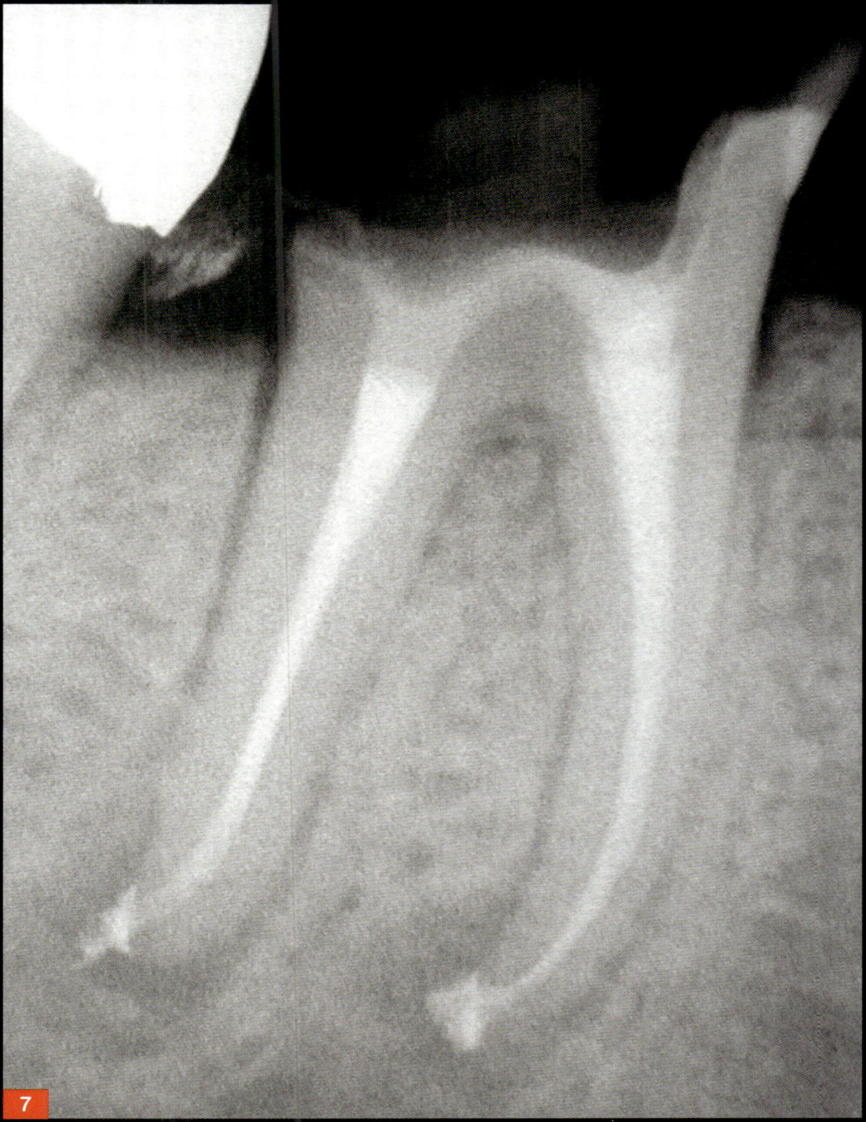

7

Figure 7: Radiographic examination in another projection.

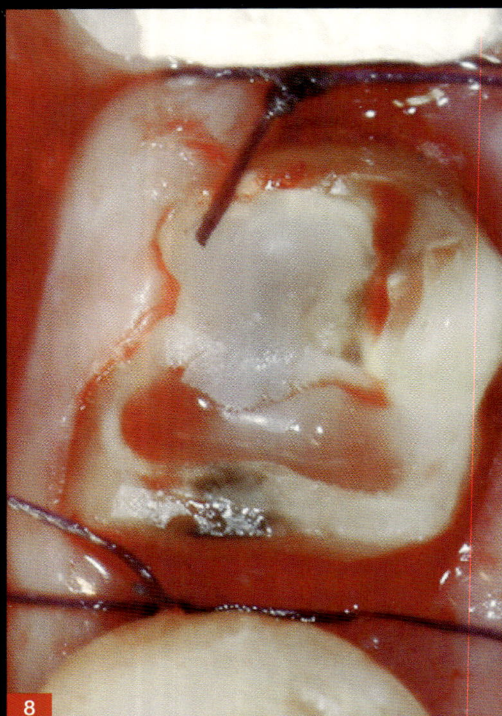

Figure 8: The apical repositioning flap to bring the margins back to the correct position the margins.

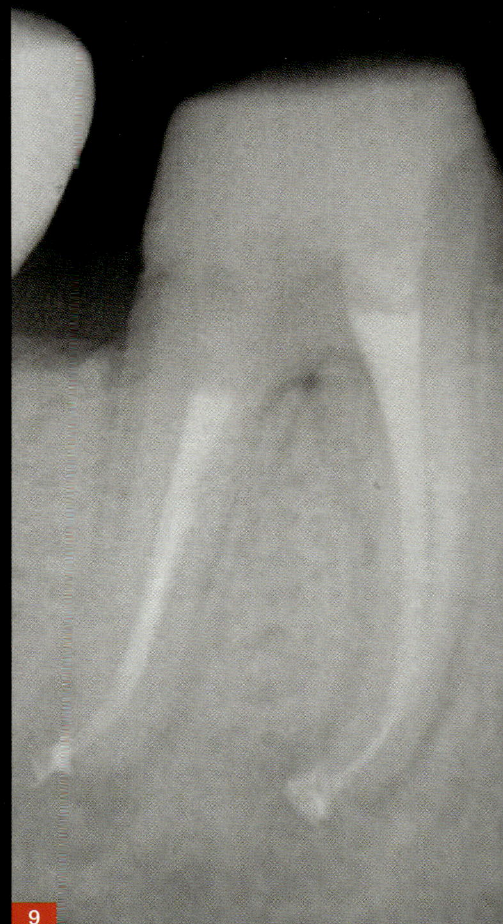

Figure 9: The 6-month follow-up x-ray provides a comforting scenario, the lesion appears to be shrinking and the patient has no symptoms.

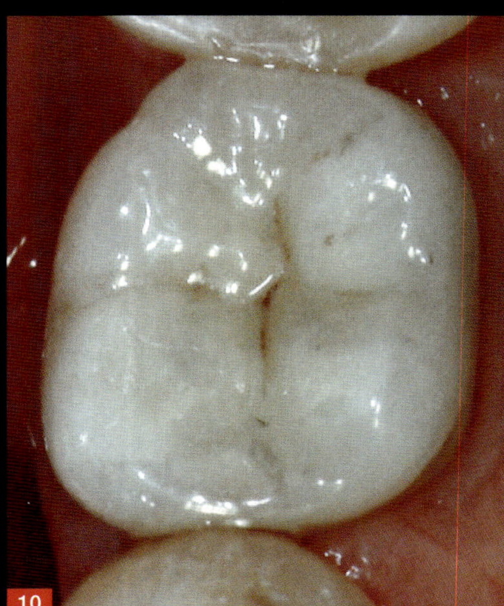

Figure 10: Occlusal aspect of the new reconstruction.

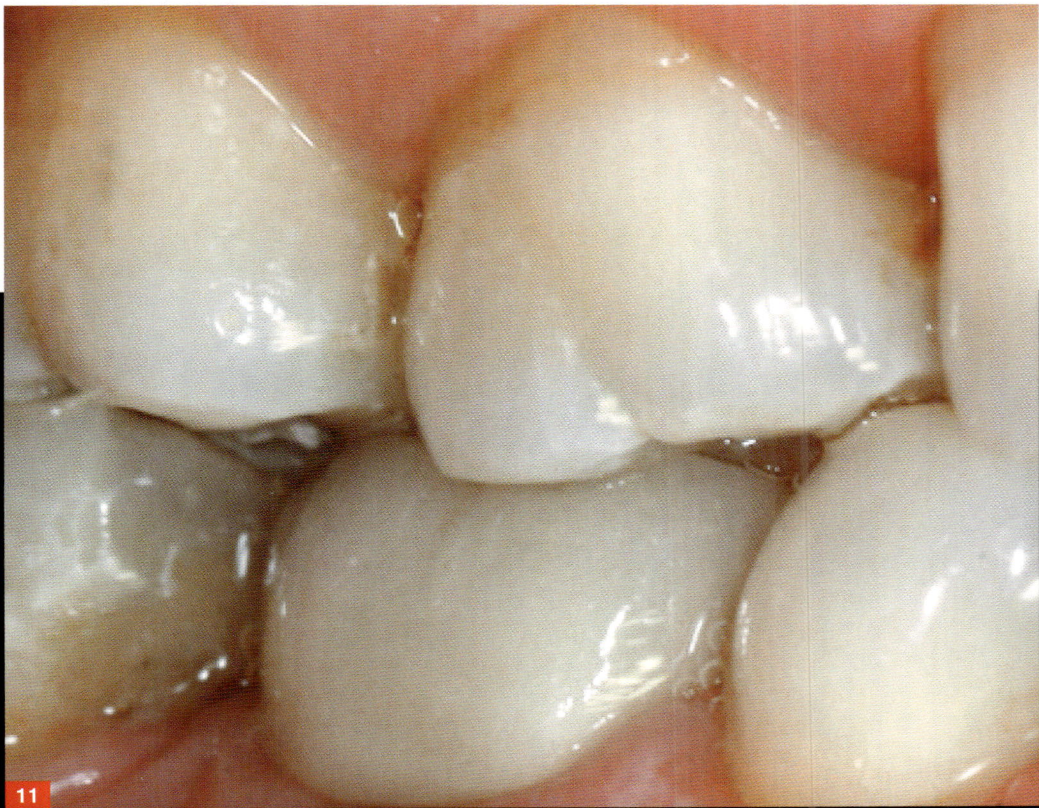

11

Figure 11: Reconstruction by means of metal-ceramic crown in vestibular view.

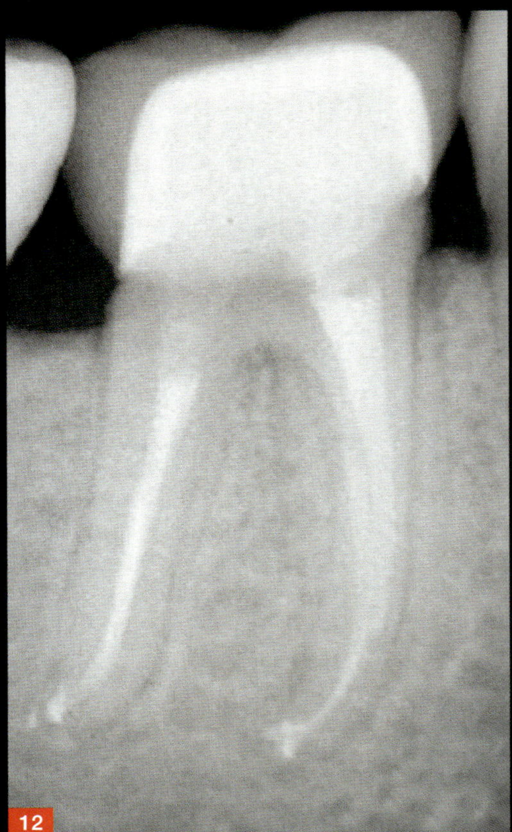

12

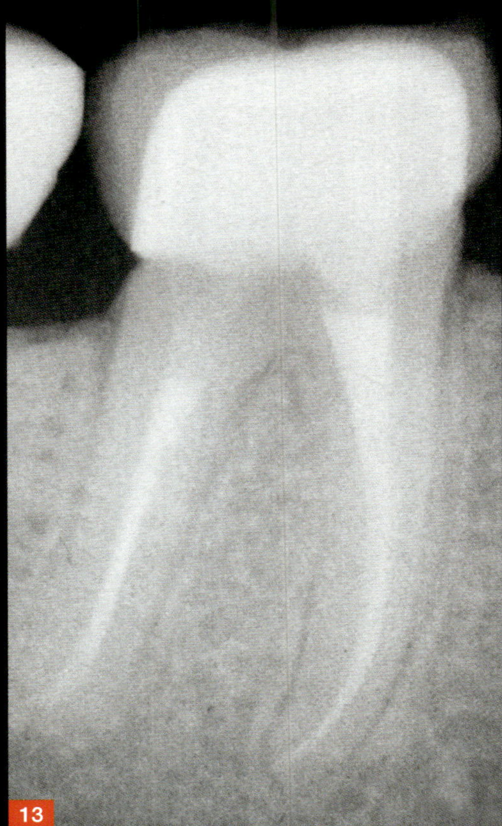

13

Figure 12-13: Follow-up x-ray at 1 and 9 years; both certify the success of the treatment despite the very critical starting condition.

POSTOPERATIVE PAIN

Nonsteroidal analgesics are used in the postoperative phases

Post–treatment drugs

Several authors have suggested using nonsteroidal analgesics to alleviate pain in the *period immediately following* endodontic treatment.
For example, Elzaki et al. [32] proposed the combination of paracetamol and ibuprofen. Naproxen is equally effective in the abovementioned combination[33]. Smith et al.[34] provided exhaustive data through a systematic review and observed that 600 mg ibuprofen combined with 1000 mg paracetamol is the most effective combination for alleviating postoperative pain.

Targeted pharmacological support seems to be the best solution. The administration of nonsteroidal anti-inflammatory drugs, with or without paracetamol, can be considered the basic rule.

In this case, adequate access preparation and pretreatment should include this strategy, i.e., the elimination of occlusal contacts and the reduction of the chewing surface; in this way, access to the endodontium becomes easier, with great benefits for the entire treatment.

ANTIBIOTICS

Reasonable antibiotic use does not encourage the **establishment of resistance**

Use of antibiotics

A different matter is the use of *antibiotics*. As resistance is to be avoided at all costs, the prescription of antibiotics (for the schemes, see Chapter 1) must be reserved for cases in which pain, symptoms, and signs of an incipient swelling occur. Pulsing pain is the first signal to be considered discriminating.
The remedy of eliminating occlusal contacts in these phases may be marginally interesting, but it must be combined with a previously devised coronal reconstruction project and, if this approach is used, this opportunity should never be present because the preferred reconstructions for these teeth are those with cuspal coverage (Chapter 9).
Studies have shown that the percentage of confirmed septic complications, such as acute alveolar abscesses, represents some of the cases treated; this percentage has been reported differently in various cases, as is verifiable in the most recent findings[5, 15].
In all cases, the use of broad-spectrum antibiotics seems to be the best choice, but dosage varies from one case to another. The general regimens for antibiotic use are summarized in Box 1.3 on page 24[35, 36].
A study carried out in a large group of American professionals[37] revealed that about 41% of professionals prescribe antibiotic therapy, primarily based on amoxicillin or similar antibiotics after endodontic surgery.

Exacerbations

The exacerbation of pain symptoms with or without swelling constitutes a different matter. The presence of swelling is consistent with a different and is the expression of a pathogenic noxa that is not controlled by retreatment or the onset of a new disease.
One of the most common problems is partial or total root fracture, which is a frequent consequence of previous shaping maneuvers and sometimes associated with the use of ultrasound, which may have induced dentinal cracks that evolve over time due to the masticatory load in established fractures.
In these cases, diagnosis is often simple given the finding of a crack at an occlusal level; however, it becomes more complex if a fracture occurs at root level (Figs. 6.4a-c).
However, the extent of the clinical scenario related to the quality of a canal treatment guides the final decision, as satisfactory endodontic treatment rarely generates very severe pain symptoms associated with swelling (see root fractures, Chapters 1 and 2; Figs. 6.4a-c).
When considering exacerbations, a non-marginal role is played by those situations in which the process of healing,

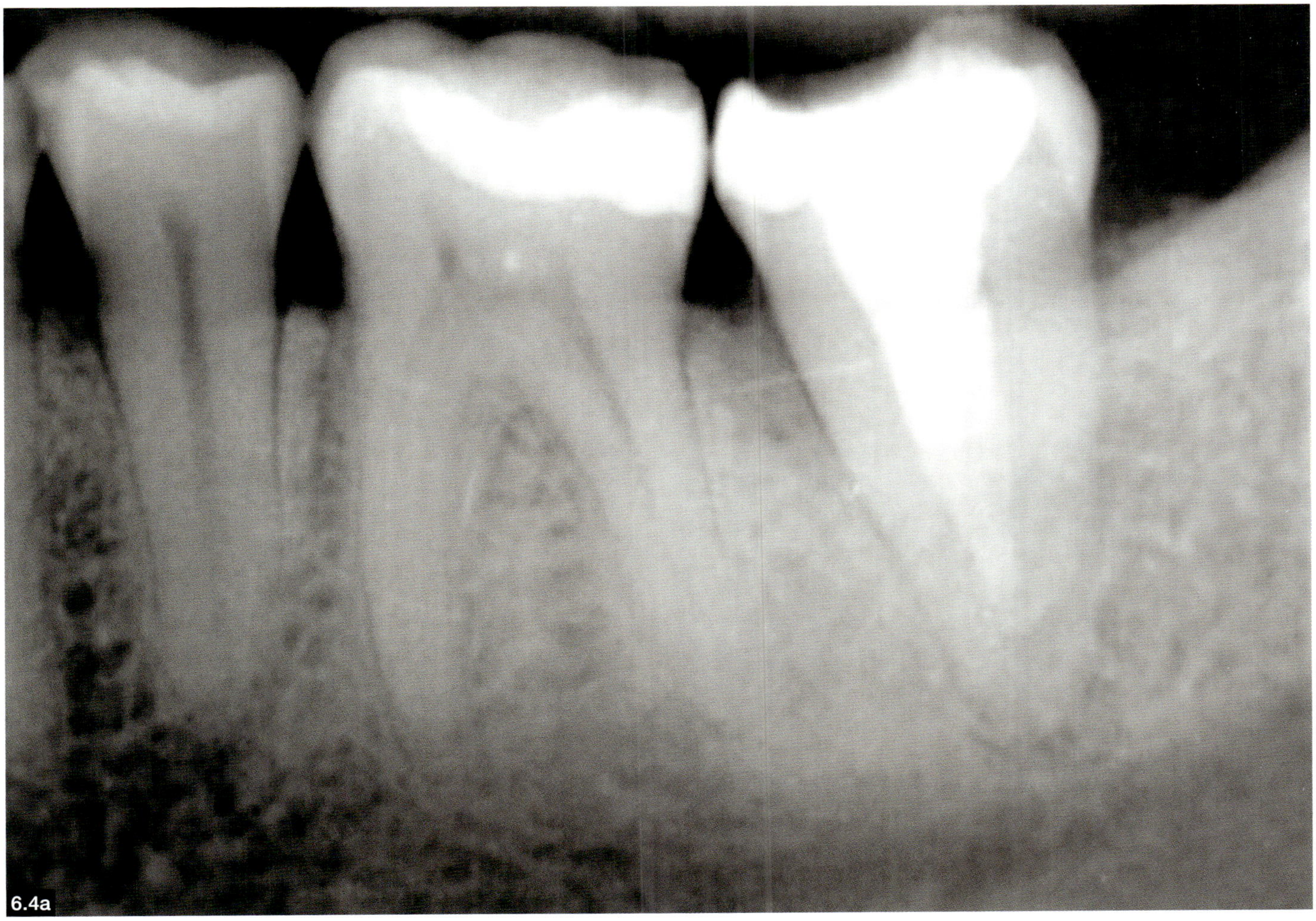

6.4a

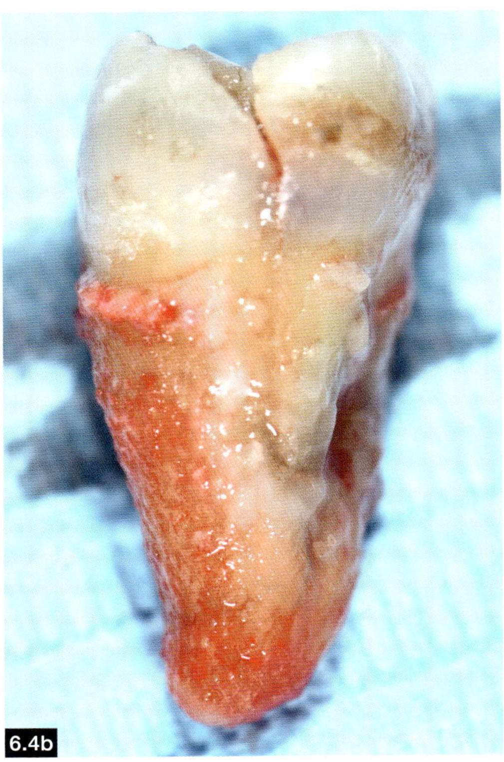

6.4b

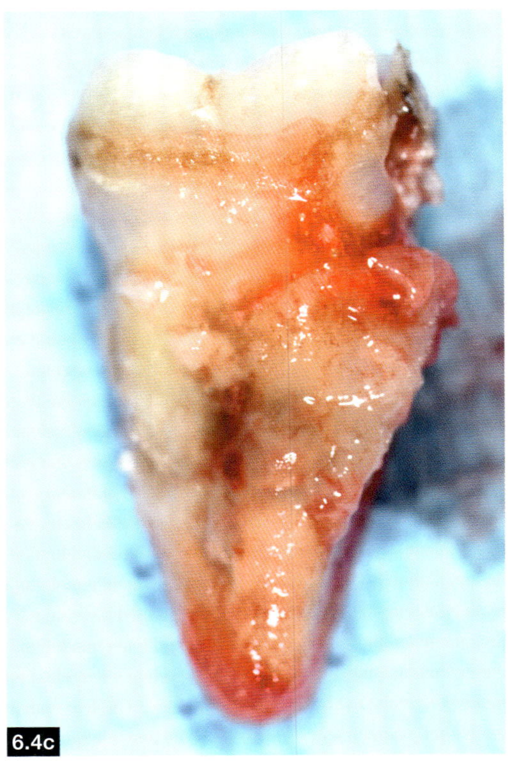

6.4c

Fig. 6.4a: Discontinuous pain during chewing determined the need for a visit; the intraoral examination led to the performance of a radiograph that did not reveal particular problems except a clearly short canal treatment; a more careful observation highlighted slight mesial coronal bone radiotransparency.

Fig. 6.4b-c: The compound fracture at coronal level extended to the most apical third and determined the need to perform an extraction.

or rather, the transformations of the radiographically visible periradicular tissues, is difficult; for instance, lesions of endodontic origin that, despite a remission of symptoms have not shown a significant evolution of the periradicular disease[38].

In all these cases, except appropriate measures to deal with painful emergencies, the use of surgical endodontics seems to be the best alternative, without waiting in vain for the course to be reversed by means of pharmacological therapies.

The follow-up of these cases should not usually exceed 4 years, but, as reported by Kirkevang et al.[39], one year after the pathological event, they should have already undergone – from a radiographic point of view – such variations as to allow a final judgment.

The cut-off is 12 months, after which the final solution may be predicted.

Fig. 6.5a: Central incisor with marked discoloration that preludes an incongruous endodontic treatment.

Fig. 6.5b: Same case checked 2 years later.

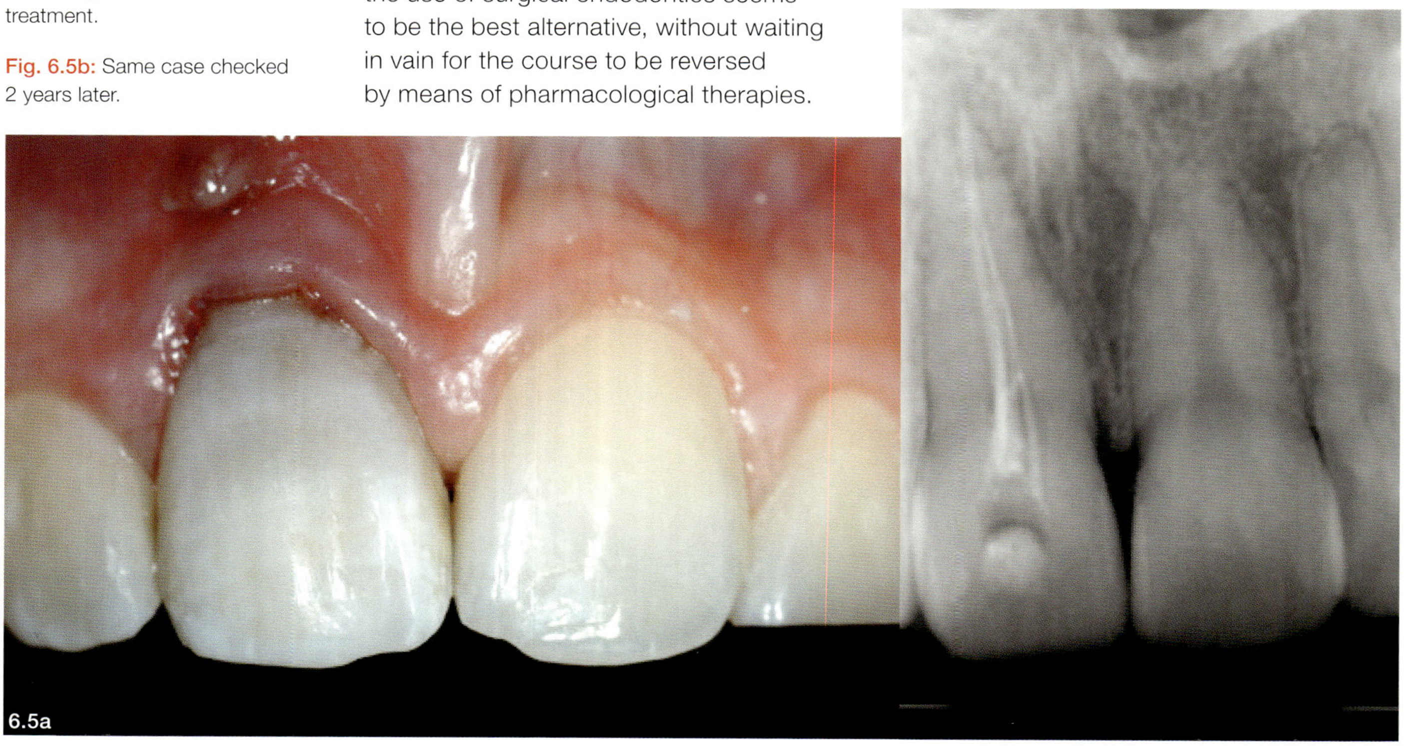

6.5a

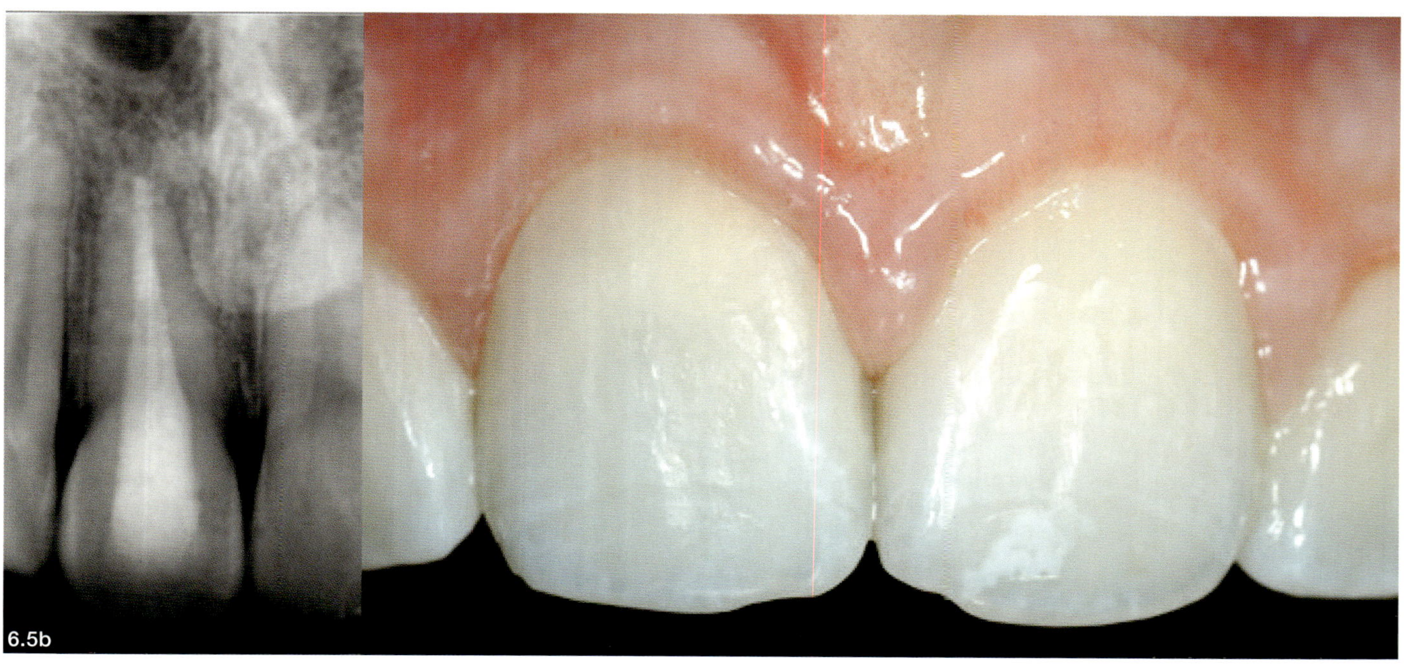

6.5b

When to define a retreatment as resolved

The time frame for determining whether symptoms are physiological or paraphysiological remains unknown. One or two weeks is a reasonable time for obtaining certain answers and the persistence of symptoms beyond this time is a clear sign that retreatment has not been successful, even in the presence of therapies with anti-inflammatory drugs or antibiotics.
A patient should be informed about the possible effects of this type of treatment in advance to prepare the necessary countermeasures.
The boundary between success and failure cannot be defined, making symptoms a key element of postoperative dynamics.
Many factors contribute to the speed of postoperative evolution and can be summarized as the "preoperative state" of the tooth and periapical tissues (Table 6.1).
In the presence of evident bacterial contamination and a confirmed periapical disease, which is possibly associated with a draining fistula, the suspicion of a longer management of the healing process leads to a more uncertain prognosis and the patient should be immediately informed of the possibility that the retreatment procedure may be followed, when conditions allow, by a surgical revision of the root apex.
The *persistence of symptoms* suggests that the treatment has failed. Vena et al.[40] described persistent pain experienced by some patients; however, this minority is still relevant for the implications of this discomfort in normal masticatory actions.
Waiting is an important factor in these cases is waiting because evolution, particularly in the most complex cases, can be extremely slow and varies between 3 months and 1 year. A period of more than 1 year should prompt dentists and surgeons to provide an alternative solution; in the same way, this proposal must be considered in all cases in which endodontic periapical lesions do not show signs of a decrease or increase in size[41].

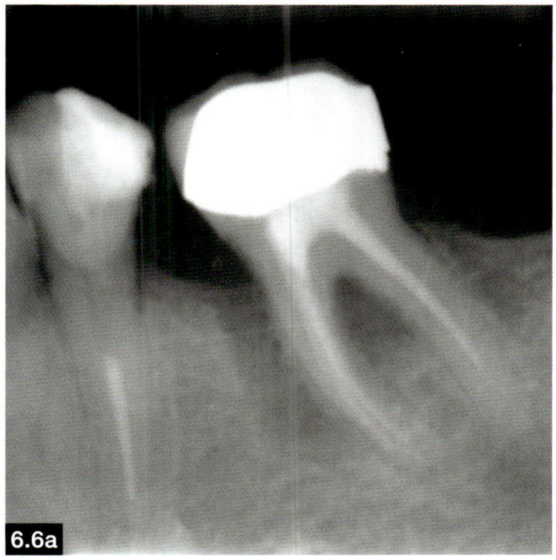
6.6a

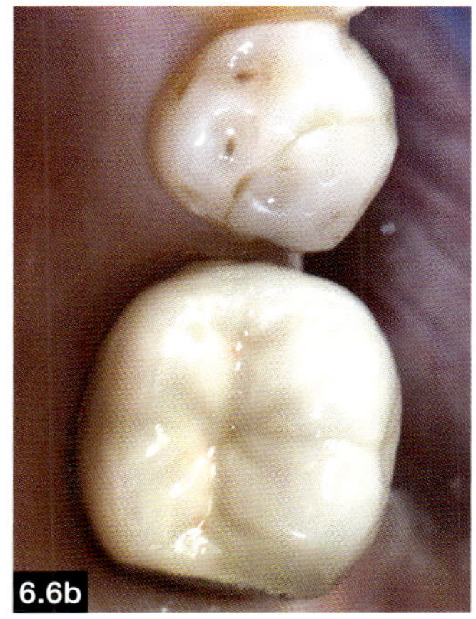
6.6b

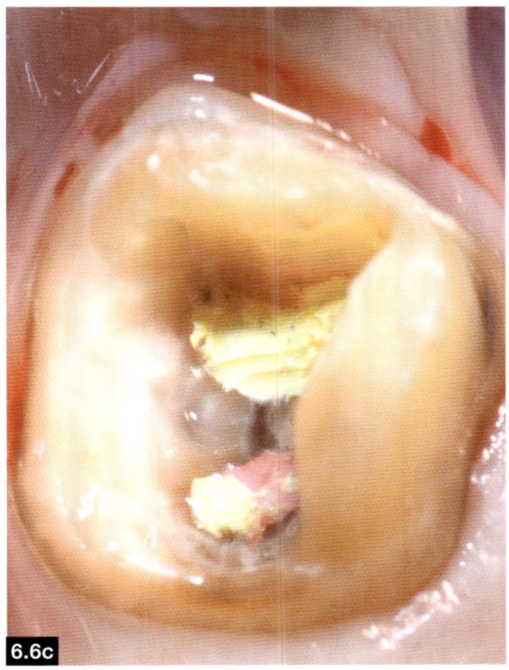
6.6c

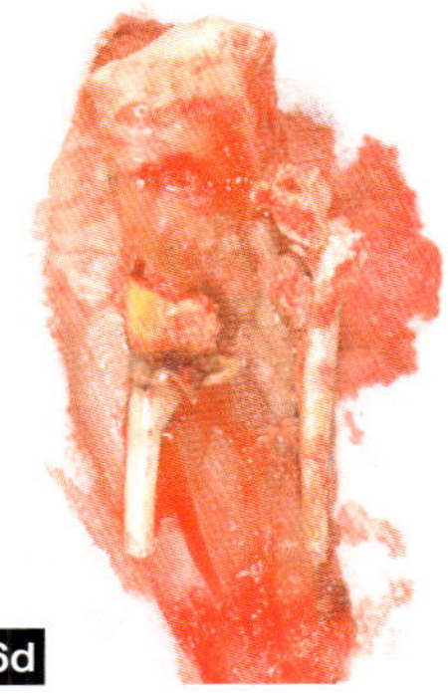
6.6d

Fig. 6.6a-d: Similar picture in the case shown in Figs. 6.4a-c complicated by the presence of a crown in the diagnostic phase. On the x-ray, the radiolucent area appears confined to the coronal third of the mesial root. The contour is barely visible (c), and the root appears to be divided into two in a way that is no longer recoverable once the tooth is removed (d).

Table 6.1 **ELEMENTS FOR DEVISING A POST-RETREATMENT FOLLOW-UP PLAN**	
A	**Analysis of the dental and periodontal health status of the treated element**
a1	Clinical aspect: periodontal tissue observation, fissure probing at follow-up appointments scheduled for 3, 6, and 12 months after the procedure
a2	Radiological aspect: x-rays 3, 6, and 12 months after surgery and 1-year CBCT when necessary
a3	Annual analysis until radiographic resolution of the disease, using CBCT in strategically relevant cases
B	**Fitting of the coronal restoration (provisional/definitive) within 15-20 days of surgery**
C	**Estimation of the alternative fate of the tooth within 1 year of retreatment**

Steps following retreatment

Radiographic follow-up of the clinical case

Although digital endodontic radiographs involve a minimal dose of radiation, monitoring endodontically induced periapical lesions cannot be obsessive; an evaluation should be made 3 or 6 months after the first retreatment procedure, and follow-up radiographs should be obtained 1 year after retreatment[41].

Depending on the type of restorative treatment to be planned, further follow-up appointments will be made with 4 years constituting the cut-off, as mentioned several times, for establishing the fate of the treated tooth.

One open question regards the use of CBCT for the long-term evaluation of endodontic periapical lesions.

Patel et al.[42] demonstrated that intraoral radiographs underestimate the extent of a problem and lead dentists or surgeons to consider cases as healed even when the inflammatory aspects are still evolving.

In the future, these examinations will require a lower dose of radiation.

At present, performing CBCT seems inappropriate for the routine monitoring of endodontic lesions except in cases that are strategically fundamental for reconstructive purposes or for the involvement of the patient's general health although radiogenic loads are progressively decreasing[43]. Directing a patient toward a more or less restrictive follow-up protocol must be based on the clinician's judgment.

Fitting of the final restoration

Gillen et al.[44] conducted a fundamental systematic review and clinically justified the assumption that a good restoration also leads to a successful endodontic treatment; therefore, the application of rapid a restoration, which has the characteristics of a suitable coronal seal, seems mandatory.

Restoration materials, whether temporary or permanent, can be variable, and their costs are associated with their quality; however, adequate restoration must be provided.

Restorations may be temporary and, as such, may be composed of direct or indirect composite materials, where indicated.

Temporary crowns made of resinous material can be an interesting temporary alternative.

No clear rule for proceeding with the final restoration has been established.

Commencing a procedure of this type should not be a concern as, if the retreatment was performed according to the state of the art, the only viable alternatives would be endodontic surgery or extraction.

In the former case, the final restoration may be saved.

In the latter, an economic agreement on the new reconstruction will be easy to formulate. Indeed, this agreement should be signed before retreatment is carried out so that it does not come as a surprise for either a dentist or a patient.

Table 6.2 **NEXT STEPS AFTER RETREATMENT**

Phase 1	Phase 2
What to tell the patient and how to tell him/her	Radiographic monitoring
Pharmacological prescription	Carrying out a temporary restoration or a final restoration
Instructions at home	Performing surgical endodontics or extraction

CASE REPORT 4

Distal apical rarefaction in endodontically treated molar

The case involves a 30-year-old man who complained of pain in quadrant 4, in the molar area. The direct observation showed only one tooth had been treated. The radiographic examination showed a rarefying lesion of the distal root of the first lower molar and ectasia of the periapical space of the mesial root.

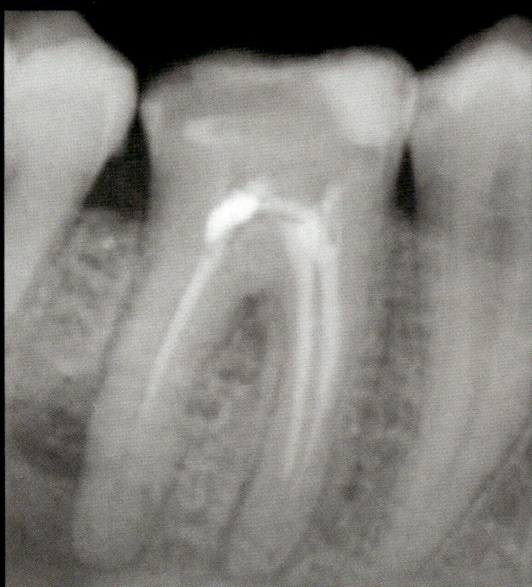

1

Figure 1: The radiographic picture at the first visit; the examination shows insufficient treatment, with an unsuitable coronal opening and an inadequate root canal filling length. The periapical lesion at the distal root extends to the middle third.

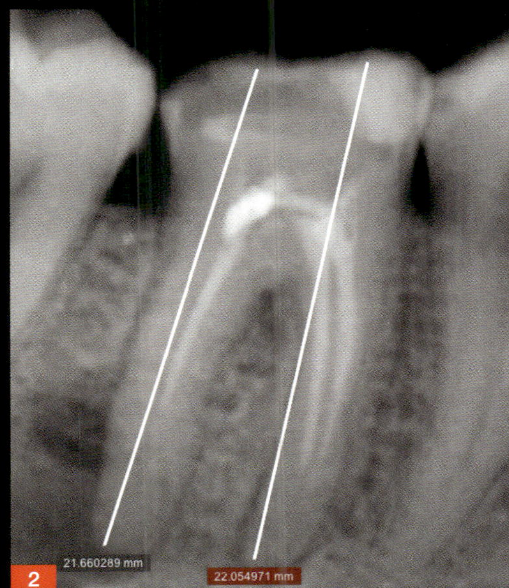

2

Figure 2: The same radiograph with the preoperative measurement; this system provides fair reliability when a centering device is used.

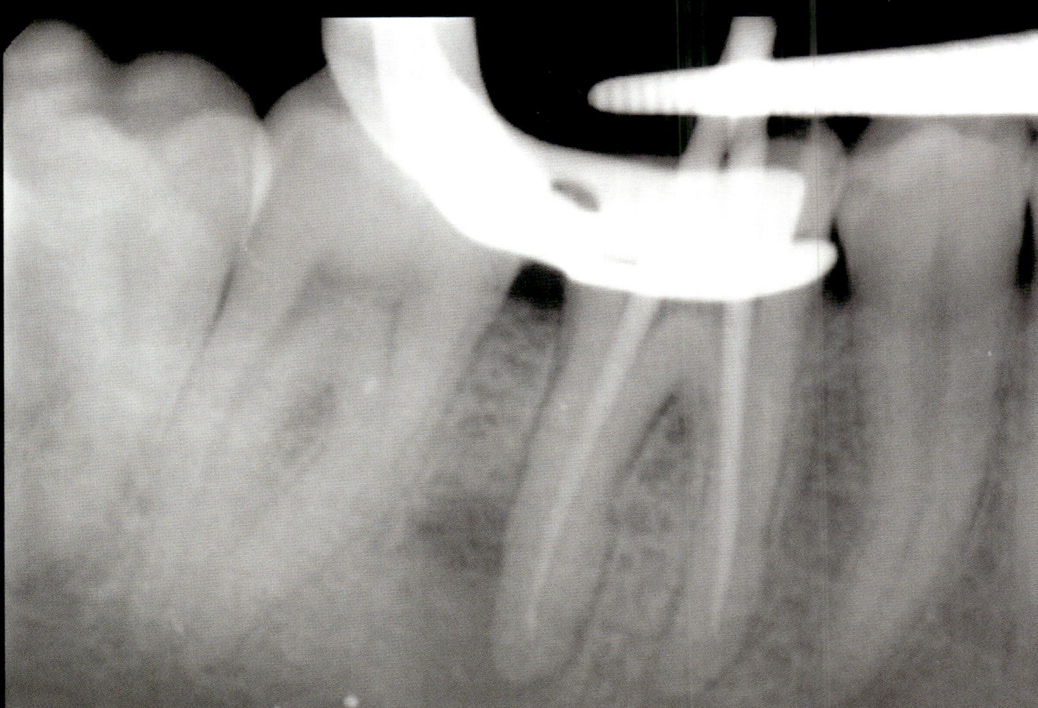

3a

Figure 3a: The cones test shows an abrupt confluence at the mesial root level and shows how narrow the residual common canal is. The previous treatment was completed in this area; the recovery of patency was particularly difficult.

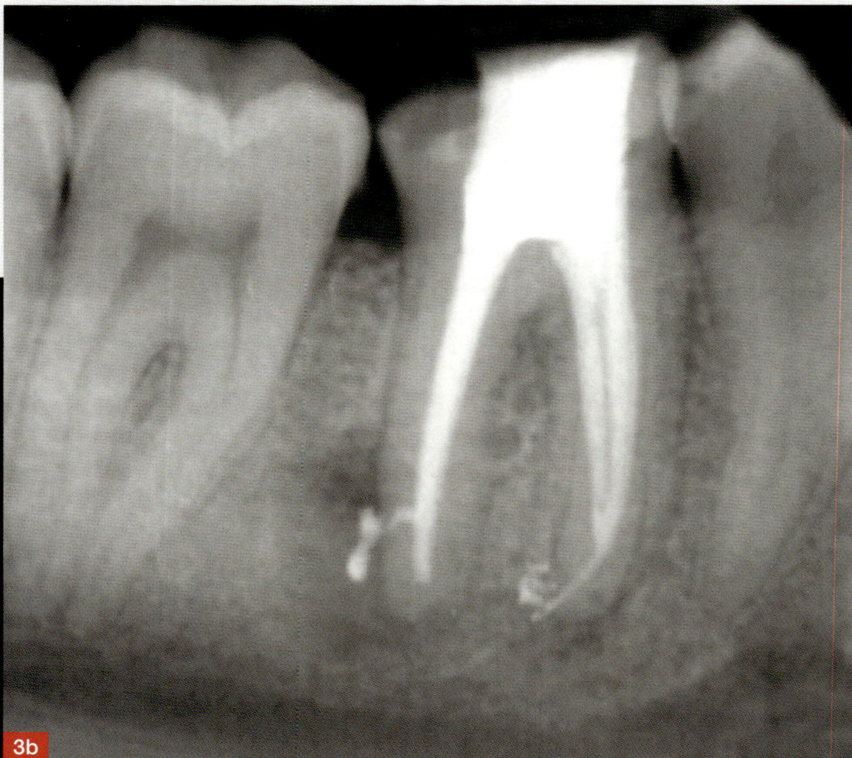

3b

Figure 4a-c: The follow-up sequence which, in this case, was quite thorough. Follow-up was performed at 1 month, 3 months, at six months, at nine months at one year, at 1 year and 6 months and 2 years. A reconstruction with ceramic-glass material milled was performed a few months later and the last check is 1 year after the placement of the ceramic onlay and about 3 years after the final closure of the endodontic space. The periapical remodelling is still present, the clinical scenario is absolutely normal.

Figure 3b: The completed case shows a very wide lateral canal distally in the homonymous root. Some slight overfilling in these canal morphologies may be acceptable as it would certify good sealing of the main endodontic space.

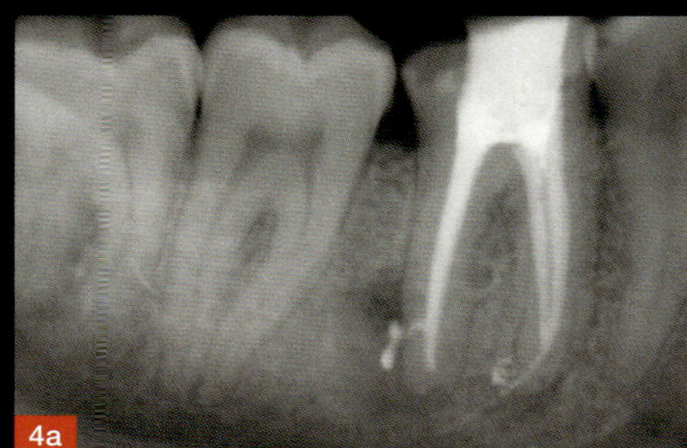

4a

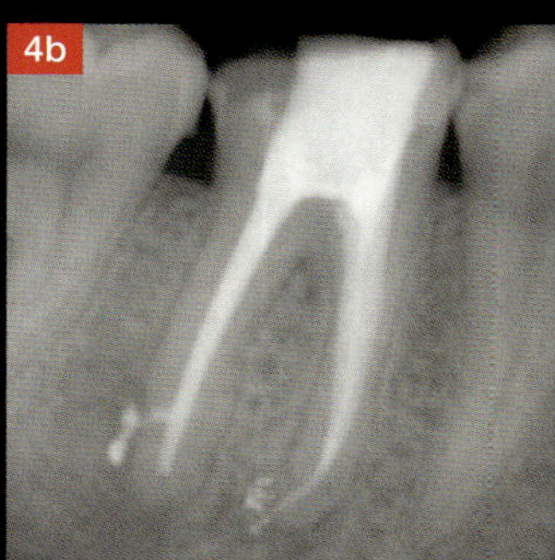

4b

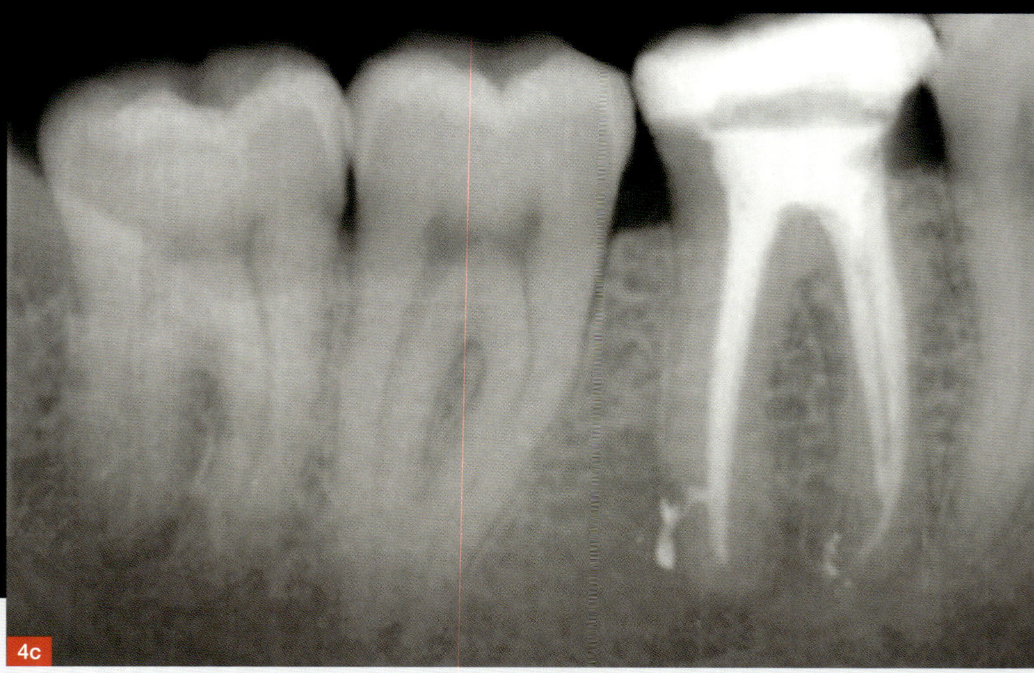

4c

Endodontic surgery extraction or implantology

The decision to recommend new clinical procedures in the absence of results in orthograde therapy is delicate. It is even more so when the most correct evaluations have not been made or the possibility of these further paths has not been shared with the patient during preoperative diagnosis. Toure et al.[45] conducted a prospective study and verified the choice to extract a tooth that has undergone unsuccessful endodontic treatment on almost half of the teeth in question.

In any case, the clinical question remains: when do I consider a case healed or how long can I wait to deem a case of retreatment healed?
The answers are the same as those that lead us at the beginning of this text (Chapter 1) to formulate a diagnosis and create a treatment plan; in this case, only the therapeutic perspective changes. In the former case, retreatment has to to be enhanced, i.e., to be better than the previous treatment. In the latter, with due exceptions, retreatment can no longer be the primary choice; instead, it must be assisted with surgery, namely, retrograde seal apicectomy, or with tooth extraction and replacement with osseointegrated implants and fixed prostheses. A randomized clinical trial (B) reported no significant differences in retreatment made with an orthograde access compared with a surgical one; the overall percentage is around 76%. A slightly higher percentage of failures due to root fractures was also reported in teeth with orthograde retreatment in which post removal is necessary.
As this choice is onerous, from many points of view, we believe the clinical situation to be decisive; in the absence of pain symptoms the clinician will be reluctant to take responsibility for carrying out operations other than those already performed.

In Chapter 10, the decision-making process has been more extensively explained, but excessive interventionism is unsuitable for this particular discipline of endodontics at this stage. This option is inevitable when the extent of endodontic lesions does not allow the functional recovery of the tooth.

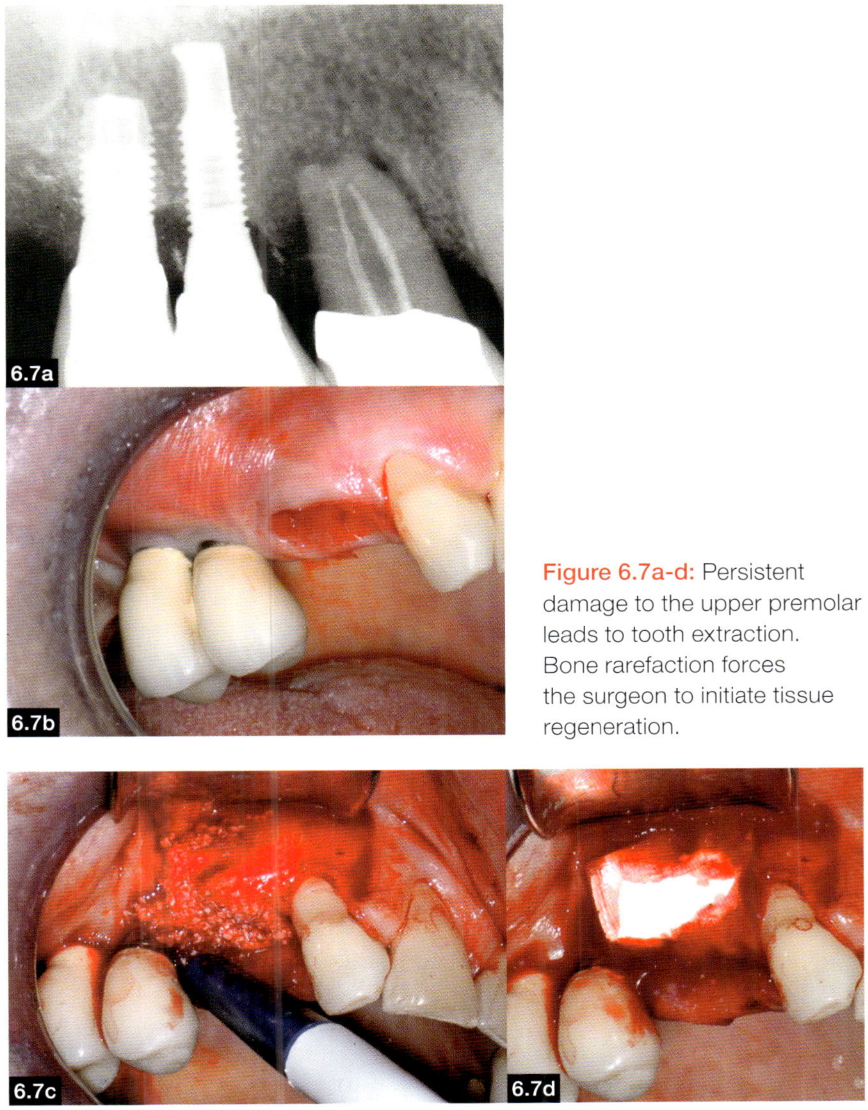

Figure 6.7a-d: Persistent damage to the upper premolar leads to tooth extraction. Bone rarefaction forces the surgeon to initiate tissue regeneration.

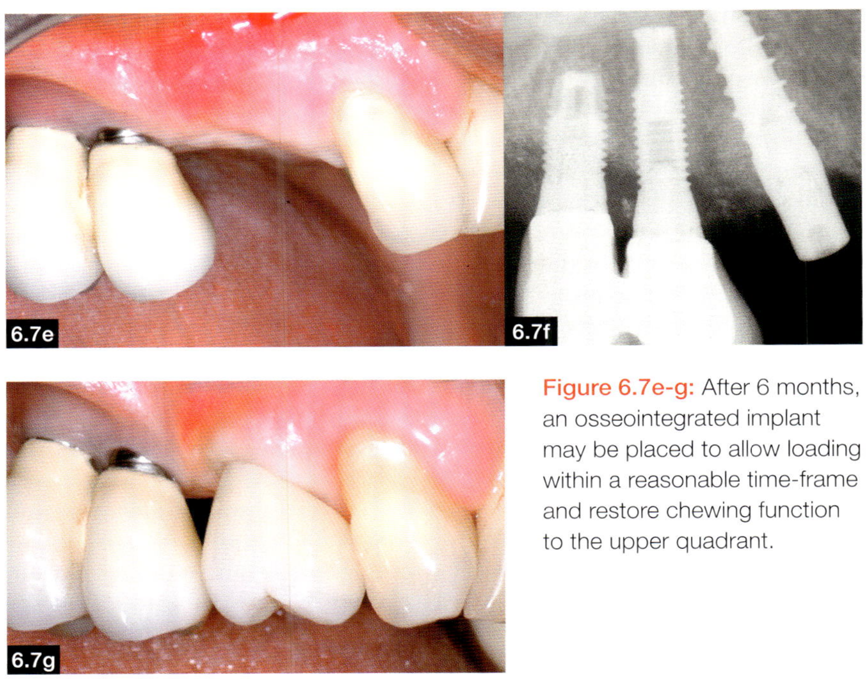

Figure 6.7e-g: After 6 months, an osseointegrated implant may be placed to allow loading within a reasonable time-frame and restore chewing function to the upper quadrant.

References

1. MonteroJ, Lorenzo B, Barrios R et al. *Patient-centered Outcomes of Root Canal Treatment: A Cohort Follow-up Study.* Journal of endodontics 2015;41(9):1456-1461.
2. Arias A, de la Macorra JC, Hidalgo JJ et al. *Predictive models of pain following root canal treatment: a prospective clinical study.* International endodontic journal 2013;46(8):784-793.
3. Liu P, McGrath C, Cheung G. *What are the key endodontic factors associated with oral health-related quality of life?* International endodontic journal 2014;47(3):238-245.
4. Pak JG, White SN. *Pain prevalence and severity before, during, and after root canal treatment: a systematic review.* Journal of endodontics 2011;37(4):429-438.
5. Gomes MS, Bottcher DE, Scarparo RK et al. *Predicting pre- and postoperative pain of endodontic origin in a southern Brazilian subpopulation: an electronic database study.* International endodontic journal 2017;50(8):729-739.
6. Nixdorf DR, Law AS, John MT et al. *Differential diagnoses for persistent pain after root canal treatment: a study in the National Dental Practice-based Research Network.* Journal of endodontics 2015;41(4):457-463.
7. Goldberg, F et al. *Relationship between unintentional canal overfilling and the long-term outcome of primary root canal treatments and nonsurgical retreatments: a retrospective radiographic assessment.* Int Endod J 2020;53(1): 19-26.
8. Alves Vde O. *Endodontic flare-ups: a prospective study. Oral surgery, oral medicine, oral pathology, oral radiology, and endodontics* 2010;110(5):e68-72.
9. Walton R, Fouad A. *Endodontic interappointment flare-ups: a prospective study of incidence and related factors.* Journal of endodontics 1992;18(4):172-177.
10. Matusow RJ. *The flare-up phenomenon in endodontics: a clinical perspective and review. Oral surgery, oral medicine, and oral pathology* 1988;65(6):750-753.
11. Tanalp J, Gungor T. *Apical extrusion of debris: a literature review of an inherent occurrence during root canal treatment.* International endodontic journal 2014;47(3):211-221.
12. Parirokh M, Rekabi AR, Ashouri R et al. *Effect of occlusal reduction on postoperative pain in teeth with irreversible pulpitis and mild tenderness to percussion.* Journal of endodontics 2013;39(1):1-5.
13. Arora M, Sangwan P, Tewari S et al. *Effect of maintaining apical patency on endodontic pain in posterior teeth with pulp necrosis and apical periodontitis: a randomized controlled trial.* International endodontic journal 2016;49(4):317-324.
14. Pasqualini D, Mollo L, Scotti N et al. *Postoperative pain after manual and mechanical glide path: a randomized clinical trial.* Journal of endodontics 2012;38(1):32-36.
15. Kherlakian D, Cunha RS, Ehrhardt IC et al. *Comparison of the Incidence of Postoperative Pain after Using 2 Reciprocating Systems and a Continuous Rotary System: A Prospective Randomized Clinical Trial*. Journal of endodontics 2016;42(2):171-176.
16. Pasqualini D, Corbella S, Alovisi M et al. *Postoperative quality of life following single-visit root canal treatment performed by rotary or reciprocating instrumentation: a randomized clinical trial.* International endodontic journal 2016;49(11):1030-1039.
17. Comparin D, Moreira EJL, Souza EM et al. *Postoperative Pain after Endodontic Retreatment Using Rotary or Reciprocating Instruments: A Randomized Clinical Trial.* Journal of endodontics 2017;43(7):1084-1088.
18. Saumya-Rajesh P, Krithikadatta J, Velmurugan N et al. *Post-instrumentation pain after the use of either Mtwo or the SAF system: a randomized controlled clinical trial. International endodontic journal 2017*;50(8):750-760.
19. Arslan H, Guven Y, Karatas E et al. *Effect of the Simultaneous Working Length Control during Root Canal Preparation on Postoperative Pain.* Journal of endodontics 2017;43(9):1422-1427.
20. Cruz Junior JA, Coelho MS, Kato AS et al. *The Effect of Foraminal Enlargement of Necrotic Teeth with the Reciproc System on Postoperative Pain: A Prospective and Randomized Clinical Trial.* Journal of endodontics 2016;42(1):8-11.
21. Silva EJ, Menaged K, Ajuz N et al. *Postoperative pain after foraminal enlargement in anterior teeth with necrosis and apical periodontitis: a prospective and randomized clinical trial.* Journal of endodontics 2013;39(2):173-176.
22. Saini HR, Sangwan P, Sangwan A. *Pain following foraminal enlargement in mandibular molars with necrosis and apical periodontitis: A randomized controlled trial.* International endodontic journal 2016;49(12):1116-1123.
23. Vera J, Ochoa J, Romero M et al. *Intracanal Cryotherapy Reduces Postoperative Pain in Teeth with Symptomatic Apical Periodontitis: A Randomized Multicenter Clinical Trial.* Journal of endodontics 2018;44(1):4-8.
24. Arslan H, Doganay E, Karatas E et al. *Effect of Low-level Laser Therapy on Postoperative Pain after Root Canal Retreatment: A Preliminary Placebo-controlled, Triple-blind, Randomized Clinical Trial.* Journal of endodontics 2017;43(11):1765-1769.
25. Figini L, Lodi G, Gorni F et al. *Single versus multiple visits for endodontic treatment of permanent teeth: a Cochrane systematic review.* Journal of endodontics 2008;34(9):1041-1047.

26. Figini L, Lodi G, Gorni F et al. *Single versus multiple visits for endodontic treatment of permanent teeth. The Cochrane database of systematic reviews* 2007(4):CD005296. Chapter 6 | Post-processing: a guided tour 319
27. Manfredi M, Figini L, Gagliani M et al. *Single versus multiple visits for endodontic treatment of permanent teeth. The Cochrane database of systematic reviews* 2016;12:CD005296.
28. El Mubarak AH, Abu-bakr NH, Ibrahim YE. *Postoperative pain in multiple-visit and single-visit root canal treatment.* Journal of endodontics 2010;36(1):36-39.
29. Su Y, Wang C, Ye L. *Healing rate and post-obturation pain of single- versus multiple-visit endodontic treatment for infected root canals: a systematic review.* Journal of endodontics 2011;37(2):125-132.
30. Jalalzadeh SM, Mamavi A, Shahriari S et al. *Effect of pretreatment prednisolone on postendodontic pain: a double-blind parallel-randomized clinical trial.* Journal of endodontics 2010;36(6):978-981.
31. Praveen R, Thakur S, Kirthiga M. *Comparative Evaluation of Premedication with Ketorolac and Prednisolone on Postendodontic Pain: A Double-blind Randomized Controlled Trial.* Journal of endodontics 2017;43(5):667-673.
32. Turner CL, Eggleston GW, Lunos S et al. *Sniffing out endodontic pain: use of an intranasal analgesic in a randomized clinical trial.* Journal of endodontics 2011;37(4):439-444.
33. Elzaki WM, Abubakr NH, Ziada HM, Ibrahim YE. *Double-blind Randomized Placebo-controlled Clinical Trial of Efficiency of Nonsteroidal Anti-inflammatory Drugs in the Control of Post-endodontic Pain.* Journal of endodontics 2016;42(6):835-842.
34. Mehrvarzfar P, Abbott PV, Saghiri MA et al. *Effects of three oral analgesics on postoperative pain following root canal preparation: a controlled clinical trial.* International endodontic journal 2012;45(1):76-82.
35. Smith EA, Marshall JG, Selph SS et al. *Nonsteroidal Anti-inflammatory Drugs for Managing Postoperative Endodontic Pain in Patients Who Present with Preoperative Pain: A Systematic Review and Meta-analysis.* Journal of endodontics 2017;43(1):7-15.
36. Segura-Egea JJ, Gould K, Sen BH et al. *European Society of Endodontology position statement: the use of antibiotics in endodontics. International endodontic journal 2018*;51(1):20-25.
37. Segura-Egea JJ, Gould K, Sen BH et al. *Antibiotics in Endodontics: a review.* International endodontic journal 2017;50(12):1169-1184.
38. Germack M, Sedgley CM, Sabbah W, Whitten B. *Antibiotic Use in 2016 by Members of the American Association of Endodontists: Report of a National Survey. Journal of endodontics 2017*;43(10):1615-1622.
39. Yu VS, Messer HH, Shen L et al. *Lesion progression in post-treatment persistent endodontic lesions.* Journal of endodontics 2012;38(10):1316-1321.
40. Kirkevang LL, Orstavik D, Wenzel A et al. *Prognostic value of the full-scale Periapical Index.* International endodontic journal 2015;48(11):1051-1058.
41. Vena DA, Collie D, Wu H et al. *Prevalence of persistent pain 3 to 5 years post primary root canal therapy and its impact on oral health-related quality of life: PEARL Network findings.* Journal of endodontics 2014;40(12):1917-1921.
42. Sathorn C, Parashos P. *Monitoring the outcomes of root canal re-treatments.* Endodontic Topics 2011;19(1):153-162.
43. Patel S, Wilson R, Dawood A et al. *The detection of periapical pathosis using digital periapical radiography and cone beam computed tomography - part 2: a 1-year post-treatment follow-up.* International endodontic journal 2012;45(8):711-723.
44. Patel S, Durack C, Abella F et al. *Cone beam computed tomography in Endodontics - a review.* International endodontic journal 2015;48(1):3-15.
45. Gillen BM, Looney SW, Gu LS et al. *Impact of the quality of coronal restoration versus the quality of root canal fillings on success of root canal treatment: a systematic review and meta-analysis.* Journal of endodontics 2011;37(7):895-902.
46. Toure B, Faye B, Kane AW et al. *Analysis of reasons for extraction of endodontically treated teeth: a prospective study.* Journal of endodontics 2011;37(11):1512-1515.
47. Riis, A., et al., *Tooth Survival after Surgical or Nonsurgical Endodontic Retreatment: Long-term Follow-up of a Randomized Clinical Trial* J Endod, 2018. 44(10): pp. 1480-1486.

Sitography

Antibiotic prophylaxis in retreatment

https://www.aae.org/specialty/wp-content/uploads/sites/2/2017/06/aae_antibiotic-prophylaxis-2017update.pdf
https://www.aae.org/specialty/wp-content/uploads/sites/2/2017/06/aae_antibiotic-prophylaxis.pdf

Antibiotics in endodontics

https://www.aae.org/specialty/wp-content/uploads/sites/2/2017/06/aae_systemic-antibiotics.pdf

- To examine all endodontic periradicular diseases with **abnormal localizations**.
- **To distinguish** between lesions of a purely endodontic nature and those caused by iatrogenic errors.
- To explore **the most suitable techniques** for coping with all these clinical situations.

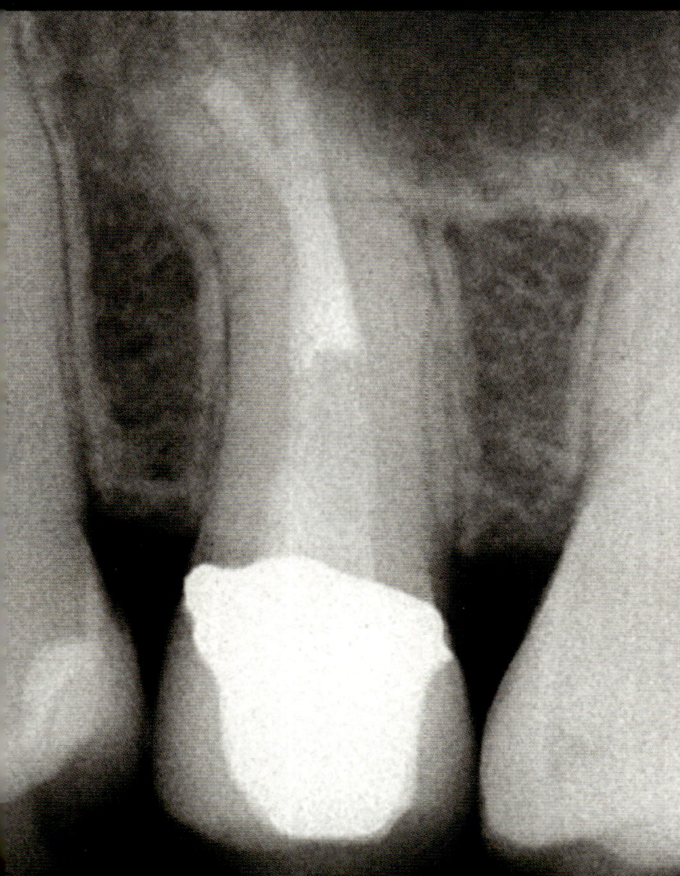

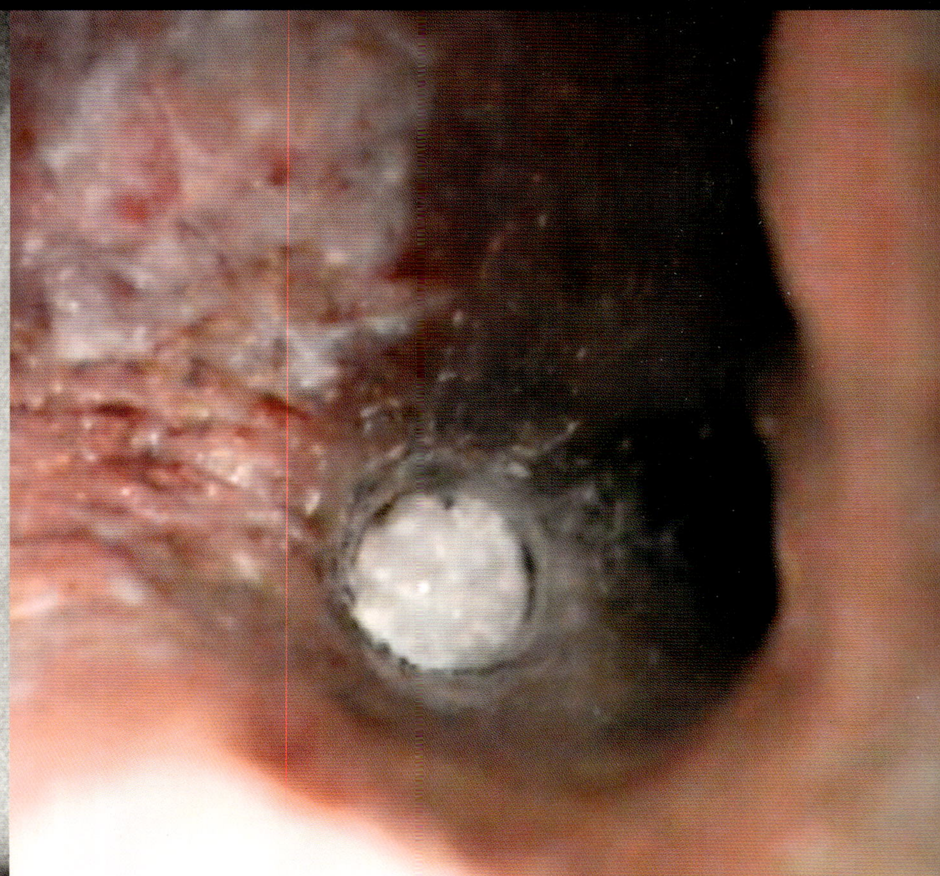

Davide Guglielmi, Riccardo Tonini, Fabio Gorni

07

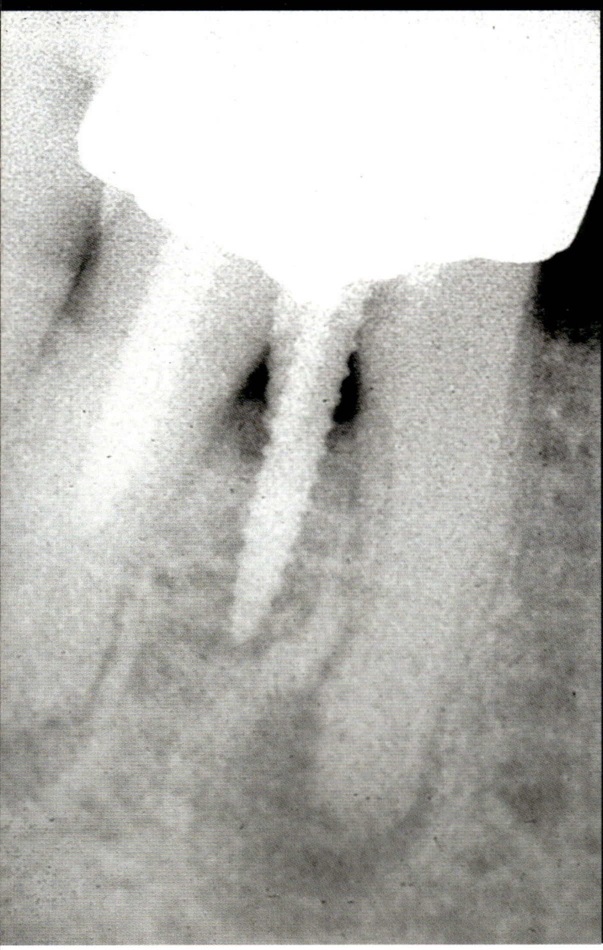

Endoperiodontal lesions and perforations

Communication between the endodontium and the periodontium: anatomical pathways and iatrogenic errors

Introduction

The treatment and prognosis of periodontal and/or endodontic diseases may vary depending on the etiology, pathogenesis, and proper recognition of each specific condition. In these cases, the clinician is faced with many doubts in order to express a correct diagnosis and prognosis; and the formulation of an adequate therapy for endoparodontal lesions is complicated. Understanding the interrelationship between endodontic and periodontal diseases will increase the clinician's ability to establish the correct diagnosis, assess the prognosis of the teeth involved in this disease, and select a treatment plan based on evidence-based literature.

Endoperiodontal communications

The dental pulp and the periodontium are connected by three main communication routes:

- exposed dentinal tubules;
- accessory canals;
- apical foramen.

Exposed dentinal tubules

Dentinal tubules that are exposed in cementless areas can serve as pathways of communication between the dental pulp and the periodontal ligament. The dentinal tubules of the root extend from the pulp to the cemento-dentinal junction with a relatively straight path and a size ranging from 1 to 3 microns in diameter. The diameter of the tubules decreases with age or in response to a chronic low-grade stimulus that causes the apposition of highly mineralized peritubular dentin[1]. The number of dentinal tubules ranges from about 8,000 near the CEJ (cemento-enamel junction) to about 57,000/mm^2 near the pulp[2, 3].

Accessory canals

The accessory canals are lateral ramifications external to the root canal system that connect the neurovascular system of the pulp to that of the periodontal ligament. They can be present at any level of the root (Fig. 7.1a–f). These accessory canals contain connective tissue and blood vessels that connect the circulatory system of the pulp to that of the periodontium.
Estimations indicate that the prevalence of accessory canal systems is around 27%, 17% of which in the apical third of the root, about 9% in the middle third, and less than 2% in the coronal third[4]. The furcation area of the pluriradicular teeth is the anatomical area that contains the most accessory canals; the incidence of these can vary from 23% to 76%[5-7]. In 2005, Vertucci distinguished various directions in which the accessory canals enter the furcation of the lower molars[8].
Although numerous clinical observations have shown the existence of this condition, the incidence of endodontic lesions

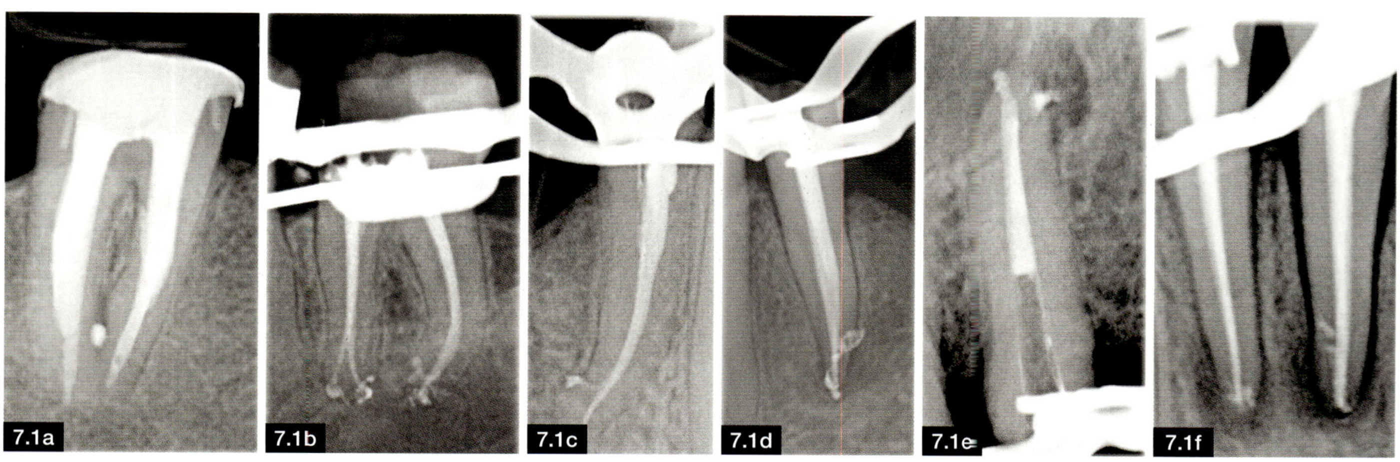

Fig. 7.1a–f: X-ray images in which, through the presence of radio-opaque canal filling materials, side canals are highlighted in different teeth.

in the marginal periodontium, deriving from accessory and furcation canals, appears to be low. Clearly, a large diameter of the accessory canals (up to 720 microns)[8] corresponds to a higher probability of developing lesions[9].

Apical foramen

The apical foramen is the main means of communication between the pulp and the periodontium. Microbial catabolites and inflammatory substances can easily escape through the apical foramen to cause periradicular disease. The apex is also a potential gateway to the pulp for inflammatory products from deep periodontal pockets[10] (Fig. 7.2a–b).

Etiology of endoparodontal lesions

The fact that periodontium and the dental pulp are anatomically interconnected also implies the possibility of an exchange of harmful agents in the opposite direction, i.e., from the environment outside the pulp to the pulp. A prerequisite for this condition is that the communication routes, which are normally protected by healthy periodontal tissue, become exposed (apical foramen, dentinal tubules, and accessory canals)[11-13]. The effect of periodontal disease on the pulp is a controversial topic, and numerous conflicting studies have been presented on the topic[14]. According to some studies, periodontal disease has no effect on the pulp, at least until it involves the apex[15]. Other studies have shown an effect of periodontal disease on the pulp that would lead to increased calcification, collagen reabsorption, and an inflammatory state[16]. However, the pulp does not seem to be severely impaired in teeth with moderate attachment loss. As long as the microvascularization of the apical foramen remains intact, the pulp retains its vitality[15]. In addition to this concept, an important detail that should be emphasized is that there may be influences related to the treatment of periodontal therapy. Although several animal studies[9, 17] support the hypothesis that subgingival cleaning procedures of pockets and/or roots do not threaten pulpal vitality, localized inflammatory changes may occur adjacent to instrumented root surfaces, followed by tissue repair in the form of hard tissue deposits on root canal walls.

Classification of endoperiodontal lesions

Colloquially defined as "endo-perio lesions," the classification system most commonly used for the diagnosis of endo-perio lesions was published in 1972 by Simon et al. and included the following categories: (1) primary endodontic lesions; (2) primary endodontic lesions with secondary periodontal involvement; (3) primary periodontal lesions; (4) primary periodontal lesions with secondary endodontic involvement; and (5) "true" combined lesions[18, 19]. (Table 7.2).
The main drawback of this classification and a recent proposed amendment is that the categories are based on the primary source of infection (root canal or periodontal pocket[20]. This seemed to be a suitable approach, as lesions of periodontal origin might have a worse prognosis than those of endodontic origin. Nonetheless, using "history of the disease" as the main criteria for diagnosis was not practical, because in the majority of cases the complete history is unavailable to the clinician[19].
Subsequently, in 1999, the classification system for Periodontal Diseases and Conditions for the first time included EPLs, which were described under Section VII – Periodontitis Associated with Endodontic Lesion, as a single category entitled "Combined Periodontal-Endodontic Lesions." This classification has an advantage over the previous ones using "history of the disease" as the main criteria.
By understanding the pathogenesis, the clinician may suggest an appropriate treatment plan after evaluating the prognosis. The main factors to be taken into consideration for the differential diagnosis of these lesions are the state of the

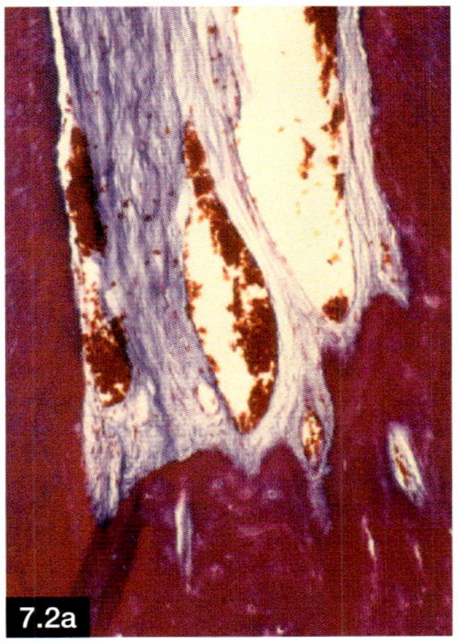
7.2a

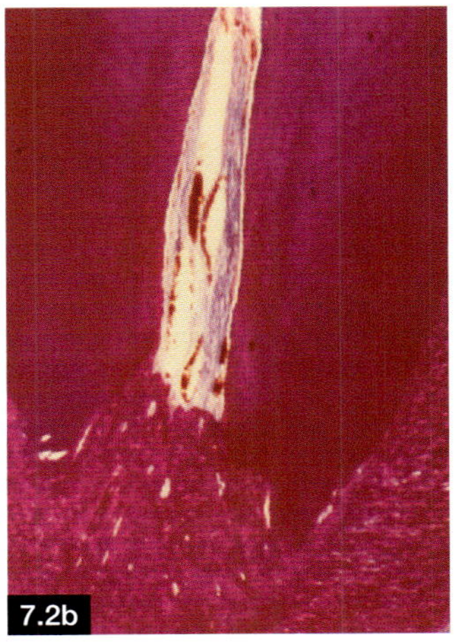
7.2b

Fig. 7.2a–b: Histological image of the apical neurovascular bundle and periapical tissues (courtesy of Prof. M. de Sanctis).

endodontium of the tooth and the type and extent of the periodontal defect.
The diagnosis of a primary endodontic lesion and of a primary periodontal lesion usually does not present difficulties. In lesions that are purely endodontic, the evaluation of the state of the endodontium is an important element of discernment.
Conversely, in a tooth with a primary periodontal lesion, the state of the endodontium may not be a key element, while probing will be more so.
Finally, primary endodontic lesions with secondary periodontal involvement and primary periodontal lesions with secondary endodontic involvement are clinically and radiographically similar, as are true combined lesions, where diagnostic doubts seem difficult to eliminate. It goes without say that these clinical situations are prone to ambiguous interpretations, and only a targeted diagnostic-therapeutic path will lead to an effective solution (Table 7.1). This is the reason why expert clinicians belonging to the America Academy of Periodontology and the European Federeration of Periodontology, during the Consensus report of workgroup 2 of the 2017 World Workshop on the Classification of Periodontal and Peri–Implant Diseases and Conditions [21] focused on different problems in these classification system (1) grouping all Endodontic–periodontal lesions under a single section entitled "Periodontitis Associated with Endodontic Lesion" was not ideal, as these lesions may occur in subjects with or without periodontitis; (2) the single category presented, "Combined Periodontal–Endodontic Lesions", was too generic and not sufficiently discriminative to help the clinician to determine the most effective treatment for a particular lesion.
Finally, Endodontic–periodontal lesions

Table 7.1 **PROPOSAL FOR ENDOPERIODONTAL LESION CLASSIFICATION**

Endoperiodontal lesion with root damage		Root fracture or cracking
		Root canal or pulp chamber perforation
		External root resorption
Endoperiodontal lesion without root damage	Endoperiodontal lesion in periodontitis patients	*Grade 1* – narrow deep periodontal pocket in 1 tooth surface
		Grade 2 – wide deep periodontal pocket in 1 tooth surface
		Grade 3 – deep periodontal pockets in more than 1 tooth surface
	Endoperiodontal lesion in non-periodontitis patients	*Grade 1* – narrow deep periodontal pocket in 1 tooth surface
		Grade 2 – wide deep periodontal pocket in 1 tooth surface
		Grade 3 – deep periodontal pockets in more than 1 tooth surface

Table 7.2 **CLASSIFICATION OF ENDOPERIODONTAL LESIONS**

Primary endodontic lesions			
Primary periodontal lesions			
Combined lesions	Primary endodontic lesions with secondary periodontal involvement (perforations)	Primary periodontal lesions with secondary endodontic involvement	True combined lesions

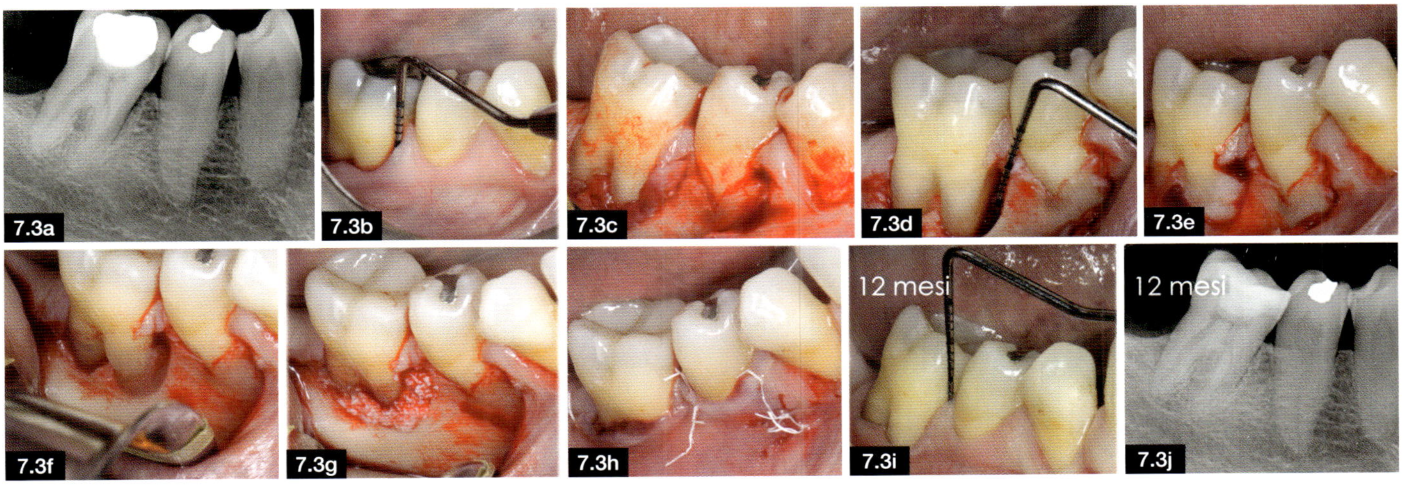

Fig. 7.3a–j: a) Initial periapical radiograph; element 4.6 is positive to the vitality test;

b) pre-surgical probing after nonsurgical periodontal therapy;

c) incision of the primary flap;

d) probing of infraosseous defects after the removal of the granulation tissue;

e) positioning of a chelating gel containing ethylene diaminotetra-acetic acid for 120 seconds;

f) positioning of a resorbable biomaterial composed of proteins derived from the enamel matrix;

g) positioning of heterologous bovine bone biomaterial to slow resorption;

h) sutures;

i) physiological probing 12 months after surgery;

j) 12-month X-ray: the amalgam reconstruction is being substituted by composite material on the same tooth.

should be classified according to signs and symptoms that can realistically be assessed at the time that the lesion is detected and that have a direct impact on their treatment, such as presence or absence of fractures and perforations, presence or absence of periodontitis, and the extent of the periodontal destruction around the affected tooth[19].

Primary endodontic lesions

A chronic apical lesion in a tooth with necrotic pulp can, occasionally, have an acute evolution, draining coronally through the periodontal ligament and thus reaching the gingival groove. This condition can clinically imitate the presence of a periodontal abscess. In primary endodontic lesions, the pulp is infected and its vitality is impaired. For diagnostic purposes, a fistogram needs to be performed, which consists of inserting a gutta-percha cone in the fistula and the simultaneous performance of one or more endodontic X-rays. The presence of the radio-opaque cone will help determine the origin of the lesion (see Chapter 2, page 81). During circumferential probing, the probe can typically be inserted into the groove only at one point, because of the fistolous path through the space of the periodontal ligament. These endodontic lesions usually heal after canal therapy[22]. An interesting topic is the differential diagnosis with root fractures, described in Chapter 2, to which we refer.

Primary periodontal lesions

These lesions are mainly caused by periodontal pathogens and are rarely isolated. In this process, chronic periodontitis progresses apically along the root surface.
In most cases, periodontitis is associated with teeth with healthy endodontium, with reactions to diagnostic tests, which indicate a clinically normal pulpal state.
The clinical examination presents the typical features of periodontal disease, with high probing depths in several points where the measurements are made.
The prognosis depends on the stage of the periodontal disease and in the effectiveness of periodontal treatment (Fig. 7.3a-j).

Combined injuries

As previously described in the section dedicated to the classification (see Table 7.2), combined lesions can be of three types: those starting from the endodontium that can then evolve, those starting from the periodontium that may affect the endodontium, and those that may involve both systems simultaneously; the latter type is much rarer than the first two[22].
The distinction is often complex (and of little interest for the purposes of this text) in the second and third types, while recognizing the first type is important for treatment purposes.

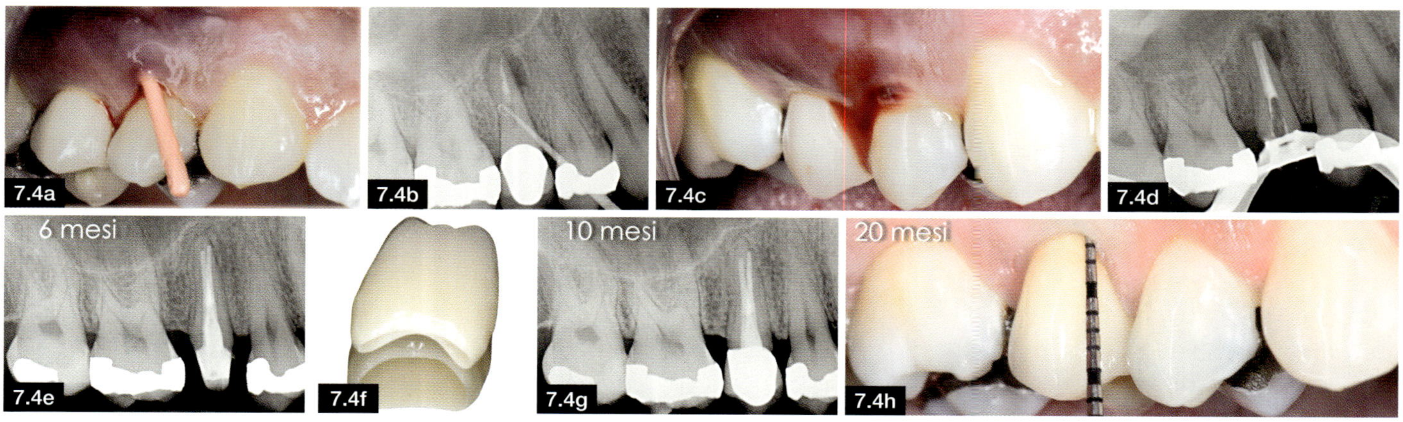

Fig. 7.4a-h: Primary endodontic lesion.
a) clinical image with a gutta-percha cone inserted in the sinus portion of the lesion;
b) fistulogram showing the origin of the lesion;
c) periodontal abscess;
d) orthodontic post-treatment X-ray;
e) follow-up X-ray 6 months after endodontic retreatments;
f) ceramic zirconium prosthesis;
g) follow-up X-ray of the prosthetic restoriation post-cementation;
h) clinical image of the physiological probing 20 months after endodontic therapy.

Primary endodontic lesion with secondary periodontal involvement

If a primary endodontic disease, which may be suppurative, remains untreated for a certain period of time, a concomitant periodontal disease may arise. In this case, the development of pathogenic plaque and tartar is the essential requirement for generating this pathological scenario and determining the need to initiate joint endodontic and periodontal therapy. Some authors have shown that the best results can be achieved by giving priority to the first of the two phases. In fact, if the endodontic treatment is adequate, then the prognosis seems more favorable, although this depends also on the severity of the marginal periodontal damage and on the effectiveness of the subsequent periodontal treatment[22].
It is therefore important to emphasize that the treatment of a primary endodontic lesion, with secondary periodontal involvement, must be reassessed after two to three months and, in the case of symptomatic and radiographic resolution, the opportunity to proceed with periodontal treatment itself can be reconsidered. This operational choice will allow sufficient time for the initial healing of the supporting tissue complex and will allow a better evaluation of the actual periodontal condition[23]. Typically, primary endodontic lesions, with secondary periodontal involvement, can occur following root perforation during canal treatment; we felt it was appropriate to focus our attention on this matter[22] (Fig. 7.4a–h).

Perforations

Root perforations are unwanted clinical complications that can lead to the failure of root canal treatment. In fact, the treatment itself is not free from adverse events, as repeatedly described in this text. The prevalence of perforations seems to increase with the number of operations carried out to manage pulp and periapical disease. As mentioned several times in this text (see Chapter 3), the deformation of root canals due to incorrect shaping (steps and stops), together with the fractures of endodontic instruments, are the major causes of failure of endodontic therapy; in addition, perforations appear to be among the most common complications[24]. Although definite data is not available in this regard, estimates suggest that perforations occur in about 20% of endodontic treatments; however, many of them are not identified and, when asymptomatic, remain silent over time[25, 26].
One study reported that during nonsurgical retreatments of teeth with an inadequate primary treatment, perforations were detected in 12% of patients[27]. In a systematic review carried out in 2010, the authors reported a prevalence of perforations ranging between 12% and 20% of nonsurgical retreatments[28]; in line with the findings reported by Gorni and Gagliani[29], who found a prevalence of around 12% in a sample of teeth intended for nonsurgical retreatments. Perforations of the root canal can occur during endodontic treatment or afterwards, i.e., during the reconstruction of the tooth. Clauder and Shin[30] reported that a high percentage (53%)

occurs following prosthetic treatment, i.e., during the placement of root canal posts, while 47% occurs during primary canal therapy (Fig. 7.5a–k).

Definition and classification of perforations

Root perforations can be defined as unnatural communications between the root canal system and the periodontal apparatus of the tooth and can be divided into:

- pathological, i.e., linked to an erosion of the dentinal component (extensive caries or resorptions);
- iatrogenic, i.e., connected to incorrect operations during canal shaping or reconstruction (for example, the execution of cavities inside the root canal for the positioning of posts).

Within this second category, which we will deal with extensively in this second part of the chapter, we can distinguish two large groups:

1. perforations related to the action of the tip of endodontic instruments or drills used during access or the shaping of the root canal;
2. erosion of the canal wall (stripping) caused by an incorrect use of instruments in relation to the canal anatomy that has to be shaped.

In the first category, the communication will have a well-defined diameter and

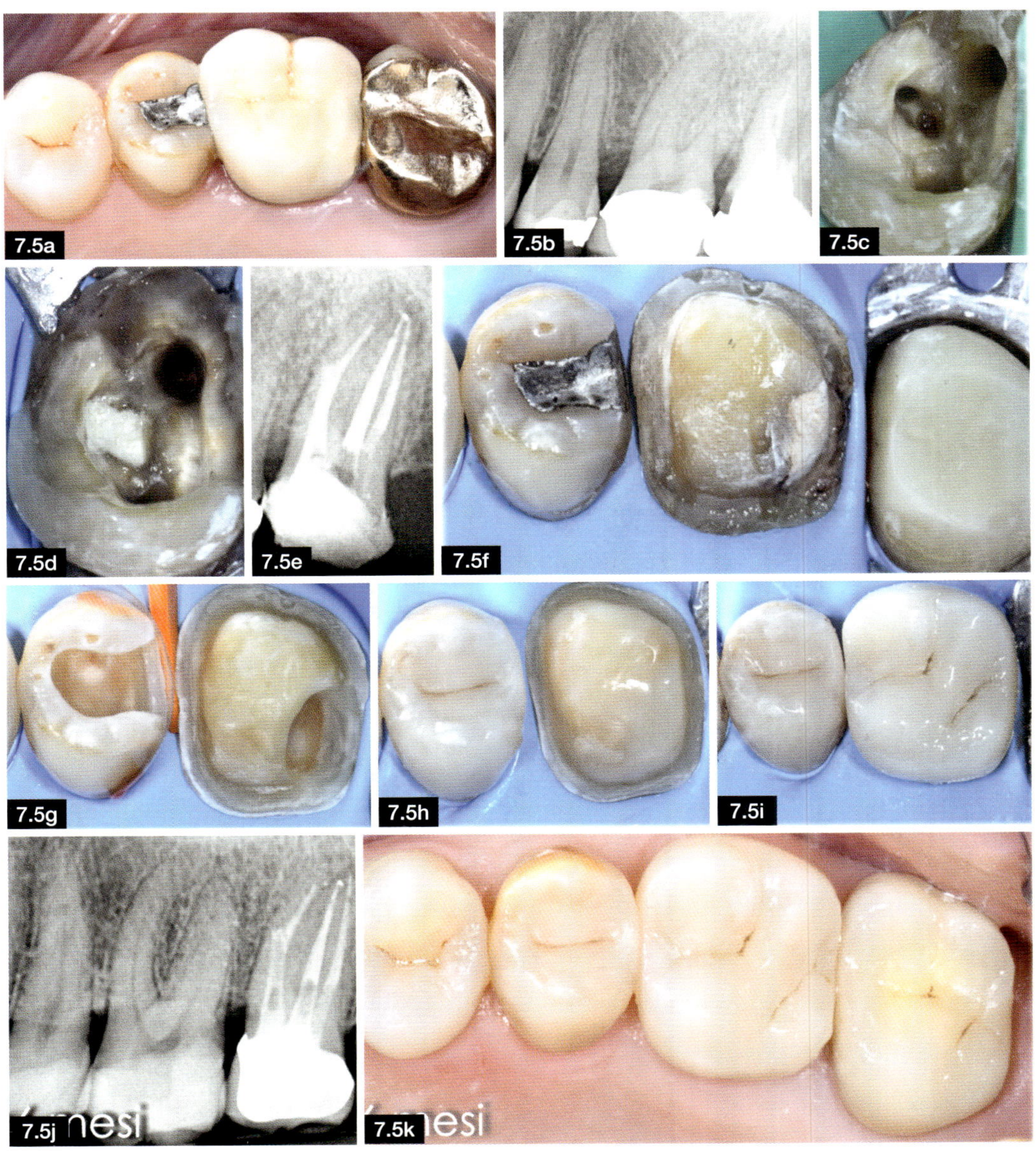

Fig. 7.5a–k: Primary endodontic lesion with secondary periodontal involvement.

a) initial clinical scenario in which the patient reports pain when chewing and when pressure is applied in the area. PSR = 4 involvement of the vestibular furcation area of tooth 2.7 of grade II A;

b) initial periapical X-ray;

c–d) clinical images in which a perforation of the chamber floor is evident and its subsequent repair by means of a mineral cement based on trioxide;

e) postoperative radiograph of orthograde retreatment;

f) clinical image of the carious lesions present on teeth 2.6 and 2.5;

g) clinical images of the cavities of 2.6 and 2.5;

h) composite resin reconstruction of 2.5 and build-up of 2.6;

i) adhesive cementation of composite overlays 4 days after build-up (and subsequent precision impression);

j) 6-month follow-up X-ray showing the direct reconstruction of 2.5, the inlay of 2.6, and the zirconium-ceramic crown on 2.7;

k) 6-month clinical image in which physiological probing is observed throughout the sextant.

Table 7.3 **FACTORS INFLUENCING THE RESOLUTION OF PERIRADICULAR DISEASE ASSOCIATED WITH A PERFORATION**[31]	
• EARLY DIAGNOSIS	• CHOICE OF TREATMENT
• DIMENSIONS	• MATERIALS USED FOR FILLING
• SHAPE	• HOST RESPONSE
• POSITION	
• NATURE OF PERFORATION	• PROFESSIONAL EXPERIENCE

contours. In the second category, both the diameter and the contours will not be uniform. Regardless of the type, a perforation, which connects the endodontium and the periodontium, is immediately filled with pathogens, generating an inflammatory reaction of the supporting structures that determines a localized loss of periodontal attachment; in the long term, this initial lesion evolves, and compromises the health of the periradicular tissues until it undermines the permanence in the oral cavity of the tooth itself. The diagnostic path to identifying perforations is not easy. However, as stated in Chapter 2, the help of a good clinical examination and the use of three-dimensional radiographic examinations can, in most cases, guide the diagnosis. It is also true that many perforations are identified during endodontic root canal retreatment actions and that these intraoperative findings place the clinician in front of operational problems that are not always within everyone's capabilities.

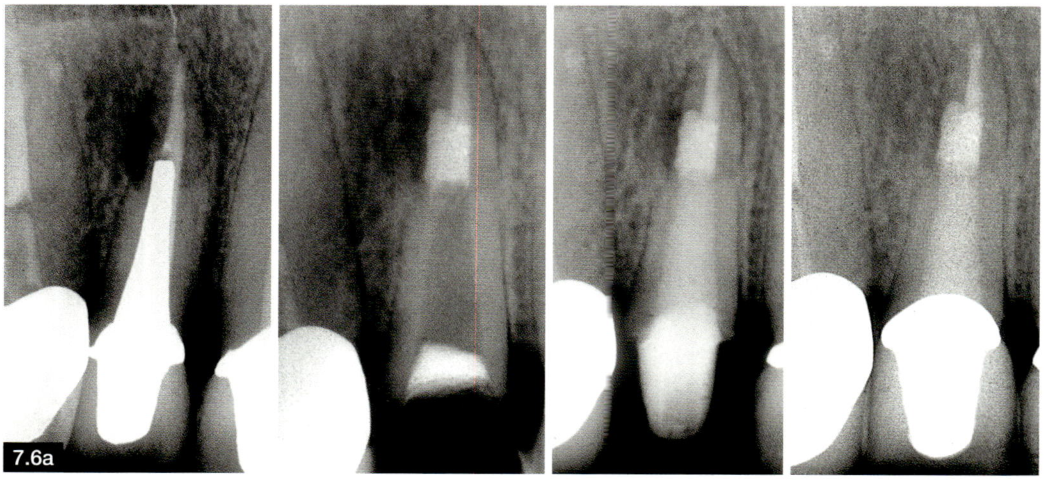

7.6a

Fig. 7.6a: Perforation of the apical third in the upper lateral incisor, probably related to the preparation for the housing of a metal post. Removal of the post and repair of the perforation with a suitable material, which allowed the functional recovery of the tooth.

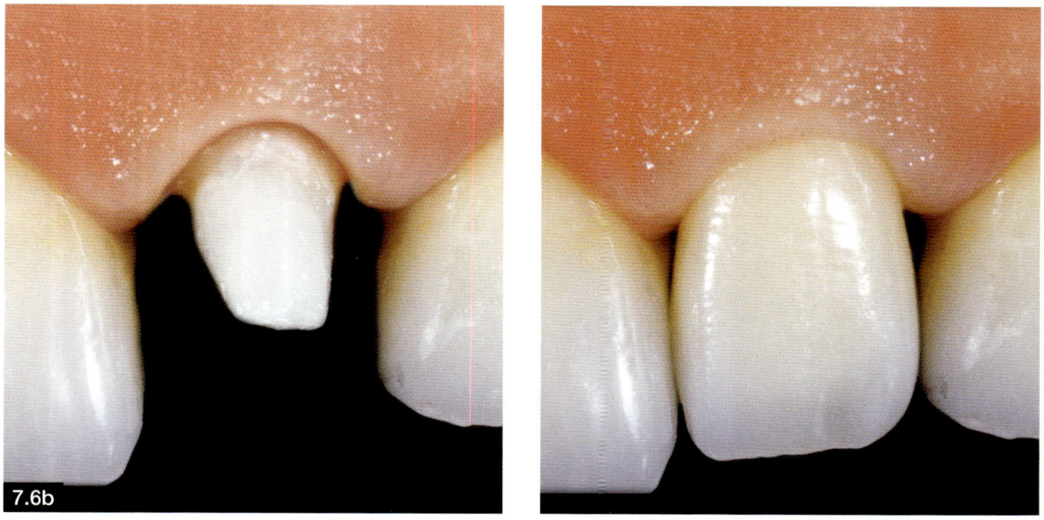

7.6b

Fig. 7.6b: Prosthetic element with core build-up made with a fiber post which is more suitable for this kind of rehabilitation.

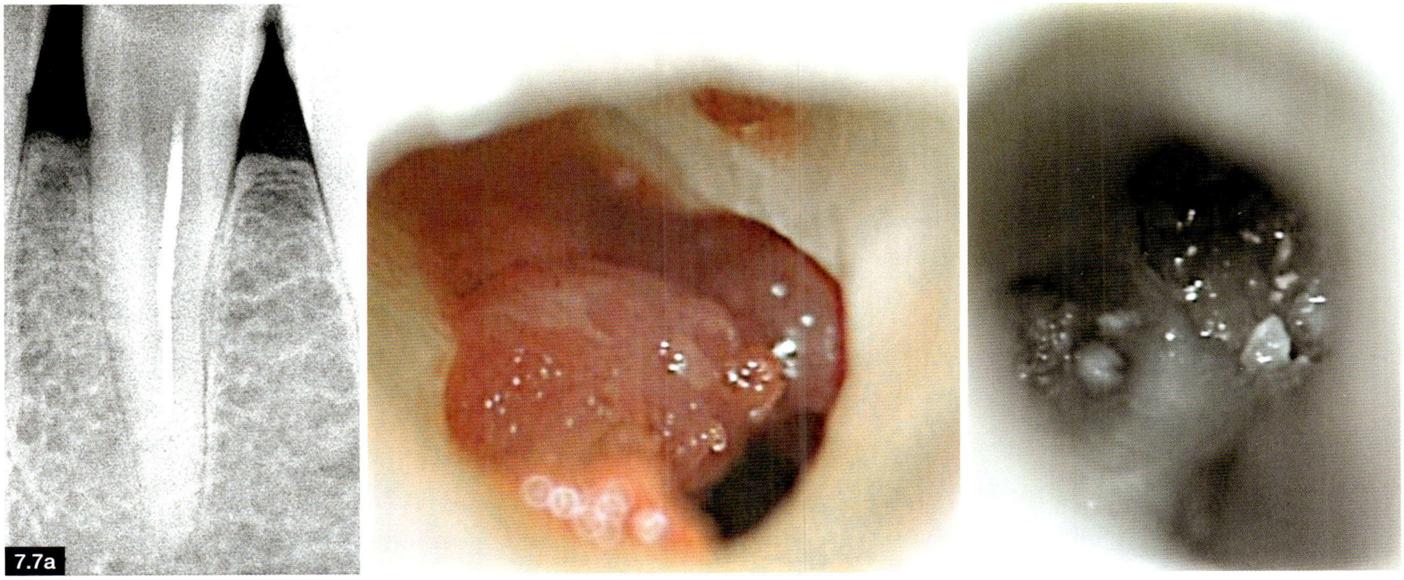

7.7a

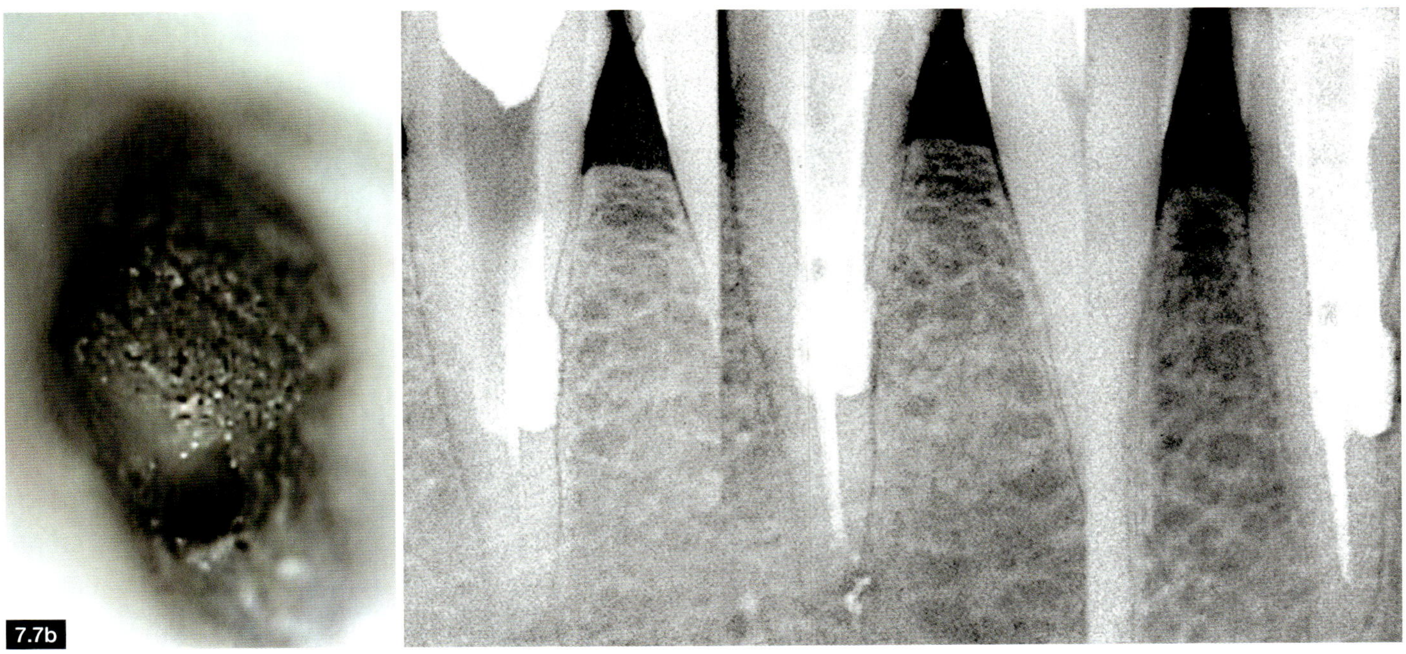

7.7b

Fig. 7.7a: Perforation of the middle third of the root in the lower premolar; note the significant proliferation of granulation tissue that must be removed in order to make the area of the perforation bloodless and reliable with specific materials.

Fig. 7.7b: Evolution of the case with 7-year follow-up.

Prognosis of perforations

When a diagnosis is performed in the preoperative clinical fase, upon finding a perforation, it makes sense to bear in mind some of the elements that determine success in repairing perforations (Table 7.3).

Fuss and Trope assigned a decisive value to the localization, which influences the prognosis, as root perforations in the crestal area are more susceptible to epithelial migration and rapid formation of a pathological periodontal pocket with evident loss of attachment[32]. Time—i.e., the immediate closure of the perforation, which would lead to an appropriate infection control—and the use of effective and biocompatible materials to seal the iatrogenic or pathological communication between endodontium and periodontium can also prevent bacterial penetration and lead to favorable treatment results[32]. The best known repair material, mineral trioxide aggregate (MTA; see Box 5.3 on page 306), allows us to look at this operation with different eyes today. Numerous studies have documented how calcium silicate derivatives promote tissue regeneration without causing inflammation and have excellent sealing

Box 7.1 **TYPES OF FOUR-WALL PERFORATIONS AND OPERATING SEQUENCES**

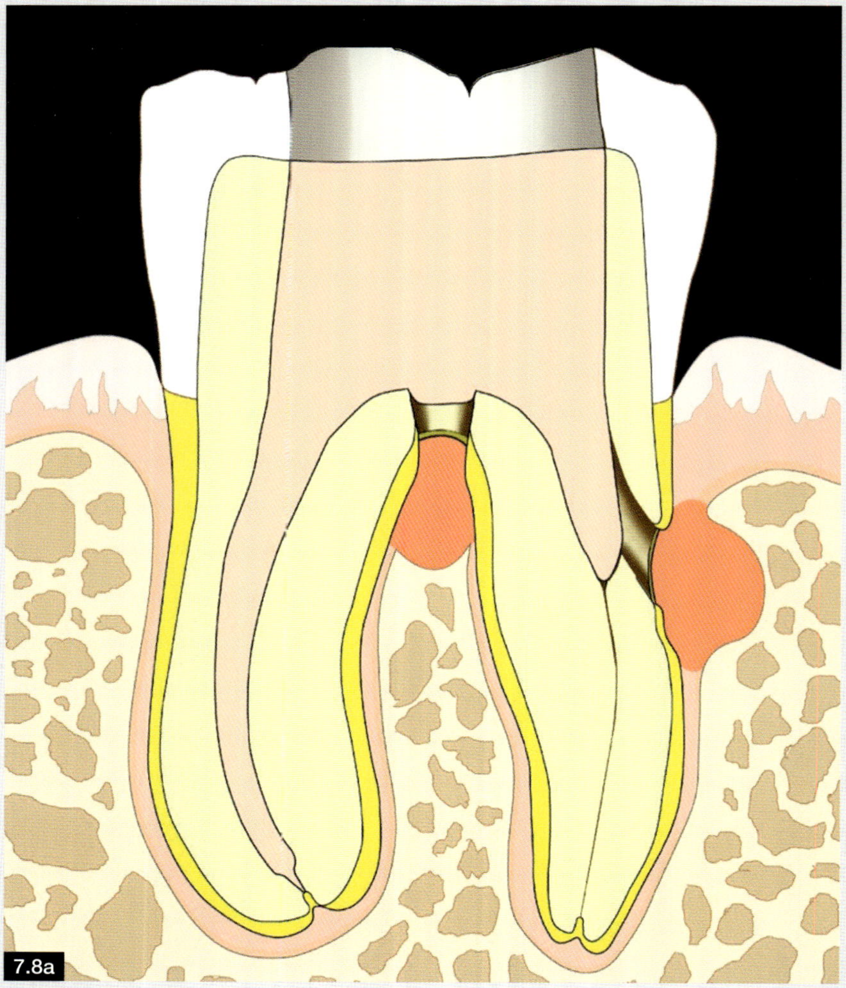

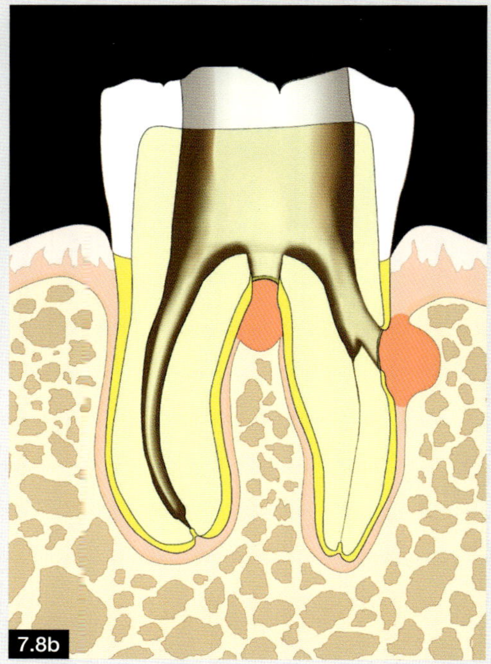

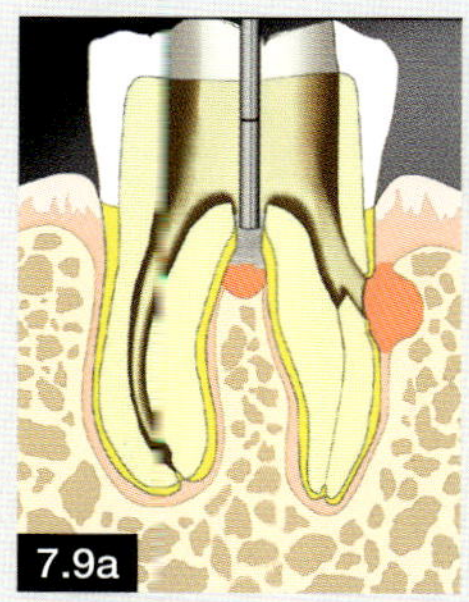

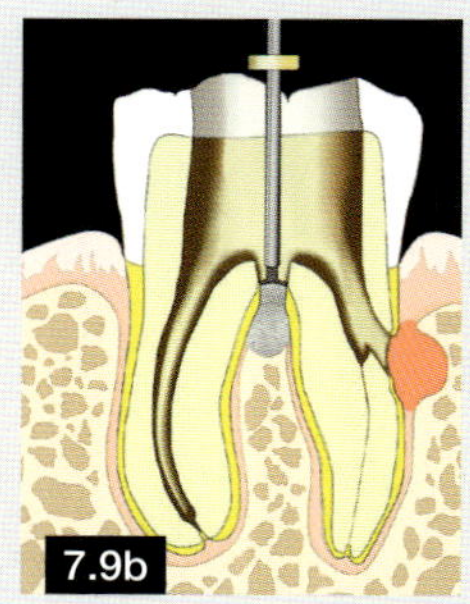

Fig. 7.8a: Types of root canal floor perforations.

Fig. 7.8b: Suitable canal shaping for filling the perforations.

Fig. 7.9a-h: Barrier positioning and filling of the perforation.
a) Insertion of collagen material to fill the lesion generated by the perforation; b) first increment of the material for filling the perforation; c) compaction of the first increment; d) second increment of the same material; e) further compaction;
f) repair of the lateral perforation completed before the root canal filling phase;
g) final filling of the root canal;
h) healing.

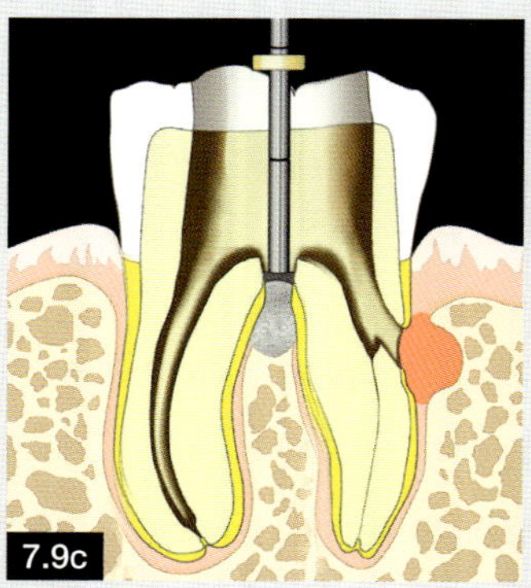

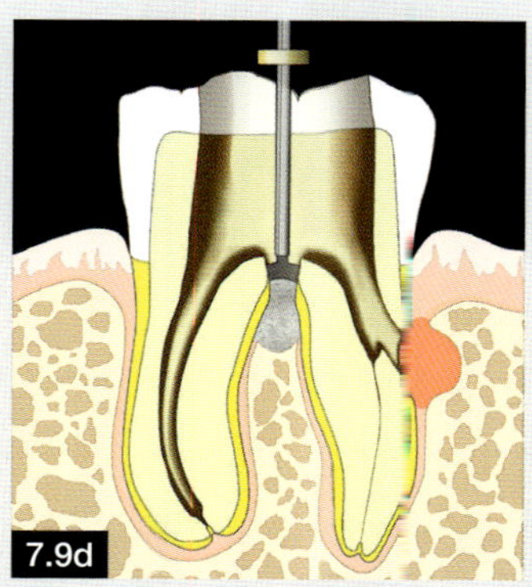

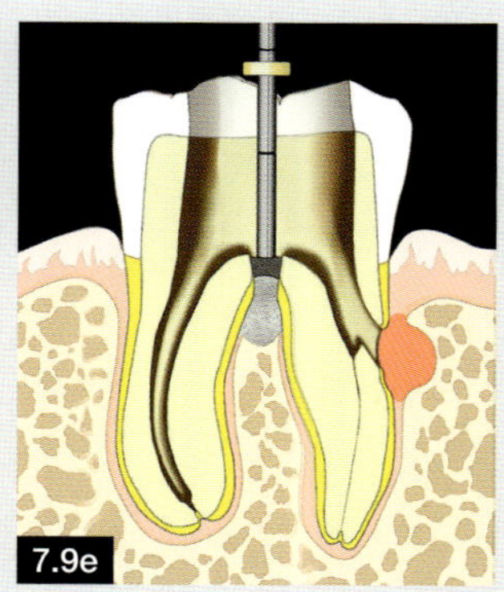

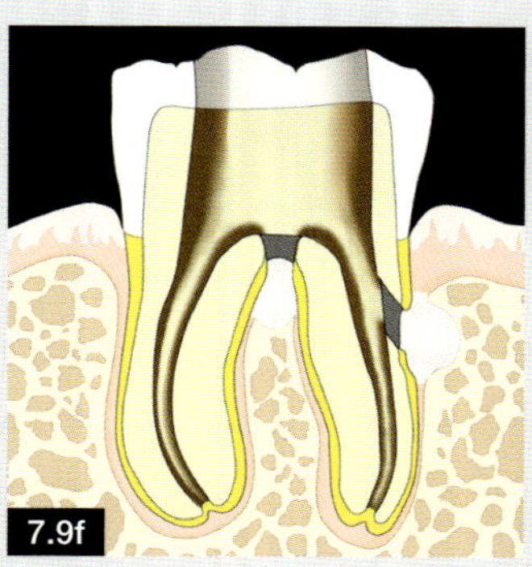

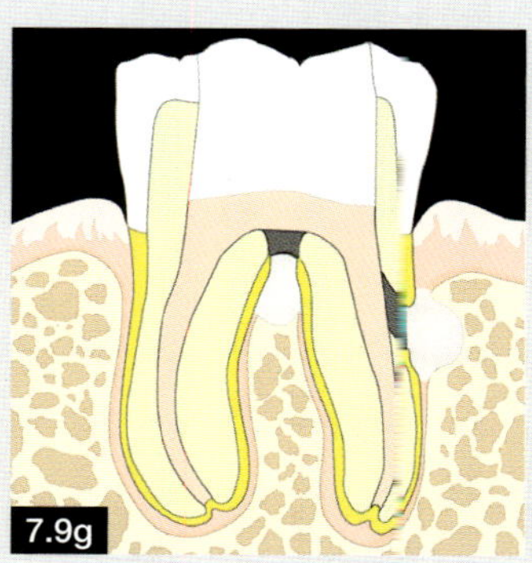

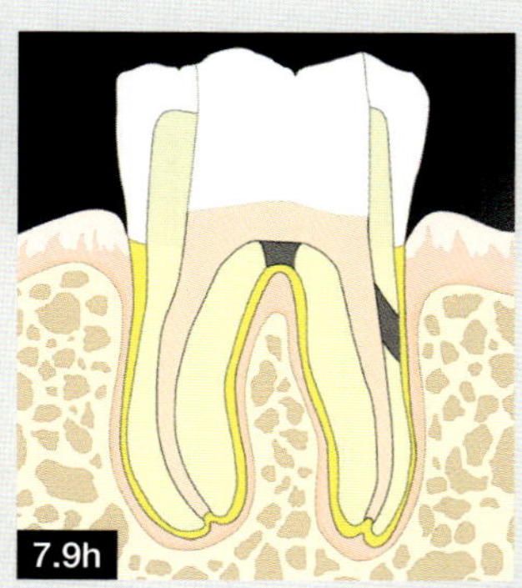

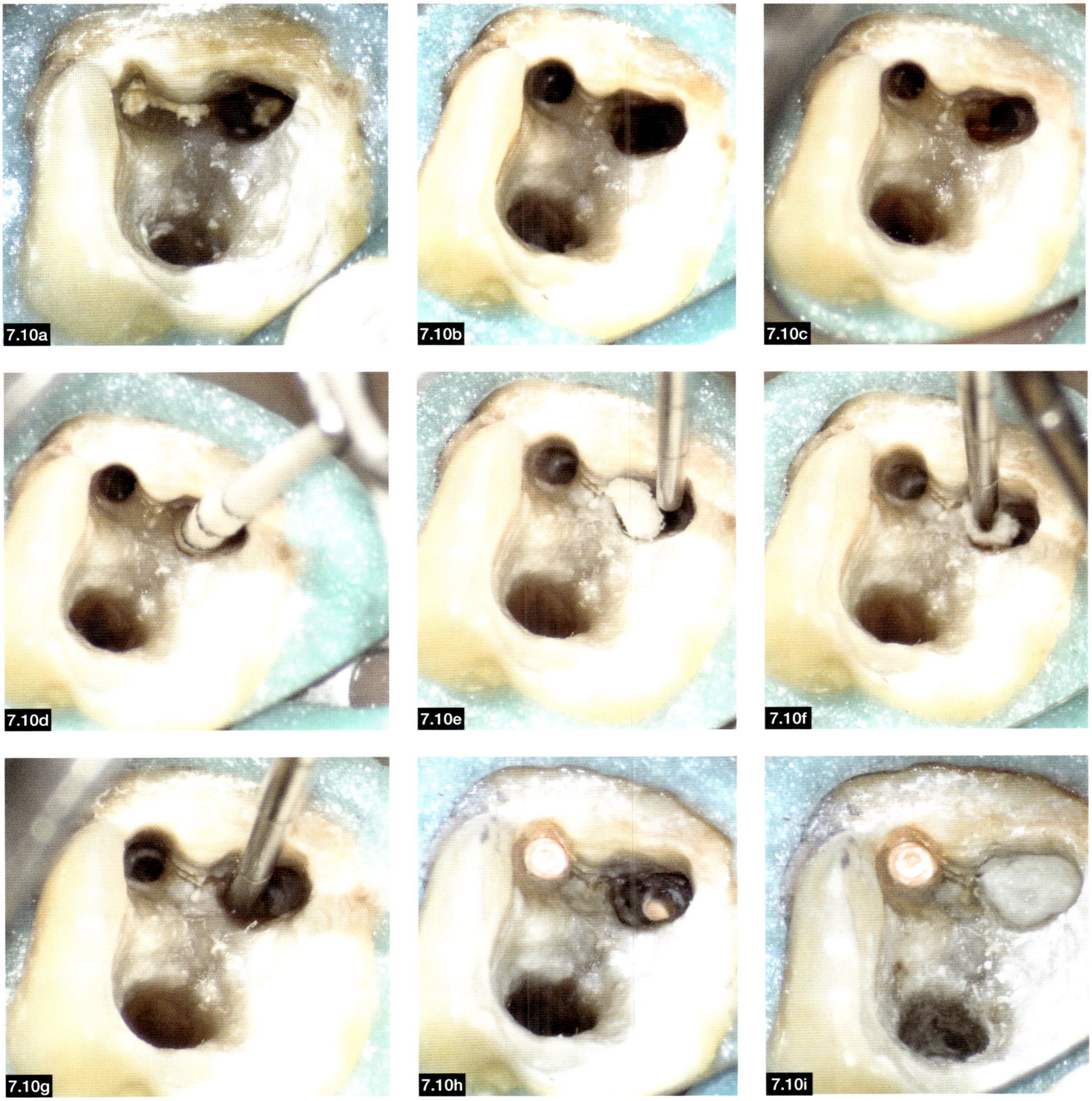

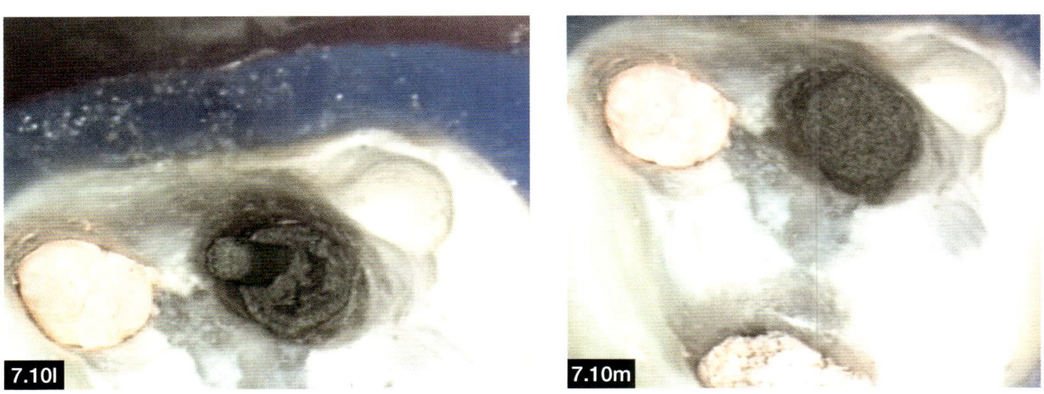

Fig. 7.10a-m: This operating sequence shows some of the key steps for repairing a perforation: a) identification; b–c) cleaning and preparation; d) drying; e–g) positioning of a barrier made of resorbable material; h) control of the canal filling; i–m) positioning of MTA to seal the perforation.

Box 7.2 LONGITUDINAL STUDY ON SUCCESS RATES IN TREATMENT OF PERFORATIONS

In a recent article, Gorni et al. observed the probability of healing after perforations are repaired with MTA, relating it to several variables[43]. The same authors, in a previous study[29], had reported a failure rate on the so-called stripping of the root canal and on the perforations of the floor of the pulp chamber in the pluriradicular teeth or of the canal itself, in the mono-radicular teeth, close to 50%.
The results were different in the prospective cohort study on 110 patients, completed with the most recent techniques.
In this study, preoperative data (periodontal visualization and probing) were clinically and radiographically recorded; perforations were diagnosed intraoperatively through direct vision or the presence of bleeding areas on paper cones.
The position (coronal, middle, and apical third) and size of each perforation (≤1, 2–3, and >3 mm) were then recorded using a calibrated periodontal probe.
Out of 110 patients with a single lesion, 101 were judged healed (92%), with 89 at the first (n = 98,89%) and 3 at the second (n = 3 3%) post-treatment control.
Only 9 (8%) showed no sign of healing during the study period (Table 7.4).
A variable number of factors have been associated with a greater or lesser probability of primary healing of the lesion caused by perforations[43]:

- Women had a higher risk of relapse than men (HR, 3.1; P = .03; Table 7.4);
- Positive periodontal probing resulted in a much higher risk of recurrence than that verified in the teeth with negative probing (HR, 21; P < .001) (Fig. 7.11a);
- A perforation in the apical or intermediate

Table 7.4 **FEATURES RELATED TO THE HEALING OF THE ENTIRE COHORT OF 110 TEETH TREATED FOR PERFORATIONS FROM 1999 TO 2009**

	Healing N (%)	Non-healing N (%)	Total N (%)	Fisher test P-value
Age (yrs)				
≤50	87 (93)	7 (7)	94 (85)	.61
>50	14 (88)	2 (12)	16 (15)	
Gender				
Male	55 (92)	5 (8)	60 (54)	1
Female	46 (92)	4 (8)	50 (46)	
Tooth localization				
Front	15 (100)	0 (0)	15 (14)	
Premolar	11 (85)	2 (15)	13 (12)	.29
Molar	75 (91)	7 (9)	82 (74)	
Test				
Negative	65 (98)	1 (2)	66 (60)	.003
Positive	36 (82)	8 (18)	44 (40)	
Perforation site				
Coronal	50 (96)	2 (4)	52 (47)	
Intermediate	48 (87)	7 (13)	55 (50)	.29
Apical	3 (100)	0 (0)	3 (3)	
Perforation size (mm)				
≤1	10 (100)	0 (0)	10 (9)	
2–3	65 (94)	4 (6)	69 (63)	.16
>3	26 (84)	5 (16)	31 (28)	
TOTAL	**101 (92)**	**9 (8)**	**110**	

zone was more likely not to heal than a similar one in the coronal zone (HR, 3.0; P = .04) (Fig. 7.11b);

- The size of the perforation was related to the risk of progression: patients with perforations >3 mm in size were more likely to show relapse or not to heal than those with smaller lesions (HR, 3.6; P = .01) (Fig. 7.11c).

These data confirm the conclusions of Fuss and Trope that report the location and size of the perforations as the most important prognostic factors[32].
The study brings to our attention another prognostic element: preoperative periodontal probing. In presence of a lesion of more than 4 mm, as indicated in Fig. 7.11a, the probability of success is reduced to the point where the intervention is not recommended.
As for the failure rate related with the perforation site, an important detail to note is that 13% of perforations in the middle third of the root did not have positive results[43].
The percentage of failure in perforations with diameter > 3 mm was 16%, that for perforations with a diameter of between 2 and 3 mm was 6%, while those with a diameter of < 2 mm did not fail. Mente et al. described how the healing rate (92%) for single-root perforated teeth was higher than for pluriradicular teeth (75%), while the healing rate (67%) was lower for perforated teeth with diameters greater than 3 mm compared with those with diameters smaller than 3 mm (88%) and those with much smaller diameters (≤1 mm) (90%)[41].
These data were then reconfirmed in a subsequent study[42].
From this examination, on the basis of the data obtained in this and other studies, the possibility of repairing perforations and of the healing of the related periradicular pathologies is clearly high. However, preoperative periodontal probing, location, and size may be elements that, together, reduce or increase the probability of success.

PROBABILITY OF NON-PROGRESSION

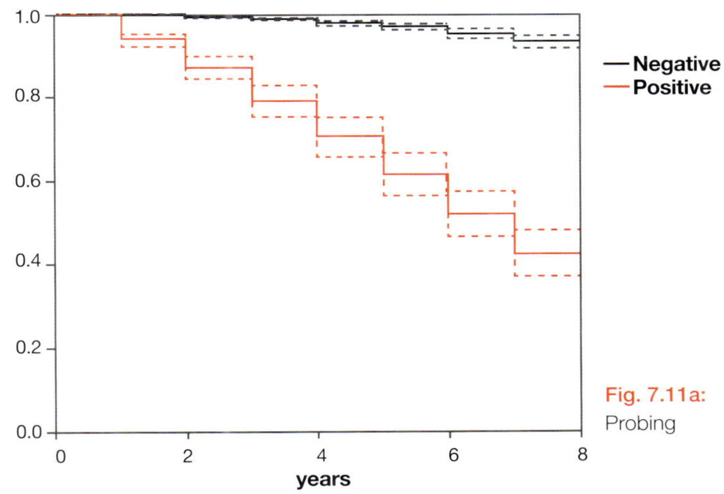

Fig. 7.11a: Probing

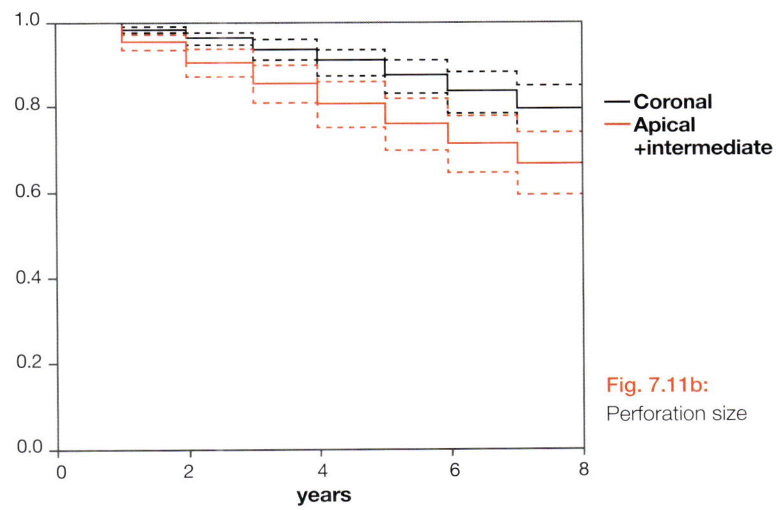

Fig. 7.11b: Perforation size

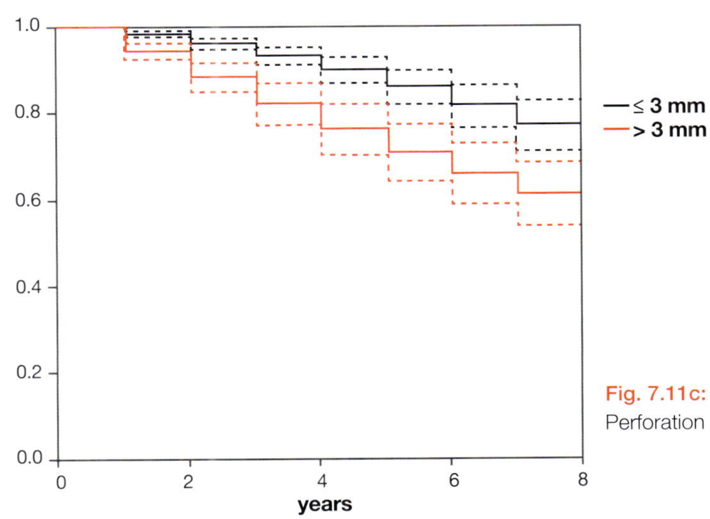

Fig. 7.11c: Perforation size

CASE REPORT 1

Iatrogenic perforation with fractured instrument

As specified in the classification, iatrogenic perforations represent a non-negligible portion of endoparodontal communications and, not infrequently lead to periodontal damage that is difficult to repair. The case shown presents a double difficulty: removing the instrument without damaging the root surface and repairing the perforation with suitable material.

Figure 1: Preoperative x-ray.

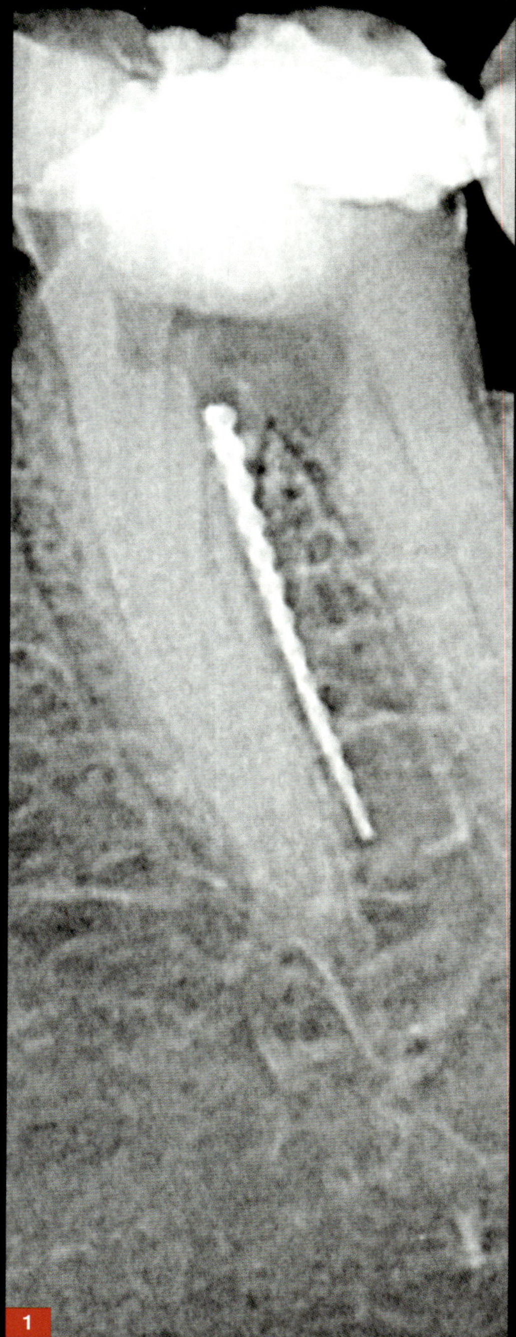

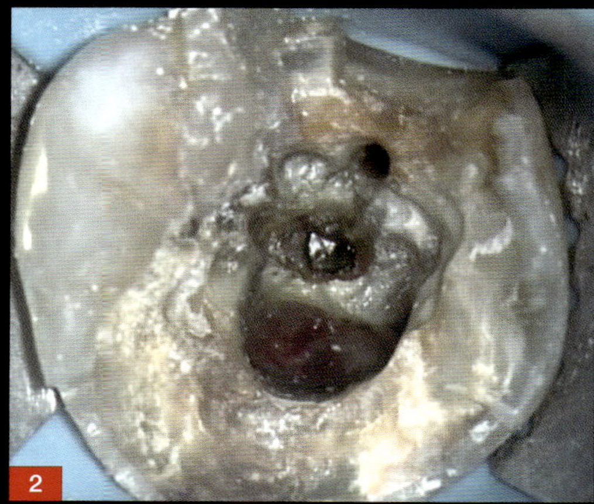

Figure 2: The fractured instrument is visible through the access cavity.

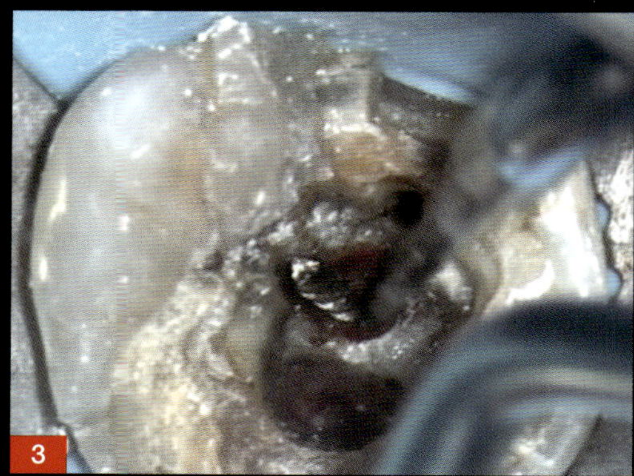

Figure 3: The ultrasonic tip transmits vibrations to the fragment in an attempt to remove it.

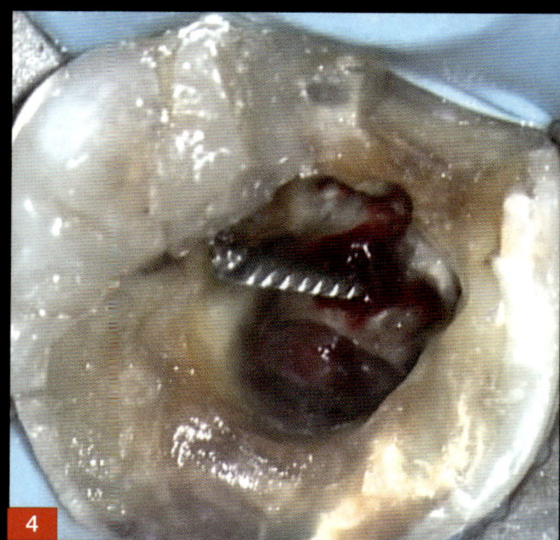

Figure 4: The fragment is now almost completely in the pulp chamber.

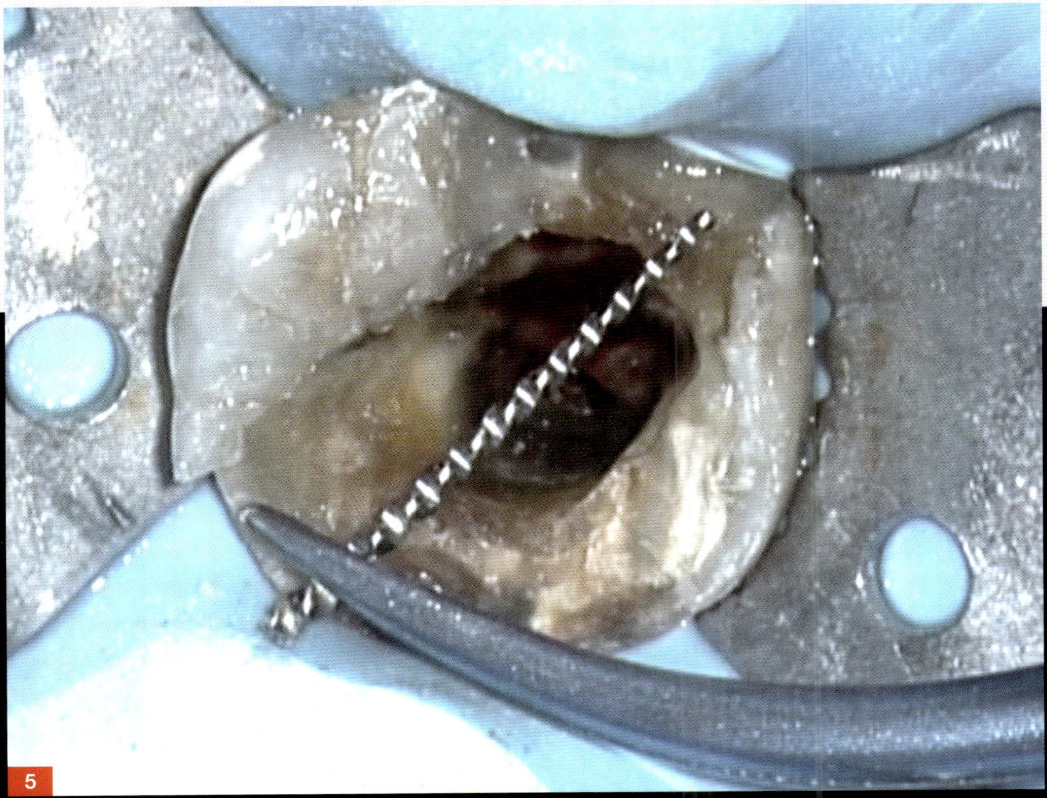

Figure 5: The fragment has been completely removed.

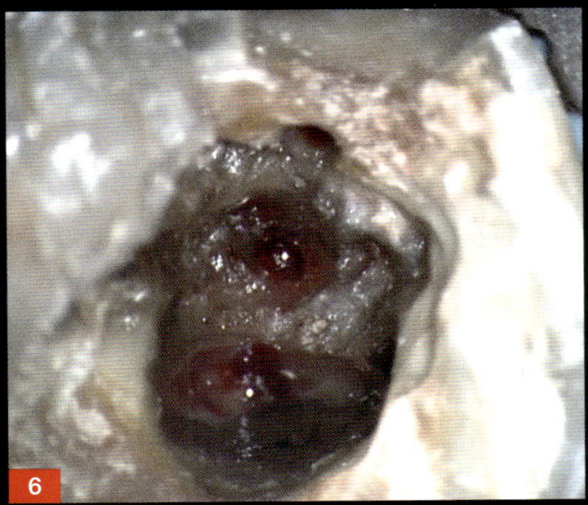

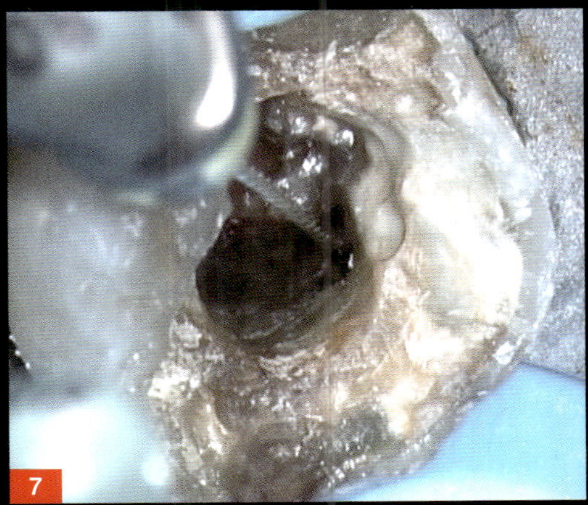

Figure 6: The chamber floor has numerous perforations.

Figure 7: The manual file has found and is probing the mesio-vestibular canal.

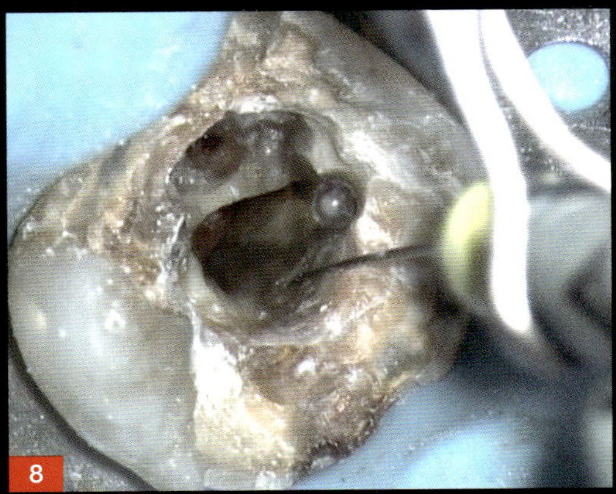

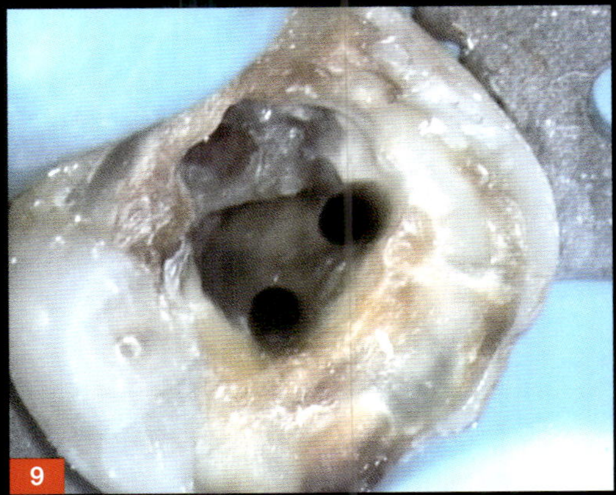

Figure 8: The manual file is now probing the mesio-lingual channel.

Figure 9: The mesial channels have been cleaned and shaped.

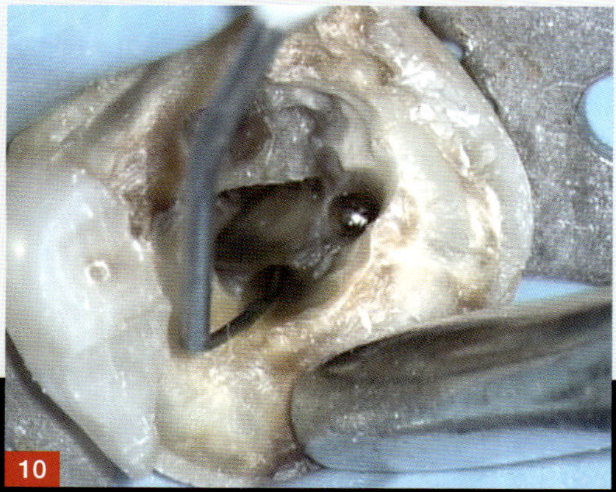

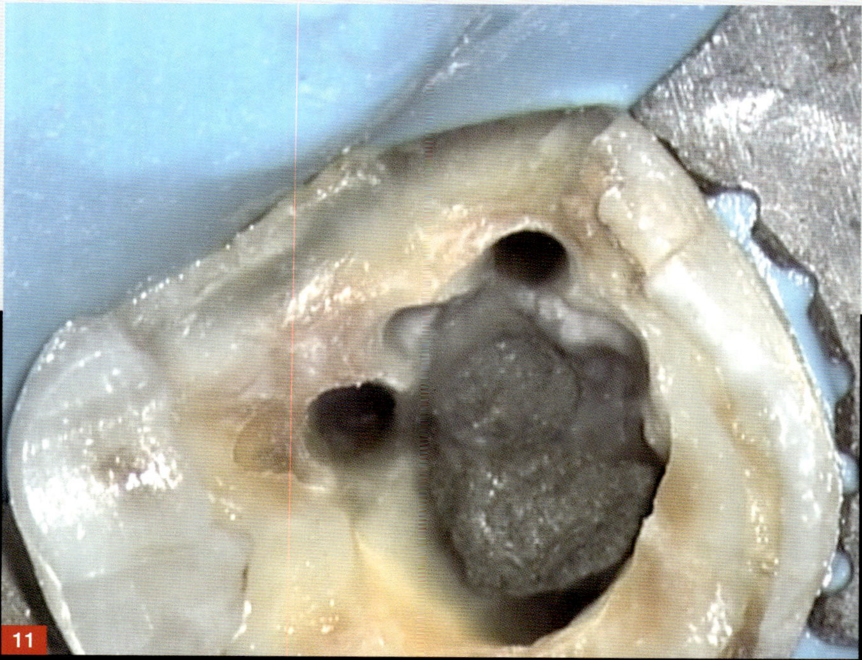

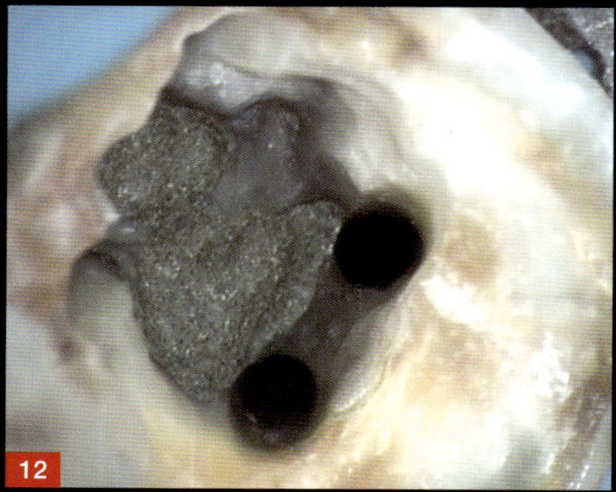

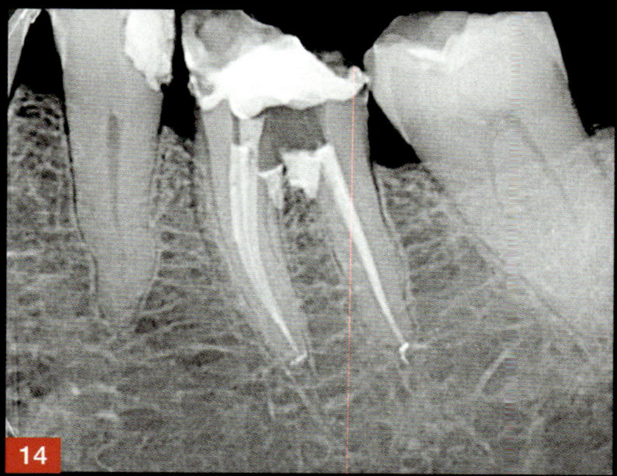

Figure 10: The irrigation system confirms the confluence of the two mesial channels.

Figure 11: The two distal channels were prepared and the distal perforation was sealed with grey MTA.

Figure 12: The two mesial channels were prepared and the mesial perforation was sealed with grey MTA.

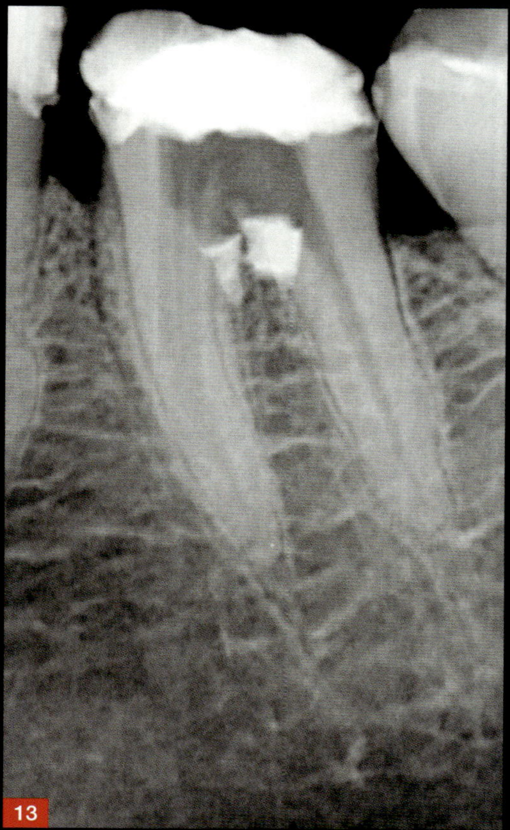

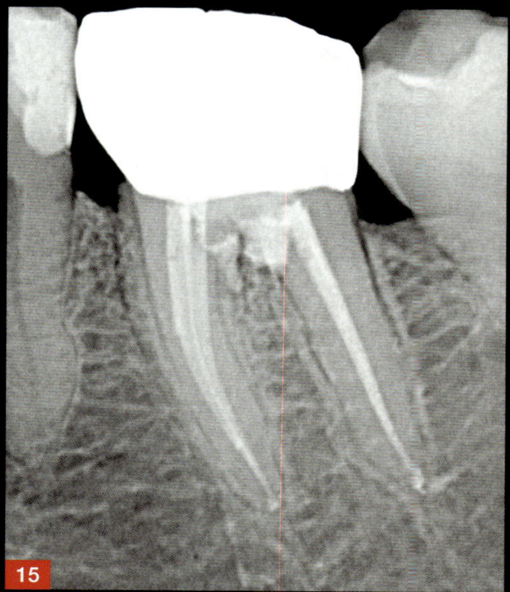

Figure 13: X-ray to check the position of the MTA.

Figure 14: Postoperative x-ray.

Figure 15: X-ray after 12 months.

properties, being biocompatible and non-toxic[33-40]. Several case studies and retrospective clinical studies reported healing rates above 80% using MTA[41, 42].
Pontius et al.[40], in a retrospective study that examined the healing rates of 70 treated perforations performed by six endodontic specialists, reported a success rate of 90%, which, they highlighted, was higher than that reported in other studies[41, 42].
At present, MTA is the most widely used material.

Perforation repair technique

Before describing the different steps for repairing a perforation using orthograde endodontic techniques, we must point out that different therapeutic options are available for perforations whose site is close to the clinical crown.
Such therapeutic options include:

- exposure of iatrogenic damage (or root defect) by resective periodontal surgery;
- orthodontic extrusion of the tooth;
- forced eruption.

The latter two alternatives to crown lengthening prevent aesthetic changes and limit the reduction of bone support in adjacent teeth[14]. These therapeutic solutions aim at positioning the perforation site above the bone crest, simplifying reparative and/or reconstructive maneuvers.

As far as the purely endodontic techniques of perforation repair are concerned, making some preliminary considerations is advisable.
The perforation requires an adequate seal to allow the healing of the supporting tissues of the tooth; the timing must be rapid and, as we will see, it will be prior to or will follow the endodontic treatment, if this is necessary. In the first instance, it is important to follow a decisional algorithm based on certain parameters that must be considered carefully when a perforation is suspected or observed, such as:

- the presence of pathological periodontal probing, i.e., more than 5 mm, in the case of suspicion, a priori, of a perforation;
- the position of the perforation: perforations of the apical or middle third of the root have a worse prognosis than those positioned at the level of the floor of the pulp chamber of the pluriradicular teeth because they are more complex to treat. If periodontal probing is found when there are perforations of the pulp chamber, then the prognosis is worse;
- size and shape: to be easily sealed, perforations must have a roundish shape and be retentive. Therefore, it is necessary to have a minimum dentinal thickness that favors the stabilization of the material;
- time: swift action is recommended, perforations should be repaired promptly, as an unrepaired perforation could result in periodontal damage over time.

Data obtained from this preliminary analysis will lead to the formulation of a prognosis, which, as seen in different studies, will be linked to the values of the individual problems, the probing data being an element of cardinal importance for the success of the treatment. Certain operating conditions are necessary for carrying out the repair of the perforations effectively.
These are:

- adequate magnification (surgical microscope) and lighting;
- the use of a material that is stable, biocompatible, and radiopaque (to facilitate radiographic control).

International literature has established that the materials of choice for filling perforations are eugenol zinc oxide cement reinforced with ethoxybenzoic acid (SuperEBA, Bosworth Co, Skokie, Illinois), MTA (Dentsply Tulsa Dental, Tulsa, Oklahoma), and all calcium silicate-based cements. In particular situations, composites associated with adhesive systems can also be used[44-47]. The choice of the most suitable material is dictated by the following clinical elements:

- position of the perforation;
- size of perforation;
- humidity control;
- control of bleeding[47].

Perforation repair procedures

As seen above, the location, shape, and size of the perforations involve different clinical approaches. Some types of clinical procedures related to different types of perforations are described below.

Repairing extraradicular lesions within the gingival groove

When the perforation does not involve the bone component and the periodontal supracrestal tissues (connective and epithelial attachment), it can be repaired with adhesive composites without changing the protocol that is normally followed from a restorative point of view. Once the perforation is closed, endodontic retreatment will begin (Fig. 7.12).

Repairing root perforations whose outlet hole is within the supracrestal tissues

When the perforation does not involve the bone component and is found in the area of periodontal supracrestal tissues (connective tissue attachment and epithelial attachment), it may be necessary to sculpt an intrasulcular flap in order to expose the lesion and be able to isolate by means of a rubber dam.
Also, in these cases it is possible to repair the perforation by using adhesive composites without changing the protocol that is normally followed from a restorative point of view. Once the perforation is closed, an endodontic retreatment can be carried out. Once the endodontic-restorative therapies have been completed, the dam can be removed and the stitches necessary to close the flap can be positioned[49].

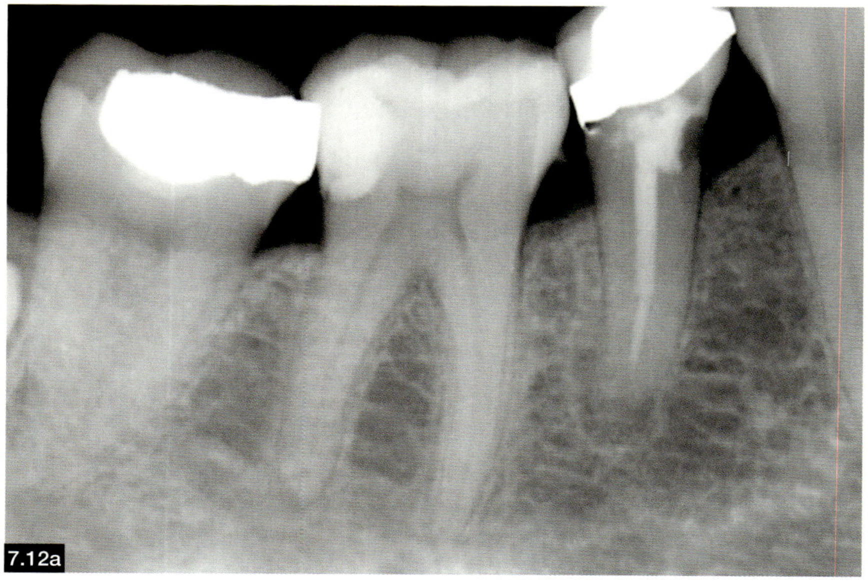
7.12a

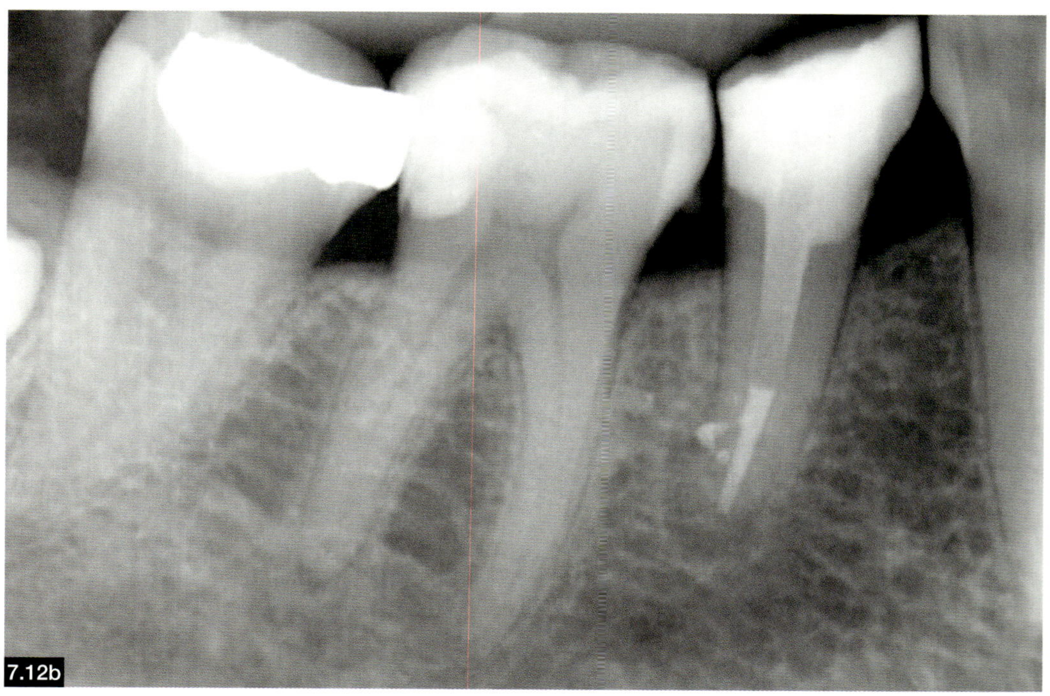
7.12b

Fig 7.12a–b: a) A perforation, clearly above the bone crest, is repaired with composite material and allows endodontic review of the previous treatment (b).

Repairing root perforations whose outlet hole is found in the area of the bone compartment

Depending on where the route, which is often oblique, starts in the intraosseous root path, we can distinguish between perforations of the coronal, middle, or apical third.

1. **Coronal third of the root**. When a perforation is found here, in monoradicular teeth, bone resection surgery or orthodontic extrusion associated or not with clinical crown lengthening can be considered as treatment options; but these will not

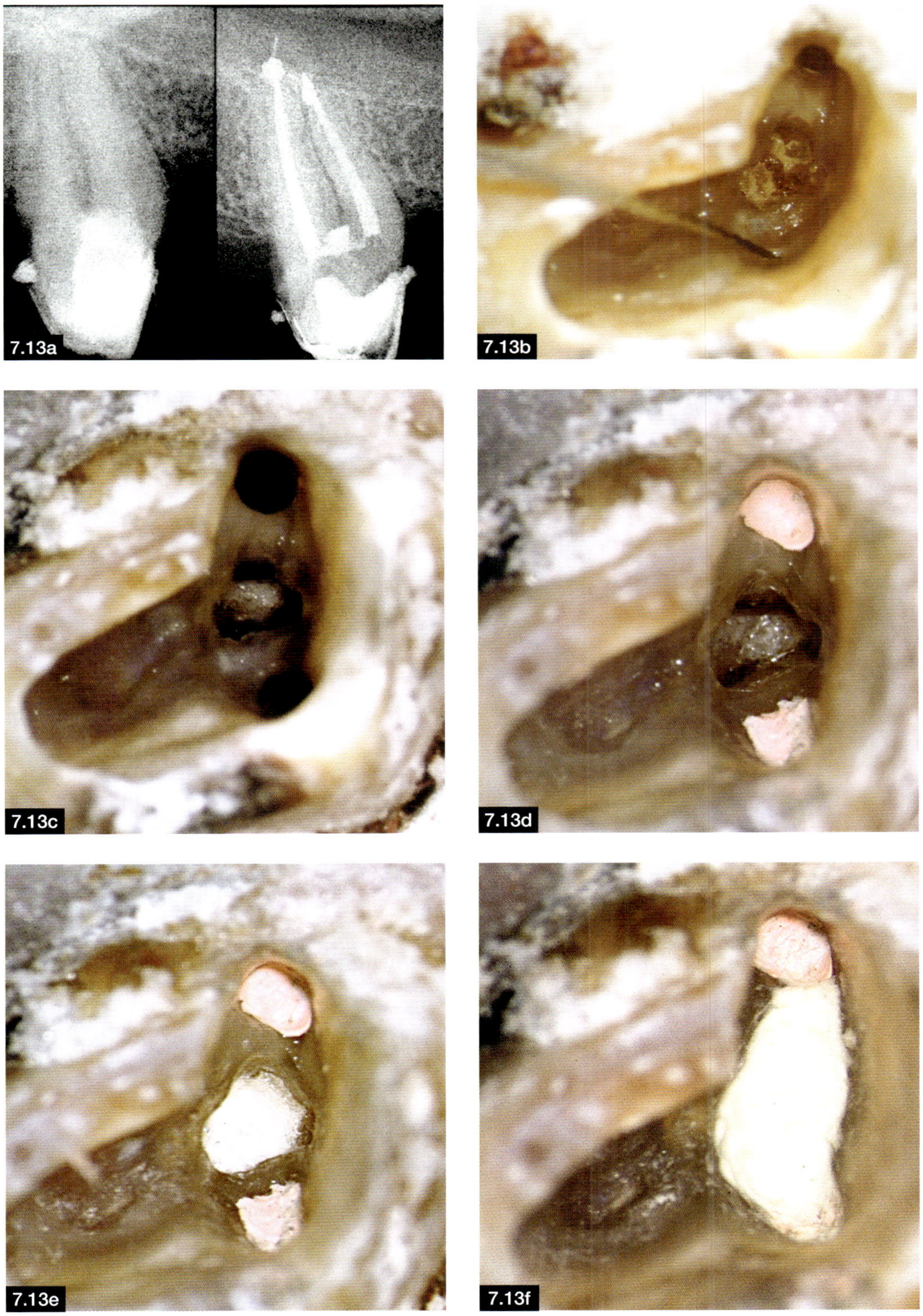

Fig 7.13a–f: a) Radiographic examination before and after the repair of the perforation; in cases such as these, the difficulty in finding the canal inlets leads to the creation of the perforations (b). The preparation of the same (c–d), once the root canals are localized, instrumented, and sealed, allows the placement of a resorbable barrier (e) and the plugging of the perforation (f).

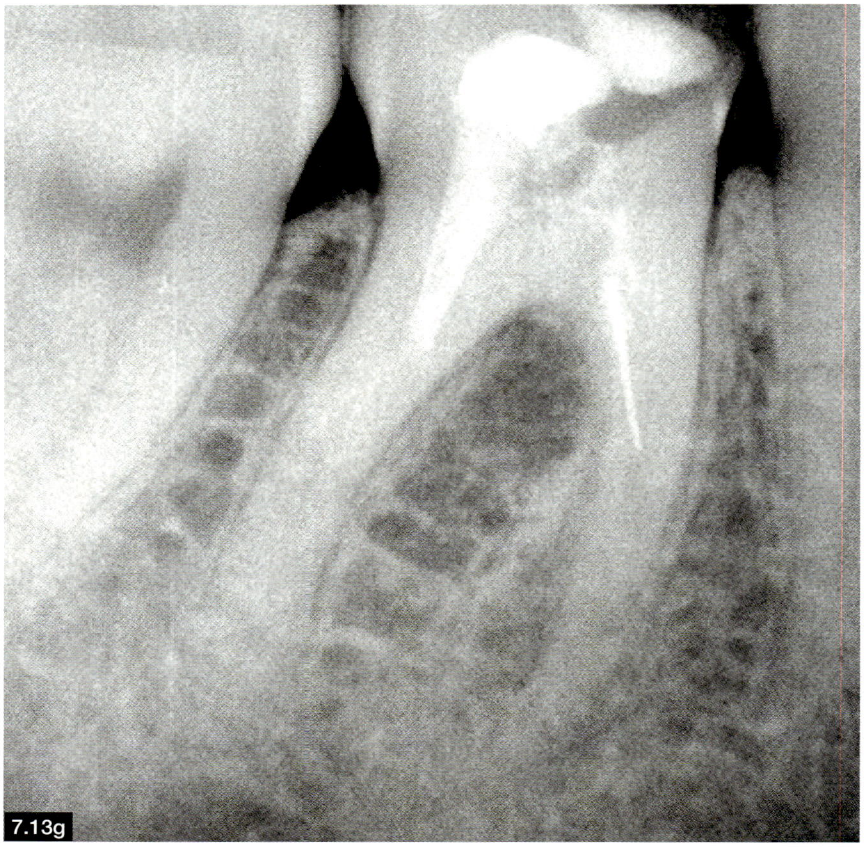

Fig 7.13g–i: A similar case, complicated by the presence of a fractured instrument (g), reveals a particular anatomy of the lower molar (h). The follow-up after 5 years (i).

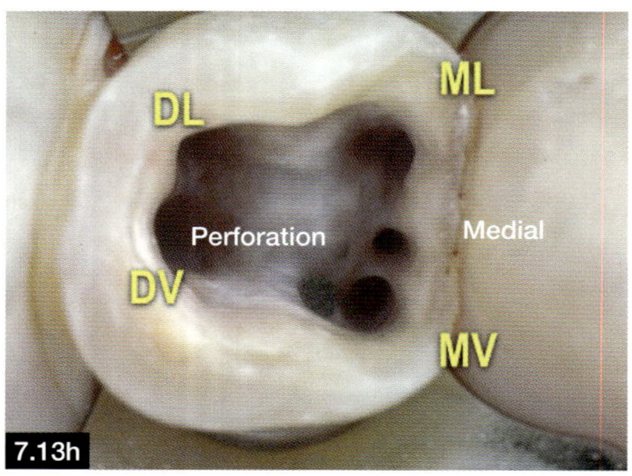

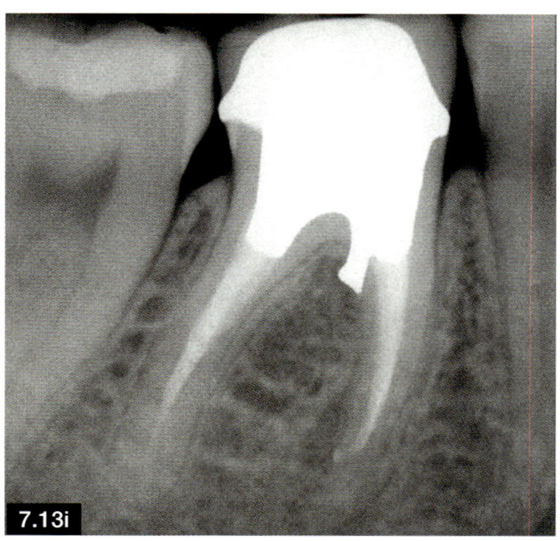

be examined in this text. If this iatrogenic lesion is found at the level of the pulp chamber floor, then it is advisable to opt for a purely endodontic treatment.
The repairment will be that typical of the so-called wall lesions, described in Figure 7.13a-f.

2. **Middle third of the root**. In cases where the perforation is in the middle of the root canal, orthograde lesion repair is recommended, and the methods of preparation for one-wall defects should be applied.
3. **Apical third of the root**. In these situations, it is always advisable to seal the perforation by retrograde means, perhaps after correctly closing the entire root canal.

Depending on the **morphology** that characterizes the perforation, we can distinguish two major types, namely:

1. four-wall perforation;
2. one-wall perforation.

Repair of four-wall perforations

If the perforation found or previously diagnosed is on the floor of the pulp chamber of a pluriradicular tooth, or at the entrance of the canal wall, then the iatrogenic communication between endodontium and periodontium will often be well bounded and defined in the contours, hence the name of circular perforation or "four-wall perforation."
In these cases, it is possible to choose whether to proceed with retreatment and then seal the perforation or vice versa. The criteria for choosing the order, with which to deal with the perforation are related to the absence of moisture. Once the granulation tissue, which may have invaded the perforated area, has been completely removed, decontamination is carried out; the area is then cleaned, disinfected, and dried. If the morphology of the perforation is not retentive, then it is possible to prepare the area with an ultrasonic tip or with a small multiblade bur.

▶ continue to page 398

Complex retreatment on upper molar with double perforation

CASE REPORT 2

Careful reading of the radiograms should lead to the diagnosis of perforation before starting treatment, where possible. In the case described in these images, once again, the presence of chamber calcifications has made it difficult to identify the canal openings and has led to the creation of two pseudo-channels that have been filled with gutta-percha.

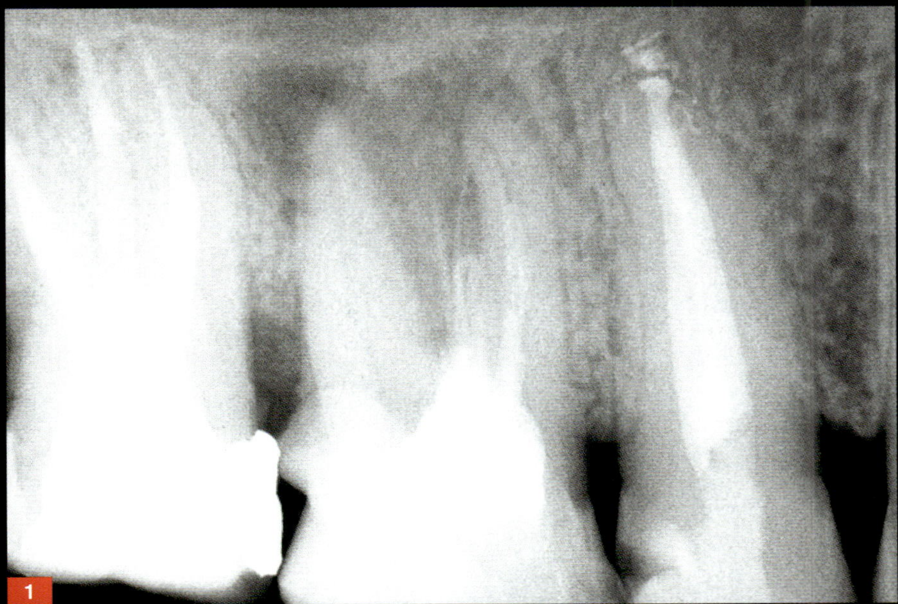

Figure 1: The radiographic image shows an incongruous treatment with clear contamination in the furcation of the root that leads to suspicion of perforation.

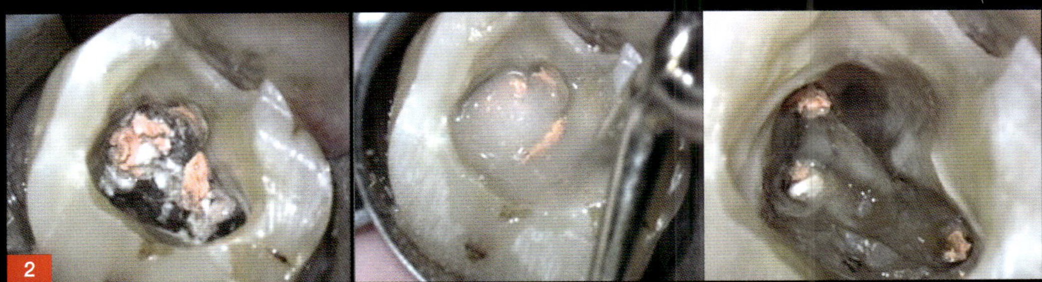

Figure 2: The appearance of the chamber: often in these cases the appearance of the pulp chamber alone should arouse the diagnostic doubt.

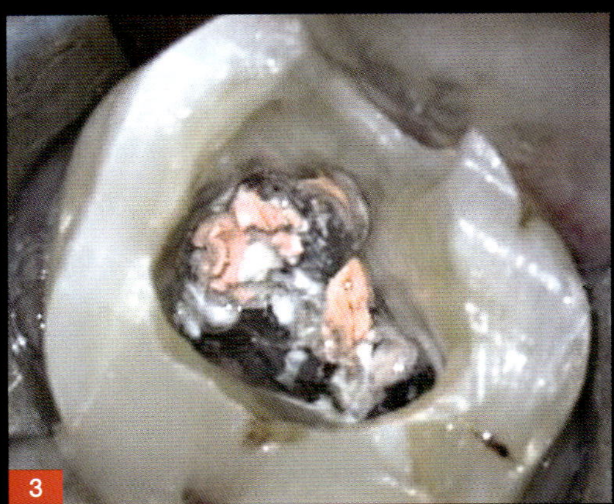

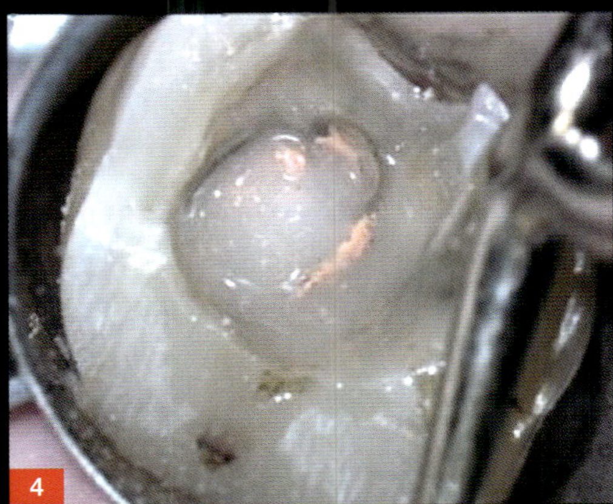

Figure 3: The contents of the chamber pulp at higher magnification.

Figure 4: The use of irrigators, disinfectants and solvents makes the material easier to remove.

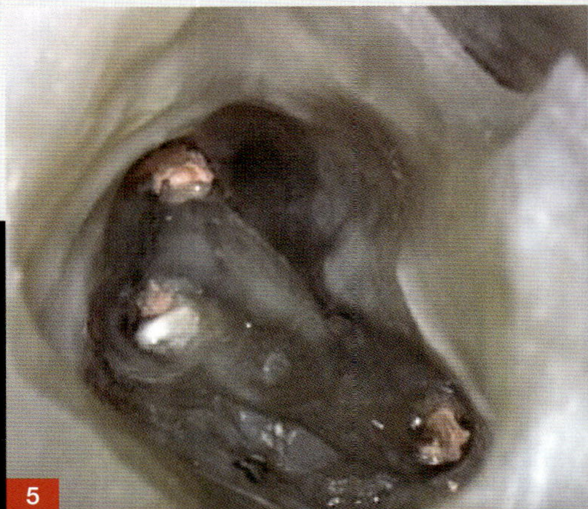

Figure 5: Once the excess material has been removed, three areas are clearly visible with relative cones of gutta-percha that seem to represent the openings of the root

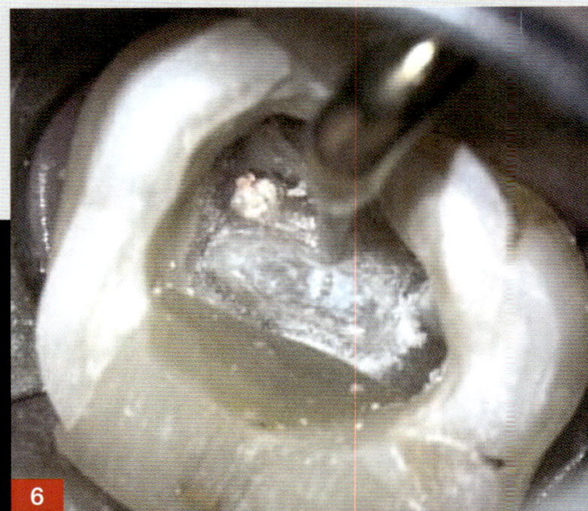

Figure 6: A closer look reveals that a dentinal roof hides the real anatomy of the root canals.

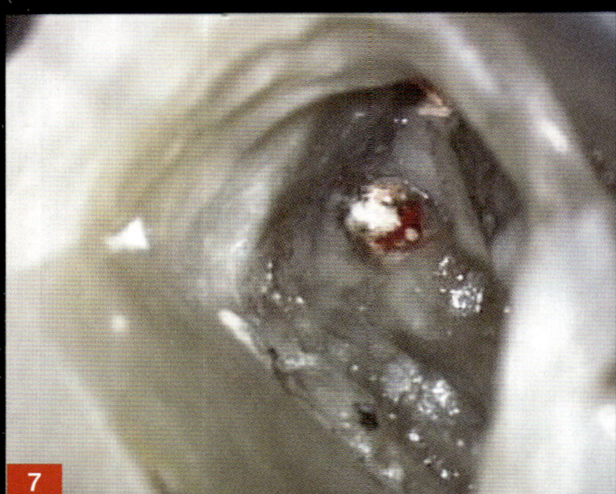

Figure 7: It becomes clear that the true canal anatomy is quite different and the "presumed" openings are nothing more than perforations of the floor.

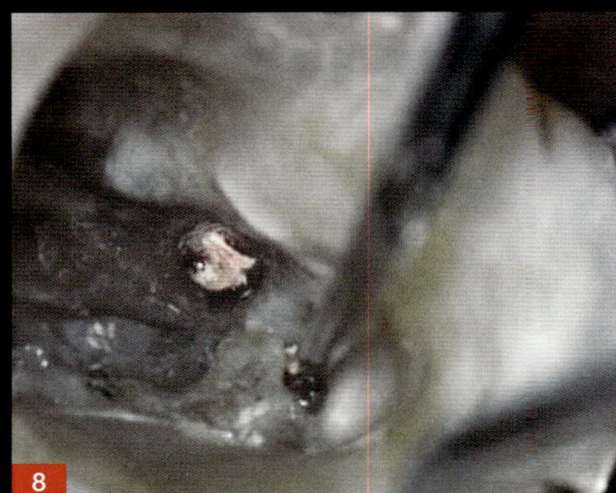

Figure 8: The vestibular perforation at higher magnification.

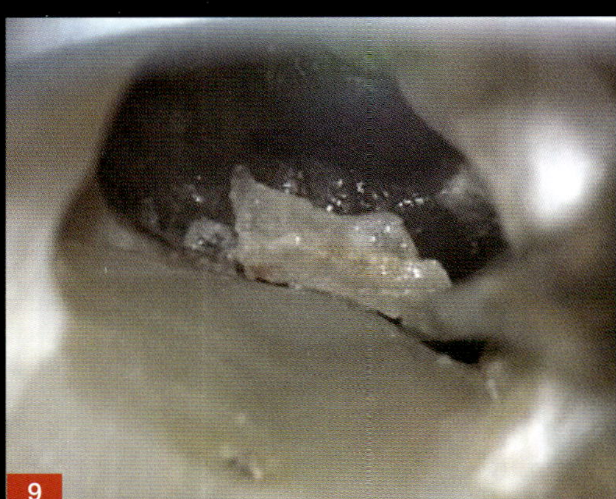

Figure 9: The perforation in the palatine area where the outermost canal of the pulp chamber is located.

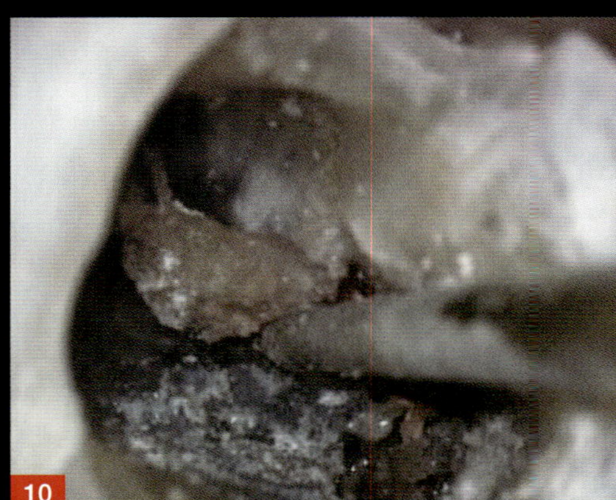

Figure 10: Further use of the dedicated ultrasonic tips makes it possible to remove a consistent block of intrapulpal dentin (pulpal calculus) that obstructs the real canal openings.

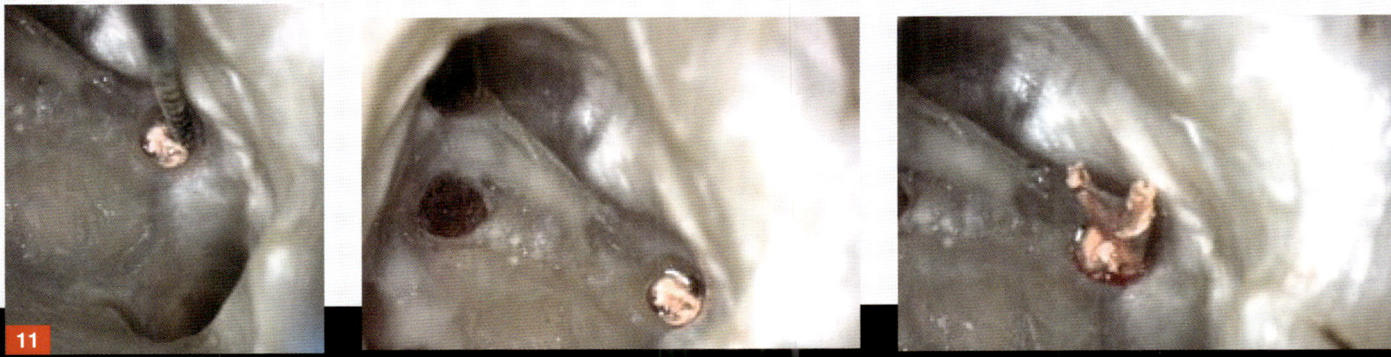

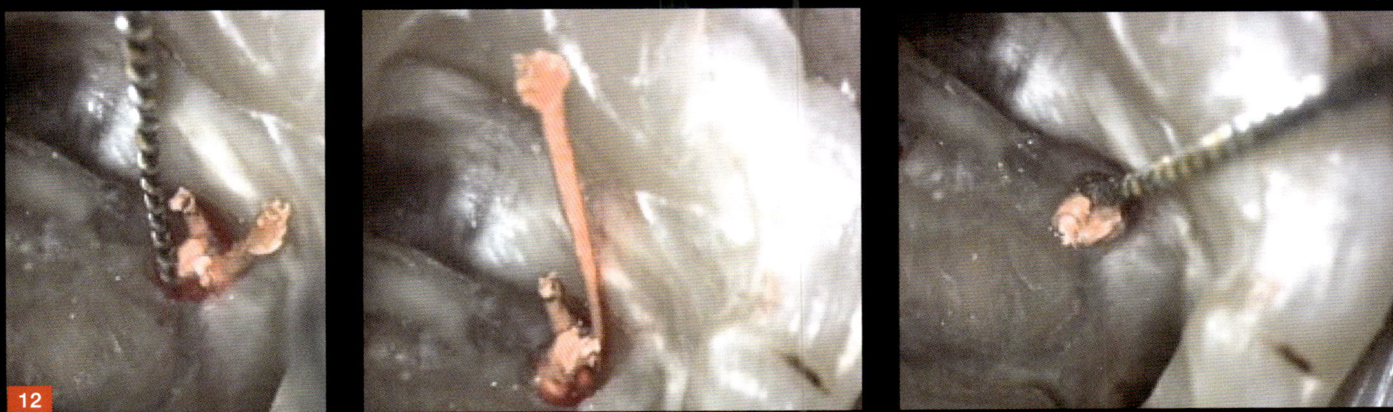

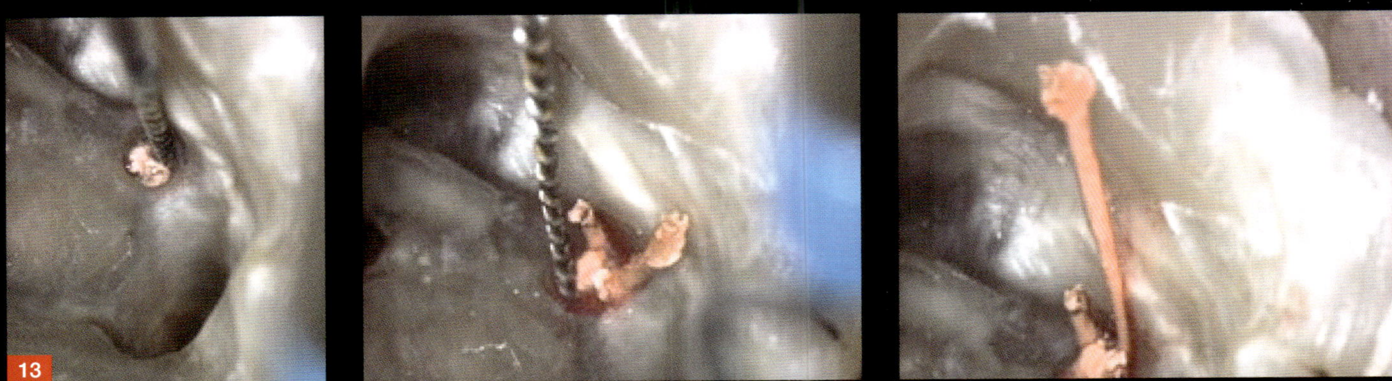

Figure 11-12: The sequence of removal of the compacted material inside the perforation.

Figure 13: The cones are gradually removed.

Figure 14: The palatine perforation is probed; it clearly has a circular appearance, which will lead to a preparation of the walls (four-wall perforation) to make it pluggable in a manner congruous with MTA.

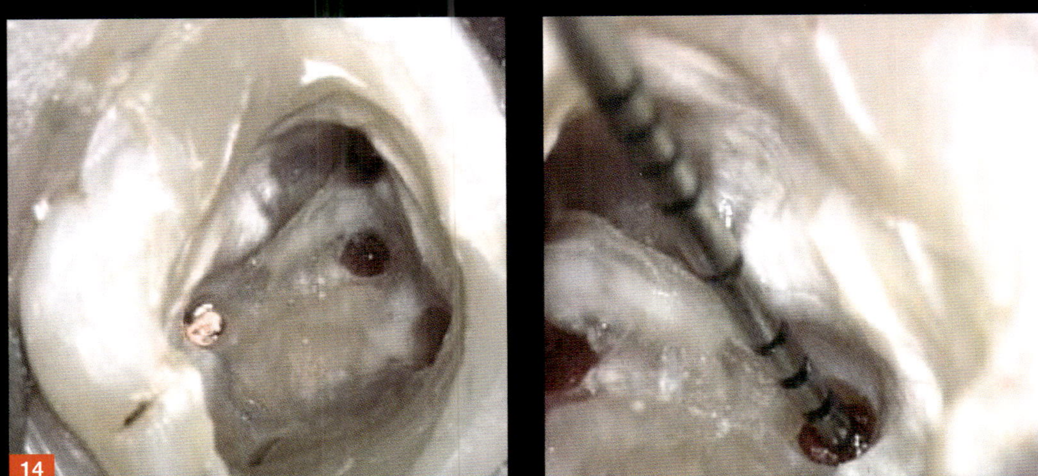

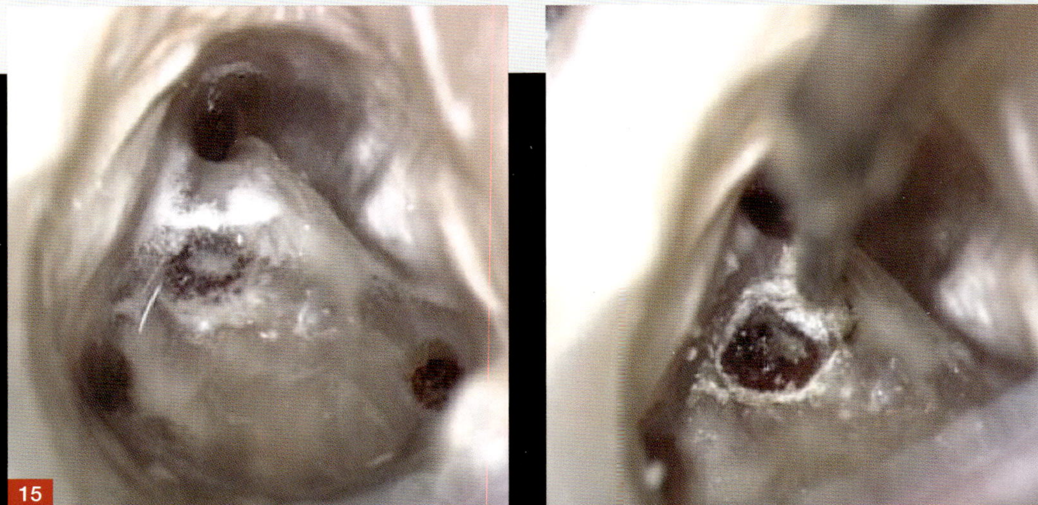

Figure 15: A preparation phase with dedicated ultrasonic tips.

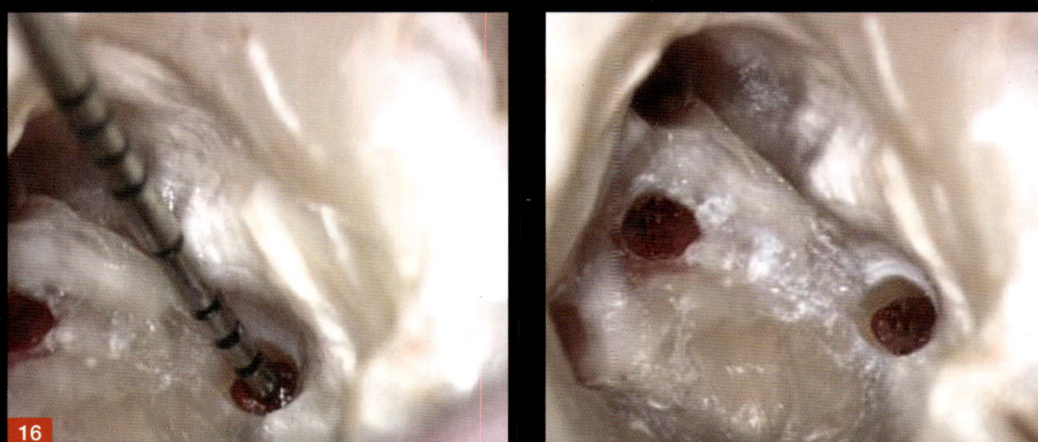

Figure 16: The two perforations are now clearly visible and can accommodate the right material.

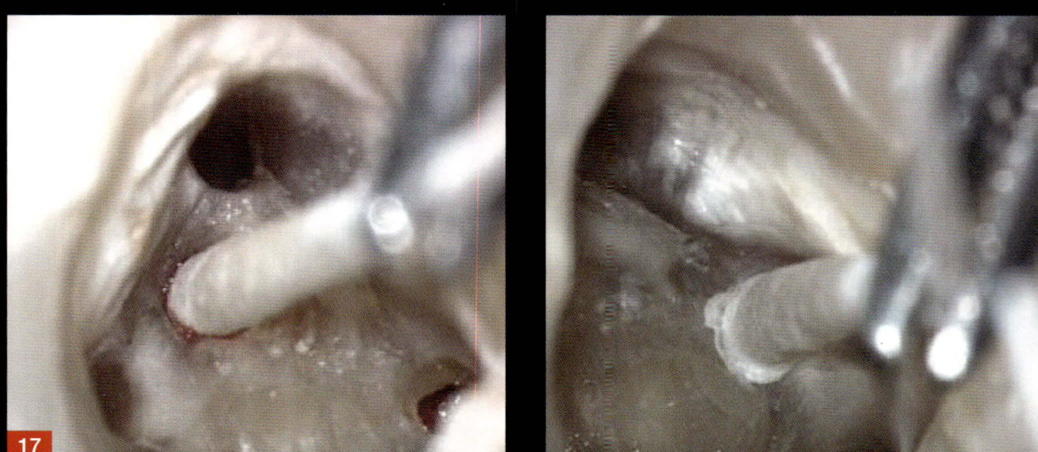

Figure 17: The drying process is very important for preventing the MTA material from dissolving.

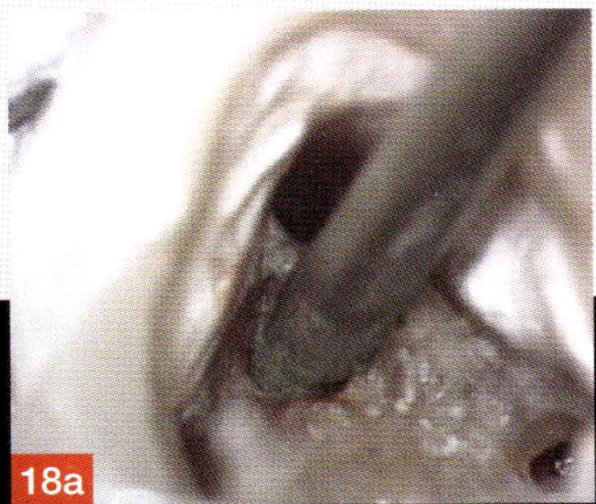

18a

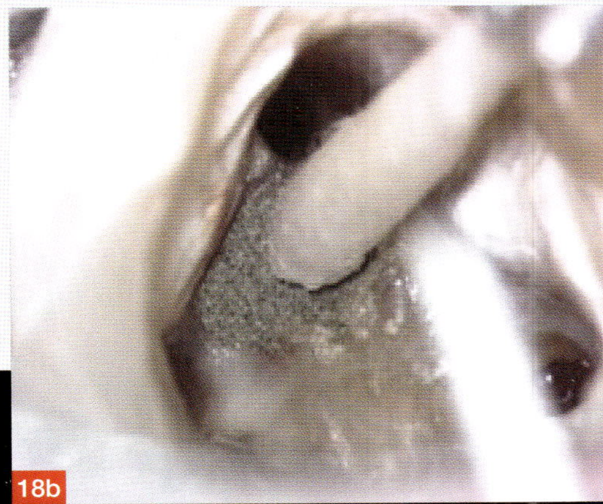

18b

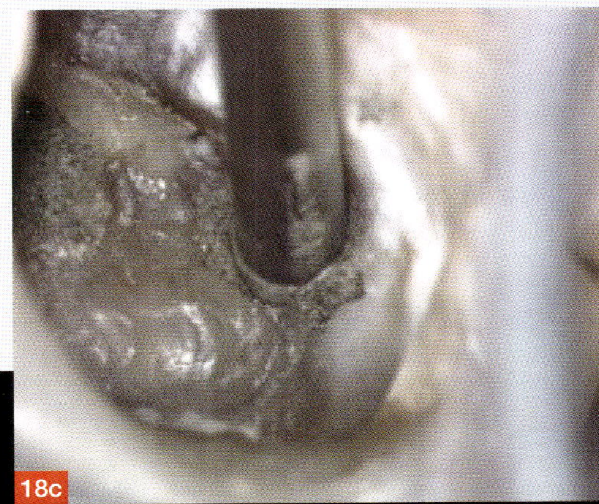

18c

Figure 18a-c: The MTA is inserted in small increments and compacted with a wet paper cone.

Figure 19: The two perforations are sealed, the channels must be instrumented.

Figure 20: The x-ray certifies the quality of the seal.

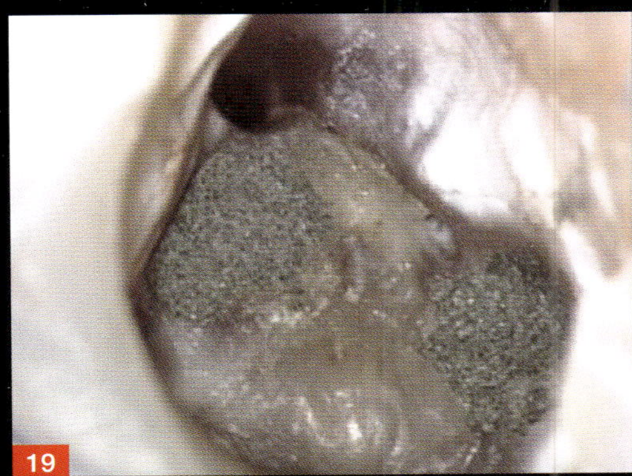

19

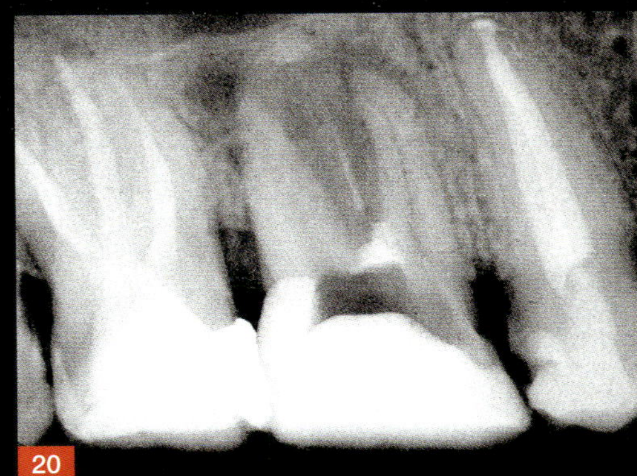

20

Figure 21: The mesial root reveals a particularly complex anatomy with several canals inside the root.

Figure 22: The appearance of the mesial canals is absolutely peculiar but not infrequent: in this case there are three openings, two of which are confluent.

Figure 23: The treatment almost one year after the end of the therapy, which certifies the success of the same.

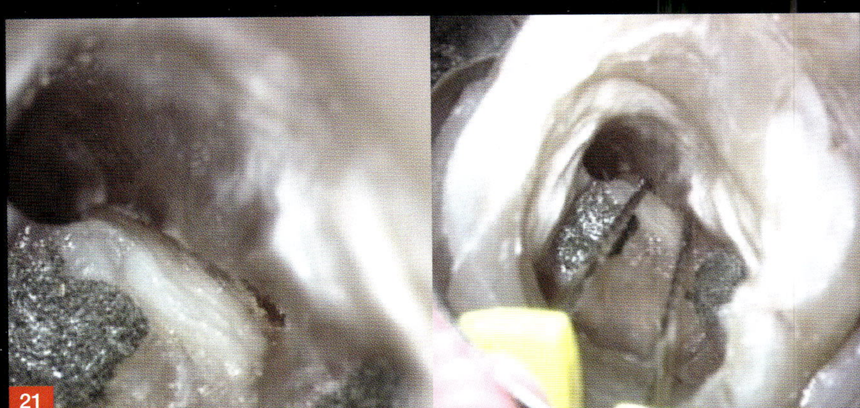

21

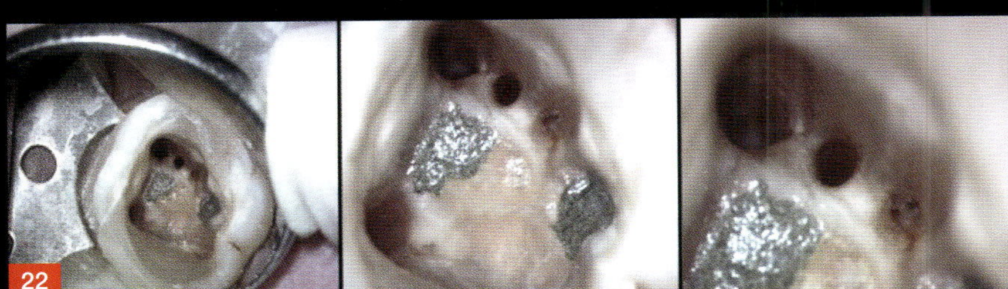

22

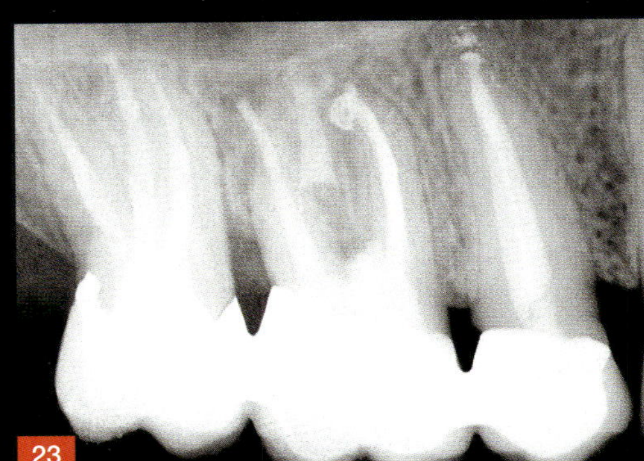

23

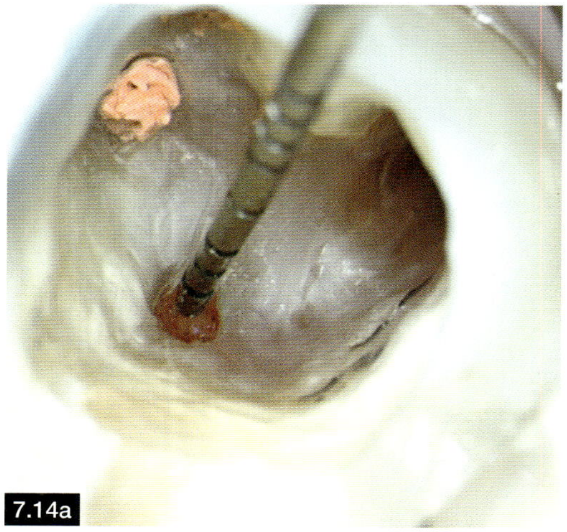

7.14a

Before proceeding with the filling, it is important to make sure good hemostasis has been established. To prevent the filling from being pushed into the periodontium, it is possible to place resorbable and biocompatible extraradicular matrices (e.g., fibrin sponges) in the defect (without these invading the walls of the perforation), after which the biocompatible cement can be compacted (Fig. 7.14a–e). To seal the perforation, MTA powder (ProRoot MTA, Dentsply Maillefer, Baillagues, Switzerland, gray and white) is used mixed with distilled water at a 3:1 ratio[50, 51]. Special tools are used to insert MTA into perforations; a sterile paper cone or cotton pellet, preferably moistened with saline solution, will improve compaction. To favor the setting of material, a damp cotton pellet is placed in the access cavity, and a temporary filling is carried out. After 48 hours, during which the material completes the setting process, the endodontic treatment can be carried out after verifying the quality of the seal obtained. MTA-like materials that set in about 20 minutes are now available. If significant bacterial contamination is found, the area can be medicated with calcium hydroxide for one week in order to eliminate the exudate before proceeding with the application of MTA[29] (Fig. 7.15a–c). The application inside the root canal, and not at the bottom of the pulp chamber, has also been defined as a "tunnel" technique (Fig. 7.16a-c).

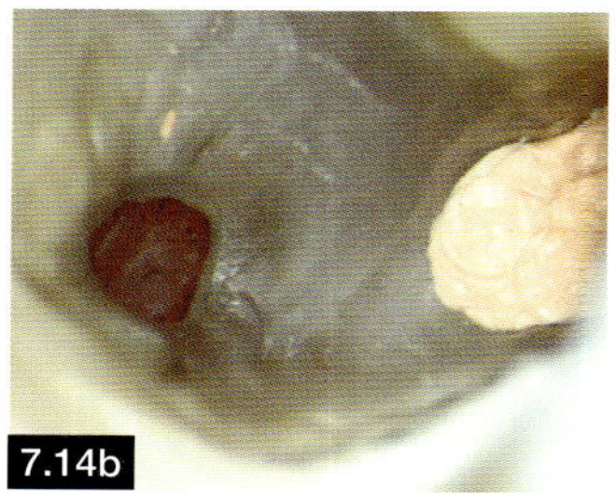

7.14b

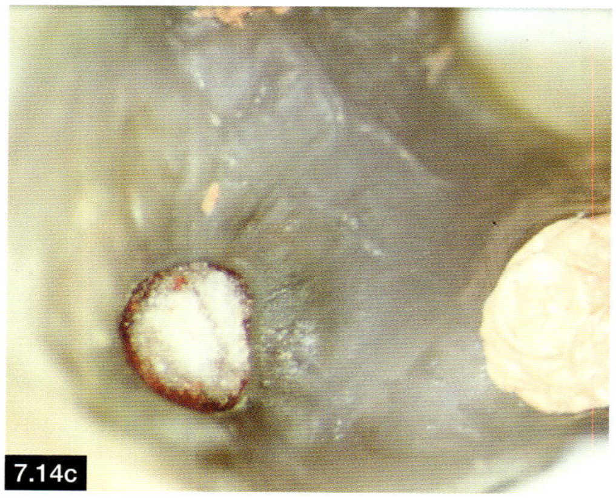

7.14c

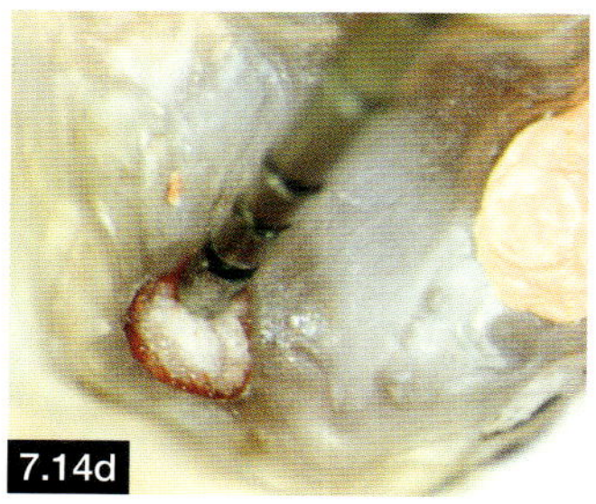

7.14d

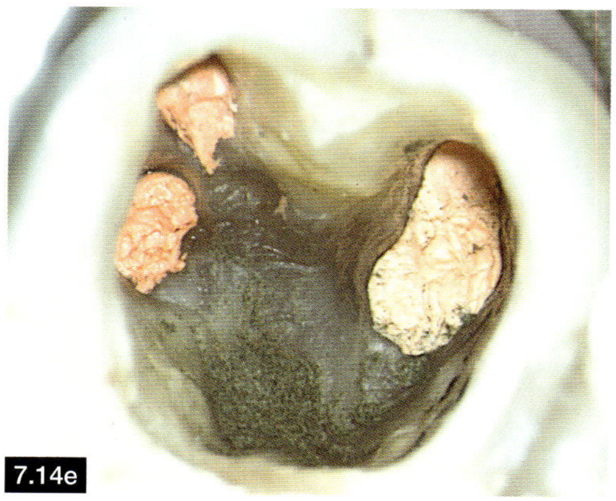

7.14e

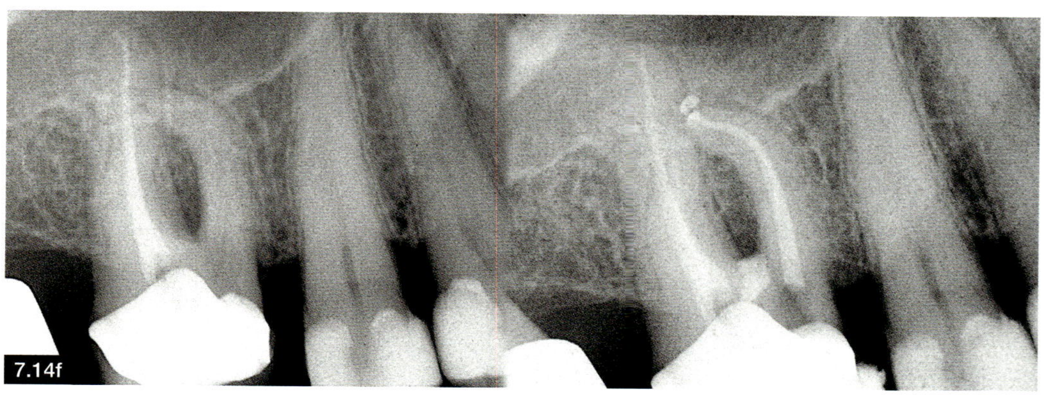

7.14f

Fig. 7.14a–f: The perforation of the floor of the pulp chamber (a) appears shallow (b) but not sufficiently retentive; a closure with gutta-percha is opted for after positioning the resorbable barrier (c-e). The follow-up x-rays (f) testify to the success of the solution.

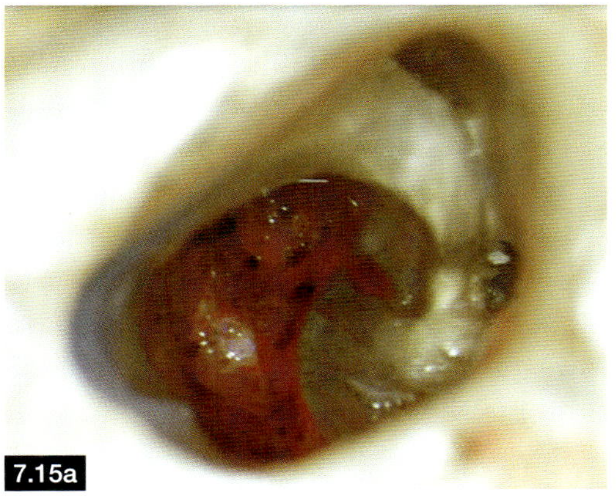
7.15a

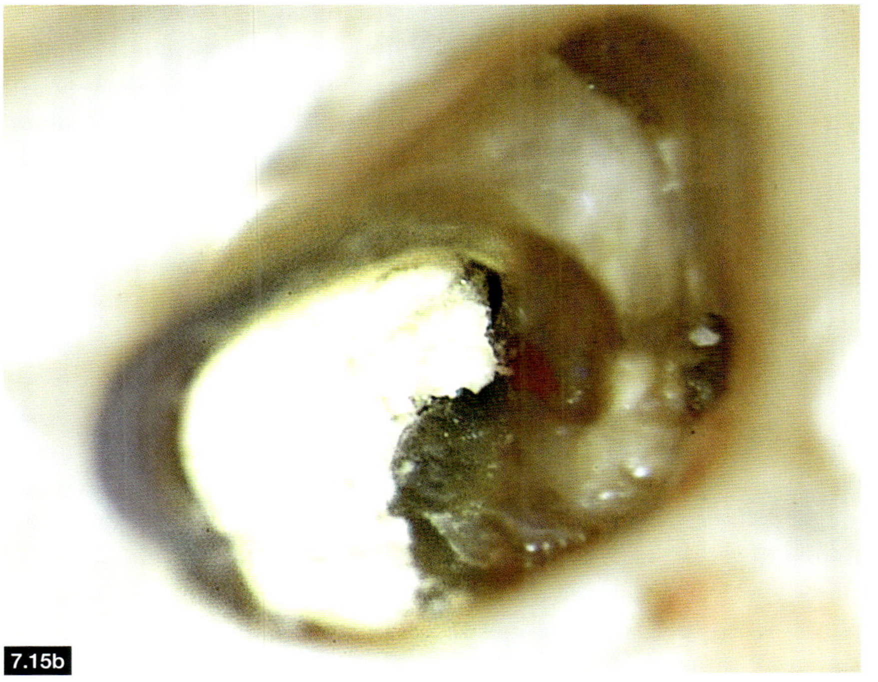
7.15b

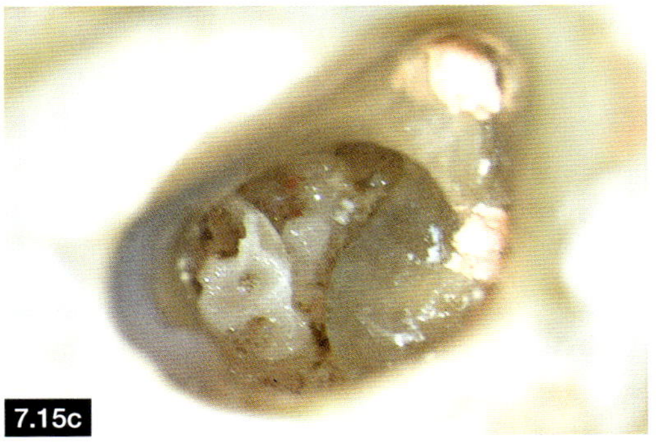
7.15c

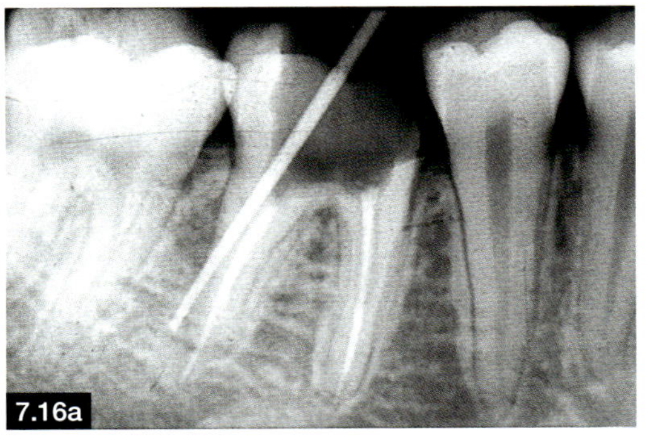
7.16a

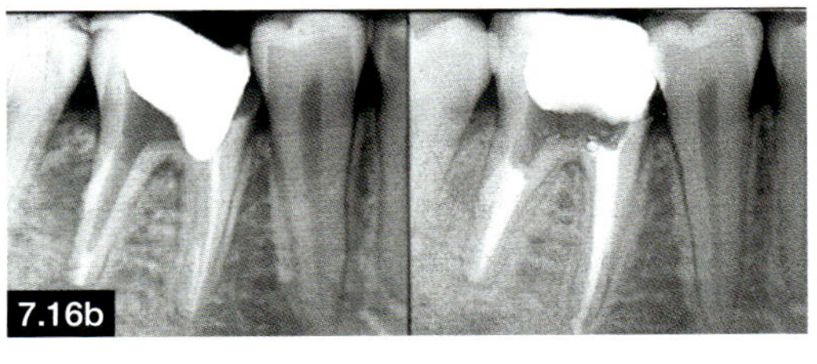
7.16b

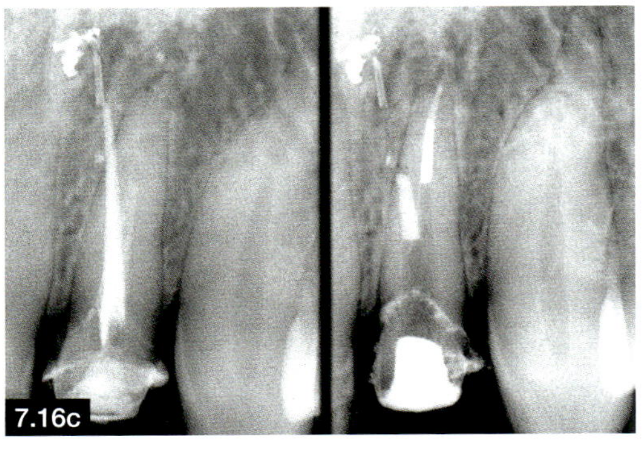
7.16c

Repair of one wall perforations

Single-wall perforations are also referred to as stripping. They can be found in the coronal, middle, or apical third of the root canal and are, in most cases, due to errors during the instrumentation phase or during the preparation of the root for housing root canal posts. They are the result of incorrect anatomical knowledge and incorrect calculation of the dentinal thicknesses present in some areas of the root canals, such as the distal part of the mesial roots of the lower and upper molars, or the medial areas of the upper premolars. When the perforation is located in the middle or coronal third, the clinician must evaluate the extent of the perforation and the contours of the same; the latter variable being a discriminating factor. If the contours are well defined, it is advisable to use the traditional technique, which is the tunnel technique (Fig. 7.17a-d). In cases where the contours are jagged and/or the dimensions do not allow a stable application of the filling material, it is advisable to use the so-called "sandwich" technique (Fig. 7.18a–b). The sandwich technique is, in any case, ideal for repairing perforations that have a corono-apical or vestibulo-lingual (palatal)

Fig. 7.15a–c: A large perforation is difficult to dry in the first instance (a); an intermediate dressing with calcium hydroxide powder (b) is necessary, which will produce a perfectly pluggable environment (c) after a few days.

Fig 7.16a–c: a) Two cases of perforation that can be repaired with the tunnel technique. The distal root of a lower molar has a false path at the middle third; b) repair carried out before the canal is closed may, depending on the clinical requirements, be postponed until the apical third is treated; (c) in order to avoid contamination of the material used to fill the perforation.

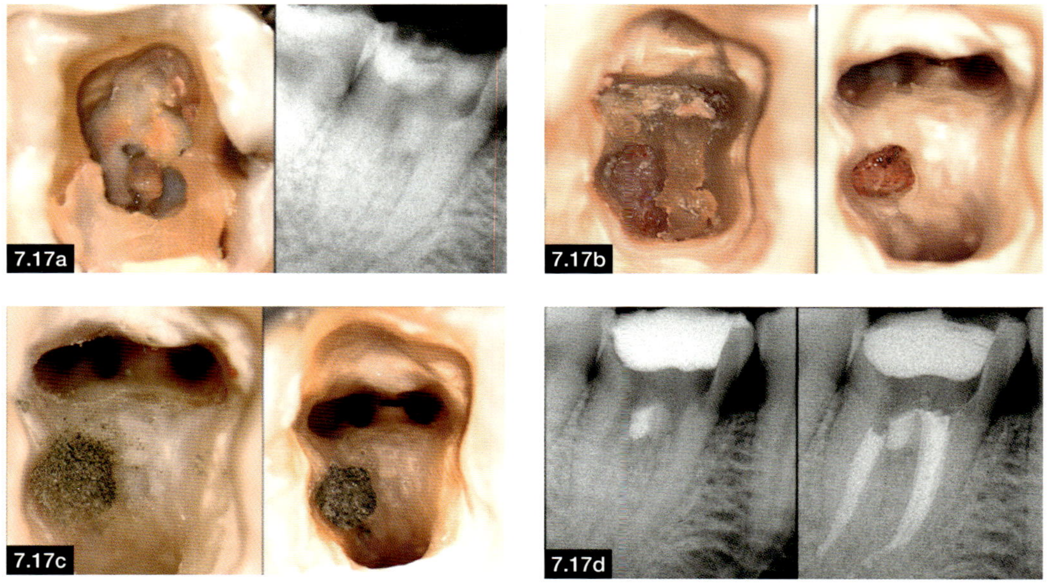

Fig. 7.17a–d: a) A significant perforation of the floor is detected; b) the cavity is also cleaned of the significant pulp calcifications; c) the perforation is sealed before the root canals are closed (d) as the filling material can be checked, filling can be carried out without any problems.

extension of less than 2 mm; in these cases, the repair material does not have enough stability to be positioned correctly.
A method of affixing different filling materials is therefore used, hence the term "sandwich." The sequence involves treating and filling the apical canal portion and subsequently filling the remaining portion of the canal with MTA, with the most apical part having the role of containing the material.
In fact, if the perforation, or rather the stripping, given the jagged contours, is on the canal wall, it is impossible to consider sealing that area with MTA without the excess material partially clogging the canal lumen, thus preventing further passages in the main canal.
With this technique, the clinician should be very careful when filling the apical portion in order to avoid contaminating the perforated area of the canal[30].
When the perforation is found in the apical third, the clinician will have to decide between the possibility of retreating the tooth in an orthograde manner or repairing the perforation in a retrograde manner. There is no written rule; only experience and access to instruments, such as the surgical microscope, make such choices possible. Furthermore, examining endoparodontal lesions, whether determined by the close anatomical connections between the pulpal system and the supporting apparatus or by pathological or iatrogenic events, is a difficult task, because the solutions to these conditions do not seem unambiguous and are extensively debated even today. However, noted when highlighted in this chapter, the elements of diagnostic-prognostic evaluation and the knowledge of the means and materials suitable for treating them now make it realistic to contemplate the long-term, certain preservation of teeth that would otherwise be lost.

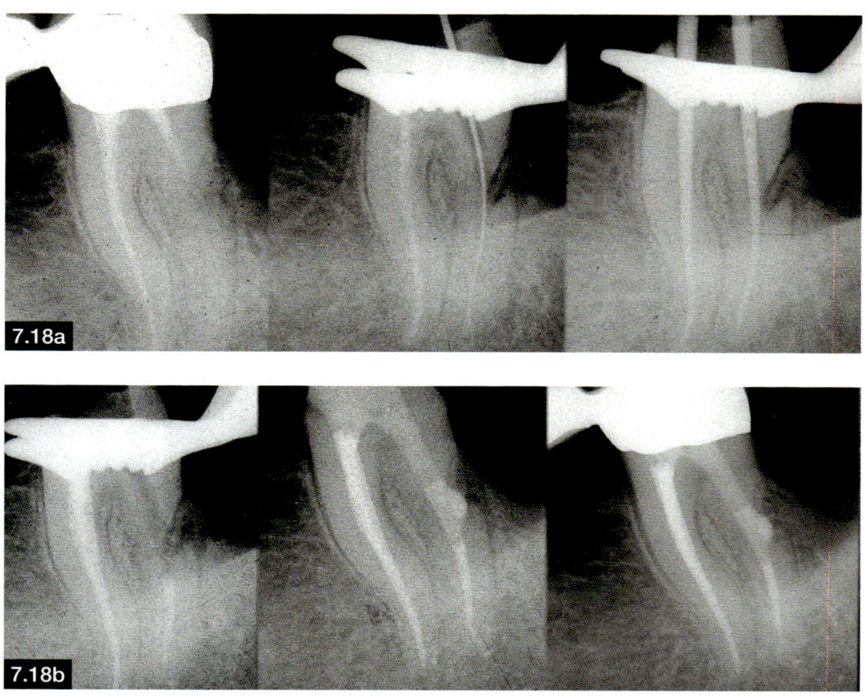

Fig. 7.18a–b: Sandwich technique. a) A perforation of middle third of the distal root is detected but not immediately sealed; b) once the root canals in the apical parts have been closed, the perforation is sealed.

Orthograde and retrograde intervention in apical perforation

CASE REPORT 3

Usually apical perforations must be solved retrospectively; in this case the presence of a fractured instrument in the apical third suggests a different approach. It was decided to close the perforation orthogonally, as the closure could be reviewed with retrograde treatment. The fractured instrument was removed by endodontic surgery. The case has been followed-up for 17 years.

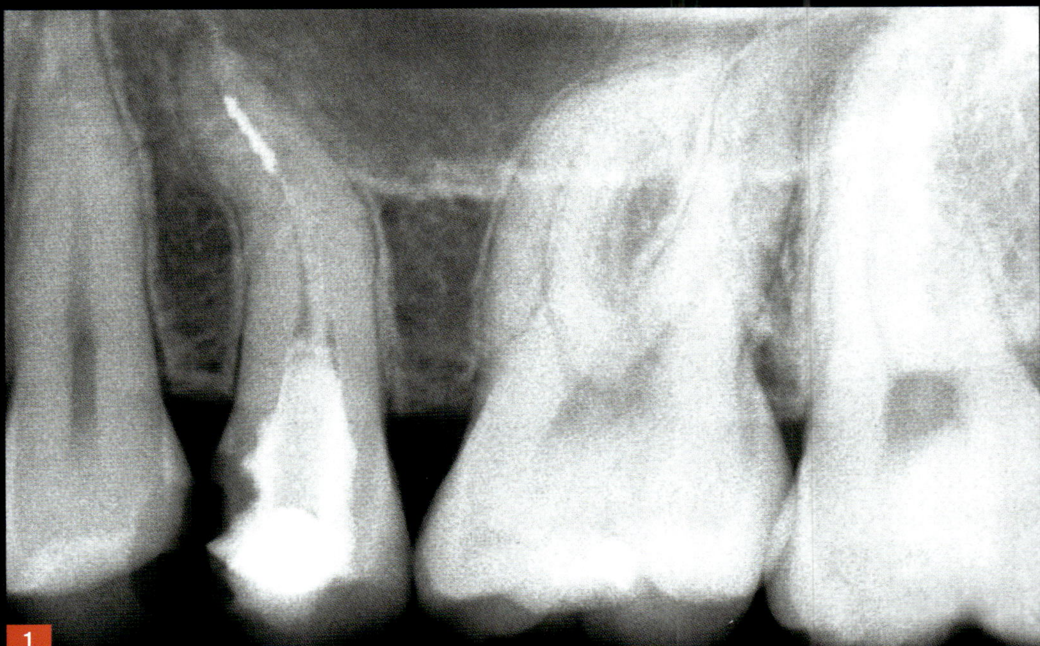

1

Figure 1: The described premolar is referred to the endodontist for observation for a broken instrument in the apical region; in these cases the approach is obviously surgical but the filling of the endodontic space is necessary.

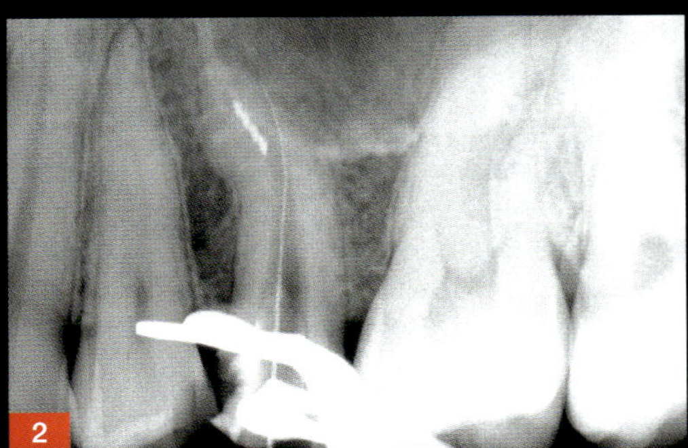

2

Figure 2: At canal probing a new exit is perceived, probably the result of a perforation created by instruments used in attempts to extract the tip of the endodontic instrument.

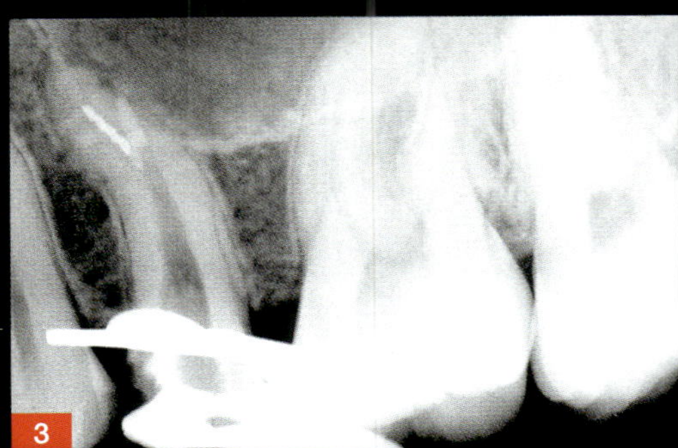

3

Figure 3: The perforation is shaped like a root canal and sealed with MTA using the "apical-plug" technique.

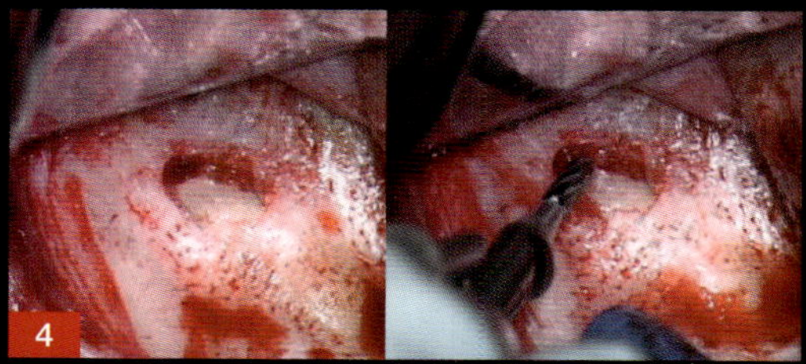

Figure 4: Surgical access is necessary to remove the instrument and to verify the quality of the orthograde seal made with MTA.

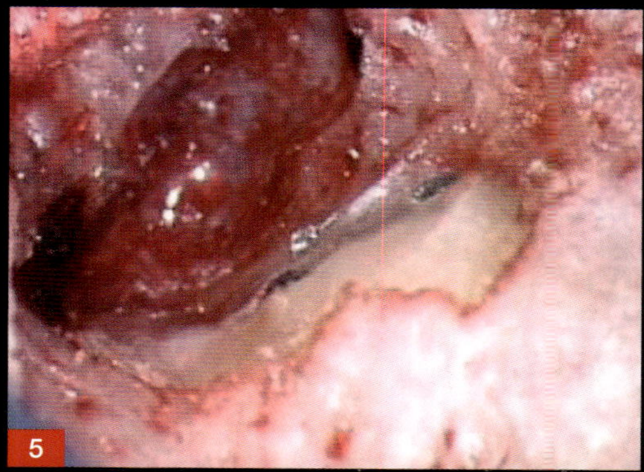

Figure 5: The apex is resected and isolated from the bone compartment.

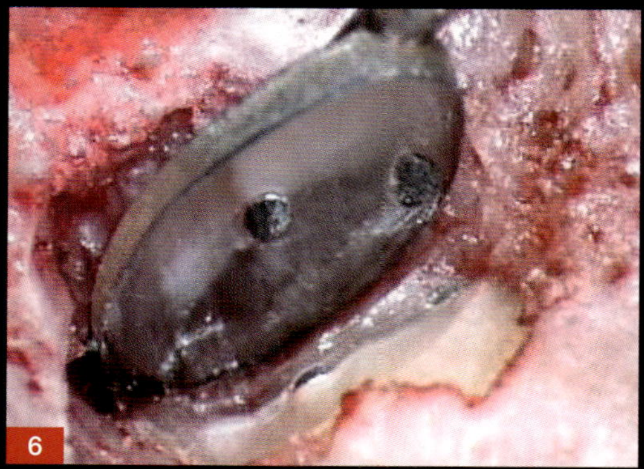

Figure 6: The fractured instrument (left) and the MTA plug are clearly visible in the mirror.

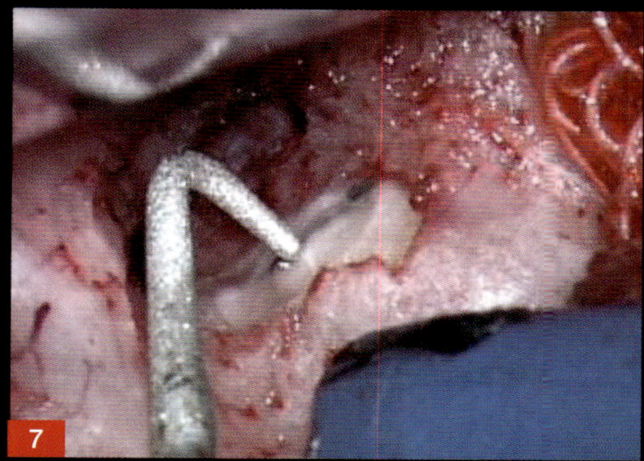

Figure 7: The instrument is removed using dedicated ultrasonic tips.

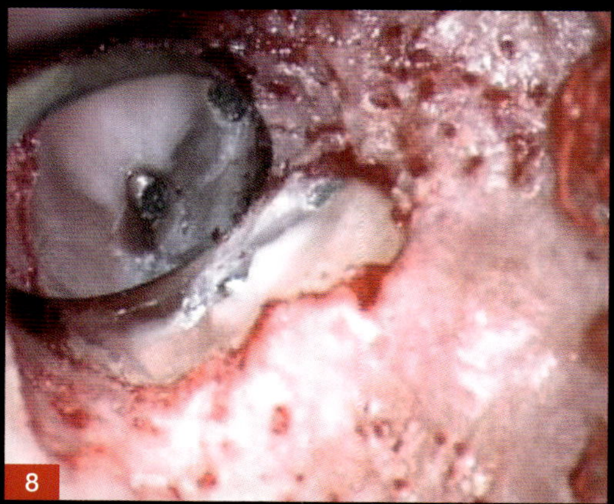

Figure 8: The instrument is isolated and ready to be removed.

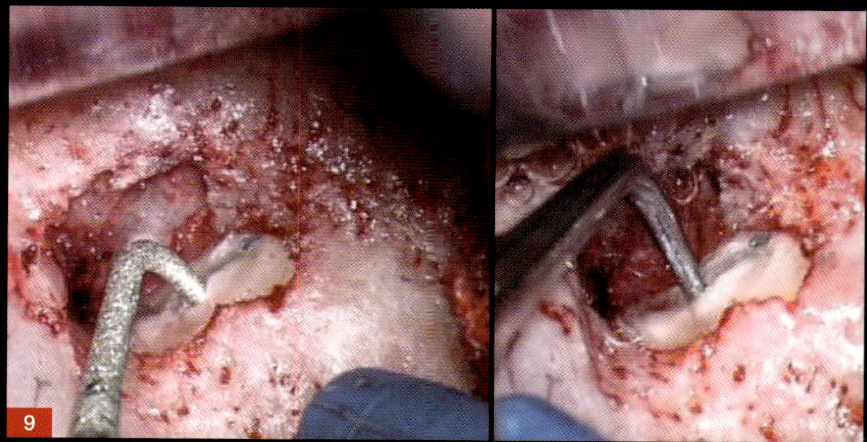

Figure 9: The retrograde cavity is finished to contain the same material used for the orthograde seal: MTA.

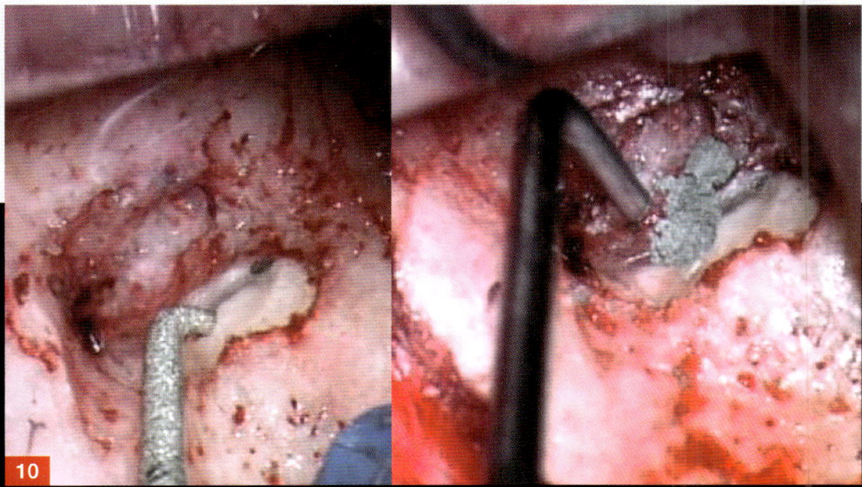

Figure 10: After further finishing, it is inserted and compacted into the retrograde cavity.

Figure 11: The double seal.

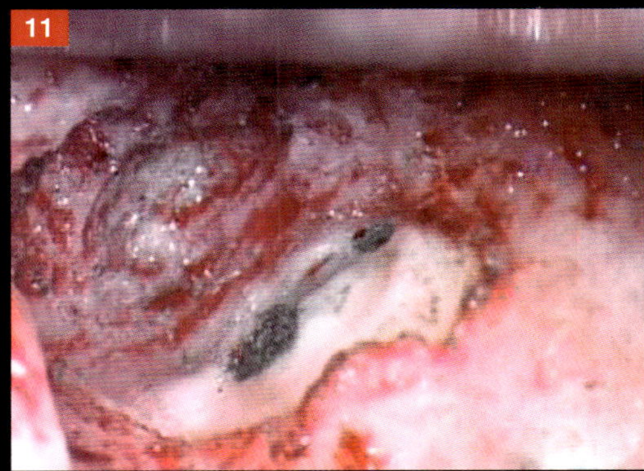

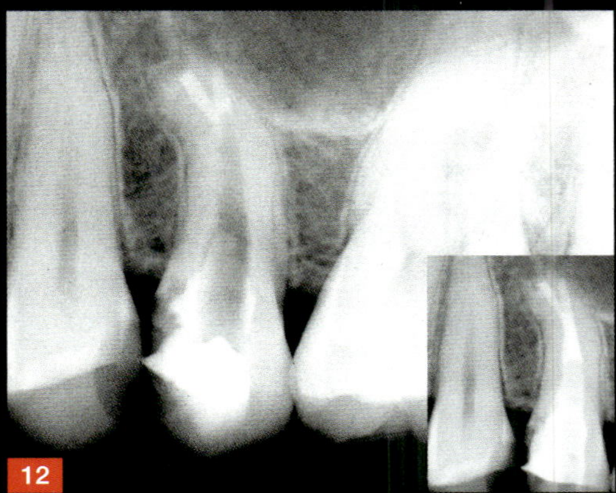

Figure 12: The emptied root canal with the double apical seal; all that remains is to fill the most coronal part of the canal.

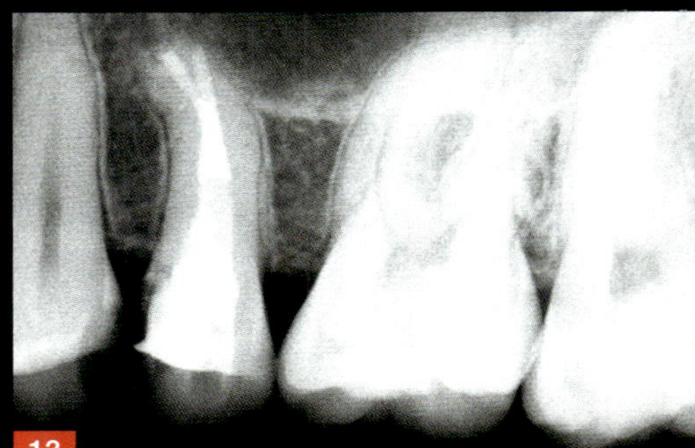

Figure 13: The treatment is complete.

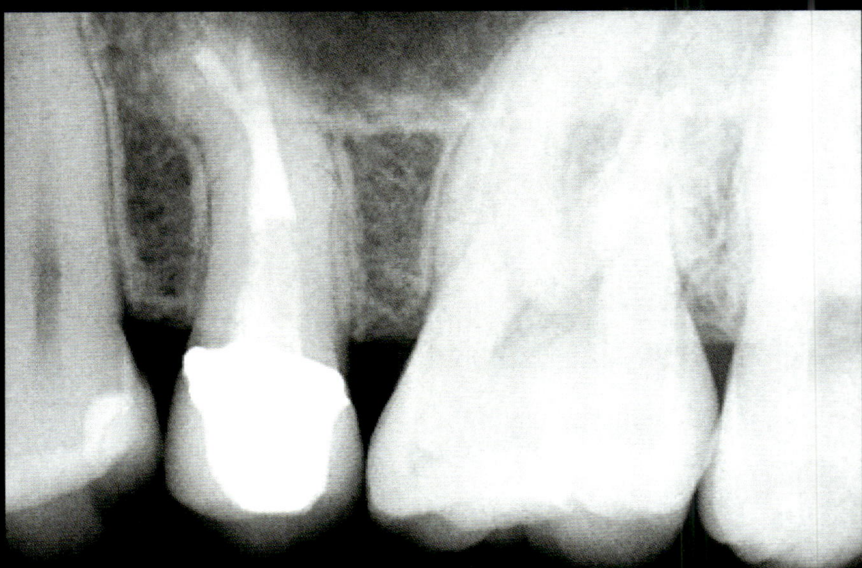

Figure 14: Follow-up 17 years later.

References

1. Mjor IA, Nordahl I. *The density and branching of dentinal tubules in human teeth*. Arch Oral Biol. 1996;41:401–12.
2. Kobayashi T, Hayashi A, Yoshikawa R, Okuda K, Hara K. *The microbial flora from root canals and periodontal pockets of non-vital teeth associated with advanced periodontitis*. Int Endod J. 1990;23:100–6.
3. Kobayashi T, Nonomura G, Watanabe LG, Marshall GWJ, Marshall SJ. *Dentin tubule numerical density variations below the CEJ*. J Dent. 2008;36:953–8.
4. De Deus QD. *Frequency, location, and direction of the lateral, secondary, and accessory canals*. J Endod. 1975;1:361–6.
5. Burch JG, Hulen S. *A study of the presence of accessory foramina and the topography of molar furcations*. Oral Surg Oral Med Oral Pathol. 1974;38:451–5.
6. Gutmann JL. *Prevalence, location, and patency of accessory canals in the furcation region of permanent molars*. . J Periodontol. 1978;49:21–6.
7. Goldberg F, Massone EJ, Soares I, Bittencourt AZ. *Accessory orifices: anatomical relationship between the pulp chamber floor and the furcation*. J Endod. 1987;13:176–81.
8. Vertucci FJ. *Root canal morphology and its relationship to endodontic procedures*. Endo Topics. 2005;10:3–29.
9. Lindhe J, Nyman S, Lang NP. T*reatment Planning. Clinical Periodontology and Implant Dentistry*. 4th Edition. Oxford: Blackwell Publishing Company; 2003. p. 414–31.
10. Ricucci D, Siqueira JF, Jr. *Fate of the tissue in lateral canals and apical ramifications in response to pathologic conditions and treatment procedures*. J Endod. 2010;36(1):1–15.
11. Seltzer S, Bender IB, Ziontz M. *The interrelationship of pulp and periodontal disease*. Oral Surg Oral Med Oral Pathol. 1963;16:1474–90.
12. Seltzer S, Bender IB, Nazimov H, Sinai I. *Pulpitisinduced interradicular periodontal changes in experimental animals. J Periodontol*. 1967;38:124–9.
13. American AAOE. *Glossary of endodontic terms*. 8th ed. Chicago: Association of Endodontists; 2012.
14. Rotstein I. *Interaction between endodontics and periodontics*. Periodontol 2000. 2017;74(1):11–39.
15. de Sanctis M, Goracci C, Zucchelli G. *Long-term Effect on Tooth Vitality of Regenerative Therapy in Deep Periodontal Bony Defects: A Retrospective Study*. Int J Periodontics Restorative Dent. 2013;33(2):151–7.
16. Mandi FA. *Histological study of the pulp changes caused by periodontal disease*. J Br Endod Soc. 1972;6:80–2.
17. Adriaens PA, Edwards CA, De Boever JA, Loesche WJ. *Ultrastructural observations on bacterial invasion in cementum and radicular dentin of periodontally diseased human teeth*. J Periodontol. 1988;59:493–503.
18. Simon JH, Glick DH, Frank AL. *The relationship of endodontic-periodontic lesions*. J Periodontol. 1972;43:202-208.
19. Herrera D, Retamal-Valdes B, Alonso B, & Feres M. *Acute periodontal lesions (periodontal abscesses and necrotizing periodontal diseases) and endo-periodontal lesions*. Journal of Clinical Periodontology. 2018;45(Suppl 1):S78-S94.
20. Al–Fouzan KS. *A new classification of endodontic-periodontal lesions*. Int J Dent. 2014;2014:919173.
21. Papapanou PN, Sanz M, Buduneli N, Dietrich T, Feres M, Fine DH, et al. *Periodontitis: Consensus report of workgroup 2 of the 2017 World Workshop on the Classification of Periodontal and Peri-Implant Diseases and Conditions*. Journal of Clinical Periodontology. 2018;45(Suppl 20):S162-S170.
22. Rotstein I, Simon JHS. T*he endo-perio lesion: a critical appraisal of the disease condition*. Endo Topics. 2006;13:34–56.
23. Chapple I, Lumley PJ. *The periodontal-endodontic interface*. Dental update. 1999;26:331–4.
24. Tawil PZ, Duggan DJ, Galicia JC. *Mineral Trioxide Aggregate (MTA): its history, composition and clinical application*. Compend Contin Educ Dent. 2015;36(4):247–52.
25. Kang JS, Rhim EM, Huh SY, Ahn SJ, Kim DS, Kim SY, et al. *The effects of humidity and serum on the surface microhardness and morphology of five retrograde filling materials*. Scanning. 2012;34(4):207–14.
26. Balachandran J, Gurucharan. *Comparison of sealing ability of bioactive bone cement, mineral trioxide aggregate and super EBA as furcation repair materials: a dye extraction study*. J Conserv Dent JCD. 2013;16(3):247–51.
27. Castellucci A. *The use of mineral trioxide aggregate to repair iatrogenic perforations*. Dentistry today. 2008;27(9):74–80.
28. Tsesis I, Rosenberg E, Faivishevsky V, Kfir A, Katz M, Rosen E. *Prevalence and associated periodontal status of teeth with root perforation: a retrospective study of 2,002 patients' medical records*. J Endod. 2010;36(5):797–800.
29. Gorni FG, Gagliani MM. *The outcome of endodontic retreatment: a 2-yr follow-up*. J Endod. 2004;30(1):1–4.
30. Clauder T, Shin S-J. *Repair of perforations with MTA: clinical applications and mechanisms of action*. Endo Topics. 2006;15:32–55.

31. Kvinnsland I, Oswald RJ, Halse A, Gronningsaeter AG. *A clinical and roentgenological study of 55 cases of root perforation*. Int Endod J. 1989;22:75–84.
32. Fuss Z, Trope M. *Root perforations: classification and treatment choices based on prognostic factors.* Endod Dent Traumatol. 1996;12:255–64.
33. Main C, Mirzayan N, Shabahang S, Torabinejad M. *Repair of root perforations using mineral trioxide aggregate: a long-term study*. J Endod. 2004;30:80–3.
34. Pace R, Giuliani V, Pagavino G. *Mineral trioxide aggregate as repair material for furcal perforation: case series*. J Endod. 2008;34:1130–3.
35. Parirokh M, Torabinejad M. *Mineral trioxide aggregate: a comprehensive literature review - Part I: chemical, physical, and antibacterial properties.* J Endod. 2010;36(1):16–27.
36. Parirokh M, Torabinejad M. *Mineral trioxide aggregate: a comprehensive literature review - Part III: clinical applications, drawbacks, and mechanism of action.* J Endod. 2010;36:400–3.
37. Torabinejad M, Parirokh M. *Mineral trioxide aggregate: a comprehensive literature review - Part II: leakage and biocompatibility investigations.* J Endod. 2010;36(2):190–202.
38. Asgary S, Motazedian HR, Parirokh M, Eghbal MJ, Kheirieh S. *Twenty years of research on mineral trioxide aggregate: a scientometric report*. Iran Endod J 2013;8:1–5.
39. Krupp C, Bargholz C, Brusehaber M, Hulsmann M. T*reatment outcome after repair of root perforations with mineral trioxide aggregate: a retrospective evaluation of 90 teeth*. J Endod. 2013;39(11):1364–8.
40. Pontius V, Pontius O, Braun A, Frankenberger R, Roggendorf MJ. *Retrospective evaluation of perforation repairs in 6 private practices*. J Endod. 2013;39(11):1346–58.
41. Mente J, Hage N, Pfefferle T, Koch MJ, Geletneky B, Dreyhaupt J, et al. *Treatment outcome of mineral trioxide aggregate: repair of root perforations*. J Endod. 2010;36(2):208–13.
42. Mente J, Leo M, Panagidis D, Saure D, Pfefferle T. *Treatment outcome of mineral trioxide aggregate: repair of root perforations-long-term results*. J Endod. 2014;40(6):790–6.
43. Gorni FG, Andreano A, Ambrogi F, Brambilla E, Gagliani M. *Patient and Clinical Characteristics Associated with Primary Healing of Iatrogenic Perforations after Root Canal Treatment: Results of a Long-term Italian Study*. J Endod. 2016;42(2):211–5.
44. Gandolfi MG, Taddei P, Tinti A, Prati C. *Apatite-forming ability (bioactivity) of ProRoot MTA*. Int Endod J. 2010;43(10):917–29.
45. Hashem AA, Wanees Amin SA. *The effect of acidity on dislodgment resistance of mineral trioxide aggregate and bioaggregate in furcation perforations: an in vitro comparative study*. J Endod. 2012;38(2):245–9.
46. Mori GG, Teixeira LM, de Oliveira DL, Jacomini LM, da Silva SR. *Biocompatibility evaluation of biodentine in subcutaneous tissue of rats*. J Endod. 2014;40(9):1485–8.
47. Silva LAB, Pieroni K, Nelson-Filho P, Silva RAB, Hernandez-Gaton P, Lucisano MP, et al. *Furcation Perforation: Periradicular Tissue Response to Biodentine as a Repair Material by Histopathologic and Indirect Immunofluorescence Analyses.* J Endod. 2017;43(7):1137–42.
48. Gorni FGM. "Endodonzia Chirurgica". In: Berutti E, Gagliani M, (editors). *Manuale di Endodonzia*. Milano: Edra. 2013. p. 2–27.
49. Gorni FGM, Cerutti F. *Il ruolo degli ultrasuoni nel ritrattamento ortogrado*. Il Dentista Moderno. 2012;1:86–93.
50. Roberts HW, Toth JM, Berzins DW, Charlton DG. *Mineral trioxide aggregate material use in endodontic treatment: a review of the literature*. Dent Mater. 2008;24:149–64.
51. Basturk FB, Nekoofar MH, Gunday M, Dummer PM. *The effect of various mixing and placement techniques on the compressive strength of mineral trioxide aggregate*. J Endod. 2013;39(1):111–4.

- Describe the main **indications** for the use of surgical endodontics to treat endodontic periapical disease.
- Explain the **techniques** and methods for an optimum approach to even the most complex cases requiring endodontic surgery.
- To provide an exhaustive picture of the clinical results that can be achieved, in the short and long term, with these surgical procedures.

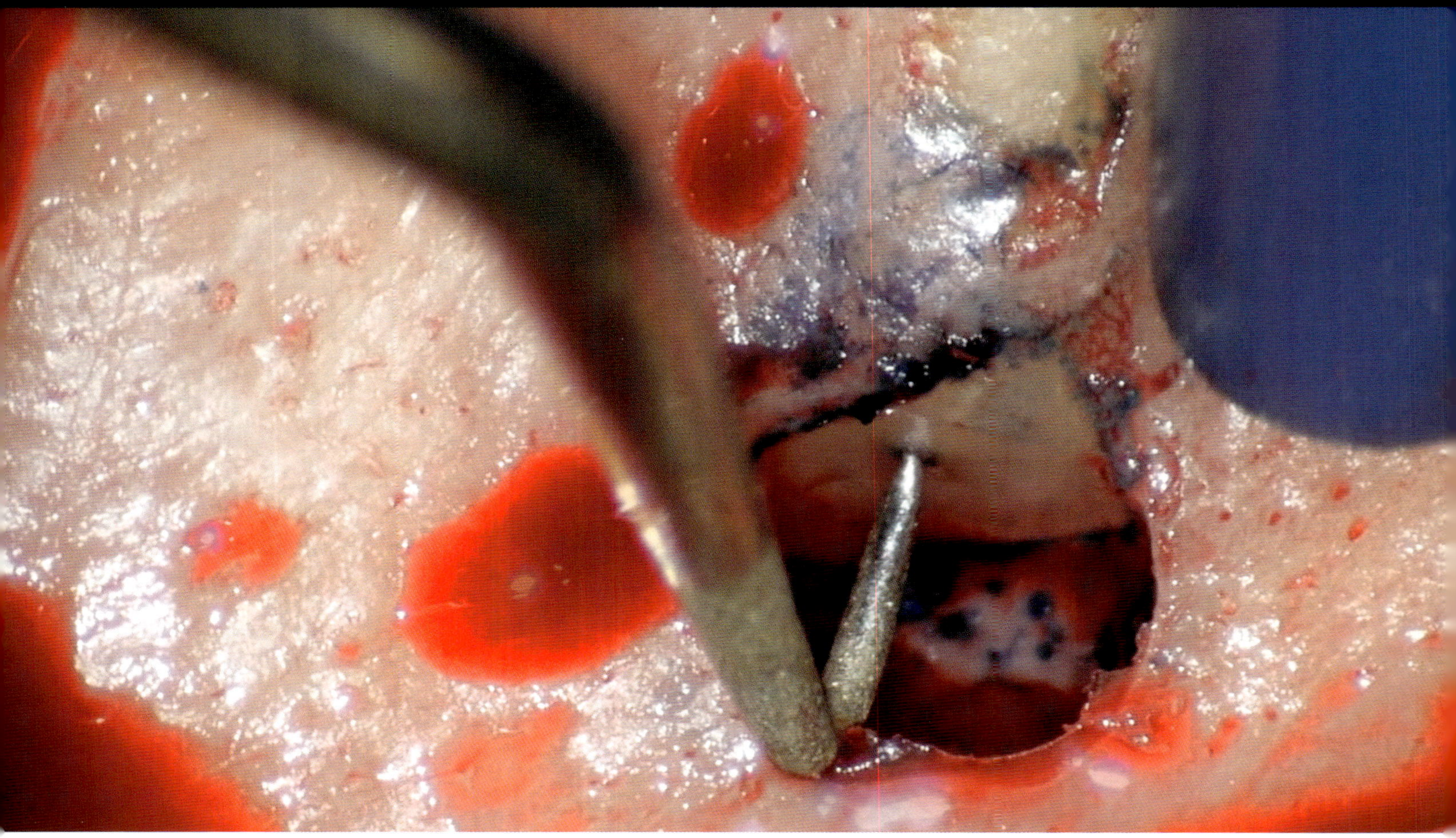

Francesca Cerutti, Fabio Gorni

08

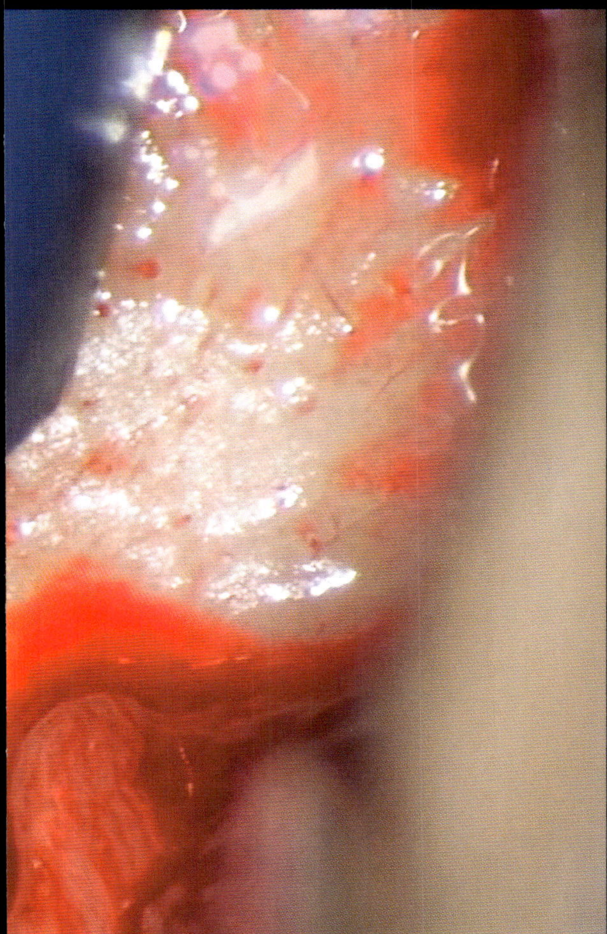

Surgical Endodontics

An alternative approach for the treatment of periapical diseases

Preliminary remarks

Surgical endodontics has its primary field of application in the treatment of teeth with lesions that cannot be solved with an orthograde approach, due to various factors, ranging from infections not reduced by previous retreatment to extraradicular infections. Among other causes, foreign body reactions, which result in cystic lesions filled with cholesterol crystals, constitute the most common conditions in this category. Finally, in some cases, such as those with non-perishable prosthetic artifacts, endocanal posts, iatrogenic obstructions or intraradicular blocks, and perforations of the apical third, orthograde access to the root canal is not possible[1, 2].

These cases are summarized in Table 8.1.

Table 8.1 **CASES THAT CAN BE RESOLVED BY SURGICAL ENDODONTICS**

Infections/Injury	Factors related to the morphology or content of the endodontium	Factors related to the reconstruction of the tooth
Persistent or refractory endodontic lesions	Perforations of the apical third	Crowns or bridges recently executed
Intraradicular infections that cannot be treated with an orthograde approach	Blocks or obliterations of the canal light	Intracanal posts
Extraradicular infections (the cement of the root surface is colonized by bacteria)	Well-executed canal treatments in which the orthograde approach cannot easily achieve positive results	
Reactions caused by foreign bodies/ periradicular cysts		

Indications

As already mentioned, primary endodontic treatments can have a negative outcome in percentages ranging from 2.7% to 17.2% in the case of vital tooth, as well as from 14% to 24.4% when considering a tooth with apical periodontitis[3, 4]. Failure is sometimes evident within a short time and can be solved in a good percentage of cases by retreatment[1, 5].
Although the criteria used to evaluate the success of endodontic therapy cannot be easily standardized[6], there is consensus that radiographically evident lesions exceeding 5 mm in size, the presence of a fistula, and the presence of iatrogenic damage to the root canal (in the middle or apical third) are factors capable of negatively influencing the success of endodontic therapy[3].
In addition, the tooth may not always be retreated with an orthograde approach or, as already mentioned, the new canal treatment may not result in success; at this point the option of surgical endodontics should be considered[1].
The reason why not all clinical situations can be managed with an orthograde approach is the complexity of the anatomy of the root canal system, which can make parts of the endodontium impossible to shape, cleanse, and fill in three dimensions. Thus, the bacteria are allowed to survive and sustain infectious and/or inflammatory processes.
The choice to perform a surgical endodontic operation frequently arises from the question as to whether a better alternative to the existing canal therapy is possible, making an appropriate cost-benefit analysis between surgical endodontics and orthograde retreatment, in the light of the success rates found in the literature[7, 8].
There is also a further possibility in which the surgical procedure is preferable to the orthograde approach: if the teeth in question have restorations that cannot be (or are not intended to be) removed or if removal would be extremely hazardous for the survival of the tooth[7] (Figs. 8.1a-8.1c).

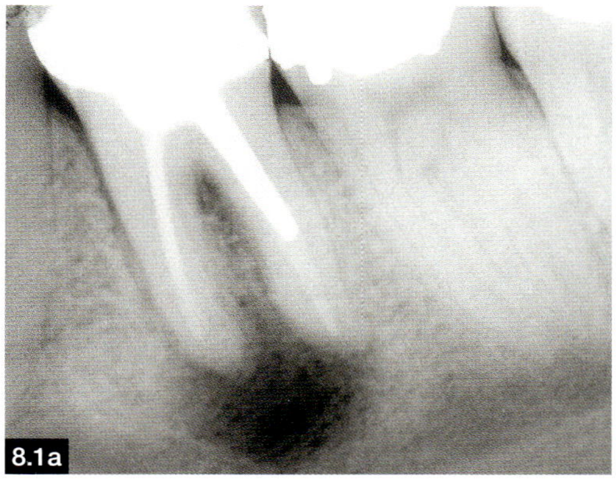

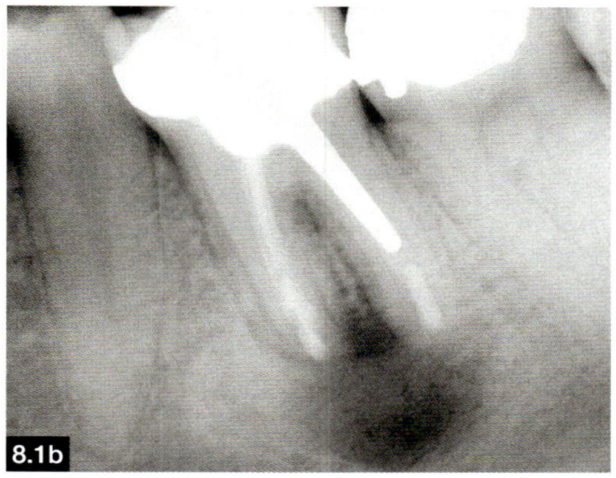

Fig. 8.1a: The X-ray shows a periapical lesion in a lower left first molar characterized by deficient endodontic treatment and a large cast post cemented in the distal root.

Fig. 8.1b: Given that the removal of the existing restoration is not an easy task and there is the risk of fracture of the tooth, direct intervention by means of surgical endodontics performed on both roots was carried out. The X-ray shows the situation immediately after surgery.

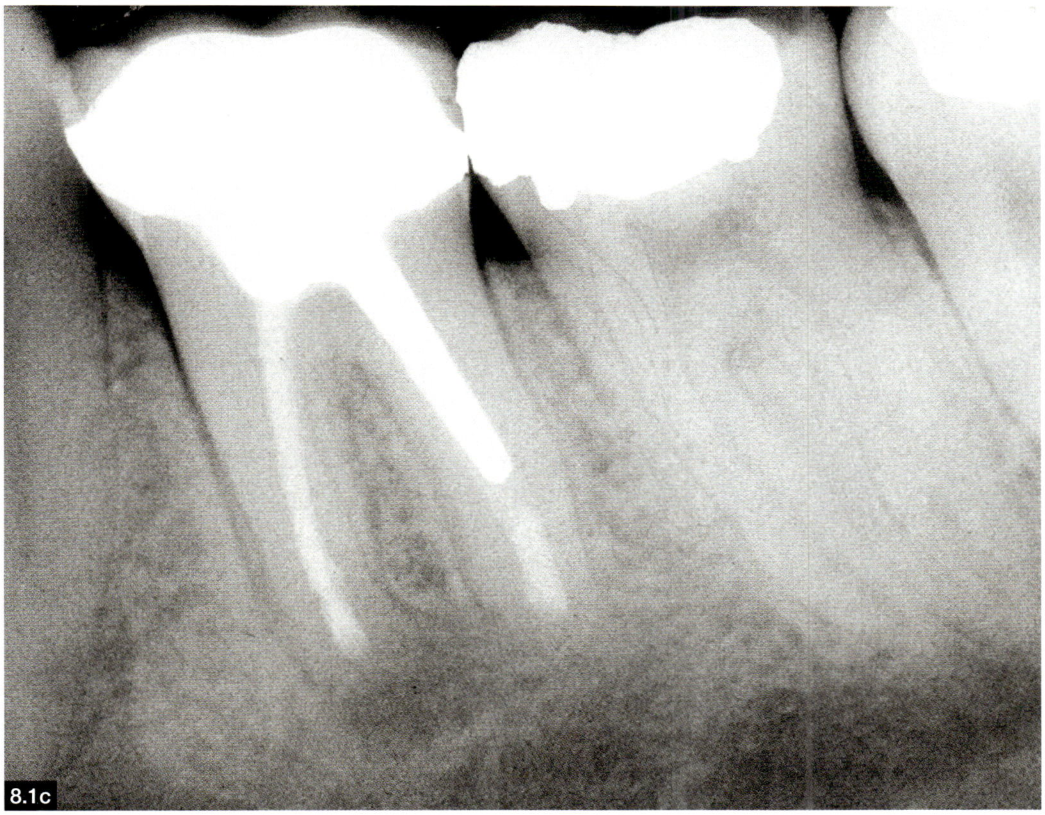

Fig. 8.1c: At 1-year follow-up the tooth was almost completely healed. The lesion on the distal root disappeared, and that on the mesial root was significantly reduced. This session will be followed by six-monthly follow-ups until the lesion is completely resolved.

Prognosis

The international literature has addressed the issue of surgical endodontics in many ways, and the data produced may seem discordant. The success rate of the surgical treatment performed in the 1990s is around 59%, while the most recent analyses show a success rate of 93%[6, 9] 1-10 years after the procedure, with the evaluation criteria being radiological and clinical data.
The enormous evolution of the surgical technique, thanks to the advent of the surgical microscope[9], use of ultrasonic instruments[11], and adoption of *biocompatible* filling materials that can harden in the presence of moisture[12, 13], has positively influenced the success rate[9, 14].
The surgical technique used until the end of the last century involved an apical resection angle of 45° and canal preparation with drills. This technique did not favor the identification of the canal anatomy and treatment was difficult from an operative point of view. Finally, filling with silver amalgam, a material with poor apical seal capacity, did not favor healing[11, 15] (Figs. 8.2a-8.2e). The current technique, thanks to the use

BIOCOMPATIBLE MATERIALS

Improve the apical seal and promote healing, thereby ensuring a successful surgical endodontic procedure.

▶ *continue to page 412*

The importance of magnifying equipment in surgical endodontics

Surgical therapy without proper magnification and lighting is strongly discouraged

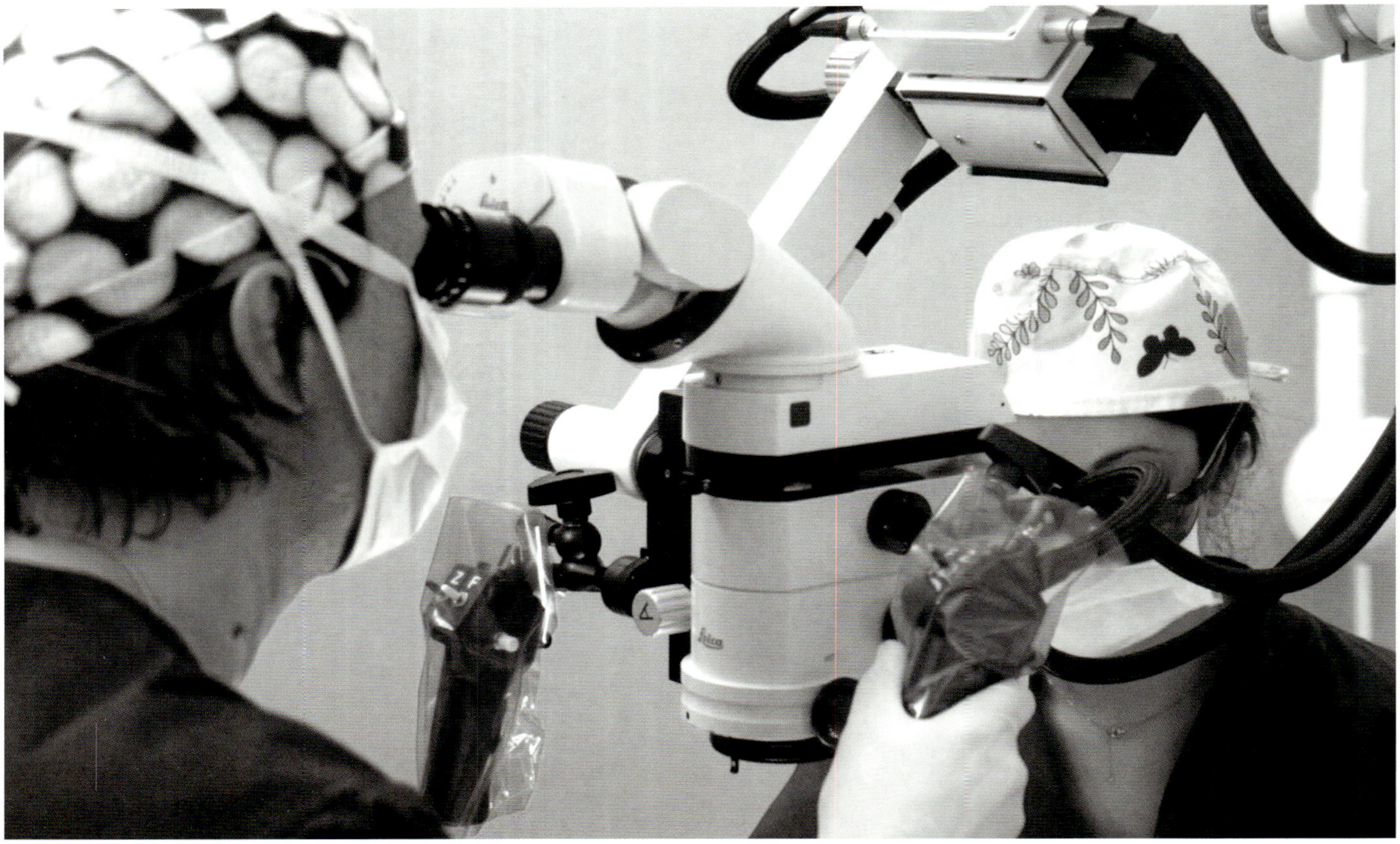

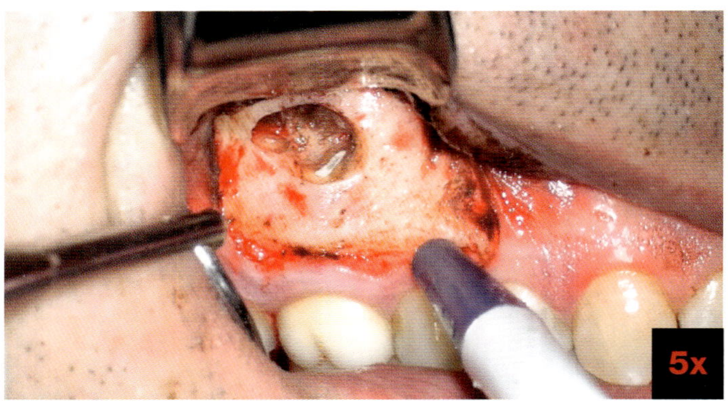

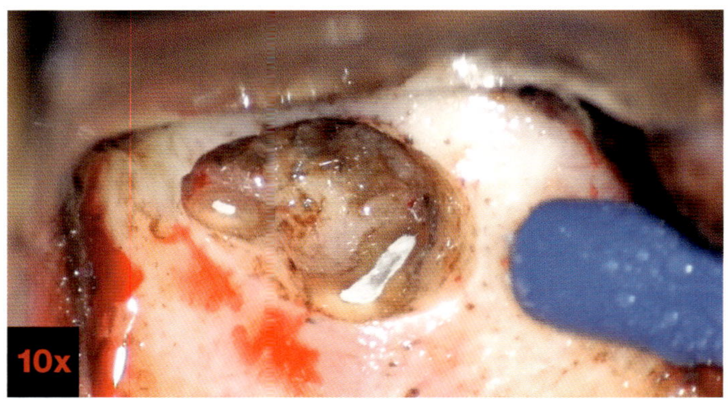

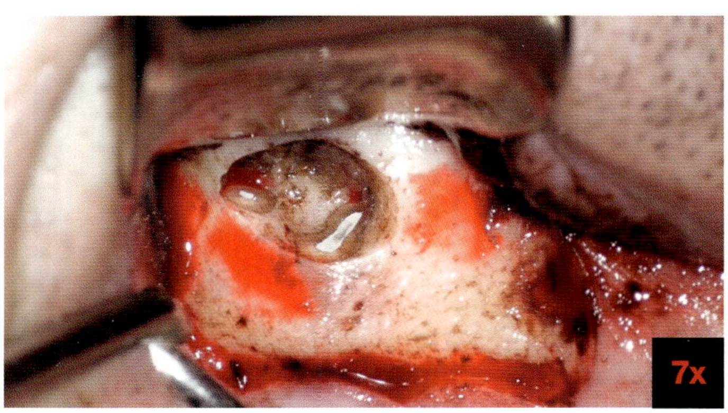

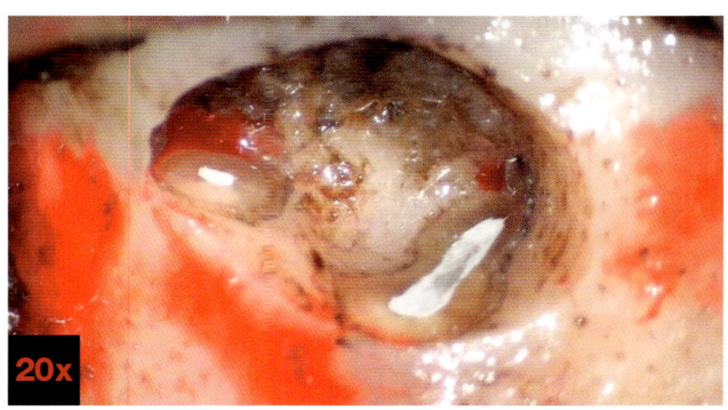

Table 8.2 **SUCCESS RATES**

Study	Follow up (years)	Cases observed	Recalls (%)	Outcome (%)		
				Healed	Healing	Functional
Zuolo et al. (2000)	1-4	102	96	91		92
Rahbaran et al. (2001)	> 4	129	61	37	33	80
Rud et al. (2001)	0.5-12.5	834	84	92	1	93
Pecora et al. (2001)		10	100	30	50	20
von Arx et al. (2001)	1	25	96	88	8	96
Rubinstein et al. (2002)	5-7	59	86	92		92
Jensen et al. (2002)	1	134	91	73	17	90
Chong et al. (2003)	2	108	59	90	6	96
Maddalone and Gagliani (2003)	0.3-3	120	82	93	3	96
Schwartz-Arad et al. (2003)	0.5-0.9	262	47	44	21	65
Wang et al. (2004)	4-8	94	85	74		91
Gagliani et al. (2005)	5	231	89	78	10	89
Lindeboom et al. (2005)		100	100	56	43	1
Taschieri et al. (2005)	1	50	46	91.3	2.2	6.5
Taschieri et al. (2006)	1	71	71	93	4.2	2.8
von Arx et al. (2007)	1	183	98,5	83	10	7
Taschieri et al. (2007)		28	100	92	4	4
Penarrocha et al. (2007)	1-10	333	100	71.7	13.9	14.4
Kim et al. (2008)	1-5	148	100	85	10	5
Taschieri et al. (2008)	2	63	100	92	3	5
		50	100	90.3	2.4	7.3
Saunders et al. (2008)	0.3-6	276	100	59.1	29.7	11.2
Taschieri and Del Fabbro (2009)	2	43	100	90.7		9.3
von Arx et al. (2010)	1	353	100	85.5		14.5
Barone et al. (2010)	4-10	106	100		72	28
Song et al. (2011)	1	42	100	78.6	16.7	4.8
Walivaara et al. (2011)	0.5-1.8	96	100	90.6		9.4
		98	100	81.6		18.4
Song et al. (2011)	1	441	100	84.8		15.2
von Arx et al. (2012)	5	170	100	70.6	16.5	12.9
Kreisler et al. (2013)	0.5-1	281	100	88		12
Song et al. (2014)	> 4	115	100	75.7	13.1	11.3
Tortorici et al. (2014)	5	206	100	71	26	3
Lui et al. (2014)	1-2	93	100	71	7.5	21.5
Çaliskan et al. (2016)	2-6	90	100		74.4	14.4

Table 8.3 **CLINICAL CIRCUMSTANCES IN SURGICAL ENDODONTICS**

Indications	Contraindications
Persistent or emerging disease following canal therapy, where orthograde retreatment is not indicated	Presence of inappropriate endodontic treatment in which the uninstrumented canal anatomy is evident
Radiological signs of apical periodontitis and/or symptoms associated with the presence of an obstructed canal (where the obstruction is not removable or its removal would entail an excessively high risk)	Radiological finding of an independent lateral lesion, indicating an untreated accessory system
Clinical or radiological signs of apical periodontitis and/or persistent symptoms in the presence of endodontic material overfill. In the case of overflow, the presence of symptoms is an indication for surgery even in the absence of radiologically visible lesions	Presence of very long root canal posts. To obtain a suitable seal, at least 2 mm of dental tissue must remain after apical resection. In these cases, once the apical part of the root has been resected, there is a risk of there not being sufficient space for an adequate retrograde filling
Perforation of the apical third of the root	Inadequacy of the clinical crown-root relationship: resecting the apex would aggravate the situation, worsening the prognosis of the tooth
Presence of unresolved injuries with orthograde retreatment, sustained by bacteria nested within the root canal system or in extraradicular sites	Inability to gain suitable surgical access
Cystic lesions – true cyst (the cyst must be surgically enucleated)	Presence of a vertical root fracture
Presence of a very extensive or recently cemented restoration	
Choice of the clinician, who considers it most likely to achieve success by intervening surgically instead of through orthograde retreatment	
Severely compromised tooth and teeth with objectively good endodontic therapies	

of ultrasonic "retro-tips," can be used to perform conservative osteotomies that do not damage the cortical bone, with angles of the root resection process close to 90°; thus, the root length is not excessively shortened[16].
The treatment is extremely accurate thanks to coaxial illumination and the high magnification factor obtained from the microscope; these features facilitate the identification of the canal anatomy and allow an ergonomically better management of the operating field[17-19].
The diversity in the success rates of the studies considered can also be attributed to the fact that many studies examined predominantly mono-radicular teeth, while very few studies considered multiradicular teeth.
This difference can significantly alter the healing rates, because multiradicular teeth present greater difficulties in treatment than monoradicular ones due to anatomical complexity and location.
Table 8.2 summarizes the success rates reported by the literature since 2000[17-49].

Correct case selection is essential to clinical success[50].
Table 8.3 summarizes the indications and contraindications for surgical endodontics[51].

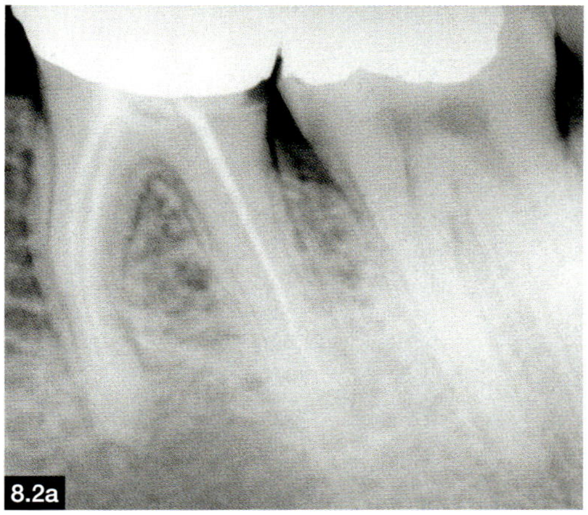

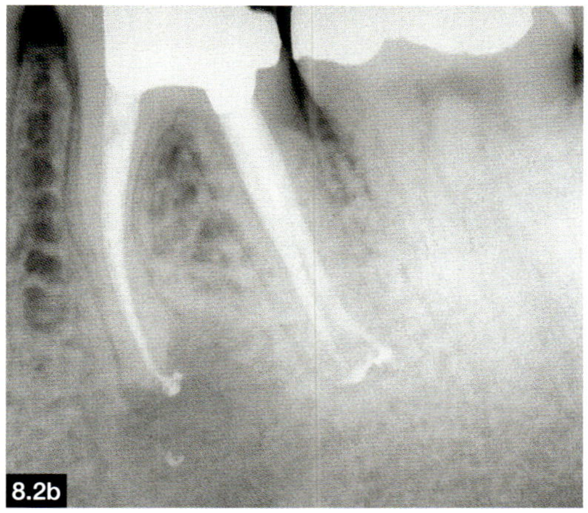

Fig. 8.2a: X-ray shows a case where the patient complained of percussion pain on tooth 3.6. Endodontic therapy was deficient, and the coronal restoration did not guarantee any seals.

Fig. 8.2b: Considering the initial situation, orthodox retreatment was deemed the appropriate solution: the X-ray shows the result of the operation on the dental tooth.

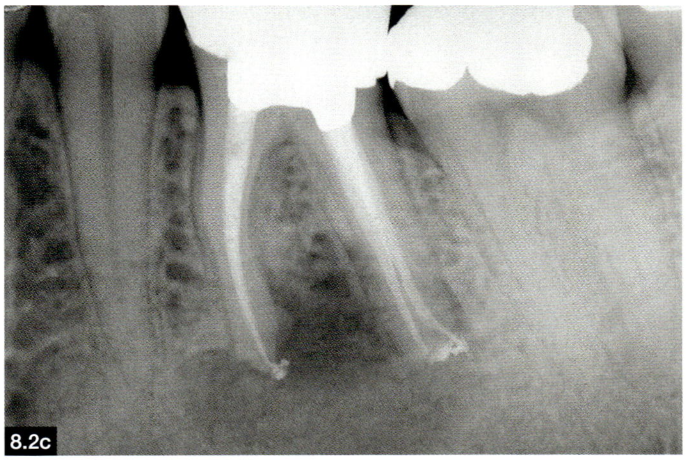

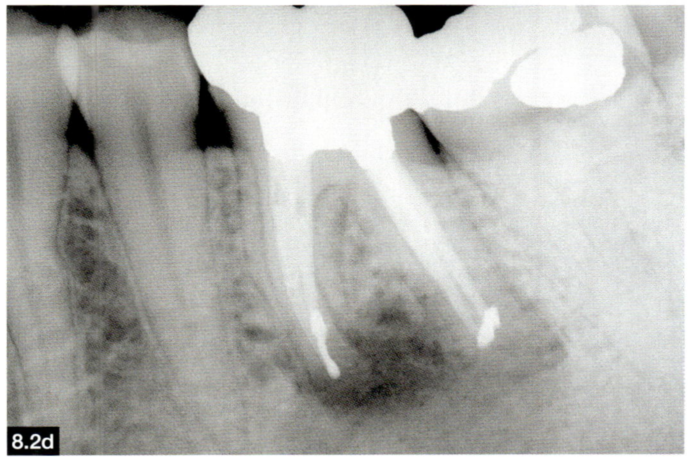

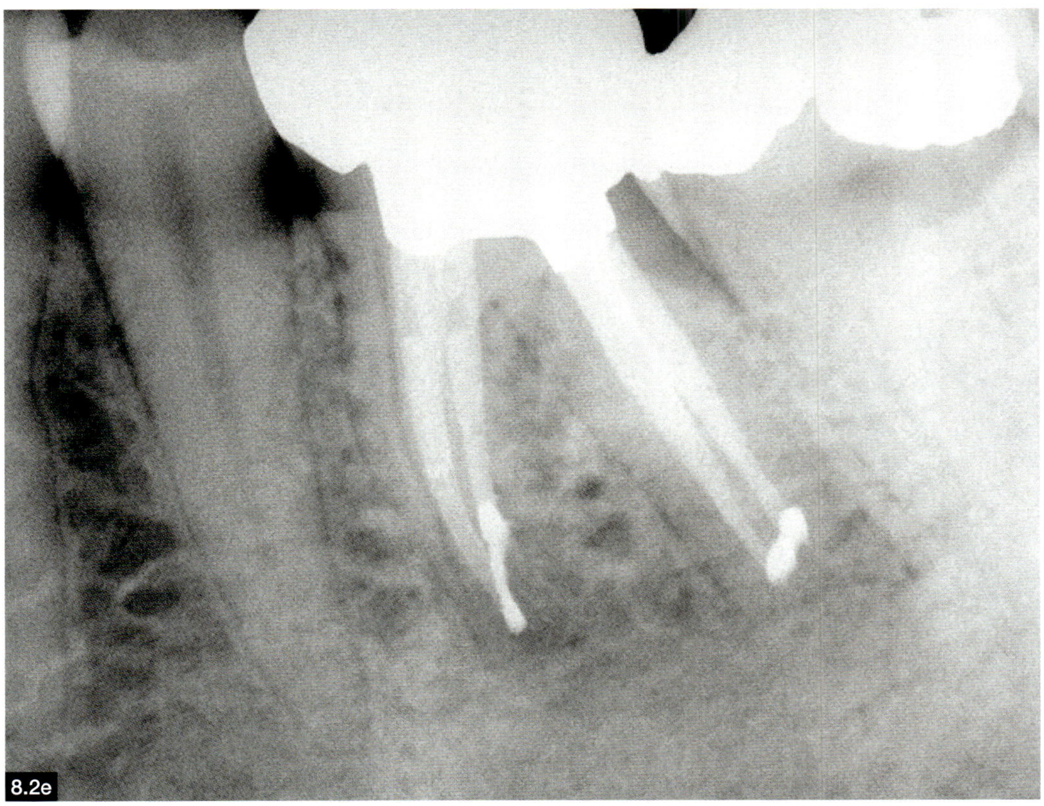

Fig. 8.2c: Two years after retreatment, the patient returned to our clinic, complaining of the same symptoms reported during the first consult. The X-ray shows a worsened clinical situation, with an increase in periapical radio-transparency.

Fig. 8.2d: As it was not advisable to attempt to improve the orthograde therapy surgical endodontics was performed. The operation was conducted in the pre-MTA era. The two mesial canals and the two distal canals could be cleansed, shaped, and sealed.

Fig. 8.2e: The x-ray after 25 years showed complete healing of the tooth and stability of the endodontic and prosthetic result.

▶ *continue to page 418*

CASE REPORT 1

Periradicular overfill and puncture injuries

This case is particularly interesting because it presents all the remarkable clinical signs that lead to the indication for a surgical treatment in this first case report.
The 47-year-old patient presented with a good oral health, with some treatments to be reviewed, but had severe spontaneous pain in area of tooth no. 46.

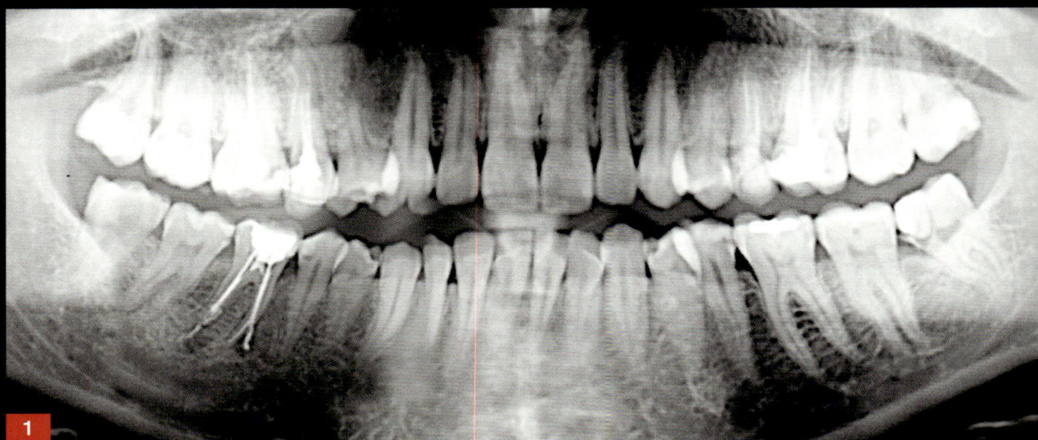

1

Figure 1: OPG showing periapical lesion on tooth no. 46 due to inappropriate treatment; note the sealed perforation with filler in the periodontal space.

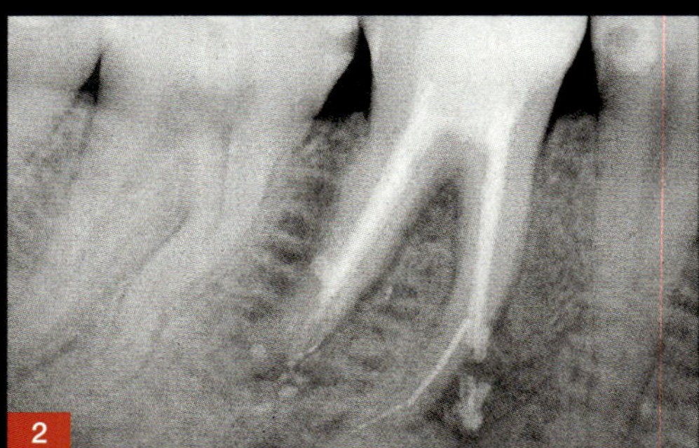

2

Figure 2: Radiographic analysis showing a fractured endodontic instrument in the mesial root.

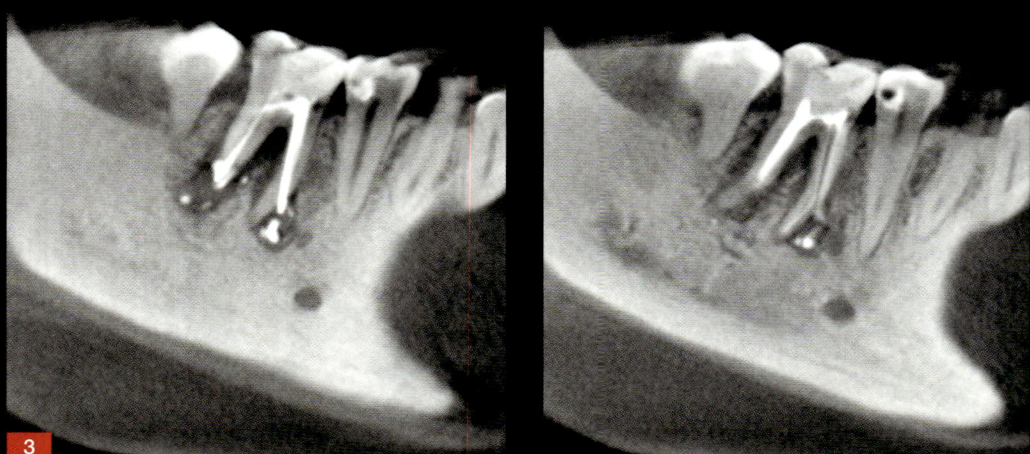

3

Figure 3: Examination with CBCT also shows a perforation at the distal root (longitudinal sections).

After the orthopanoramic X-ray, the case was examined by CBCT in order to more thoroughly assess the relationship between the lesion and the soft tissues, i.e. the inferior alveolar nerve. Having established the extent and position of the lesion, it was decided to perform endodontic surgery with a retrograde seal in reinforced eugenol zinc oxide cement (Super EBA, Bosworth, USA).

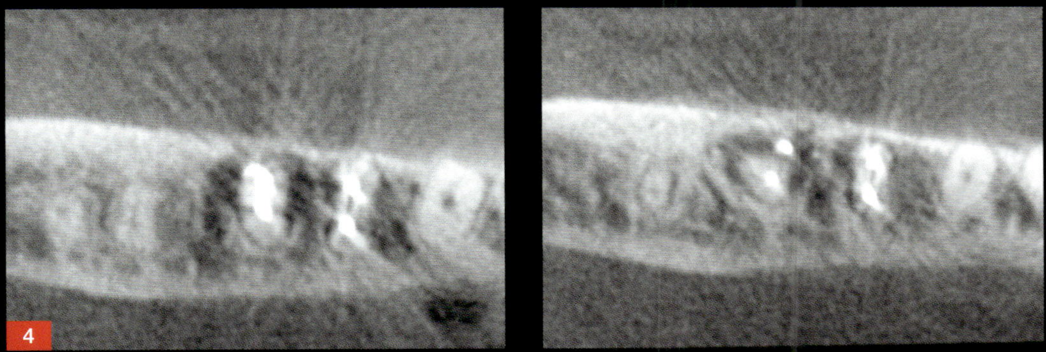

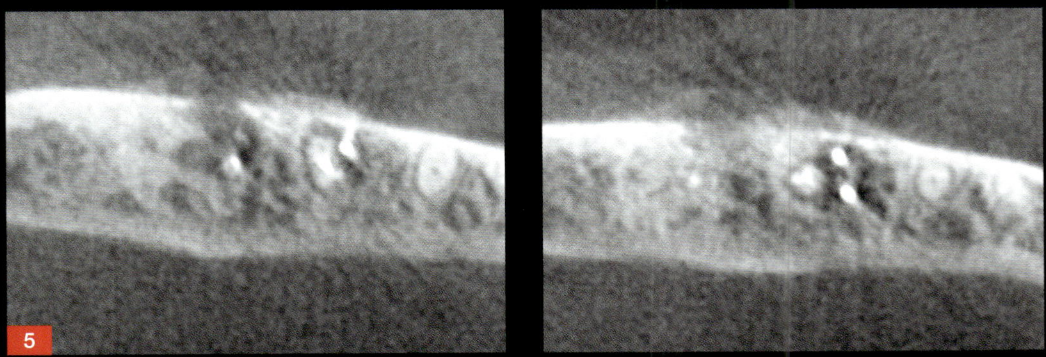

Figure 4 and 5: The CBCT analysis verifies, by means of the axial sections, the possible relationships with the inferior alveolar nerve and highlights the complete demolition of the vestibular cortical, which makes the intervention more precise but no less difficult.

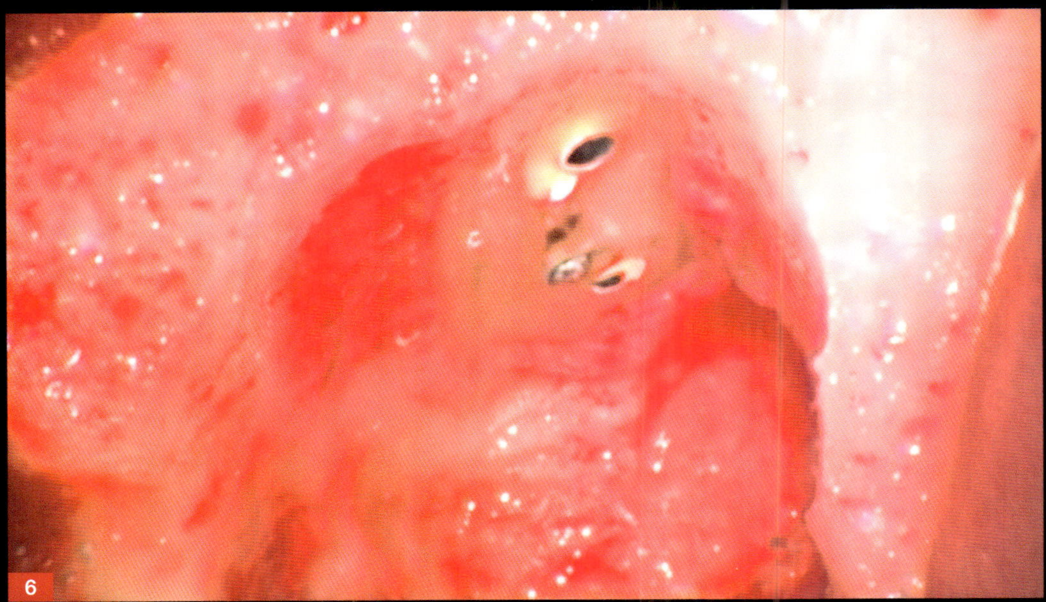

Figure 6: Intraoperative image of the cut mesial root (14x magnification).

Figure 7: Intraoperative image with ultrasonic tip to perform the retrograde cavity.

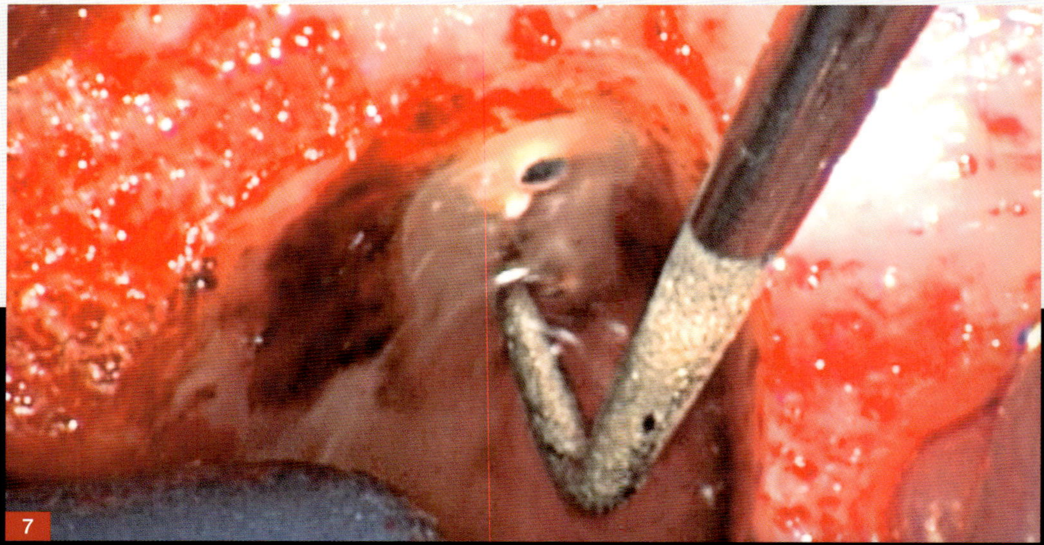

Figure 8: Retrograde cavity performed.

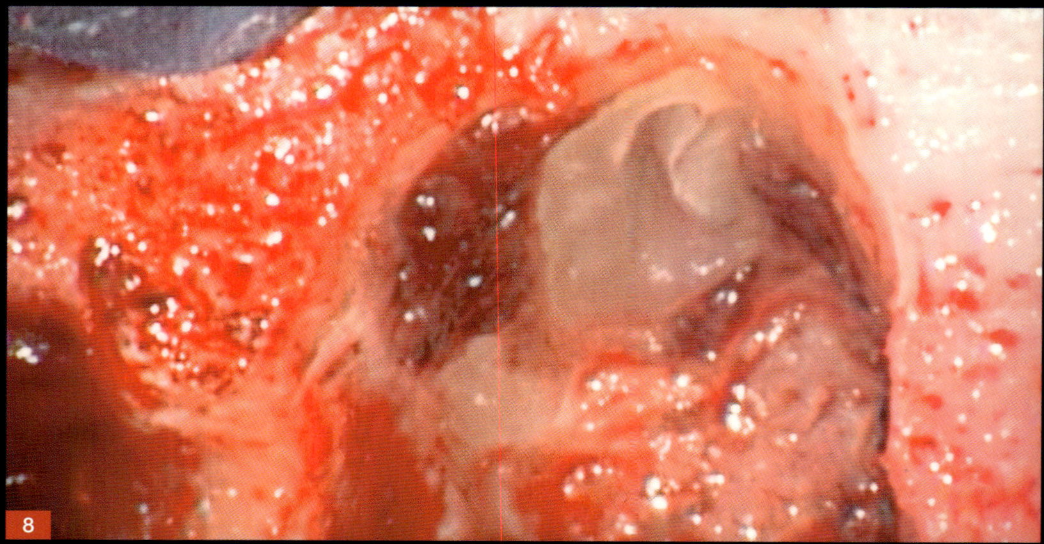

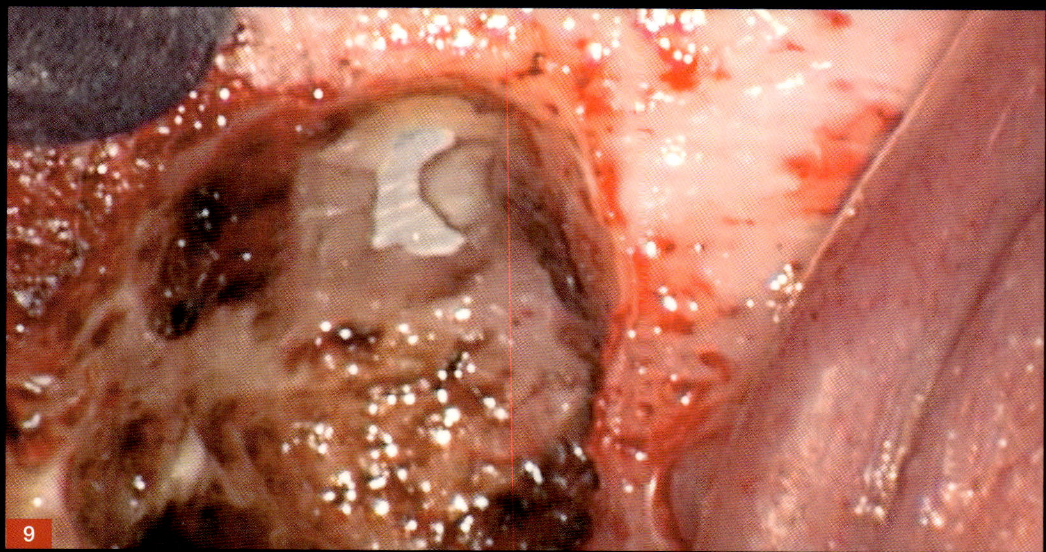

Figure 9: Seal performed with reinforced eugenol zinc oxide cement.

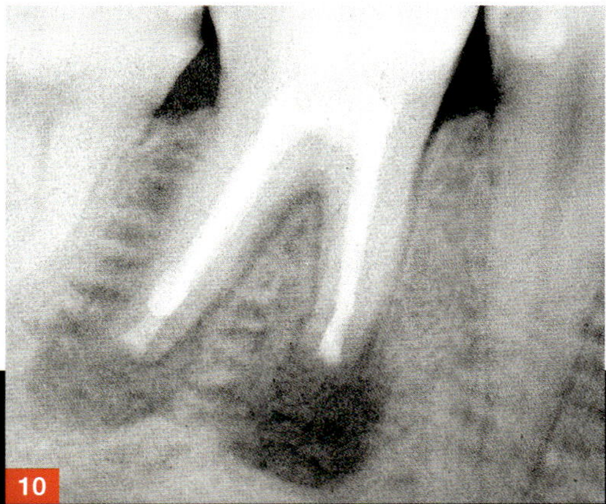

10

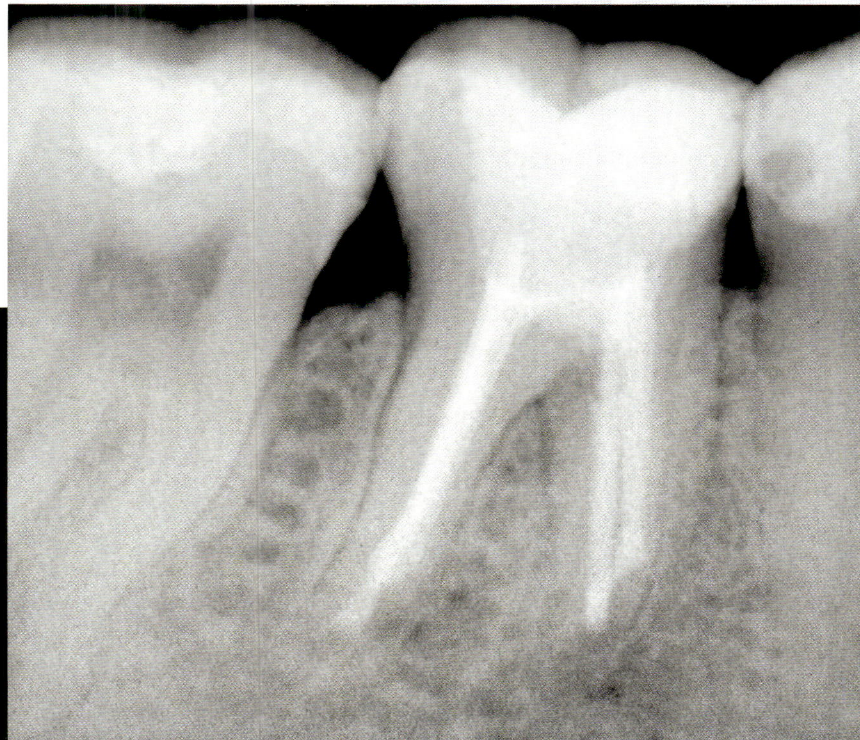

Figure 10: Radiograph of the completed case and follow-up two years later. Notice the reappearance of the periodontal ligament all around the contour of the mesial and distal root, sign of a perfect healing of the periradicular bone.

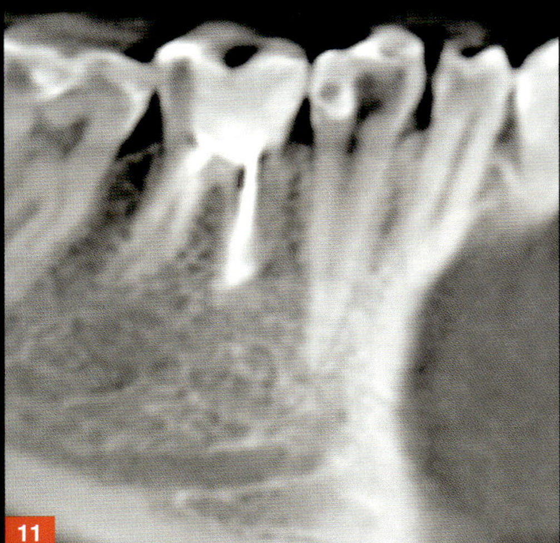

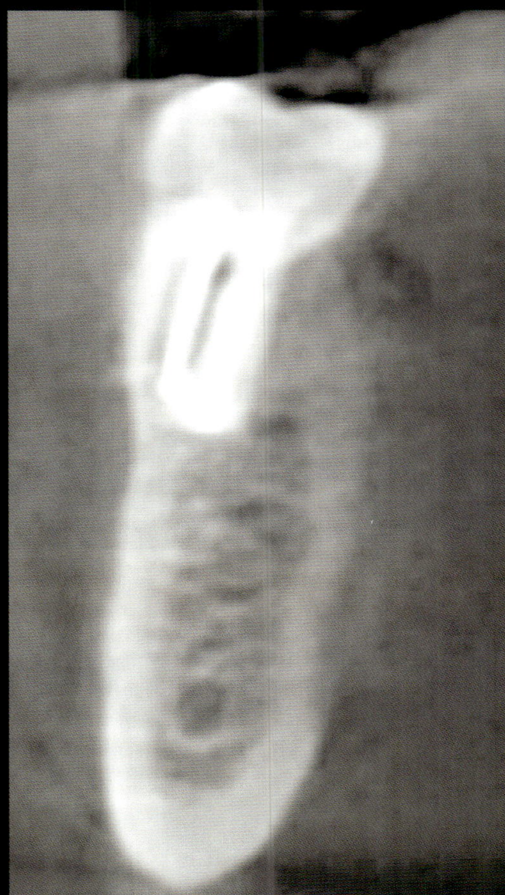

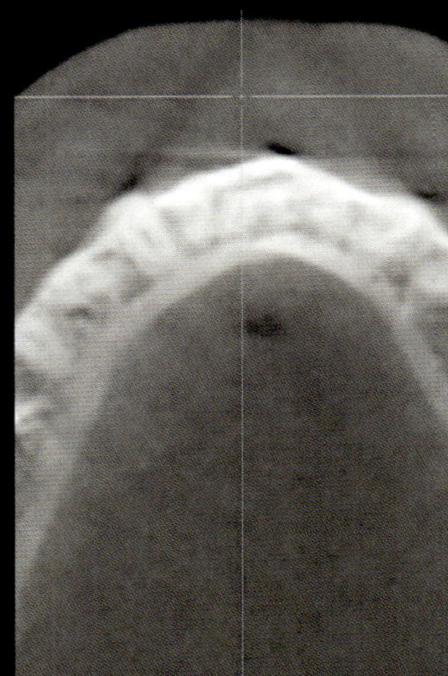

11

Figure 11: The confirmation of the achievement of full periodontal health comes from three-dimensional radiographic examination (CBCT) as the absence of periradicular radiotransparent areas and the recomposition of the cortical bone adjacent to the tooth further supports this result.

Phases of endodontic surgery

The surgical approach can be summarized in the following steps:

1. Preoperative planning and evaluation
2. Premedication and anesthesia
3. Realization of mucosal and bone access to the area to be treated
4. Root apex resection and enucleation of inflamed and/or infected periapical tissue
5. Retrograde identification and shaping of the endodontic space
6. Shaped space cleaning
7. Root canal system filling
8. Suture

❶ Intervention planning

Beyond the investigations carried out for diagnostic purposes, knowing the location and extent of the inflammatory lesion and its bone location is the first essential step for the correct planning of surgical endodontic therapy. Traditionally, one or more endodontic X-rays from different angles give an idea of the clinical case. However, we must not forget the objective limits of endodontic radiography which, by representing a three-dimensional structure two-dimensionally, has three main problems:

1. it does not make it possible to appreciate the labio-lingual dimension of the lesions (although it is able to give the clinician a fairly faithful representation of the mesio-distal extension of the defect);
2. in some cases, especially for multiradicular teeth, the exact location of an injury cannot be determined;
3. the radiopacities and radio-transparencies on which clinicians base their radiological diagnosis are not always univocally distinguishable from the surrounding anatomical structures.

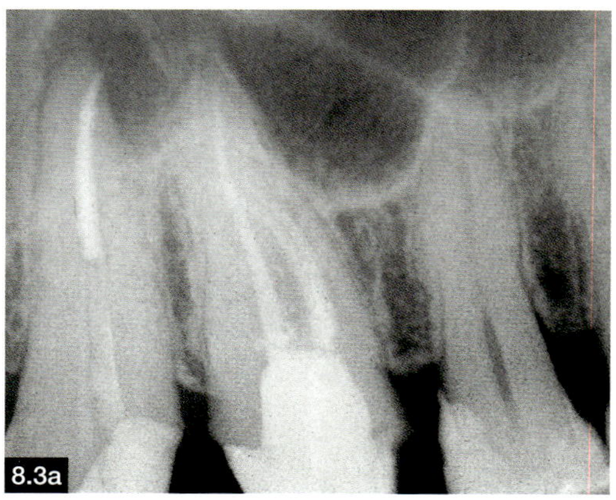

Fig. 8.3a: The endodontic X-ray showed an area of periapical radiotransparency at tooth 1.7.

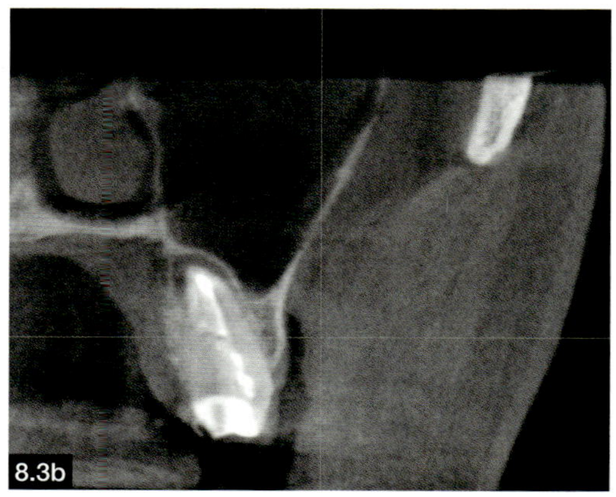

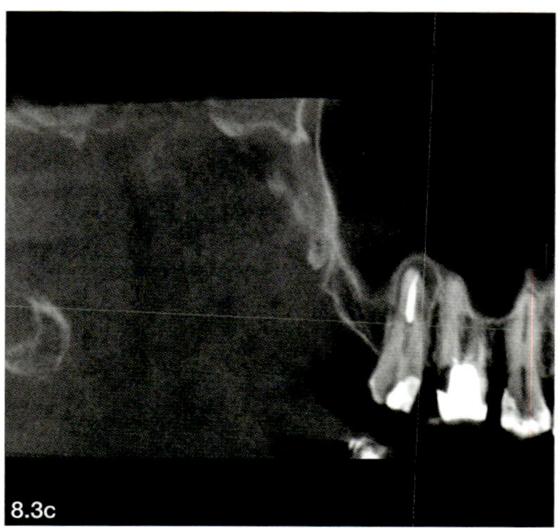

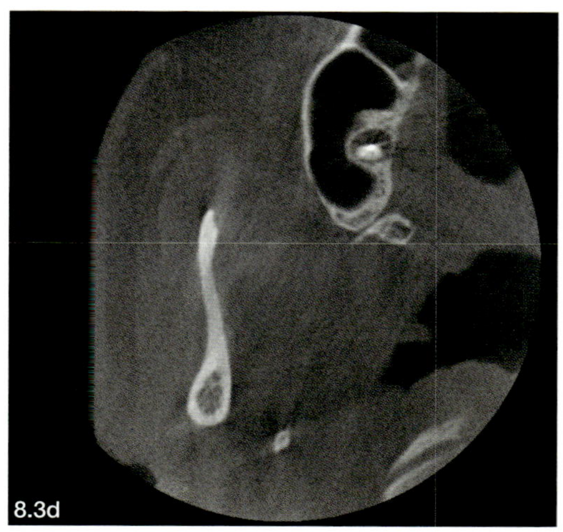

Fig. 8.3b-e: The CBCT beam enables the clinician to visualize the lesion in the three dimensions of the space, allowing precise planning of the intervention.

The possibility of using high-resolution 3D images of cone beam computed tomography (CBCT) has improved diagnosis in dentistry, allowing the precise identification of the extent and location of a lesion, or diagnosis of the presence of lesions in asymptomatic tooth[52]. In endodontic surgery, this examination is widely used in planning the procedure due to the speed of execution and the limited dose of radiation to which the patient is exposed[53-55] (Figs. 8.3a-8.3i).

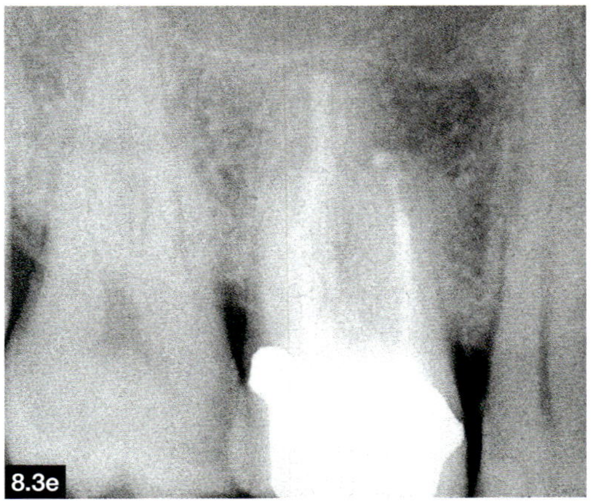

8.3e

Fig. 8.3e: Patient complains of percussion pain at tooth 1.6; endodontic radiography did not allow the clinician to clearly highlight the problem within the tooth.

Fig. 8.3f-i: CBCT clearly displayed the lesion of the mesial root of 16, proving its fundamental value when formulating diagnosis and devising the treatment plan for the patient.

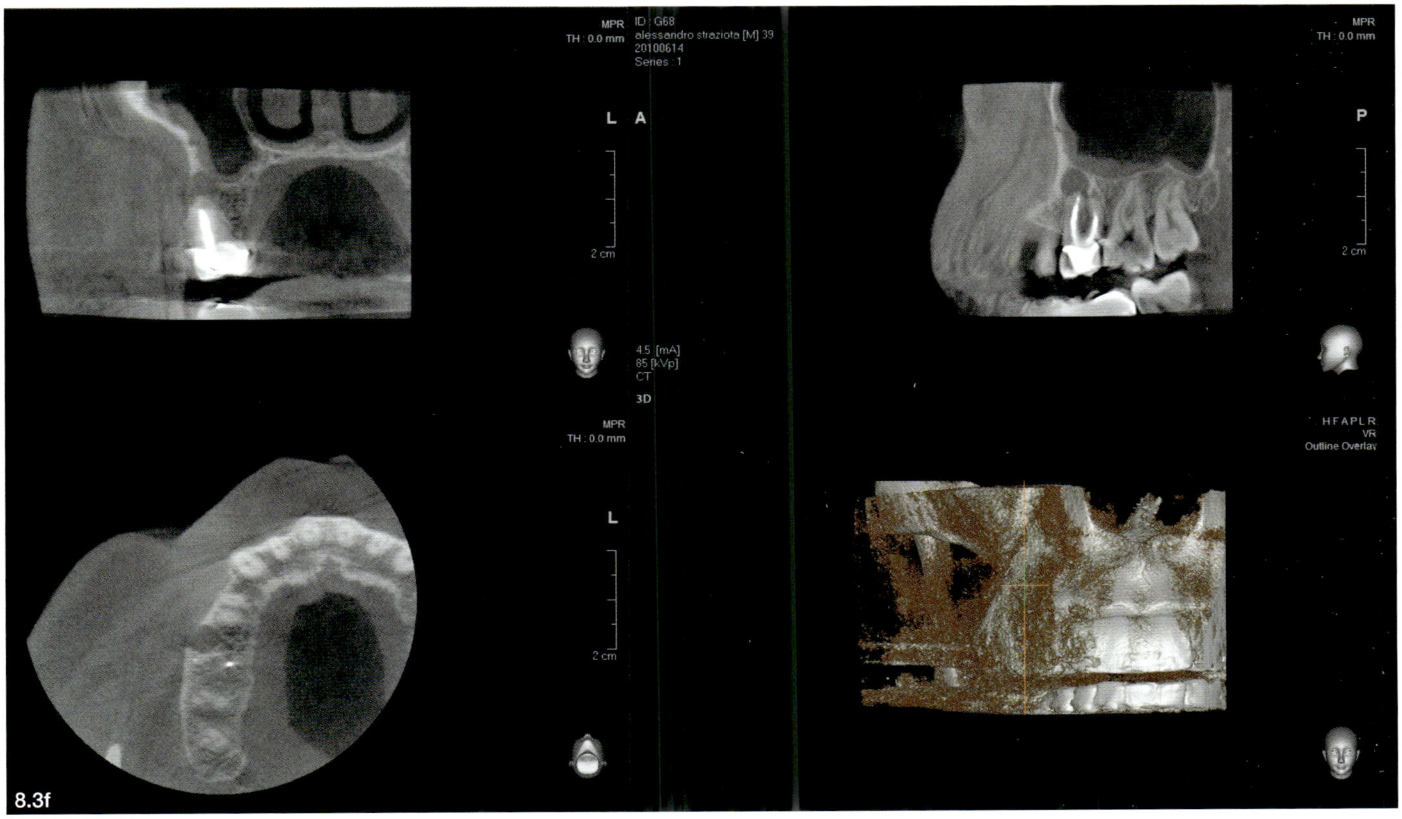

8.3f

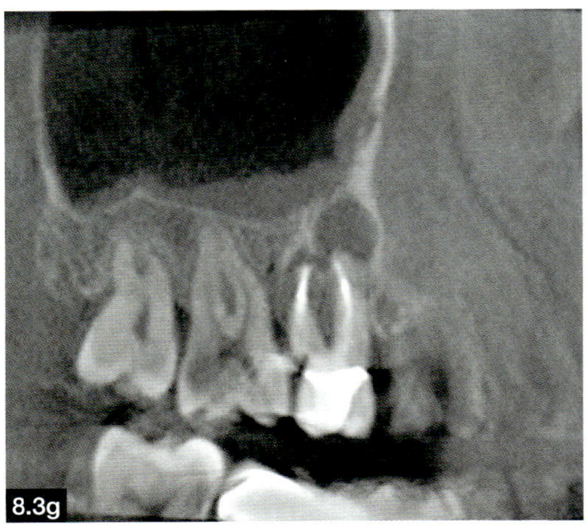

8.3g

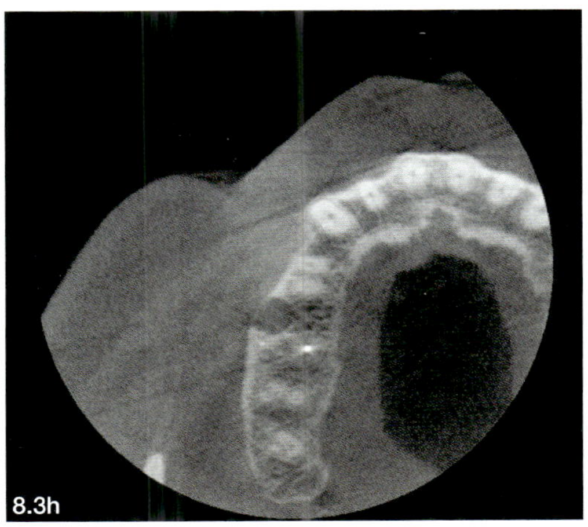

8.3h

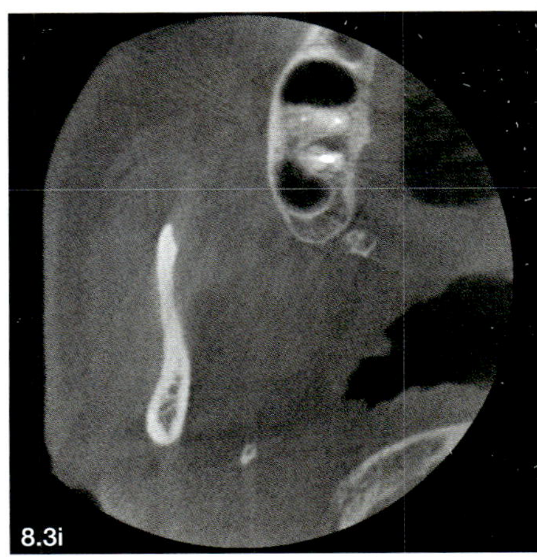

8.3i

Before proceeding with the surgery, adequate surgical access must be ensured: the patient must be observed with his mouth closed and cheeks wide apart, and the area of the operation must be visible and accessible.

The other features of the tooth to be evaluated are as follows:

1. fornix depth and bone thickness. The difficulty of surgical access depends on the inclination of the alveolar process. The operation will be more complex as the depth of the fornix decreases and as the parallelism between cortical bone and root axis decreases;
2. position and rotation of the teeth. In addition to the teeth involved in the operation, adjacent teeth should always be considered, as excessive proximity can cause damage to adjacent teeth during the operation. The more distal the position of the surgery area, the more difficult the task becomes for the operator;
3. relationship of apexes with at-risk structures (e.g., maxillary sinus and inferior alveolar nerve). An accurate diagnostic phase enables the operator to know the anatomy of the area concerned, to predict and prevent possible complications, and to avoid iatrogenic damage;
4. root length;
5. position and extent of the lesion.

❷ Premedication and anesthesia

In general, anesthesia is performed by infiltrating the vestibular fornix using an anesthetic with vasoconstrictor (articaine or mepivacaine with epinephrine 1:100,000-1:50,000) at room temperature. Injections should be slow (1 min per milliliter of liquid) to decrease patient discomfort, to prevent the formation of wheals in the area of surgery, and to promote diffusion of the molecule into deep tissues.
Thus, vasoconstriction is controlled, and an anesthesia adequate to the duration of the intervention is obtained[7].

❸ Mucosal access

Choice of flap type

The flaps used in surgical endodontics have a trapezoidal shape, with the major base arranged apically, and clean margins. The design usually includes a tooth anterior and posterior to the tooth to be treated. Some exceptions in this area of the mouth where the anatomy imposes variations are as follows:

1. in the upper and lower anterior segments, the flaps involve a greater number of teeth, because the presence of the interincisal frenum conditions

Table 8.4 **FLAPS FOR SURGICAL ACCESS**

Flap type	Features	Advantages	Disadvantages
Paramarginal flap	Good periodontal management of tissues Allows you not to expose the margins of any prosthetic restorations Can **only** be performed in the presence of at least 2-3 mm of adherent gingiva Must not involve periodontal pockets and fistulous routes	Cosmetic result	Limited vision of the operating area with consequent increase in the difficulty of the operation
Intrasulcular flap	Can be performed under all anatomical conditions	Improves the view of the operating area	Complex periodontal tissue management Less predictable healing in the presence of prosthetic margins
Combined flap	Combines an intrasulcular incision with another paramarginal incision	Allows the periodontium to be kept partially intact Excellent tissue stabilization	

the position of the releasing incisions which often fall between the lateral incisor and the canine[56, 57];

2. the area of the lower premolar, where the design of the flap is conditioned by the position of the mental foramen: the anterior incision must be positioned mesially or distally to the foramen to avoid damage to the inferior alveolar nerve.

The choice of flap type is influenced by periodontal and clinical factors. The most commonly used flaps in surgical endodontics are listed in Table 8.4.

Incision and detachment

Flap design is carried out by mapping the incision area and checking the depth of any pockets and the thickness of the adherent gingiva.
The flap should be precisely designed by using very small, sharp blades on both sides to allow first intention tissue healing once the surgery has been performed[57, 58].
Normally, when drawing the flap, the blade of the scalpel does not touch the bone plane; this makes it possible to keep the edge of the blade unaltered until the completion of the incision.
Only now can the full-thickness flap be detached using sharp blades (Ruddle or Pritchard curettes)[7] (Figs. 8.4a-8.4h).
Flap retraction can be performed with the most suitable instrument for the position of the flap itself, e.g., Columbia, Seldin, Pritchard, Henan, Carr, and Minnesota type retractors.

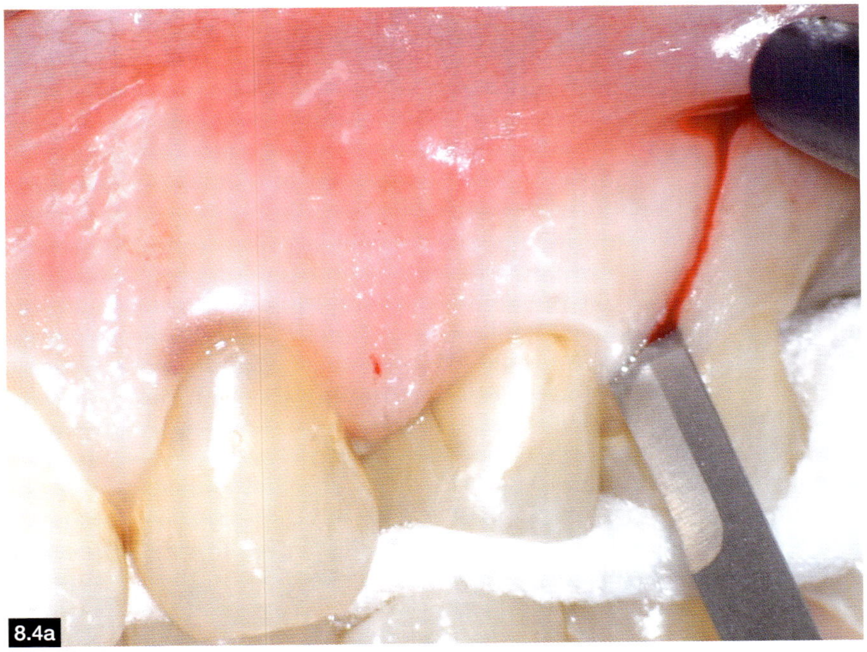

Fig. 8.4a: The flap is carved with a very sharp beaver scalpel, starting from the most distal portion.

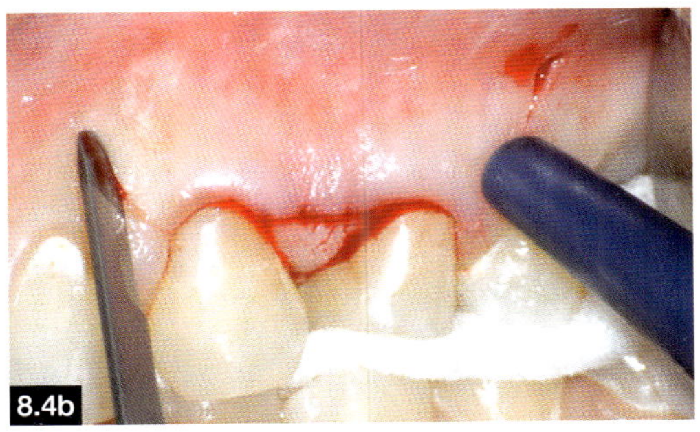

Fig. 8.4b: The flap extends for several teeth, preserving the papillae of teeth 23 and 24.

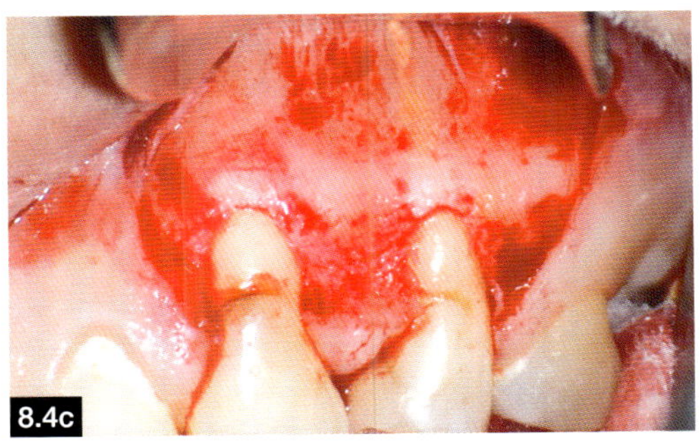

Fig. 8.4c: A periosteal elevator is used to separate the full-thickness flap and expose the root surfaces.

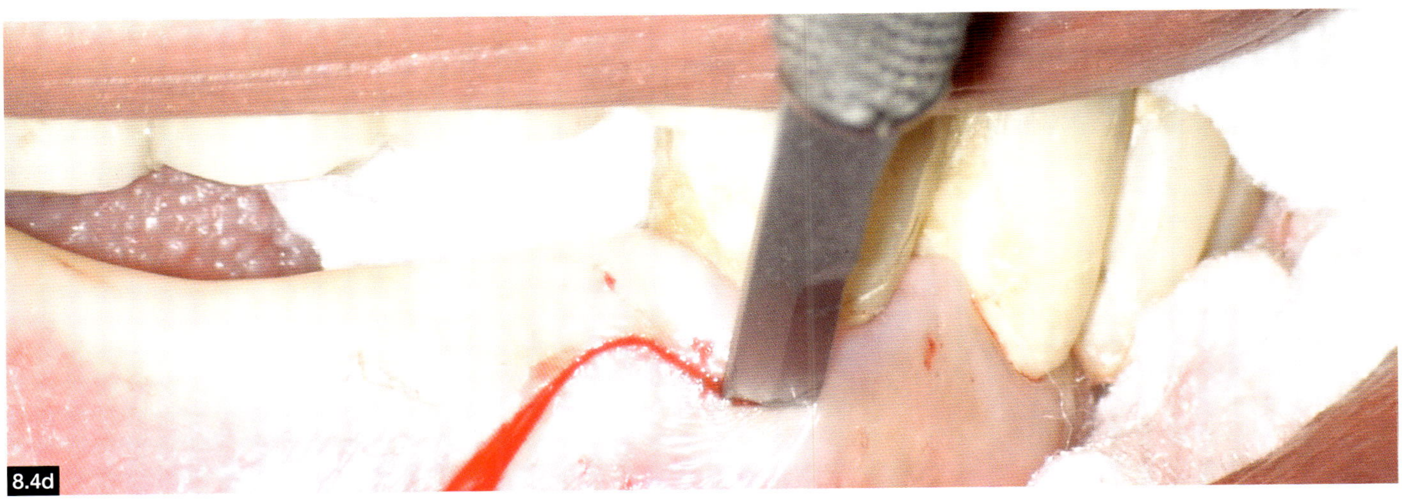

Fig. 8.4d: The scalpel never touches the bone plane to avoid blunting the blade.

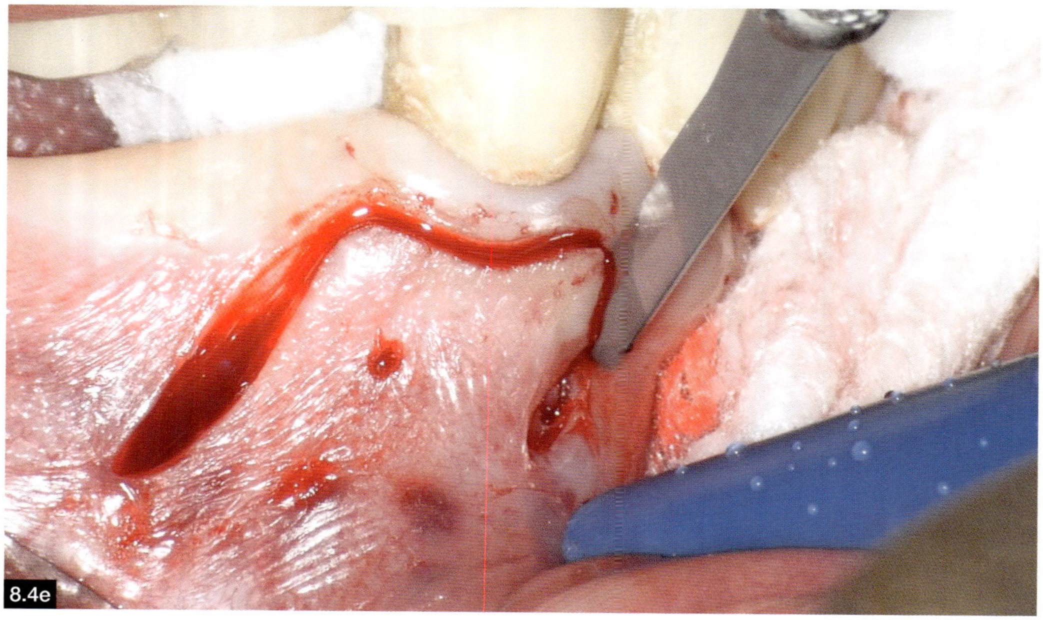
8.4e

Fig. 8.4e-h: The same principle applies to small flaps, where detachmentn is performed with a Ruddle curette.

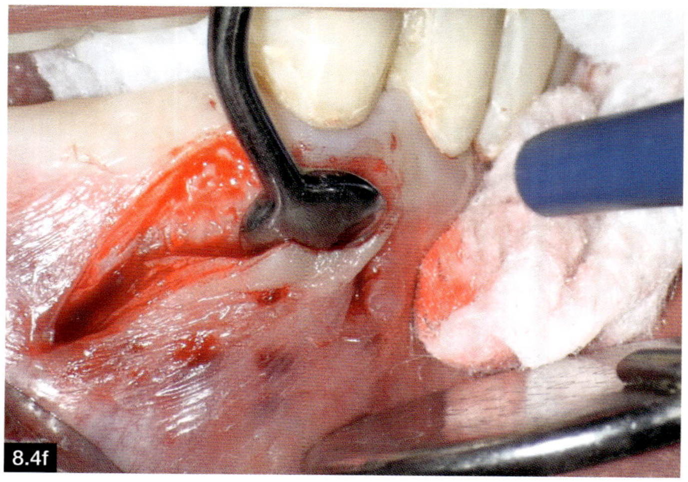
8.4f

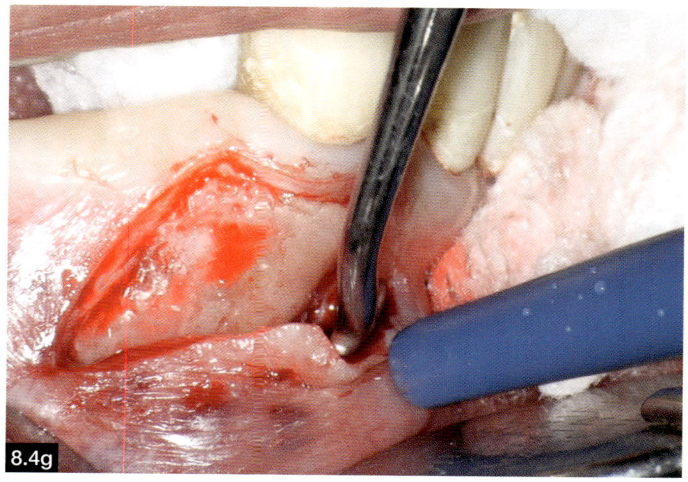
8.4g

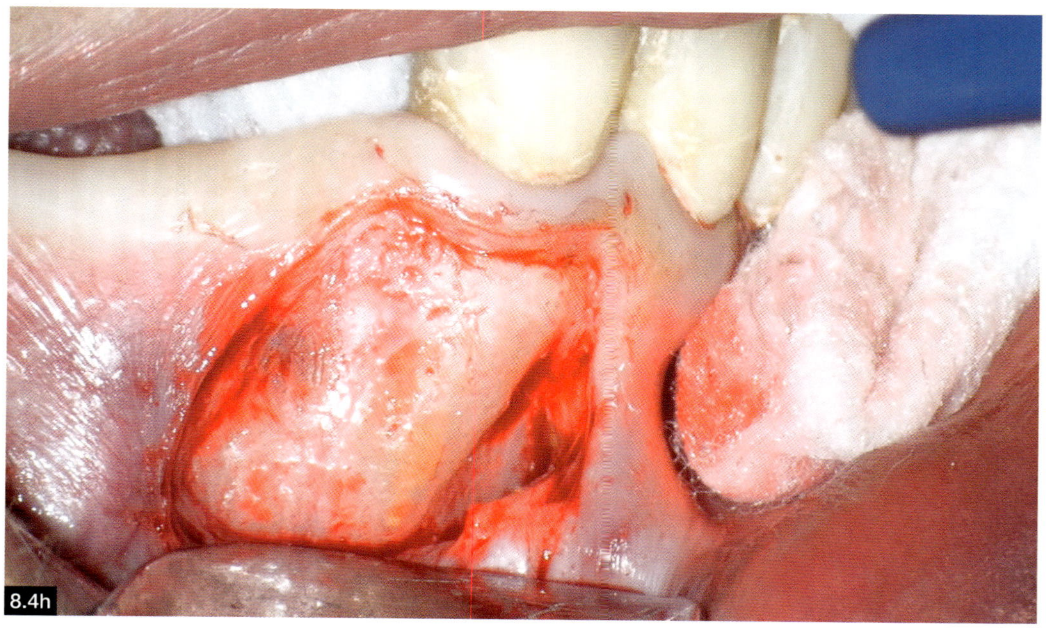
8.4h

Bone Breach

The bone breach is performed a couple of millimeters coronally of the estimated position of the apex of the root to be treated, using a straight hand piece and extra-long tungsten carbide burs with uncut blades (to achieve a smooth surface without disrupting the gutta-percha placed inside the root canals). When the bone breach is located near sensitive structures, the straight hand piece can be replaced with the *piezoelectric technique* (Figs. 8.5a-8.5m). In the first case, osteotomy and apical resection are performed simultaneously. In cases where piezoelectric surgery is used (when the cavity is very large), apical resection is performed later. Any cystic lesions or granulation tissues are enucleated by the use of surgical spoons (Figs. 8.5n and 8.5o). When the bone is being breached, the flap must be properly separated and the cheek must retracted and protected, so at least one assistant is necessary[59].

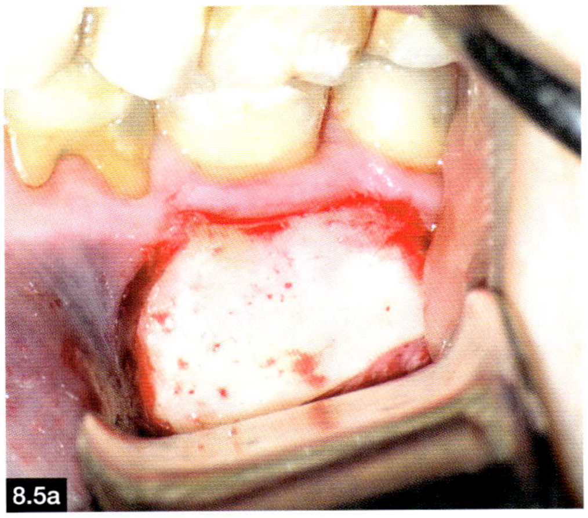

8.5a

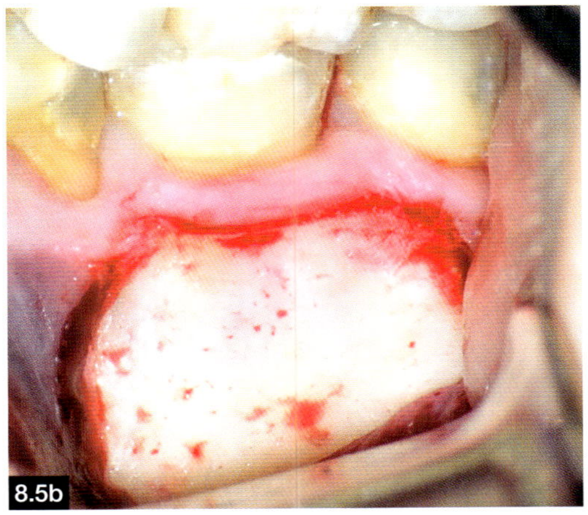

8.5b

Fig. 8.5a-b: The planning of surgical endodontics. The flap is sculpted and detached. On the basis of the evaluations carried out in the preoperative phase, it is possible to establish the position of the bone breach.

Fig. 8.5c: The bone breach is performed with burs mounted on a straight hand piece, with abundant irrigation.

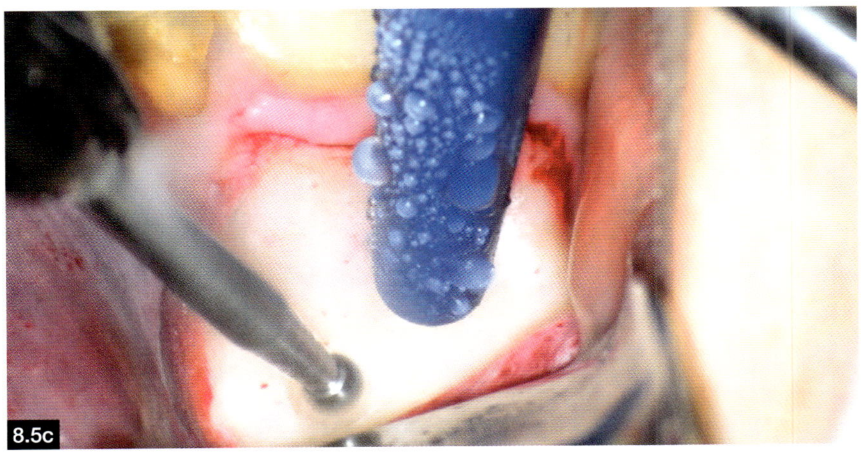

8.5c

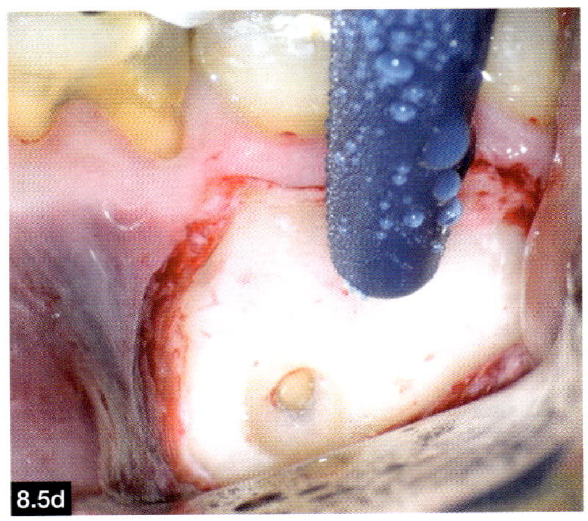

8.5d

Fig. 8.5d: After the first phase the apex of the mesial root is exposed.

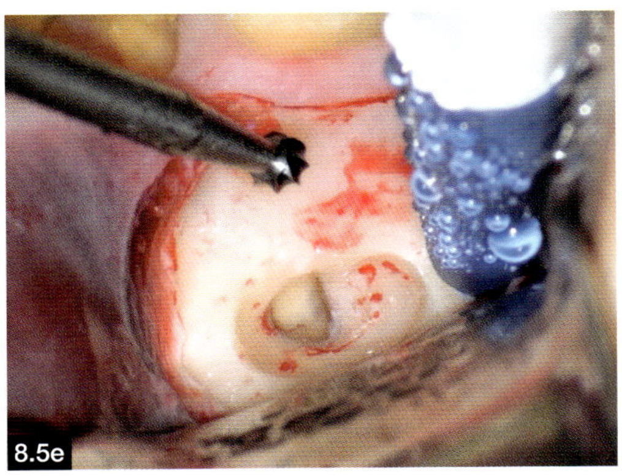

8.5e

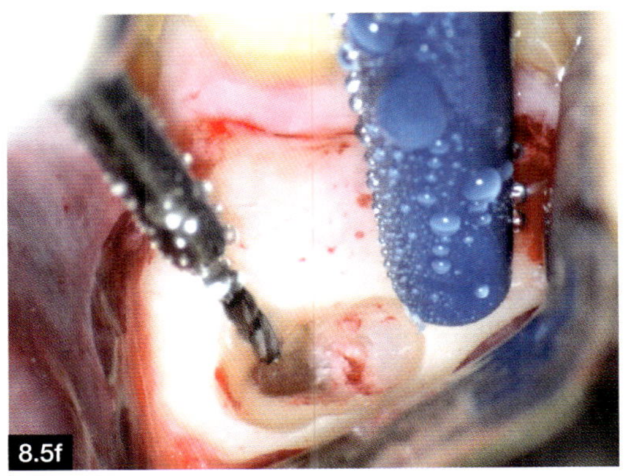

8.5f

Fig. 8.5e: The bone breach is extended for sufficient space to insert tools and allow them to work.

Fig. 8.5f: With a multi-blade bur, the resection phase of the apex begins.

Fig. 8.5g: Total apical resection is carried out on both the mesial and distal roots.

Fig. 8.5h: Methylene blue dye helps identify the canal anatomy.

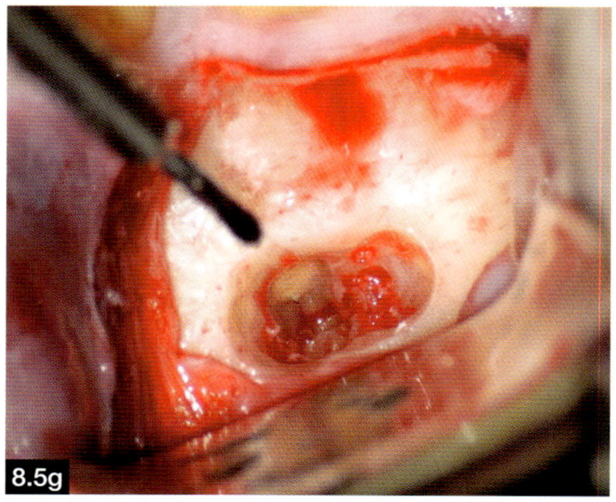

8.5g

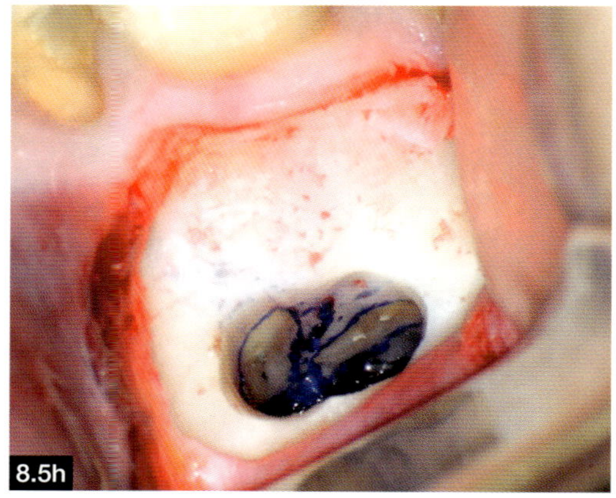

8.5h

Fig. 8.5i: Once the canal preparation has been carried out using ultrasonic inserts, the filling is completed with super EBA.

Fig. 8.5l: Bleeding control is essential to verify the efficiency of the work.

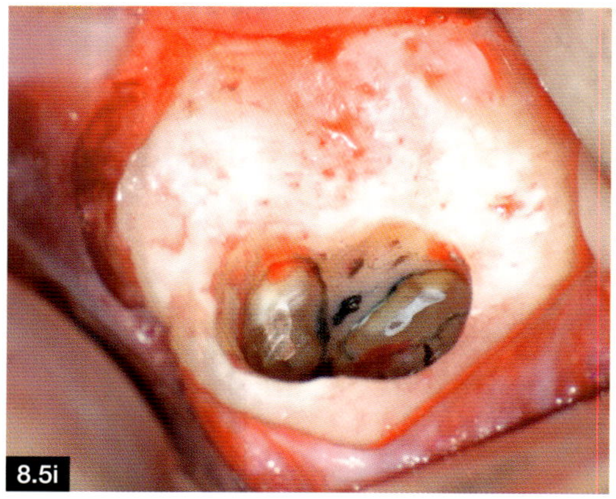

8.5i

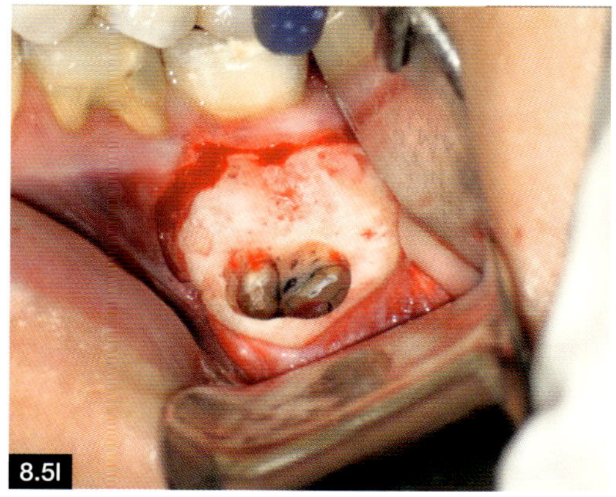

8.5l

Fig. 8.5m: The presence of a true cyst makes surgery on the tooth necessary.

Fig. 8.5n: Once the bone breach has been made, the enucleation of the cyst is carried out.

Fig. 8.5o: The cavity is evaluated, taking care to remove all the granulation tissue.

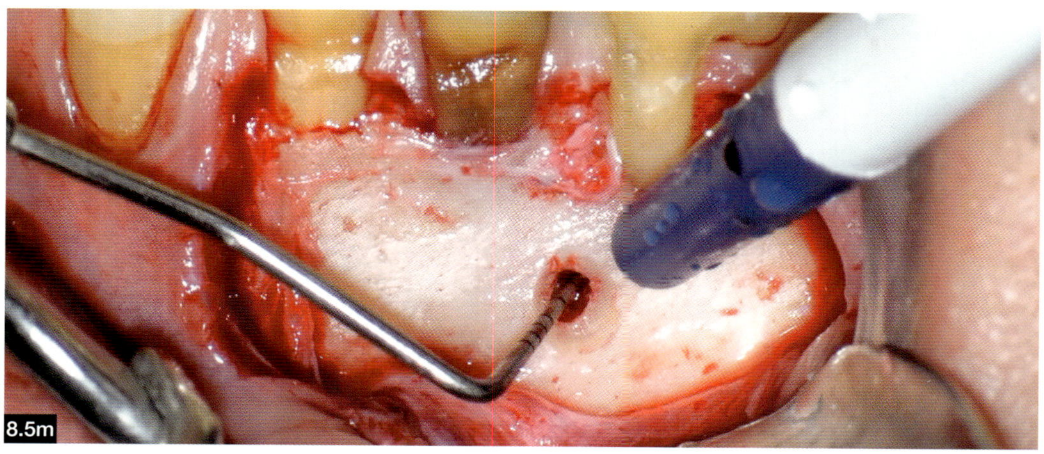

8.5m

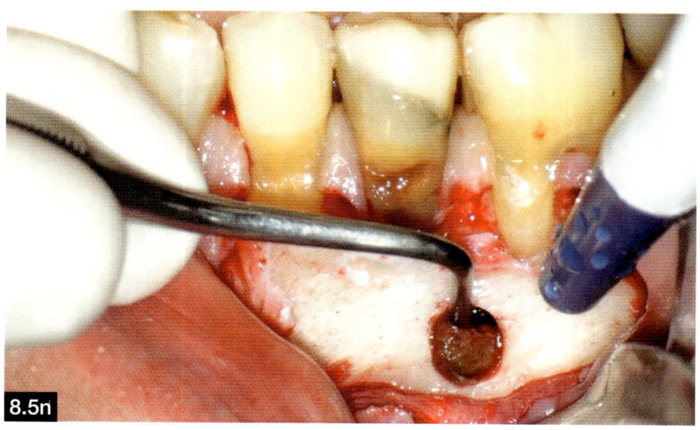

8.5n

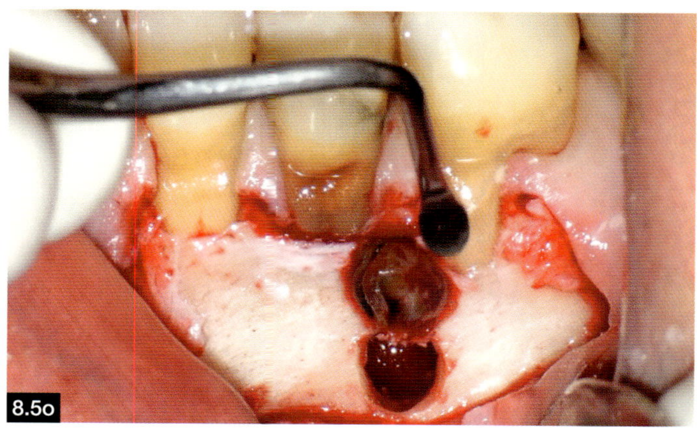

8.5o

❹ Apical resection

Normally, apical resection involves 2-3 mm of dental tissue. Ideally, to achieve favorable future prognosis, the root should be resected until healthy bone is obtained circumferentially around it.
There are clinical situations where this is not possible, such as in the presence of very large lesions or an unfavorable crown/root ratio. Performing apical resection at the same time as the osteotomy has the advantage of facilitating the subsequent phases, because the lesion is intimately attached to the root apex and removed with it as a whole.
Complete removal of the granulation tissue results, thereby facilitating the achievement of a clean surgical cavity[7].

❺ Retrograde cavity

Retrograde cavity design

Methylene blue provides a valuable aid to the clinician in identifying endodontic anatomy and selectively staining the endodontic system and periodontal ligament (Figs. 8.6a-8.6d). Once the canal system has been identified, the clinician must select the appropriate ultrasonic tip for the retrograde cavity; the choice of tip will depend on the position of the tooth, length, and angle of the root. There should be space between the osteotomy roof and the ultrasound tip to allow the latter to work optimally[7]. A correct retrograde cavity is parallel to the root axis (both mesio-distally and labio-lingually), respectful of the endodontic anatomy

Fig. 8.6a: Once the cavity has been made and the apex has been resected, the canal anatomy must be identified.

Fig. 8.6b: A micro brush is used to stain the cavity with methylene blue dye to highlight the organic component.

Fig. 8.6c-d: After washing and drying the cavity, the root canal is clearly visible at the center of the root.

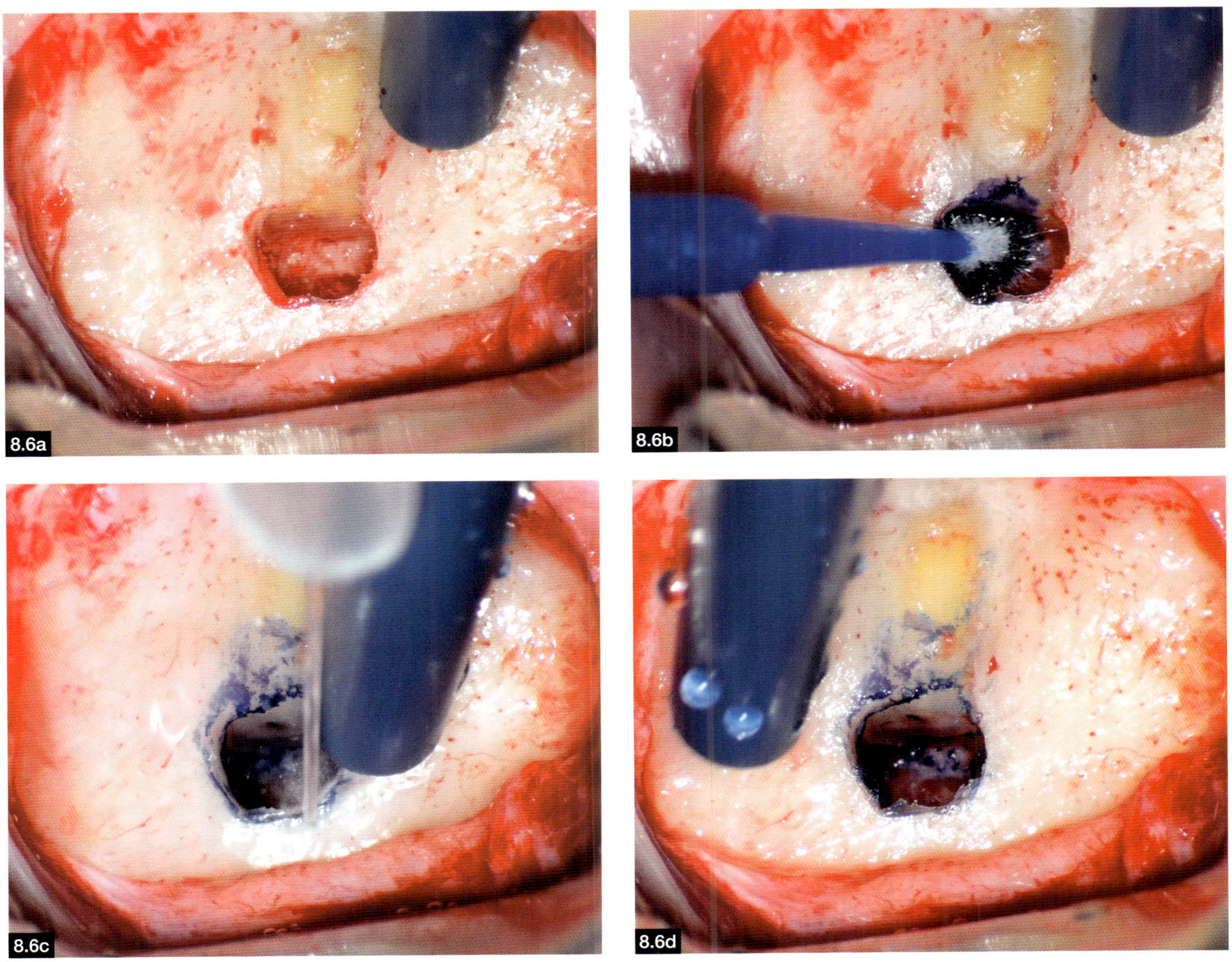

and as small as possible based on the extent of the endodontium (Figs. 8.7a and 8.7b). In general, the ultrasonic diamond tips used in this phase make it possible to obtain cavities 3-4 mm deep, with a cut slope between 0° and 10°, combining the action of the ultrasound with that of irrigation. Very precise and well-cleaned cavities are achieved, with a few exposed dentin tubules that are easy to fill, increasing the predictability of the therapy and reducing the risk of marginal infiltration[33]. For an optimal view of the treated area, we use micro-mirrors in sapphire glass or polished steel, which is an ergonomic and space-saving technique.

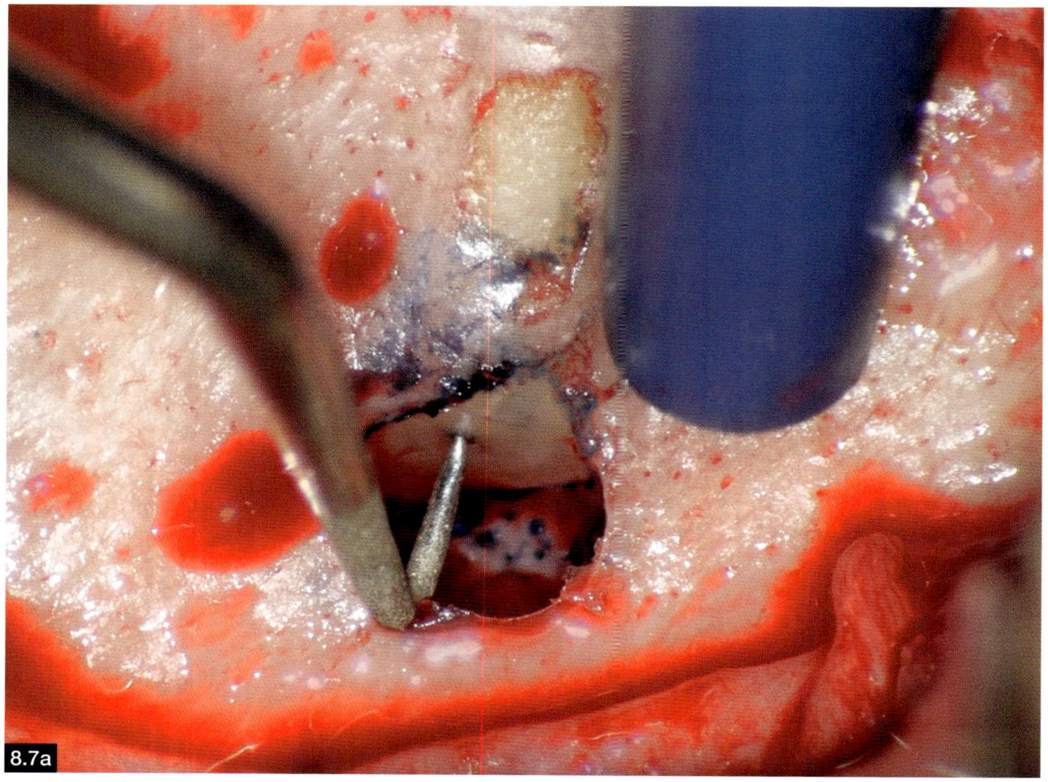

Fig. 8.7a: The cavity must be large enough to allow the ultrasonic retro tip to be inserted easily and to work without touching the edge of the bone breach.

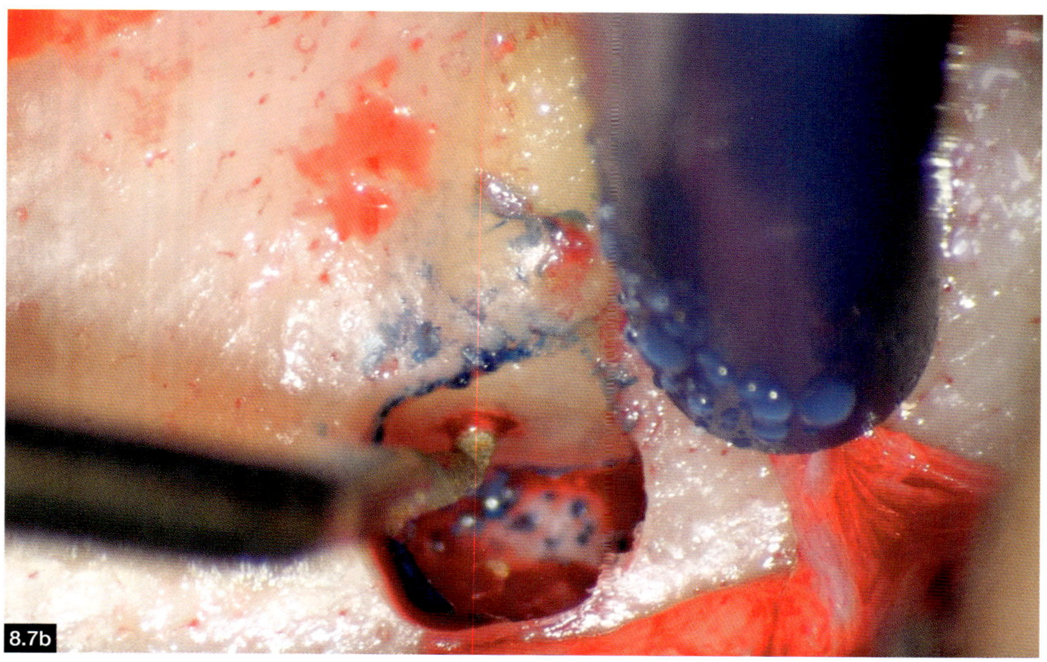

Fig. 8.7b: The ultrasonic insert penetrates the root canal, cleansing and shaping it in the same operational phase.

❻ Cleaning of the shaped space

Drying of the cavity and control of bleeding

Controlling bleeding is crucial for a good view of the root cavity and the preparation carried out and for positioning the filling material. The steps that allow adequate control of bleeding are

1. an effective anesthesia;
2. thorough elimination of the granulation tissue;
3. use of micro-suction;
4. use of small sterile gauzes and/or micro brushes soaked in ferric sulfate or aluminum chloride to cushion the area.

Before placing the filling, the clinician must ensure that the cavity has been properly prepared and dried.
The most effective system for drying a retrograde cavity is the Stropko irrigator, an insert to be fixed on an air-water syringe which, through an etching needle, allows air to be blown into the cavity, drying it in a few seconds (Figs. 8.8a and 8.8b).

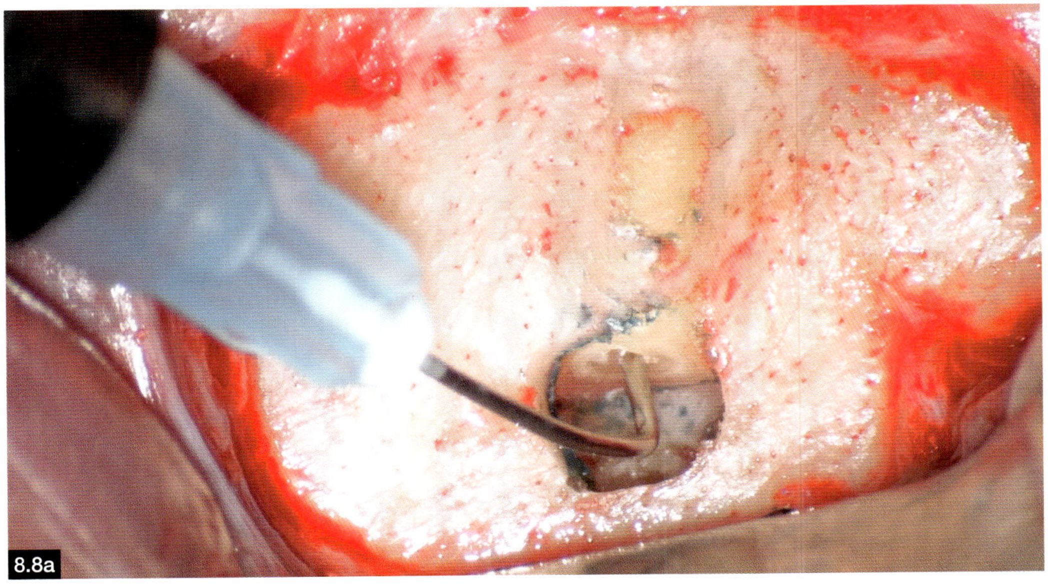

8.8a

Fig. 8.8a: The cavity should be dried to achieve a good seal. The use of the Stropko irrigator is essential for this.

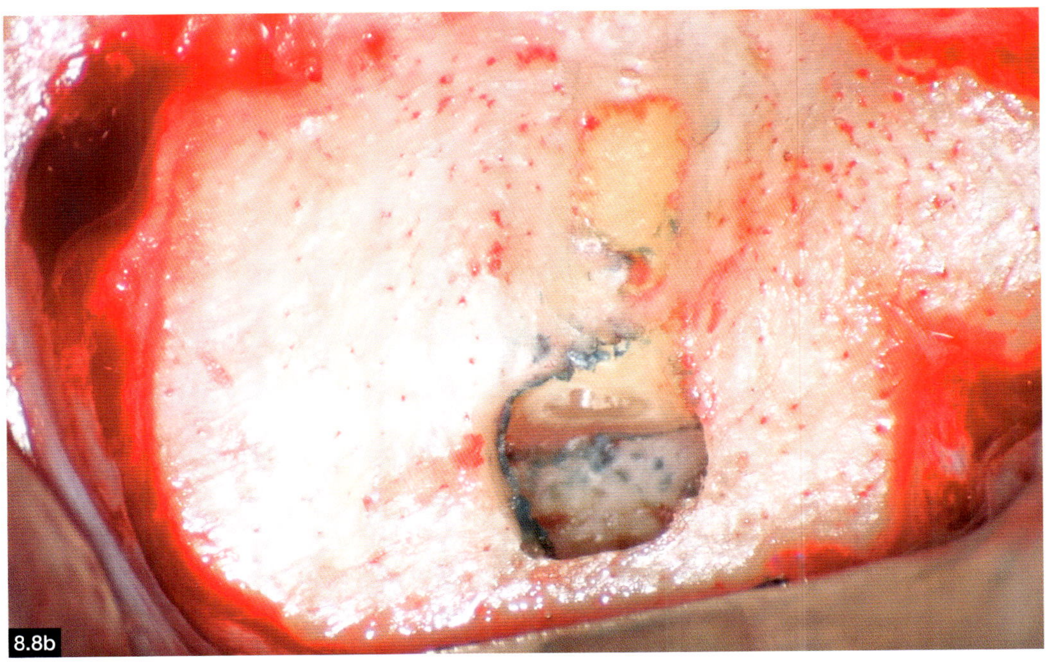

8.8b

Fig. 8.8b: Once it has been, cleansed and dried, the cavity is ready to receive the filling.

7 Retrograde filling

Retrograde seal

Materials for retrograde sealing

The quality and depth of the retrograde seal strongly influence the success rate of the therapy, especially the type of material used to perform retrograde filling. Currently, both Super EBA (zinc oxide eugenol cement, reinforced with alumina and enriched with ortho-ethoxybenzoic acid) and mineral trioxide aggregate (MTA) are used in surgical endodontics. Readers are referred to chapter 5 for an extensive description of their specific characteristics. From a strictly clinical point of view, the slightly different characteristics of the two cements direct their use: in extremely large cavities and where bleeding is difficult to control, Super EBA is more suitable. It is positioned by means of micro spatulas and condensed and burnished by means of pluggers until it hardens completely (which takes 4-5 min). The excesses are then removed, and the surface of the retrograde cavity can be finished with a multi-blade bur (Figs. 8.9a-8.9i). If, on the contrary,

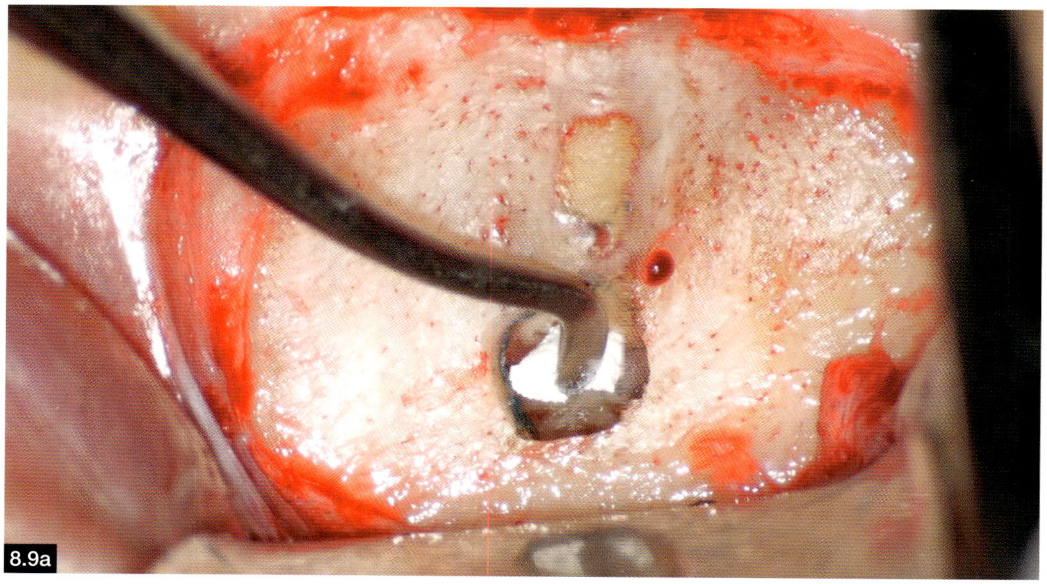

8.9a

Fig. 8.9a: Super EBA is positioned inside the cavity with the help of a small spatula.

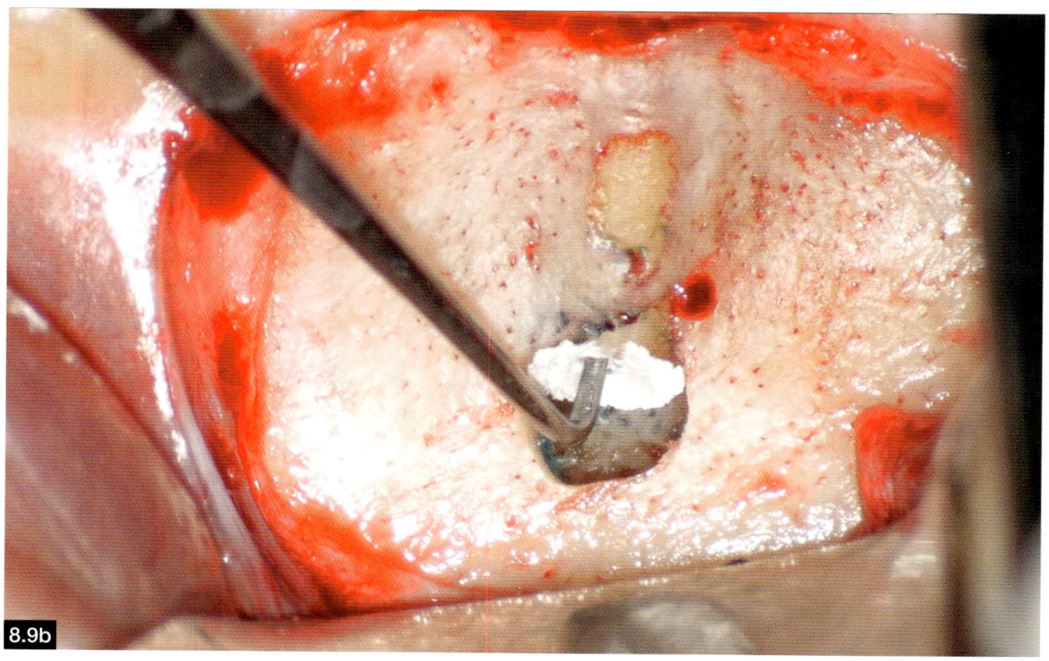

8.9b

Fig. 8.9b: During this phase, care must be taken to compact the material well for sufficient thickness of the retrograde filling.

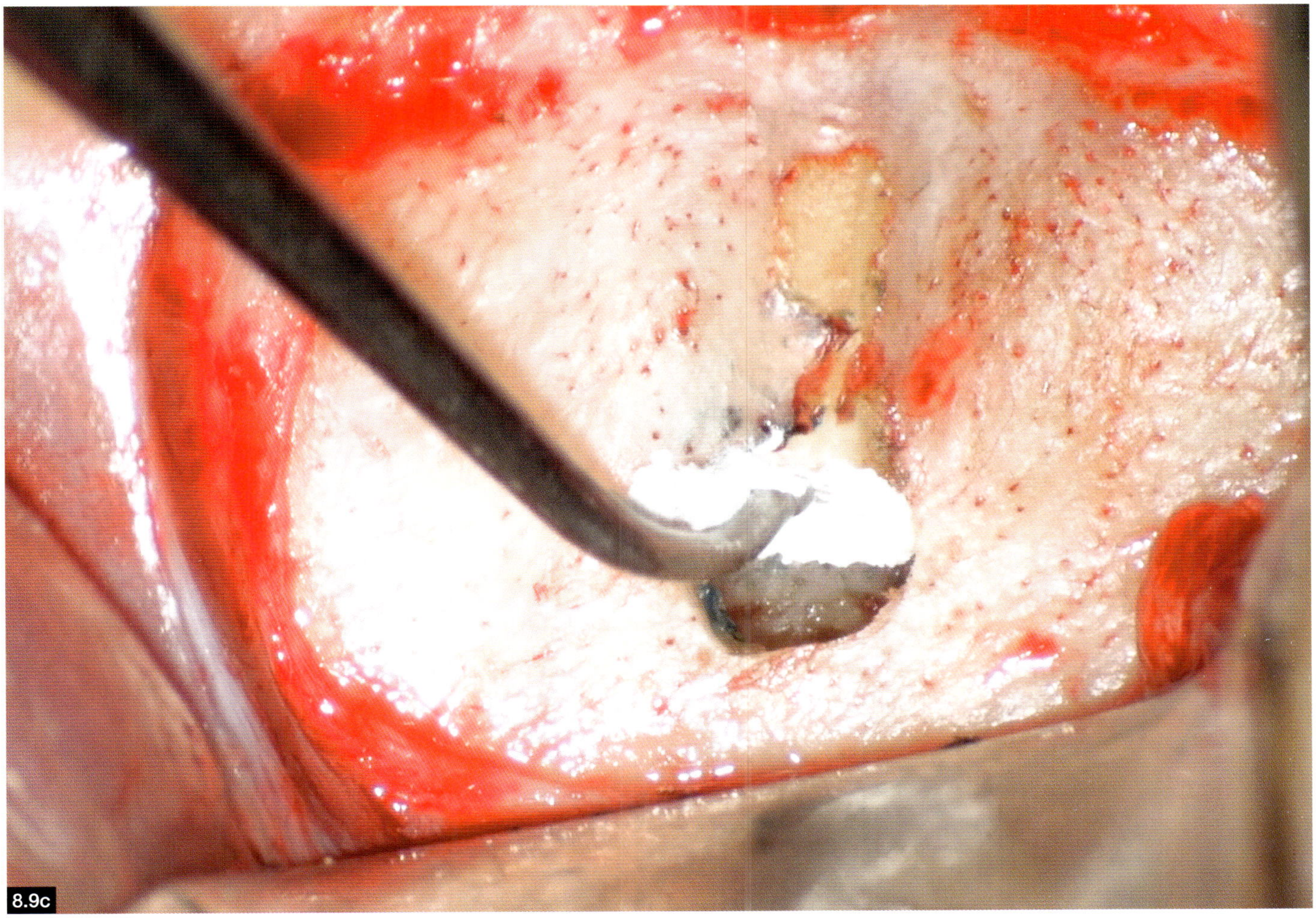

8.9c

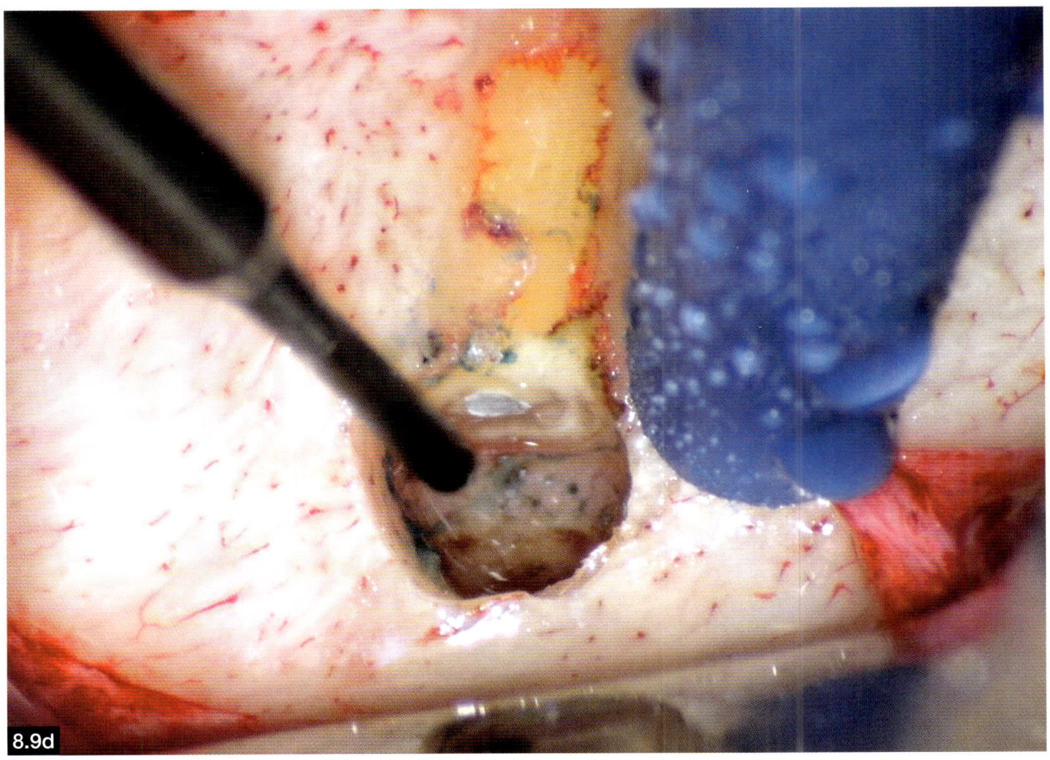

8.9d

Fig. 8.9c: It is necessary to continue compacting the material until the cavity margin is reached.

Fig. 8.9d: The filling is then burnished with the help of a multi-blade bur.

Fig. 8.9e-h: The cavity seen at different magnifications.
The apical seal the edges of the bone cavity and the general appearance of surgical access are visible. Having performed a correct filling, we may proceed to suture.

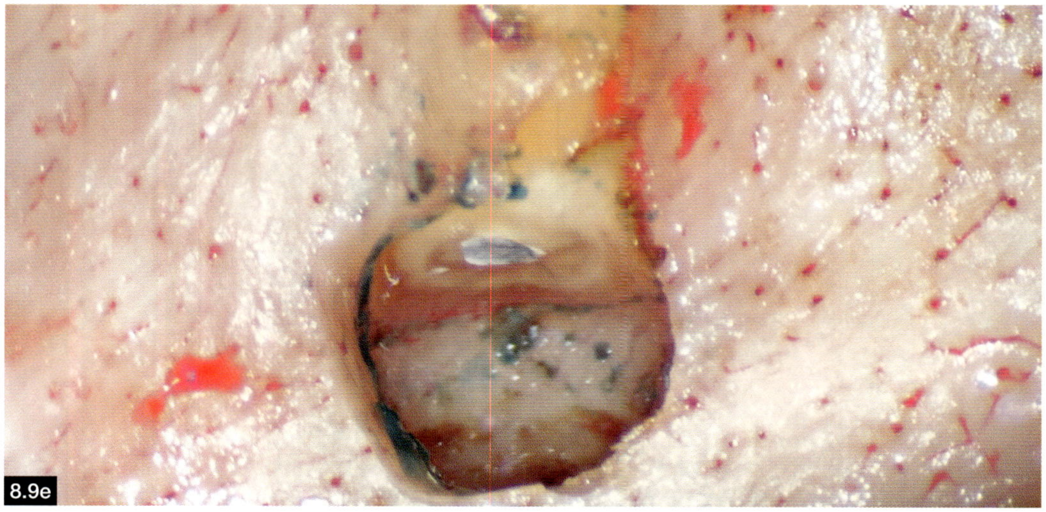

8.9e

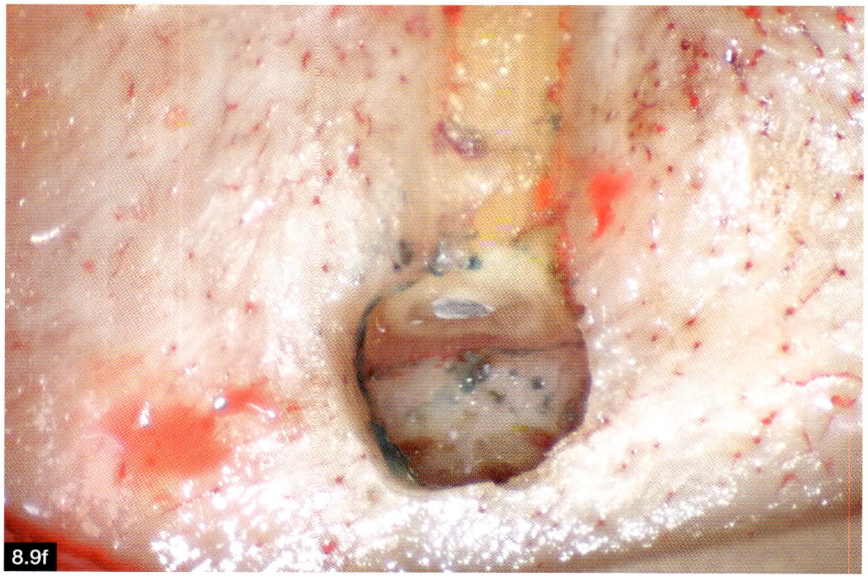

8.9f

the control of bleeding is good, it is possible to use MTA, which cannot be compacted in the presence of bleeding.
The latter condenses by placing small increments of cement in cavities using dedicated tools and compressing them with small pluggers.
Once the operation is complete, a cotton pellet soaked in sterile saline is used to moisten the material and adapt it to the cavity walls. A time between 3 and 48 h will be sufficient for the material to harden, depending on the type chosen[27, 49] (Figs. 8.9l and 8.9m).
Before suturing, the cavity should be allowed to bleed to remove material residues and facilitate the healing process.

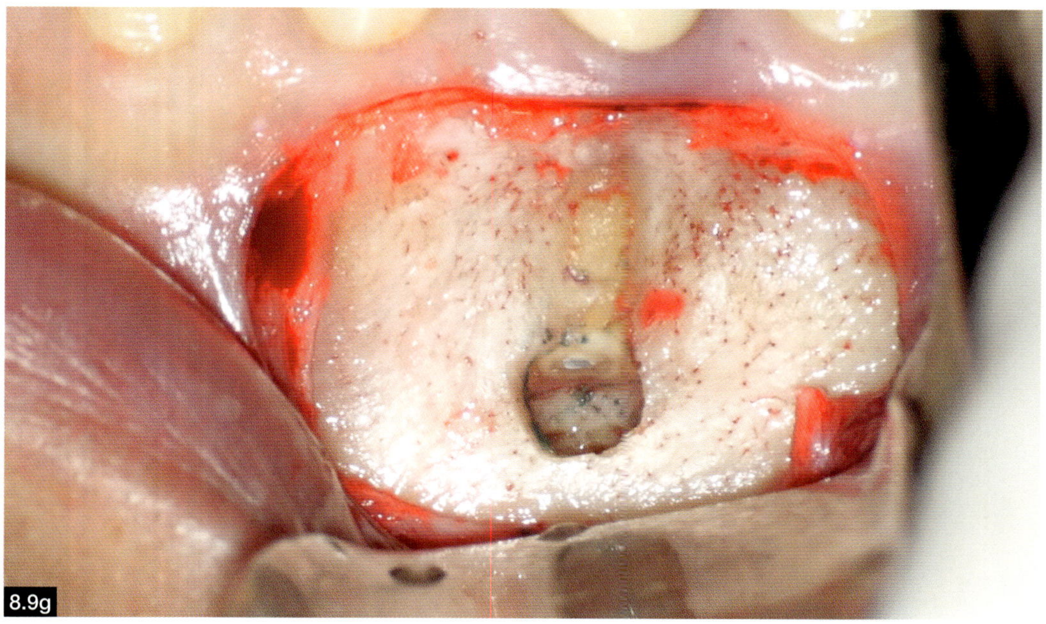

8.9g

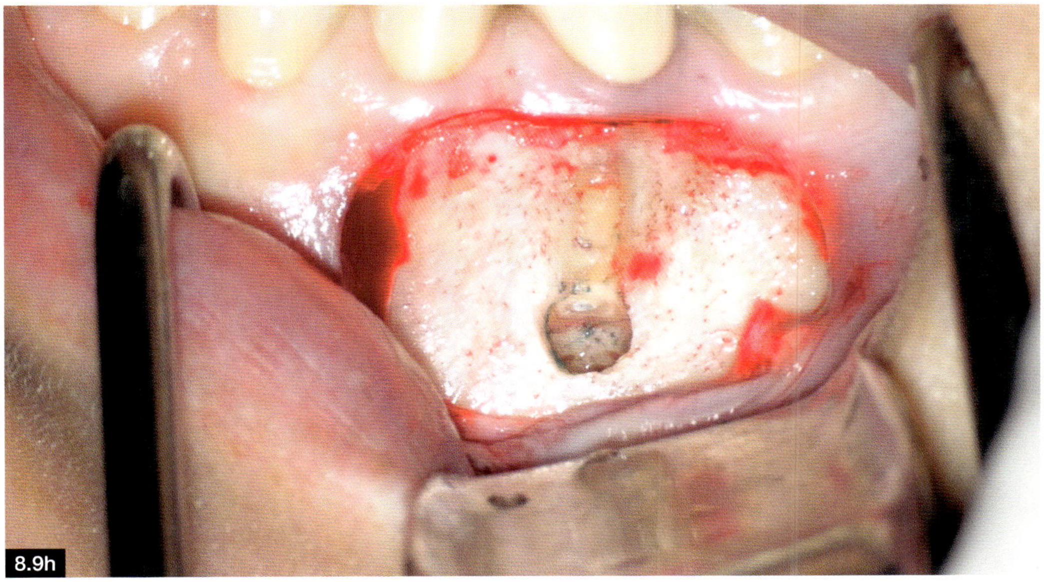

8.9h

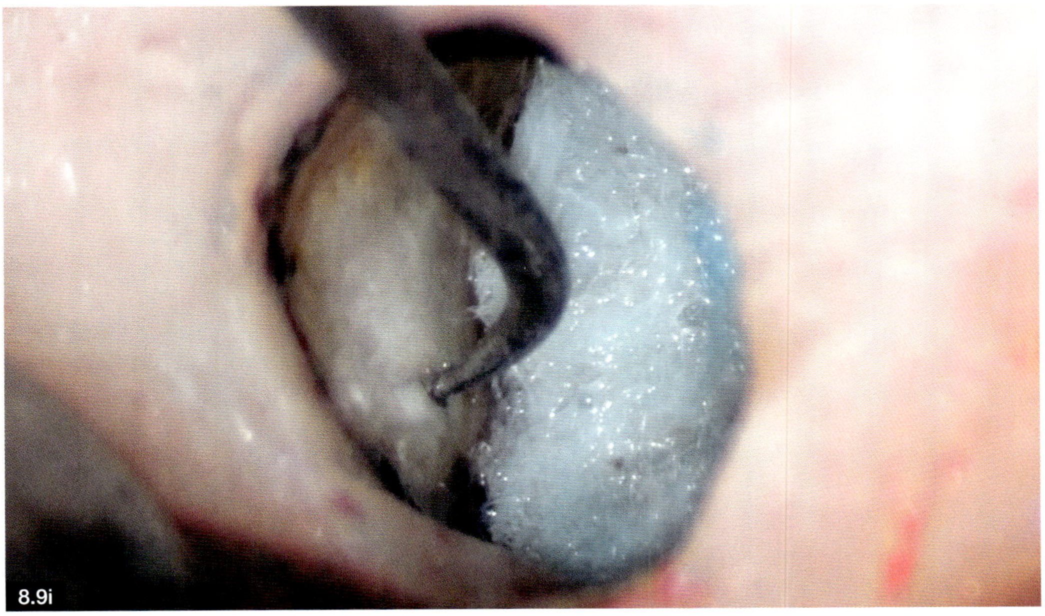

8.9i

Fig. 8.9i: The bone breach confirms the presence of two lateral canals, which are probably responsible for the endodontic lesion.

Fig. 8.9l: The canals are shaped and cleaned with the use of a diamond ultrasonic retro tip.

Fig. 8.9m: The two canals are then filled with Super EBA.

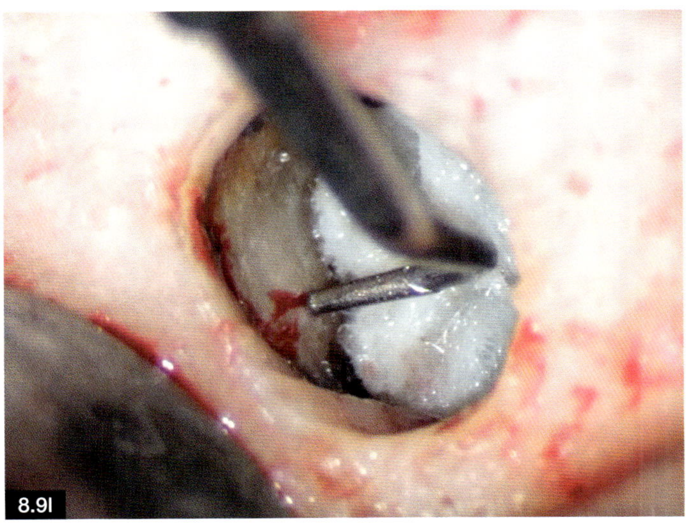

8.9l

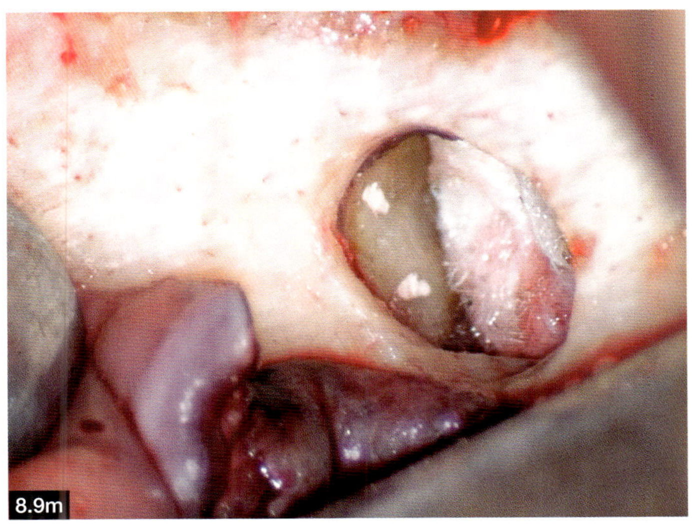

8.9m

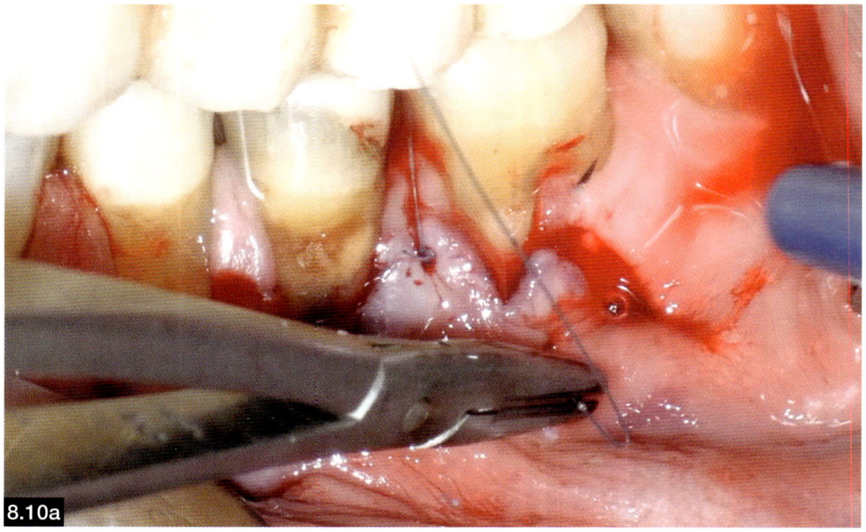

8 Suture

A correct suture is crucial for the success of the operation: we recommend a very thin monofilament, 5/6 0, to perfectly match the flap.

To achieve first intention healing, start suturing at the top of the vertical incision and then continue coronally (Figs. 8.10a-8.10d).

When using a thin, extremely rigid synthetic suture, you can round off the ends of the wire with a heat carrier to avoid traumatizing the patient. Normally, the suture is removed after 7-10 days, but early removal is advisable in esthetically relevant areas[7].

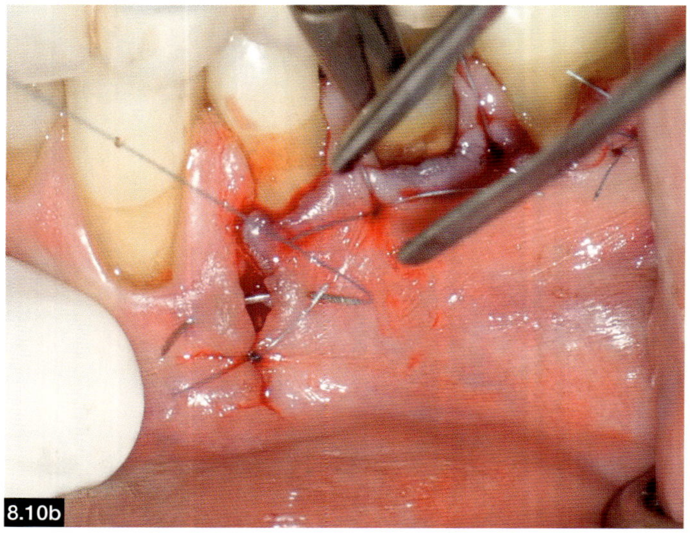

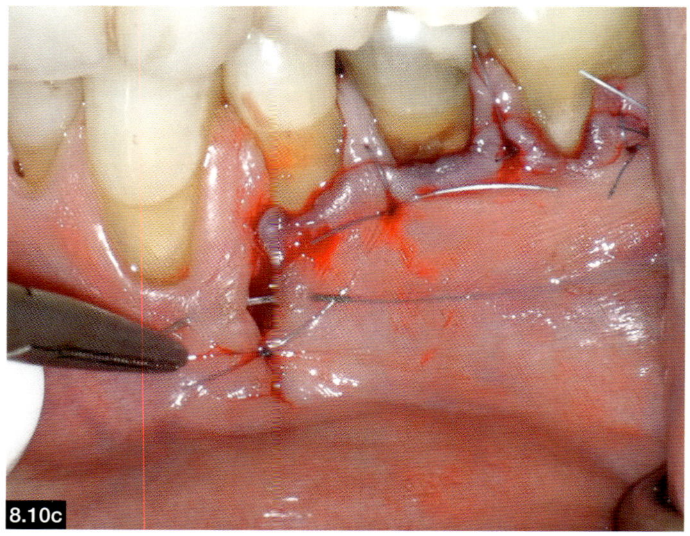

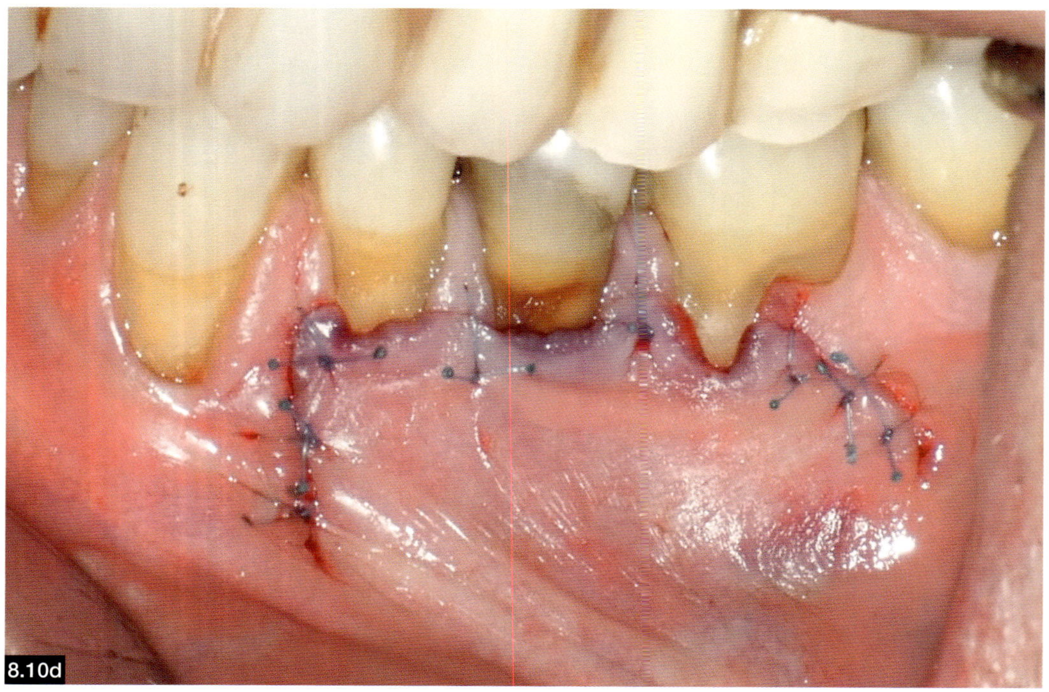

Fig. 8.10a: Suturing is a delicate step of therapy, because the goal is to achieve first intention healing without scars. A thin monofilament, 5/6 0, is used, with an interrupted stitch technique. The first suture is generally located in the most distal part of the incision.

Fig. 8.10b: We proceed with the suture with interrupted stitches, after repositioning the edges of the flap.

Fig. 8.10c: We then focus on the release incision.

Fig. 8.10d: Once suturing is completed, the ends of the wire may be rounded with a heat carrier to ensure greater postoperative comfort for the patient.

Follow-up and evaluation of success

A first indication of the success of the therapy is a total lack of symptoms or fistulas. Follow-up evaluations are generally performed by periapical radiographs carried out at 4, 8, and 12 months after surgery.

Surgical endodontics is a therapeutic procedure of proven efficacy for treating teeth with or without periapical lesions, particularly when the case is complex or it is impossible to intervene endodontically[23, 24, 26, 31]. The considerable improvements made to the technique, thanks to the advent of new technologies, have contributed to making the procedure more conservative, predictable, and rapid[7, 16, 20] through the use of ultrasonic tips that allow the execution of conservative preparations and the use of biocompatible cements, which allow us to achieve a good seal even in a moist environment.

A study has highlighted the factors that positively influence the success of endodontic surgery, including the filling material, the type of tooth treated, and the sex of the patient. Table 8.5 summarizes the most significant factors that contribute to the success of endodontic surgery[60].

The skill of the operator, the use of the operating microscope, and the correct clinical indication for the use of surgery should not be overlooked.

Table 8.5 **FACTORS ASSOCIATED WITH A SIGNIFICANT INCREASE IN THE HEALING RATE[56]**

Absence of preoperative pain	
Good material density in the canal filling	
No periapical lesions or lesion size less than or equal to 5 mm	
Use of magnifying devices	These improve the vision of the operating field and facilitate the recognition of the canal system, accessory systems, and any fracture paths. There is no article in the literature that indicates a statistically significant difference between the outcome of a therapy performed with or without magnifying devices, but the healing rates using the surgical microscope are higher than those of treatments performed without the aid of this instrument.
Use of ultrasound inserts	These allow precise preparations to be made that respect the endodontic anatomy, making it easier for the clinician to carry out the treatment
Filling materials	Super EBA and MTA, when used according to the indications, have similar reported results but they are far better than those obtained with other filling materials (e.g., silver amalgam and glass ionomer) due to their biocompatibility and the peculiarity of hardening even in the presence of moisture

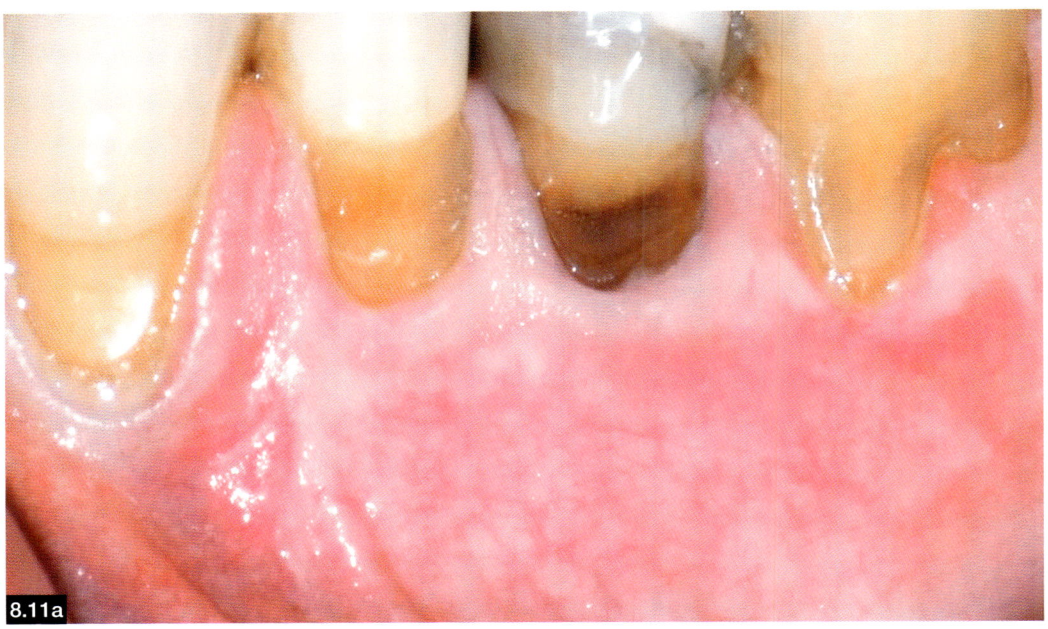

8.11a

Fig. 8.11a: Stability one year after the operation, showing the maturation of the tissues.

Fig. 8.11b: Healing of the soft tissues occurred by first intention.

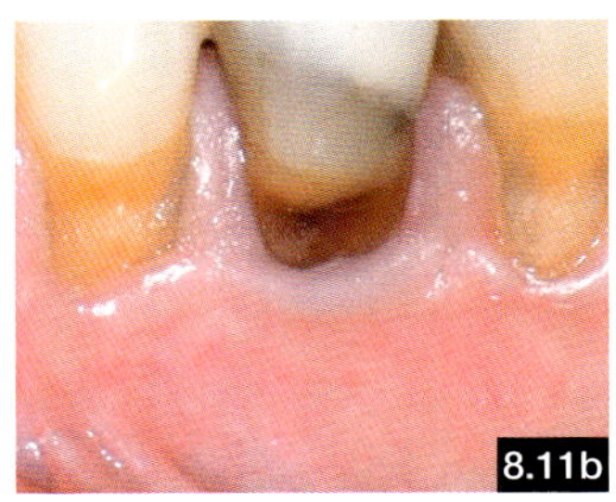

8.11b

CASE REPORT 2

Surgical retreatment

As already mentioned in the initial part of this chapter, several studies have reported the success rate of primary surgical endodontic treatments; however, there is a possibility that an unsuccessfully treated tooth can be retreated using the same surgical approach. On teeth in which there has been no success, we can retreat following another surgical procedure. This method, if carried out with suitable techniques and materials, has a success rate that is almost identical to that reported for primary treatments.

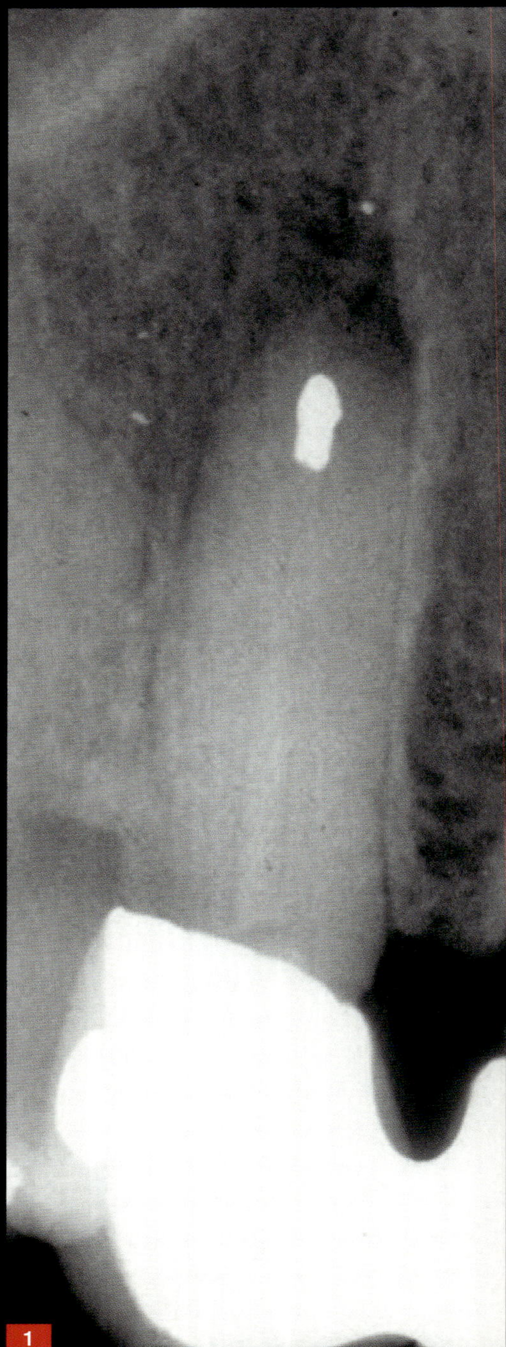

1

Figure 1: An old endodontic surgery performed with the use of silver amalgam resulting in a periapical lesion.

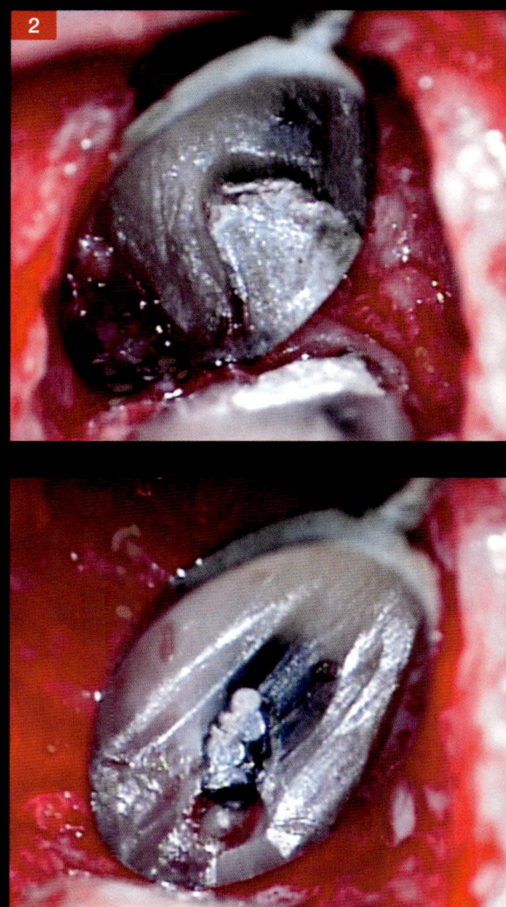

2

Figure 2: After opening the bone breach and isolating the root apex, the amalgam cap is exposed and progressively removed until the root canal is visible.

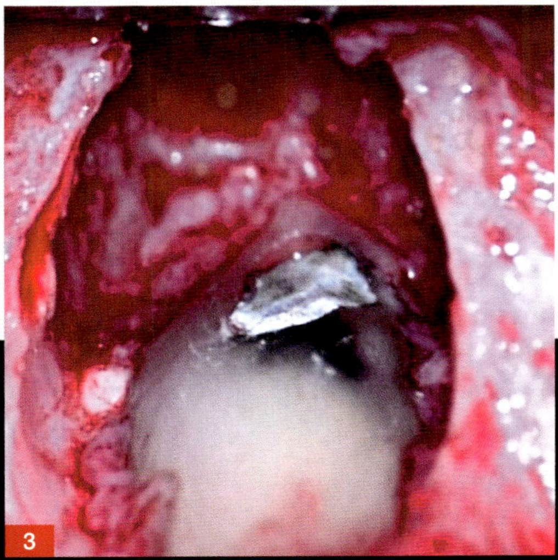

3

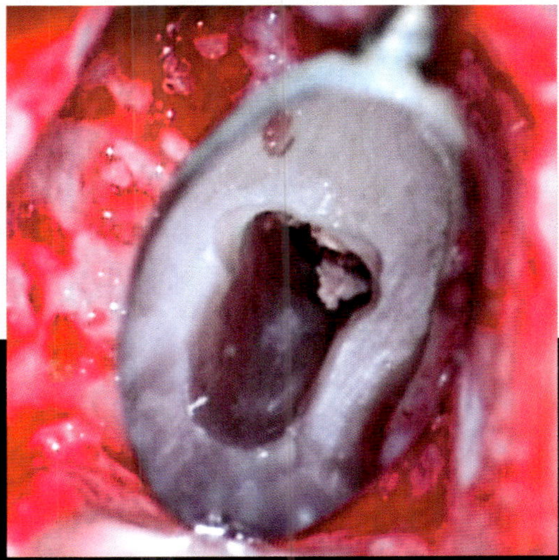

Figure 3: The complete elimination of the previous retrograde filling has resulted in the creation of a new very large cavity that must be completely cleaned before filling.

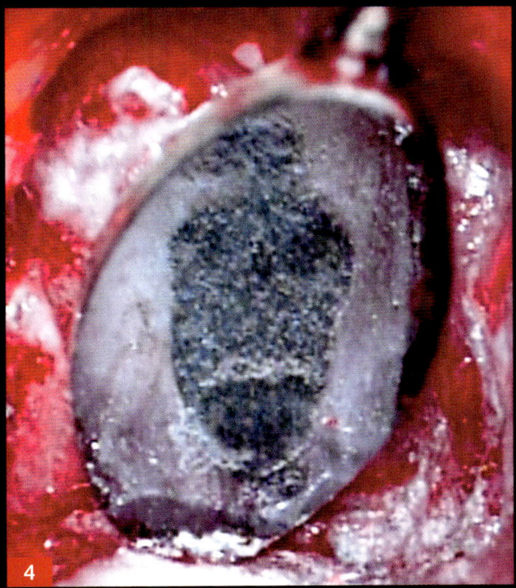

4

Figure 4: Detail of the apical filling performed with MTA, the material of choice, which is highly biocompatible, and has ideal sealing properties for this type of treatment.

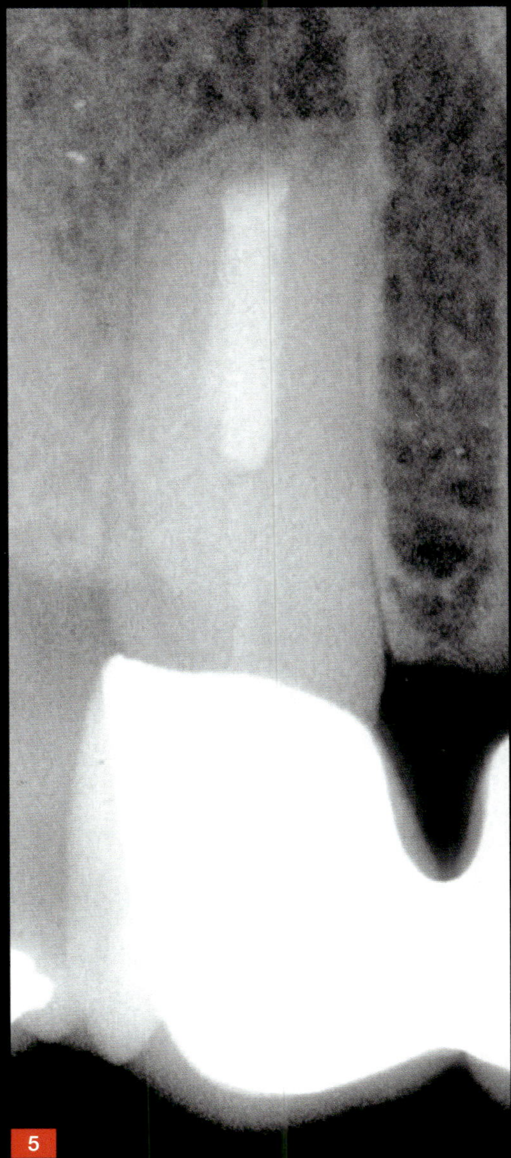

5

Figure 5: Follow-up appointments confirmed the perfect healing of the periapical tissues.

CASE REPORT 3

Surgical treatment of a lesion supported by lateral canals

The presence of a lateral lesion is often associated with the presence of large lateral canal but are frequently sustained by an incomplete shaping, cleaning and filling of the principal canal. When a large lateral canal is part of the endodontic pace it may permit the survival of bacteria and maintain a periapical lesion of endodontic origin. In this case a clear radiolucency was

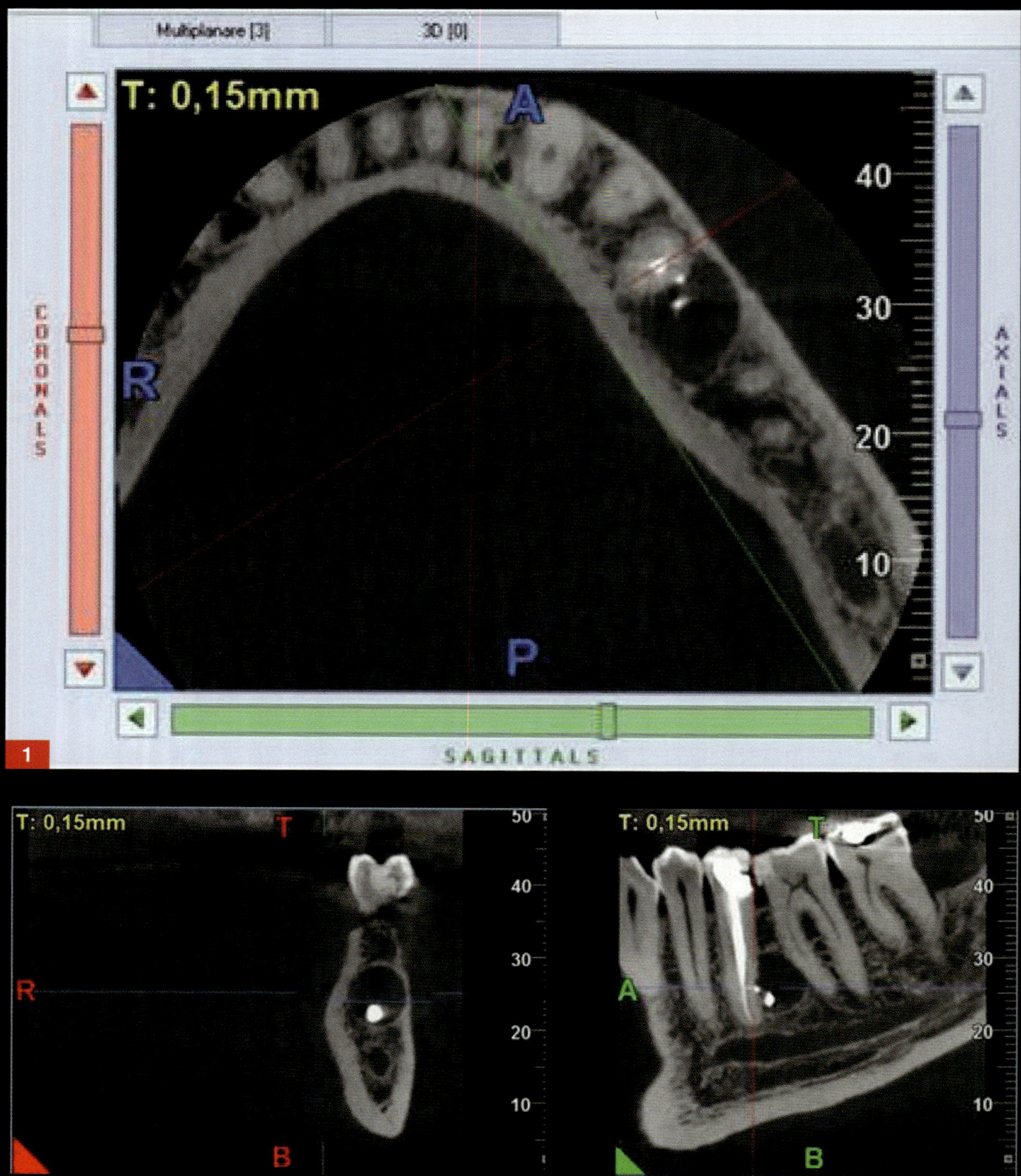

Figure 1: Preoperative CBCT shows that the lesion only affects the distal portion of the root and that the existing endodontic treatment is objectively good.
Given the particular location of the lesion, the presence of a foreign body inside it and the probable presence of an untreated lateral canal, it is decided to perform endodontic surgery only on the distal portion of the tooth, without apical resection.

detected in the lateral aspect of a premolar. The root canal treatment was well-executed and both an orthograde retreatment or a classic surgical endodontic treatment were considered not suitable. For this reason, a surgical approach has been adopted to cover the area affected by the lesion, curetting the radicular surface and the surrounding bone.

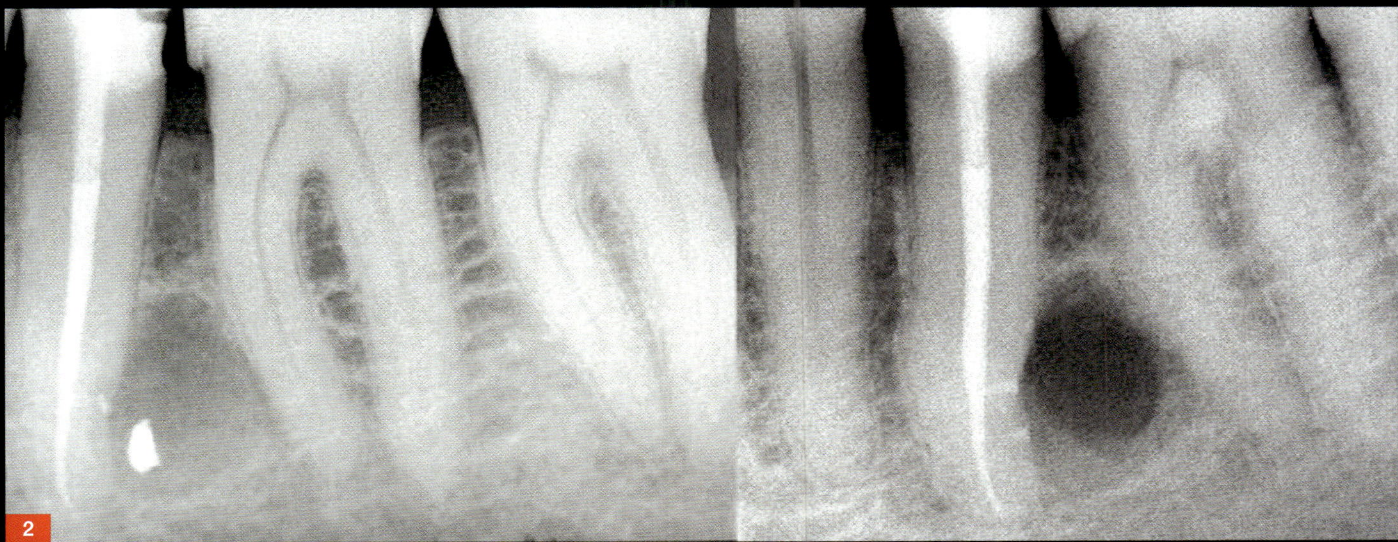

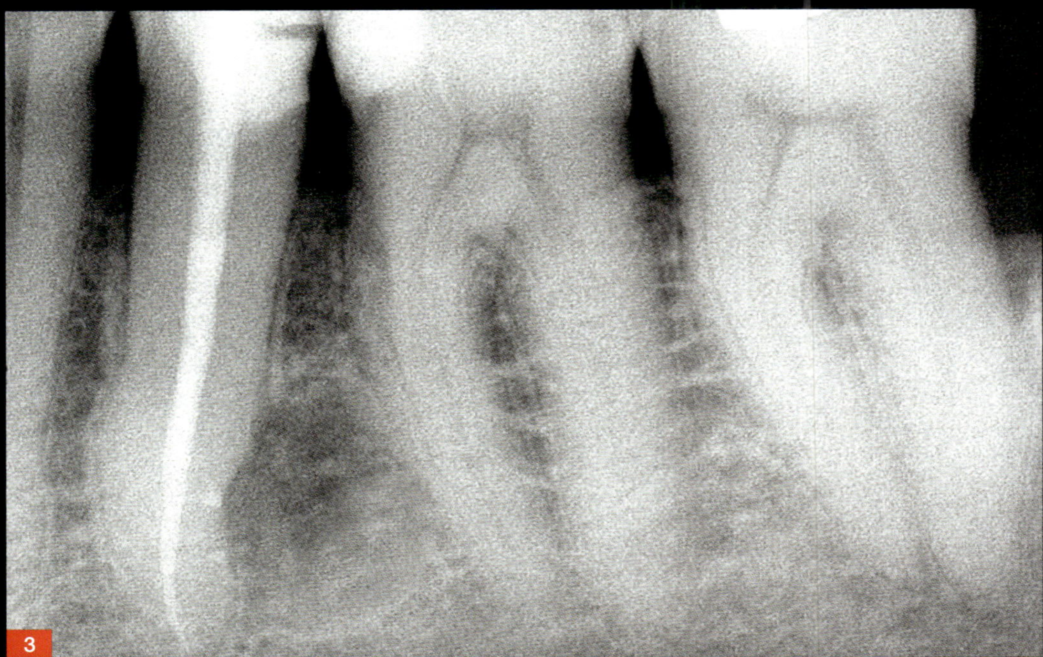

Figure 2: The pre- and postoperative x-rays show that the foreign body was removed and that two lateral canals were shaped, cleansed and filled.

Figure 3: The follow-up x-ray at 6 months shows that the tooth is healing and the lesion has disappeared almost completely.

References

1. Gutmann J, Harrison J. *Surgical endodontics. Boston: Blackwell Scientific Publications;* 1991.
2. Kim S, Pecora G, Rubinstein R. *Microsurgery in endodontics. Philadelphia: WB Saunders Company*; 2001.
3. Ng Y, Mann V, Rahbaran S, et al. *Outcome of primary root canal treatment: systematic review of the literature - part 1. Effects of study characteristics on probability of success.* Int Endod J. 2007;40(12):921-339.
4. Fleming C, Litaker M, Alley et al. *Comparison of classic endodontic techniques versus contemporary techniques on endodontic treatment success*. J Endod. 2010;36:414-418.
5. Peterson J, Gutmann J. *The outcome of endodontic surgery: a systematic review*. Int Endod J. 2001;34(3):169-175.
6. Chércoles-Ruiz A, Sánchez-Torres A, Gay-Escoda C. *Endodontics, Endodontic Retreatment, and Apical Surgery Versus Tooth Extraction and Implant Placement: A Systematic Review*. J Endod. 2017;43(5):679-686.
7. Gorni FGM. *Manuale di Endodonzia.* In: Berutti E, Gagliani M, editors.: Edra; 2013. pp 2-27.
8 Ogutlu F, Karaca I. Clinical and Radiographic Outcomes of Apical Surgery: A Clinical Study. J Maxillofac Oral Surg. 2018;17(1):75-83.
8. Tsesis I, Rosen E, Schwartz-Arad D et al. *Retrospective evaluation of surgical endodontic treatment: traditional versus modern technique*. J Endod. 2006;32(5):412-416.
9. Rubinstein R. *Endodontic microsurgery and the surgical operating microscope: Compendium*; 1997.
10. Setzer F, Shah S, Kohli M et al. *Outcome of endodontic surgery: a meta-analysis of the literature--part 1: Comparison of traditional root-end surgery and endodontic microsurgery*. J Endod. 2010;36(11):1757-1765.
11. Wang Z, Zhang M, Wang J et al. *Outcomes of Endodontic Microsurgery Using a Microscope and Mineral Trioxide Aggregate: A Prospective Cohort Study*. J Endod. 2017;43(5):694-698.
12. Zhou W, Zheng Q, Tan X et al. *Comparison of Mineral Trioxide Aggregate and iRoot BP Plus Root Repair Material as Root-end Filling Materials in Endodontic Microsurgery: A Prospective Randomized Controlled Study*. J Endod. 2017;43(1):1-6.
13. Riis, A., S. Taschieri, M. Del Fabbro and T. Kvist (2018). "Tooth Survival after Surgical or Nonsurgical Endodontic Retreatment: Long-term Follow-up of a Randomized Clinical Trial." J Endod 44(10): 1480-1486.
14. Yoon J, Cho BH, Bae J, Choi Y. Anatomical analysis of the resected roots of mandibular first molars after failed non-surgical retreatment. Restor Dent Endod. 2018;43(2):e16.
13. von Arx T, Janner S, Jensen S et al. *The resection angle in apical surgery: a CBCT assessment*. Clin Oral Investig. 2016;20(8):2075-2082.
14. Taschieri S, Del Fabbro M, Testori T et al. *Endoscopic periradicular surgery: a prospective clinical study*. Br J Oral Maxillofac Surg. 2007;45:242-424.
15. Taschieri S, Del Fabbro M. *Endoscopic endodontic microsurgery: 2-year evaluation of healing and functionality*. Braz Oral Res. 2009;23:23-30.
16. von Arx T, Jensen S, Hänni S et al. *Five-year longitudinal assessment of the prognosis of apical microsurgery*. J Endod. 2012;38:570-579.
17. Zuolo M, Ferreira M, Gutmann J. *Prognosis in periradicular surgery: a clinical prospective study*. Int Endod J. 2000;33(2):91-98.
18. Pecora G, De Leonardis D, Ibrahim N et al. *The use of calcium sulphate in the surgical treatment of a 'through and through' periradicular lesion*. Int Endod J. 2001;34(3):189-197.
19. Rahbaran S, Gilthorpe M, Harrison S et al. *Comparison of clinical outcome of periapical surgery in endodontic and oral surgery units of a teaching dental hospital: a retrospective study*. Oral Surg Oral Med Oral Pathol Oral Radiol Endod. 2001;91(6):700-709.
20. Rud J, Rud V, Munksgaard E. *Periapical healing of mandibular molars after root-end sealing with dentine-bonded composite*. Int Endod J. 2001;34(4):285-292.
21. von Arx T, Gerber C, Hardt N. *Periradicular surgery of molars: a prospective clinical study with a one-year follow-up*. Int Endod J. 2001;34(7):520-525.
22. Jensen S, Nattestad A, Egdø P et al. *A prospective, randomized, comparative clinical study of resin composite and glass ionomer cement for retrograde root filling*. Clin Oral Investig. 2002;6(4):236-243.
23. Rubinstein R, Kim S. *Long-term follow-up of cases considered healed one year after apical microsurgery*. J Endod. 2002;28(5):378-383.
24. Chong B, Pitt Ford T, Hudson M. *Prospective clinical study of Mineral Trioxide Aggregate and IRM when used as root-end filling materials in endodontic surgery*. Int Endod J. 2003;36(8):520-526.
25. Maddalone M, Gagliani M. *Periapical endodontic surgery: a 3-year follow-up study*. Int Endod J. 2003 Mar;36(3):193-198.
26. Schwartz-Arad D, Yarom N, Lustig J et al. *A retrospective radiographic study of root-end surgery with amalgam and intermediate restorative material.* Oral Surg Oral Med Oral Pathol Oral Radiol Endod. 2003;96(4):472-477.
27. Wang N, Knight K, Dao T et al. *Treatment outcome in endodontics-The Toronto Study. Phases I and II: apical surgery*. J Endod. 2004;30(11):751-761.
28. Gagliani M, Gorni F, Strohmenger L. *Periapical resurgery versus periapical surgery: a 5-year longitudinal comparison*. Int Endod J. 2005;38(5):320-327.

29. Lindeboom J, Frenken J, Valkenburg P et al. *The role of preoperative prophylactic antibiotic administration in periapical endodontic surgery: a randomized, prospective double-blind placebo-controlled study*. Int Endod J. 2005;38(12):877-881.
30. Taschieri S, Del Fabbro M, Testori T et al. *Endodontic surgery with ultrasonic retrotips: one-year follow-up*. Oral Surg Oral Med Oral Pathol Oral Radiol Endod. 2005;100(3):380-387.
31. Taschieri S, Del Fabbro M, Testori T et al. *Endodontic surgery using 2 different magnification devices: preliminary results of a randomized controlled study*. J Oral Maxillofac Surg. 2006;64(2):235-242.
32. Peñarrocha M, Martí E, García B et al. *Relationship of periapical lesion radiologic size, apical resection, and retrograde filling with the prognosis of periapical surgery*. J Oral Maxillofac Surg. 2007;65(8):1526-1529.
33. von Arx T, Hänni S, Jensen S. *Correlation of bone defect dimensions with healing outcome one year after apical surgery*. J Endod. 2007;33(9):1044-1048.
34. Kim E, Song J, Jung I et al. *Prospective clinical study evaluating endodontic microsurgery outcomes for cases with lesions of endodontic origin compared with cases with lesions of combined periodontal-endodontic origin*. J Endod. 2008;34(5):546-551.
35. Saunders W. *A prospective clinical study of periradicular surgery using mineral trioxide aggregate as a root-end filling*. J Endod. 2008;34:660-665.
36. Taschieri S, Del Fabbro M, Testori T et al. *Microscope versus endoscope in root-end management: a randomized controlled study*. Int J Oral Maxillofac Surg. 2008;37:1022-1026.
37. Barone C, Dao T, Basrani B et al. *Treatment outcome in endodontics: the Toronto study*. Phases 3, 4, and 5: apical surgery. J Endod. 2010;36(1):28-35.
38. von Arx T, Hänni S, Jensen S. *Clinical results with two different methods of root-end preparation and filling in apical surgery: mineral trioxide aggregate and adhesive resin composite*. J Endod. 2010;36(7):1122-1129.
39. Song M, Jung I, Lee S et al. *Prognostic factors for clinical outcomes in endodontic microsurgery: a retrospective study*. J Endod. 2011;7(37):927-933.
40. Song M, Shin S, Kim E. *Outcomes of endodontic micro-resurgery: a prospective clinical study*. J Endod. 2011;37:316-320.
41. Wälivaara DA, Abrahamsson P, Fogelin M et al. *Super-EBA and IRM as rootend fillings in periapical surgery with ultrasonic preparation: A prospective randomized clinical study of 206 consecutive teeth*. Oral Surg Oral Med Oral Pathol Oral Radiol Endod. 2011;112:258-263.
42. Kreisler M, Gockel R, Aubell-Falkenberg S et al. *Clinical outcome in periradicular surgery: effect of patient- and tooth-related factors-a multicenter study*. Quintessence Int. 2013;44:53-60.
43. Lui J, Khin M, Krishnaswamy G et al. *Prognostic factors relating to the outcome of endodontic microsurgery*. J Endod. 2014;40:1071-1076.
44. Song M, Nam T, Shin S et al. *Comparison of clinical outcomes of endodontic microsurgery: 1 year versus long-term follow-up*. J Endod. 2014;40:490-494.
45. Tortorici S, Difalco P, Caradonna L et al. *Traditional endodontic surgery versus modern technique: a 5-year controlled clinical trial*. J Craniofac Surg. 2014;25:804-807.
46. Çalışkan M, Tekin U, Kaval M et al. *The outcome of apical microsurgery using MTA as the root-end filling material: 2- to 6-year follow-up study*. Int Endod J. 2016;49(3):245-254.
47. Serrano-Giménez M, Sánchez-Torres A, Gay-Escoda C. *Prognostic factors on periapical surgery: A systematic review*. Med Oral Patol Oral Cir Bucal. 2015;20(6):e715-722.
48. European Society of E. *Quality guidelines for endodontic treatment: consensus report of the European Society of Endodontology*. Int Endod J. 2006;39(12):921-930.
49. Kruse C, Spin-Neto R, Wenzel A, Vaeth M, Kirkevang LL. *Impact of cone beam computed tomography on periapical assessment and treatment planning five to eleven years after surgical endodontic retreatment*. Int Endod J. 2018;51(7):729-37.
49. Ahlowalia MS, Patel S, Anwar HM, Cama G, Austin RS, Wilson R, et al. *Accuracy of CBCT for volumetric measurement of simulated periapical lesions*. Int Endod J. 2013;46(6):538-546.
50. D'Addazio PS, Carvalho AC, Campos CN et al. *Cone beam computed tomography in Endodontics*. Int Endod J. 2016;49(3):311-312.
51. Davies A, Patel S, Foschi F et al. *The detection of periapical pathoses using digital periapical radiography and cone beam computed tomography in endodontically retreated teeth - part 2: a 1 year post-treatment follow-up*. Int Endod J. 2016;49(7):623-635.
52. Kramper B, Kaminski E, Osetek E et al. *A comparative study of the wound healing of three types of flap design used in periapical surgery*. J Endod. 1984;10:17-25.
53. Velvart P, Peters C, Peters O. *Soft tissue management: flap design, incision, tissue elevation, and tissue retraction*. Endo Topics. 2005;11:78-97.
54. Lubow R, Wayman B, Cooley R. *Endodontic flap design: analysis and recommendations for current usage*. Oral Surg Oral Med Oral Pathol. 1984;58:207-212.
55. Craig K, Harrison J. *Wound healing following demineralization of resected root ends in periradicular surgery*. J Endod. 1993;19:339-347.
56. von Arx T, Jensen S, Hänni S. *Clinical and radiographic assessment of various predictors for healing outcome 1 year after periapical surgery*. J Endod. 2007;33:123-128.

- Describe the **relevant features** related to the restoration of the retreated tooth.
- Illustrate the **timing** for optimizing the stages of reconstruction.
- Present the **techniques** useful for the reconstructive treatment.

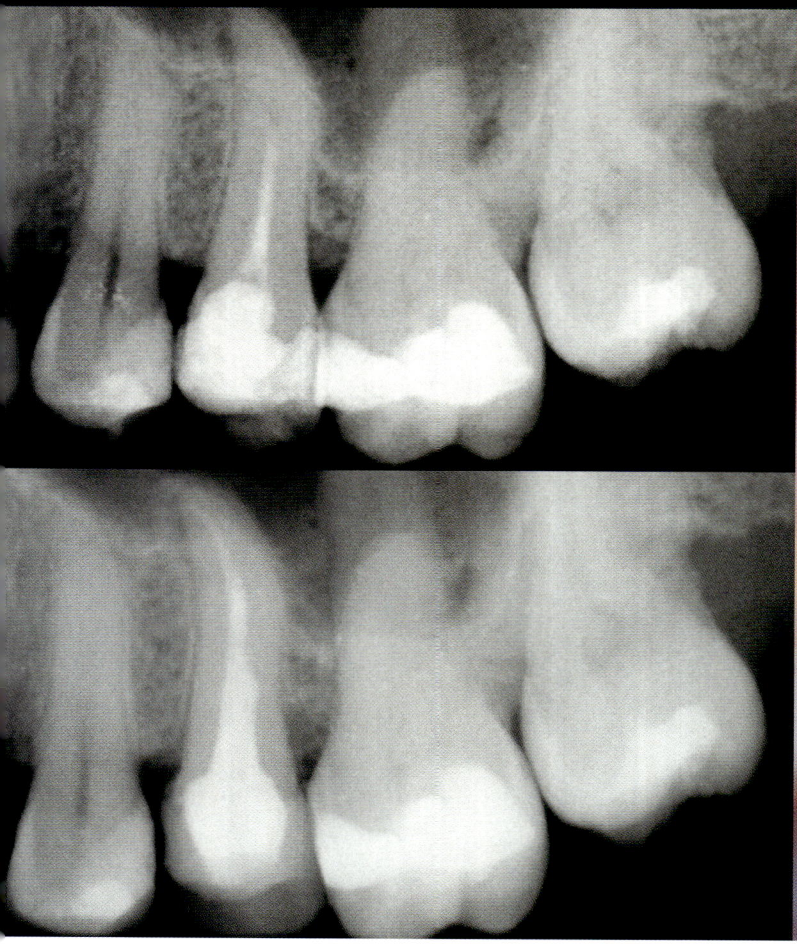

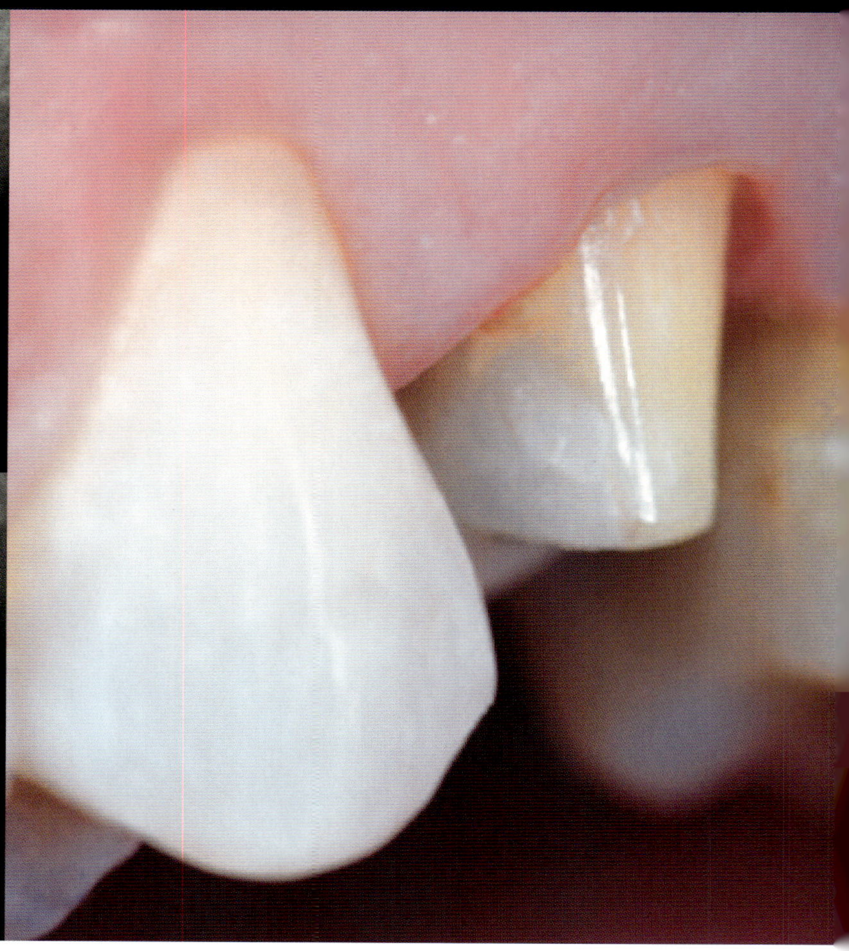

Pio Bertani, Paolo Generali

09

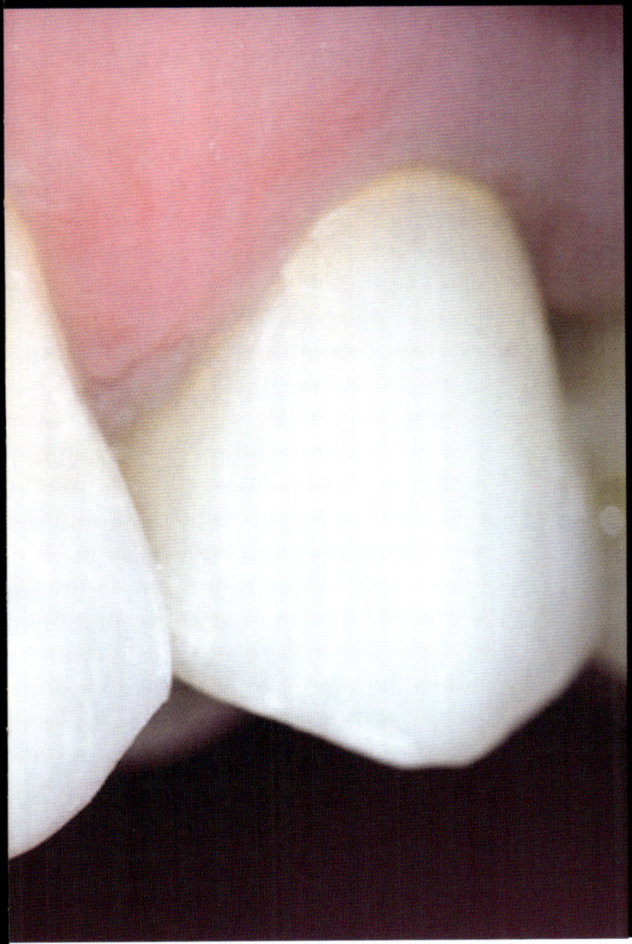

Restoration of the endodontically retreated tooth

Peculiarities and operating techniques

Preliminary remarks

The issue of endodontically retreated tooth reconstruction has not been the subject of much attention in the literature, probably because of the widespread belief that protocols and techniques used for endodontically treated tooth reconstruction can be directly applied to the retreated tooth. The retreated tooth has certain peculiarities that are worthy of attention for reconstructive purposes.
In the retreated tooth, the need to remove existing restorations, the loss of tissue due to caries or fractures, and the preparation of the access cavity determine the amount of residual dentin[1]. An in vivo study showed that retreated teeth with less than 30% residual dentin have a significantly lower success rate than less damaged ones[2].

Fig. 9.1a-d: The reconstruction phase is essential for restoring shape and function to a retreated tooth.

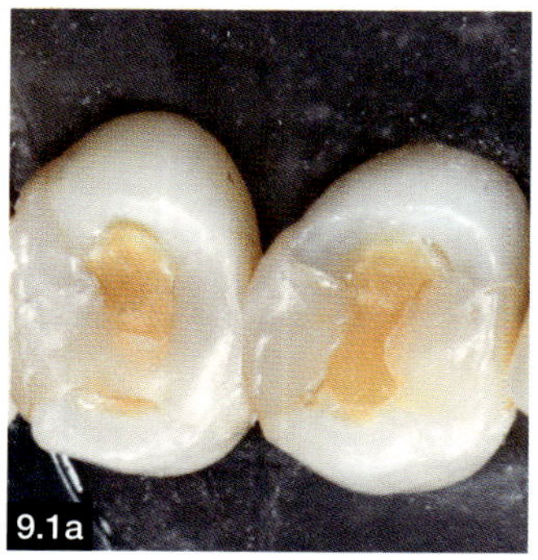

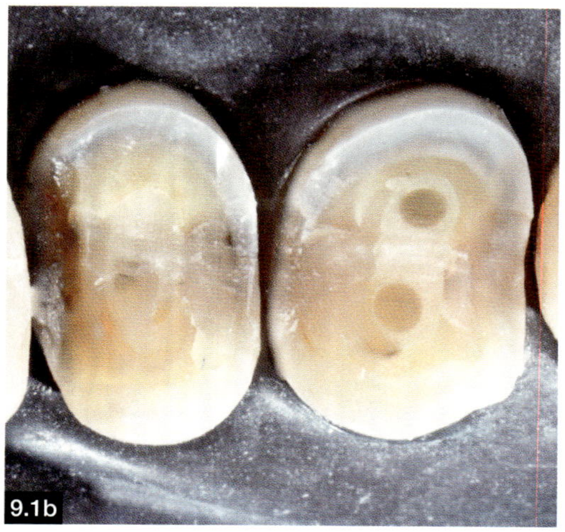

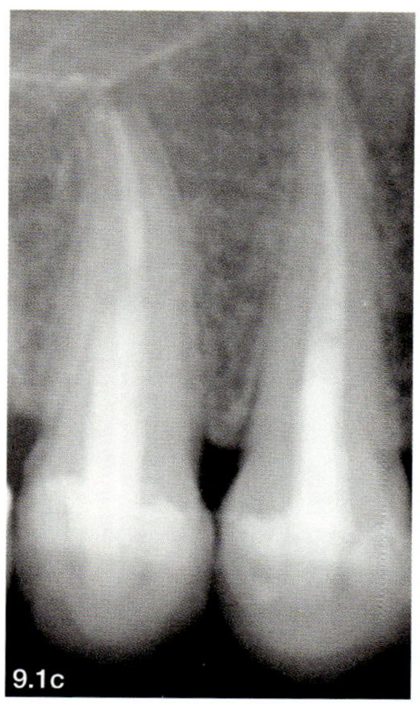

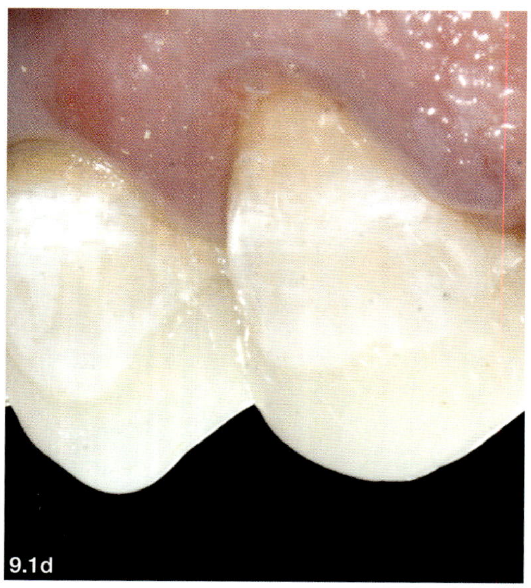

Endodontic retreatment is necessary in the event of failure to heal, or the appearance of disease, after primary endodontic treatment.
This is true in most cases, because of the persistence of infection in the root canal system[3], which may occur in the case of sub-standard treatment[4], and technical errors that prevent the control and prevention of infection.
However, sometimes a state-of-the-art endodontic treatment may fail. Reinfection may occur due to treatment failure. Microorganisms can find a way to contaminate the endodontic space through the loss of coronal seal, following the failure of the post-endodontic restoration. Therefore, retreatment may be made necessary due to reconstructive failures and requires adequate reconstruction to succeed.
Another aspect concerns the presence of pre-existing restorations, which may be worthy of preservation, through access cavity repair procedures.
Occasionally, the retreated tooth is part of a prosthetic rehabilitation that must be restored due to the patient's unwillingness to face the demands of another prosthetic treatment. However, the maneuvers required for the removal of build-up materials and root canal filling affect the quantitative and qualitative characteristics of the residual dentin.
Careful evaluation of the amount of residual healthy dentin before undertaking retreatment is important.
The most frequent cause of extraction of an endodontically treated tooth is the severe loss of healthy dental tissue[5]; in addition, endodontic and reconstructive procedures generate additional stress that can be among the causes of failure[6].

This chapter will first examine the effects of retreatment procedures on the tooth structure to provide useful information for reconstructive purposes.
Subsequently, techniques capable of repairing or restoring pre-existing prosthetic artifacts will be examined.

The effects of retreatment procedures

The objective of endodontic retreatment is the removal of existing materials from the endodontic space and the correction of any pathological or iatrogenic defects present[7]. In addition, retreatment procedures allow the detection of mechanical failures, forgotten canals, and subcrestal root fractures; enable the shaping of the canal; and permit the cleaning and the three-dimensional filling of the endodontic space[8, 9].
These procedures should be performed under the best aseptic conditions, and a final coronal restoration should be placed as soon as possible, ideally within the first week after treatment[10]. The outcome of endodontic retreatment is generally favorable, although it shows a lower success rate than primary treatment[11]. However, retreatment procedures subject the dental tissue to further stress, which will be analyzed below.

Resistance of the retreated tooth

By investigating the fracture resistance of extracted, treated, and retreated teeth in vitro, Marianna De Carlo Bello et al.[12] excluded in their experimental model that retreatment procedures may result in reduced tooth strength. These results were confirmed by Missau et al. (including the aforementioned De Carlo Bello)[13]. These studies, which were mostly performed on perfectly healthy teeth with a straight root, confirmed that endodontic procedures on an intact tooth do not reduce its resistance.

Gutta percha removal

Endodontic instrumentation with NiTi instruments and subsequent root canal filling can cause dentinal damage and create defects in the root canal walls[14, 15]; thus, the need to repeat these procedures will induce further defects. Removal of the gutta percha can be facilitated by dissolving it with chloroform; however, this solvent can cause a significant softening of the dentin after 5 min of application[16] and reduce the mineral component of dentin[17].
The use of rotary or manual instruments, in combination with chloroform, for the removal of the gutta percha, results in the formation of a significantly higher number of dentinal defects in the retreated tooth compared with the endodontically treated tooth; defects and fractures were found to be more frequent in samples treated with manual instruments such as Hedstroem files than those treated with rotary instruments (e.g., ProTaper Retreatment Files) according to a 2011 study by Shemesh et al.[18] In 2014, Topçuoğlu et al.[19, 20] demonstrated the possibility of inducing apical cracks following the use of various rotary instruments; in these cases, the use of manual instruments was safer than the use of rotary instruments. These results were confirmed by Capar et al. in 2015[21, 22] and by Ozyurek et al. in 2017[23] in a similar study, which included the most recently introduced rotary instruments. In addition to the gutta percha, various other materials are used (or have been used) for the closure of root canals. The effects of the mechanical removal of one of these materials, a resin containing resorcinol and formaldehyde, on the residual dentin formed the subject of research that revealed the formation of dentinal cracks[24].

DENTIN INTEGRITY

The **mechanical and chemical effects** of repeated endodontic procedures can damage the integrity of the dentin tissue.

Effect of solvents

The use of chloroform as a solvent for gutta-percha has already been discussed. Other substances are used to remove or resin-based cements.
The use of these solvents is often necessary for the complete removal of the existing root canal filling, but they can lead to the formation of a layer of debris on the canal walls[25] or other alterations in the dentin that may result in a poorer effectiveness of the adhesion techniques[26].
Most in vitro studies agree that solvents have a negative effect on adhesion[27, 28], with the sole exception of one study by Topçuoğlu et al.[29].

Post removal and use of ultrasound

Removing root canal posts can also damage the residual dentin. In vitro studies showed that the use of ultrasonic vibration can result in the formation of dentin cracks[30] more frequently than the use of a Gonon-type extractor[31]. The increase in temperature due to the use of ultrasonic instruments inside the canal, in the absence of adequate irrigation and for a sufficiently long time, can increase the temperature of the dentin to levels considered dangerous for the integrity of the periodontium[32].

In short...

To conclude, from the review of the relevant literature, the majority of in vitro studies highlight the possibility that retreatment procedures may induce damage to residual dentin. As far as fracture resistance is concerned, studies on retreated teeth confirmed what is already known for teeth undergoing primary endodontic treatment, i.e., endodontic procedures do not reduce the strength of a structurally intact tooth[33]. In the scarcity of scientific evidence, a randomized and controlled clinical study by Esposito et al.[34] reported that endodontic retreatment remains the least invasive option and the first therapeutic option to be considered in the case of teeth treated endodontically with periapical lesions and/or symptoms, even in the presence of an uncertain prognosis.

Techniques for retreated tooth reconstruction

Reconstruction of endodontically treated teeth

Teeth requiring endodontic retreatment are often severely damaged by destructive or recurrent caries, fractures, or previous restorations.

FLOW CHART OF ENDODONTICALLY TREATED TOOTH RESTORATION

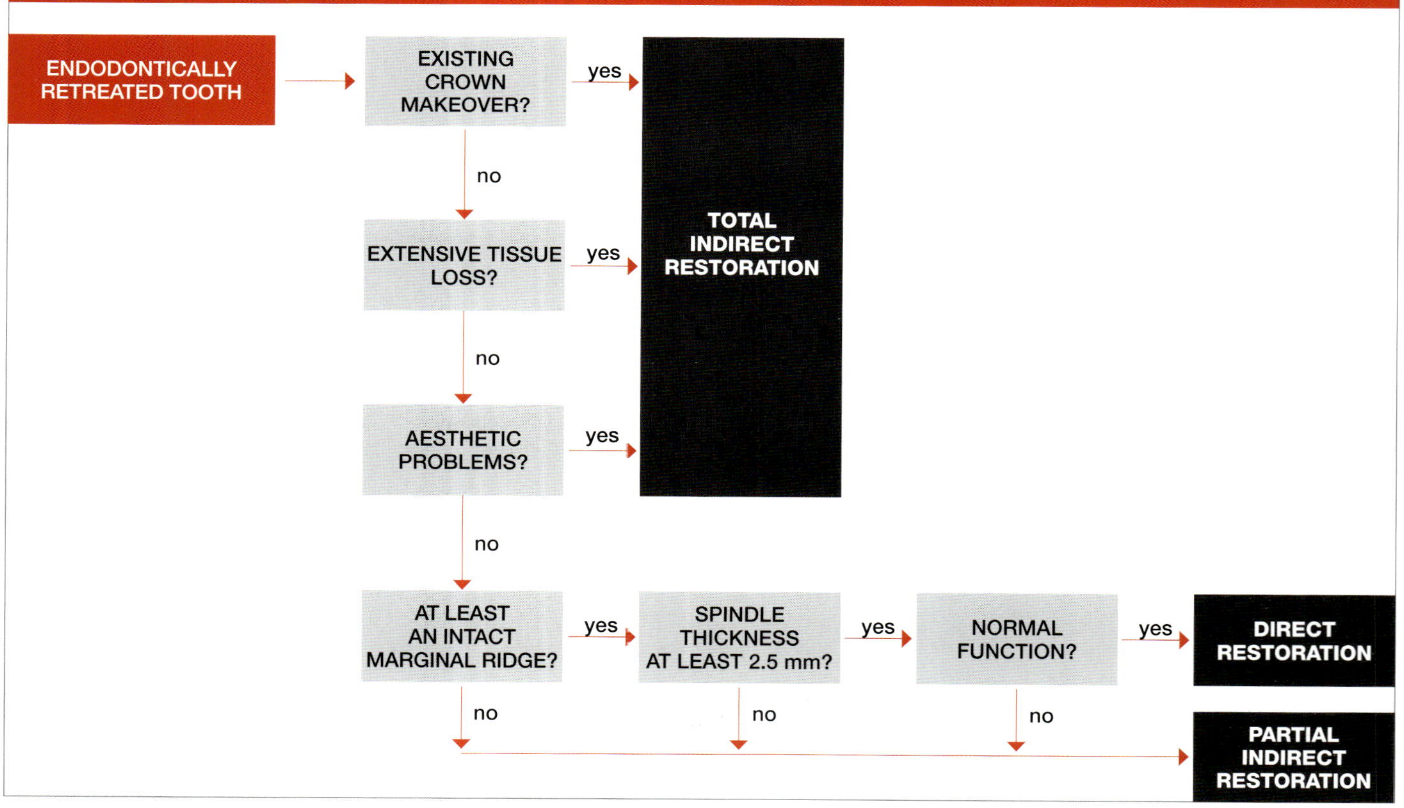

Retreatment is often difficult due to isolation problems, the need to overcome various obstacles, the management of any perforations, or changes in the endodontic anatomy; all these factors influence the prognosis of the tooth[35].
The final restoration is another factor that can influence prognosis, as reported in the prevailing literature; the quality of the restoration and the quality of endodontic treatment have the same influence on successful outcome[36].
In line with today's prevailing opinions on endodontic tooth restoration, the use of adhesive techniques, composite materials, non-metallic posts, and partial ceramic restorations may be considered in the restoration of the retreated tooth for the maximum preservation of residual dentin, thereby reducing the need for further removal of healthy tissue for retention purposes.
The preservation of healthy dentin and the use of adhesive techniques and materials with characteristics similar to natural tissues are considered to be the most significant success factors for the restoration of endodontically treated teeth[37, 38].
Despite the biomechanical, structural, and aesthetic advantages of these techniques, they are still underused in clinical practice in favor of the classic full crown approach, with or without a post[39].
Others in the field are not sufficiently familiar with the procedures of adhesive dentistry, and complete crowns are a proven reconstructive modality that is still afforded attention in scientific literature[40].

Special features of the retreated tooth

In the case of a retreated tooth, a wide variety of situations can be encountered from a reconstructive point of view.
When examining a prosthetic tooth, one should establish whether the situation presents a prosthetic restoration that is to be preserved, requires a total or partial crown through which an access cavity has been made, or whether the restoration is to be replaced. In any case, evaluation of the marginal integrity of a restoration is not easily achieved through X-ray images and inspection of the margins of closure.
After opening an access cavity in a clinically acceptable crown, micro-fractures, caries, incoherent substances related to non-polymerized materials, small posts from radiological examinations, empty spaces, cotton balls, and much more may be detected.
In addition, the preparation of the access cavity itself can, albeit rarely, induce the formation of cracks that can irreparably undermine the integrity of the crown; for the same material, the methods of manufacture can also have an influence, given that the preparation of an access cavity reduces the resistance of die-cast disilicate but not that obtained by milling[41].
However, in a 2004 study by Abbot[42], after removal of a crown, 56% of abutments had caries, fractures, or other defects that were not detected by physical examination with the crown in situ.
Therefore, we must not take it for granted that it will be possible simply to repair each crown, even when apparently in good condition, after having made an access cavity. Moreover, written consent specifying that the crown may prove *to be irreparable* should be provided, and replacement may be necessary.
The possibility of surgical retreatment, in the case of well executed restorations that deserve to be preserved, must be examined and discussed with the patient.

CROWN PRESERVED

Retreatment procedures may irreparably **damage the existing restoration**.

Possibility of preserving the existing restoration

In spite of these considerations, in the event that the existing restoration is preserved, the access cavity must be sealed by repairing the crown.
The increasing use of all-ceramic crowns has led several researchers to experiment the effects of preparing an access cavity with monolithic crowns made of zirconia, layered zirconia, lithium disilicate, and other materials[43-45].
The factors to be considered lie in the nature of the material, the possibility of adhesion,

the cementation technique (adhesive or not), the grain size of the diamond bur used to prepare the cavity, the relationship between the size of the crown and the size of the access cavity, and a thorough inspection of the interior of the cavity to identify infiltrations or micro-fractures. The data available in the literature are scarce, making it impossible to devise clinical protocols of certain effectiveness. The repair possibilities of various materials will be analyzed below.

REPAIR OF THE RESTORATION

Repairing a **prosthetic restoration** through which an access cavity has been created is often possible. The use of **appropriate techniques** for each material is essential to obtaining a seal that is stable over time.

Metal crowns

Metal crowns in which an access cavity has been made can be sealed with composite through mechanical retention. A rough surface, capable of providing micromechanical retention, can be obtained with coarse-grained drills or with air abrasion[46], while silane has no effect on metal adhesion[47]. Tinning is an effective method for increasing mechanical retention[48]. Despite the availability of intraoral devices, this procedure has not had extensive clinical use. Commercial primers are available to improve the bond between metal and resin[49-51].
The use of glass fiber-reinforced composite can increase the strength of repaired metal-ceramic crowns[52].

Etchable ceramics: metal-ceramic or all-ceramic

Access cavities prepared from etchable metal-ceramic or all-ceramic crowns can be repaired using ceramic etching[53] and salinization techniques[54].
Etched ceramic forms a solid and lasting bond with the resin[55], with a bond strength of more than 13 MPa; any failure of the bond is usually cohesive in the context of ceramic[56].
Silane acts as a surfactant to reduce surface tension and forms double bonds with the hydroxyl groups of the ceramic. The preparation of access cavities made of lithium disilicate crowns or can result in the formation of radial cracks and surface chipping, as well as other forms of damage to the surface[57]. These defects, especially in the presence of an unfavorable ratio between the size of the access cavity and the size of the crown, can occur in the anterior teeth and result in catastrophic failure[58].
Failure is reported in up to 50% of cases in the lower incisors. The preparation of access cavities made of integral feldspar or leucite-reinforced ceramics greatly reduces their strength[59].
These materials are susceptible to hydrofluoric acid etching, salinization, and application of adhesives, which leads to effective adhesion capable of preventing infiltration.
The use of coarse-grained diamond burs (150–180 μm) appears to have a negative influence on the strength of ceramic crowns after preparation of the access cavity, whereas the use of medium-grained burs on lithium disilicate crowns does not reduce their strength[60].
Hydrofluoric acid acts by dissolving the glassy component of the ceramic; it is supplied in various concentrations, usually between 5% and 10%, and the manufacturer's instructions must be precisely followed, because the application time and the concentration required vary depending on the type of ceramic. A short time is ineffective and does not lead to a proper bond, whereas an excessively long time weakens the ceramic[61].
After the adhesive procedures, the composite material is applied to seal the access cavity. Achieving a good aesthetic result is not easy, because most composites are too low in value compared with the surrounding ceramic. Therefore, a very opaque composite that may be layered on the surface with a translucent material should be selected, and pigments should be applied in the grooves[62].
The metal component of metal-ceramic crowns is normally not significant in the closure of the access cavity (Figs. 9.2–9.16).

Box 9.1 CREATION OF ENDODONTIC ACCESS THROUGH CERAMIC CROWNS AND ENDODONTIC RESTORATION

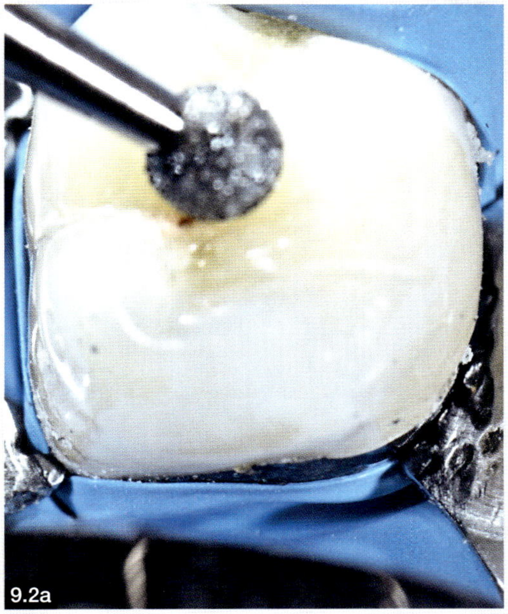

9.2a

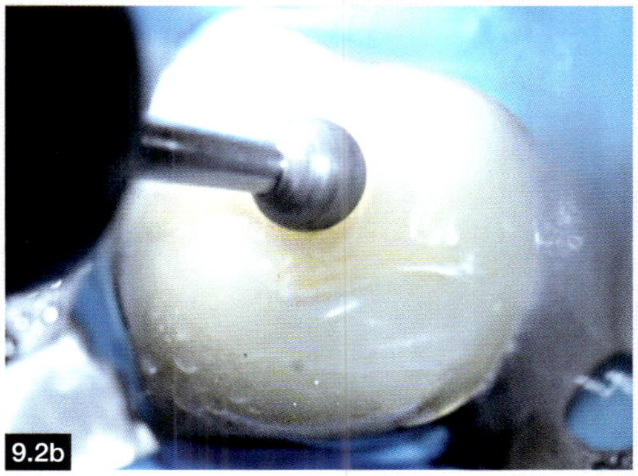

9.2b

Fig. 9.2a-b: Ceramic veneer is abraded with a diamond ball bur.

Fig. 9.3: Metal structure is treated with a milling bur in tungsten carbide.

Fig. 9.4: Once the dentin has been reached, a truncated cone diamond bur can be used.

Fig. 9.5: After the retreatment, the dentin is etched first as in a normal post-endodontic restoration.

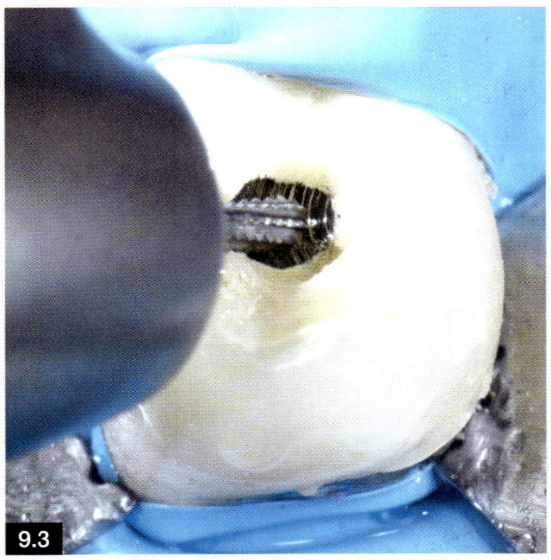

9.3

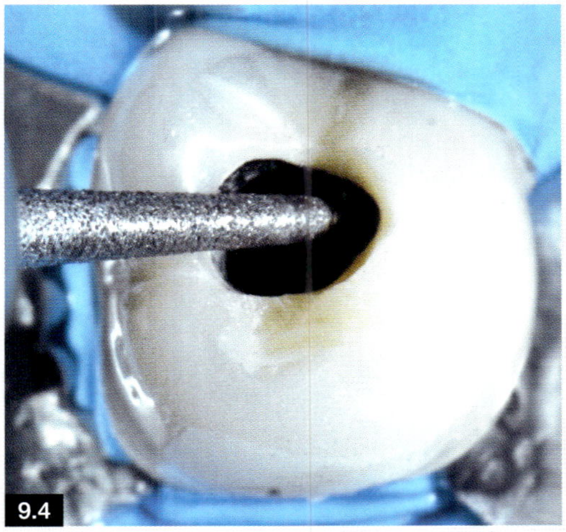

9.4

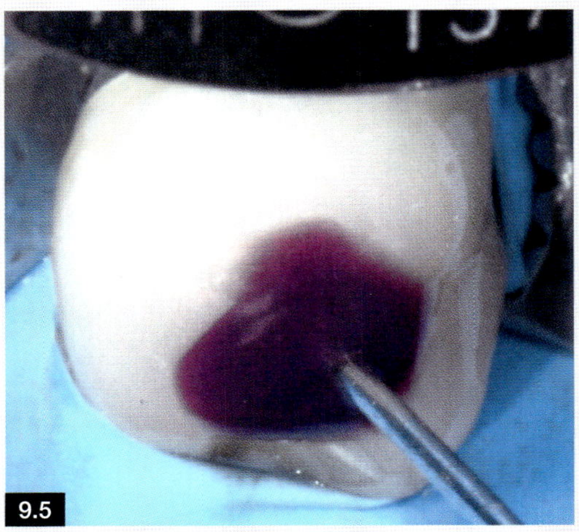

9.5

Fig. 9.6: A post should be inserted into the restoration of a retreated and prosthetic tooth.

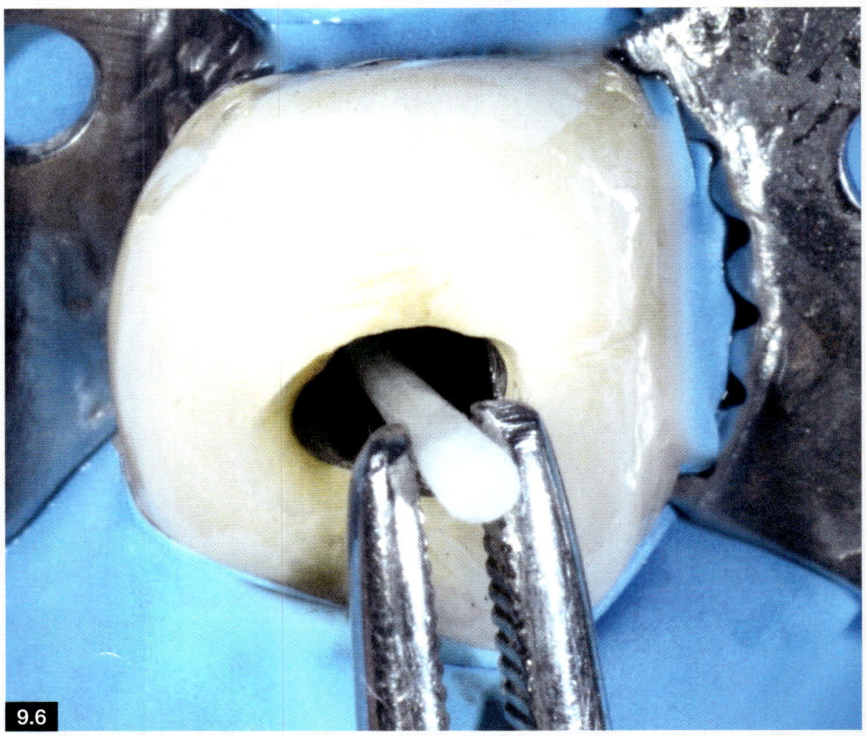

9.6

Fig. 9.7a-b: The adhesive procedures are performed, and the cement is extruded from the deepest portion.

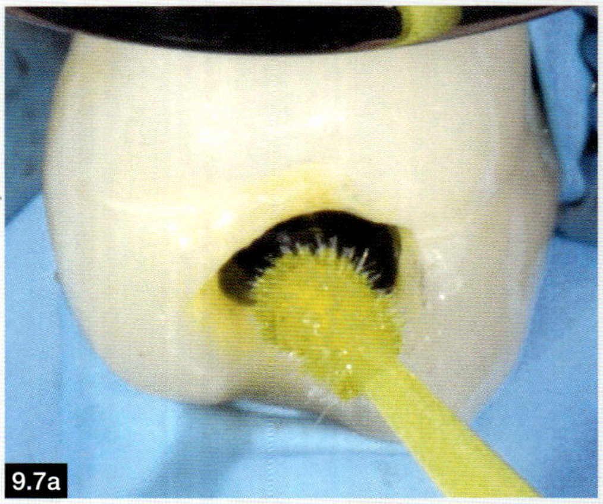

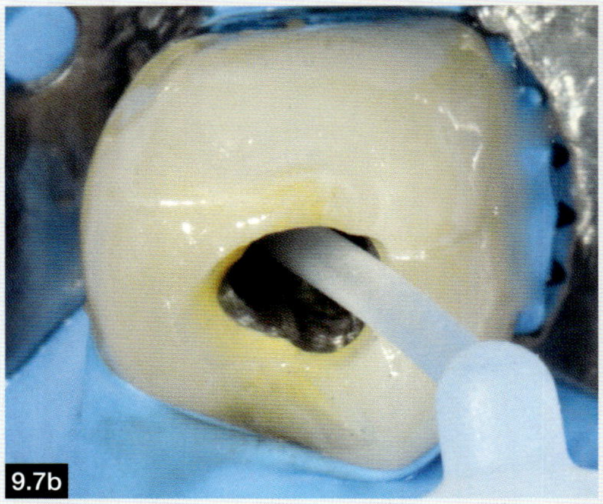

Fig. 9.8: The ceramic is bevelled around the access cavity for effective adhesion.

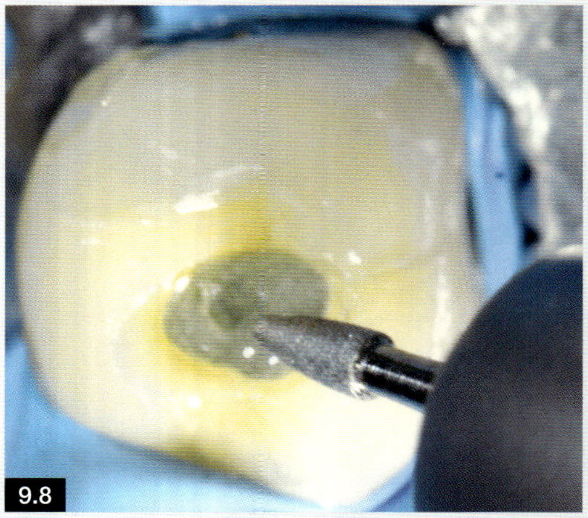

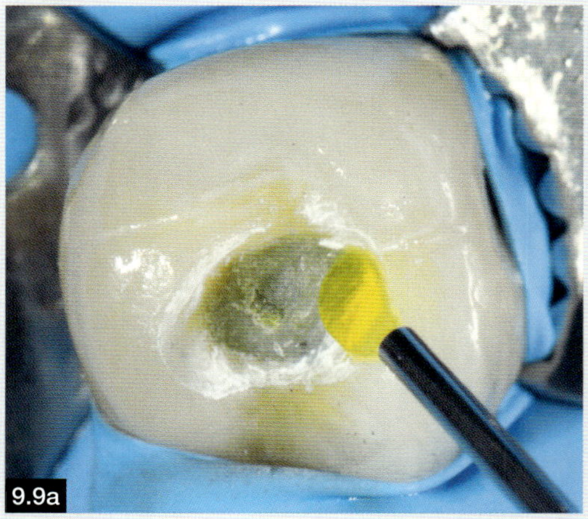

Fig. 9.9a-b: Feldspar ceramic is etched with 9.6% hydrofluoric acid for 3 min.

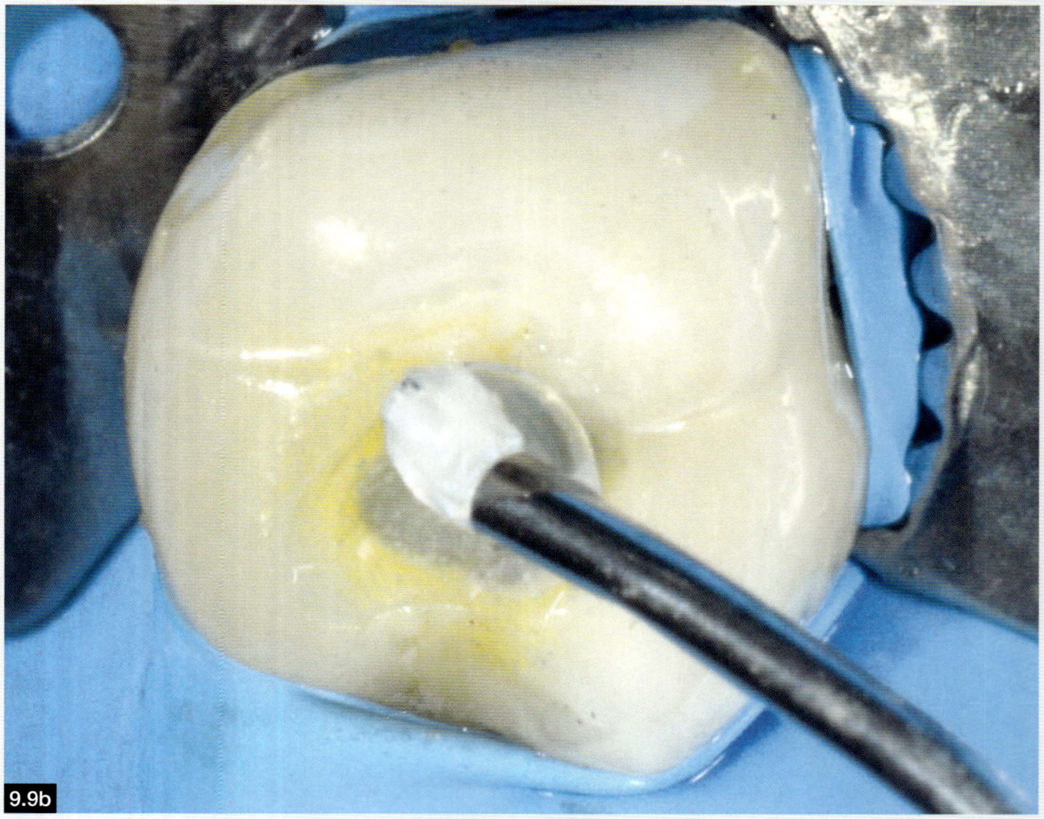

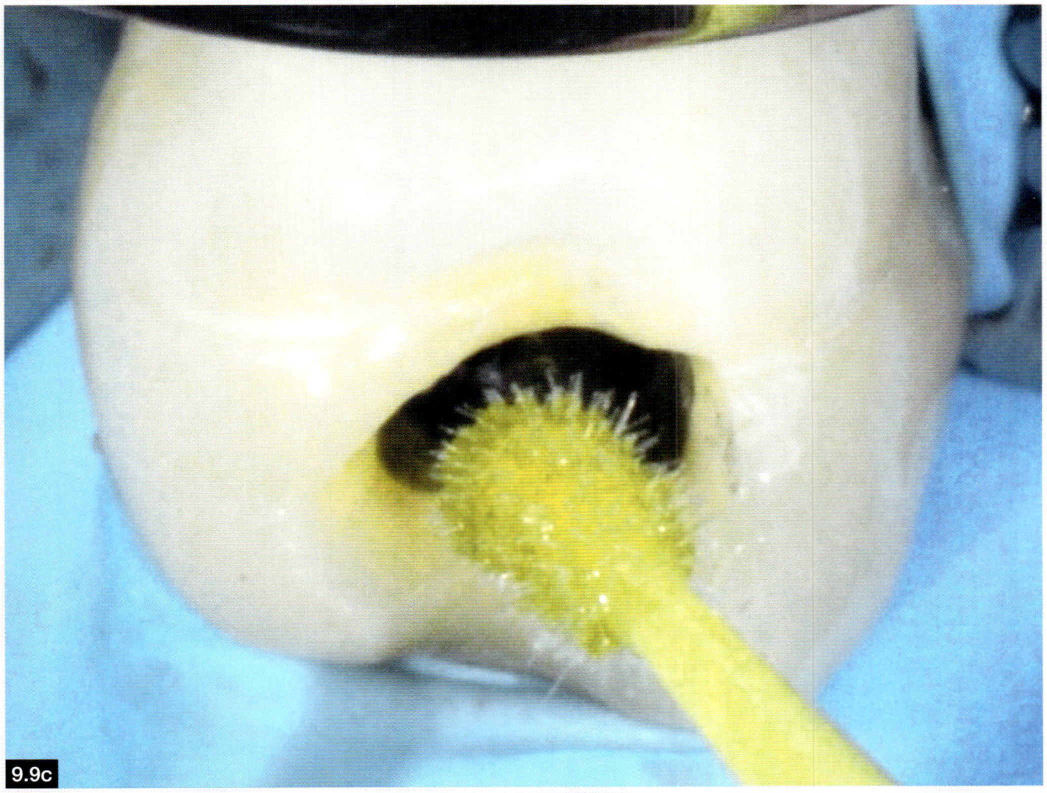

9.9c

Fig. 9.9c: It silanizes the ceramics, and the adhesive procedure is realized.

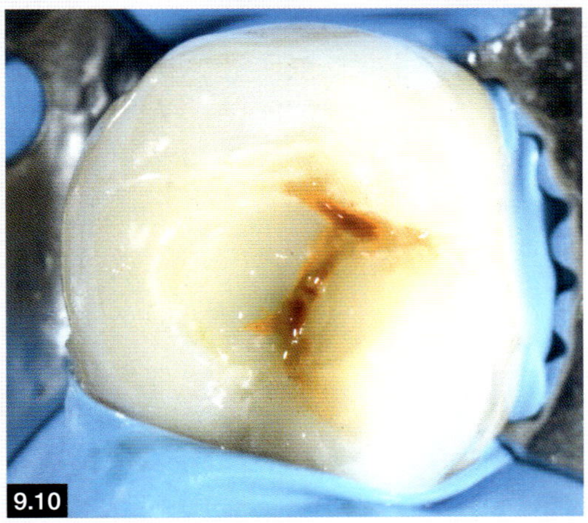

9.10

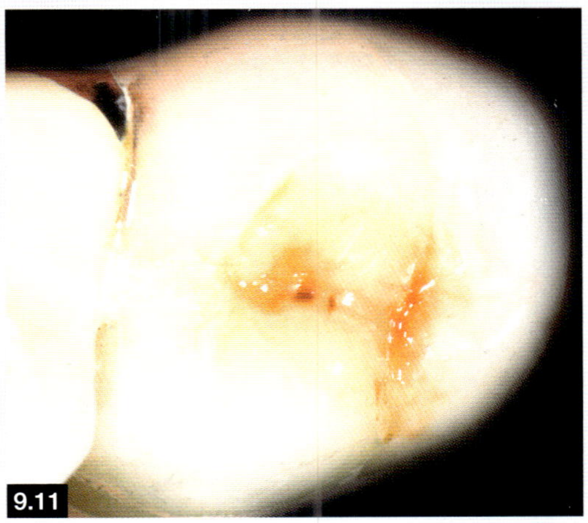

9.11

Fig. 9.10: After the reconstruction, camouflage helps to make the restoration more natural.

Fig. 9.11: Good functional and aesthetic restoration of the existing crown.

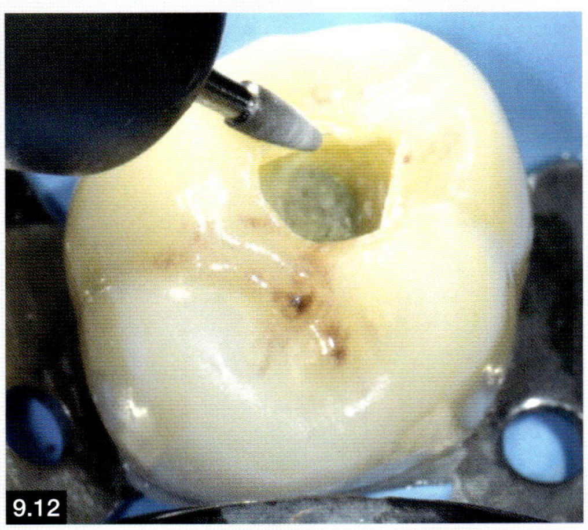

9.12

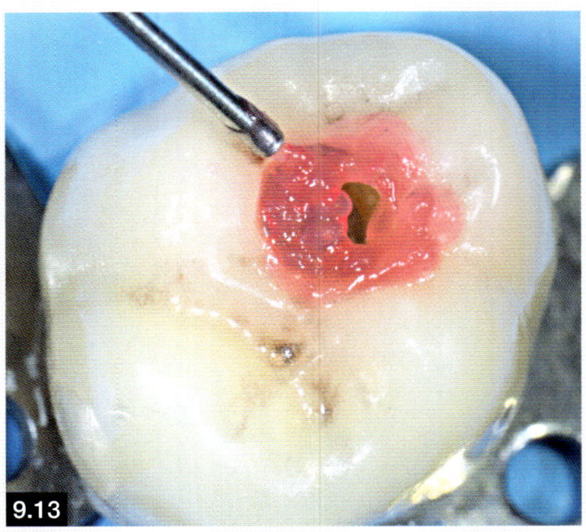

9.13

Fig. 9.12: In all-ceramic restorations that can be etched, the restorative procedures are identical to those on a metal-ceramic crown up to the beveling.

Fig. 9.13: In an all-ceramic etchable, etching is performed with 5% hydrofluoric acid for a short time, following the manufacturer's directions.

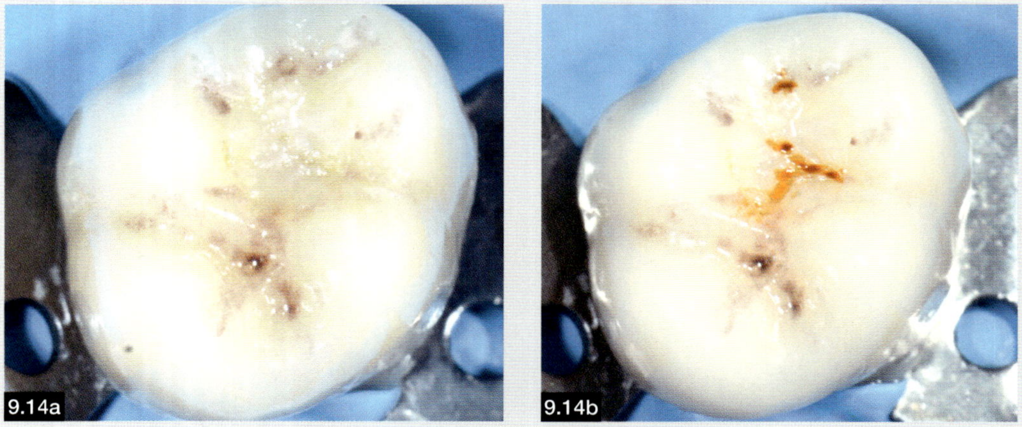

Fig. 9.14a-b: Once the restoration is finished, the camouflage helps mask repair better.

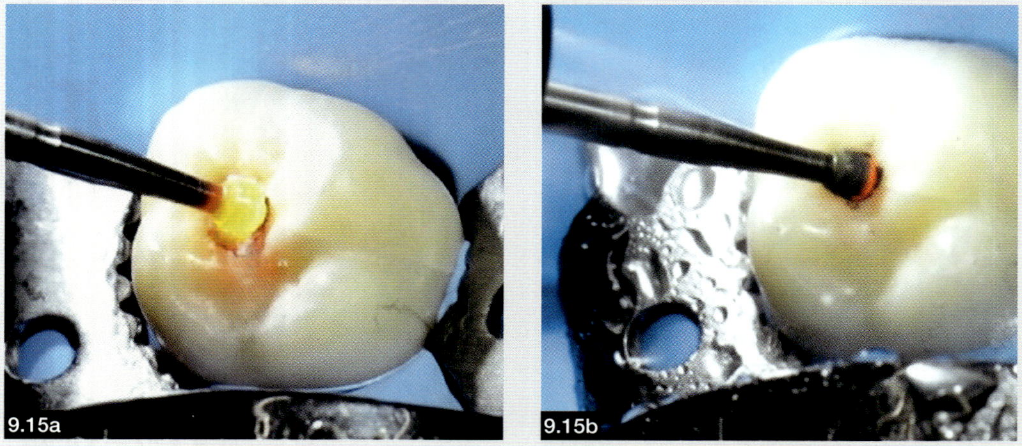

Fig. 9.15a-b: In zirconia crowns, the friction of the milling bur causes a dangerous rise in temperature, which is not off-set by an abundant jet of water. Dedicated cutters are available to reduce this problem.

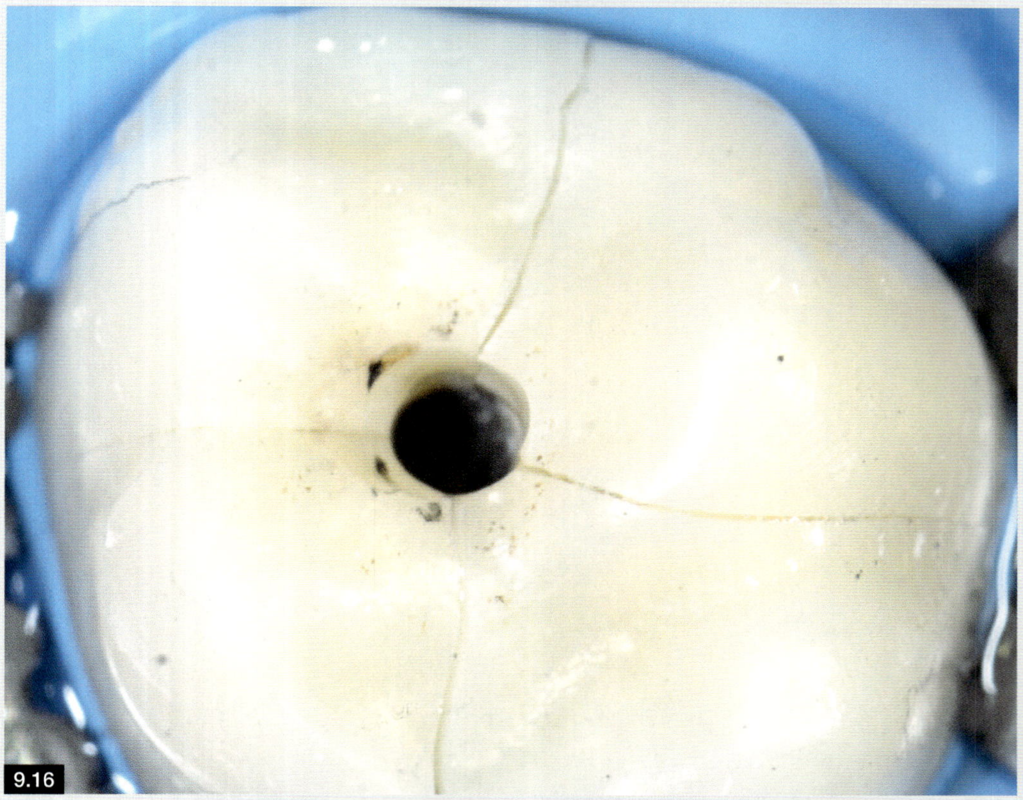

Fig. 9.16: Mechanical and thermal shock can have disastrous effects.

Zirconia crowns

Opening an access cavity in a zirconia crown takes seven times longer than opening a leucite crown for the same operation[63]; monolithic restorations are less susceptible to damage than layered zirconia[44].
The preparation of an access cavity in a zirconia crown reduces its strength[64] and can adversely affect its retention[65], as is the case with ceramic on metal crowns[66]. Zirconia resists etching, and other surface treatments have been tested with varying results to achieve adhesion; the use of phosphate monomers (MDPs) can improve adhesion, but the bond is susceptible to degradation in in vitro models over time[67]. Therefore, zirconia crowns can be repaired with good mechanical sealing possibilities but with some concerns regarding microleakage. Beveling the edges of zirconia is not recommended, contrary to the case for etchable ceramics[68].

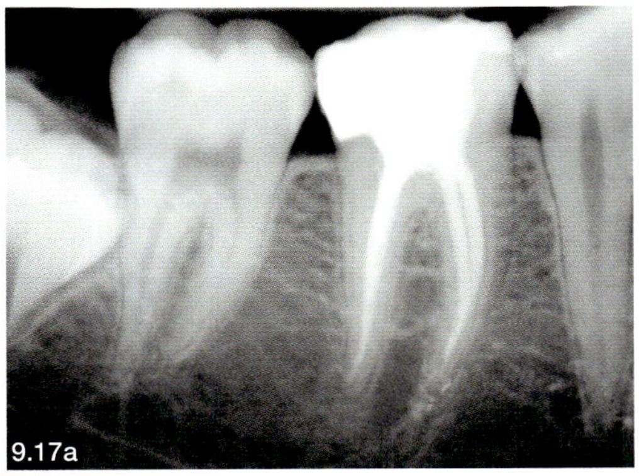
9.17a

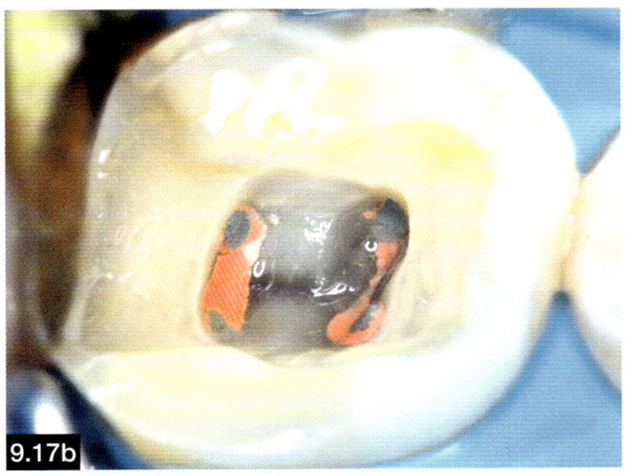
9.17b

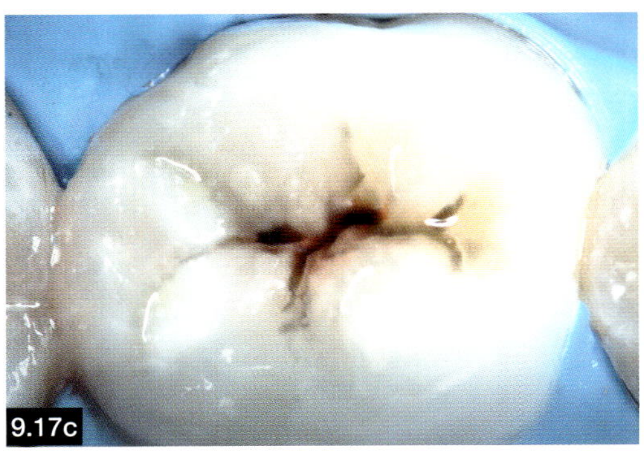
9.17c

Positioning a post

The alternative of placing a post in an endodontically treated tooth through an existing crown has been discussed; this topic is relevant to the restoration of a retreated tooth where the prosthetic crown is to be preserved. At a conference at the annual meeting of the American Association of Endodontics in 2011[69], Marga Ree reported that the prevailing literature supports the appropriateness of placing a fiber post in endodontically treated teeth through a prosthetic crown, if they constitute the abutment of a bridge or if they are small in size.

Replacing the restoration: conventional or adhesive techniques

If a replacement of the restoration after retreatment is considered necessary, then the usual procedures for endodontically treated teeth, for which an extensive description is available in the literature, will be applied. In a retreated tooth, the result will be a considerable loss of dental substance, which will guide the choice toward an indirect type of restoration. Total cusp cover in the posterior teeth will be necessary due to the loss of tissue and probable consequences of the various manual skills associated with the phases of endodontic retreatment.
The conventional approach based on a cast abutment post (or a reconstruction anchored to a prefabricated post) and a total crown (Fig. 9.17a-c) is still widespread but increasingly losing ground in favor of a restoration that fully exploits the possibilities offered by adhesive dentistry (Fig. 9.18a-d).

Fig. 9.17a-c: Direct restoration.

CASE REPORT 1

Bleaching of an upper lateral incisor

Dyschromic variation in endodontically treated teeth is quite common; however, unpleasant dark discoloration can be avoided by thorough removal from the pulp chamber of pulp remnants, sealing cement and gutta-percha before and after the root canal treatment. In this case bleaching procedures could be adopted immediately after careful cleaning of the endodontic access, removing all the filling materials and infected dentin below the cement-enamel junction.

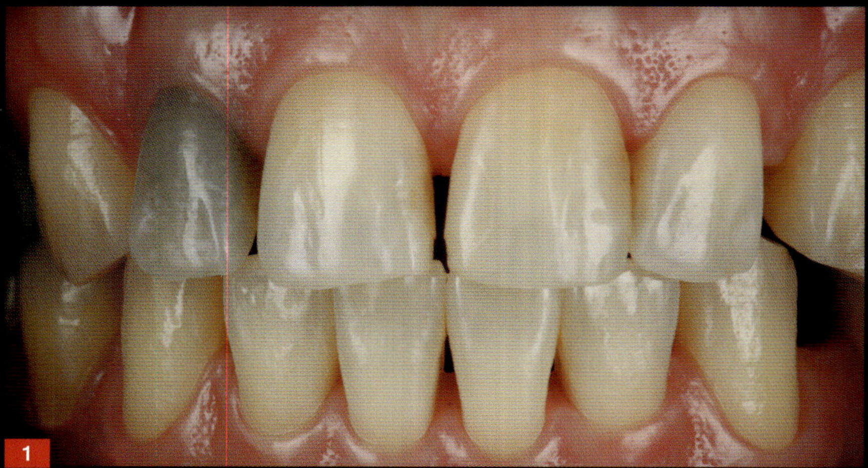

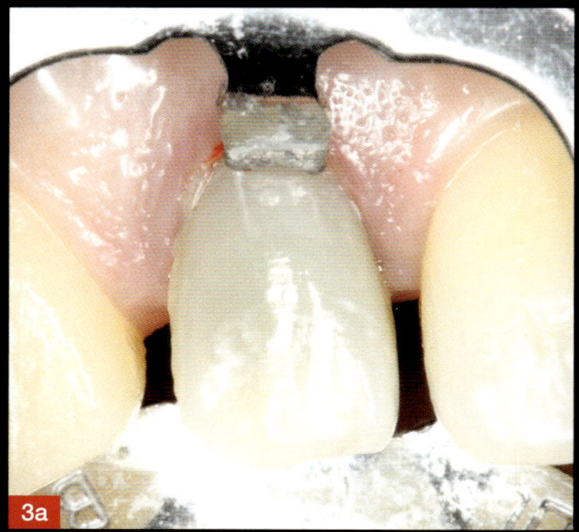

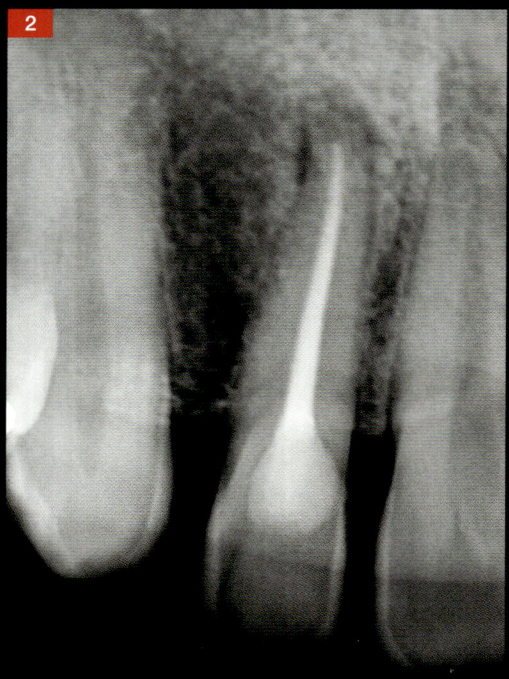

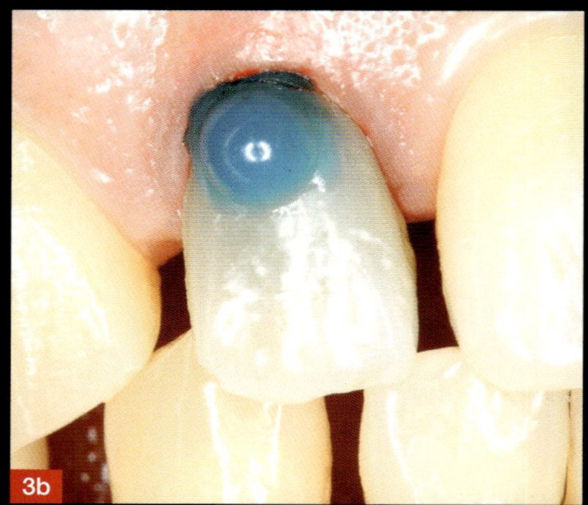

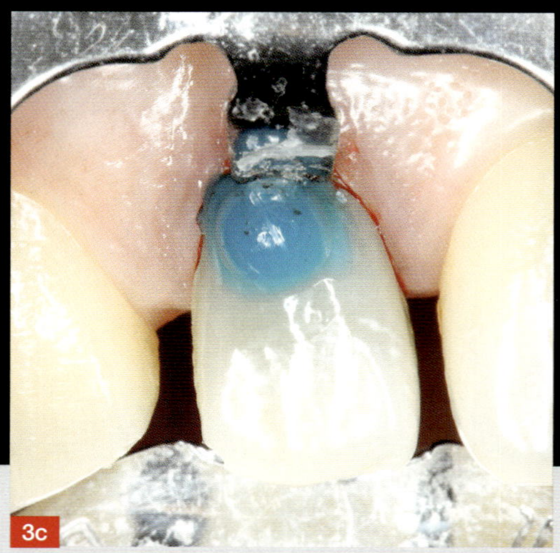

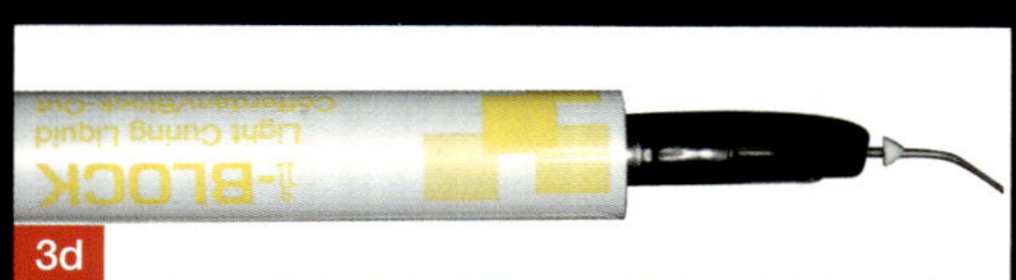

Figure 1: A frontal view of the upper and lower anterior teeth; the dark colour of the lateral upper incisor was a concern for the patient.

Figure 2: X-ray showing an incomplete root canal treatment with periapical radiolucency.

Figure 3a-d: To obtain a stable stop for the rubber dam clamp a spot of liquid dam was firmly fixed to the vestibular part of the lateral incisor.

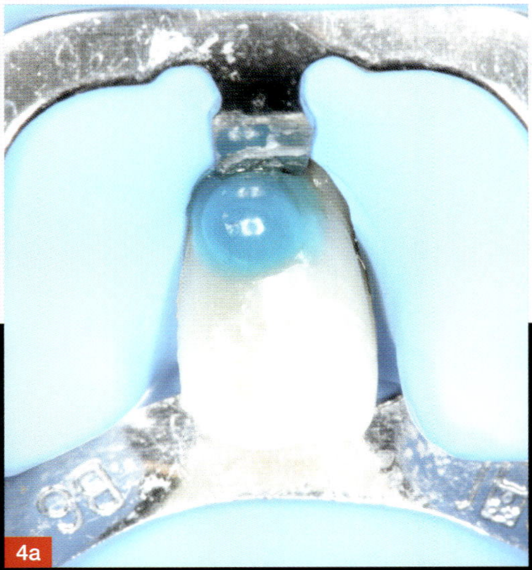

4a

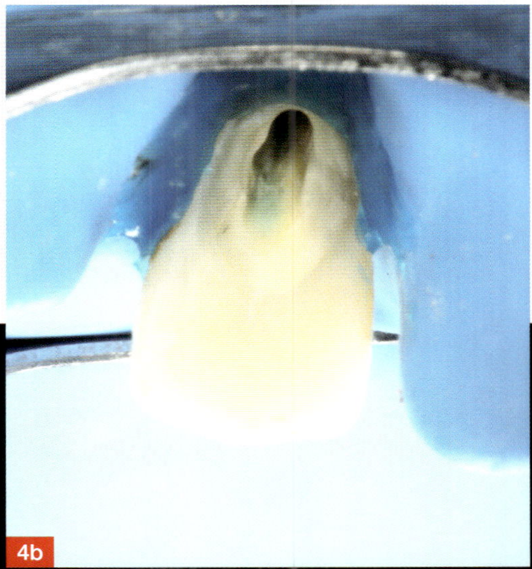

4b

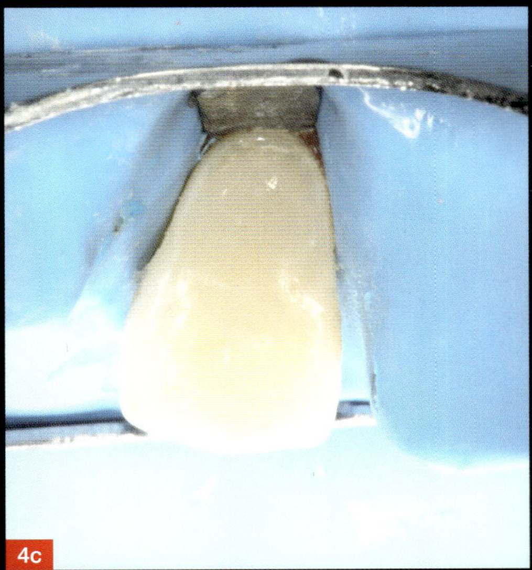

4c

Figure 4a-c: The rubber dam was fixed and the pulp chamber cleaning process was followed by the root canal retreatment.

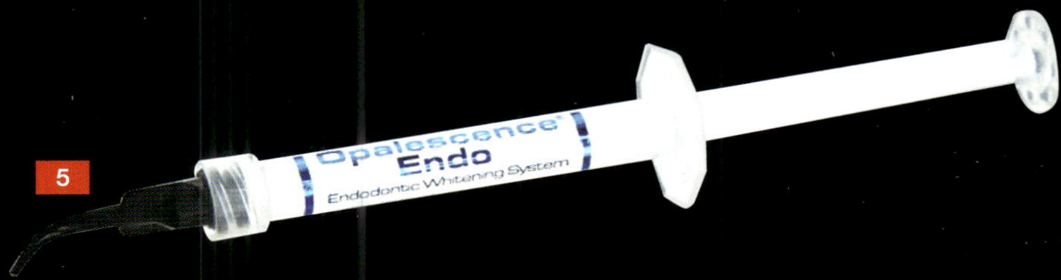

5

Figure 5: At the end of the retreatment, a bleaching agent (Opalescence, Ultradent, USA) was utilized.

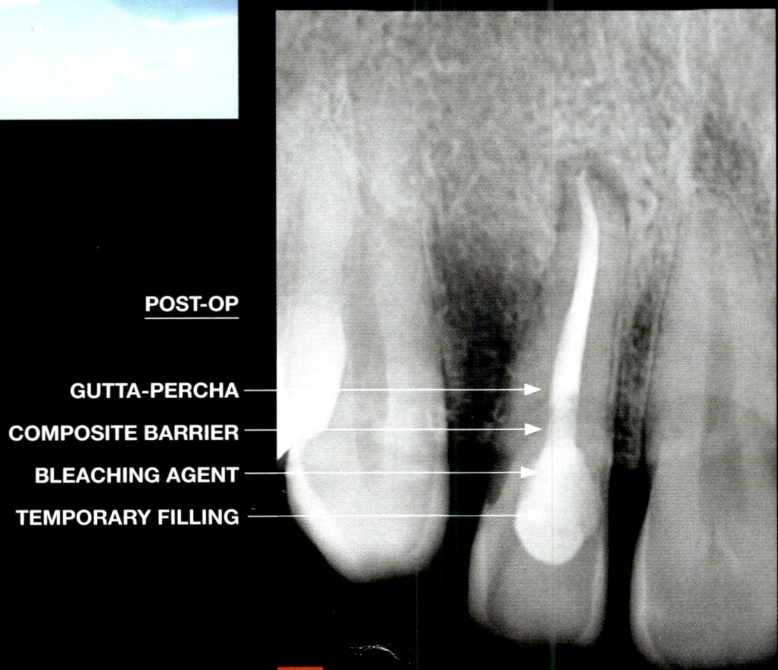

6

Figure 6: The final X-ray and the strategy employed to prevent contaminations of the pulp chamber and of the bleaching agent.

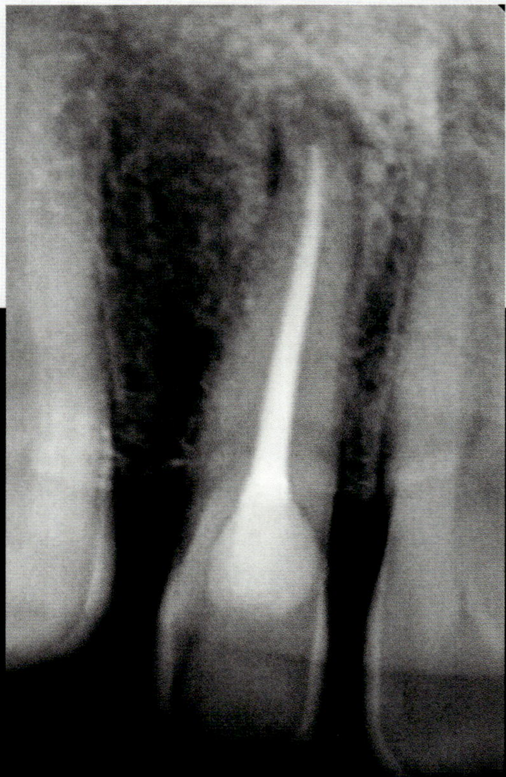
7a

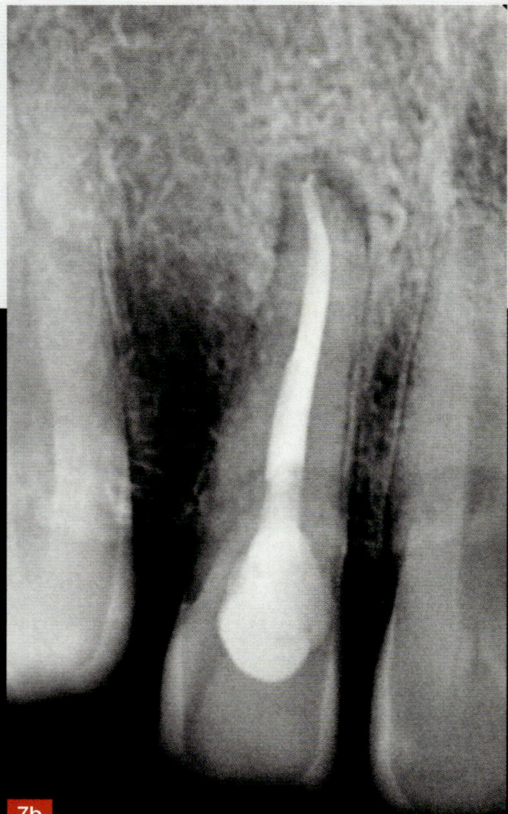
7b

Figure 7a-b: The progression of the periapical reparation procedure is noticeable.

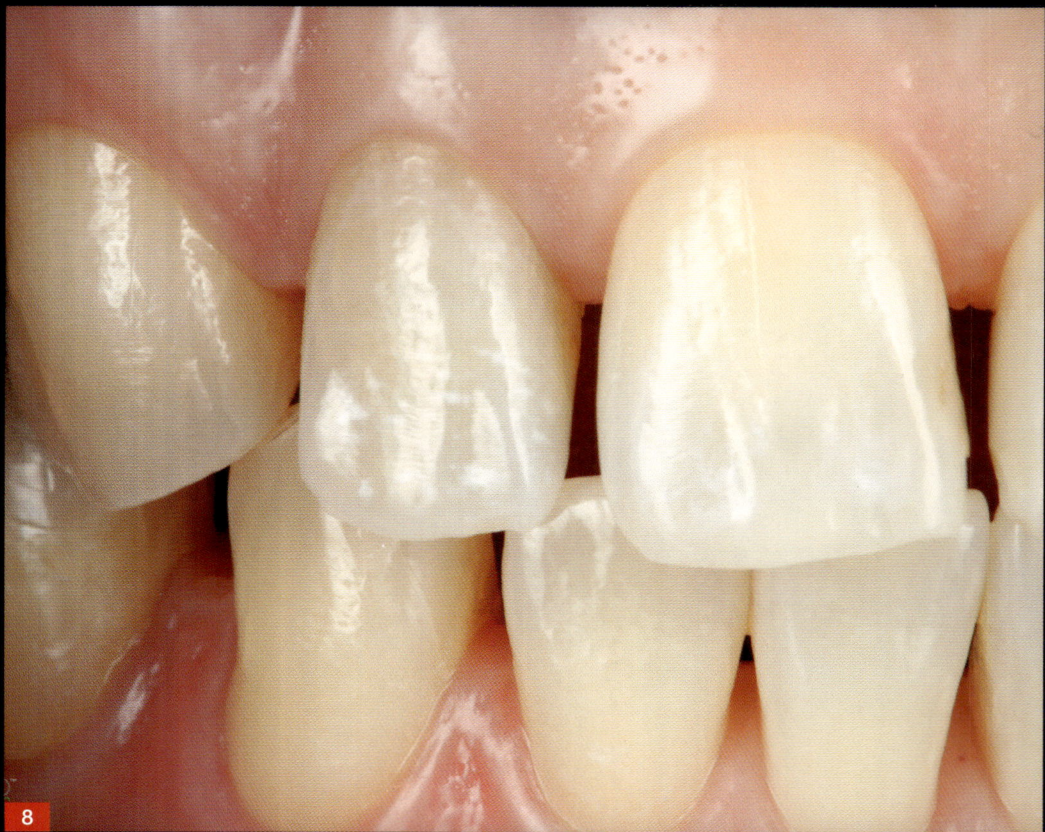
8

Figure 8: The frontal view of the lateral incisor is returning to normality; the slightly gray appearance can be improved by further external bleaching.

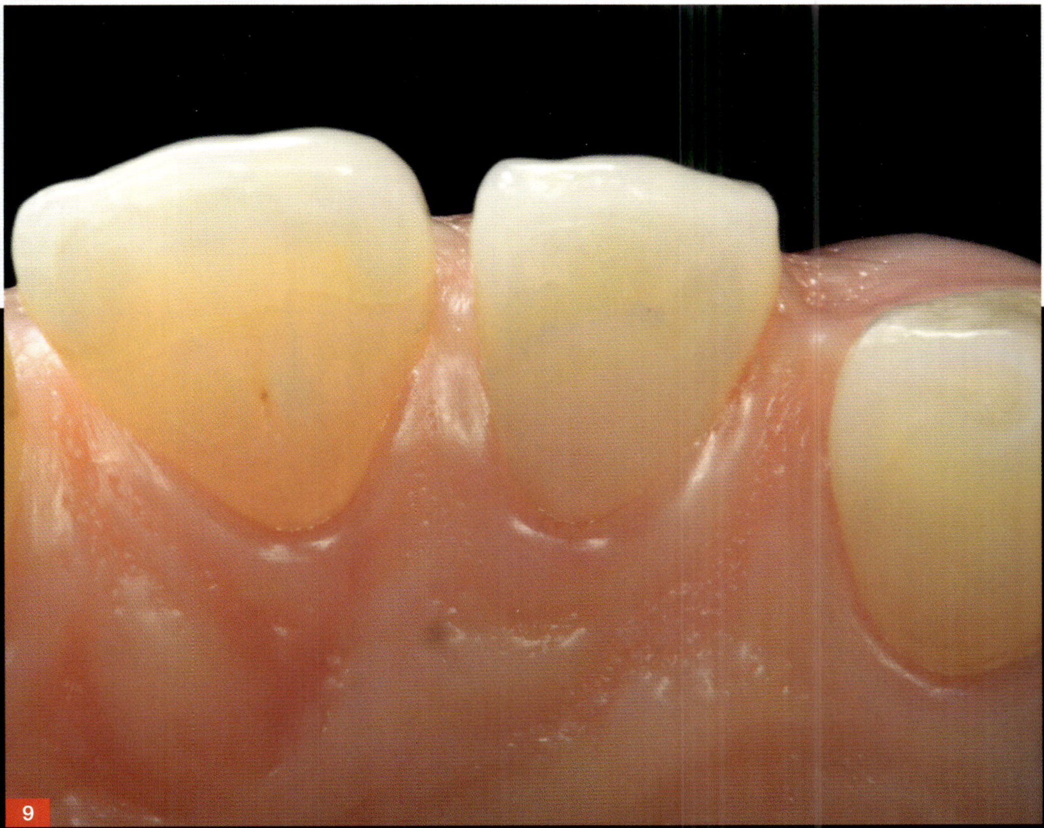

9

Figure 9: Palatal view showing the filling material is perfectly integrated with the enamel.

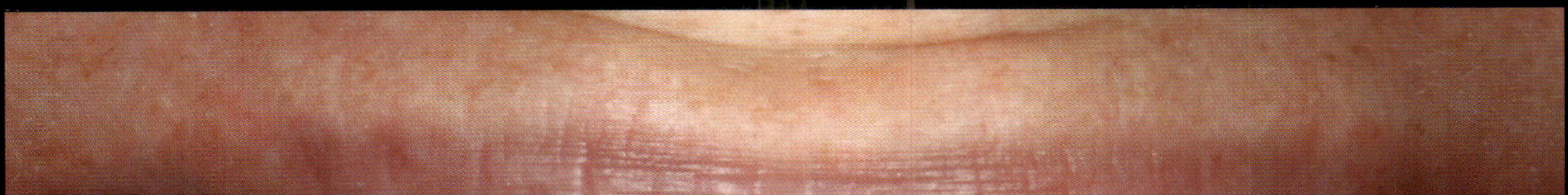

10

Figure 10: The whole mouth and the satisfactory esthetical aspect of the tooth in the patient's smile.

CASE REPORT 2

Postendodontic reconstruction by CAD/CAM overlay

The tooth was endodontically treated approximately 2 years previously. The patient came in with some concerns as a small part of the old filling was broken. The initial x-ray revealed that the tooth had a inefficient root canal filling, in the mesial and distal root (Fig. 1).
There was no sign of disease in the periapical region and the tooth was asymptomatic.

Figure 1: Initial X-ray

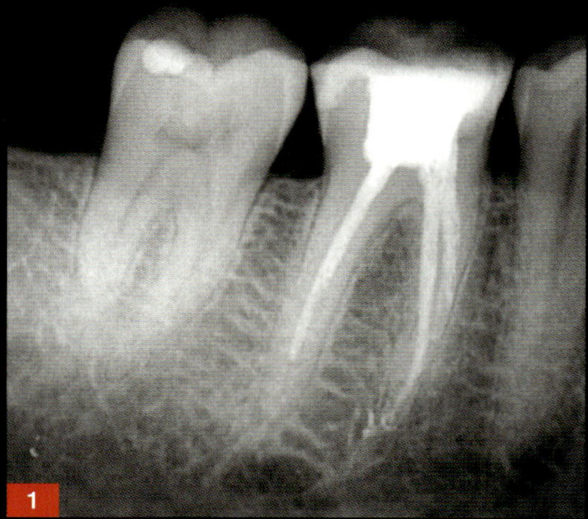

Figures 2-5: The first session started with the isolation and the removal of the old filling using the MTWO retreatment file (VDW) and Gutasolv (Septodont), a product to soften the gutta percha and which enables it to be easily removed. After removing the gutta percha, we detected the second distal canal, the mechanical instrumentation of all canals is performed with Reciproc blue file. For the chemical irrigation in this case we used 5.25% NaOCl, EDTA, citric acid and the activation was performed with Eddy (VDW). Canal filling was performed with Guttafusion and Ah+.

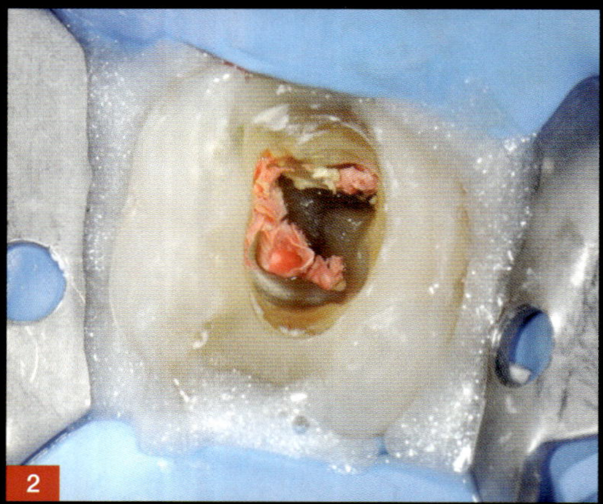

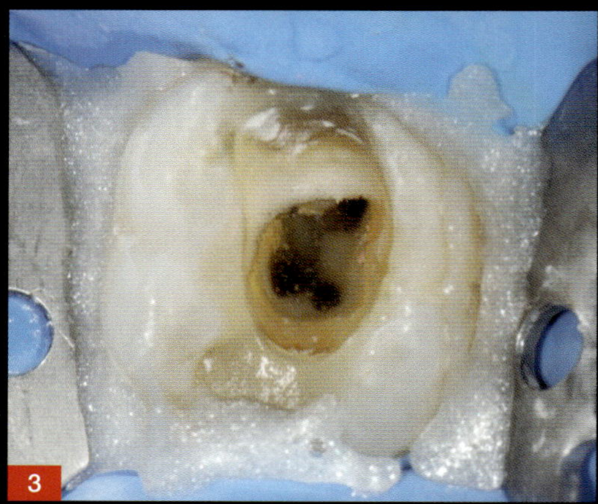

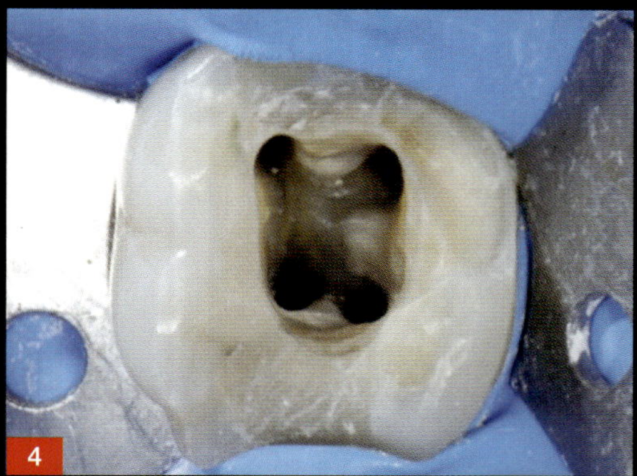

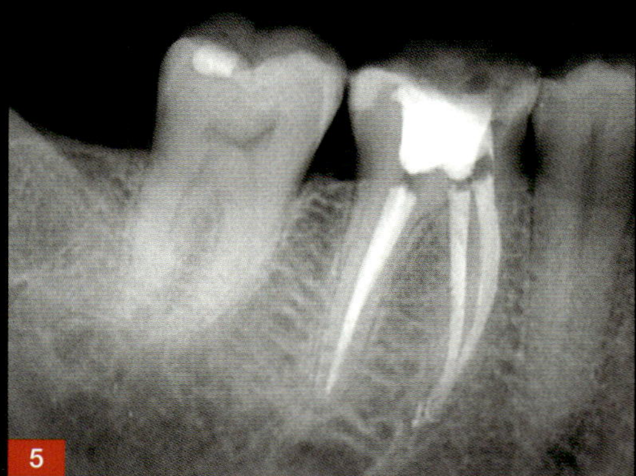

Owing to the poor quality of the previous post-endodontic restoration, an indirect partial restoration was planned; an overlay was preferred to a crown because the tooth was endodontically treated and a cuspal protection should be provided, particularly in molar teeth, which are to prevent cuspal or coronal fractures, more frequent when composite direct fillings have been used.

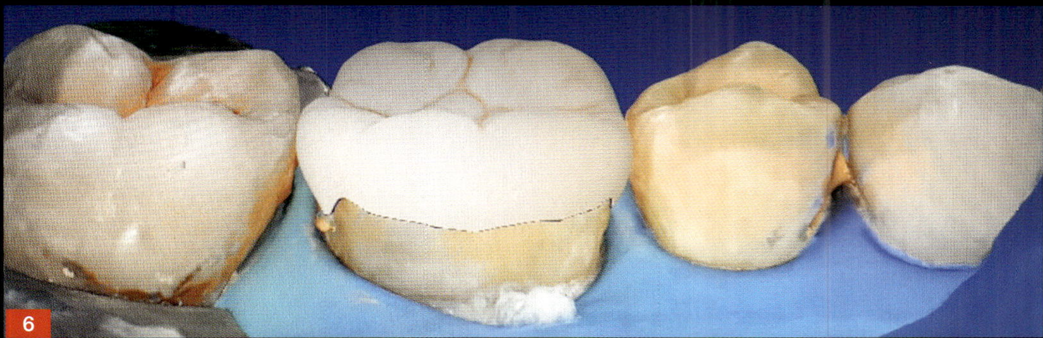

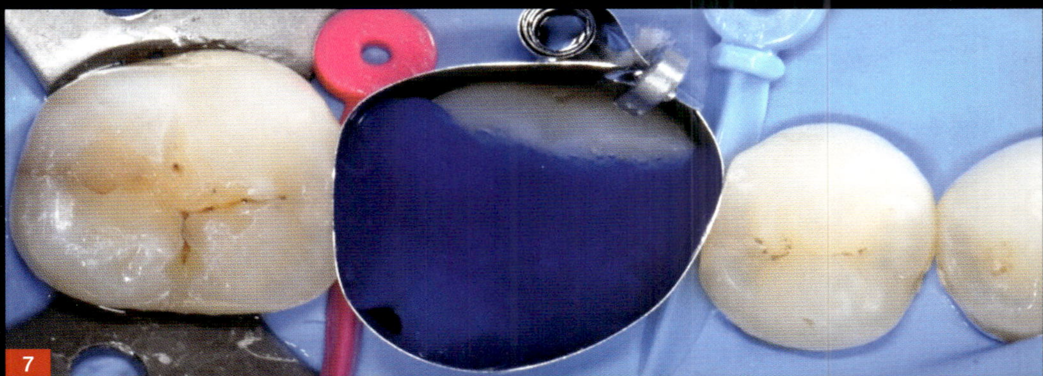

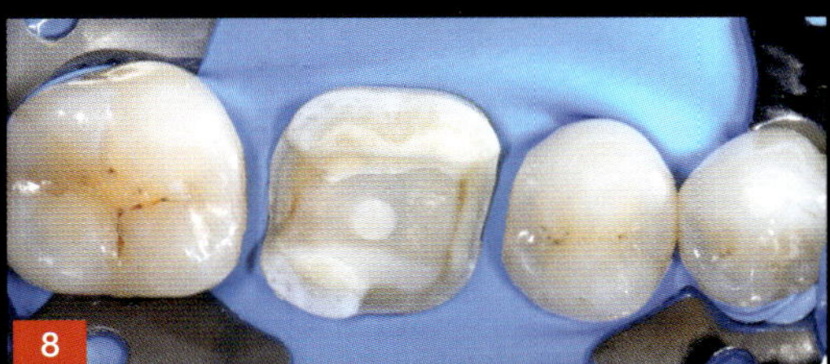

Figures 6-8: For the final restoration a fiber post and an indirect partial restoration were choosen. The cavity was filled with composit and then prepared for an overlay.

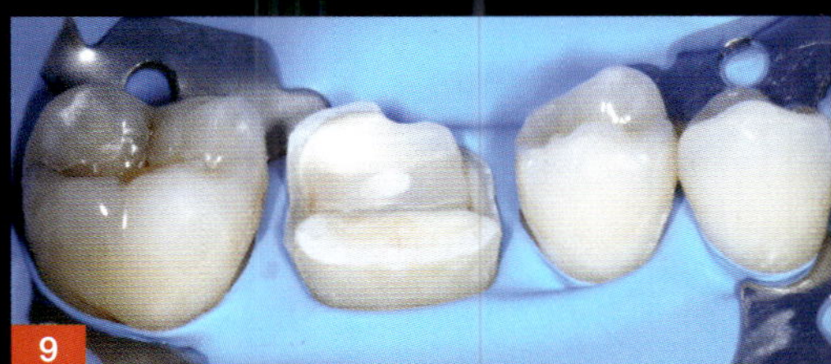

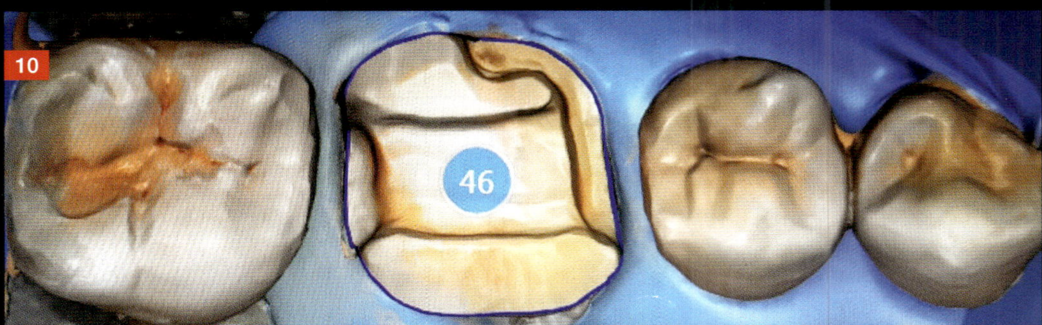

Figures 9-10: The overlay preparation made the optical impression by intraoral scanner (Cerec, Dentsplay Sirona) easier, although the tooth is still isolated by the rubber dam. The optical impression, with this strategy, facilitated the identification of the preparation lines during the overlay design phase.

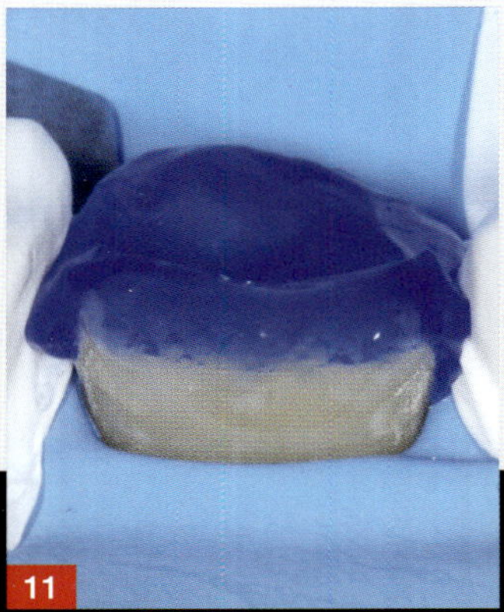

11

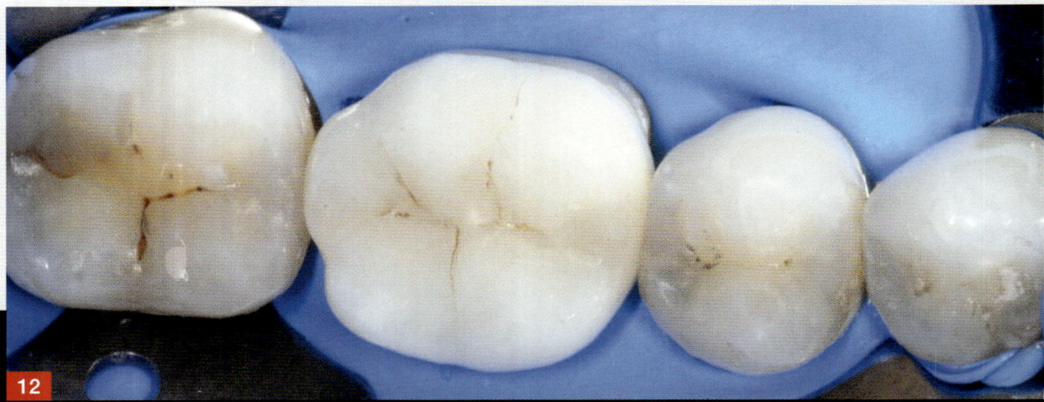

12

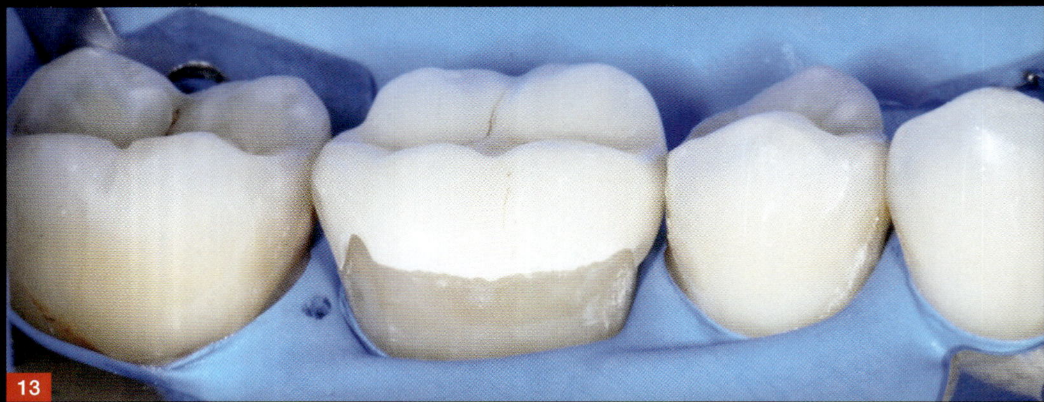

13

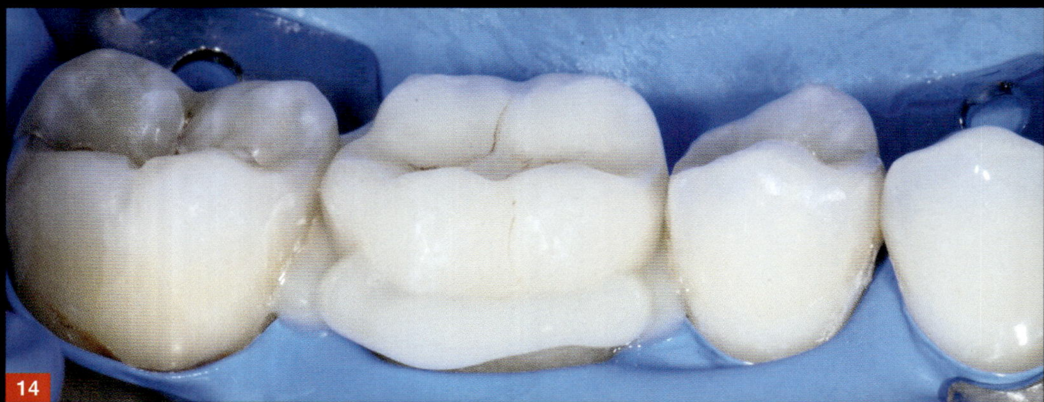

14

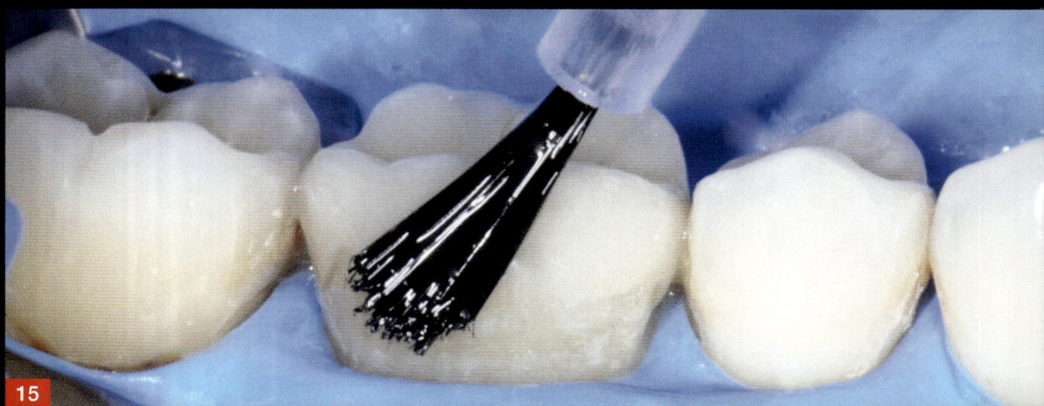

15

Figures 11-15: We chose a lithium disilicate crown (ips e.max) for better chemical adhesion. Multiple tooth isolation is very important for cleaning the interdental spaces after cementation. The cementation of the crown was performed with Multilink. The use of a brush to remove the excess cement is more practica in order I to avoid micropremises between the tooth and the marginal part of the crown.

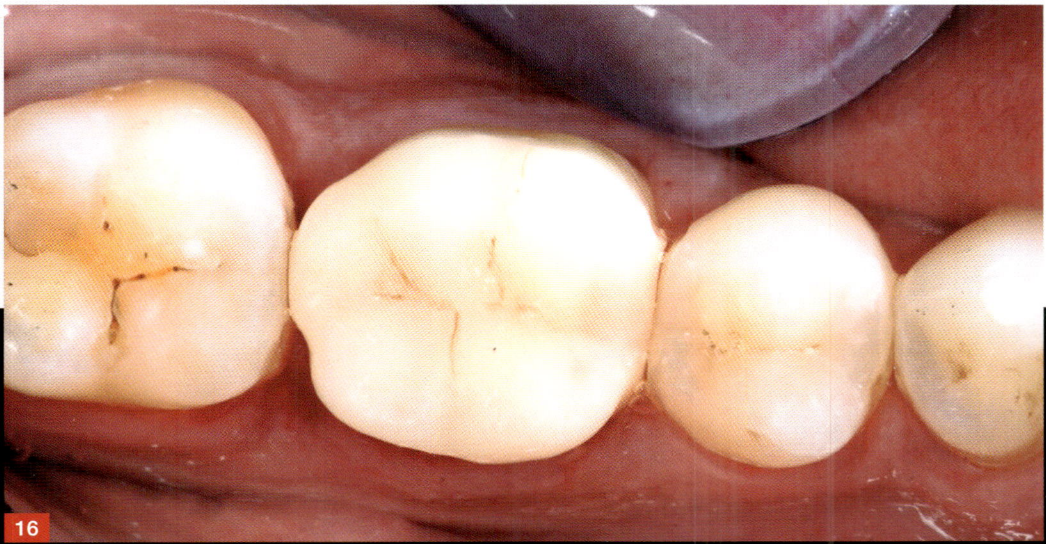

16

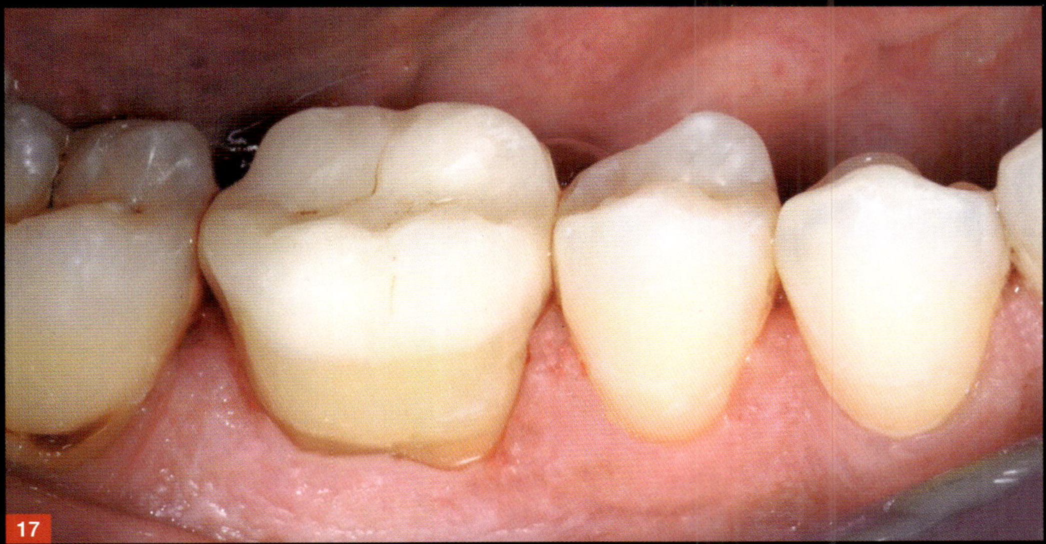

17

Figures 16 -17: The occlusal view and the lateral view of the final lithium disilicate restoration; this type of restoration has the extraordinary advantage of preserving much of the tooth structure.

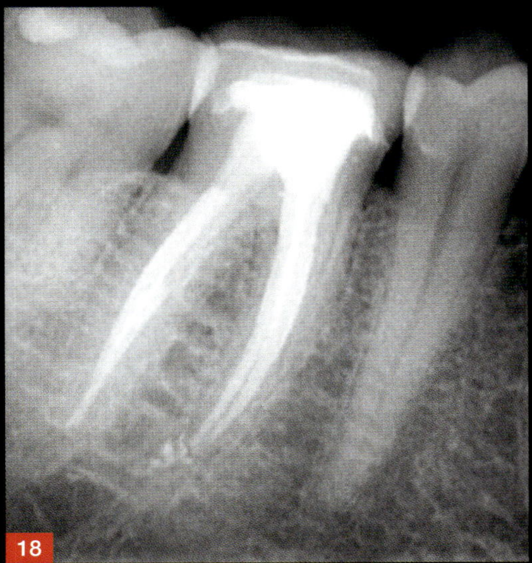

18

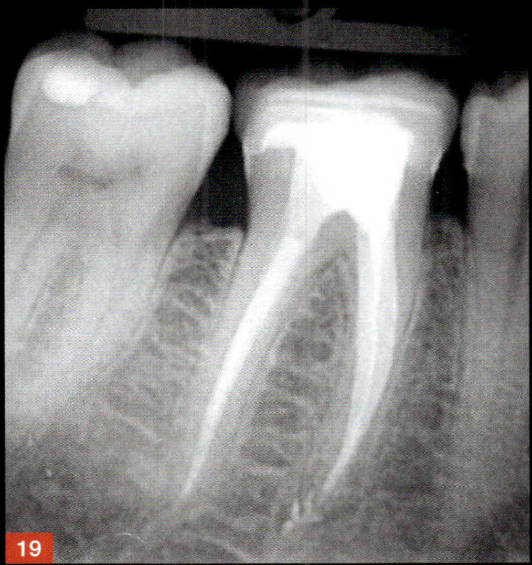

19

Figures 18-19: After 18 months the x-ray shows a complete healing of periapical tissues and the patient has no complaints.

CASE REPORT 3

Proximal lesions and retreatments: a restorative approach

A 22-year-old patient who came in with pain localized at the interdental papilla between teeth 15 and 16. Clinical and radiographical examination (Figs.1-2) revealed the presence of carious lesions on teeth 17-16-15-14. The second upper premolar had an incorrect root canal treatment, so a root canal retreatment was indicated. The treatment plan was split over three appointments.

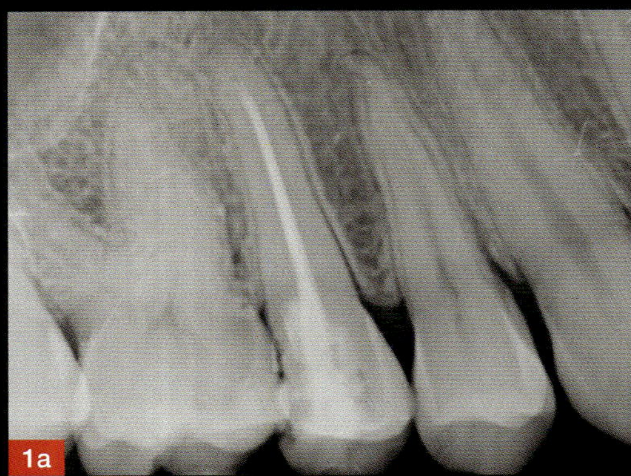

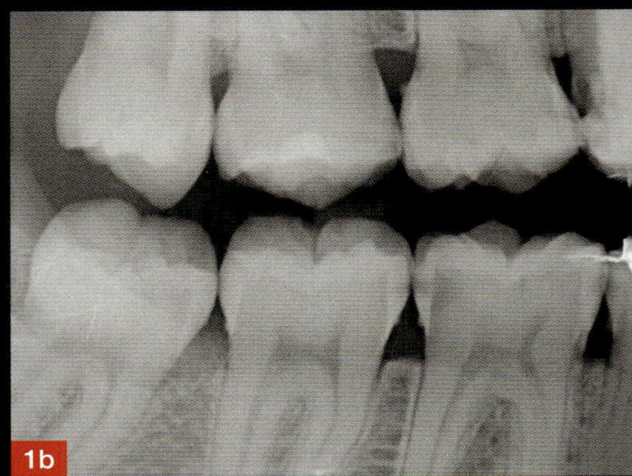

Figure 1a-b: Radiographic examination.

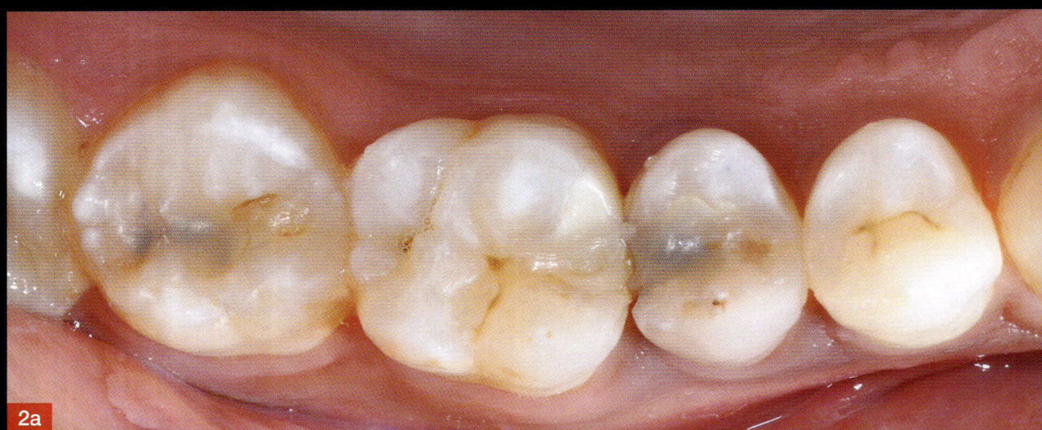

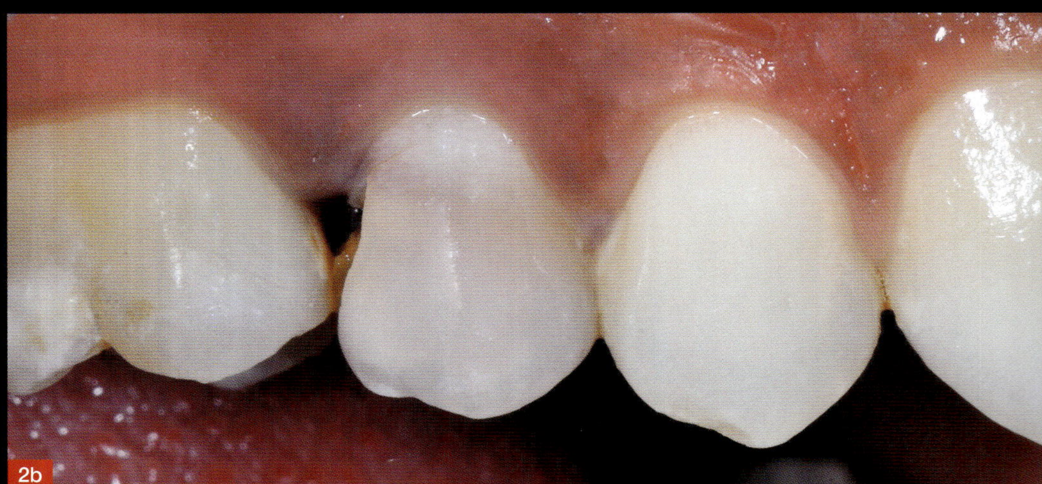

Figure 2a-b: Clinical examination.

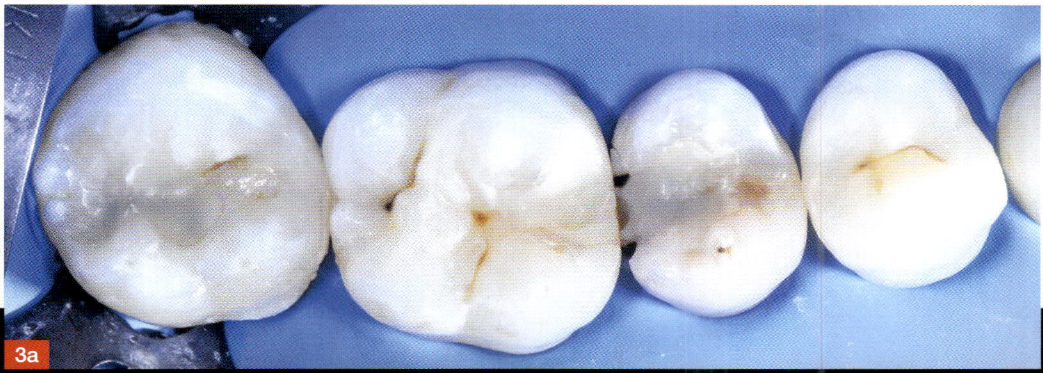

3a

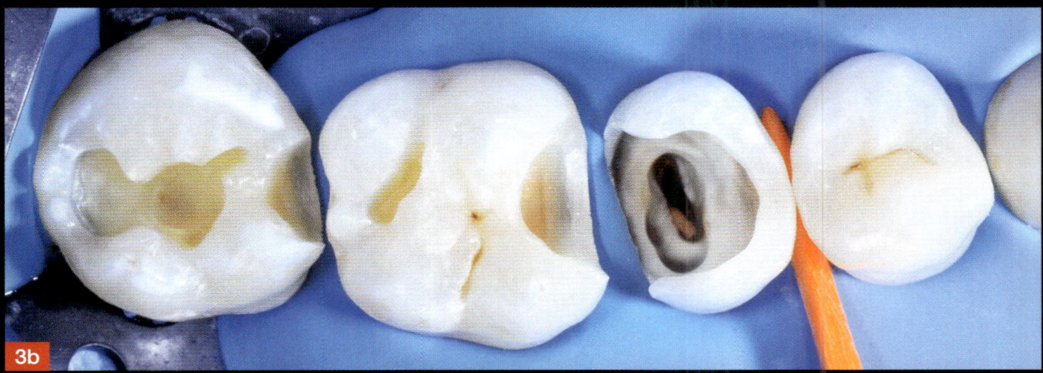

3b

Figure 3a-b: During the first appointment direct restorations of teeth 17-16-14 and a pre-endo build-up of tooth 15 were performed. After the isolation of the quadrant (Fig. 3a), the cavities were cleaned with diamond and tungsten carbide burs, then the margins were finished with ultrasonic tips (Fig. 3b).

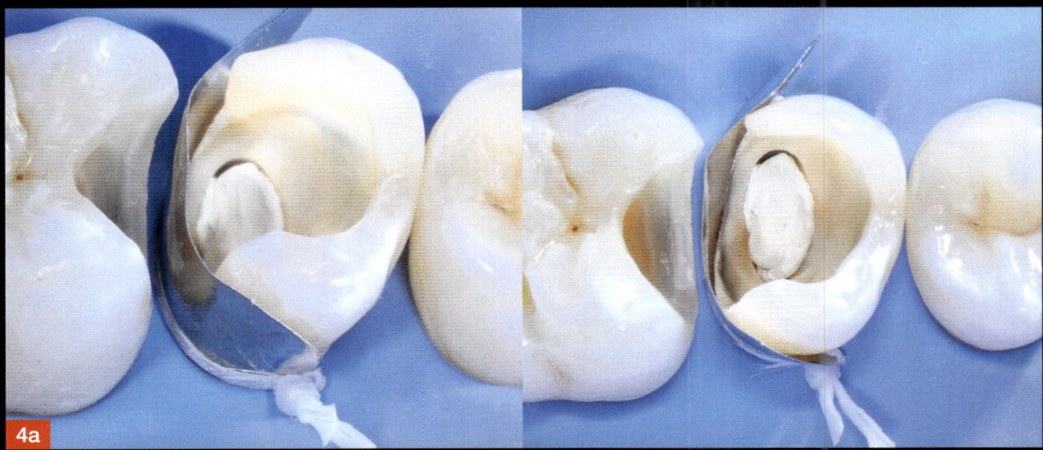

4a

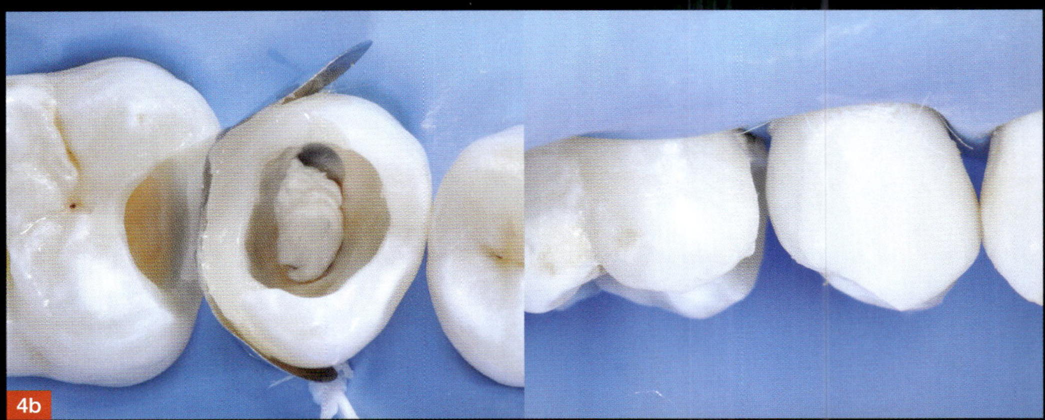

4b

Figure 4a-b: The direct restoration and the pre-endo build up were performed with a 3 step etch and rinse adhesive system and a nanofilled composite material.

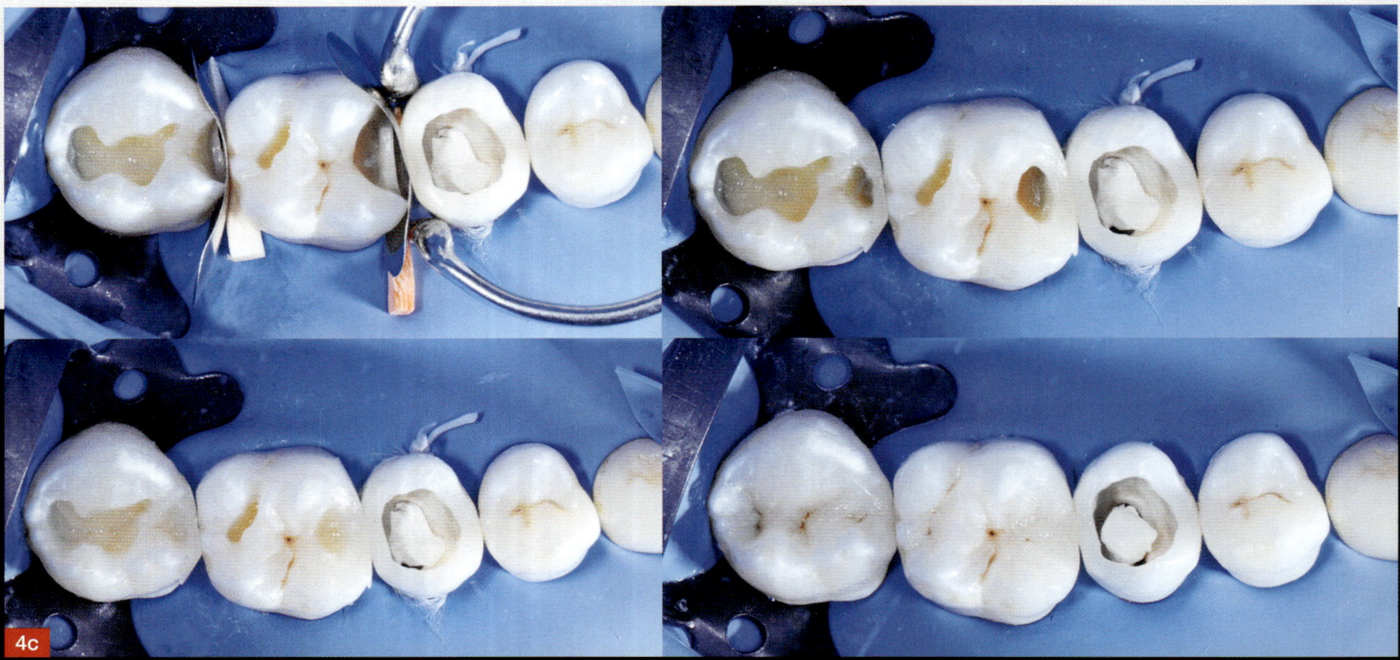

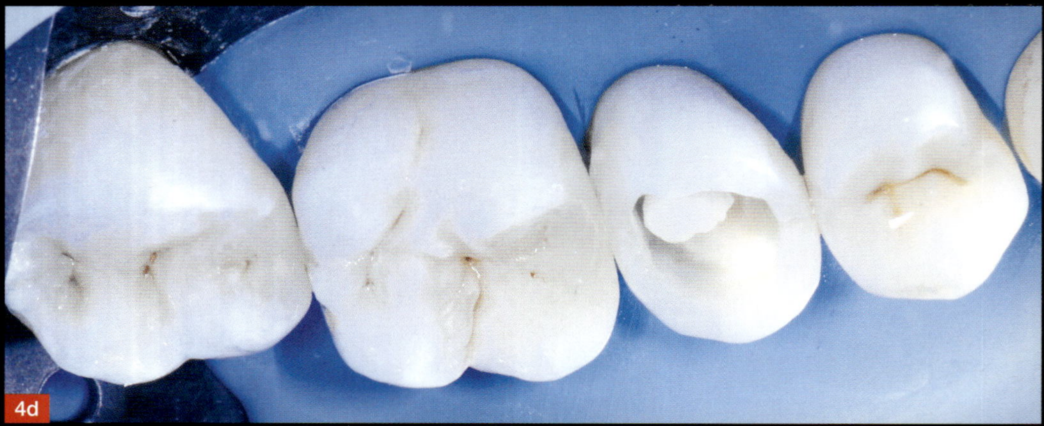

Figure 4c-d: Some of the clinical procedures to restore the occlusal and mesial caries in the molars and the posterior build-up in retreated premolar.

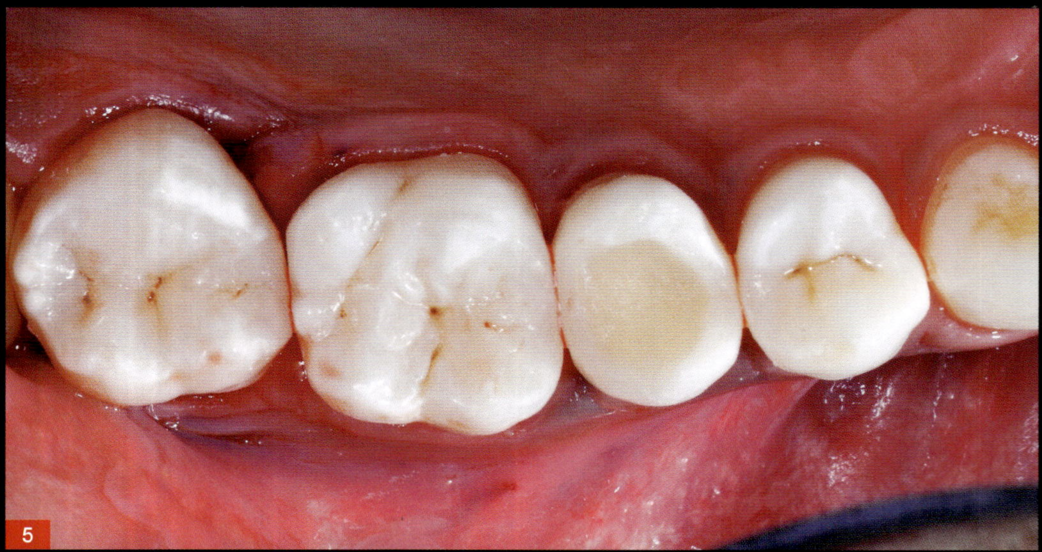

Figure 5: The occlusal cavity of tooth 15 was closed with a temporary material.

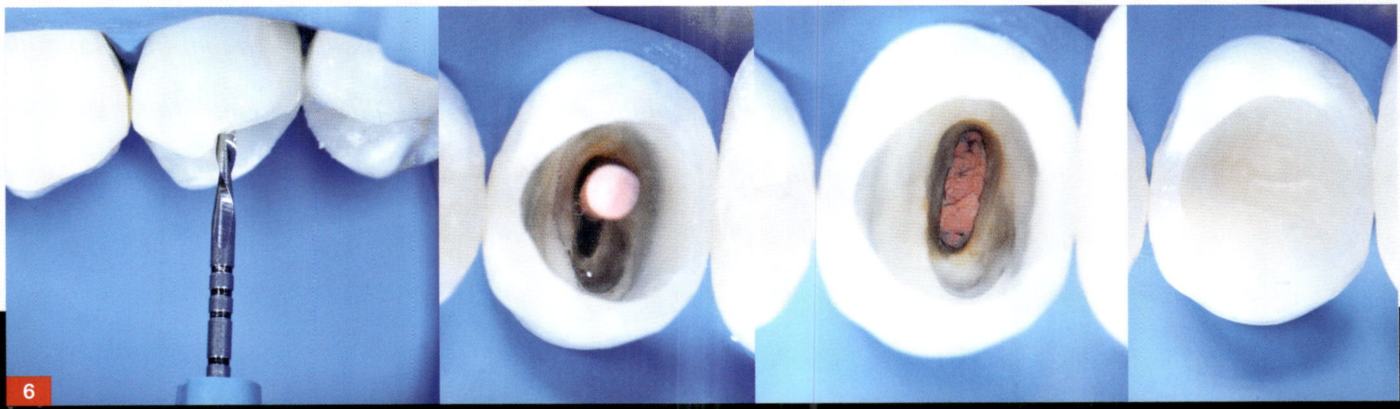

6

Figure 6: During the second appointment the root canal was retreated and restored and tooth 15 was prepared for a lithium disilicate veneer. The preparation of a veneer was necessary for esthetic reasons. A single canal was present and it was shaped with M2 to a size of 25 and 0.06 conicity, then the apical portion of the canal was finished with protaper gold until F3.

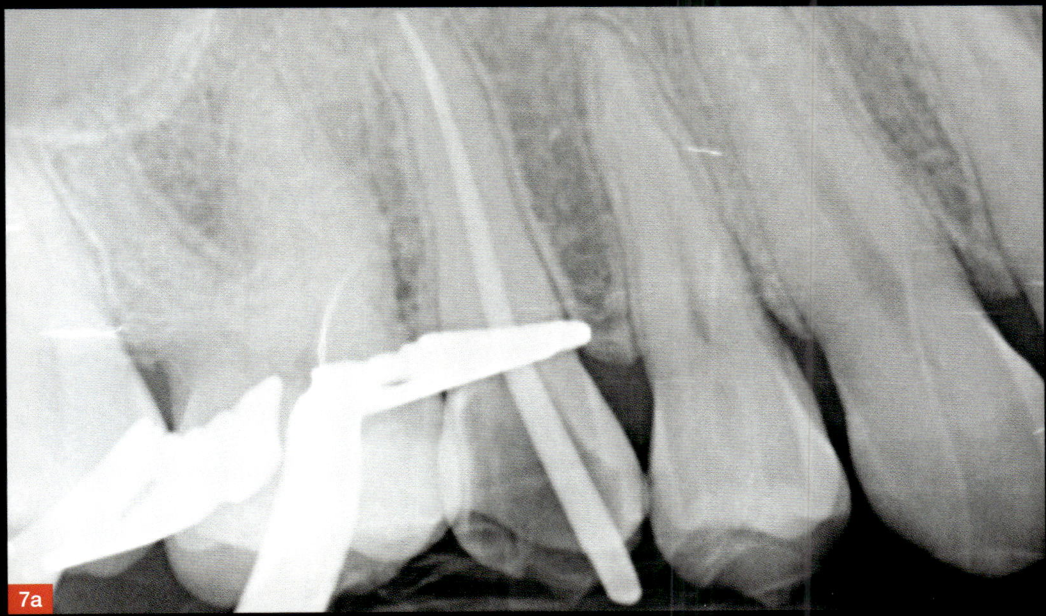

7a

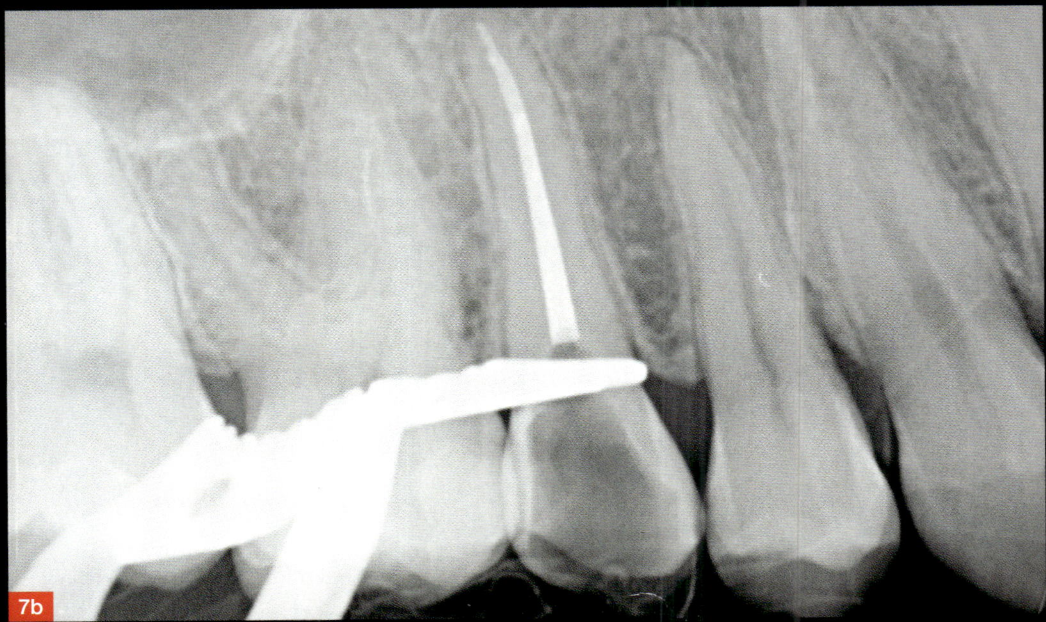

7b

Figure 7a-b: The working length was checked radiographically and the subsequent irrigation protocol consisted in 5.25% NaOCl and 17% EDTA. The canal was dried and the filling was performed with warm vertical condensation. The restoration was performed with a 3 step etch and rinse adhesive system and a nanofilled composite material (see Fig. 6).

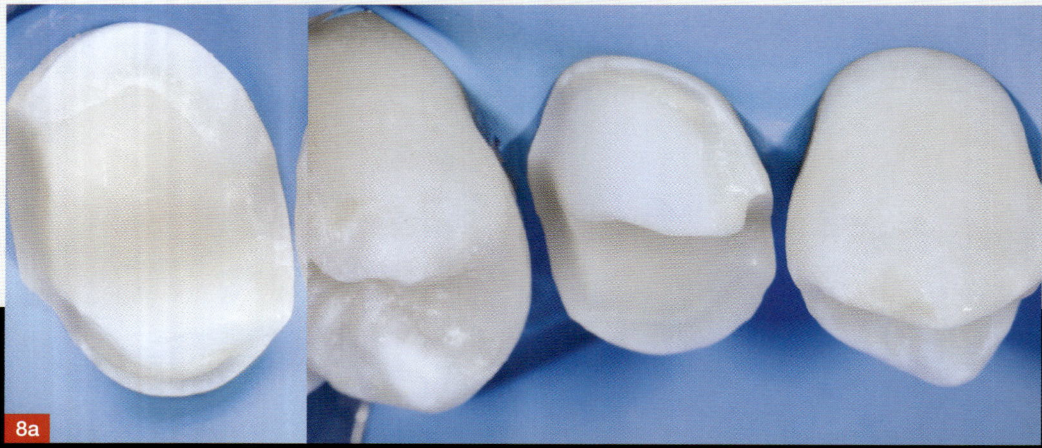

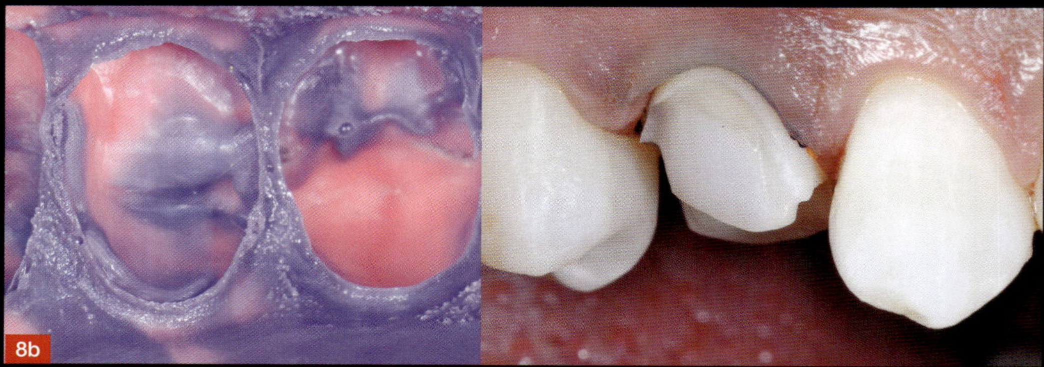

Figure 8a-b: The tooth was prepared with diamond burs (a) and the impression was taken with a polyether (b).

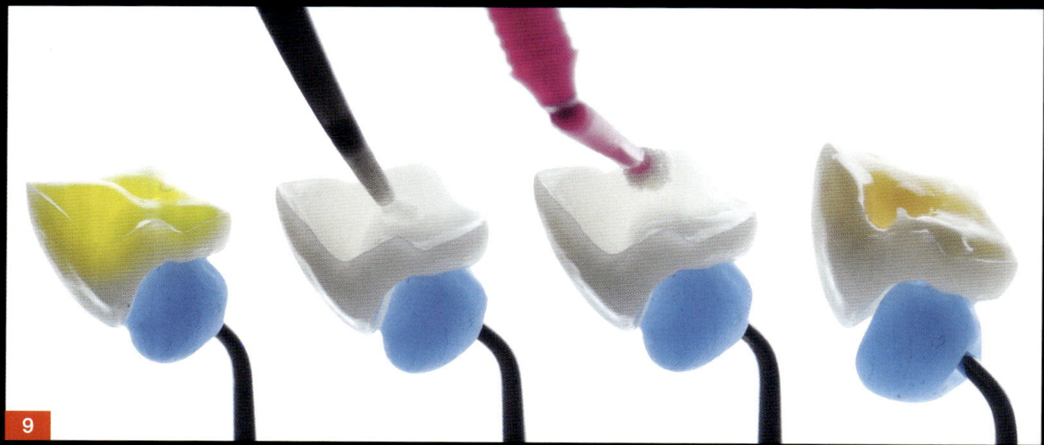

Figure 9: During the third appointment the veneer was cemented. The tooth surface was treated with air abrasion and a 3 step etch and rinse adhesive system, the lithium disilicate surface was treated with hydrofluoric acid, orthophosphoric acid, silane and bonding.

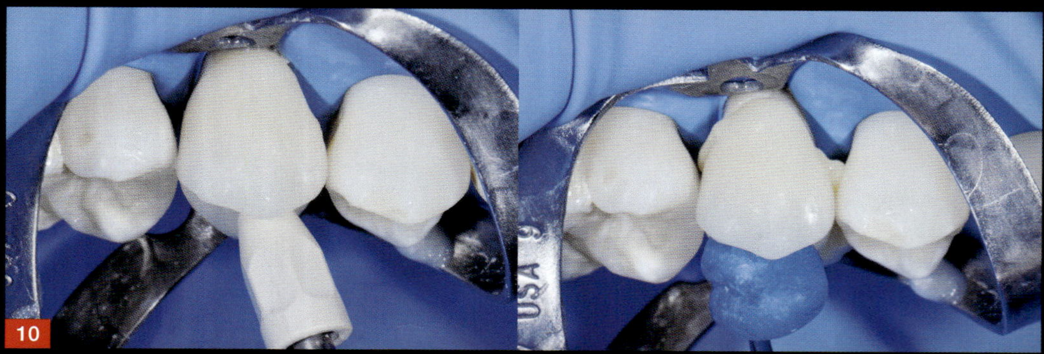

Figure 10: The veneer was cemented with a nanofilled composite material.

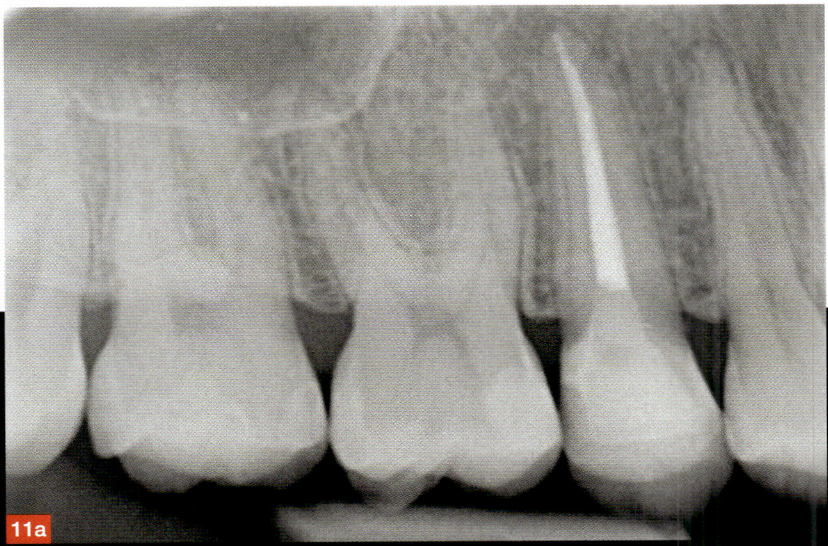

Figure 11a: The radiographic examination after one year demonstrates a perfect sealing of both restoration and root canal filling with no apical signs of post treatment disease.

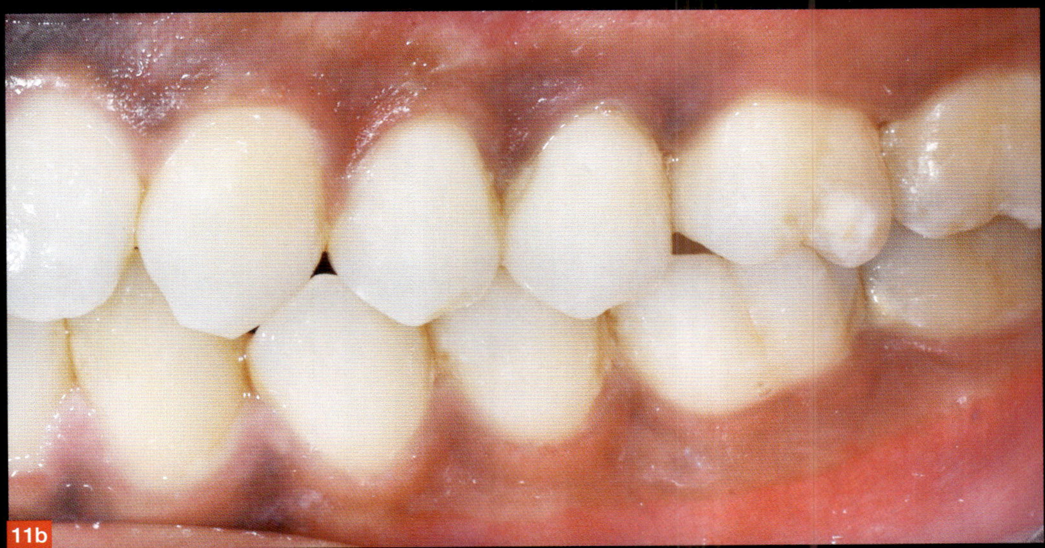

Figure 11b: Buccal aspect of the restored teeth.

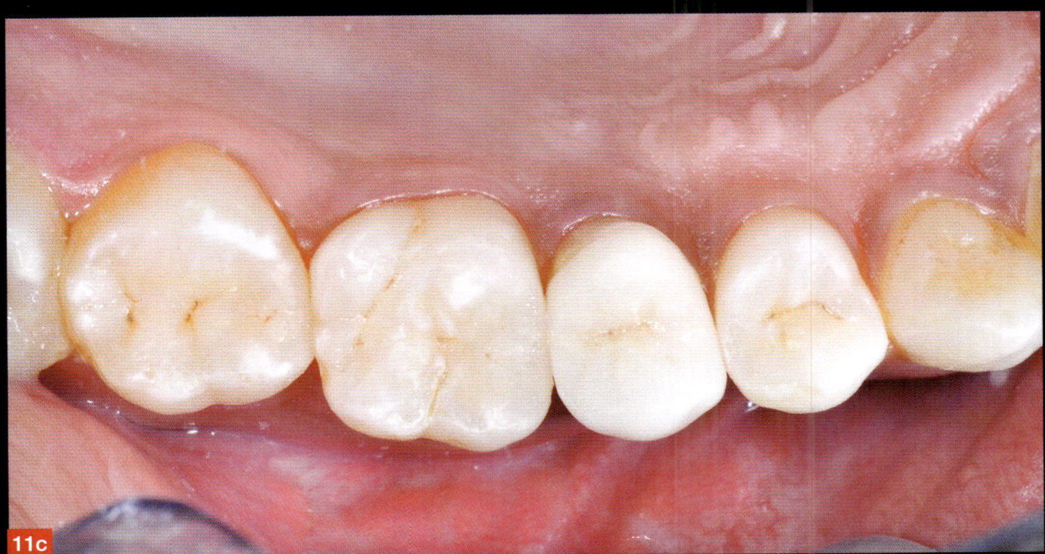

Figure 11c: Occlusal aspect of the teeth restored by direct and indirect restorations.

From the perspective of materials, research suggests the use of materials mechanically similar to dentin, namely, fiber posts and composite materials, and discourages use of stiff (e.g., metallic) materials. Adhesive techniques are indicated for the cementation of a root canal post, reconstruction of the abutment, and cementation of an indirect composite or ceramic restoration.

Useful techniques for the reconstruction of retreated teeth

The operating methods, largely borrowed from those used in the era of non-adhesive dentistry, have been enhanced in recent years by new proposals aimed at achieving the best performance from metal-free ceramic restorations. These choices are motivated by the fact that the biomechanical characteristics and wear of restorative materials are similar to those of teeth.
The endocrown, margin reallocation, "Morphology-driven Preparation Technique," and "Outcome-based Preparation Design" techniques yield good findings in retreated teeth.

Endocrown

The endocrown (Figs. 9.19-9.21), which was proposed in 1999 by Bindl and Mormann[70], whose work was based on the concepts expressed by Pissis in 1995[71] as an alternative to the classic abutment post and crown, is a monolithic ceramic adhesive restoration. The endocrown is characterized by a flat shoulder supragingival closure, possibly on enamel, which finds retention inside the pulp chamber without invading the canals. It can be manufactured by Cad/Cam milling or die-casting.
The type of preparation and the adhesive cementation are highly favorable from a biomechanical point of view[72, 73].
This technique should be counted among the reconstruction options for retreated teeth[74].

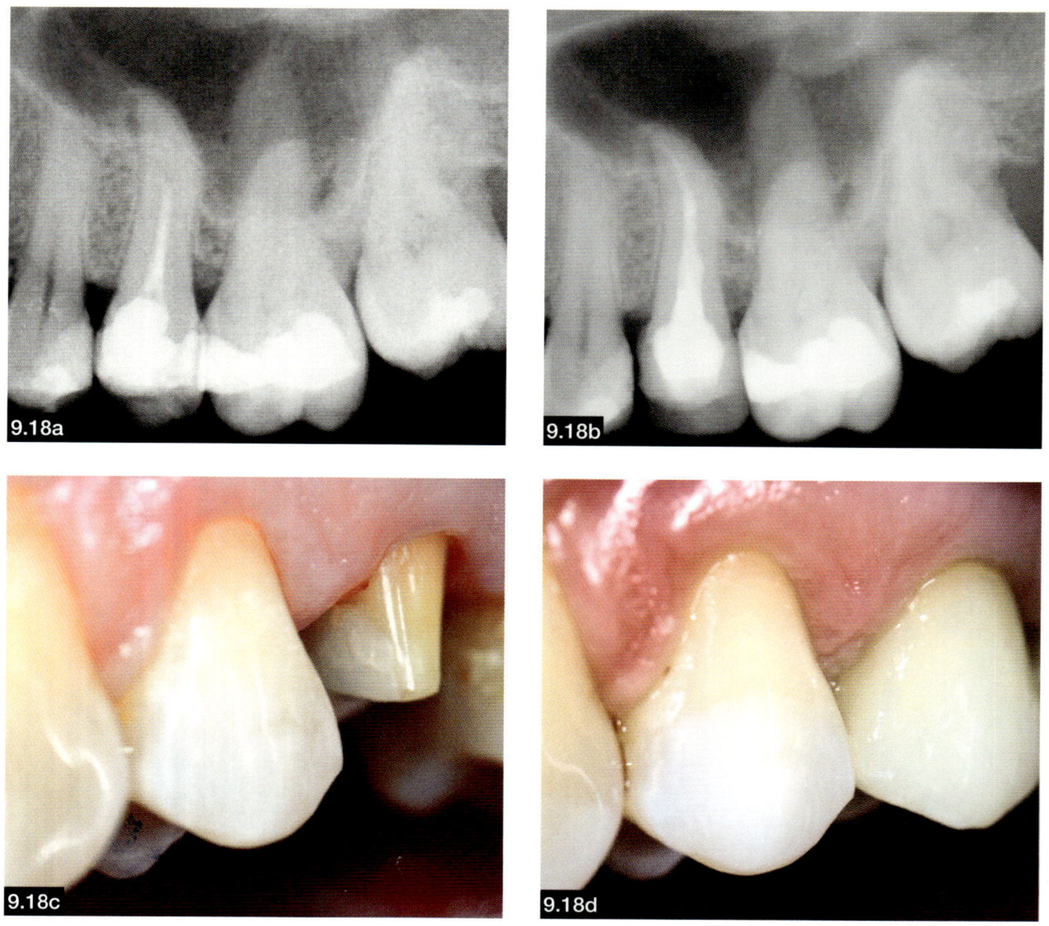

Fig. 9.18a-d: Total indirect restoration. In a premolar with a failed endodontic treatment a new canal therapy is carried out and has the desired effect. A complete crown is made due to the destruction of the tooth.

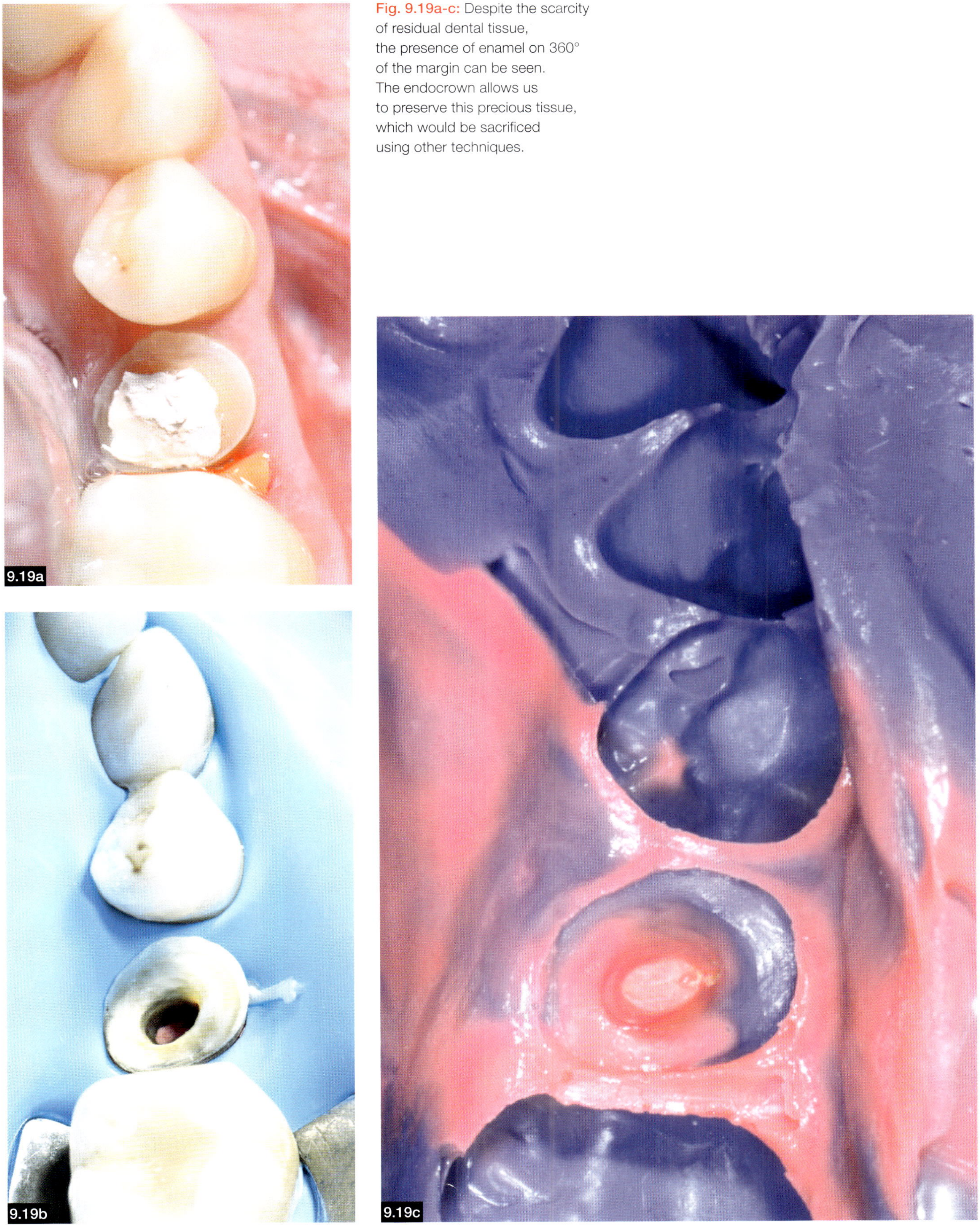

Fig. 9.19a-c: Despite the scarcity of residual dental tissue, the presence of enamel on 360° of the margin can be seen. The endocrown allows us to preserve this precious tissue, which would be sacrificed using other techniques.

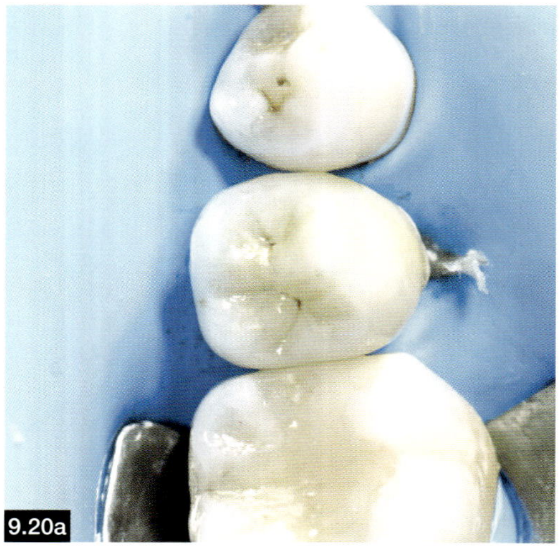
9.20a

Margin reallocation

The technique of reallocating the reconstructive margin may be frequently indicated in the restoration of a retreated tooth. In cases of deep caries, when a rubber dam can be positioned and in the absence of an invasion of the biological space, the prosthetic margin can be made to emerge or be "reallocated" to a more coronal site, simplifying subsequent maneuvers[75]. This procedure can also be performed early in the endodontic pre-treatment stages[76].
This will greatly facilitate all endodontic procedures required in such complex cases.

Fig. 9.20a-c: The adaptation of the endocrown is checked and cemented with an adhesive technique.

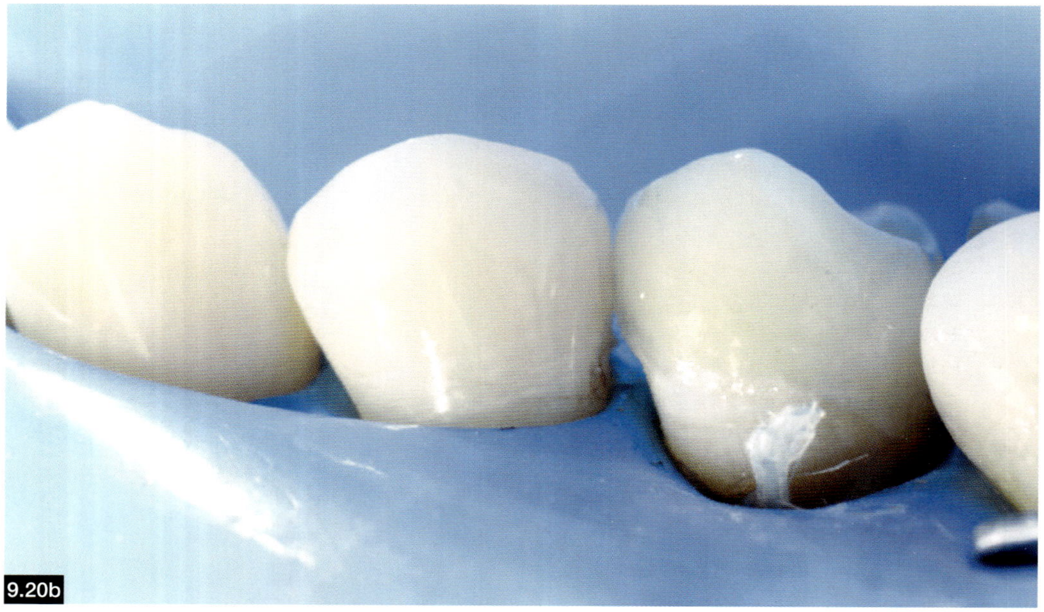
9.20b

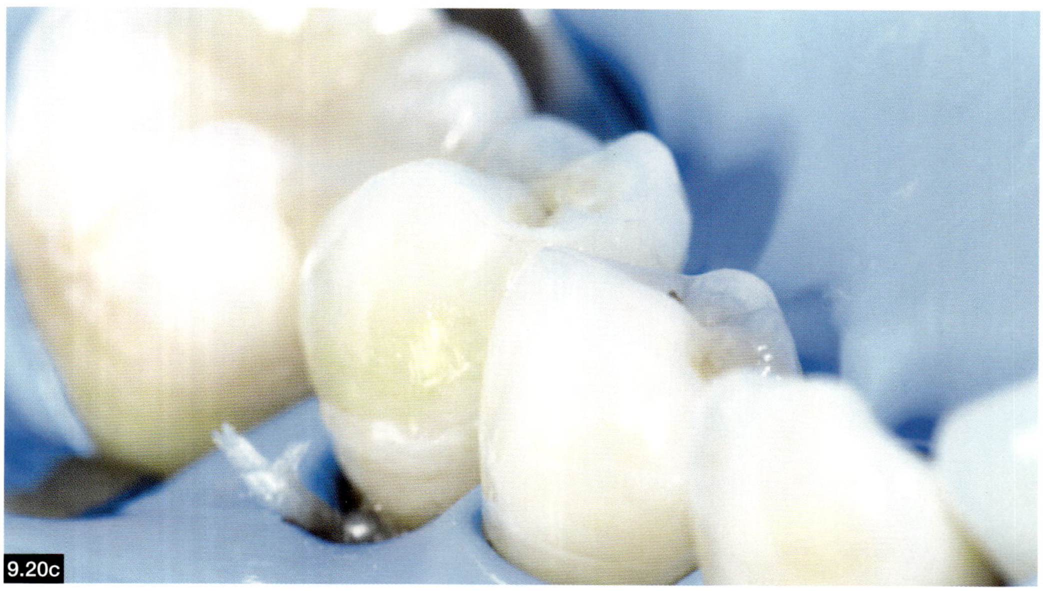
9.20c

Morphology-driven Technique Preparation

The "Morphology-driven Preparation Technique"[77] is a technique that describes types of preparation intended for adhesive ceramic restorations on the posteriors, with maximum savings in dental tissue and with strong possibility of adhesion to residual structures. This technique is an alternative option to the other categories of indirect partial adhesive restorations that are used in retreated teeth, namely *overlay-veneer, long-wrap overlay*, and *adhesive crown* (Figs. 9.22–9.28).

Outcome-Based Preparation Design

With similar aims, the "Outcome-based Preparation Design"[78] describes a differentiated anterior preparation protocol aimed at restoring structurally compromised teeth. As is often the case in retreated teeth, the thicknesses needed to achieve good aesthetic and functional outcome and the various types of materials indicated must be identified. In this technique, three types of preparations are used, namely, "minimal," "conventional," and "extended."

Readaptation (retrofitting) of an existing crown

If an endodontically treated tooth rehabilitated with a complete crown needs to be retreated, it is possible to decement the crown, dismantle the abutment, perform endodontic procedures, reconstruct the abutment, and recement the existing crown. Ideally, this procedure requires a perfect marginal fit and at least 2 mm of circumferentially present coronal dentin. Numerous techniques have been proposed. In 1970, Goldrich described two techniques for the construction of posts under existing crowns and even used part of a paperclip[79]. In 1982, Brady[80] described a procedure based on the use of copper rings, parapulpal posts, and thermoplastic paste.

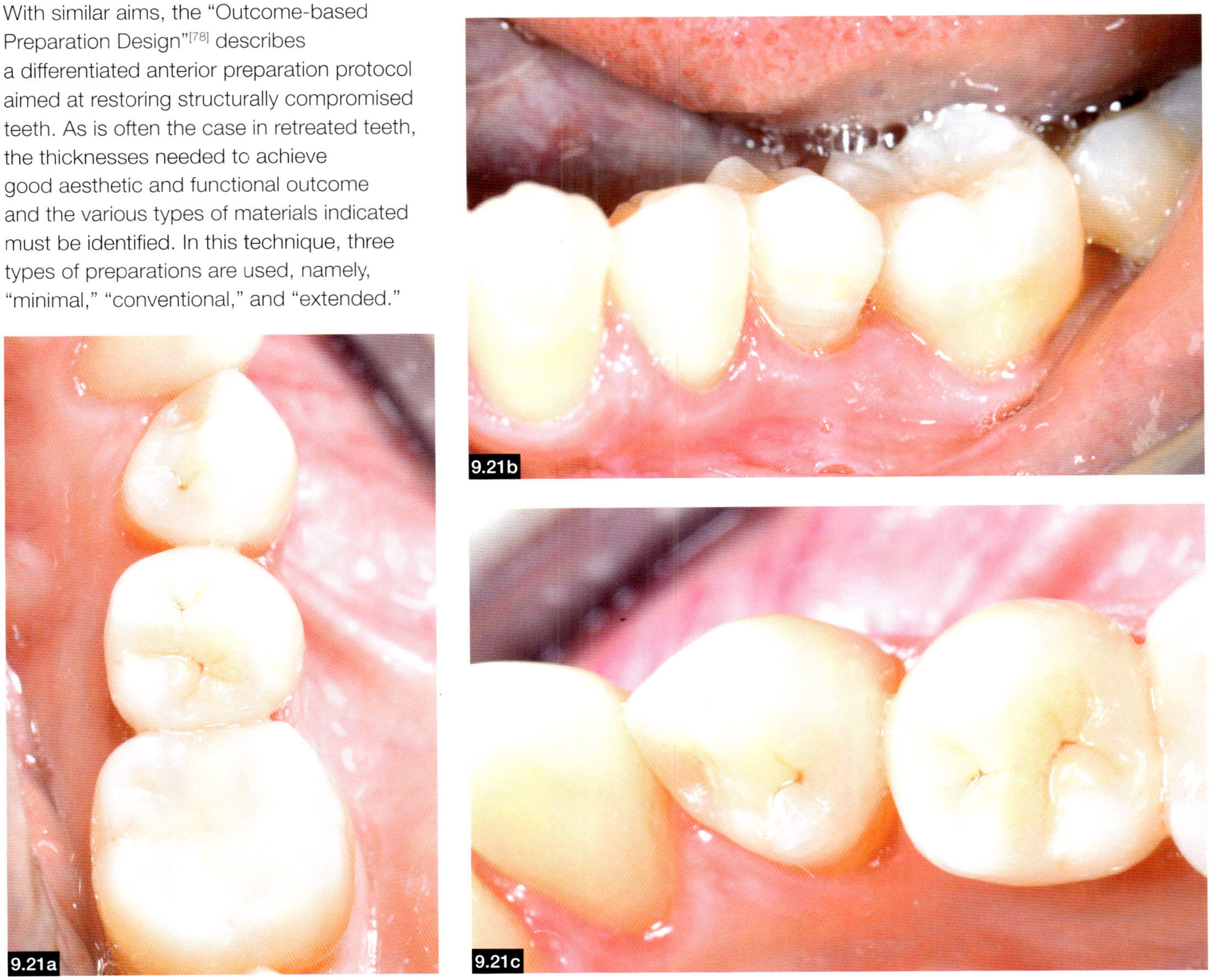

Fig. 9.21a-c: After removal of the rubber dam, the accuracy of the occlusal contacts is checked. Functional and aesthetic integration in the natural teeth is good.

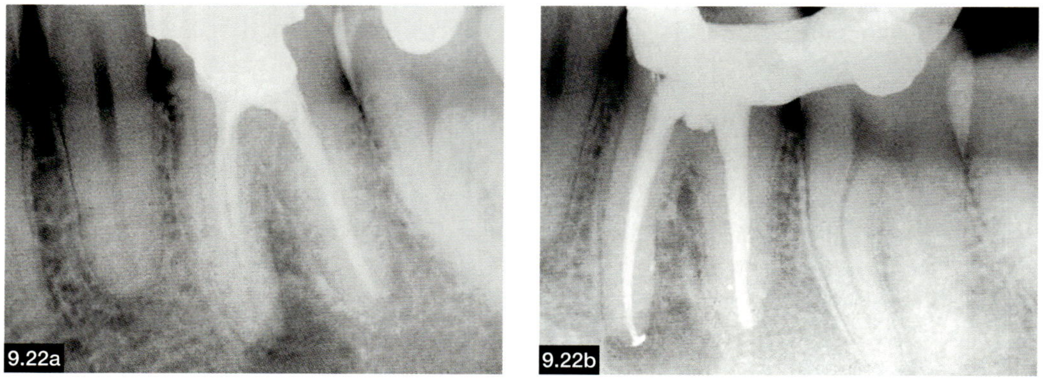

Fig. 9.22a-b: Endodontic retreatment allows the healing of a periradicular lesion arising after ineffective treatment.

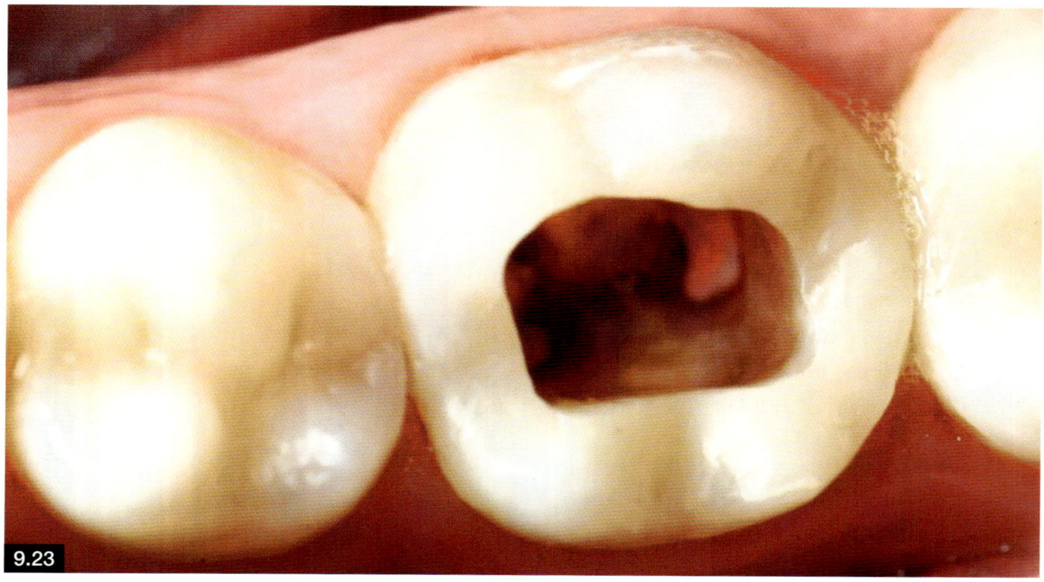

Fig. 9.23: Residual dentin tissue is scarce; an indirect restoration is necessary.

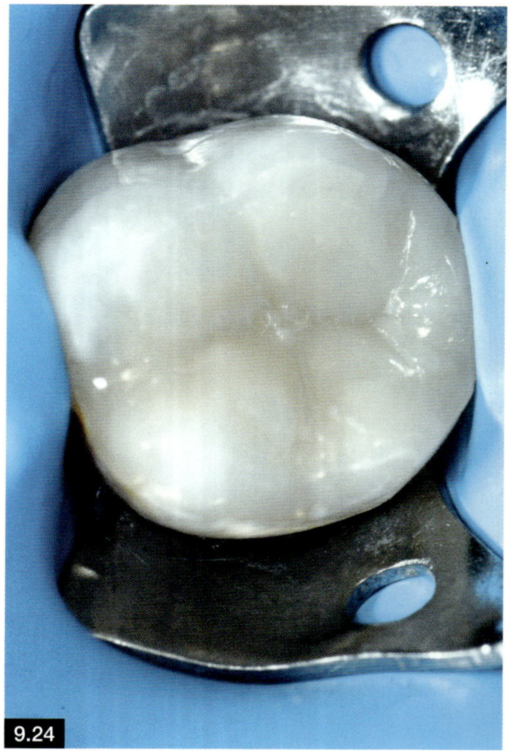

Fig. 9.24: The cavity is filled with composite, and an adhesive technique is carried out for the build-up.

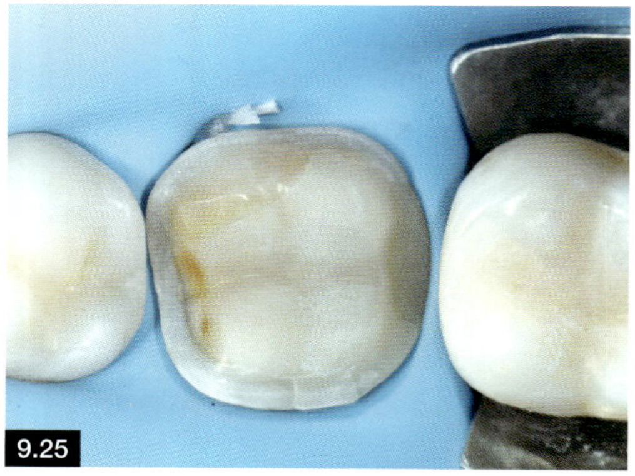

Fig. 9.25: A minimally invasive partial preparation allows for the maximum preservation of the residual healthy tissue.

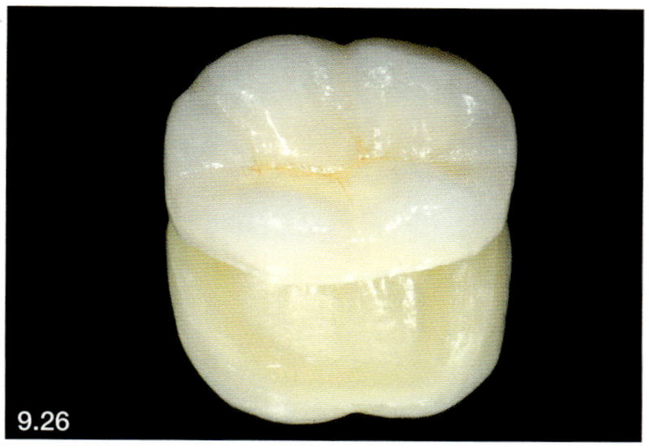

Fig. 9.26: Restoration is carried out using lithium disilicate ceramic.

In 2017, Lee[81] demonstrated the use of digital Cad/Cam technology for the reconstruction of an abutment under a prefabricated crown. The use of the existing crown as a mold for rebuilding the abutment is often proposed, both with direct and indirect techniques. However, the possibility of introducing distortions and voids, the lack of space for cement, and the impossibility of using light-curing materials make this technique unpredictable. Some variations were subsequently introduced, such as the interposition of a thin Teflon tape[82, 83] or aluminum foil[84], or the use of elastomeric matrices obtained from the existing model (obviously if this is available)[85], or the use of a transparent thermoformed template on a replica of the inside of the crown to be readjusted[86].
Each of these techniques can be used directly, with the use of prefabricated and composite posts, or indirectly, by constructing a burn-out resin post to be cast into an individual gold alloy post.

Retrofitting of an existing cast post

In the past, the only viable method for retaining a core in severely damaged teeth was to insert a cast post or to use prefabricated posts or screws. Prefabricated posts, despite their simple use, present a major problem in that the root canal must be prepared to house the post. Sound dentinal tissue has to be removed to place them, unnecessarily weakening the root.
By contrast, custom cast posts have a long history of clinical success. The traditional custom cast post and core can adapt to flared or elliptical canals and require minimal tooth structure removal. A common drawback of metallic posts (custom or prefabricated) is their modulus of elasticity, which can be as high as 10 times or more that of natural dentin. This feature can create stress concentration, resulting in catastrophic failure, according to the literature, which mainly contains data from in vitro studies. Custom-cast posts are supposed to have higher failure loads than posts with a low modulus of elasticity, but failure is often unrestorable. Favorable failures occur with posts with low modulus of elasticity[87]. Clinical studies on posts present a different story. Studies with lengthy follow-up (between

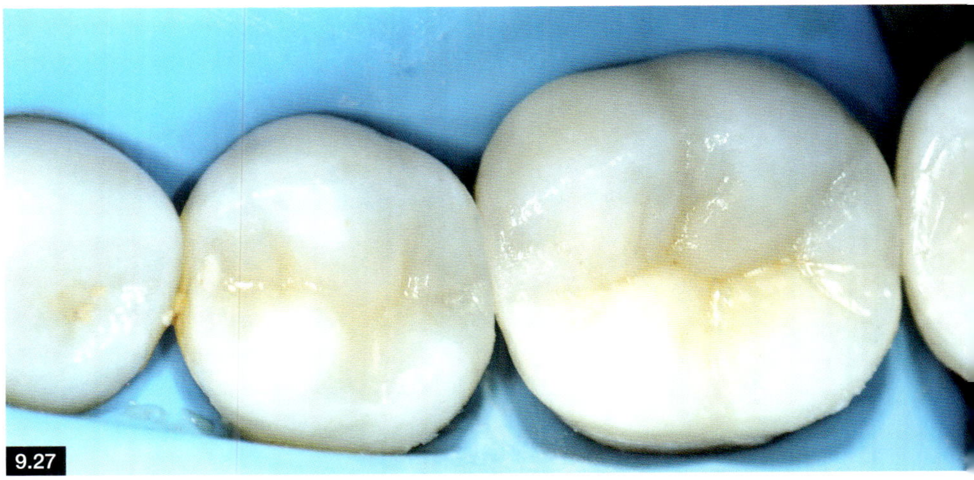

Fig. 9.27: After evaluating the internal and marginal fit, the restoration is cemented using an adhesive and composite technique.

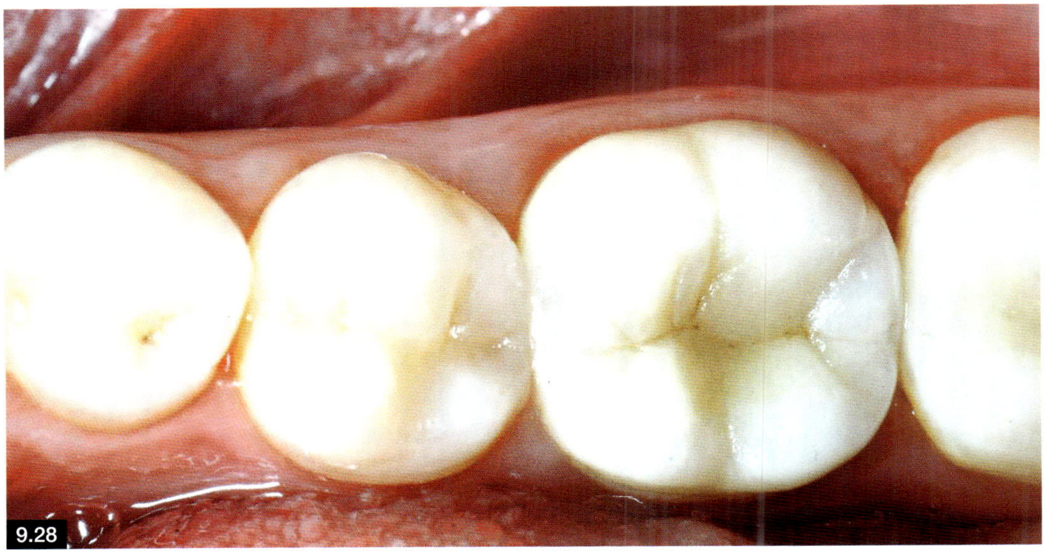

Fig. 9.28: Restoration after the removal of excess and the occlusion check.

CASE REPORT 4

Retrofitting of an existing cast post in an upper central incisor

In this clinical case, a patient presented with complaints about an upper central incisor, treated more than 20 years previously with root canal treatment, cast post and core, and a porcelain-fused-to-metal crown. The tooth eventually developed a sinus tract and became esthetically unacceptable. The treatment plan, which was decided with the patient, was endodontic

Figure 1: The initial clinical situation, a clear chromatic mismatch can be observed in the upper right central incisors.

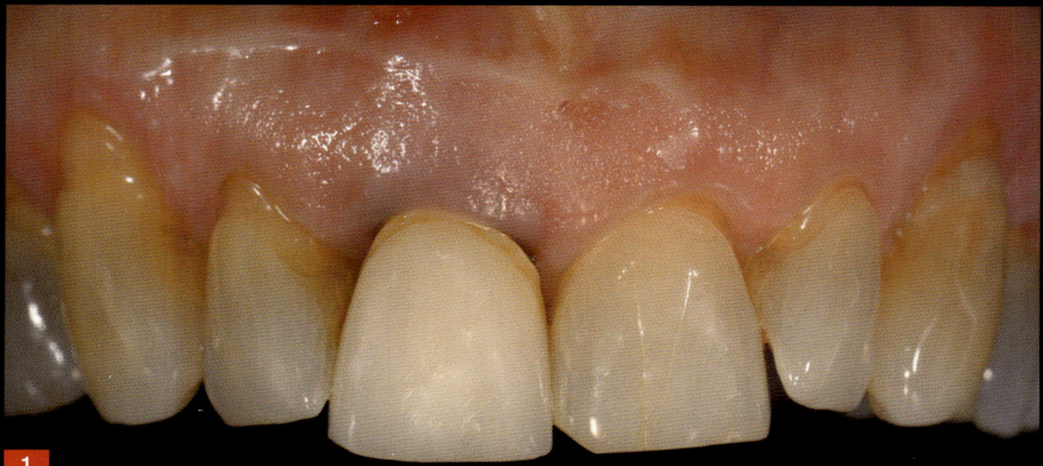

1

Figure 2: After the removal of the crown a metallic post and brown radicular dentin was present in the cervical part.

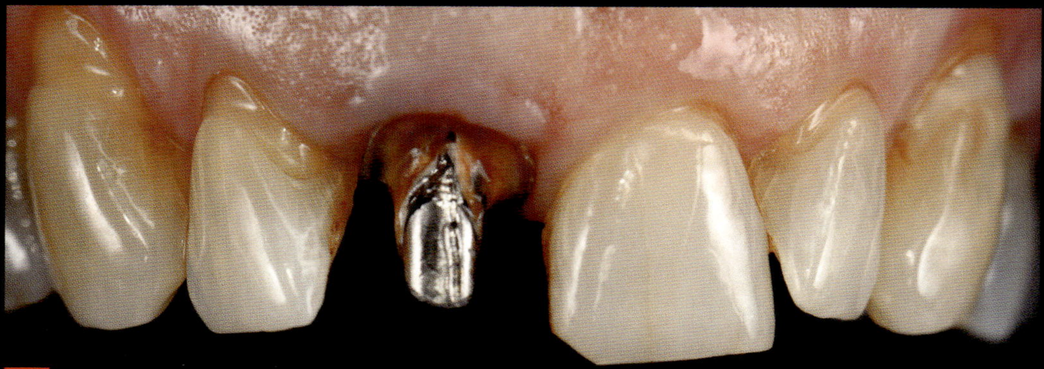

2

Figure 3: The removal of the cast post was easily accomplished by ultrasound and post-extractor devices.

Figure 4: Once the root canal retreatment had been performed a fiber post with composite was luted inside the root canal.

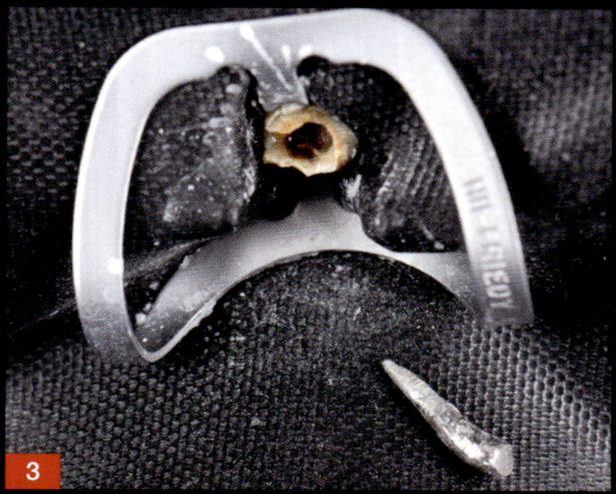

3

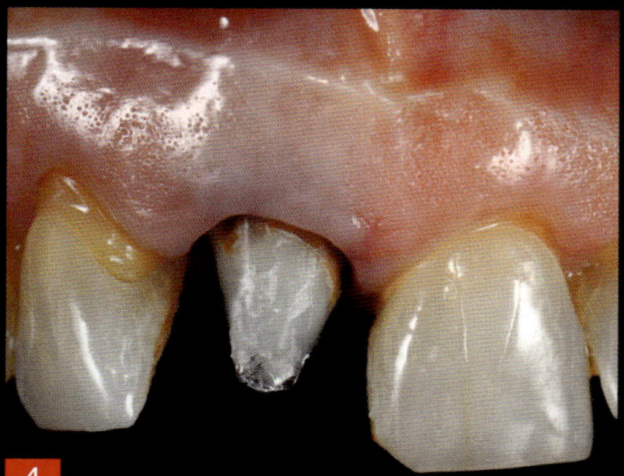

4

retreatment, post, core, and a new full ceramic crown. The post was easily removed, the root was retreated, and the old post was used again and cemented using an adhesive technique. The tooth was prepared and scanned, and a new ceramic crown was cemented.

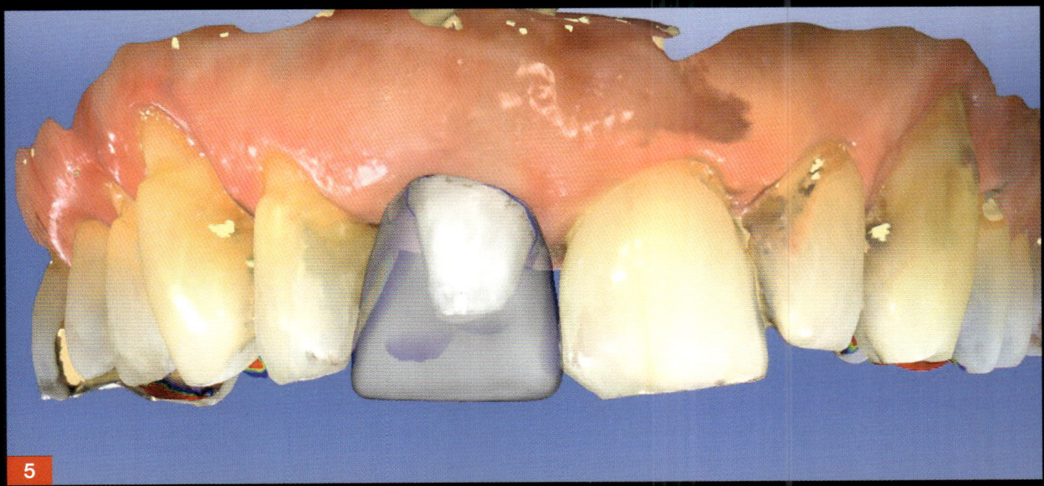

5

Figure 5: The digital impression obtained by intraoral scanner was utilized to project a suitable full ceramic crown.

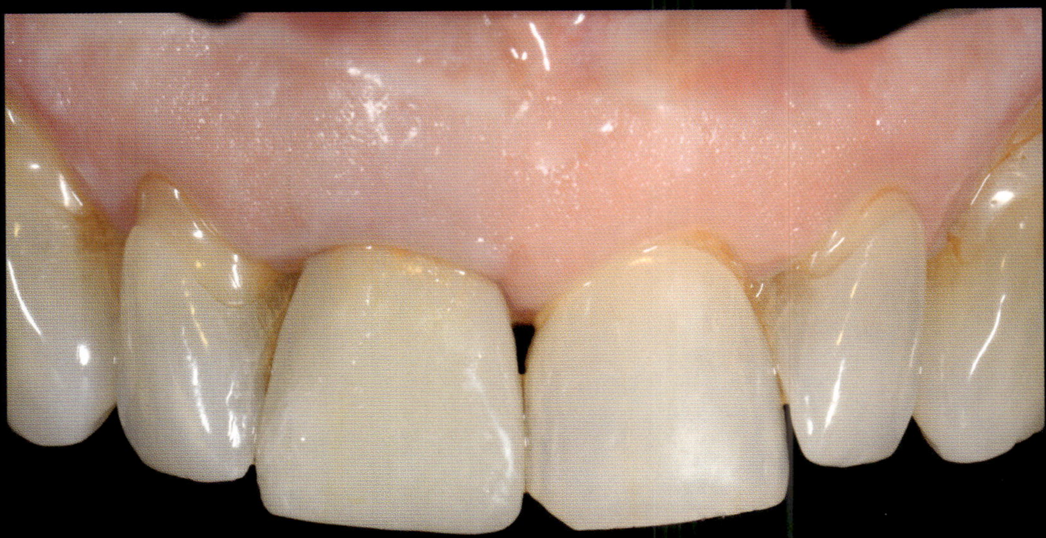

6

Figure 6: The luted ceramic crown.

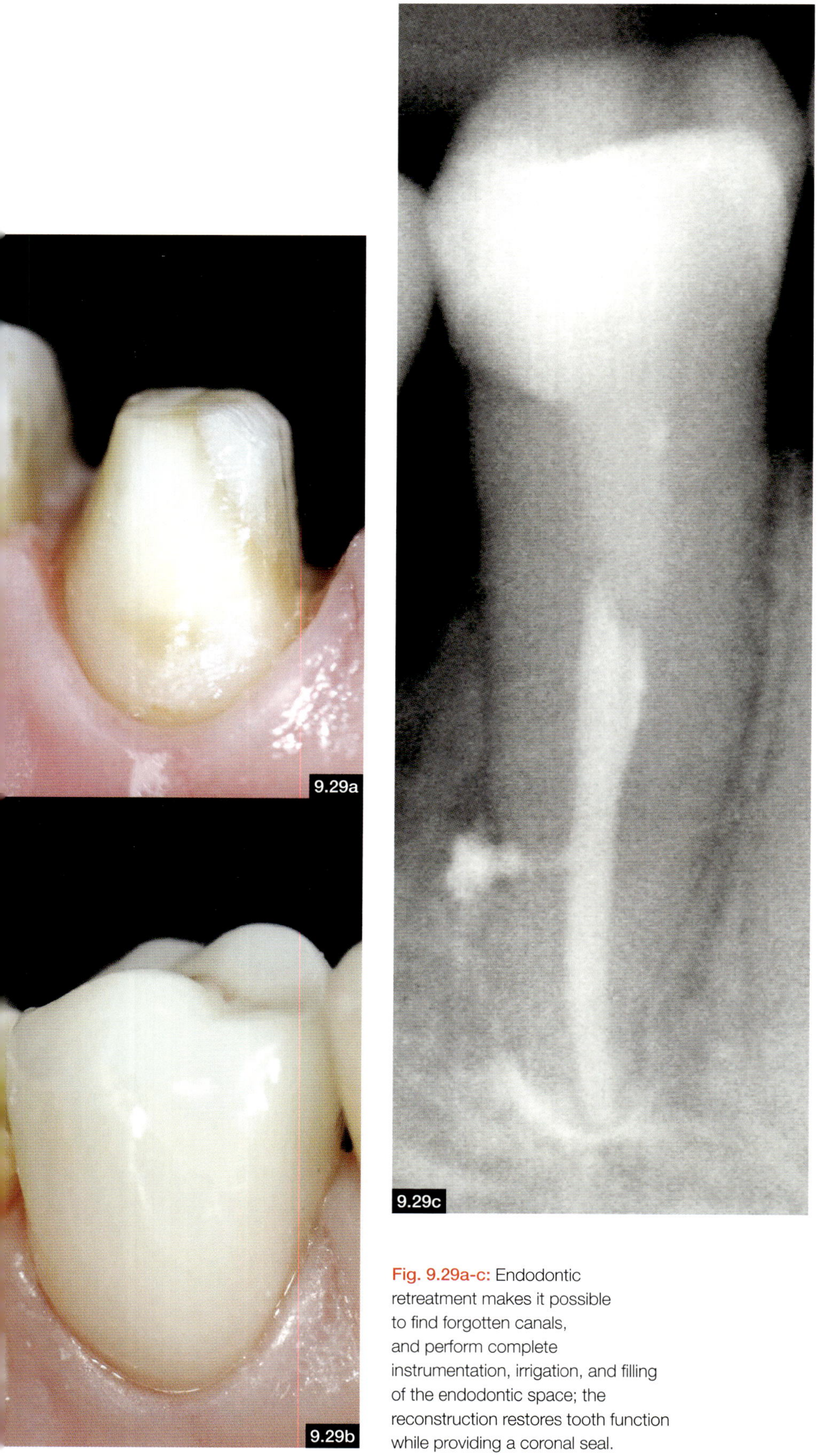

Fig. 9.29a-c: Endodontic retreatment makes it possible to find forgotten canals, and perform complete instrumentation, irrigation, and filling of the endodontic space; the reconstruction restores tooth function while providing a coronal seal.

10 and 17 years)[88, 89] and evaluations on posts with high values of elastic modulus reported good performance. By contrast, a long follow-up period of up to 6 years has been reported for posts with low modulus of elasticity[90]. A recent systematic review confirmed that a high modulus of elasticity post is preferred in the absence of adequate ferrule, because long follow-up studies are necessary to analyze the performance of posts with low elastic modulus[91]. Endodontically treated teeth restored with metallic posts sometimes need to be retreated, and posts are often easily removed. These posts have had a successful clinical performance for decades and can be retrofitted in the new restoration with the help of adhesive techniques.

Conclusion

The theme of the reconstruction of the retreated tooth stems from prognostic considerations regarding the restorability of the tooth and develops with the manual skills to be implemented during the various phases of operation. Clinical, economic, and appropriateness-related considerations guide the choice between preserving the existing restoration and replacing it. The general criterion (taken from the reconstruction of the treated tooth) of the maximum conservation of healthy enamel and dentin, and the use of adhesive techniques must be combined with knowledge of the characteristics of the materials used for the primary restoration, through which the access cavity has been made when the existing restoration is preserved. The reuse of a restoration removed with non-destructive techniques is often possible with adhesive or traditional techniques. Each of these reconstructive assessments, with their implications in terms of time, invasiveness of procedures, risks, prognosis, and economic commitment, should be properly assessed with the patient before undertaking the retreatment procedure. The patient should also be informed of possible alternatives, so that the patient can choose the solution that best suits his individual needs and possibilities.

References

1. Mannocci F, Bhuva B, Stern S. *Restoring teeth following root canal re-treatment*. Endod Topics. 2008;19(1):125–152.
2. Al-Nuaimi N, Patel S, Austin RS et al. *A prospective study assessing the effect of coronal tooth structure loss on the outcome of root canal retreatment*. Int Endod J. 2017;50(12):1143–1157.
3. Nair PNR, Sjögren U, Krey G et al. *Intraradicular bacteria and fungi in root-filled, asymptomatic human teeth with therapy-resistant periapical lesions: a long-term light and electron microscopic follow-up study*. J Endod. 1990;16(12):580–588.
4. Sundqvist G, Figdor D. *Endodontic treatment of apical periodontitis*. In: Orstavik D, Pitt Ford T. Essential Endodontology, pp. 242–77, Blackwell Science Ltd, Oxford, UK, 1998.
5. Tzimpoulas NE, Alisafis MG, Tzanetakis GN et al. *A prospective study of the extraction and retention incidence of endodontically treated teeth with uncertain prognosis after endodontic referral*. J Endod. 2012;38(10):1326–1329.
6. Tang W, Wu Y, Smales RJ. *Identifying and reducing risks for potential fractures in endodontically treated teeth*. J Endod. 2010;36(4):609–617.
7. Ruddle CJ: Ch. 25, *Nonsurgical endodontic retreatment*. In Cohen S, Burns RC: Pathways of the Pulp, pp. 875–929, 8th ed., Mosby, St. Louis, 2002.
8. Ruddle CJ: Ch. 8, *Cleaning and shaping root canal systems*. In Cohen S, Burns RC: Pathways of the Pulp, pp. 231–291, 8th ed., Mosby, St. Louis, 2002.
9. Ruddle CJ: Ch. 9, *Three-dimensional obturation: the rationale and application of warm gutta percha with vertical condensation*, In Cohen S, Burns RC: Pathways of the Pulp, pp. 243–247, 6th ed., Mosby Co., St. Louis, 1994.
10. Siqueira Jr JF. *Aetiology of root canal treatment failure: Why well-treated teeth can fail*. Int Endod J. 2001;34(1):1–10.
11. De Chevigny C, Dao TT, Basrani BR et al. *Treatment outcome in endodontics: the Toronto study-phases 3 and 4:orthograde retreatment*. J Endod. 2008;34(2):131–137.
12. De Carlo Bello M, Pillar R, Mastella Lang P et al. *Incidence of Dentinal Defects and Vertical Root Fractures after Endodontic Retreatment and Mechanical Cycling*. Iran Endod J. 2017;12(4):502–507.
13. Missau T, De Carlo Bello M, Michelon C et al. *Influence of Endodontic Treatment and Retreatment on the Fatigue Failure Load, Numbers of Cycles for Failure, and Survival Rates of Human Canine Teeth*. J Endod. 2017;43(12):2081–2087.
14. Bier CA, Shemesh H, Tanomaru-Filho M et al. *The ability of different nickel-titanium rotary instruments to induce dentinal damage during canal preparation*. J Endod. 2009;35(2):236–238.
15. Shemesh H, Bier CA, Wu MK et al. *The effects of canal preparation and filling on the incidence of dentinal defects*. Int Endod J. 2009;42(3):208–213.
16. Rotstein I, Cohenca N, Teperovich E et al. *Effect of chloroform, xylene, and halothane on enamel and dentin microhardness of human teeth*. Oral Surg Oral Med Oral Pathol Oral Radiol Endod. 1999;87(3):366–368.
17. Erdemir A, Eldeniz AU, Belli S. *Effect of gutta-percha solvents on mineral contents of human root dentin using ICP-AES technique*. J Endod. 2004;30(1):54–56.
18. Shemesh H, Roeleveld AC, Wesselink PR et al. *Damage to root dentin during retreatment procedures*. J Endod. 2011;37(1):63–66.
19. Topcuoglu HS, Demirbuga S, Tuncay O et al. *The effects of Mtwo, R-Endo, and DRaCe retreatment instruments on the incidence of dentinal defects during the removal of root canal filling material*. J Endod. 2014;40(2):266–270.
20. Topçuoğlu HS, Düzgün S, Kesim B et al. *Incidence of apical crack initiation and propagation during the removal of root canal filling material with ProTaper and Mtwo rotary nickel-titanium retreatment instruments and hand files*. J Endod. 2014;40(7):1009–1012.
21. Çapar İD, Uysal B, Ok E et al. *Effect of the size of the apical enlargement with rotary instruments, single-cone filling, post space preparation with drills, fiber post removal, and root canal filling removal on apical crack initiation and propagation*. J Endod. 2015;41(2):253–256.
22. Capar ID, Saygili G, Ergun H et al. *Effects of root canal preparation, various filling techniques and retreatment after filling on vertical root fracture and crack formation*. Dent Traumatol. 2015;31(4):302–307.
23. Özyürek T, Tek V, Yılmaz K et al. *Incidence of apical crack formation and propagation during removal of root canal filling materials with different engine driven nickel-titanium instruments*. Restor Dent Endod. 2017;42(4):332–341.
24. Nedzinskienė E, Pečiulienė V, Aleksejūnienė J et al. *Potential to induce dentinal cracks during retreatment procedures of teeth treated with "Russian red": An ex vivo study*. Medicina. 2017;53(3):166–172.
25. Gu LS, Ling JQ, Wei X Huang XY. *Efficacy of ProTaper Universal rotary retreatment system for gutta-percha removal from root canals*. Int Endod J. 2008;41(4):288–295.
26. Shokouhinejad N, Sabeti MA, Hasheminasab M et al. *Push-out bond strength of Resilon/Epiphany self-etch to intraradicular dentin after retreatment: a preliminary study*. J Endod. 2010;36(3):493–496.
27. Erdemir A, Adanir N, Belli S. *In vitro evaluation of the dissolving effect of solvents on root canal sealers*. J Oral Sci. 2003;45(3):123–126.
28. Palhais M, Sousa-Neto MD, Rached-Junior FJA et al. *Influence of solvents on the bond strength of resin sealer to intraradicular dentin after retreatment*. Braz Oral Res. 2017;31,e11.

29. Topçuoğlu HS, Demirbuga S, Tuncay Ö et al. *The bond strength of endodontic sealers to root dentine exposed to different gutta-percha solvents*. Int Endod J. 2014;47(12):1100–1106.
30. Satterthwaite JD, Stokes AN. *Dentinal crack incidence following ultrasonic vibration to intra-radicular posts*. N Z Dent J. 2004;100(4):105–109.
31. Altshul JH, Marshall G, Morgan LA et al. *Comparison of dentinal crack incidence and of post removal time resulting from post removal by ultrasonic or mechanical force*. J Endod. 1997;23(11):683–686.
32. Huttula AS, Tordik PA, Imamura G et al. *The effect of ultrasonic post instrumentation on root surface temperature*. J Endod. 2006;32(11):1085–1087.
33. Reeh ES, Messer HH, Douglas WH. *Reduction in tooth stiffness as a result of endodontic and restorative procedures*. J Endod. 1989;15(11):512–516.
34. Esposito M, Tallarico M, Trullenque-Eriksson A et al. *Endodontic retreatment vs dental implants of teeth with an uncertain endodontic prognosis: 1-year results from a randomised controlled trial*. Eur J Oral Implantol. 2017;10(3):293–308.
35. Gorni FGM, Gagliani MM. *The outcome of endodontic retreatment: a 2-yr follow-up*. J Endod. 2004;30(1):1–4.
36. Gillen BM, Looney SW, Gu LS et al. *Impact of the quality of coronal restoration versus the quality of root canal fillings on success of root canal treatment: a systematic review and meta-analysis*. J Endod. 2011;37(7):895–902.
37. Dietschi D, Duc O, Krejci I et al. *Biomechanical considerations for the restoration of endodontically treated teeth: a systematic review of the literature - Part 1. Composition and micro- and macrostructure alterations*. Quintessence Int. 2007;38(9):733–743.
38. Dietschi D, Duc O, Krejci I et al. *Biomechanical considerations for the restoration of endodontically treated teeth: a systematic review of the literature - Part II (Evaluation of fatigue behavior, interfaces, and in vivo studies)*. Quintessence Int. 2008;39(2):117–129.
39. Jackson RD. *The role of modern composites and ceramics in clinical practice*. Dent Today. 2011;30(6):58–62.
40. Peroz I, Blankenstein F, Lange KP et al. *Restoring endodontically treated teeth with posts and cores-a review*. Quintessence Int. 2005;36(9):737–746.
41. Bompolaki D, Kontogiorgos E, Wilson JB et al. *Fracture resistance of lithium disilicate restorations after endodontic access preparation: An in vitro study*. J Prosthet Dent. 2015;114(4):580–586.
42. Abbott PV. *Assessing restored teeth with pulp and periapical diseases for the presence of cracks, caries and marginal breakdown*. Aust Dent J. 2004 Mar;49(1):33–39.
43. Wood K.C., Berzins D.W., Luo Q. et al. *Resistance to fracture of two all-ceramic crown materials following endodontic access*. J Prosthet Dent. 2006;95:33–41.
44. Grobecker-Karl T, Christian M, Karl M. *Effect of endodontic access cavity preparation on monolithic and ceramic veneered zirconia restorations*. Quintessence Int. 2016;47(9):725–729.
45. Gorman CM, Ray NJ, Burke FM. *The effect of endodontic access on all-ceramic crowns: A systematic review of in vitro studies*. J Dent. 2016;53:22–29.
46. Verzijden CW, Feilzer AJ, and Watanabe LG. *The influence of polymerization shrinkage of resin cements on bonding to metal*. J Dent Res. 1992;71:410–413.
47. Umemoto K and Kurata S. *Effects of mixed silane coupling agent on porcelain tooth material and various dental alloys*. Dent Mater J. 1995;14:135–142.
48. Imbery TA and Davis RD. *Evaluation of tin plating systems for a high-noble alloy*. Int J Prosthodont. 1993;6:55–60.
49. Antoniadou M, Kern M, and Strub JR. *Effect of a new metal primer on the bond strength between a resin cement and two high-noble alloys*. J Prosthet Dent. 2000;84:554–560.
50. Matsumura H, Shimoe S, Nagano K et al. *Effect of noble metal conditioners on bonding between prosthetic composite material and silver-palladium-copper-gold alloy*. J Prosthet Dent. 1999;81:710–714.
51. Watanabe I, Hotta M, Watanabe E et al. *Shear bond strengths of laboratory-cured prosthetic composite to primed metal surfaces*. Am J Dent. 2003;16:401–403.
52. Ozcan M, van der Sleen JM, Kurunmäki H et al. *Comparison of repair methods for ceramic-fused-to-metal crowns*. J Prosthodont. 2006;15(5):283–288.
53. Calamia JR. *Etched porcelain facial veneers: a new treatment modality based on scientific and clinical evidence*. NY J Dent. 1983;53:255–259.
54. Rochette AL. *A ceramic restoration bonded by etched enamel and resin for fractured incisors*. J Prosthet Dent. 1973;33:287–293.
55. Kato H, Matsumura H, Tanaka T et al. *Bond strength and durability of porcelain bonding systems*. J Prosthet Dent. 1996;75:163–168.
56. Thurmond JW, Barkmeier WW, and Wilwerding TM. *Effect of porcelain surface treatments on bond strengths of composite resin bonded to porcelain*. J Prosthet Dent. 1994;72:355–359.
57. Song XF, Yin L. *Subsurface damage induced in dental resurfacing of a feldspar porcelain with coarse diamond burs* J. Biomech. 2009 Feb; 42(3):355–360.
58. Sutherland JK, Teplitsky PE, Moulding MB. *Endodontic access of all-ceramic crowns* J Prosthet Dent. 1989;61(2):146–149.
59. Kelly RD, Palin WM, Tomson PL et al. *The impact of endodontic access on the biaxial flexure strength of dentine-bonded crown substrates – an in vitro study*.Int Endod J. 2017;50(2):184–193.

60. Qeblawi D, Hill T, Chlosta K. *The effect of endodontic access preparation on the failiure load of lithium disilicate glass-ceramic restorations* J Prosthet Dent. 2011 Nov;106(5):329–335.
61. Barghi N. *To silanate or not to silanate: making a clinical decision. Compend Contin Educ Dent*. 2000;21:659–662.
62. Schwartz RS, Fransman R. *Adhesive Dentistry and Endodontics: Materials, Clinical Strategies and Procedures for Restoration of Access Cavities: A Review. J Endod*. 2005;31(3):151–165.
63. Nakamura K, Katsuda Y, Ankyu S et al. *Cutting Efficiency of Diamond Burs Operated with Electric High-Speed Dental Handpiece on Zirconia*. European Journal of Oral Sciences. 2015;123:375–380.
64. Wood KC, Berzins DW, Luo Q et al. *Resistance to fracture of two all-ceramic crown materials following endodontic access*. J Prosthet Dent. 2006;95(1):33–41.
65. Cohen BD, Wallace JA. *Castable glass ceramic crowns and their reaction to endodontic therapy Oral Surg Oral Med Oral Pathol Oral Radiol Endod. 1991*;72(1):108–110.
66. McMullen AF 3rd, Himel VT, Sarkar NK. *An in vitro study of the effect endodontic access preparation has upon the retention of porcelain fused to metal crowns of maxillary central incisors*. J Endod. 1989;15(4):154–156.
67. De Souza G, Hennig D, Aggarwal A et al. *The use of MDP-based materials for bonding to zirconia*. J. Prosthet. Dent. 2014;112(4):895–902.
68. Salcetti MA, *Closing Endo Access Openings*, Spear Digest 2016, http://www.speareducation.com/spear-review/2014/11/closing-endo-access-openings accessed 14/01/2018.
69. Ree MH. *The Endo-Restorative Interface: Current Concepts. Educational Session. Presented at the Meeting of American Association of Endodontics*, San Antonio, TX, 2011.
70. Bindl A, Mörmann WH. *Clinical evaluation of adhesively placed Cerec endo-crowns after 2 years – preliminary results*. J Adhes Dent. 1999;1(3):255–265.
71. Pissis P. *Fabrication of a metal-free ceramic restoration utilizing the monobloc technique*. Pract Periodontics Aesthet Dent. 1995;7(5):83–94.
72. Slangen P, Corn S, Fages M et al. *Prosthodontic crown mechanical integrity study using Speckle Interferometrie In: Osten W, Kujawinska M, editors. Fringe 2009: 6th International Workshop on Advanced Optical Metrology*. Berlin Heidelberg: 2009: 734–738.
73. Zaslansky P, Friesem AA, Weiner S. *Structure and mechanical properties of the soft zone separating bulk dentin and enamel in crowns of human teeth: insight into tooth function*. J Struct Biol. 2006;153(2):188–199.
74. Sedrez-Porto JA, Rosa WL, da Silva AF et al. *Endocrown restorations: A systematic review and meta-analysis*. J Dent. 2016;52:8–14.
75. Magne P, Spreafico R. *Deep Margin Elevation: A Paradigm Shift*. Am J Esthet Dent. 2012;2(2):86–96.
76. Nicheva S, Lyubomir St. Vangelov, DMD and Ivan Filipov, DMD, PhD. *Endodontic retreatment and adhesive restoration of structurally compromised second premolar*. Roots C.E. Magazine. 2013;9(3):6–10.
77. Veneziani M. *Posterior indirect adhesive restorations: updated indications and the Morphology Driven Preparation Technique*. Int J Esthet Dent. 2017;12(2):204–230.
78. Winter R. Outcome-Based Preparation Design: Part IV. Da: http://www.speareducation.com/spear-review/2016/03/outcome-based-preparation-design-part-iv. Consultato il 10/01/2018.
79. Goldrich N. *Construction of posts for teeth with existing restorations*. J Prosthet Dent 1970;23(2):173–176.
80. Brady WF. *Restoration of a tooth to accommodate a preexisting cast crown*. J Prosthet Dent. 1982;48(3):268–270.
81. Lee JH. *A Digital Approach to Retrofitting a Post and Core Restoration to an Existing Crown*. J Prosthodont. 2017 Nov 30. [Epub ahead of print.]
82. Arabolu M, Nair KC, Raheel SA et al. *Using an existing crown to repair a damaged cast post and core restoration*. J Int Oral Health. 2014;6(5):111–113.
83. Chan DNC. *Technique for repair of multiple abutment teeth under preexisting crowns*. J Prosthet Dent. 2003;89(1):91–92.
84. Abubakkar P, Katheesa P, Shamshad M. *Simplified technique for rebuilding a fractured abutment tooth with post and core with a pre-existing crown*. Guident. 2014;7(9)24–26.
85. Jahangiri L, Feng J. *A simple technique for retrofitting a post and core to a crown*. J Prosthet Dent. 2002;88(2):234–235.
86. Patil PG, Tay K. *Modified technique to retrofit the crown on fractured core*. J Interdiscip Dentistry. 2016;6(1):50–53.
87. Fokkinga WA, Kreulen CM, Vallittu PK, Creugers NH. *A structured analysis of in vitro failure loads and failure modes of fiber, metal, and ceramic post-and-core systems*. Int J Prosthodont. 2004;Jul-Aug;17(4):476–82.
88. Fokkinga WA, Kreulen CM, Bronkhorst EM, Creugers NH. *Up to 17-year controlled clinical study on post-and-cores and covering crowns*. J Dent. 2007 Oct;35(10):778–86.
89. Ellner S, Bergendal T, Bergman B. *Four post-and-core combinations as abutments for fixed single crowns: a prospective up to 10-year study*. Int J Prosthodont. 2003;16:249–254.
90. Ferrari M, et al. *A Randomized Controlled Trial of Endodontically Treated and Restored Premolars*. J Dent Res. 2012;91:72S–78S.
91. Sarkis-Onofre R, Fergusson D, Cenci MS, Moher D, Pereira-Cenci T. *Performance of Post-retained Single Crowns: A Systematic Review of Related Risk Factors*. J Endod. 2017 Feb;43(2):175–183.

- Evaluate the most predictable **clinical indications** and the contraindications to the performance of post-extraction implantation.
- Identify the correct timing for **implant insertion**, especially in areas of high aesthetic value.
- Illustrate the correct **surgical techniques** to optimize clinical and aesthetic results.
- Provide a procedural algorithm for **immediate implant placement** in the anterior and posterior sectors.

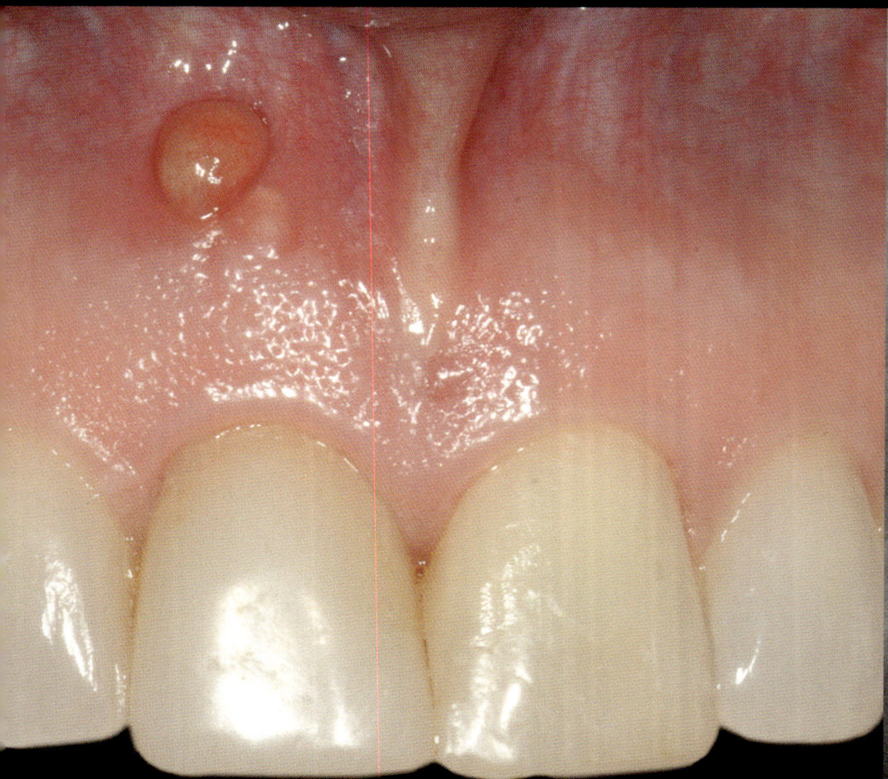

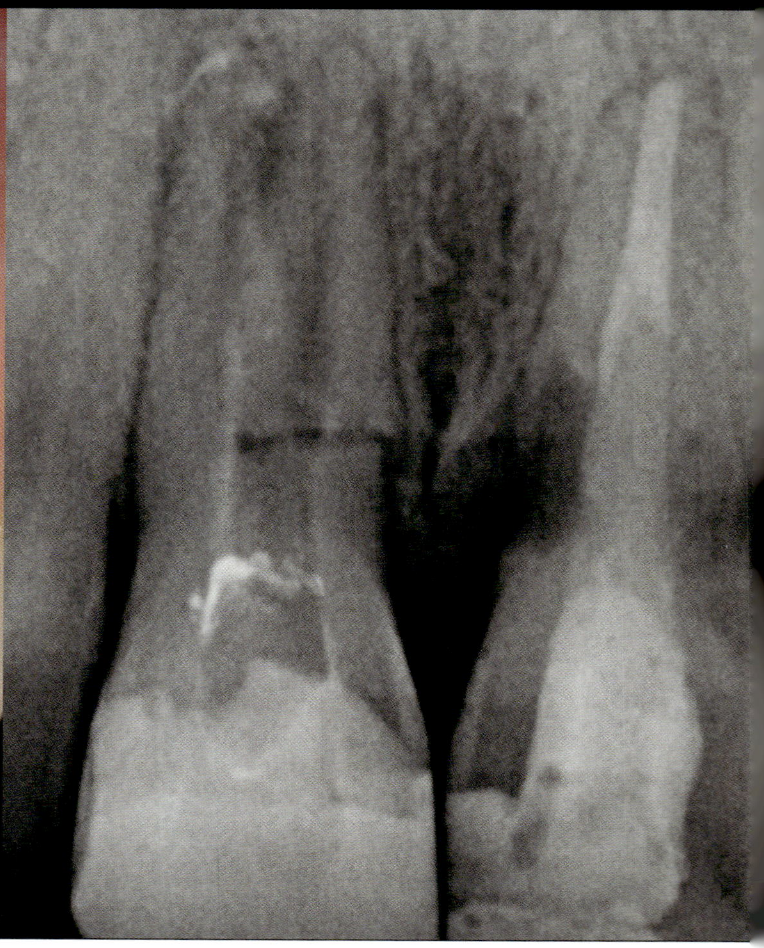

Tiziano Testori, Matteo Deflorian, Riccardo Scaini, Silvio Taschieri, Massimo Del Fabbro

10

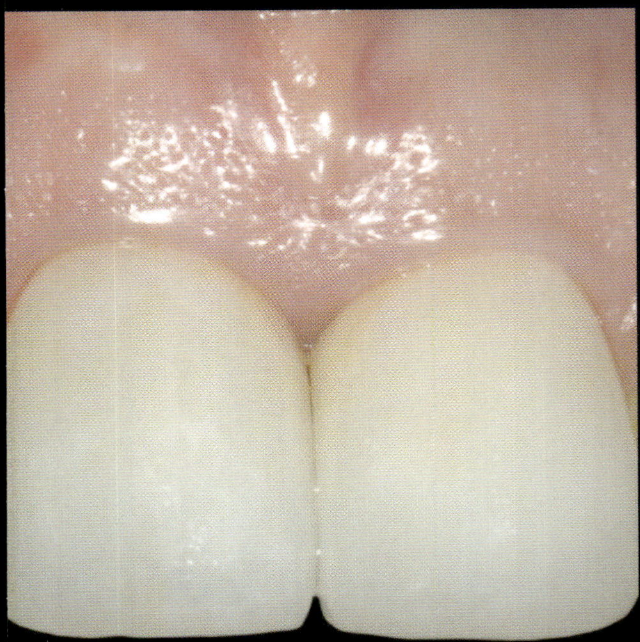

Tooth or implant: criteria for solving the dilemma

Clinical indications and operating procedures for post-extraction implant placement

Introduction

The insertion of post-extraction implants has met with great success among clinicians as it offers unquestionable advantages: it reduces the number of surgical sessions and treatment times and allows the exploitation of a wider bone crest.[1] Although there is consensus in the literature that these protocols are highly reliable in terms of implant survival, there is no common view on how to achieve satisfactory aesthetic results and how to manage the dimensional discrepancy between the alveolar walls and the inserted implant.[2-6] The first studies that analyzed the process of bone healing following the extraction of the teeth were conducted on an animal model in 1952[7] and with human biopsies in 1969.[8] Morphological changes resulting from tooth extraction have only recently been analyzed on study models and by measurements performed during implant placement.[9] However, post-extractive implant insertion does not change the physiological resorption process that the socket undergoes after extraction of the tooth. After tooth loss, there is resorption of the alveolar bone, which is greater at buccal level than at the lingual and palatal sides. In addition, the horizontal component is prevalent.[10,11] In summary, during the first year, about 50% of the initial crestal thickness is resorbed; two-thirds of this resorption is concentrated in the first 3 months. For these reasons, the insertion of immediate post-extraction implants requires careful diagnosis and correct surgical management of the clinical case to obtain predictable and long-lasting results.[12-14] Anatomically, the fibers of the periodontal ligament find their bone insertion in a portion of the alveolar bone called the fibrillar bone. Araujo et al.[15] demonstrated on an animal model that the structure of fibrillar bone plays a decisive role in post-extractive morphological alterations. The fibrillar bone receives vascularization from the periodontal ligament and periosteum; the endosteum is not present because of the limited bone thickness of the post-extractive alveolus in its coronal areas. Once the tooth has been extracted, the vascular support provided by the periodontal ligament is removed, and the first step in the process of resorption of the fibrillar bone begins.

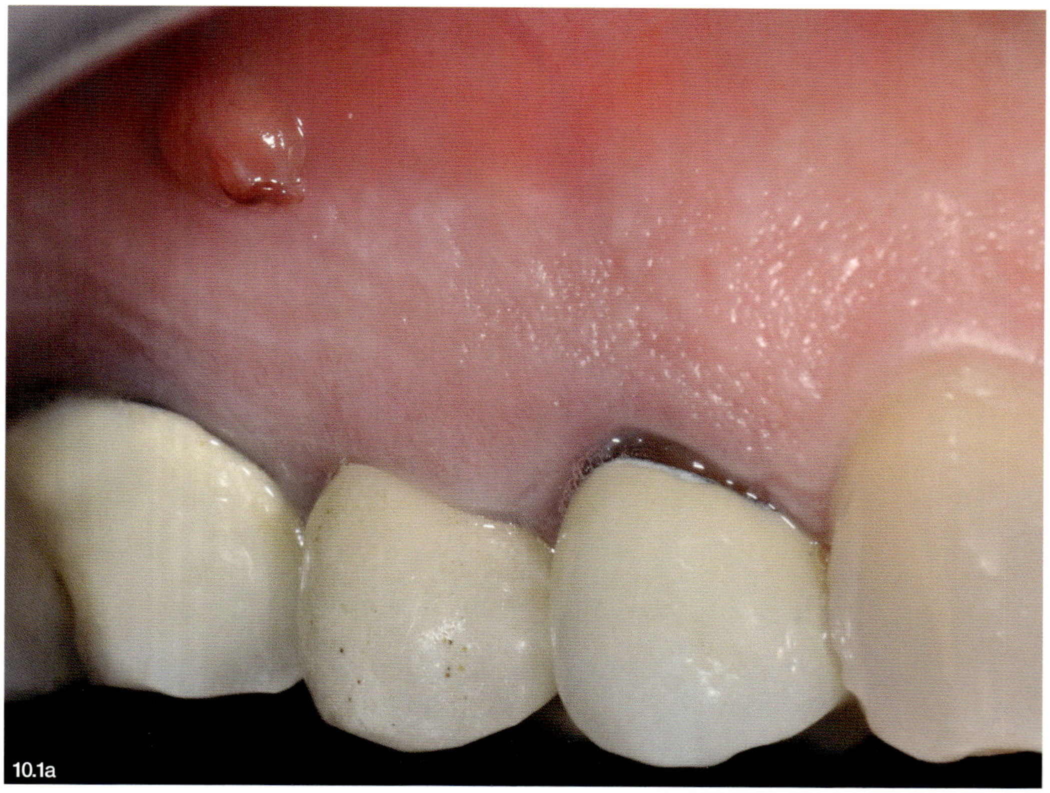

Fig. 10.1a-c: a-b) The initial clinical situation with vestibular fistula in the first sextant. (c) CBCT images show a lesion at tooth 14 with loss of vestibular hard tissue.

The vascularization offered by the periosteum is not sufficient to completely preserve the fibrillar bone. In patients with a thin biotype, the fibrillar bone may be the only mineralized vestibular structure, giving rise to significant horizontal post-extraction resorptions.
A careful preoperative diagnosis is therefore essential to allow the operator to identify the ideal cases, in which to schedule the insertion of immediate post-extraction implants, and the cases at risk, in which it is advisable to implement a deferred loading protocol by combining regenerative techniques.

General principles of post-extraction implantology

Diagnosis and prognosis of the tooth concerned

Regardless of the area of intervention, it is essential that the inauspicious prognosis and the clinical decision to extract the tooth come at the end of a diagnostic process that takes into account all conservative therapeutic alternatives and assesses the costs and biological benefits of each option.
Once an element has been deemed nonmaintainable, according to the guidelines of conservative and prosthetic practice, it is, therefore, necessary to establish the treatment plan for rehabilitation.
The presence of subacute, subchronic and chronic *periapical and periodontal lesion*, if managed correctly from a medical point of view, is not to be considered as an absolute contraindication to immediate implant positioning (Figs. 10.1–10.8).[16]
A recent retrospective study of 369 patients and 527 implants placed in infected and noninfected sites with an average follow-up of 54 months found no statistically significant differences in two approaches in terms of implant survival.
However, the authors emphasized the importance of a thorough alveolar inspection.[17]
This is achieved by a good intra-alveolar view by means of magnification, such as surgical goggles with a dedicated light and alveolar spoons, together with instruments such molt curettes of various sizes.

NONACUTE PERIODONTAL AND PERIAPICAL LESIONS

are not a contraindication to implant placement because no bacteria have been detected at bone level.

▸ to be continued on page 486

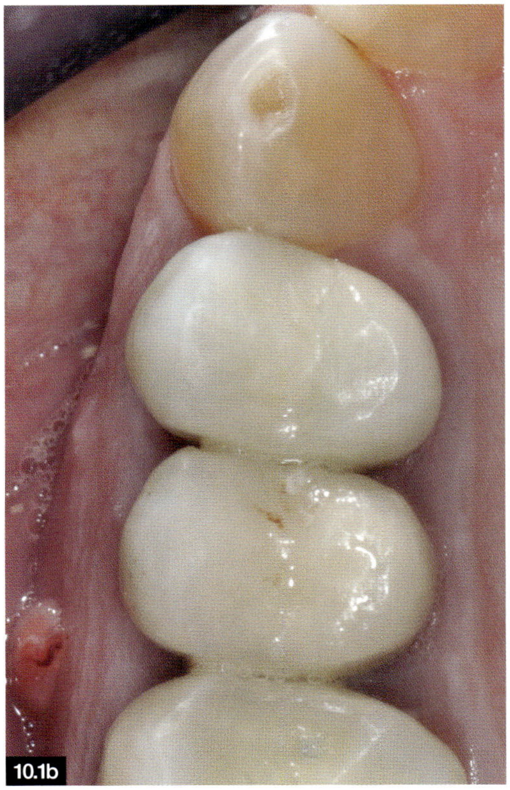

10.1b

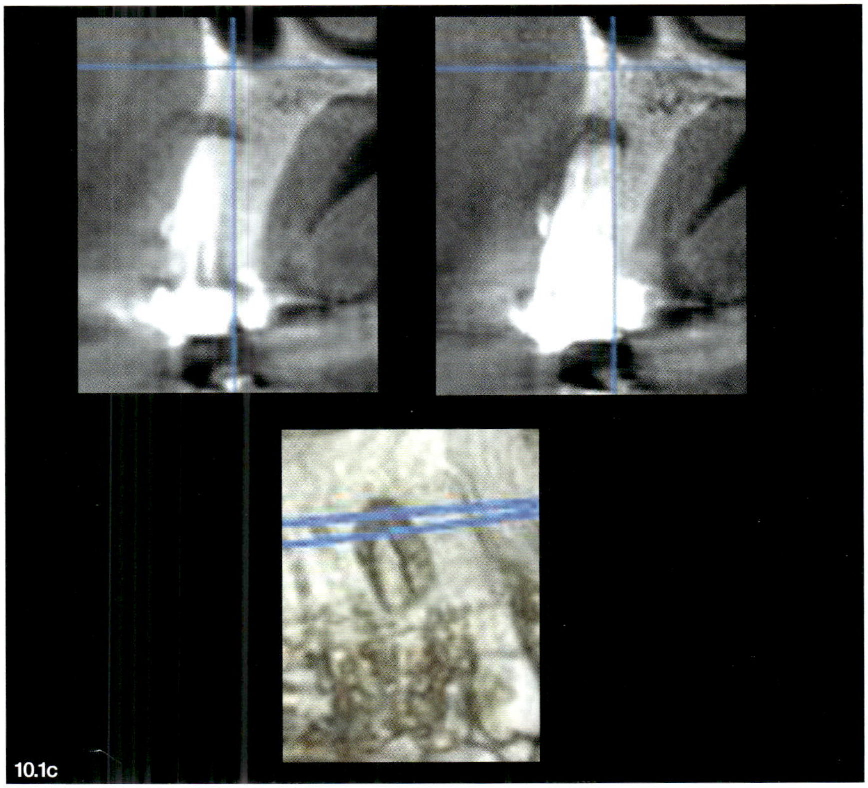

10.1c

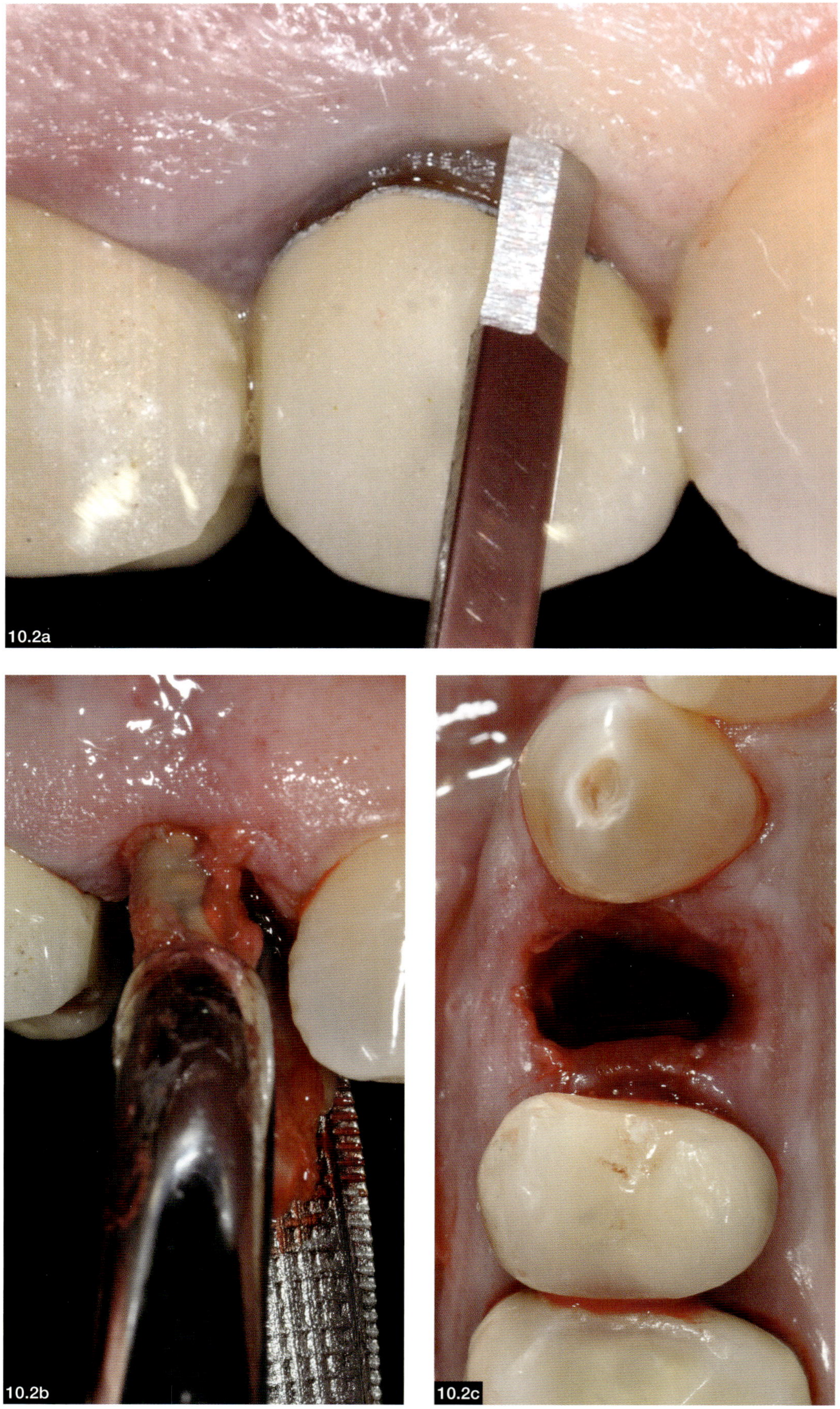

Fig. 10.2a-c: Periotomy with all-around microblade and extraction of tooth 14 exerting axial forces at the root.

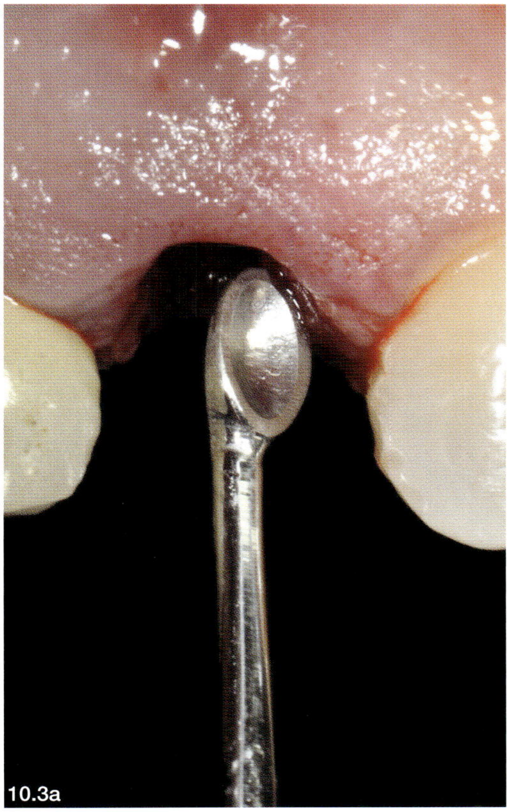

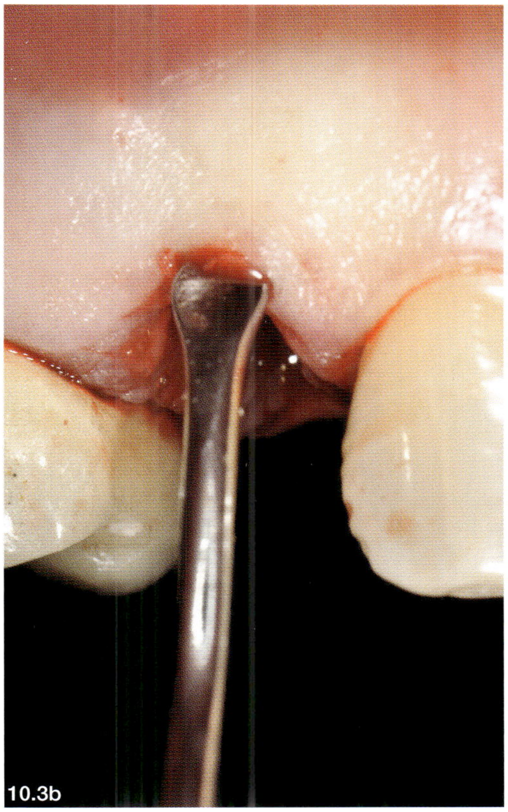

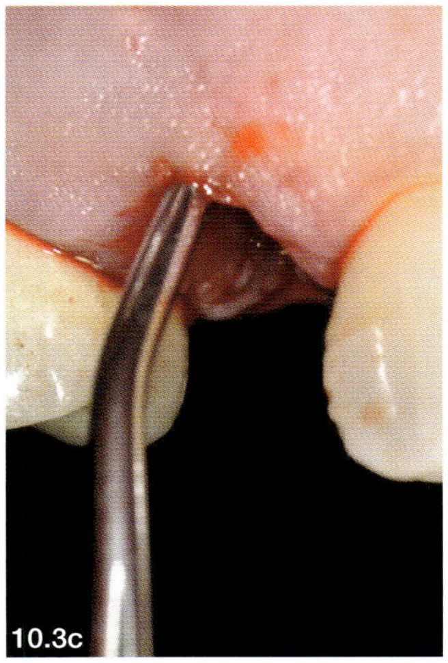

Fig. 10.3a-c: After extraction, alveolar review will be carried out with a surgical spoon and the use of micro-cutter to perform soft tissue dissection.
The micro-sculptor works on the bone plane without affecting the interdental papillae to keep the marginal soft tissues intact.

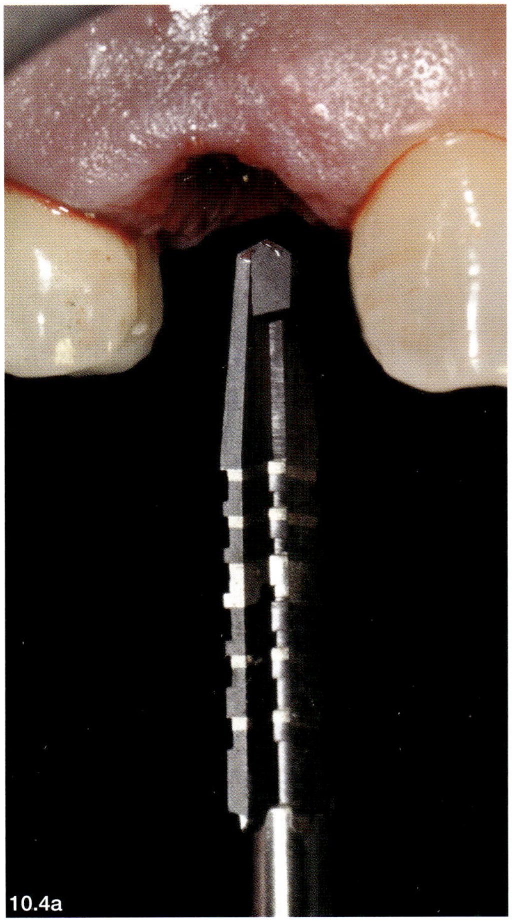

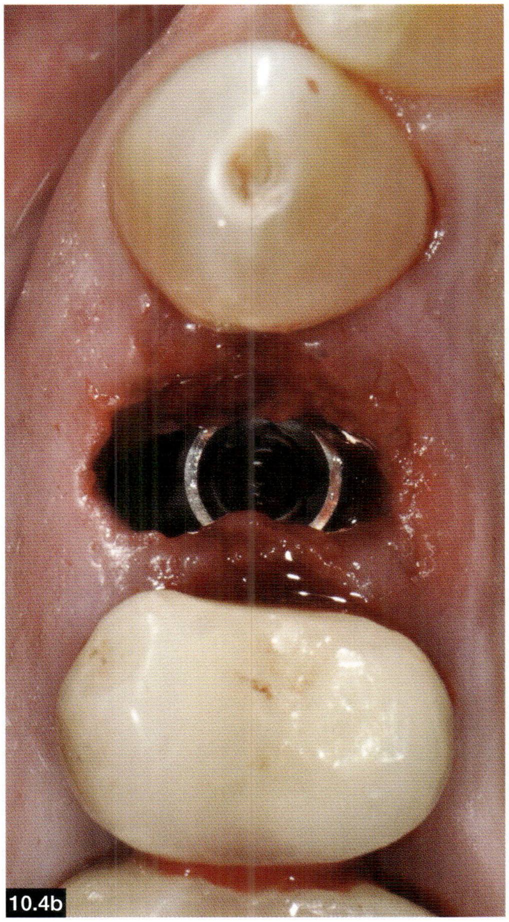

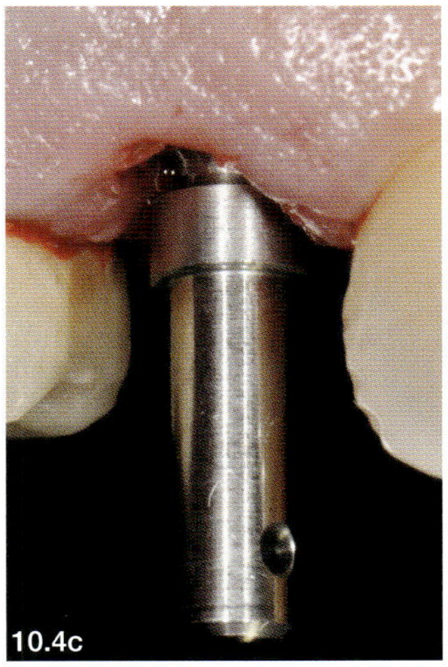

Fig. 10.4a-c: Flapless preparation of the implant site and prosthetically guided implant placement. Because of the high primary stability achieved, an intraoperative impression is performed before regenerative maneuvers are carried out to prepare an immediate loading screw-retained temporary crown.

Fig. 10.5a-c: Regenerative operations are carried out without an open view. Therefore, a resorbable membrane shaped vestibularly to fit the operated site and a slow-resorbing biomaterial graft are inserted. At the end of the procedure, a sponge of collagen type I is placed to protect the graft.

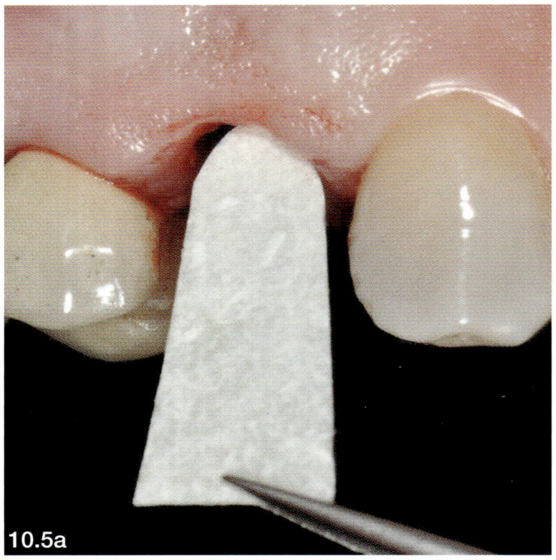
10.5a

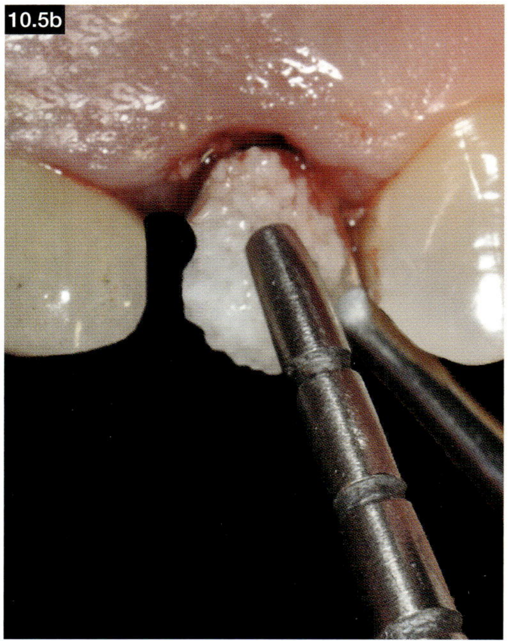
10.5b

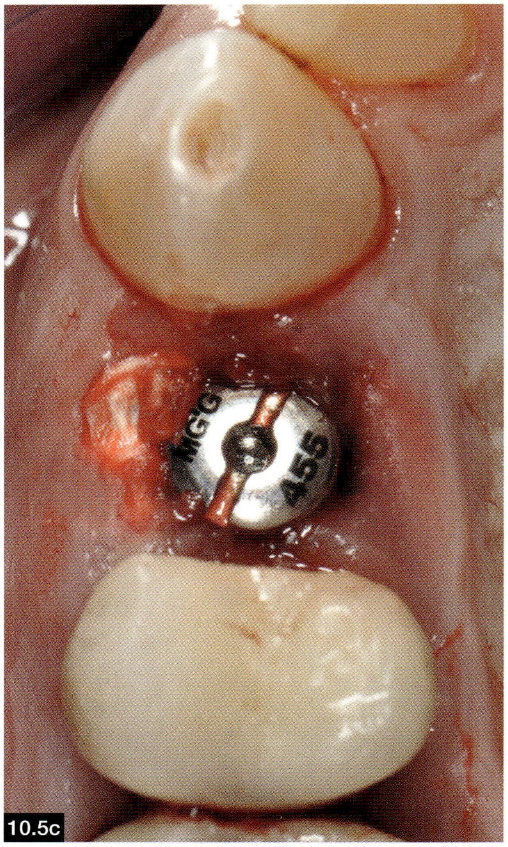

10.5c

Fig. 10.6a-b: Four hours after the end of the surgical phase, the temporary crown is immediately loaded and screwed directly to the implant, and intraoral radiographic control is performed.

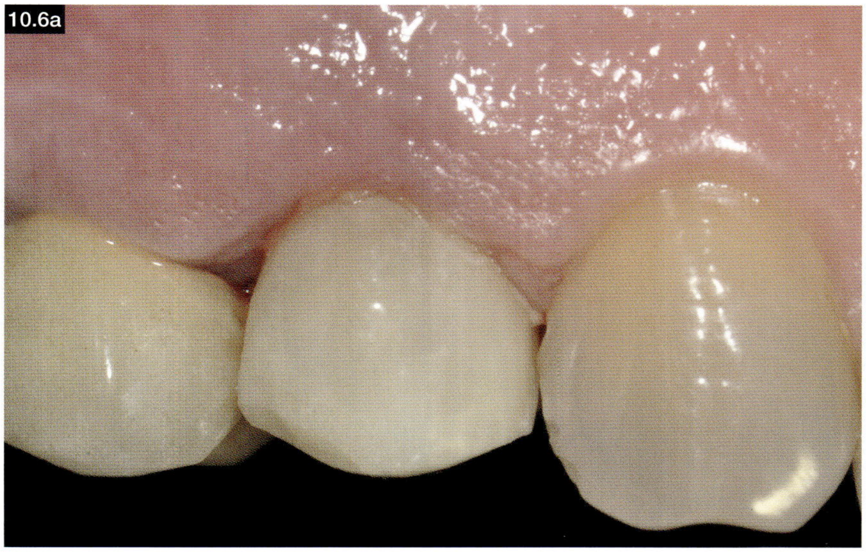
10.6a

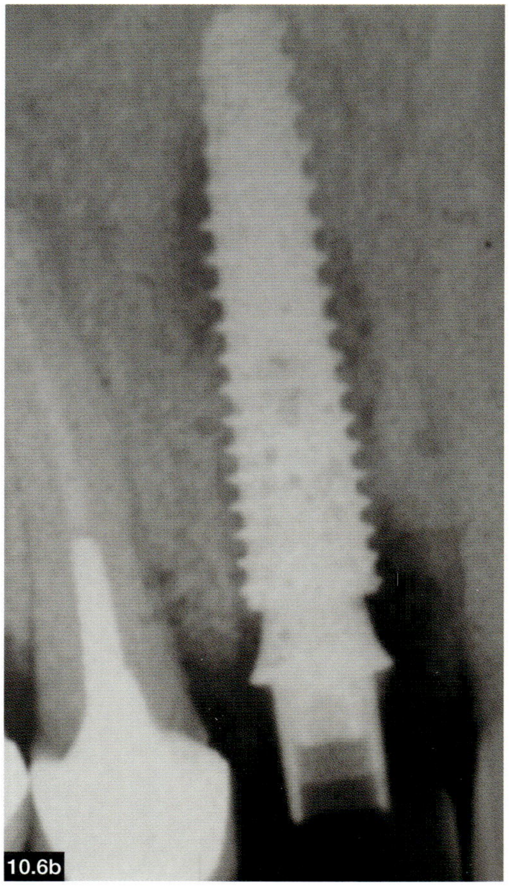
10.6b

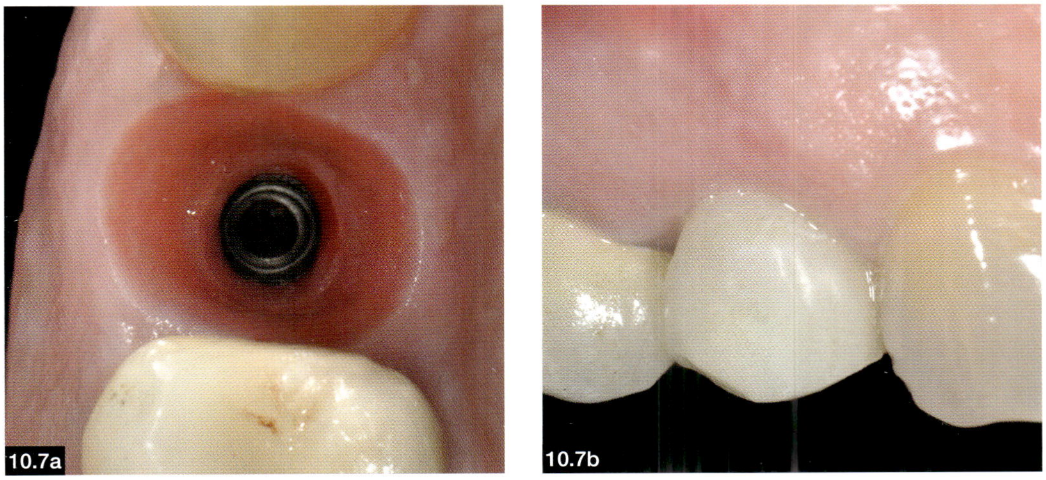

Fig. 10.7a-b: Twelve months after the surgical phase, implant integration, good peri-implant tissue health and natural integration of the temporary restoration with adequate tissue conditioning are observed, allowing us to proceed with the definitive prosthetic phase.

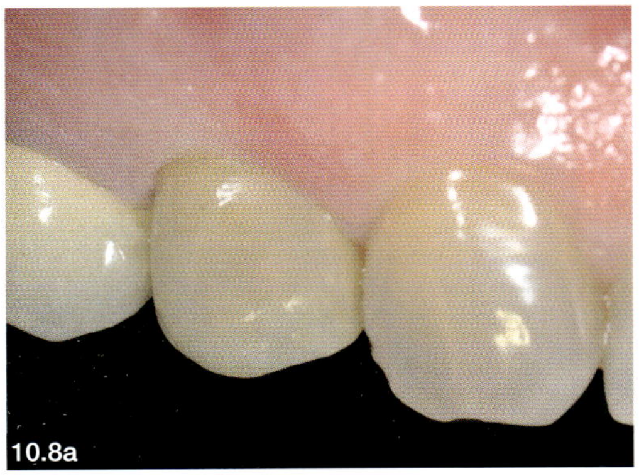

Fig. 10.8a-b: Screw-retained zirconium-ceramic final crown and endodontic x-ray follow-up. Note the volumetric stability of the tissues that allows optimal aesthetic integration of the implant-prosthetic rehabilitation.

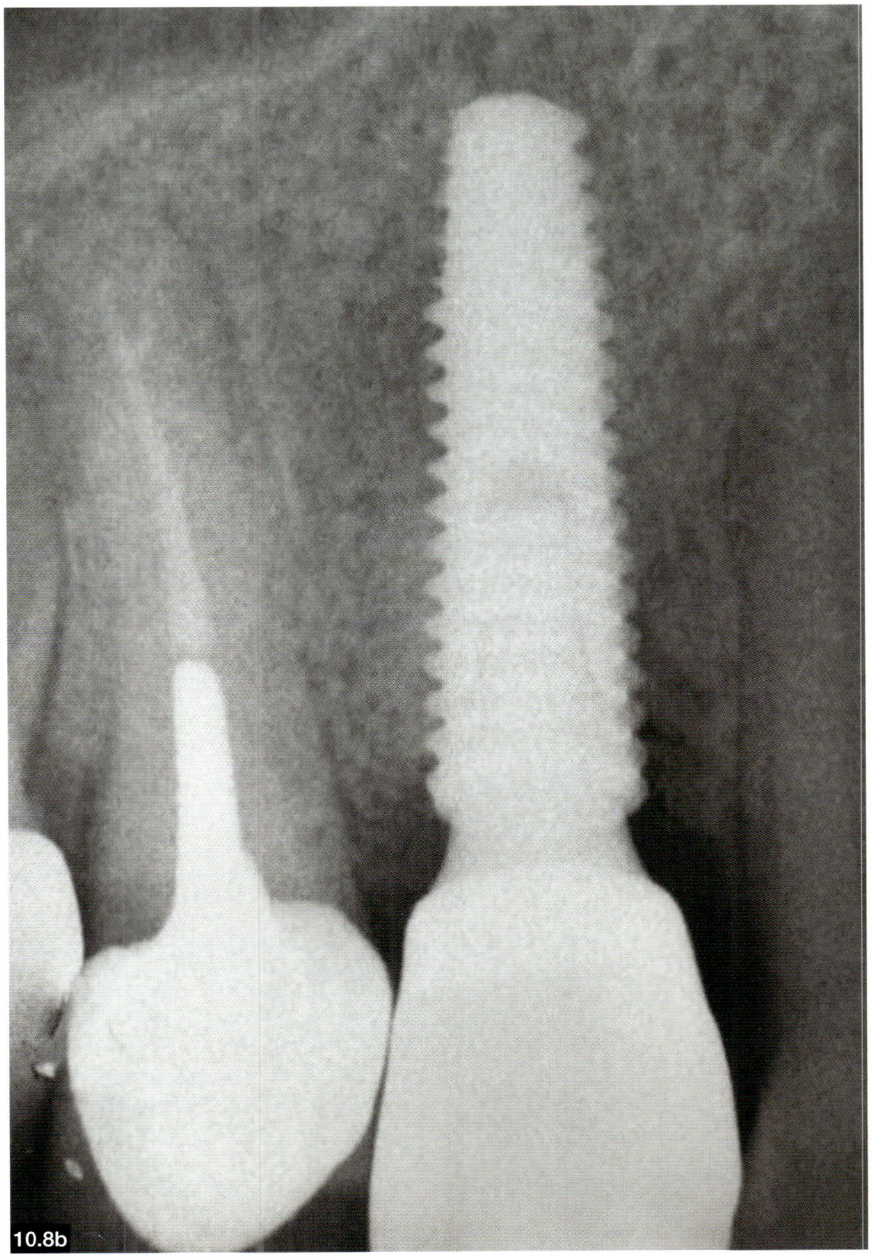

The cleaning of the alveolar cavity with an antibiotic solution is not scientifically validated.[16] If all risk factors for failure are analyzed,[18] an implant solution is chosen, and the clinician must evaluate the timing of insertion, any surgical techniques for the management of peri-implant hard and soft tissues, and the type of provisional restoration.
We refer to specific texts regarding the basic principles of prosthetically guided implant placement.[19]

Timing of insertion

An immediate post-extraction approach cannot be considered as the treatment of choice in every clinical situation.
The classification of the technique related to the implant insertion timing to which we refer was proposed by Hämmerle et al. and provided four types of intervention:

- TYPE 1: Immediate post-extraction implants (positioning at the same time as extraction);

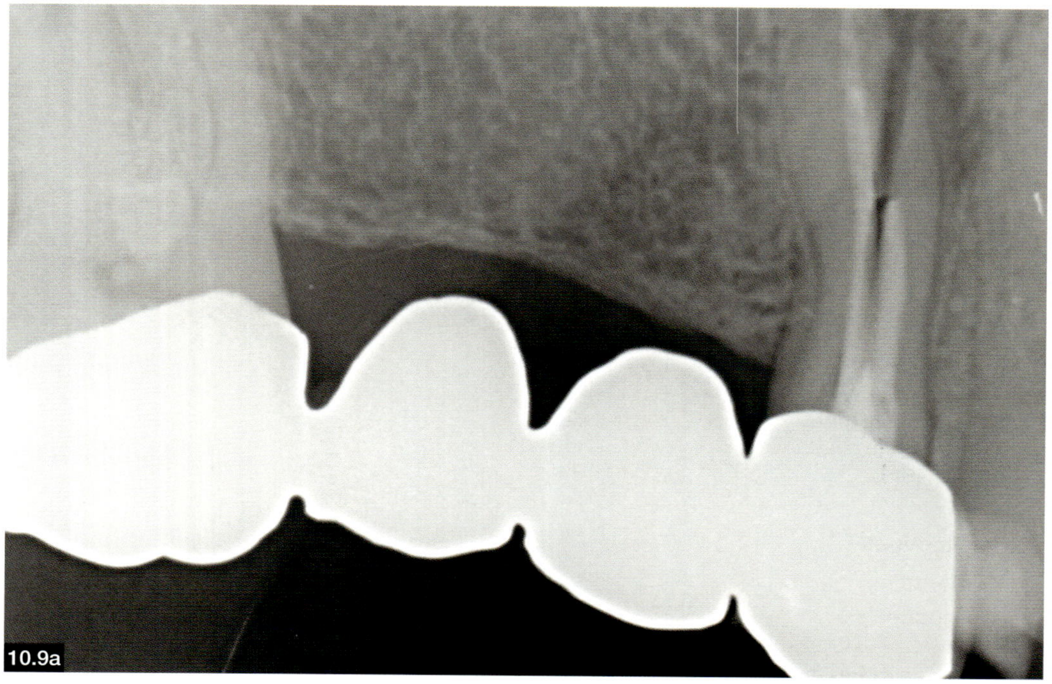

10.9a

Fig. 10.9a-b: Periapical radiographic examination, evidence of fracture in tooth 14. Conical beam computed tomography examination to evaluate the possibility, later confirmed, of immediate implant placement.

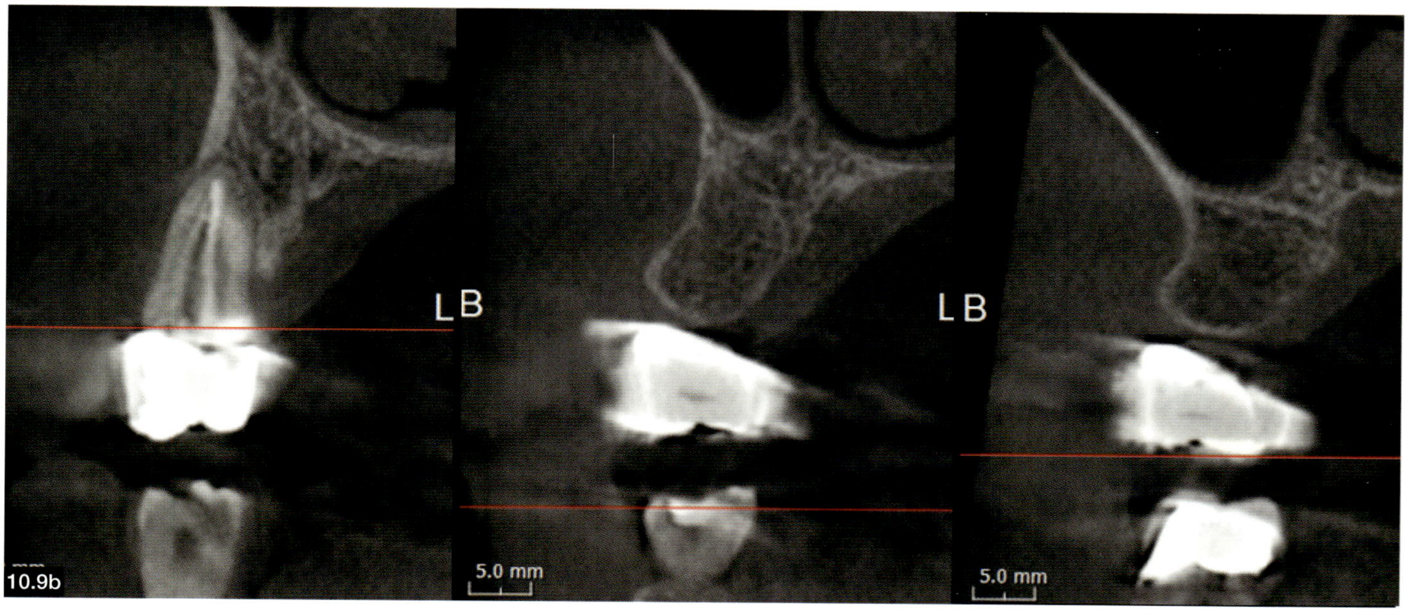

10.9b

ANALYSIS OF RISK FACTORS IN THE PLACEMENT OF POST-EXTRACTION IMPLANTS/PROSTHETIC RESTORATIONS			
Score	**0 pt.**	**1 pt.**	**2 pt.**
Aesthetic expectations of the patient	Low	Medium	High
Dental exposure	Low	Medium	High
Gingival phenotype	Often flat	Medium, with medium festooning	Thin festooned
Shape of dental crowns	Rectangular	Triangular	
Bone level at the adjacent tooth	≤ 5 mm at the point of contact	5.5 to 6.5 mm at point of contact	≥ 7 mm at the point of contact
Edentulous saddle size	1 tooth (≥ 7 mm)	1 tooth (≤ 7 mm)	2 teeth or more
Soft tissue anatomy	Preserved		Altered
Gingival parables of adjacent elements	Harmonious		Non-harmonious
Anatomy of the alveolar crest	Intact alveolar crest	Horizontal defect	Vertical defect
Thickness of the vestibular cortical bone	Sufficient ≥ 1 mm		Insufficient ≤ 1 mm
Number of surgical procedures (simultaneous or in stages)	Implant placement without additional surgical procedures	Additional surgical procedures at the time of implant placement	Need for multiple surgical interventions to perform implant-prosthetic rehabilitation
Parafunctions	Absent		Present
Implant site	Posterior		Anterior (14-24)
Passive eruption impaired (adjacent teeth)	Absent		Present
Vestibular bone probing (mm)	< 3		> 3
Possibility of obtaining primary stability	Apical		Mesio-distal
Position of the root in the socket*	Types 1 and 2		Types 3 and 4

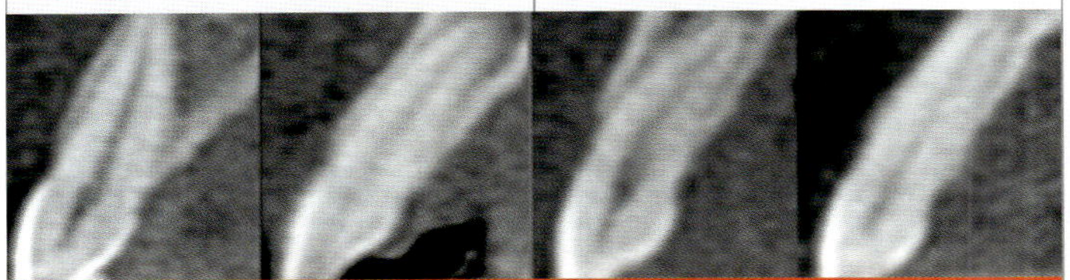

Type 1 Type 2 Type 3 Type 4

* Kan JYK, Rungcharassaeng K, Deflorian M, Weinstein T, Wang HL, Testori T. *Immediate implant placement and provisionalization of maxillary anterior single implants*. Periodontology 2000. 2018;77(1):197-212.

UNCOMPLICATED **ADVANCED** **COMPLICATED**

0 7 16 34

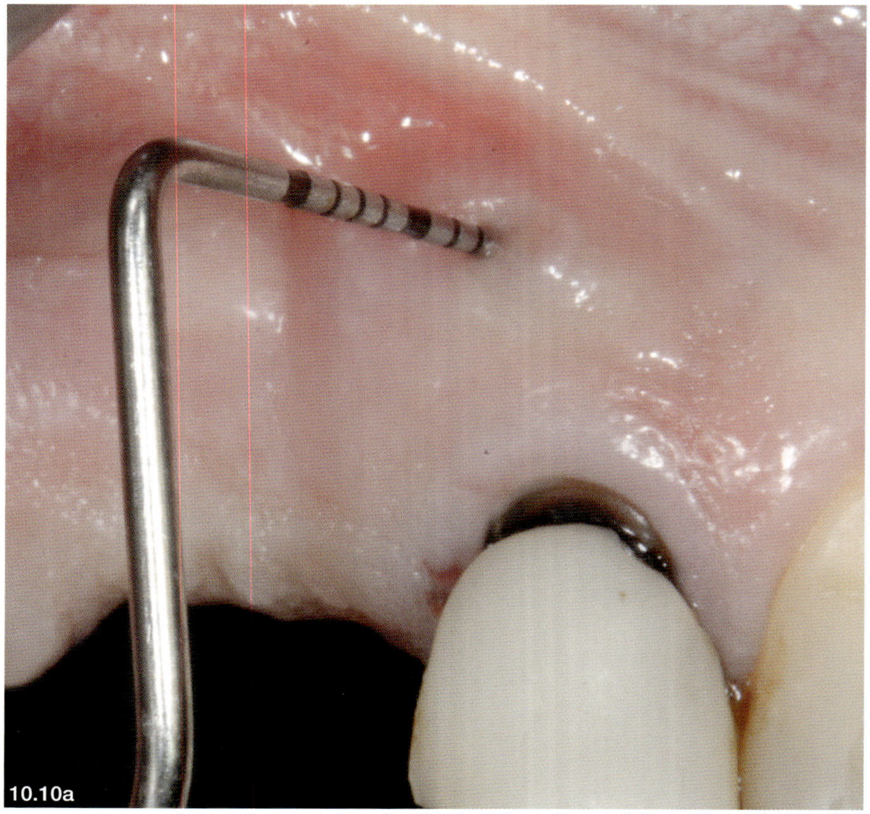

10.10a

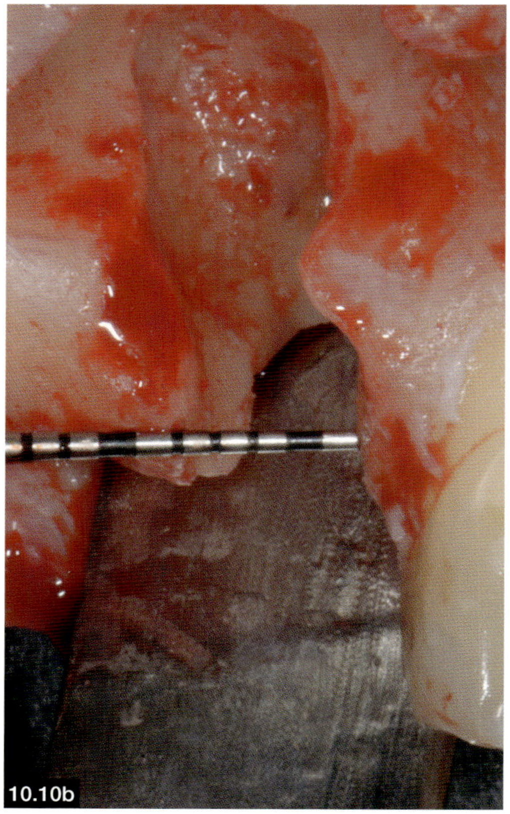

10.10b

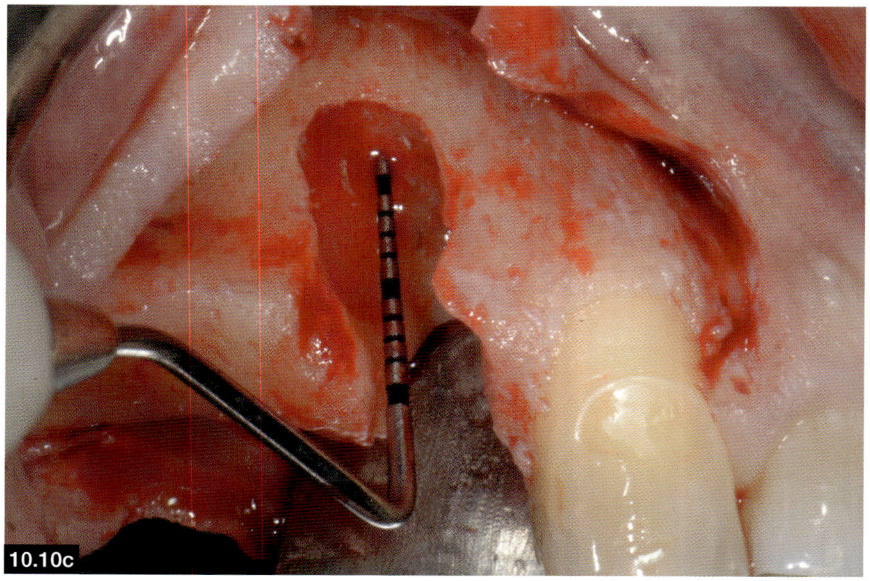

10.10c

Fig. 10.10a-c: Intraoral view: evidence of a fistula at tooth 14, elevation of a muco-periosteal flap, extraction of tooth 14 and review of the defect. The bone lesion is seen to have a full-thickness morphology.

- TYPE 2: Early post-extraction implantation (positioning within 4–8 weeks of extraction),
- TYPE 3: Deferred implantation (positioning between 12 and 16 weeks after extraction, in the healed bone), and
- TYPE 4: Deferred implantation (positioning 16 weeks after extraction, in the healed bone).

Hard and soft peri-implant tissue management

Contrary to the postulations proposed proposed in the past,[2] post-extraction implants do not make it possible to halt the post-extraction bone resorption mechanism. The extent of bone remodeling is therefore determined both by purely surgical post-extractive biological factors and by factors linked to the implant position in the apico-coronal and buccolingual directions[20] and may have negative effects on the aesthetic result. The use of grafts within the alveolar sites has been proposed to reduce the volumetric contraction of the post-extraction site regardless of the periodontal biotype of the patient.[6,12] Artzi et al.[21] inserted deproteinized bovine bone grafts into 15 human post-extraction alveoli and performed biopsy samples 9 months after their insertion. The study concludes that this type of graft is able to preserve the bone crest. The use of deproteinized bovine bone was analyzed by preoperative computed tomography (CT) analysis and at 30 and

90 postoperative days, evaluating the degree of resorption of the vestibular bone portion.[5] The authors found a lower bone reduction (20%) at the test sites compared with the sites where the biomaterial had not been grafted (79%).
Compensating for the inevitable volumetric contraction makes it possible to obtain an optimal aesthetic result. In addition, increasing the thickness of the soft tissue ensures long-term stability of gingival levels. The problem is less pressing in the treatment of patients with thick biotypes, as they are less prone to develop gum recessions.[22,23] For this reason, there is no indication of increased soft tissue thickness in these cases.[24] On the other hand, in patients with thin periodontal biotypes, it is highly probable that after dental extraction the vestibular bone, which is generally thin,[25] will undergo resorption followed by clinically relevant soft tissue contraction.[1]
A recent literature review establishes that the combination of immediate loading implant and connective graft could contribute to the stability of the gingival margin level and to an increase in peri-implant soft tissue.[26] However, most of the selected studies do not include a "control group" that directly demonstrates the advantages of a connective graft at the same time as implant placement.[26]

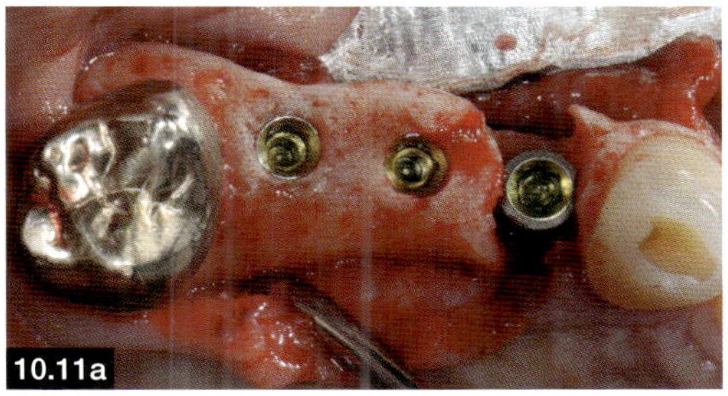

10.11a

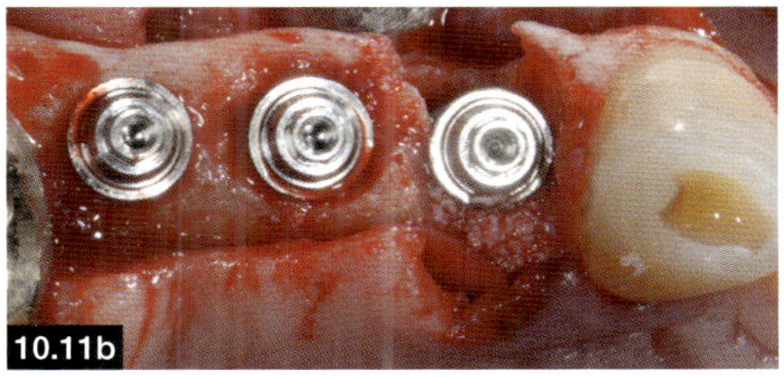

10.11b

Fig. 10.11a-d: Implant insertion. The residual palatal and vestibular defect of tooth 14 is managed with guided bone regeneration.

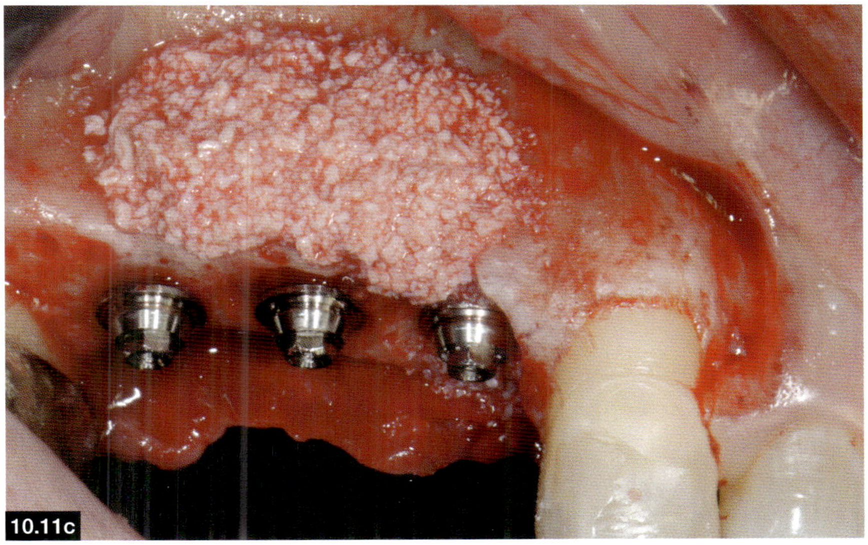

10.11c

Soft tissue healing and provisional adjustments

In areas of high aesthetic value, the temporary prosthetic phase is critical for both the patient, who must exert an adequate chewing function and lead an acceptable social life, and the clinician, who can protect and guide the healing of hard and soft tissues as is most appropriate for the aesthetic-functional success of the case.
In this case, immediate loading is a fundamental option but not the only one.[27] In cases in which – for surgical, mechanical, or aesthetic reasons – it is not possible to carry out temporary restorations with implant support, it is possible to proceed with fixed adhesive or removable solutions.

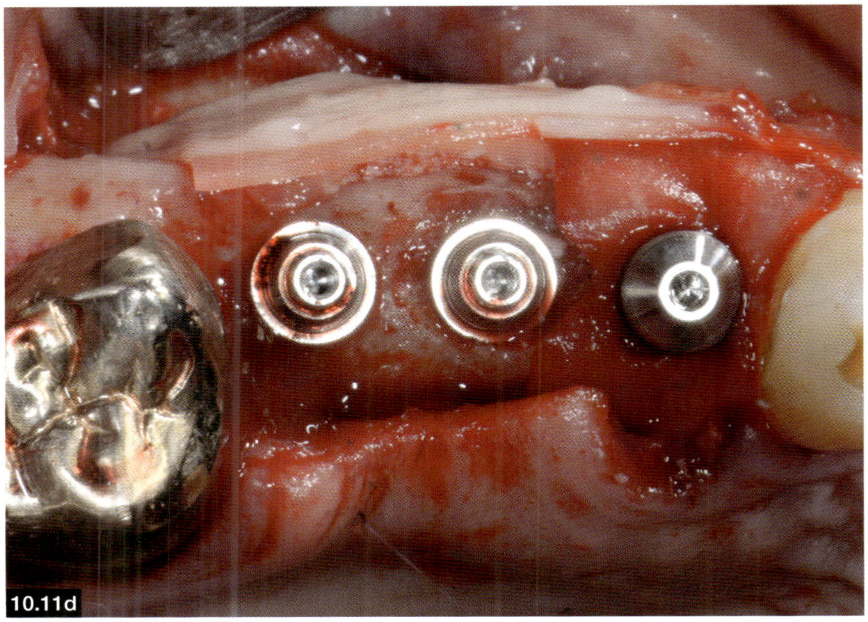

10.11d

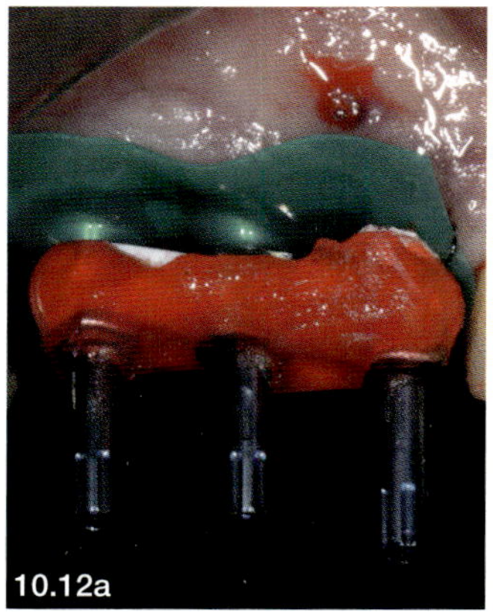
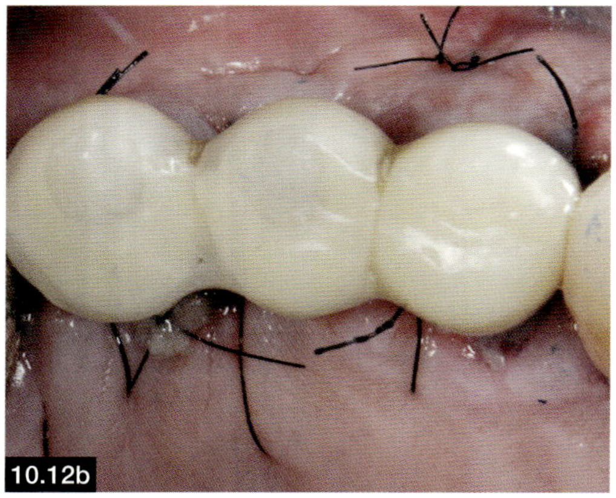
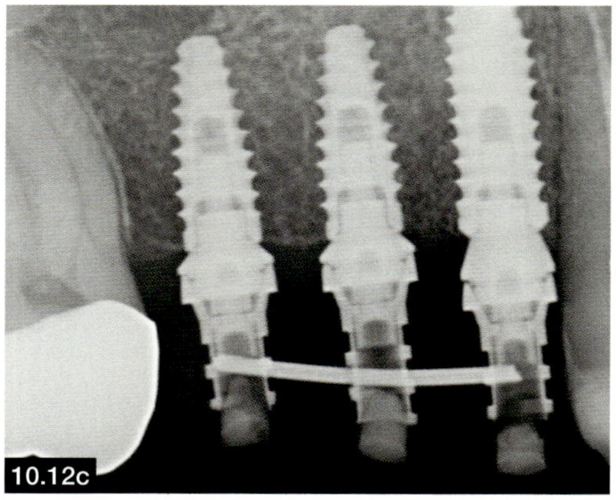

Fig. 10.12a-c: Detection of the implant position and delivery of the temporary immediate-loading implant.

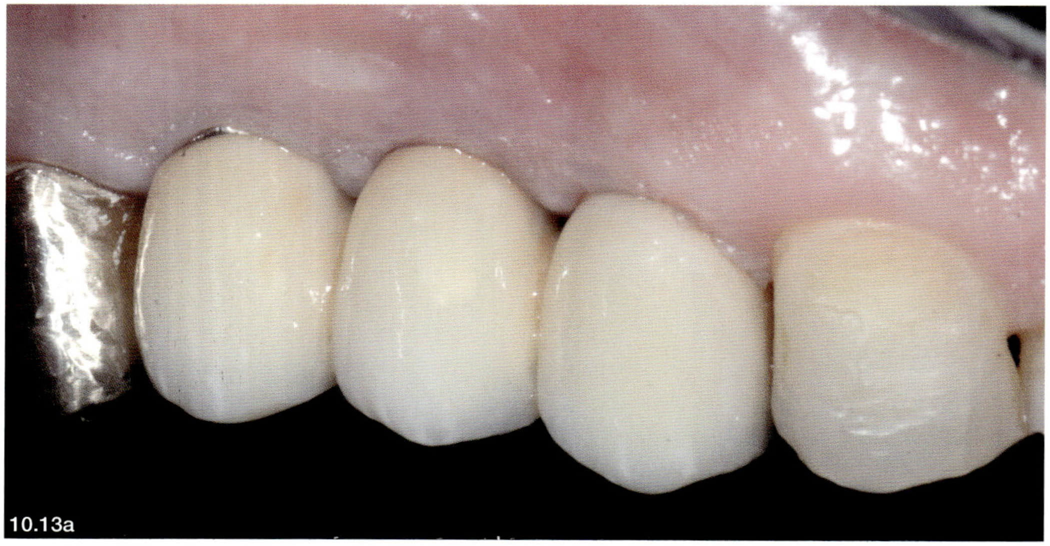

Fig. 10.13a-c: Delivery of the final prosthetic restoration and periapical x-ray inspection.

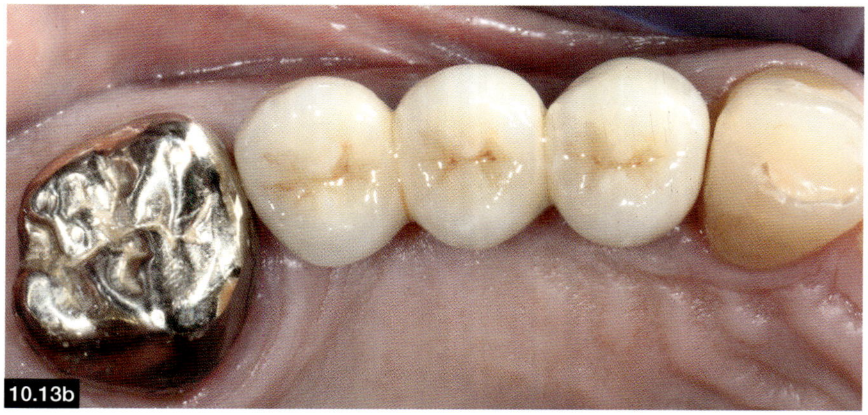
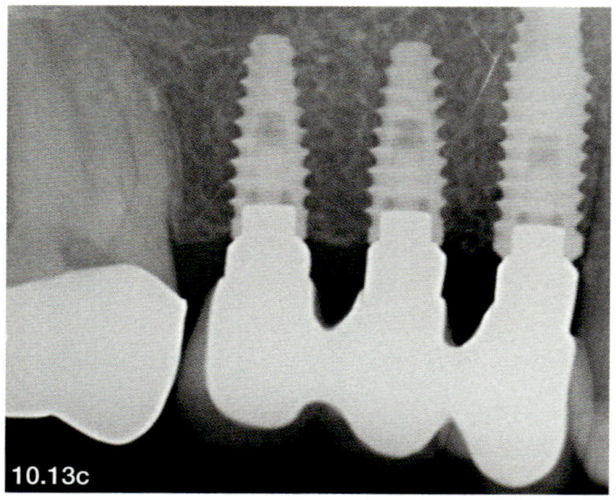

Fig. 10.13d-f: On the cone-beam computed tomography axial image, one can see there is a distance of 1.5 mm between the natural tooth and the implant. The area of inter-implant radiotransparency is due to *beam hardening*. The paraxial images show the restoration of the vestibular cortical bone.

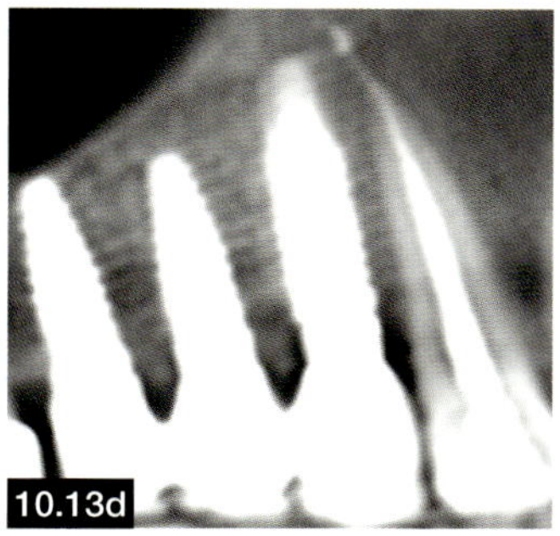
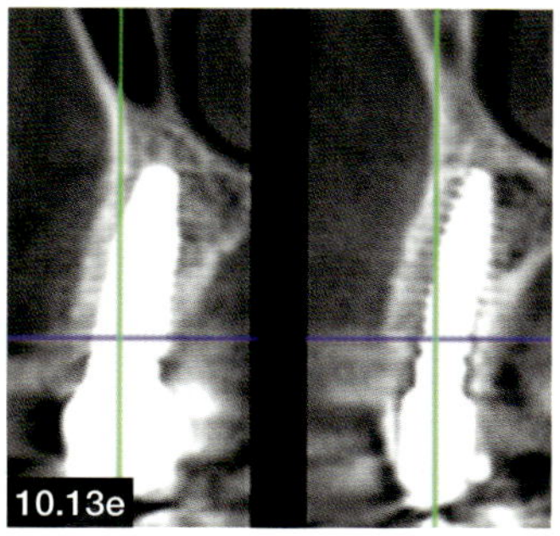
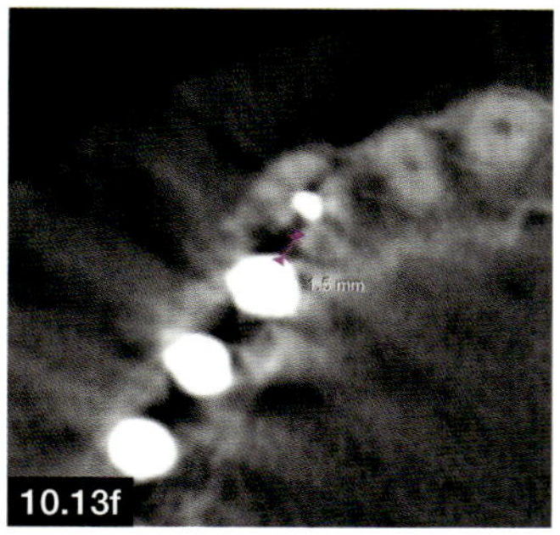

Diagnosis and procedural algorithms

The diagnostic phase in the case of post-extraction implants must evaluate the site (posterior-side sectors or aesthetic sector) that will be affected by the treatment and must be considered stratified on several levels:

- diagnosis and prognosis of the tooth concerned;
- clinical objective evaluation of the state of the hard and soft supporting tissues;
- bidimensional and/or three-dimensional radiographic evaluation of hard tissues.

Aesthetic sector (from 14 to 24)

Analysis of diagnostic parameters

According to our analysis, the factors to be considered in the diagnostic phase to draw up a rational treatment plan in case of a doomed tooth in a frontal sector are the following:

- predictability of obtaining adequate primary stability;
- presence/absence of the vestibular bone;
- periodontal biotype;
- absence/presence of recessions.

Predictability of achieving adequate primary stability

To achieve primary stability in a post-extraction site at the level of the anterior portion of the jaw, it is essential to observe the anatomical characteristics of the site to be treated and relate them to the prosthetically guided placement of the implant.

The anatomical characteristics to be considered include the following:

1. the parallelism between the long axis of the tooth and alveolar process or whether there is a more or less important degree of disparallelism;
2. the presence/absence of a bone portion of at least 4 mm apical to the root apex of the tooth to be extracted;
3. the amount of palatal bone at the post-extractive alveolus[28];
4. the extent of vestibular concavity of the premaxilla between the two canine pillars at both radiological and clinical levels (through palpatory examination).

We can expect to achieve *primary stability* when:

1. there is the possibility of anchoring the apical/palatal implant to the post-extractive socket for at least 4 mm;
2. surgical techniques are performed that involve under-preparation of the osteotomy site;
3. implants with a conical morphology and sharp turns should be used rather than implants with a cylindrical morphology;
4. in the absence of adequate palatal/apical bone volumes, larger diameter implants should be used, seeking stability in the mesiodistal portions of the alveolus. In this case, an adequate distance must be maintained between the implant shoulder and the vestibular bone theca[12] and between the implant shoulder and the root of the adjacent teeth (Figs. 10.9–10.13).[29]

ANATOMICAL CHARACTERISTICS

The morphology of the alveolar process, the amount of apical (3–4 mm) and palatal bone at the root of the tooth to be extracted, and the bone quality are important **factors to consider** to place an implant that has adequate primary stability.

Presence/absence of vestibular bone theca

It has been demonstrated in the literature that the presence of the intact *vestibular bone theca* is a fundamental requirement for the stability of the vestibular soft tissue at the site to be treated.[30] If there is a vestibular bone defect in the tooth to be extracted, a careful analysis of the morphology of the defect becomes fundamental to establish the correct therapeutic approach. In fact, a study shows that in the case of immediate post-extraction implants, facial defects limited to the facial component of the vestibular bone theca are associated with a gingival recession rate >1.5 mm in 8.3% of cases.

VESTIBULAR BONE THECA

Immediate post-extraction implants in the **absence of vestibular bone theca** are clinical situations to be tackled with **extreme caution** assessing cost-benefit; in cases of high aesthetic value, a deferred approach is more predictable.

Conversely, defects involving the mesial and distal components of the element to be extracted, or even involving the mesial and distal aspects of the adjacent elements, lead to a recession rate >1.5 mm of 42.8% and 100%, respectively, of the cases treated.[31] For this reason, an immediate post-extraction approach should be carefully considered in the case of absence of the vestibular bone theca, even in the light of the periodontal biotype.
An innovative technique was recently introduced to preserve the buccal bone crest in situations where it is particularly thin and can easily fracture during root extraction. Hürzeler et al. were the first to describe this technique called the "socket-shield technique" in an experiment performed on Beagle dogs. The technical note describes the hemisection of a premolar and the preservation of a portion (the shield) at the buccal level due to wear. This is maintained 1 mm coronal to the buccal bone crest. The implant placed immediately after the creation of the palatal/lingual shield should not be placed in contact but in close proximity to it. No complications were found, and the subsequent histology showed cement formation in the area between the implant surface and the remaining root portion.[32] Further histological confirmations were proposed by Schwimer.[33]
Some changes to the technique were made by different authors without, however, varying the biological principles.[34-36]
The promising results currently urge us to try to further improve this technique and to make it more predictable.[37]
The possibility of leaving this portion of the root, often resulting from an endodontically pathological tooth, is given by the fact that the remaining portion is essentially external root cement, where the dentin tubules, potential bacterial, can be cleansed and treated intrasurgically with low surface tension products and ethylenediaminetetraacetic acid and then undergo a bactericidal treatment with 0.2% chlorhexidine.[38,39]
The surgical technique described requires a specific learning curve of the operator (Figs. 10.14–10.17).

Periodontal biotype

Over the years, an attempt has been made to classify the population simply according to a series of morphological characteristics of the gum tissue. These morphological characteristics are linked both to genetic traits and to local factors such as shape, size, and position of the teeth.
In the literature, it has been observed that there are gingival phenotypes characterized, among other factors, by different thicknesses of soft tissues.[22,40] It has been shown that there is a certain correlation between gingival biotype and vestibular bone thickness of the alveolar process, analyzed both intraoperatively and by cone-beam CT examinations.[25] It has also been described how the different periodontal biotypes have an important clinical significance.[41] Specifically, implantology has shown that patients with a reduced thickness (<1 mm) of the vestibular cortical sites treated with immediate post-extraction

PROCEDURAL ALGORITHM FOR IMPLANT PLACEMENT IN THE FRONT SECTORS

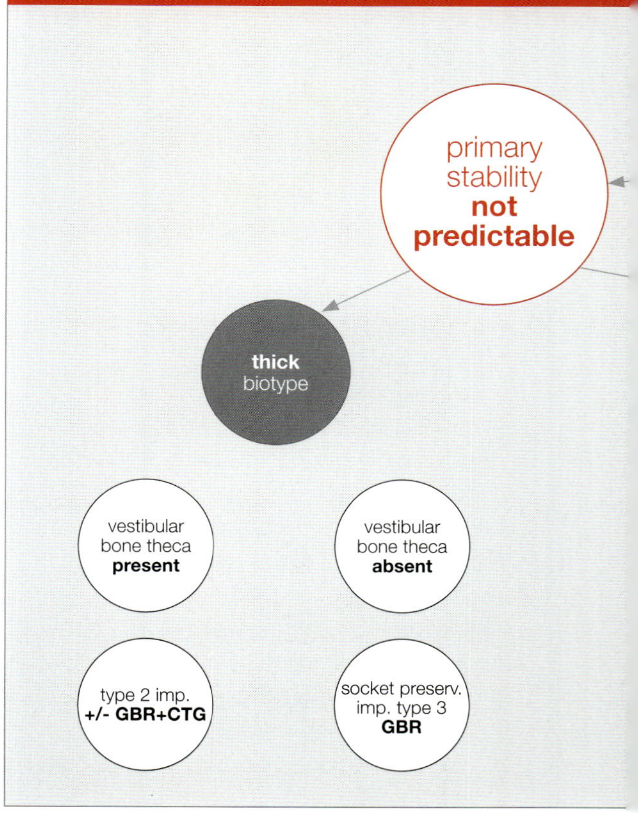

implants have a greater degree of vestibular recession in the medium term.[42,43]
There is, therefore, an association between thin periodontal biotype and vestibular recession in immediate post-extraction implants performed with both a flapless technique[44] and flap procedures.[45]
Despite the unfavorable clinical course of post-extraction implant treatment of thin periodontal biotypes, it is possible to modify the prognosis of the onset of vestibular recessions by performing vestibular connective grafts at the treated site, modifying the thickness of the soft tissue itself.[46]

Absence/presence of recessions

Gingival recession is defined as the pathological displacement of gingival tissues in an apical direction with root surface exposure.[47] The diagnostic importance of the presence of a recession in determining the treatment plan is linked to the anatomical alteration due to the recession itself.
In the first analysis, the recession is characterized by loss of clinical attachment, resulting in the loss of a more or less large portion of the vestibular bone theca.
In addition, gingival recession can also be defined as a loss of keratinized tissue.
Consequently, a tooth to be extracted with a *gingival recession* has several aesthetically unfavorable prognostic factors in the case of an immediate post-extraction approach.[30] In these cases, a deferred approach may be more effective than an immediate post-extraction approach.[48]

GUM RECESSION

A gum recession, in the absence of an adequate band of keratinized tissue, may represent a **contraindication** to the insertion of a post-extraction implant.

Procedural algorithm

The following procedural algorithm aims to schematically illustrate the various possible scenarios to facilitate the clinician in the choice of surgical treatment.

▸ *to be continued on page 496*

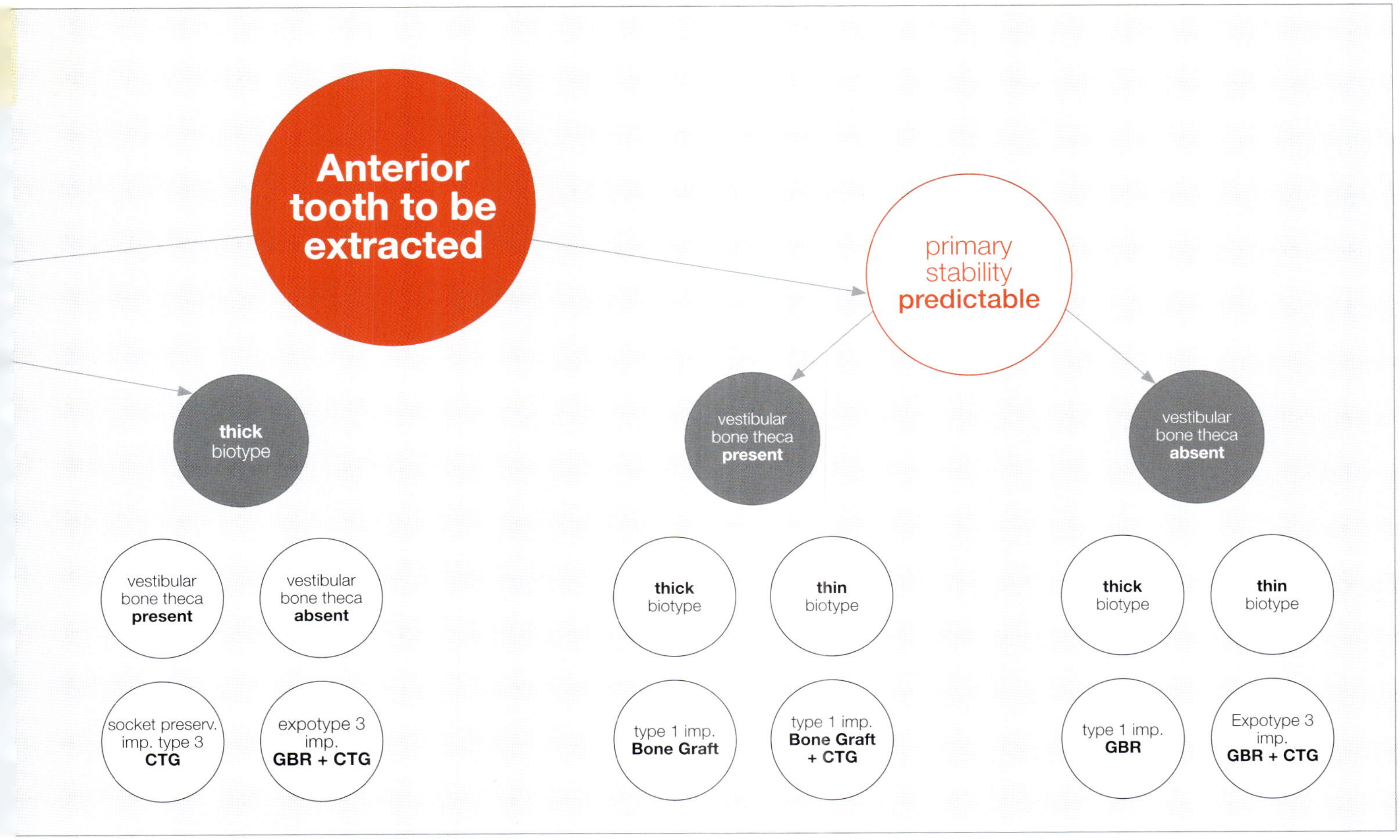

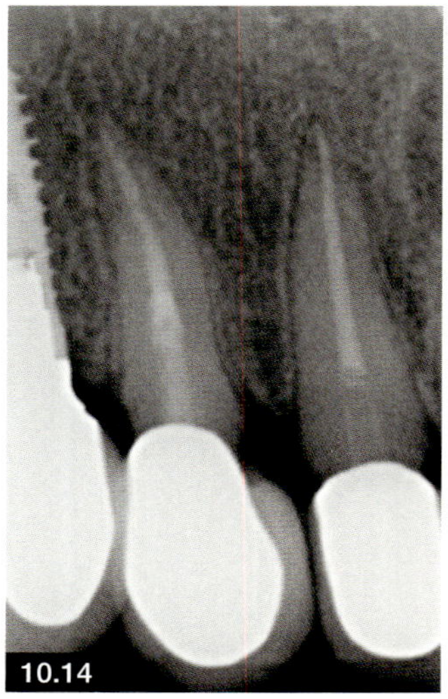

10.14

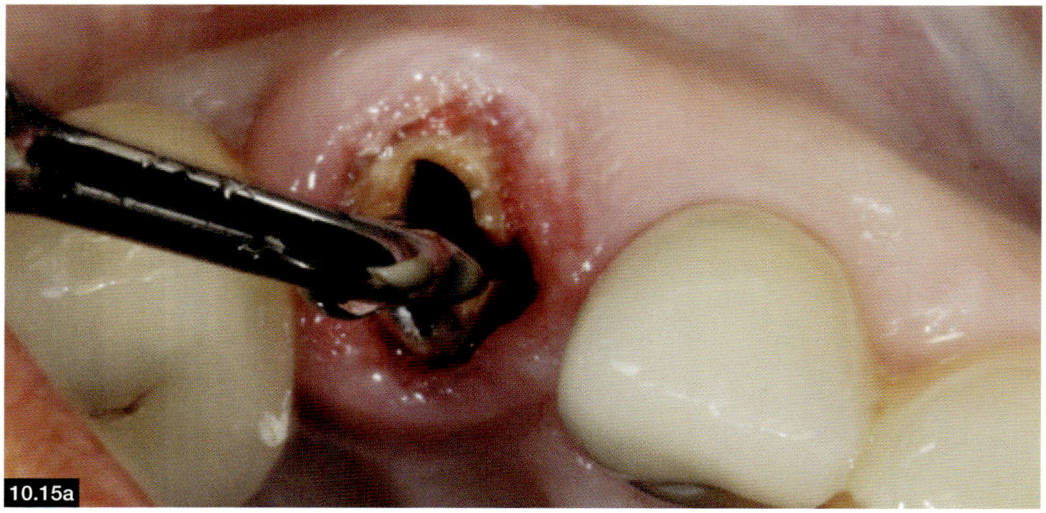

10.15a

Fig. 10.14: Preoperative periapical X-ray following a certain diagnosis of root fracture of tooth 13.

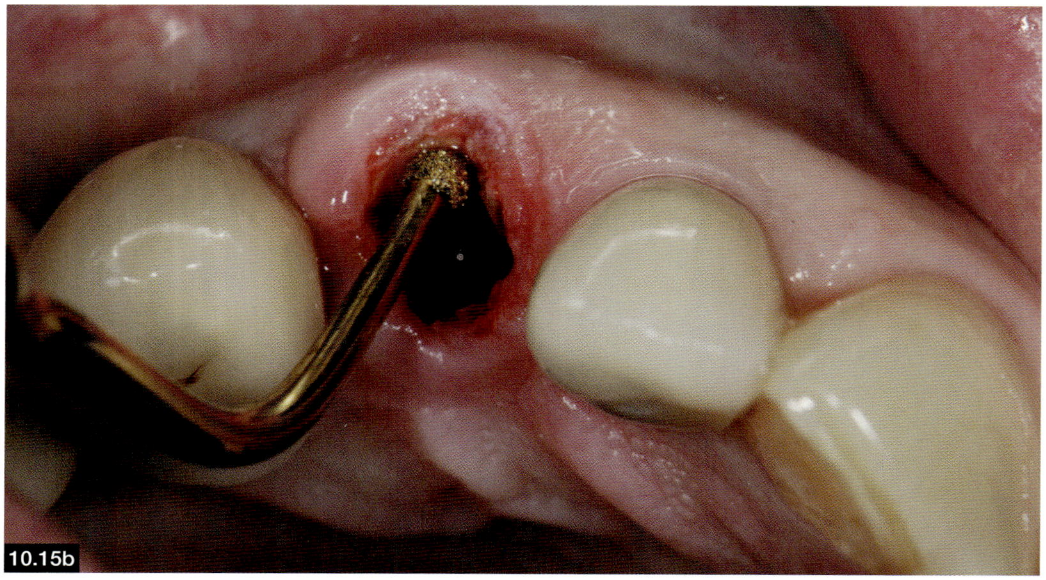

10.15b

Fig. 10.15a-c: Partial extraction of tooth 13: the tooth is sectioned in mesiodistal direction, and the palatal portion of the root is extracted. At this stage, it is essential to also remove the apex of the tooth without removing the vestibular fragment.
The *shield*, whose coronal margin must be positioned 1 mm coronal to the vestibular bone crest, is shaped using ultrasonic instruments.

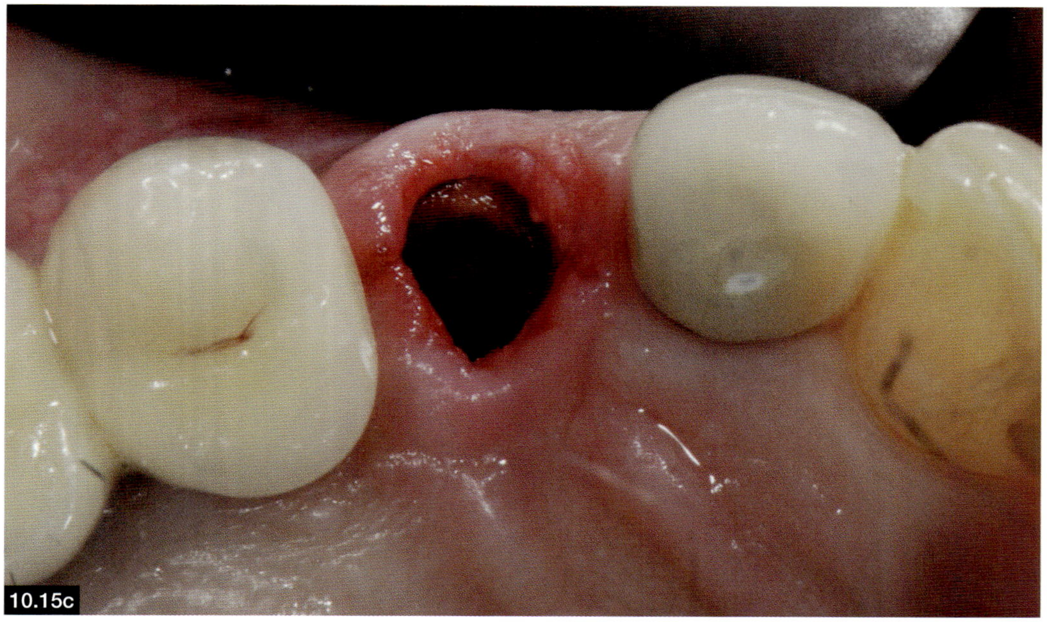

10.15c

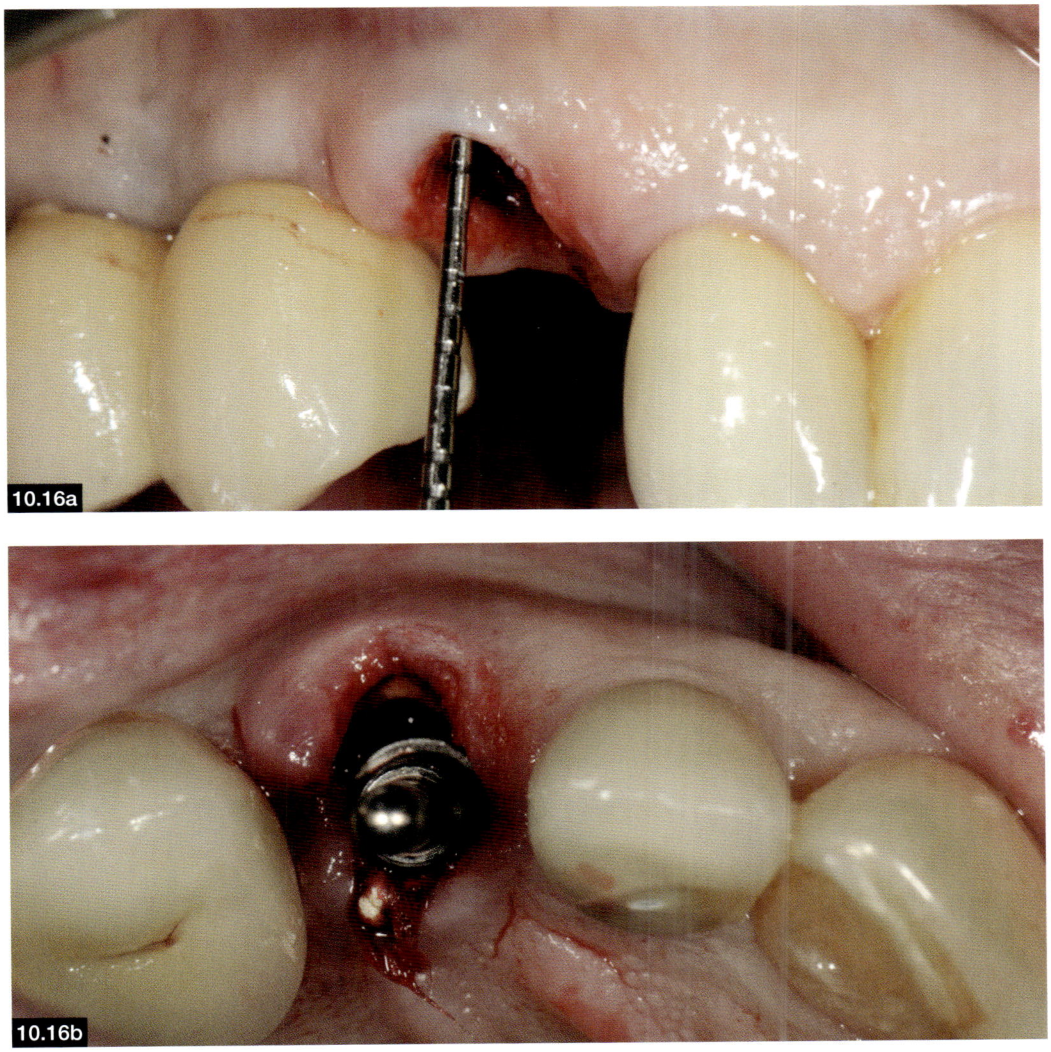

Fig. 10.16a-b: Occlusal view of the *shield*, implant insertion.

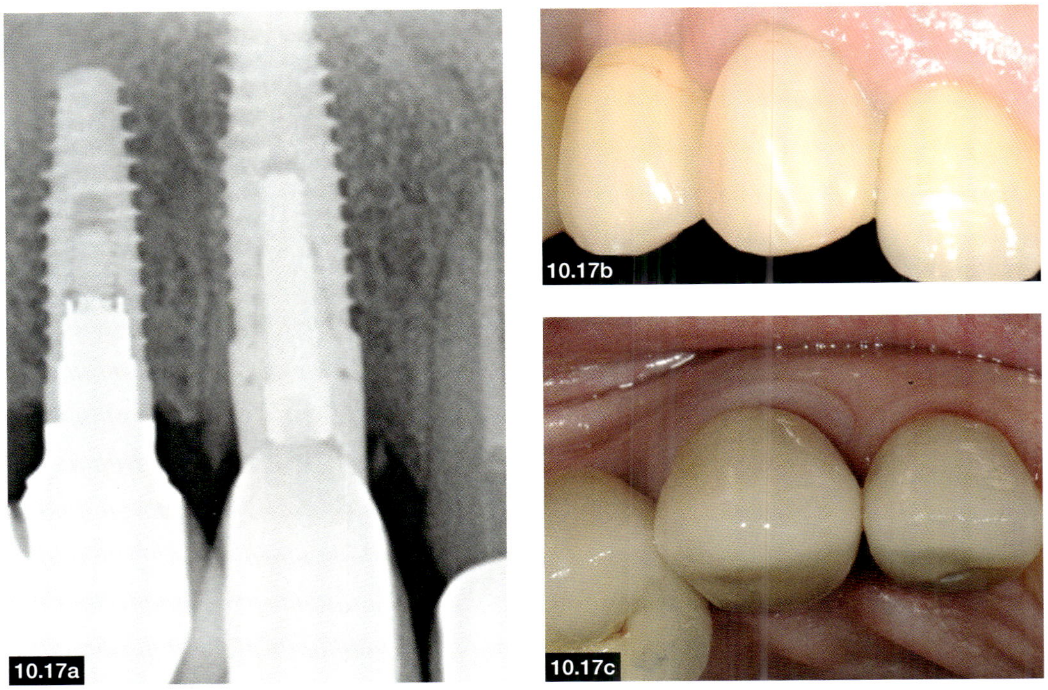

Fig. 10.17a-c: Final restoration: clinical and radiographic examination 5 years after implant placement.

Once a tooth in the frontal sector has been evaluated nonmaintainable, the fundamental question that the clinician must ask himself is: "After the extraction of the tooth, will I be able to stabilize the implant?" If the answer is negative, the implant placement must automatically be postponed. Consequently, the first surgical step will be represented only by the extraction of the tooth, taking care to carry out a procedure that is as atraumatic and as conservative as possible. Subsequently, the situation of the alveolar bone should be evaluated to predict the morphological changes it will undergo during the early stages of healing. The fundamental clinical aspects to be analyzed simultaneously are as follows:

- the thickness of hard and soft tissues;
- the presence/absence of the vestibular cortical.

More specifically, a number of clinical situations can be observed:

1. If we find a thick biotype and the simultaneous presence of the entire vestibular cortical tissue, we can predict that physiological bone resorption will be limited and contained in the thickness of the bone theca with the consequent maintenance of vestibular tissue levels. In this case, the clinician only has to wait for a sufficient amount of bone (even immature) to be formed to guarantee the achievement of primary stability acceptable for implant survival. For these reasons, the clinical protocol provides for a type 2 implant placement (4–8 weeks) associated or not with maneuvers to increase in hard and/or soft tissue in relation to the actual degree of resorption to which the extraction site has been subjected.
2. A second less favorable scenario may present a thick biotype but absent or partially absent cortical bone (typical case of a vertical fracture). The potential for spontaneous regeneration is limited and, in addition, part of the vestibular bone support is missing, so marked bone resorption partially masked by the initial thickness of the soft tissue will be inevitable. To avoid this eventuality, at the same time as the extraction, it is advisable to carry out maneuvers that favor alveolar regeneration, limiting atrophy and facilitating the subsequent correct implant positioning, with biomaterial grafts and resorbable membranes (socket preservation).[49,50] After a standard healing period (beyond 12 weeks), implant placement (type 3/4) can be performed, inevitably associated with a further horizontal bone regeneration maneuver to obtain a vestibular bone thickness at the implant that favors long-term success.
3. If, on the contrary, the patient's biotype is classified as thin, the scenario becomes much more complex to manage. In fact, the blood supply to the soft and hard tissues is lower, and consequently, even an atraumatic extraction sees its invasiveness increased. For this reason, a high degree of resorption of both hard and soft tissue is to be expected. If not managed properly, this reabsorption will result in atrophy, which may also be vertical. Our school, therefore, suggests always combining bone regeneration maneuvers with both the extraction (socket preservation) and the implant positioning (guided bone regeneration [GBR]) carried out no earlier than after 12 weeks of healing. In addition, soft tissue augmentation maneuveres with connective grafts will be performed during implant placement.
4. In the event of a thin periodontal biotype, in which the vestibular cortical bone is partially resorbed, we will also find a recession that will result in post-extraction vertical resorption. In these cases, we recommend proceeding with the extraction, letting the soft tissues heal, and then positioning an implant, combined with maneuvers to regenerate both hard and soft tissues.

In all these cases, a traditional prosthetic protocol should be used, using adhesive techniques and/or adjacent teeth.
If, on the other hand, the amount of residual bone present after extraction offers

the possibility of stabilizing the implant in the correct position, the clinician should consider making a simultaneous implant placement or managing the extraction site and then inserting the implants.
Again, in this case, the presence of the vestibular bone and the periodontal biotype must be evaluated.
More specifically, the following clinical situations can be observed:

1. In the case of a thick biotype, simultaneous implant placement (type 1) is often used. If the thick biotype is associated with complete cortical bone, then no flaps will be made, and additional maneuvers will aim to fill only the post-extraction gap with biomaterials, limiting surgical invasiveness (clinical case 1).
2. If, on the contrary, the cortical bone is insufficient, it would be necessary to perform a procedure, with or without a flap, to perform GBR with the placement of a resorbable membrane and a biomaterial graft (clinical case 2).
3. Simultaneous positioning is also possible with a thin periodontal biotype with no recession (a clinical sign of vestibular cortical bone integrity). This scenario is managed with a mandatory minitraumatic extraction, favored by the use of micro-blades, periotomes, and axial tractions to be performed with the extraction forceps, implant placement, insertion of biomaterial in the alveolar gap, and connective graft with tunneling or flap techniques.
4. Finally, in the case of a thin biotype and recession (a sign of the absence of the vestibular cortical bone), although implant placement is possible, our school prefers a prudent attitude, and the clinical protocol is transformed into a deferred placement with simultaneous correction of hard tissues (with GBR) and soft tissues (with connective tissue graft [CTG]).

The prosthetic protocols in these situations can be different.
It is recommended to carry out immediate temporary restorations only in the most favorable cases, that is, in situations where there are a thick periodontal biotype and no gingival recession.

Lateral-posterior sector

Analysis of diagnostic parameters

For the insertion of post-extraction implants in the lateral and posterior sectors, the evaluation of periodontal criteria is the same as for the teeth of the anterior group; in the diagnostic phase, the possibility of obtaining adequate primary stability dictated by bone morphology must be considered.

Procedural algorithm

In cases where a post-extraction approach is required in the molar area, the morphology of the root complex must be carefully assessed (Page 498). In addition to the number, shape, and length of the roots, the presence of inter-radicular septa of adequate volume should be investigated with the help of three-dimensional radiographic examinations to obtain good primary stability.
It is also necessary to assess the presence and extent of any periapical lesions of the tooth to be extracted and of the adjacent teeth. In the lower molars, the presence of lingual undercuts and the position of the inferior alveolar neurovascular bundle should be assessed to avoid iatrogenic neurological lesions or important hemorrhagic complications.
In the clinical situation in which it is necessary to rehabilitate the lower premolars, it is essential to investigate in advance the position and the relationship to the mentalis foramen with the root apexes.
In the lateral and posterior areas of the upper jaw (molars and premolars), the number and shape of the roots, the presence of wide interradicular septa, and the relationship between root apexes

and contiguous anatomical structures (maxillary sinus and anatomical morphology of the same) must be evaluated.
This evaluation will allow the clinician to choose between different treatment plans; in the case of apical bone availability at the socket, a two-step approach can be followed, with or without alveolar preservation techniques. If adequate bone volumes are not present, a deferred approach is recommended. The introduction of diagnostic algorithms can help the clinician to formulate the appropriate treatment plan for the patient based on objective data collected during the physical examination.

Conclusion

Implant prosthetic rehabilitation of unmaintainable teeth is a delicate procedure that certainly requires surgical and prosthetic skills but that cannot be separated from an important diagnostic sensitivity. Knowing how to perform the correct protocol in the right situation is the real discrimination between a successful procedure and a treatment plan that will lead to complications and failures.[52,53]. The clinician, before determining the therapeutic timing, should evaluate the following:

- predictability of an adequate primary stability;
- presence/absence of the vestibular bone theca;
- periodontal biotype;
- absence/presence of recessions.

Only after these assessments can the clinician choose the most rational and predictable treatment plan.

PROCEDURAL ALGORITHM FOR POSTERIOR IMPLANT PLACEMENT

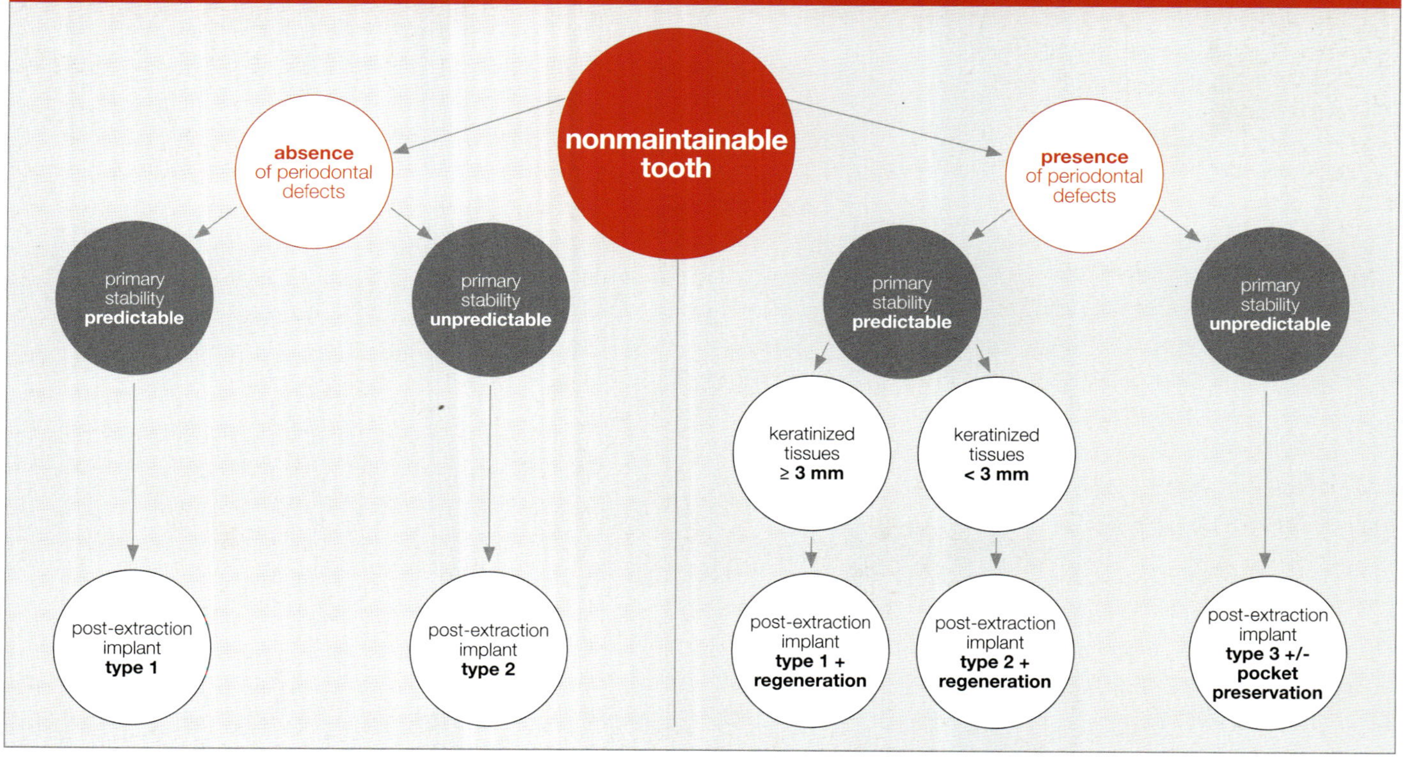

Immediate post-extraction implant of upper right lateral incisor

CASE REPORT 1

The patient was referred for spontaneous pain at tooth 11 and reported previous trauma of the tooth. Clinically, a microinclination of the upper interincisal line was observed. In addition, failed prosthetic rehabilitation of teeth no. 11-21 was observed with evident marginal tissue inflammation that cannot be resolved with causal therapy alone (Figure 1a-c).

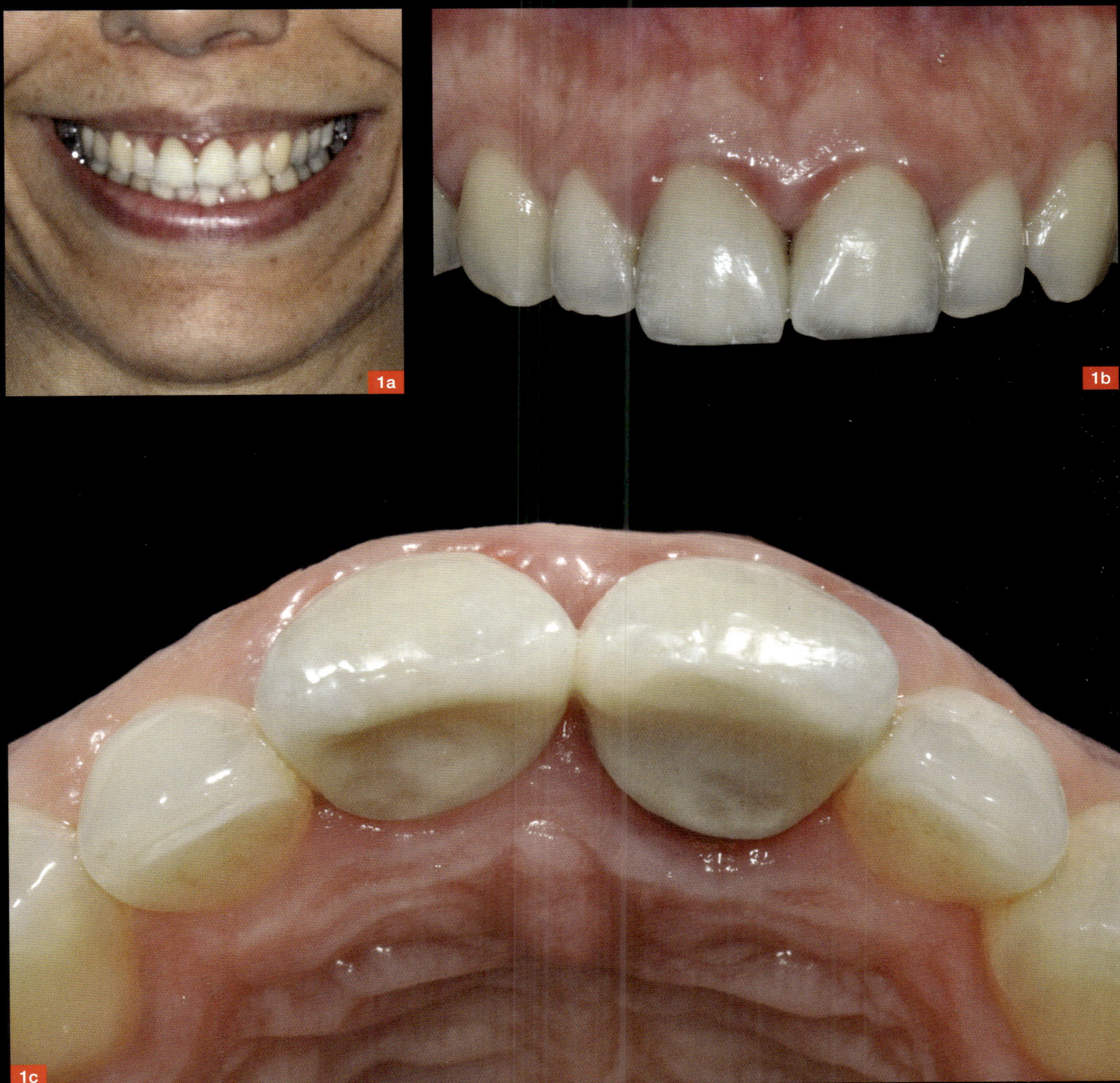

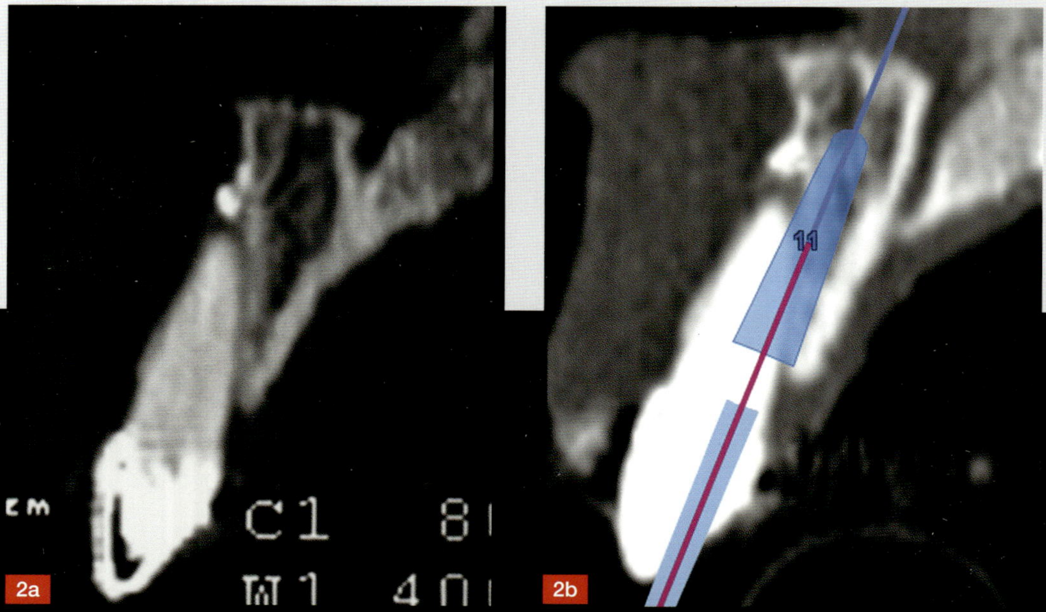

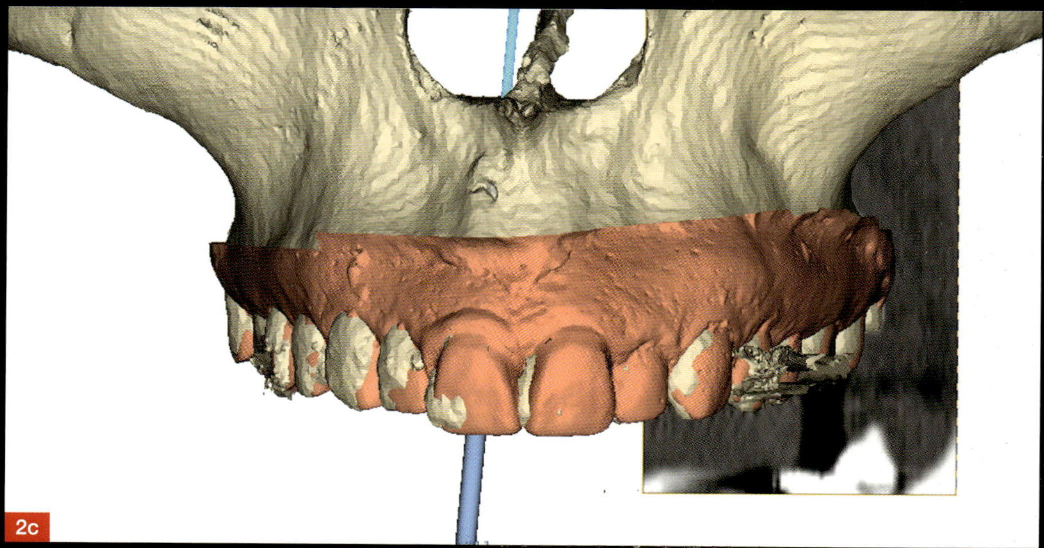

Figure 2a-d: Radiographic examinations showed corono-radicular fracture of tooth 11 and extruded endodontic material beyond apex also at tooth 11. Therefore, on the basis of clinical and radiographic examination, tooth no. 11 is considered unmaintainable. Computerized surgical programing performed with the aid of dedicated software, superimposing the scan of the diagnostic wax-up with the CT for the insertion of an immediate post-extraction implant.

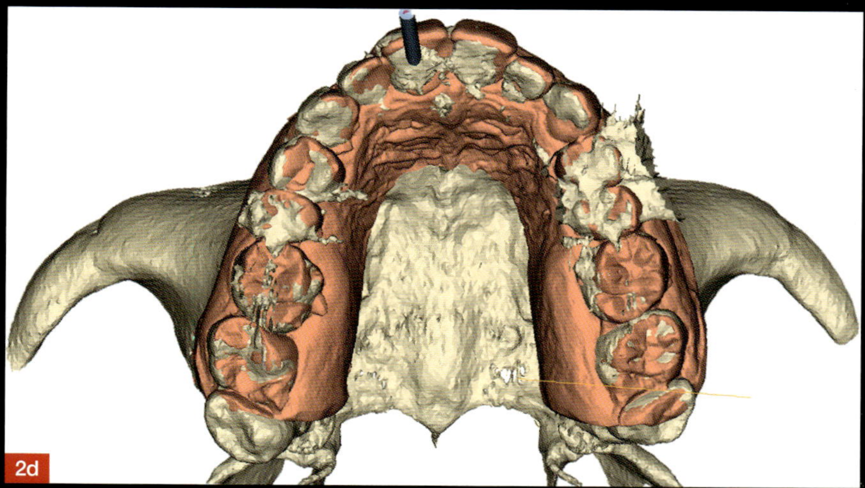

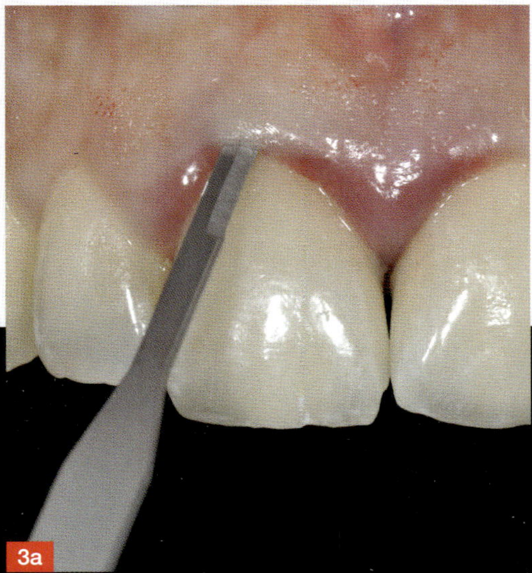

3a

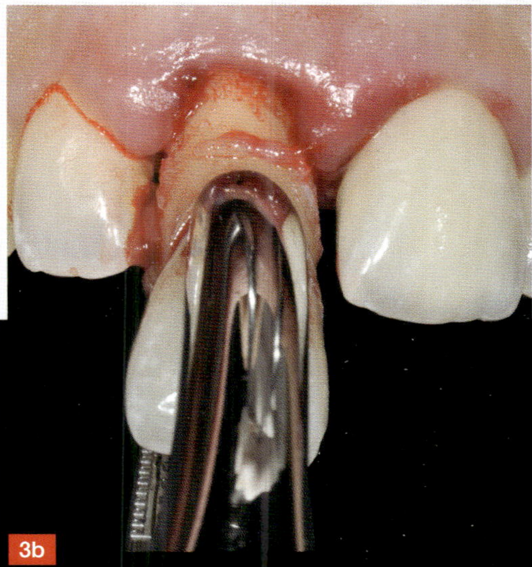

3b

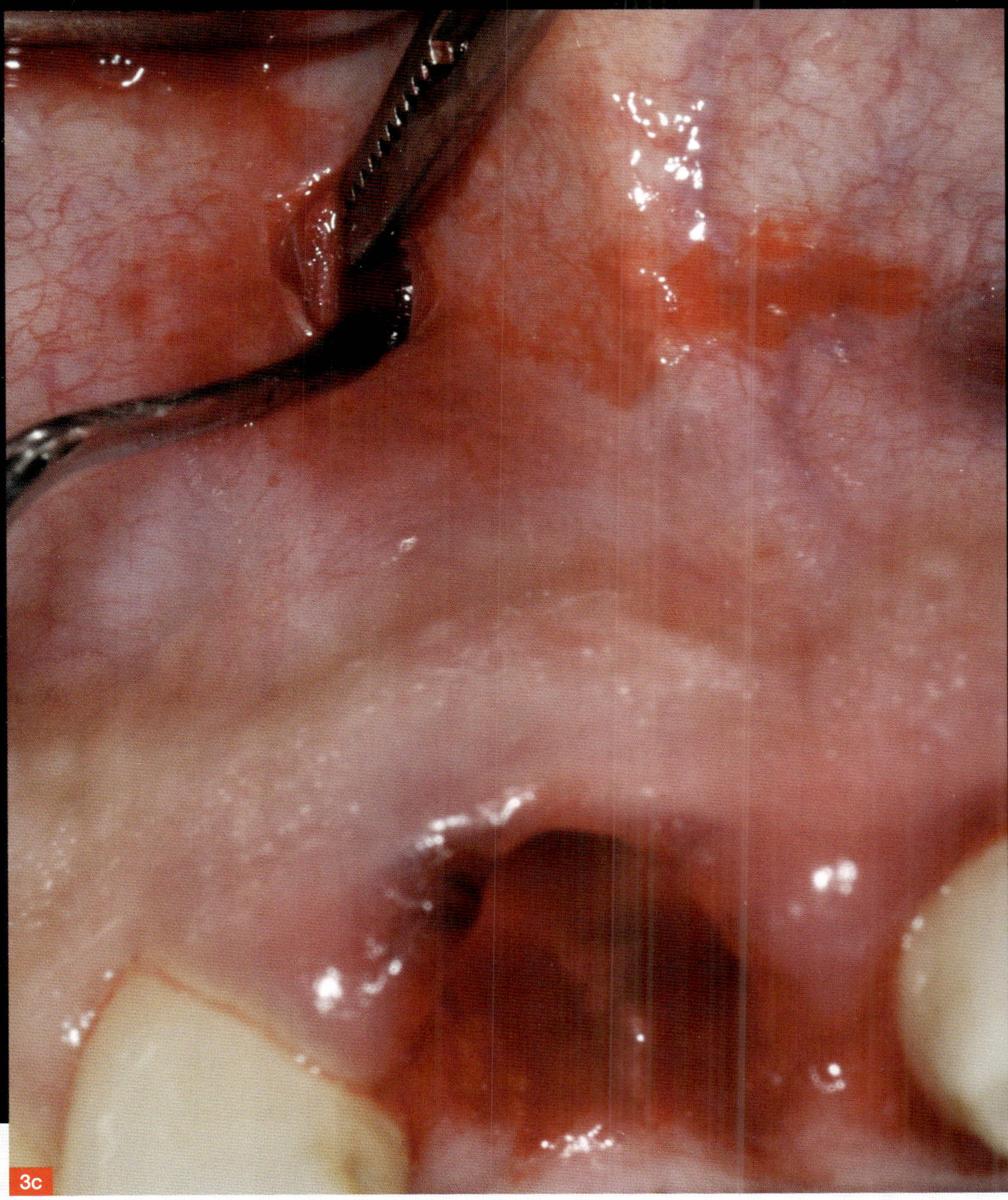

3c

Figure 3a-c: Intra-sulcular incision with microsurgery blade. The atraumatic extraction using pliers with forces developed axially at the root. The extruded material beyond the apex is removed through an incision of about 4 mm at the alveolar mucosa so as not to affect the marginal soft tissue.

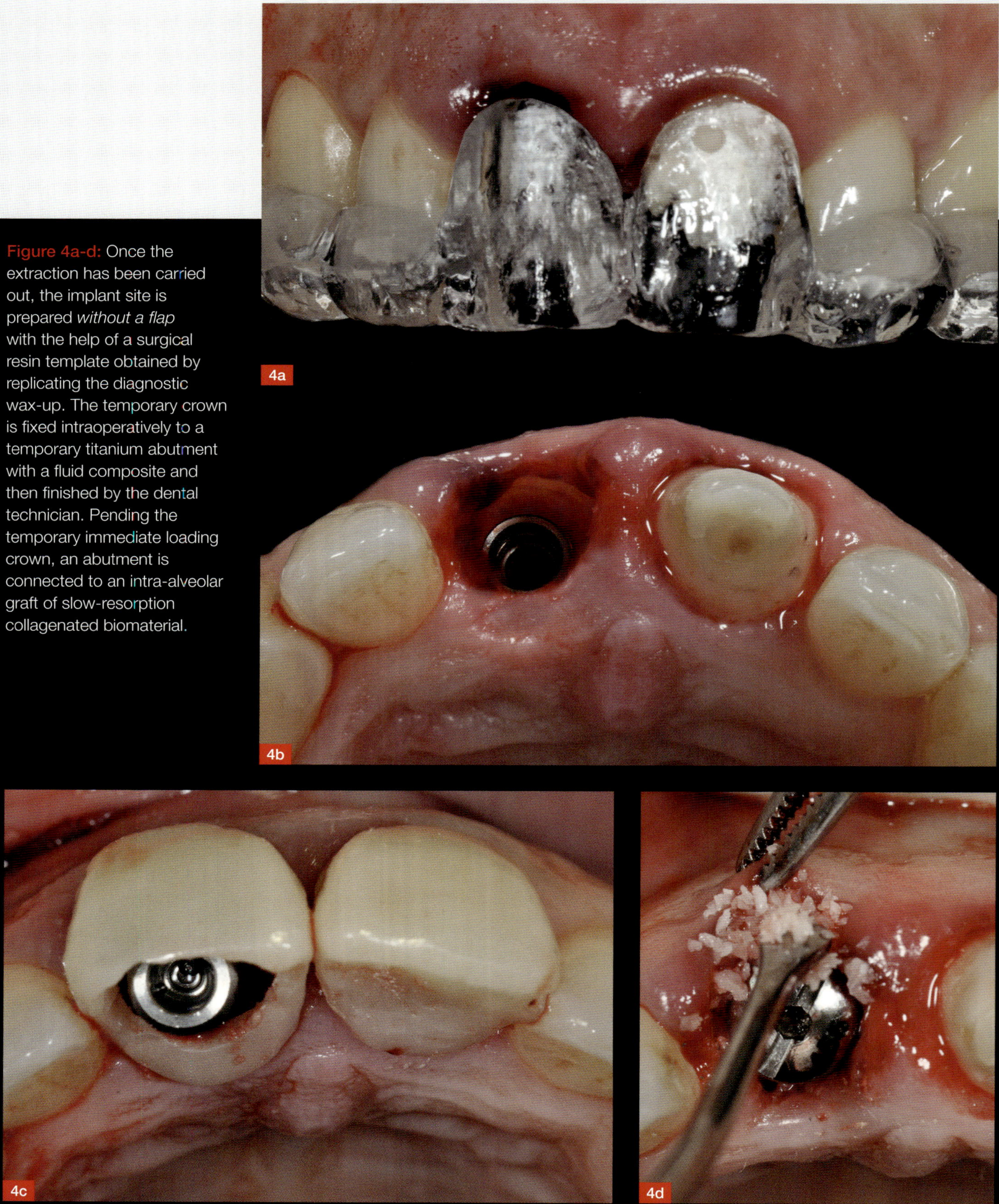

Figure 4a-d: Once the extraction has been carried out, the implant site is prepared *without a flap* with the help of a surgical resin template obtained by replicating the diagnostic wax-up. The temporary crown is fixed intraoperatively to a temporary titanium abutment with a fluid composite and then finished by the dental technician. Pending the temporary immediate loading crown, an abutment is connected to an intra-alveolar graft of slow-resorption collagenated biomaterial.

Figure 5a-b: Temporary immediate-loading screw-retained crown without centric and protrusive occlusal contacts and endodontic radiographic image.

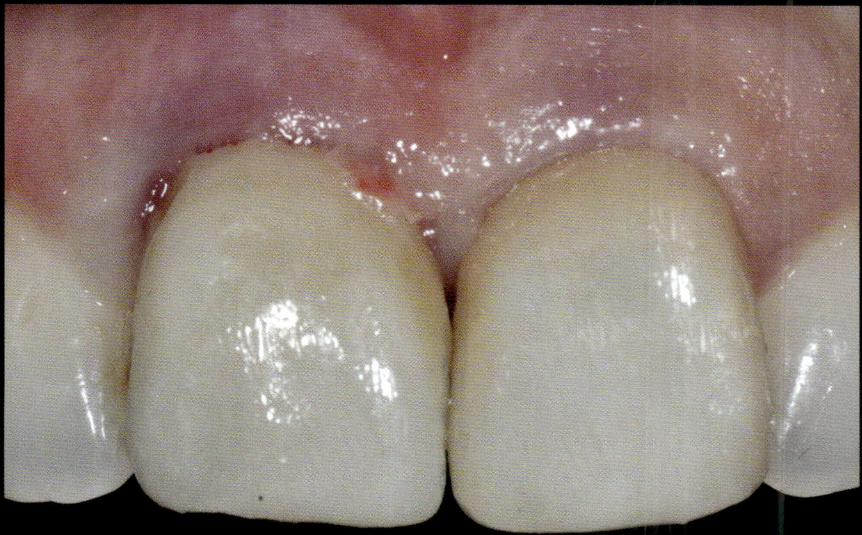

5a

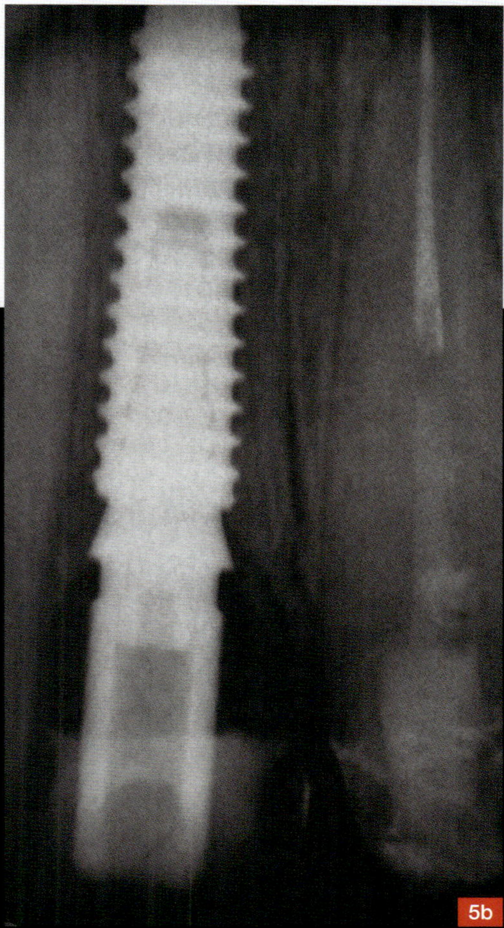

5b

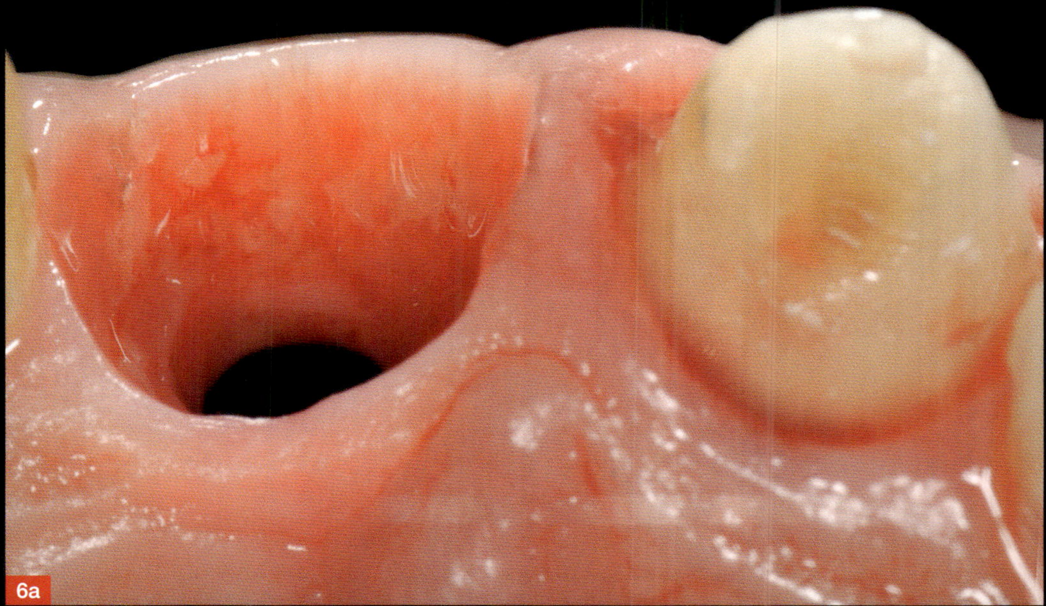

6a

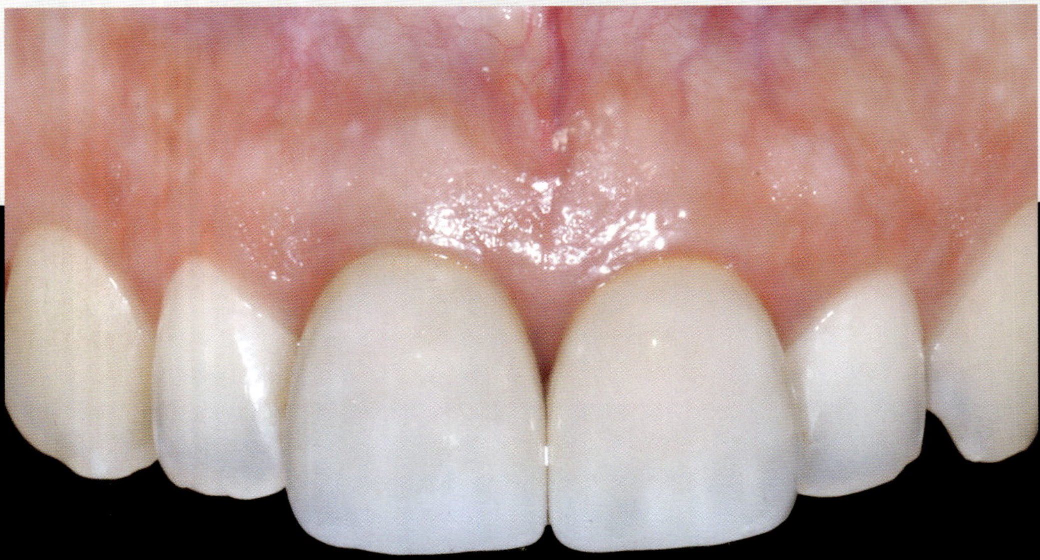

6b

Figure 6a-d: Soft tissue healing 12 months after loading. Definitive crowns in zirconium-ceramic of teeth no. 11 and 21. For the tooth no. 11 a screw-retained crown that was adhesively cemented in the laboratory on a titanium pillar was chosen. Endodontic clinical and radiographic images. Note the total filling of the interdental papilla between teeth no. 11 and 21, the stability of the vestibular soft tissue and the emergence profiles of the crown of no. 11, one 1 year after delivery of the final restorations (24 months after loading).

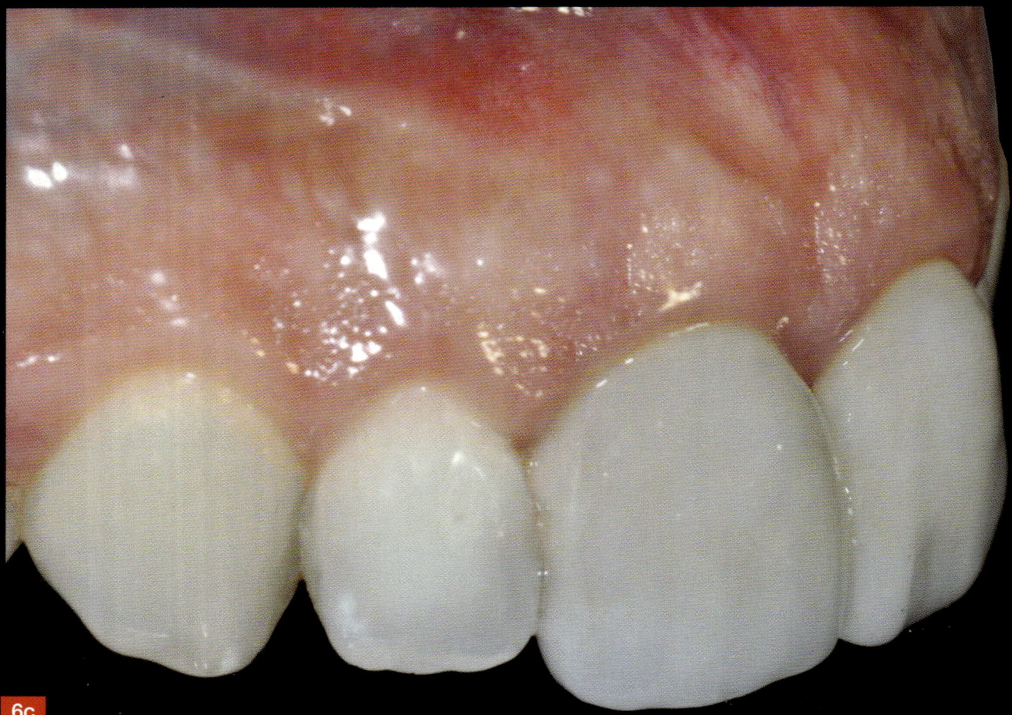

6c

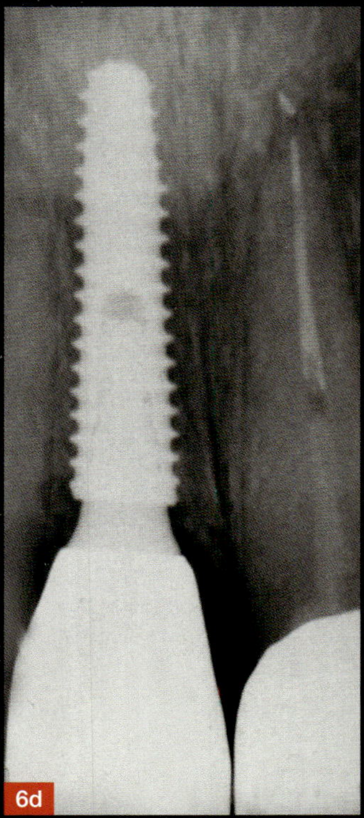

6d

Immediate post-extraction treatment plan for upper left incisor

CASE REPORT 2

The patient was referred for spontaneous pain, the presence of a fistula and dyschromia of the soft tissues in tooth no. 21. The endodontic radiographic examination shows the presence of a reconstruction with a failed metal post and prosthetic restoration made of ceramic metal. A presumed diagnosis of root fracture is made (Figure 1a-c).

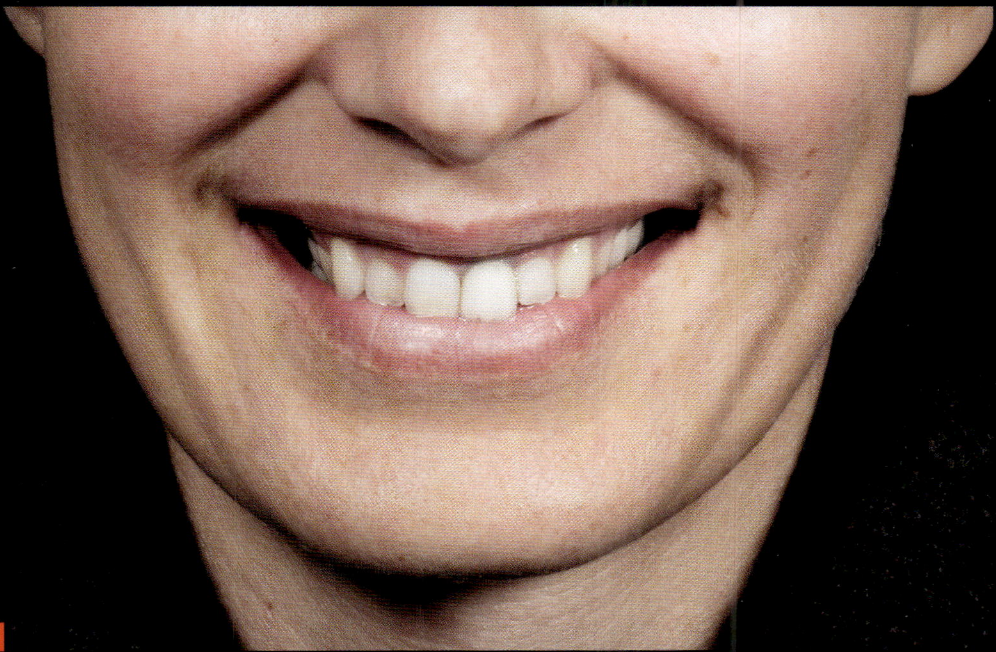

1a

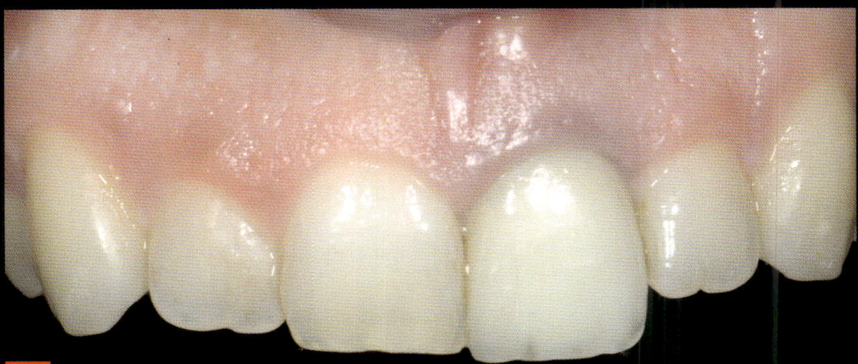

1b

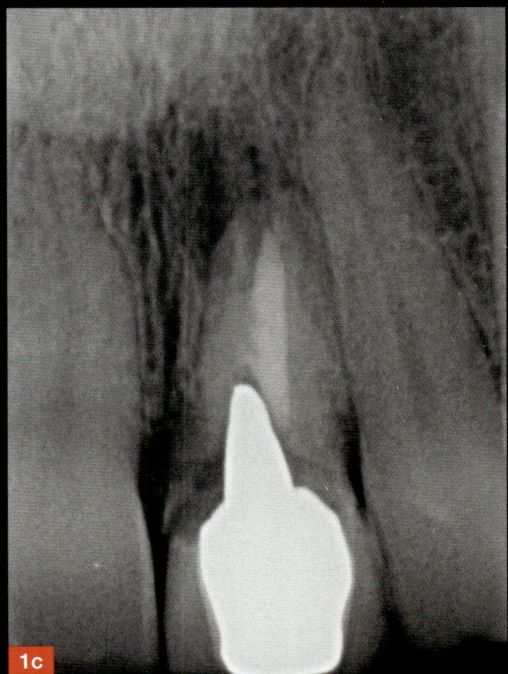

1c

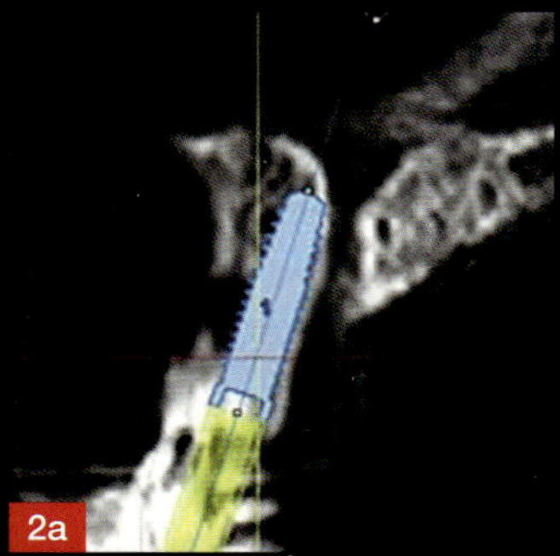

2a

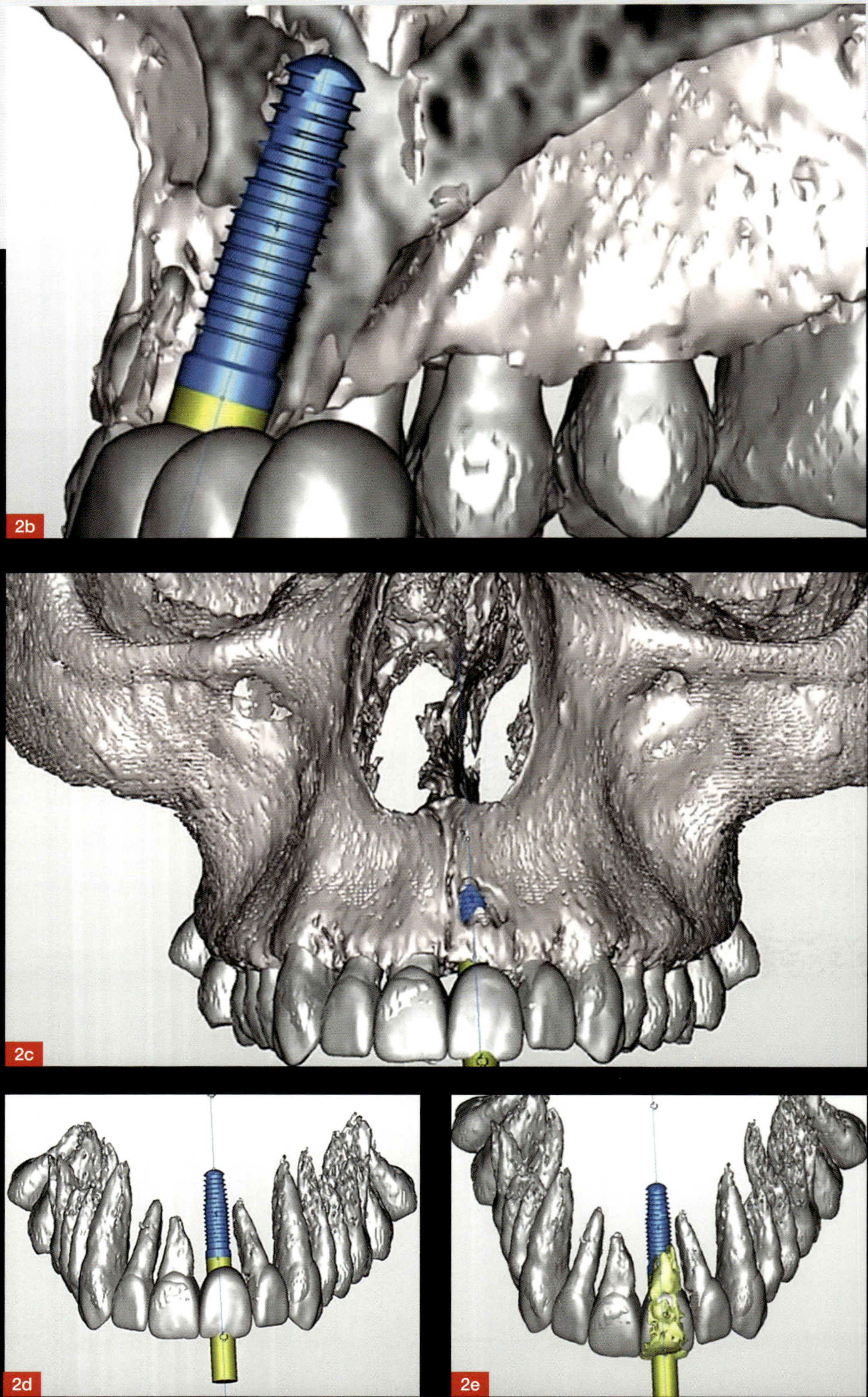

2b 2c 2d 2e

Figure 2a-e: Three-dimensional radiographic examination showing the presence of a bone lesion compatible with root fracture. On the basis of the clinical information and the results of the X-ray examination, tooth no. 21 is considered not to be maintainable. Immediate post-extraction implant placement is therefore planned.

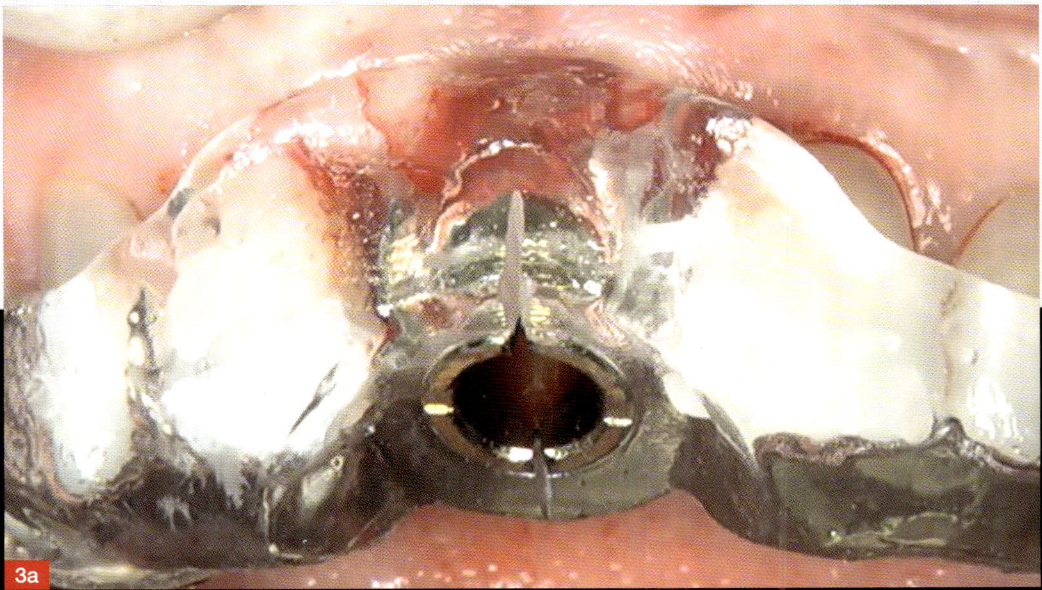

3a

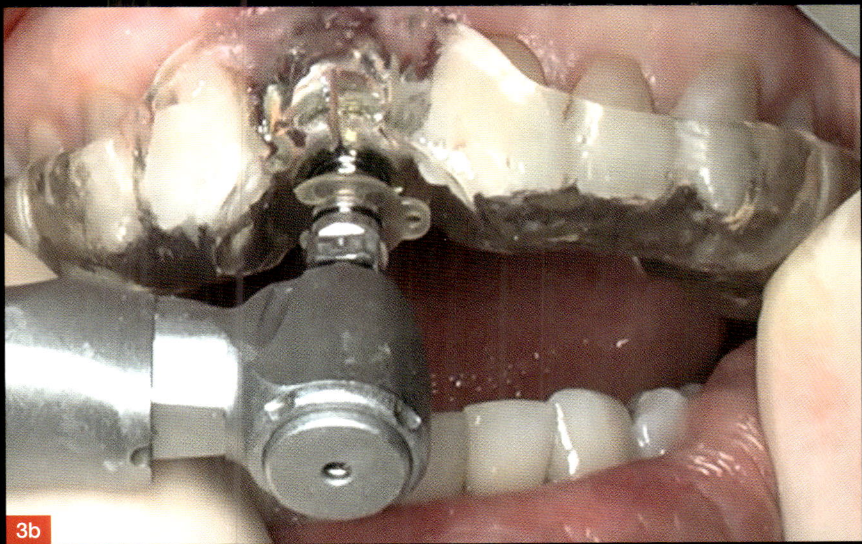

3b

Figure 3a-b: Computer-guided flapless implant insertion is performed.

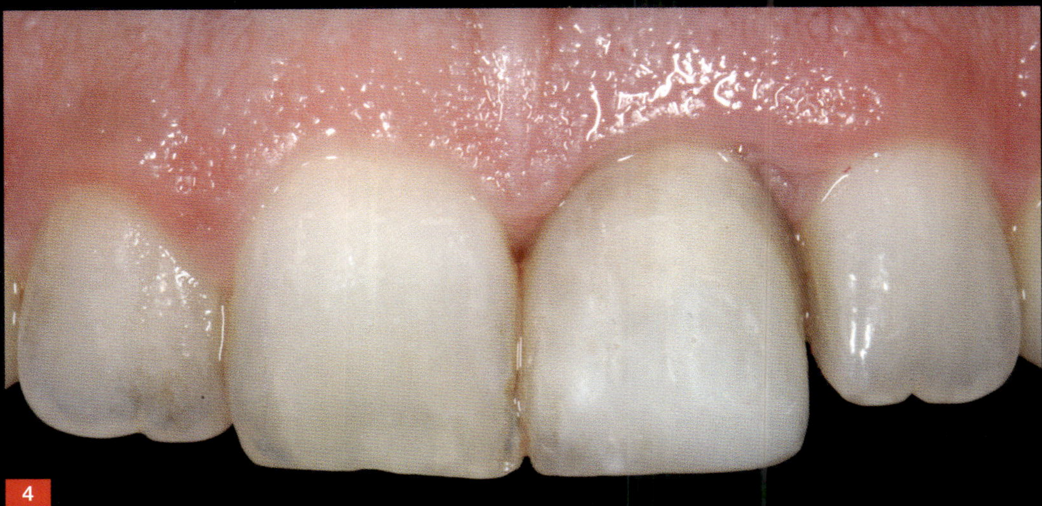

4

Figure 4: Temporary immediate-loading implant.

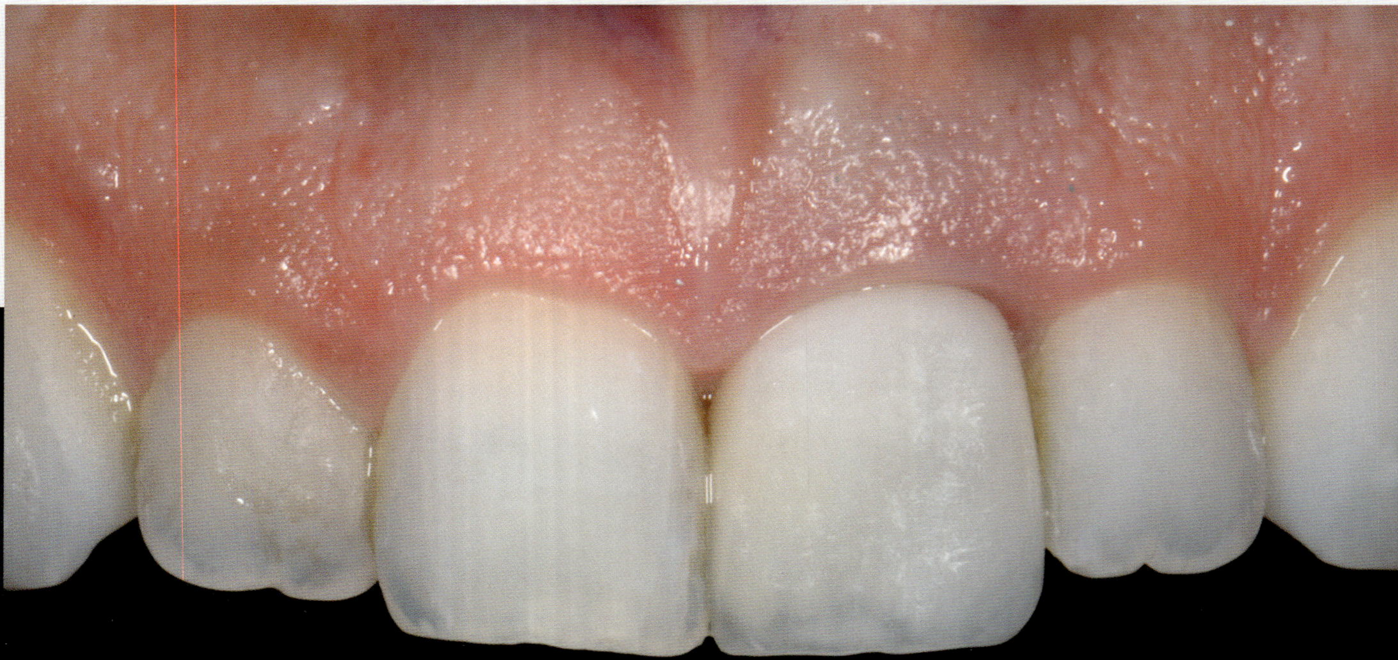

5a

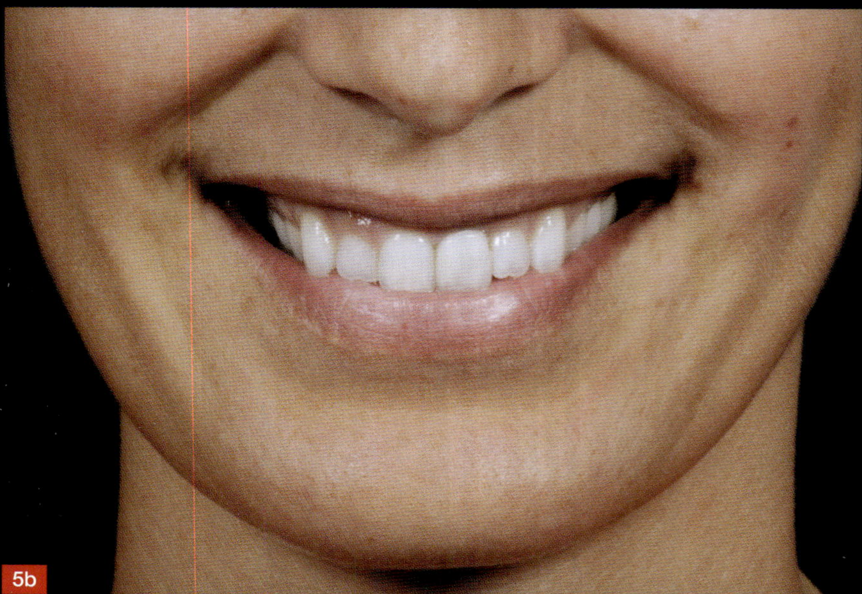

5b

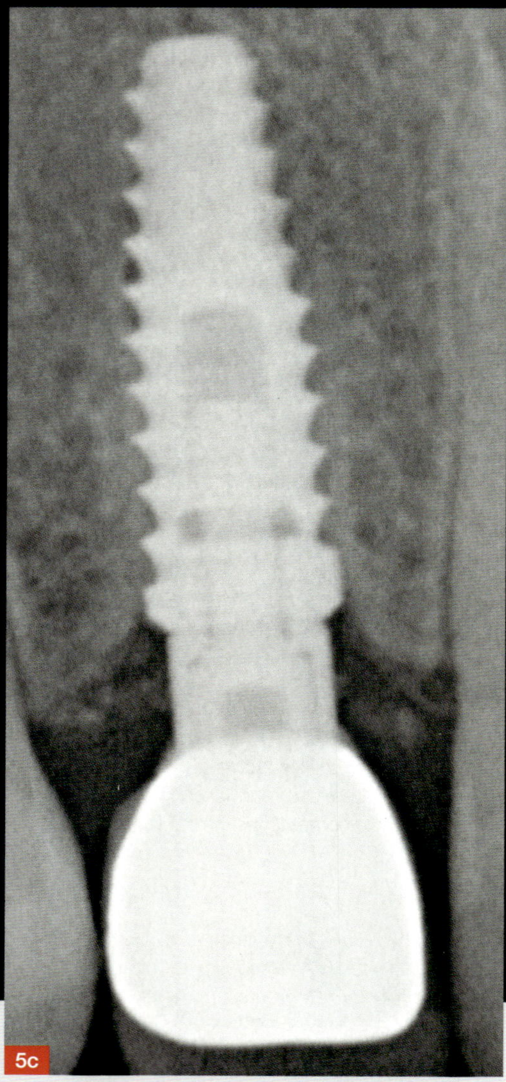

5c

Figure 5a-c: Final prosthetic restoration, periapical x-ray.

References

1. Hämmerle CH, Chen ST, Wilson TG Jr. *Consensus statements and recommended clinical procedures regarding the placement of implants in extraction sockets*. Int J Oral Maxillofac Implants. 2004; 19 Suppl:26-8.
2. Lazzara R.J. *Immediate implant placement into extraction sites: surgical and restorative advantages*. Int. J. Period. Rest. Dent. 1989; 9:332-343.
3. Lekovic V, Kenney EB, Weinlaeder M et al. *A bone regenerative approach to alveolar ridge maintenance following tooth extraction*. Report of 10 cases. J. Period. 1997; 68:563-570.
4. Lekovic V, Camargo PM, Klokkevold PR et al. *Preservation of alveolar bone in extraction sockets using bioabsorbable membranes*. J. Period. 1998; 69: 1.044-1.049.
5. Nevins M, Camelo M, De Paoli S et al. *A study of the fate of the buccal wall of extraction sockets of teeth with prominent roots*. Int. J. Period. Rest. Dent. 2006; 26:19-29.
6. Zuffetti F, Esposito M, Capelli M et al. *Socket grafting with or without buccal augmentation with anorganic bovine bone at immediate post-extractive implants: 6-month after loading results from a multicenter randomised controlled clinical trial*. Eur J Oral Implantol. 2013; 6(3):239-250.
7. Huebsch R.F., Caleman R.D., Frandsen A.M. *The healing process following molar extraction*. Oral Surg. 1952; 5:864-876.
8. Amler M.H. *The time sequence of tissue regeneration in human extraction wounds*. Oral Surg. Oral Med. Oral Pathol. 1969 Mar; 27(3):309-318.
9. Schropp L., Wenzel A., Kostopolulos L et al. *Bone healing and soft tissue contour changes following single-tooth extraction: a clinical and radiographic 12-month prospective study*. Int. J. Period. Rest. Dent. 2003; 23:313-323.
10. Cardaropoli G., Araujo M., Lindhe J. *Dynamics of bone tissue formation in tooth extraction sites. An experimental study in dogs*. J. Clin. Period. 2003; 30: 809-818.
11. Araujo M., Lindhe J. *Dimensional ridge alterations following tooth extraction. An experimental study in dogs*. J. Clin. Periodontol. 2005; 32:212-218.
12. Capelli M, Testori T, Galli F et al. *Implant-buccal plate distance as diagnostic parameter: a prospective cohort study on implant placement in fresh extraction sockets*. J Periodontol. 2013; 84:1768-1774
13. Deflorian M, Parenti A, Fumagalli L. *Impianti post estrattivi nei settori latero posteriori*. Quintessenza Internazionale & JOMI 2014;30(2):76-81.
14. Parenti A, Fumagalli L, Capuzzo C et al. *Razionale per un corretto posizionamento implantare*. Settori anteriori. Dental Cadmos 2004; 5:57-62.
15. Araujo M., Wennstrom J.L., Lindhe J. *Modeling of the buccal and lingual bone walls of fresh extraction sites following implant installation*. Clin. Oral Impl. Res. 2006; 17:606-614.
16. Chrcanovic BR, Martins MD, Wennerberg A. *Immediate placement of implants into infected sites: a systematic review*. Clin Implant Dent Relat Res. 2015 Jan;17 Suppl 1:e1-e16.
17. Zuffetti F, Capelli M, Galli F et al. *Post-extraction implant placement into infected versus non-infected sites: A multicenter retrospective clinical study.Clin Implant Dent Relat Res*. 2017;19:833-840.
18. Testori T, Clauser C, Deflorian M et al. A *Retrospective Analysis of the Effectiveness of the Longevity Protocol for Assessing the Risk of Implant Failure*. Clin Implant Dent Relat Res. 2016;18:1113-1118.
19. Testori T, Weinstein T, Scutellà F et al. *Implant placement in the esthetic area: criteria for positioning single and multiple implants*. Periodontology 2000.2018;77:176-196.
20. Siegenthaler D.W., Jung R.E., Holderegger C et al. *Replacement of teeth exhibiting periapical pathology by immediate implants. A prospective, controlled clinical trial*. Clin. Oral Impl. Res. 2007; 18:727-737.
21. Artzi Z., Tal H., Davan D. *Porous bovine bone mineral in healing of human extraction sockets. Part 1: histomorphometric evaluations at 9 months*. J. Periodontol. 2000; 21:1015-1023.
22. Müller HP, Eger T. *Gingival phenotypes in young male adults*. J Clin Periodontol. 1997; 24:65-71.
23. Müller HP, Eger T, Schorb A. *Gingival dimensions after root coverage with free connective tissue grafts*. J Clin Periodontol. 1998;25:424-430.
24. Kan JYK, Rungcharassaeng K, Deflorian M et al. *Immediate implant placement and provisionalization of maxillary anterior single implants. Periodontology 2000*. 2018; 77:197-212.
25. Jia-Hui Fu, Chu-Yuan Yeh, Hsun-Liang Chan et al. *Tissue Biotype and Its Relation to the Underlying Bone Morphology*. J. Periodontol. 2010; 81:569-574.
26. Chun-Teh Lee, Chih-Yun Tao, Stoupel J. *The Effect of Subepithelial Connective Tissue Graft Placement on Esthetic Outcomes After Immediate Implant Placement: Systematic Review*. J Periodontol 2015; 87:156-167.
27. Saito H, Chu SJ, Reynolds MA et al. *Provisional Restorations Used in Immediate Implant Placement Provide a Platform to Promote Peri-implant Soft Tissue Healing: A Pilot Study*. Int J Periodontics Restorative Dent. 2016;36:47-52.
28. Kan JYK, Roe P, Rungcharassaeng K, Patel R et al. *Classification of Sagittal Root Position in Relation to the Anterior Maxillary Osseous Housing for Immediate Implant Placement: A Cone Beam Computed Tomography Study*. Int J Oral Maxillofac Implants 2011; 26:873-876.

29. Tarnow DP, Magner AW, Fletcher P. *The effect of the distance from the contact point to the crest of bone on the presence or absence of the interproximal dental papilla*. J Periodontol. 1992; 63(12):995-996.
30. Kois JC, Kan JYK. *Predictable peri-implant gingival esthetics: surgical and prosthodontic rationales*. Pract Proced Aesthet Dent 2001; 13:711-715.
31. Kan JYK, Rungcharassaeng K, Sclar A et al. *Effects of the facial osseous defect morphology on gingival dynamics after immediate tooth replacement and guided bone regeneration: 1-year results*. J Oral Maxillofac Surg 2007; 65:13-19 Suppl 1.
32. Hürzeler MB, Zuhr O, Schupbach P et al. *The socket-shield technique: A proof-of-principle report*. J Clin Periodontol. 2010; 37:855-862.
33. Schwimer C, Pette GA, Gluckman H et al. *Human Histologic Evidence of New Bone Formation and Osseointegration Between Root Dentin (Unplanned Socket-Shield) and Dental Implant: Case Report*. Int J Oral Maxillofac Implants. 2018 Jan/Feb;33(1):e19-e23.
34. Kan JY, Rungcharassaeng K. *Proximal socket shield for interimplant papilla preservation in the esthetic zone*. Int J Periodontics Restorative Dent. 2013; 33:24-31.
35. Gluckman H, Salama M, Du Toit J. Partial Extraction Therapies (PET) *Part 1: Maintaining Alveolar Ridge Contour at Pontic and Immediate Implant Sites. Int J Periodontics Restorative Dent. 2016*; 36(5):681-687.
36. Gluckman H, Salama M, Du Toit J.Partial Extraction Therapies (PET) *Part 2: Procedures and Technical Aspects.* Int J Periodontics Restorative Dent. 2017; 37:377-385.
37. Gharpure AS, Bhatavadekar NB. *Current evidence on the socket shield technique: a systematic review*. J Oral Implantol. 2017; 43:395-403.
38. Eswar K, Venkateshbabu N, Rajeswari K et al. *Dentinal tubule disinfection with 2% chlorhexidine, garlic extract, and calcium hydroxide against Enterococcus faecalis by using real-time polymerase chain reaction: In vitro study*. J Conserv Dent, 2013 May. 16(3):194-198.
39. Kandaswamy D, Venkateshbabu N, Gogulnath D et al. *Dentinal tubule disinfection with 2% chlorhexidine gel, propolis, morinda citrifolia juice, 2% povidone iodine, and calcium hydroxide*. Int Endod J, 2010 May. 43(5):419-423.
40. Müller HP, Heinecke A, Schaller N et al. *Masticatory mucosa in subjects with different periodontal phenotypes*. J Clin Periodontol. 2000; 27:621-626.
41. Rasperini G, Acunzo R, Cannalire P et al. *Influence of Periodontal Biotype on Root Surface Exposure During Orthodontic Treatment: A Preliminary Study*. Int J Periodontics Restorative Dent. 2015; 35:665-675.
42. Chen ST, Darby IB, Reynolds EC. *A prospective clinical study of non-submerged immediate implants: clinical outcomes and esthetic results*. Clin Oral Implants Res. 2007; 18:552-562.
43. Ferrus J, Cecchinato D, Pjetursson EB et al. *Factors influencing ridge alterations following immediate implant placement into extraction sockets*. Clin Oral Implants Res. 2010; 21:22-29
44. Chen ST. *Immediate implant placement postextraction without flap elevation*. J Periodontol 2009;80:163-172.
45. Evans CD, Chen ST. *Esthetic outcomes of immediate implant placements*. Clin Oral Implants Res. 2008; 19:73-80.
46. Kan JY, Rungcharassaeng K, Morimoto T et al. *Facial gingival tissue stability after connective tissue graft with single immediate tooth replacement in the esthetic zone: consecutive case report*. J Oral Maxillofac Surg. 2009; 67 Suppl:40-8.
47. Zucchelli G, *Eziologia delle recessioni gengivali*. In: Zucchelli G. (ed.) Chirurgia estetica mucogengivale. Milano: Quintessenzaedizioni, 2012: 13-60.
48. Buser D, Chen ST, Weber HP et al. *Early implant placement following single-tooth extraction in the esthetic zone: biologic rationale and surgical procedures*. Int J Periodontics Restorative Dent. 2008; 28:441-451.
49. Rasperini G, Canullo L, Dellavia C et al. *Socket grafting in the posterior maxilla reduces the need for sinus augmentation*. Int J Periodontics Restorative Dent. 2010; 30:265-273.
50. Pagni G, Pellegrini G, Giannobile WV, Rasperini G. *Postextraction alveolar ridge preservation: biological basis and treatments*. Int J Dent. 2012; 151030.
51. Lin MH, Mau LP, Cochran DL et al. *Risk assessment of inferior alveolar nerve injury for immediate implant placement in the posterior mandible: a virtual implant placement study*. J Dent. 2014; 42(3):263-270.
52. Deflorian M, Galli F, Parenti A et al. *La tempistica di inserimento implantare nei settori anteriori: algoritmo diagnostico*. I&J. 2017; 33:12-23.
53. Galli F, Deflorian M, Parenti A. *La tempistica dell'inserimento implantare nei settori latero-posteriori: algoritmo decisionale*. I&J. 2015; 31:11-18.